Annual Update in Intensi
Emergency Medicine 201

SHIVA THIPPAIAH
16/11/2013

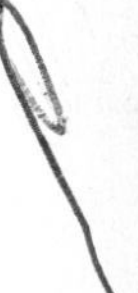

The series *Annual Update in Intensive Care and Emergency Medicine* is the continuation of the series entitled *Yearbook of Intensive Care Medicine* in Europe and *Intensive Care Medicine: Annual Update* in the United States.

Jean-Louis Vincent
Editor

Annual Update in Intensive Care and Emergency Medicine 2013

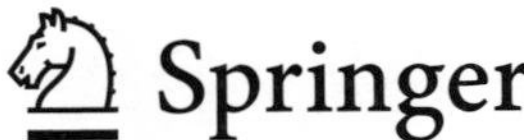

Editor

Prof. Jean-Louis Vincent
Erasme Hospital, Université libre de Bruxelles
Brussels, Belgium
jlvincen@ulb.ac.be

ISSN 2191-5709
ISBN 978-3-642-35108-2 ISBN 978-3-642-35109-9 (eBook)
DOI 10.1007/978-3-642-35109-9
Springer Heidelberg New York Dordrecht London

Cover design: WMXDesign GmbH, Heidelberg

Printed on acid-free paper

Springer is part of Springer Science+Business Media
www.springer.com

Contents

Part IX Monitoring

Part X Transthoracic Monitoring

Part XI Lung Cells

Common Abbreviations

AKI	Acute kidney injury
ALI	Acute lung injury
ARDS	Acute respiratory distress syndrome
BAL	Bronchoalveolar lavage
CABG	Coronary artery bypass graft
CI	Cardiac index
COPD	Chronic obstructive pulmonary disease
CPB	Cardiopulmonary bypass
CRRT	Continuous renal replacement therapy
CT	Computed tomography
DO_2	Oxygen delivery
ECMO	Extracorporeal membrane oxygenation
EEG	Electroencephalogram
EKG	Electrocardiogram
GFR	Glomerular filtration rate
ICP	Intracranial pressure
ICU	Intensive care unit
IL	Interleukin
LPS	Lipopolysaccharide
LV	Left ventricular
MAP	Mean arterial pressure
MRI	Magnetic resonance imaging
NO	Nitric oxide
OR	Odds ratio
PEEP	Positive end-expiratory pressure
PPV	Pulse pressure variation
ROS	Reactive oxygen species
RRT	Renal replacement therapy
SIRS	Systemic inflammatory response syndrome
SOFA	Sequential organ failure assessment
SVR	Systemic vascular resistance
SVV	Stroke volume variation
TBI	Traumatic brain injury
TNF	Tumor necrosis factor
VAP	Ventilator-associated pneumonia
VILI	Ventilator-induced lung injury

Part I

Emergencies

Analgesia in the Emergency Department: A GRADE-based Evaluation of Research Evidence and Recommendations for Practice

C. Lipp, R. Dhaliwal, and E. Lang

Introduction

Emergency physicians care for patients with pain on an extremely frequent basis [1–20]. The prevalence of pain as the presenting complaint of patients seeking emergency department (ED) care ranges from 38 % [3] to as high as 78 % [1]. As a result, evidence-based use of analgesics should be a foundational skill of emergency physicians. However, the literature consistently reports that emergency physicians are often poor at treating pain [1, 2, 8, 13, 14, 16, 19, 20]. Notwithstanding the prevalence of pain in the ED, many patients often report that their pain was not properly treated [3, 7, 20]. In addition to a compromised patient experience, sub-optimal treatment of pain will result in decreased department flow, increased wait times, more return visits to the ED, and increased hospitalization rates.

Very few evidence-based resources and guidelines exist to inform emergency physicians on how to treat pain. One recent guideline on acute pain management compiled by the college of Anaesthetists of Australia and New Zealand [21] was focused primarily on treating pain perioperatively and did not include stratified or graded recommendations based on the literature, highlighting the paucity of emergency medicine-specific guidance. Emergency physicians need an effective, evidenced-based approach to analyze and apply the options available for acute pain management.

C. Lipp
University of Calgary, Faculty of Medicine, Alberta Health Services, Calgary, Canada

R. Dhaliwal
University of Calgary, Faculty of Medicine, Alberta Health Services, Calgary, Canada

E. Lang (✉)
University of Calgary, Faculty of Medicine, Alberta Health Services, Calgary, Canada
E-mail: Eddy.Lang@albertahealthservices.ca

J.-L. Vincent (Ed.), *Annual Update in Intensive Care and Emergency Medicine 2013*,
DOI 10.1007/978-3-642-35109-9_1, © Springer-Verlag Berlin Heidelberg
and BioMed Central Ltd. 2013

The objective of this article is to synthesize and evaluate the quality of medical literature surrounding analgesia delivery in the adult ED using the Grading Assessment, Development and Evaluation (GRADE) framework. We further strived to provide emergency physicians with graded recommendations upon which analgesics should be used to treat adults with acute pain in the ED.

Question Formulation

Prior to searching the literature we developed seven clinically-oriented questions based on a scoping of the literature and a review of locally utilized ED analgesic order sets. This initial surveying of medical literature and our local practice environment allowed us to identify the most commonly prescribed intravenous and oral analgesics used in adult EDs in our health care region.

Table 1 The seven questions developed for analysis

Question (PICO format: Population-Intervention-Comparison-Outcome)		Route
1.	For adults accessing the emergency department with acute pain, should parenteral morphine or fentanyl be used to manage acute moderate-severe pain based on reported change in pain using the visual analog scale?	Intravenous
2.	For adults accessing the emergency department with acute pain, should parenteral hydromorphone or morphine be used to manage acute severe pain based on reported change in pain using the visual analog scale?	Intravenous
3.	For adults accessing the emergency department with acute pain, should a parenteral hydromorphone 1 + 1 mg patient-driven protocol or other intravenous opioids at any dose (physician-driven protocol) be used to manage acute pain based on reported change in pain using the visual analog scale?	Intravenous
4.	For adults accessing the emergency department with acute pain who do not need parenteral analgesia but request an analgesic for outpatient pain management, should oral hydromorphone or oxycodone be used to treat acute pain based on patient reported efficacy (change in pain) and adverse side effects?	Oral
5.	For adults accessing the emergency department with acute pain who do not need parenteral analgesia but request an analgesic for outpatient pain management, should non-specific NSAIDs (e. g., ibuprofen) or codeine-acetaminophen be used for mild-moderate acute pain based on patient reported efficacy (change in pain) and adverse side effects?	Oral

Table 1 *Continued*

	Question (PICO format: Population-Intervention-Comparison-Outcome)	Route
6.	For adults accessing the emergency department with acute pain who do not need parenteral analgesia but request an analgesic for outpatient pain management, should COX-2 specific NSAIDs (e. g., celecoxib) or codeine-acetaminophen be used for mild-moderate acute pain based on patient reported efficacy (change in pain) and adverse side effects?	Oral
7.	For adults accessing the emergency department with acute pain who do not need parenteral analgesia but request an analgesic for outpatient pain management, should oxycodone-acetaminophen or codeine-acetaminophen be given to patients with acute pain based on patient reported efficacy (change in pain) and adverse side effects?	Oral

NSAID: non-steroidal anti-inflammatory drug; COX: cyclooxygenase

We then used the patient-intervention-comparison-outcome (PICO) approach to develop our seven research questions (Table 1). This approach has been adopted by many authors of systematic reviews and guideline panels, including the International Liaison Committee on Resuscitation (ILCOR) and the American College of Chest Physicians (ACCP) [22–24]. It involves identifying a specific population or setting to which recommendations may be applied. Subsequently each question compares two specific management strategies (intervention and comparison). Finally, we defined important patient oriented outcomes (e. g., change in pain) as well as any adverse effects of the medication or other safety concerns.

All seven draft questions were reviewed and revised through an iterative process involving all authors. These seven clinically-based PICO questions compared analgesics (morphine, fentanyl, hydromorphone, non-steroidal anti-inflammatory drugs [NSAIDs], codeine, oxycodone) commonly used in the management of adult acute pain in the ED. The primary critical outcome across all PICO questions was a clinically significant change in pain using validated instruments, such as a visual analog (VAS) or numeric rating scale (NRS). The time frame used to assess change in pain varied from 30 minutes to two hours, depending on the medication route of administration. Secondary patient-oriented outcomes included serious adverse events, patient satisfaction, and side effects. Serious adverse events were defined as respiratory depression (less than 12 breaths per minute), decline in pulse oximetry oxygen saturation to less than 92 %, decline in systolic blood pressure below 90 mmHg, or the need for administration of naloxone after opioid administration.

Search Strategy

After developing the seven PICO questions we conducted searches for each question using PubMed, Ovid MEDLINE, EMBASE, the Cochrane Database of Systematic Reviews, and the TRIPdatabase. These databases were systematically

Table 2 Search keywords, inclusion and exclusion criteria for literature searches

Search Terms	Inclusion Criteria	Exclusion Criteria
Pain* Therapy Treatment Emergency medicine* Emergency service hospital* Adult* Analgesia Therapeutics*	Randomized controlled trials Systematic reviews Meta-analyses Clinical trials Cohort studies Published from year 1990–present Adults (18 years and older)	Case studies, primary research Published prior to the year 1990 Oncology-related treatments

* MeSH search terms

searched following consultation with a professional health sciences librarian who assisted us in our search methodology and use of specific keywords including Medical Subject Headings (MeSH) terms (Table 2). Our search took place over a six-month period of time, from January to June 2011. We conducted seven unique searches using the same search keywords as well as the various names of the intervention and comparison drugs in each question. When possible, we used MeSH terms for searching the U.S. National Library of Medicine. Prior to searching the databases we also developed inclusion and exclusion criteria (Table 2) to assist us in focusing each literature search.

The results of each literature search were saved and a single reviewer screened titles, flagging articles that met the inclusion criteria based on the search keywords and terms.

Articles flagged as relevant in the initial screen were selected for abstract review. Abstracts for each PICO question were screened by the same reviewer and when abstracts met the inclusion criteria, a full text copy of the article was retrieved.

Use of GRADE

In our analysis of the situation we decided to use the GRADE framework, which is becoming the benchmark for communicating evidence-based medicine throughout the world [25]. Numerous prominent health organizations, including the World Health Organization (WHO), the ACCP, the Society of Critical Care Medicine (SCCM), the National Institute for Clinical Excellence (NICE, UK), and the European Respiratory Society (ERS) have endorsed or adopted the GRADE approach as a means of analyzing medical evidence and developing guidelines.

We used the GRADE system and its quality of evidence criteria as well as GRADE-Pro software to analyze the articles for each PICO question. This software-supported approach is used in the GRADE methodology and enables clinician-researchers to succinctly analyze structured clinical questions using the GRADE methodology [26, 27]. GRADE classifies evidence into four categories (high, moderate, low and very low) based on a body of evidence related to a specific outcome. This classification is based on an assessment of the research studies in question, including assessing for bias, indirectness, imprecision, inconsistency, and publication bias. Subsequently, the software assists the researcher through a multifactorial process of compiling the results of each study for the outcomes studied in the research question. The software then summarizes all the pertinent details of the research question and each outcome in a summary of findings (SoF) table. Each SoF table outlines the level of evidence for each question (high, moderate, low, or very low) and serves as the basis for making recommendations on each clinical question.

Following the grading of the evidence for each of the seven PICO questions, seven separate SoF tables were developed by the first author using the GRADE-Pro software. Subsequently the first author drafted recommendations for each of the seven PICO question using the data in the SoF tables. Once these drafts were complete, the second and third authors reviewed the SoF tables and reviewed the recommendations in an iterative process. These recommendations were then compiled into a succinct table.

Results

A total of 153 abstracts were screened for eligibility and 26 articles met eligibility criteria. Three articles compared fentanyl and morphine (PICO #1); five articles assessed hydromorphone (PICO #2), two of which analyzed the 1 + 1 hydromorphone protocol (PICO #3); three articles compared oral hydromorphone and oxycodone (PICO #4); eight articles compared non-specific NSAIDs and codeine-acetaminophen (PICO #5); two articles compared specific NSAIDs and codeine-acetaminophen (PICO #6); and five articles compared oxycodone and codeine (PICO #7).

The same reviewer assessed the full text articles and determined that 14 of the 26 offered quantitative results that could be analyzed using the GRADE-pro software [28–41]. The remaining 12 articles were excluded because they did not compare both drugs assessed in a PICO question [42–47], compared analgesics not addressed in the seven PICO questions (such as acetaminophen alone) [48, 49], used unconventional medication dosing [50, 51], used non-validated pain measurement scales [52, 53], and/or unusual study designs [50].

The 14 articles evaluated using the GRADE approach included eight randomized clinical trials, four systematic reviews, one retrospective cohort study, and one prospective clinical trial. An example of a SoF table developed for PICO number two is included (Table 3). Similar SoF tables were developed for each PICO question. Overall, the grading process supported the use of intravenous hydromorphone and fentanyl as superior to intravenous morphine for rapid and effective pain relief (weak recommendation, moderate quality evidence). Oral NSAIDs, oxycodone, and hydromorphone are generally superior to codeine-acetaminophen combinations (weak recommendations, very-low quality evidence; due to bias, indirectness, and imprecision).

Table 3 The summary of findings table for PICO #2: Hydromorphone (i.v.) vs. morphine (i.v.) for acute severe pain in the emergency department

Outcomes	No of patients (studies) Follow-up	Quality of the evidence (GRADE)	Relative effect (95 % CI)	Anticipated absolute effects Time frame is 30 min	
				Risk with morphine	Risk difference with hydromorphone (95 % CI)
Change in pain score Mean change in numeric rating scale (NRS) [0 = no pain; 10 = worst pain possible]; scale from 0–10	374 (2 studies) 2 h	⊕⊕⊕O MODERATE[2,3] due to indirectness		The mean change in pain score ranged across control groups from 3.3–4.1 NRS	The mean change in pain score in the intervention groups was 0.9 higher (0.35 to 1.75 higher)[1]
Serious adverse events respiratory depression (RR < 12) or SpO_2 < 95 % or systolic blood pressure (SBP) < 90 mmHg or administration of naloxone after opioid administration	374 (2 studies) 2 h	⊕⊕OO LOW[3,4] due to indirectness, imprecision	RR 0.96 (0.91–1.02)	54 per 1,000	2 fewer per 1,000 (from 5 fewer to 1 more)[4]
Adverse effects Nausea or vomiting or pruritus	374 (2 studies) 2 h	⊕⊕OO LOW[3,4] due to indirectness, imprecision	RR 0.96 (0.83–1.1)	299 per 1,000	12 fewer per 1,000 (from 51 fewer to 30 more)
The basis for the assumed risk (e. g., the median control group risk across studies) is provided in footnotes. The corresponding risk (and the 95 % confidence interval [CI]) is based on the assumed risk in the comparison group and the relative effect of the intervention. RR: risk ratio					
GRADE Working Groups grades of evidence					
High quality:	Further research is very unlikely to change our confidence in the estimate of effect				
Moderate quality:	Further research is likely to have an important impact on our confidence in the estimate of effect and may change the estimate				

Table 3 *Continued*

Outcomes	No of patients (studies) Follow-up	Quality of the evidence (GRADE)	Relative effect (95 % CI)	Anticipated absolute effects Time frame is 30 min	
				Risk with morphine	Risk difference with hydromorphone (95 % CI)
Low quality:	Further research is very likely to have an important impact on our confidence in the estimate of effect and is likely to change the estimate				
Very low quality:	We are very uncertain about the estimate				

[1]At 30 min, one study had a between-group NRS difference of 1.3 (0.5–2.2) in favor of hydromorphone.

[2]One of the studies did not do a Mini Mental State Examination (MMSE) on the elderly patients; and the other cited that the hydromorphone group had a higher baseline pain score.

[3]Both studies were conducted in an underserviced inner city hospital with 45–60 % of the patients of Hispanic descent.

[4]the confidence interval from the calculated relative risk is quite wide.

Discussion

Using the GRADE framework, we have synthesized and evaluated the medical literature surrounding analgesia delivery in the adult ED and developed clear and actionable recommendations for analgesic use based on graded recommendations. Despite using a thorough, systematic approach to reviewing the literature on each PICO question we identified only 14 articles that met our inclusion criteria. However, although the number of studies used to make our recommendations may seem low, our recommendations take into consideration the quality of evidence of the studies. Pragmatic derivations of the seven PICO questions, their recommendations, and the rationale for these recommendations are listed in Table 4 [28–41]. Furthermore, we also developed a flowchart as a suggested approach to analgesia in the ED (Fig. 1).

Table 4 The intravenous and oral analgesics analyzed in this study: Associated recommendations and rationale

Intravenous analgesics	Oral analgesics
1. Should morphine or fentanyl be used for acute moderate-severe pain? We recommend fentanyl (1 mcg/kg, then ~30 mcg q 5 min) over morphine *(weak recommendation, low quality evidence)* If morphine is used to treat acute pain, we suggest giving 0.1 mg/kg, then 0.05 mg/kg at 30 min, with the maximum suggested dose of 10 mg ***Rationale*** [28–30] • People with morphine allergies do not have allergies to fentanyl • Fentanyl has a shorter onset of action as well as being 100 times more potent than morphine, and thus is better suited to treat acute moderate to severe pain. (Fentanyl is more lipid soluble and thus has higher bioavailability) • There is no substantial cost difference between the two medications • Fentanyl is reported to be less pro-emetic than morphine and does not produce a histamine release like morphine does. This leads to less hypotension and less pruritus, facial flushing, or urticaria • Fentanyl with its 2–3 min onset and 30–60 min duration is less likely to cause prolonged sedation, and may encourage more frequent reassessment of ill patients • Fentanyl has less of a dose stacking risk than morphine. This is especially relevant in patients with renal failure in whom morphine's metabolite accumulates,	**4. Should hydromorphone or oxycodone be used for acute pain?** We are unable to comment on the superiority/inferiority of either of these drugs in treating acute pain The only studies we identified that compared these drugs assessed the extended release forms of hydromorphone (Exalgo®) and oxycodone Further research is needed to assess the immediate release forms of hydromorphone (e. g., Dilaudid®) and oxycodone, and whether they have a role in treating acute pain in the emergency department ***Rationale*** [34, 35] • We only identified two studies comparing hydromorphone and oxycodone. They assessed the extended release forms. Both studies suggested no difference between the drugs in either pain relief or adverse effects • We are unable to make recommendation about hydromorphone (PO) and oxycodone (PO) in treating acute pain. Extended release forms appear to be equal in terms of pain relief and side effect profile (when dosed in an equal analgesic way 2:5) based on two RCTs *(strong recommendation, very low quality evidence)*.

Table 4 *Continued*

Intravenous analgesics	Oral analgesics
whereas fentanyl does not. Currently the order sets have general doses of morphine at 2.5 mg or 5 mg, and fentanyl at 50 mcg. Because adults vary in weight, ED physicians may be well served to estimate the patient's weight and dose based on that For example a 70 kg patient should be given 7 mg of morphine or 70 mcg of fentanyl as an initial loading dose (assuming there is no contraindication to a high loading dose) **2. Should hydromorphone or morphine be used for acute severe pain in the emergency department?** We recommend hydromorphone (0.015 mg/kg i.v.) as a comparable, potentially superior, analgesic to morphine (0.1 mg/kg i.v.) *(strong recommendation, moderate quality evidence)* ***Rationale*** [28, 31, 32] • Hydromorphone has a quicker onset of action, when compared with morphine • Hydromorphone is comparable in cost to morphine • Morphine, with a longer onset of action and greater risk for dose stacking, places patients at a higher risk for toxicity (in the context of renal failure) and hypoventilation or, on the other hand oligoanalgesia • Because hydromorphone is more potent, at a much smaller milligram dose, physicians may be more likely to adequately treat pain by giving a dose of 1.5 mg of hydromorphone vs. 10 mg of morphine • Hydromorphone causes little or no histamine release, and may be safely administered to patients who report a type 2 allergy to morphine (urticaria, pruritis, and facial flushing) **3. Should hydromorphone 1 + 1 mg patient-driven protocol or other intravenous opioids at any dose (physician-driven protocol) be used for acute pain management?** We recommend a 1 mg + 1 mg patient-driven protocol over other intravenous opioids in the emergency department *(weak recommendation, low quality evidence)* This may be especially helpful for patients who are unable to clearly communicate their level of pain (acute mental status change, non-	**5. Should non-specific NSAIDs (e. g., ibuprofen) or codeine-acetaminophen be used for mild-moderate acute pain?** We recommend non-COX specific NSAIDs over codeine-acetaminophen combinations *(weak recommendation, moderate quality evidence)* ***Rationale*** [36–38] • The reported numbers needed to treat for naproxen and ibuprofen are 2.7 vs. 4.4 for codeine-acetaminophen • NSAIDs have been shown to have a longer time to re-medication with a safer side effect profile. The number needed to treat for codeine-acetaminophen was 6 • NSAIDs do not have the CNS depressing effects of codeine • Certain genotypes may not metabolize or may hyper-metabolize codeine into morphine (due to a CYP2D6 polymorphism) **6. Should COX-2 specific NSAIDs (e. g., celecoxib) or codeine-acetaminophen be used for mild-moderate acute pain?** We recommend COX-specific NSAIDs over codeine acetaminophen combinations (*weak recommendation, moderate quality evidence)* ***Rationale*** [36] • This is based on a Cochrane systematic review that compared NSAIDs and codeine-acetaminophen combinations with placebo in treating acute postoperative pain • The number needed to treat for 400 mg of celecoxib was 2.5 whereas that for 600 mg/60 mg of acetaminophen/codeine was 3.9 • The average time to re-medication with celecoxib was 8.4 h, whereas patients who used acetaminophen/codeine re-medicated in 4.1 h • The relative risk between these two drugs is 1 **7. Should oxycodone-acetaminophen or codeine-acetaminophen be given to patients with acute pain in the ED?** We recommend oxycodone-acetaminophen as marginally superior to codeine-acetaminophen (*weak recommendation, low quality evidence)*

Table 4 *Continued*

Intravenous analgesics	Oral analgesics
English speaking patients) ***Rationale*** [28, 31–33] • Hydromorphone has a quicker onset of action compared with morphine • Hydromorphone is comparable in cost to morphine • Morphine, with a longer onset of action and greater risk for dose stacking, places patients at a higher risk for toxicity (in the context of renal failure) and hypoventilation or, on the other hand, oligoanalgesia • Because hydromorphone is more potent, at a much smaller milligram dose, physicians may be more likely to adequately treat pain by giving a dose of 1.5 mg of hydromorphone vs. 10 mg of morphine • Hydromorphone causes little or no histamine release, and may be safely administered to patients who report a type 2 allergy to morphine (urticaria, pruritis, and facial flushing) • This is superior to standard morphine and fentanyl dosing for a few reasons: Physicians tend to be concerned about giving patients more morphine than 5 mg and often give small doses, e. g., 2.5 mg. A 1 + 1 approach not only allows physicians to appropriately treat pain, but also requires fewer repeat orders	***Rationale*** [39–41] • This recommendation is based on two Cochrane reviews that compared each of these drugs with placebo • There are few studies that directly compare these two drugs, especially in an adult emergency department setting • However, the Cochrane reviews and single studies consistently show that oxycodone with acetaminophen is slightly better at relieving pain than acetaminophen-codeine

Despite the synthesis of information in this study there are also some limitations to consider. First, there is a limited body of literature analyzing the use and efficacy of analgesics in the ED setting. Even after searching multiple databases there were few studies conducted in the ED setting that compared one oral analgesic with another oral analgesic. As a result, many of our recommendations were limited by the fact that some studies were conducted in postoperative settings and subsequently downgraded due to indirectness. Second, there were difficulties making comparisons between different studies that compared the various oral agents. In particular, it was difficult to properly compare studies in which codeine-acetaminophen combinations were used as there is a significant amount of variability in the codeine to acetaminophen ratio in the various combinations of this oral analgesic. As a result, we were unable to clearly compare two studies if they differed in their codeine to acetaminophen ratios. Third, while the authors collaborated extensively throughout this project, only one author was responsible for analyzing the article titles and abstracts. Finally, this review did not include the pediatric population in the literature search, and our recommendations do not extend to treating acute pain in children.

Fig. 1 Suggested approach to acute pain in the emergency department. NSAID: non-steroidal anti-inflammatory drug; IV: intravenous ▶

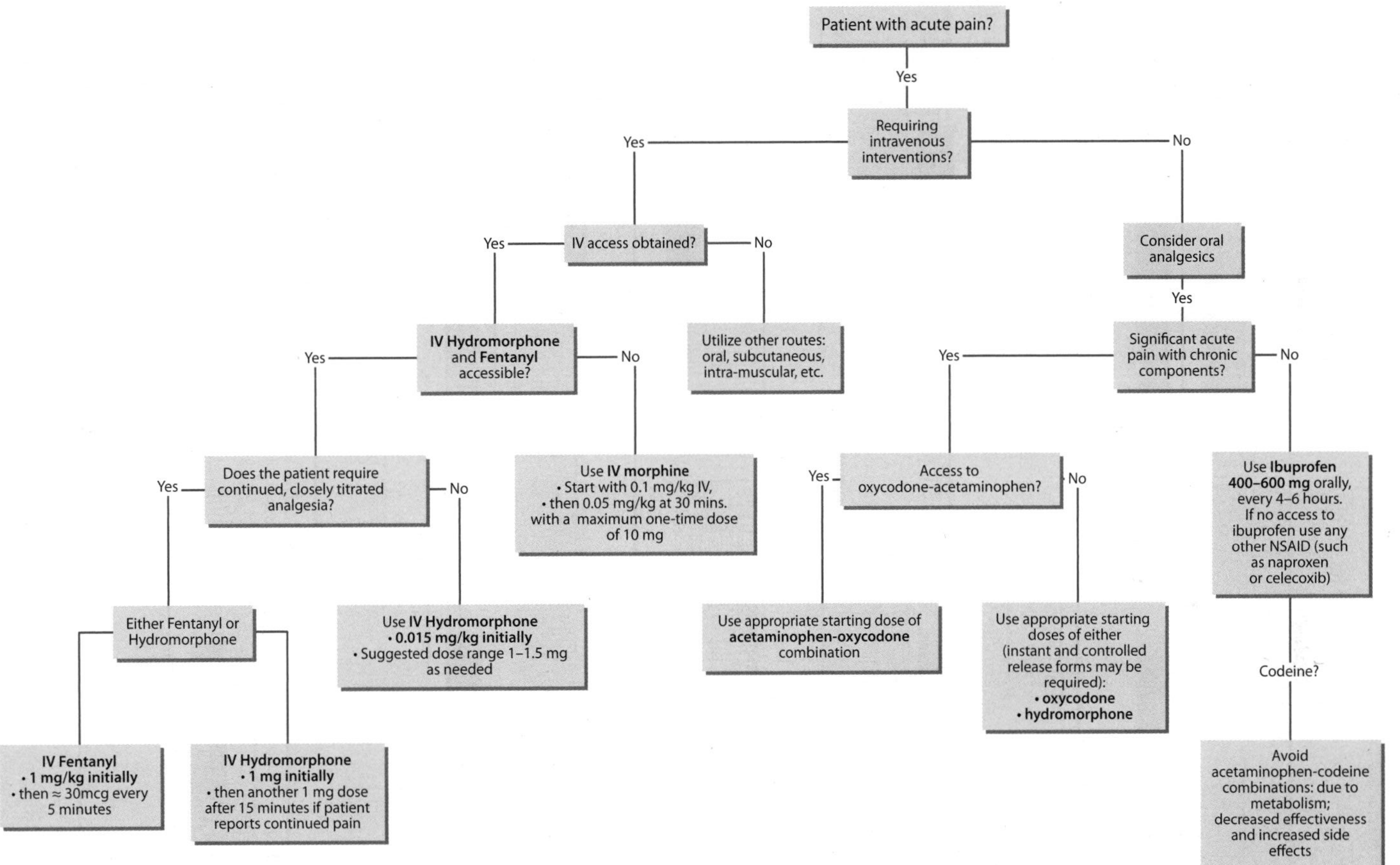
Patient with acute pain?
Yes
Requiring intravenous interventions?
Yes
IV access obtained?
Yes
IV Hydromorphone and Fentanyl accessible?
Yes
Does the patient require continued, closely titrated analgesia?
Yes
Either Fentanyl or Hydromorphone
IV Fentanyl
• 1 mg/kg initially
• then ≈ 30mcg every 5 minutes
IV Hydromorphone
• 1 mg initially
• then another 1 mg dose after 15 minutes if patient reports continued pain
No
Use IV Hydromorphone
• 0.015 mg/kg initially
• Suggested dose range 1–1.5 mg as needed
No
Use IV morphine
• Start with 0.1 mg/kg IV,
• then 0.05 mg/kg at 30 mins. with a maximum one-time dose of 10 mg
No
Utilize other routes: oral, subcutaneous, intra-muscular, etc.
No
Consider oral analgesics
Yes
Significant acute pain with chronic components?
Yes
Access to oxycodone-acetaminophen?
Yes
Use appropriate starting dose of acetaminophen-oxycodone combination
No
Use appropriate starting doses of either (instant and controlled release forms may be required):
• oxycodone
• hydromorphone
No
Use Ibuprofen 400–600 mg orally, every 4–6 hours. If no access to ibuprofen use any other NSAID (such as naproxen or celecoxib)
Codeine?
Avoid acetaminophen-codeine combinations: due to metabolism; decreased effectiveness and increased side effects

Despite these limitations this study also has a number of strengths. First, this study is extremely relevant to emergency physicians and health care workers who must treat acute pain, and to our knowledge it is the first GRADE-based evaluation of ED analgesia. Furthermore, this study serves as a model for clinician-researchers and administrators who want to promote evidence-based medicine in their clinical context. By conducting similar PICO question based analyses, successful knowledge translation from medical literature into clinical practice may be accomplished and, thereby, insure that treatments at the bedside remain current.

Conclusion

Despite the frequent occurrence of pain in ED patients, there are no ED-based syntheses and guidelines that compare analgesics commonly used in the ED. We have developed the first GRADE based recommendations for improving analgesia in the ED. Going forward, these findings can be used by ED clinicians and guideline panels to evaluate and develop analgesic order sets based on specific clinical presentations as well as drive the research agenda in ED analgesia.

These evidence-based guidelines have the potential to not only impact on patient morbidity, but also on health care costs and ED efficiency. As health care professionals with the role of treating emergent health problems, it is crucial that all emergency physicians have up-to-date, evidence-based knowledge to adequately treat acute pain.

Acknowledgement: We thank Dr Helen Lee-Robertson, librarian at the University of Calgary Health Sciences Center, for her contributions to this study.

References

1. Todd KH, Ducharme J, Choiniere M et al (2007) Pain in the emergency department: Results of the pain and emergency medicine initiative (PEMI) multicenter study. J Pain 8:460–466
2. Silk J, Baird L, Ahern M, Holdgate A, Fry M (1999) An emergency department's analysis of pain management patterns. Australian Emerg Nurs J 2:31–36
3. Pines JM, Hollander JE (2008) Emergency department crowding is associated with poor care for patients with severe pain. Ann Emerg Med 51:1–5
4. Allione A, Melchio R, Martini G et al (2011) Factors influencing desired and received analgesia in emergency department. Intern Emerg Med 6:69–78
5. Ducharme J (1996) Proceedings from the first international symposium on pain research in emergency medicine: Foreword. Ann Emerg Med 27:399–403
6. Cordell WH (1996) Pain-control research opportunities and future directions. Ann Emerg Med 27:474–478
7. Afilalo M, Tselios C (1996) Pain relief versus patient satisfaction. Ann Emerg Med 27:436–438

8. Lee G, Smith S, Jennings N (2008) Low acuity abdominal pain in the emergency department: Still a long wait. Int Emerg Nurs 16:94–100
9. Finckh A, Robertson F, McDonell K, Welch S, Gawthorne J (2010) Implementation of a guideline to improve prescription of analgesia for adult trauma patients in an emergency department. Australas Emerg Nurs J 13:25–29
10. Wilson JE, Pendleton JM (1989) Oligoanalgesia in the emergency department. Am J Emerg Med 7:620–623
11. Singer A, Chisum E, Stark M (2003) An educational intervention to reduce oligoanalgesia in the emergency department. Ann Emerg Med 42:S41–S41
12. Decosterd I, Hugli O, Tamchès E et al (2007) Oligoanalgesia in the emergency department: Short-term beneficial effects of an education program on acute pain. Ann Emerg Med 50:462–471
13. Calil AM, MattosPimenta CA, Birolini D (2007) The "oligoanalgesia problem" in the emergency care. Clinics 62:591–598
14. Motov SM, Khan AN (2008) Problems and barriers of pain management in the emergency department: Are we ever going to get better? J Pain Res 2:5–11
15. Chen EH, Shofer FS, Dean AJ et al (2008) Gender disparity in analgesic treatment of emergency department patients with acute abdominal pain. Acad Emerg Med 15:414–418
16. Rupp T, Delaney KA (2004) Inadequate analgesia in emergency medicine. Ann Emerg Med 43:494–503
17. Arendts G, Fry M (2006) Factors associated with delay to opiate analgesia in emergency departments. J Pain 7:682–686
18. Cordell WH, Keene KK, Giles BK et al (2002) The high prevalence of pain in emergency medical care. Am J Emerg Med 20:165–169
19. Ducharme J (1995) A prospective blinded study on emergency pain assessment and therapy. J Emerg Med 13:571–575
20. Tcherny-Lessenot S, Karwowski-Soulié F, Lamarche-Vadel A et al (2003) Management and relief of pain in an emergency department from the adult patients' perspective. J Pain Symptom Manag 25:539–546
21. Macintyre P, Scott DA, Schug SA, Visser EJ, Walker SM (2010) Acute Pain Management: Scientific Evidence. Available at: http://www.anzca.edu.au/resources/college-publications/pdfs/Acute%20Pain%20Management/books-and-publications/acutepain.pdf. Accessed October 2012
22. Morley PT, Atkins DL, Billi JE et al (2010) Part 3: Evidence evaluation process: 2010 International Consensus on Cardiopulmonary Resuscitation and Emergency Cardiovascular Care Science With Treatment Recommendations. Circulation 122:S283–S8290
23. Schunemann HJ, Cook D, Guyatt G (2008) Methodology for antithrombotic and thrombolytic therapy guideline development: American College of Chest Physicians Evidence-based Clinical Practice Guidelines (8th edition). Chest 133(Suppl 6):110S–112S
24. Guyatt GH, Oxman AD, Kunz R et al (2011) GRADE guidelines: 2. Framing the question and deciding on important outcomes. J Clin Epidemiol 64:395–400
25. Guyatt G, Vist G, Falck-Ytter Y et al (2006) An emerging consensus on grading recommendations? Evid Based Med 11:2–4
26. The GRADE Working Group (2012) Organizations that have endorsed or that are using GRADE. Available at: http://www.gradeworkinggroup.org/society/index.htm. Accessed October 2012
27. Guyatt G, Oxman AD, Akl EA et al (2011) GRADE guidelines: 1. introduction-GRADE evidence profiles and summary of findings tables. J Clin Epidemiol 64:383–394
28. Patanwala AE, Keim SM, Erstad BL (2010) Intravenous opioids for severe acute pain in the emergency department. Ann Pharmacother 44:1800–1809
29. Galinski M, Dolveck F, Borron SW et al (2005) A randomized, double blind study comparing morphine with fentanyl in prehospital analgesia. Am J Emerg Med 23:114–119

30. Fleischman RJ, Frazer DG, Daya M, Jui J, Newgard CJ (2010) Effectiveness and safety of fentanyl compared with morphine for out-of-hospital analgesia. Prehosp Emerg Care 14:167–175
31. Chang AK, Bijur PE, Gallagher EJ (2011) Randomized clinical trial comparing the safety and efficacy of a hydromorphone titration protocol to usual care in the management of adult emergency department patients with acute severe pain. Ann Emerg Med 58:352–359
32. Chang AK, Bijur PE, Campbell CM, Murphy MK, Gallagher EJ (2009) Safety and efficacy of rapid titration using 1 mg doses of intravenous hydromorphone in emergency department patients with acute severe pain: The "1 + 1" protocol. Ann Emerg Med 54:221–225
33. Chang AK, Bijur PE, Davitt M, Gallagher EJ (2009) Randomized clinical trial comparing a patient-driven titration protocol of intravenous hydromorphone with traditional physician-driven management of emergency department patients with acute severe pain. Acute Pain 11:152–153
34. Binsfeld H, Szczepanski L, Waechter S, Richarz U, Sabatowski R (2010) A randomized study to demonstrate non-inferiority of once-daily OROS hydromorphone for moderate to severe chronic non-cancer pain. Pain Pract 10:404–415
35. Hale M, Tudor IC, Khanna S, Thipphawong J (2007) Efficacy and tolerability of once-daily OROS hydromorphone and twice-daily extended-release oxycodone in patients with chronic, moderate to severe osteoarthritis pain: results of a 6-week, randomized, open-label, noninferiority analysis. Clin Ther 29:874–888
36. Moore RA, Derry S, McQuay HJ, Wiffen PJ (2011) Single dose oral analgesics for acute postoperative pain in adults. Cochrane Database Syst Rev CD008659
37. Drendel AL, Gorelick MH, Weisman SJ et al (2009) Randomized clinical trial of ibuprofen versus acetaminophen with codeine for acute pediatric arm fracture pain. Ann Emerg Med 54:553–560
38. Innes GD, Croskerry P, Worthington J, Beveridge R, Jones D (1998) Ketorolac versus acetaminophen-codeine in the ED treatment of acute low back pain. J Emerg Med 16:549–556
39. Gaskell H, Derry S, Moore RA, McQuay HJ (2009) Single dose oral oxycodone and oxycodone plus paracetamol for acute postoperative pain in adults. Cochrane Database Syst Rev CD002763
40. Toms l, Derry S, Moore RA, McQuay HJ (2009) Single dose oral paracetamol with codeine for post-operative pain in adults. Cochrane Database Syst Rev CD001547
41. Marco CA, Plewa MC, Buderer N, Black C, Roberts A (2005) Comparison of oxycodone and hydrocodone for the treatment of acute pain associated with fractures: a double-blind randomised clinical trial. Acad Emerg Med 12:282–288
42. Larijani GE, Pharm D, Goldberg MD et al (2004) Analgesic and hemodynamic effects of a single 7.5 mg intravenous dose of morphine in patients with moderate-to-severe postoperative pain. Pharmacotherapy 24:1675–1680
43. Kanowitz A, Dunn T, Kanowitz EM et al (2006) Safety and effectiveness of fentanyl administration for pre-hospital pain management. Prehosp Emerg Care 10:1–7
44. Chang AK, Bijur PE, Napolitano A et al (2009) Two milligrams intravenous hydromorphone is efficacious for treating pain but is associated with oxygen desaturation. J Opioid Manag 5:75–80
45. Pergolizzi J, Böger RH, Budd K et al (2008) Opioids and the management of chronic severe pain in the elderly: consensus statement of an International Expert Panel with focus on the six clinically most often used World Health Organization Step III opioids (buprenorphine, fentanyl, hydromorphone, methadone, morphine, oxycodone). Pain Pract 8:287–313
46. Clark E, Plint AC, Correll R et al (2007) A randomized, controlled trial of acetaminophen, ibuprofen, and codeine for acute pain relief in children with musculoskeletal trauma. Pediatrics 119:460–467
47. Derry S, Barden J, McQuay HJ, Moore RA (2008) Single dose oral celecoxib for acute postoperative pain in adults. Cochrane Database Syst Rev CD004233

48. McNicol ED, Strassels S, Goudas L et al (2011) NSAIDS or paracetamol, alone or combined with opioids for cancer pain. Cochrane Database Syst Rev CD005180
49. Holdgate A, Pollock T (2004) Nonsteroidal anti-inflammatory drugs (NSAIDS) versus opioids for acute renal colic. Cochrane Database Syst Rev CD004137
50. Miner JR (2009) Randomized double-blind placebo controlled crossover study of acetaminophen, ibuprofen, acetaminophen/hydrocodone, and placebo for the relief of pain from a standard painful stimulus. Acad Emerg Med 16:911–911
51. White PF, Joshi GP, Carpenter RL et al (1997) A comparison of oral ketorolac and hydrocodone-acetaminophen for analgesia after ambulatory surgery. Anesth Analg 85:37–43
52. Gimbel JS, Brugger A, Zhao W, Verburg KM, Geis GS (2001) Efficacy and tolerability of celecoxib versus hydrocodone/acetaminophen in the treatment of pain after ambulatory orthopedic surgery in adults. Clin Ther 23:228–241
53. Litkowski LJ, Christensen SE, Adamson DN et al (2005) Analgesic efficacy and tolerability of oxycodone 5 mg/ibuprofen400 mg compared with those of oxycodone 5 mg/acetaminophen 325 mg and hydrocodone 7.5 mg/acetaminophen 500 mg in patients with moderate to severe postoperative pain: A randomized, double-blind, placebo-controlled, single-dose, parallel-group study in a dental pain model. Clin Ther 27:418–429

Postpartum Hemorrhage

N. Kiefer and S. Weber

Introduction

Peripartum maternal death is a tragedy that claims lives of young women and leaves behind a devastated family. Postpartum hemorrhage (PPH) is the leading cause of maternal mortality worldwide, and it is all the more tragic as, among causes of maternal mortality, death from PPH appears preventable in many, if not most cases, at least in resource rich countries [1–3]. Management of PPH involves an interdisciplinary team of midwives, obstetricians, anesthetists and transfusion specialists. The scope of this review is to highlight current trends in epidemiology, medical treatment and the current controversy on transfusion protocols, blood component therapy or specific pharmacological interventions on the coagulation system.

A Symptom, Not a Diagnosis: Pathophysiological Considerations

The gravid uterus receives some 350 ml/min of maternal blood [4], thus PPH can be extremely severe and then easily diagnosed. For initial stages of PPH or less than severe bleeding diagnosis may be more difficult. There are several different definitions for PPH, mostly relying on arbitrary thresholds in terms of ml of blood loss, either separated for vaginal and Cesarean delivery, or, as the in the case of the UK's Royal College of Obstetrics and Gynecology, combined, statistically coupling increasing rates of Cesarean delivery to an increased incidence of PPH. Additionally, in many countries, there are varying definitions of 'severe PPH', which is

N. Kiefer (✉)
Department of Anesthesiology and Intensive Care Medicine, University of Bonn, Bonn, Germany
E-mail: dr.nicholas.kiefer@gmail.com

S. Weber
Department of Anesthesiology and Intensive Care Medicine, University of Bonn, Bonn, Germany

J.-L. Vincent (Ed.), *Annual Update in Intensive Care and Emergency Medicine 2013*,
DOI 10.1007/978-3-642-35109-9_2, © Springer-Verlag Berlin Heidelberg 2013

mostly defined by functional thresholds like the need for transfusion of more than four packed red blood cell (RBC) units or hemodynamic stigmata of hemorrhagic shock. However, most PPH thresholds are not well defined, as they rely on estimation of blood loss, which is known to be inaccurate [5]. Underestimation of actual blood loss can be substantial, even by experienced obstetricians and midwives [6]. Interestingly, the actual average peripartal blood loss exceeds 500 ml when measured with Cr51-tagged erythrocytes [7], thus really most vaginal deliveries would have to be considered as being followed by PPH. It is, therefore, not surprising that reported incidences of PPH vary with the technique of assessment of blood loss [8, 9]. These shortcomings have led to a call for an international revision of definitions and initiation of an international database [3]. Another general issue is that the term 'postpartum hemorrhage' suggests a diagnosis, which it is definitely not. Contrarily, if the syndrome of PPH occurs, a diagnosis must be aggressively sought [10]. The authors of this review prefer 'peripartum' to 'postpartum' hemorrhage, because it semantically does not exclude bleeding prior to delivery and its subterms open the path to a differential diagnosis of the underlying cause of hemorrhage: Antepartum hemorrhage, primary PPH and secondary PPH, which typically have distinct pathophysiological causes and therapeutic consequences.

Antepartum Hemorrhage

The most common causes for antepartum hemorrhage (bleeding after 24 weeks of gestation until delivery) are placenta previa, placental abruption and uterine rupture. All conditions can be very severe, with a mortality of 22 % and 37 % for placenta previa and abruption [11, 12]. Uterine rupture following uterine scaring or obstructed labor very often results in catastrophic fetal outcome and, in developing countries, it is a major cause of maternal mortality [13], whereas in Europe it rarely contributes to maternal mortality, but to maternal morbidity by a high hysterectomy rate [14]. The most difficult issue in all of these patients is, of course, that they have not yet delivered, thus there are two lives at stake; the well known difficulties in resuscitation during pregnancy have recently been reviewed by Farinelli and Hameed [15]. Another important feature is that placental abruption may be chronic, with ongoing coagulation and fibrinolysis in the tear between placenta and decidua, triggering disseminated intravascular coagulation (DIC) in up to 50 % of cases [16].

Primary Postpartum Hemorrhage

Defined as hemorrhage within the first 24 hours following delivery, primary PPH is the most common subtype of PPH. The reason for this is that the most frequent cause of PPH, uterine atony, presents as primary PPH. Other differential diagnoses

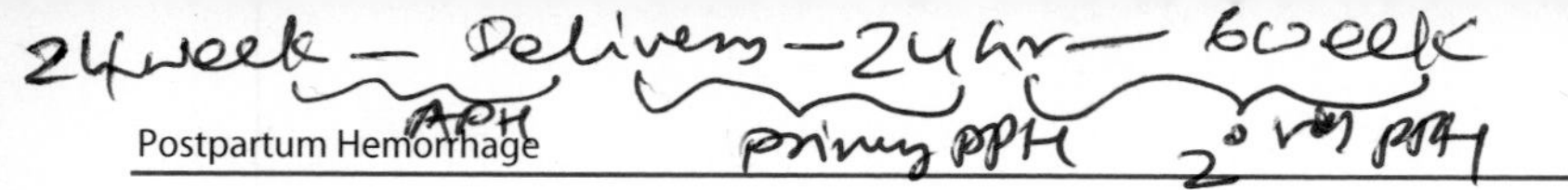

include: Retained placenta, cervical or genital tract lacerations, and inverted uterus as a consequence of severe atony or vigorous chord traction and, rarely, preexisting defects of coagulation like HELLP (hemolysis, elevated liver enzymes and low platelets), acute fatty liver of pregnancy or innate defects. The reason why coagulation disorders play a minor role in primary PPH is that uterine contraction plays the pivotal role in hemostasis at first. Myometrium fibers, running in all directions, mechanically clamp spiral arteries; only later, does coagulation become more important.

Secondary Postpartum Hemorrhage

Bleeding with an onset later than 24 hours until 6 weeks after birth is termed secondary PPH. In addition to coagulopathy, as pointed out earlier, other factors become important that develop only after birth, like intrauterine sepsis.

Thus, the onset of PPH before, early after or late after delivery already provides very important first steps in differential diagnosis that anesthetists in the medical emergency team or ICU must be aware of.

Epidemiology: A Clear Trend but No Clear Risk Profile

PPH accounts for roughly 100,000 maternal deaths per year [17], one every 5 minutes. Sequelae of PPH include infertility, neurological deficit or persistent organ failure, accounting for a large proportion of about 15 million cases of severe acute maternal morbidity. In Canada, 25 % of cases of severe acute maternal morbidity or 1 in 1,000 live births is attributed to PPH [18]. In the UK, severe PPH complicates 0.1 % of live births, and 2/3 of those result in severe acute maternal morbidity [19]. PPH is a paradigm of extreme global inequality in healthcare: Compared to Western Europe or the United States maternal mortality from PPH is about 100 times more frequent in developing countries, in some of them even 200 times [20], so that 99 % of the deaths occur in developing countries. Within the 'high resource' countries, PPH occurs significantly more often among members of racial or ethnic minorities [21] or in circumstances of social-economic disadvantage [22]. However, the global trend in maternal mortality is favorable, with a decrease by a third from 1990 [17], following a worldwide effort of the United Nations and several other organizations (millennium development goal 5A). Surprisingly, in that interval, the rate of PPH in developed countries rose, almost exclusively due to a rise in atonic PPH [3, 22–25]. The reasons for this rise remain unclear. Some of the increase has been attributed to a rise in certain risk factors, such as Cesarean section, maternal age, maternal obesity or multiple gestations following reproductive interventions [3].

Table 1 Risk factors for development of postpartum hemorrhage (PPH)

	Prepartum	Peri-/postpartum
Placenta/fetus	**anomalous insertion of the placenta** hypertensive diseases of pregnancy chorioamnionitis	**morbidly adherent placenta/retained placenta** **macrosomy**/large for gestational age baby
Uterus/birth channel	history of surgery of the uterus, including Cesarean section myoma uterine overdistension (polyhydramnion, **multiple gestations**, non-cephalic presentation) multiparity (>5)	induced/**prolonged labor** instrumental birth trauma of the birth channel (**uterine rupture, cervical laceration**, vaginal trauma)
Coagulation	innate or acquired coagulopathy, including HELLP syndrome and pregnancy associated thrombocytopenia/**thrombocytopathy**	amniotic fluid embolism
Other	**antenatal bleeding** **history of PPH**/retained placenta nicotine abuse age <20/>35 anemia	elective Cesarean section **emergency Cesarean section**, inhaled anesthetics

modified from [26], risk factors with an odds ratio >3 in **bold**

A logical way to reduce maternal morbidity and mortality from PPH should be to identify patients at risk for PPH and schedule their delivery in a tertiary center with an appropriate infrastructure to handle severe PPH efficiently. However, this approach is currently impossible. Large efforts have been undertaken to identify risk factors (Table 1) [26], develop scores or nomograms for the risk of PPH [9, 19, 27–29], but, even though an odds ratio of 18.4 has been found for certain risk constellations [28], 90 % of PPHs remain unpredicted [29], and in parturients with scheduled vaginal delivery (thus, absence of abnormal placentation, abnormal fetal position, etc.), predicted probability of PPH in presence of all remaining risk factors stays below 1 % [9]. The main reason is that well known antepartum risk factors are relatively frequent compared to the incidence of PPH, hence their low positive predictive probability. Stronger risk factors, like prolonged labor and retained placenta develop only during labor and delivery, making primary admission to a specialized center impossible. Thus, PPH mostly remains an unpredicted event, or, *vice versa*, the inability to predict PPH makes delivery for all women with risk factors in a tertiary center impossible. As a consequence, PPH will continue to occur in settings with a less than optimal infrastructure. It should thus be the aim to develop and validate protocols for prevention of morbidity and mortality from PPH that can be adopted in clinical settings outside large medical centers (and possibly in low resource countries), like the obstetric AMTSL (active management of the third stage of labor) protocol, a bundle of low cost and easily feasible measures for the management of a parturient after childbirth until the placenta is expelled:

- Administration of a uterotonic agent (oxytocin is the drug of choice) within one minute after birth
- Controlled cord traction
- Uterine massage after delivery of the placenta

Adherence to AMTSL has been shown to substantially reduce the incidence and severity of PPH [30–32].

Causal Treatment and Resuscitation

As for many medical situations, the Pareto-Principle also applies for reduction of mortality and morbidity from PPH: A small proportion of measures and interventions will have the most important impact on outcome, and failure in the timely initiation of these cannot be compensated for by other, even more sophisticated measures. The single most important factor in preventing adverse maternal outcome, of course, is early recognition of imminent or actual PPH [33], a factor, which anesthetists and intensivists cannot influence. In this respect, underestimation of blood loss is a key issue leading to late initiation of therapy [2, 5, 6]. The second most important factor is early onset of resuscitation, a factor that will be largely determined by the hospital's infrastructure and organization of medical emergency teams, activation pathways and ultimately by staff training [34]. A problem of staff competence to handle severe PPH is that in a single institution, PPH is a relatively rare complication affecting 1 in 1,000 live births [35]. Only because childbirth itself is such a frequent event, does the total number sum up to a high burden. As a consequence, it is simply impossible to develop routine skills in handling severe PPH, especially in smaller delivery units. On the other hand, within European countries, PPH regularly occurs in a setting where virtually all resources for sufficient initial resuscitation are readily available, including staff experienced in resuscitation (e. g., a medical emergency team), laboratory testing and blood products. A clear aim must, therefore, be to avoid underresuscitation, including hypothermia, coagulopathy and acidosis, what has been referred to as the "lethal triad" [36]. To succeed, clear standard procedures and massive transfusion protocols, team drills and simulation are valuable, if not essential tools [10, 37–40], and have been clearly advocated by an international expert panel [3]. After each case of severe PPH, a multidisciplinary debriefing session should be organized in a timely manner, in order to identify any problems in the local management of PPH, so that they can be addressed [41].

Medical Treatment: Uterotonics, Volume and Hemostatic Resuscitation

Uterotonics

Most cases of PPH will be primary PPH due to atony of the uterus, which is failure of the uterus to contract sufficiently to clamp the vascular bed of the decidua. Atony will occur in about 5 % of live births, but substantially more often in complicated births. Usually, it presents with painless vaginal bleeding and develops slowly at the beginning. A boggy uterus can easily contain more than 1,000 ml of blood, adding to the underestimation or underrecognition of PPH. An overview of commonly used uterotonics is given in Table 2, and although these drugs may be rarely used by anesthetists, knowledge of their properties is important as, in the setting of acute, massive PPH, obstetricians may have to rely on the anesthetist for medical treatment while surgically managing the patient. Currently, oxytocin is the drug of choice as first line uterotonic for prophylaxis and initial treatment of atonic PPH [42]. However, its efficacy may be limited and repeated doses may produce no further effect, which has been attributed to receptor desensitization [43]. The most important untoward effects of oxytocin are vasodilation and reflex tachycardia via calcium-dependent activation of the nitric oxide (NO) pathway, leading to an increase in cardiac output in healthy patients, but to a decrease if the physiologic cardiac response is impaired, such as in the setting of PPH [44]. Thus, extreme caution is warranted with the use of oxytocin in the setting of unresuscitated PPH. The German Society for Anesthesiology and Intensive Care Medicine recommends not to administer oxytocin as a bolus [45]; the Confidential Enquiry into Maternal and Child Health (CEMACH) reported at least one maternal death following administration of a bolus of oxytocin in a hypovolemic patient [46]. In pre-eclamptic patients, the cardiovascular effects may be stronger and less predictable, so in these patients it must be used with special caution [47]. Some years ago, carbetocin, an oxytocin analog was introduced into clinical practice. Its main advantage is the longer duration of action compared to oxytocin (plasma half-life around 40 min [48] vs. less than 180 s for oxytocin [49]). Use of 100 mcg carbetocin is equivalent to oxytocin for prevention of PPH, with a reduced need for uterine massage [50]. However, no data exist for the treatment of manifest PPH, so this new drug cannot be recommended for that use, especially as, from a mechanistic point of view, it shares the problem of a ceiling effect and possibly untoward hemodynamic effects of oxytocin. If oxytocin agonists fail as first line treatment, use of alternative uterotonics should not be delayed. Prostaglandin derivates are widely used, especially PGE_1 (misoprostol), which can be administered vaginally, rectally and sublingually. It is usually the drug of choice in low-resource countries, and has limited cardiovascular side-effects. However misoprostol is associated with a higher blood loss than oxytocin [51, 52]. Currently, many delivery units use misoprostol in addition to oxytocin, as this combination appears to have fewer side-effects than other combinations, though conclusive data are lacking. Other prostaglandins and ergot derivates are used as second line uterotonics; their

Table 2 Uterotonic drugs

	Dosage	Cautions
Oxytocin Analogs		
Oxytocin	Bolus: 3–10 IU i.v/10 IU i.m. continuous: 10 IU/h titrated	Vasodilation, tachycardia, hypotension (especially with hypovolemia), antidiuresis (fluid overload), caution in preeclampsia, nausea, vomiting
Carbetocin	100 mcg i.v.	
Ergot Derivates		
Ergometrine	0.25 mg i.m/i.v.; can be repeated every 5 min, max. 5 doses	Potent vasoconstrictor: contraindicated in hypertensive diseases of pregnancy, extreme caution for use in combination with other uterotonics, myocardial ischemia, pulmonary arterial hypertension nausea/vomiting/dizziness
Methergonovine	0.20 mg i.m.; every 5 min, max. 5 doses	
Prostaglandin Derivates		
Sulprostone	8.3 mcg/min (≙ 500 mcg/h), max 1,500 mcg/24 h, deescalation of dosing necessary	Careful in hypertensive/hypovolemic patients, gastrointestinal disturbance, shivering, pyrexia, hypotension with PGF$_{2\alpha}$. Bronchospasm (extreme caution in patients with asthma), pulmonary arterial hypertension
Carboprost (15-methyl-PGF$_{2\alpha}$)	0.25 mg i.m./i.my.; every 15 min., max. 2 mg.	
Dinoprostone	2 mg p.r. every 2 h	
Dinoprose	0.5–1 mg i.my or 20 mg + 500 ml NaCl 0.9 % infused into uterine cavity	
Gemeprost	1–2 mg i.u./1 mg p.r.	
Misoprostol (PGE$_2$)	600–1,000 mcg p.r.//i.u./s.l.	

i.m: intramuscular; i.my: intramyometrically; i.v: intravenously; p.r: per rectum; s.l: sublingually; modified from [33]

dosing is summarized in Table 2 [33]. All may cause severe adverse effects and should not be administered as a bolus. Their combination can lead to unpredictable cardiovascular effects, especially in the setting of ongoing bleeding. In our department, the combination of any two uterotonic drugs except oxytocin and misoprostol is discouraged. However, a fixed combination of oxytocin and ergometrine (Syntometrine™) is commercially available.

Fluid Resuscitation and Hemostatic Interventions

Without doubt, mass transfusion protocols can improve the outcome of patients with massive bleeding [53, 54]. Although these protocols have been derived from combat medicine, and their adoption for PPH ignores some very important differences, they have been advocated repeatedly for that indication [10, 55, 56] and may be useful in severe PPH [57]. One key factor in mass transfusion protocols is the fixed ratio of blood products given, with the aim of avoiding a delay in hemostatic resuscitation while waiting to receive laboratory results. Another factor is that such mass transfusion protocols are tailored to the local circumstances and resources. They are usually developed by multidisciplinary teams, involving (obstetric) surgeons, anesthetists, hematologists, blood bank and transportation staff, so that they are locally feasible. However, it must be kept in mind that PPH occurs in a setting where resuscitation can be initiated from the moment of the diagnosis, in contrast to trauma victims, who may reach the emergency room already severely exsanguinated and having undergone prolonged resuscitation with crystalloids or colloids. This event is, however, exactly what must and can be avoided in PPH [58], and concerns about overtriage to mass transfusion protocols have been raised [59]. It would be desirable to develop, validate, adopt and enforce mass transfusion protocols specific for PPH, because they may help to avoid the most common reason for insufficient therapy: Blood products administered too late in insufficient quantities [60]. It is not unlikely that vigorously enforced interdisciplinary PPH emergency protocols, continuous staff training, drills and scrupulous quality management will save more lives at a lower cost than any pharmacological intervention.

The main difference between traumatic bleeding and PPH is an altered hematological profile of pregnant women compared to trauma victims. PPH occurs in an already activated coagulation system: The activity of coagulation factors is increased, fibrinolysis is activated and antifibrinolysis impaired; additionally cross-link formation between fibrin monomers is diminished, making fibrin less stable and less resistant to fibrinolysis. The resulting hypercoagulable and hyperfibrinolytic state has been interpreted as a chronic, low grade DIC [61]. Other authors have used the term "pelvic consumption coagulopathy" [62], suggesting that this preexisting latent disorder can rapidly evolve to massive DIC and, as a consequence, consumption coagulopathy, which is indeed a frequent and early feature of PPH (review of physiological changes during pregnancy and their consequences: [58]). In contrast, the coagulopathy of trauma victims has typically been described as a dilutional coagulopathy. Only recently, early changes in trauma victims' coagulation status and the significance of these changes have come into focus [63, 64]. Whether that "acute coagulopathy of trauma" actually relates to the situation in early PPH is unclear.

Tranexamic Acid

Levels of D-dimers and fibrinogen degradation products are regularly elevated during pregnancy and are further increased directly postpartum because of placental derived plasminogen activator inhibitor (PAI) type 2 [65] as a sign of activated fibrinolysis [66]. This makes therapy with antifibrinolytic drugs, like tranexamic acid, attractive in the setting of PPH. Additionally there is very convincing evidence for the use of tranexamic acid in bleeding trauma patients [67] and in surgical patients [68]. Antifibrinolytic drugs are recommended in current European guidelines for trauma care [69]. In obstetrics, tranexamic acid has been found to reduce blood loss after vaginal and Cesarean delivery in a Cochrane review and two recent randomized trials [70–72]. However, the evidence for tranexamic acid as a treatment for manifest PPH has been poor [73]. Last year, a first randomized study in 144 women diagnosed with peripartum blood loss > 800 ml showed a significant reduction in blood loss with a high dose of tranexamic acid (4 g), albeit only 50 ml difference [74]. Several other surrogate parameters, e. g., efficacy of first line uterotonic treatment, were also significantly improved. The study, however, did not show any significant differences in major outcome parameters, e. g., hysterectomy rate or ICU stay. A concern with the use of antifibrinolytic drugs is the risk of vascular occlusive events, a complication to which pregnant patients are prone. Aprotinin, another antifibrinolytic drug, has been withdrawn after a large trial was stopped prematurely [75]. A meta-analysis of available data on thrombotic side effects after prophylactic use of tranexamic acid [73] showed no increase in such events (none occurred in 461 patients included in the meta-analysis). Another meta-analysis, including case reports and non-randomized trials, identified two cases of pulmonary embolism, but stated that a causal relationship was not clear [76]. In the study by Ducloy-Bouthors et al. more vascular occlusive events occurred after administration of 4 g tranexamic acid than in the control group [74], albeit far from statistically significant, but the study was underpowered to assess this parameter. In bleeding trauma patients, however, the risk for occlusive vascular events has been found to be reduced with the use of tranexamic acid [67]. The results of a large international, randomized and controlled trial expected to enroll 15,000 parturients, initiated from members of the CRASH collaborator group, are thus of outstanding interest, but will not be available before 2015. Until then, the potential benefit has to be weighed against the risk of ongoing bleeding on an individual basis. Keeping in mind that a parturient regularly has increased fibrinolysis, that the effect of tranexamic acid on blood loss after delivery without PPH has been documented, and the strong evidence for tranexamic acid in bleeding trauma and surgical patients, it may be appropriate to administer 1–2 g tranexamic acid in cases of severe, life-threatening bleeding, even without laboratory evidence of hyperfibrinolysis. Further administration can then be guided by detailed laboratory analyses. Several authors and the current World Health Organization (WHO) guidelines have endorsed the use of tranexamic acid in severe PPH [55, 60, 77, 78] although they acknowledge the limited evidence. Moreover, this endorsement should not prompt the use of this drug as a routine prophylactic. In uncomplicated vaginal and Cesarean delivery, the blood sparing effect may be as little as 50 ml, and the risk of adverse events prompted by pregnancy-induced hypercoagulability has not yet been adequately assessed [60].

Fibrinogen

Fibrinogen levels have recently come into focus, after they were found to be a valuable laboratory parameter to predict progress from mild to severe PPH [79]. Fibrinogen levels are usually elevated at term (4.8 g/l vs. 1.8–4 g/l in non-pregnant individuals [80]) and may decrease rapidly with ongoing PPH. Laboratory testing shows that clot formation depends on fibrinogen levels being above 0.7 g/l [81]. A cut-off value of 4 mg/dl has a negative predictive value of 79 % and the positive predictive value of a concentration below 2 g/l (thus within the normal range of a non-pregnant population) was 100 %. These findings have recently been confirmed [82] and have sparked a debate as to whether this decrease in plasma fibrinogen levels plays a pathophysiological role in the development of severe PPH or is rather an epiphenomena of ongoing bleeding. An undisputed advantage of commercially available fibrinogen (Haemocomplettan P™) is that: (a) it can be stored in the delivery unit as an immediately available rescue drug; and (b) only small volumes, which can be administered as a bolus, are necessary to restore fibrinogen levels. Although 1,000–2,000 ml of fresh frozen plasma are needed to elevate the fibrinogen plasma concentration by 1 g/l, 2 g of fibrinogen will accomplish the same result [83]. As for tranexamic acid, we will have to await the results of randomized studies addressing the use of fibrinogen in PPH. One medium sized study in patients meeting criteria for mild PPH is currently enrolling patients and is expected to be completed in autumn 2013 (clinicaltrials.gov identifier: NCT01359878). Until these data are available, the reasonable approach to fibrinogen (or cryoprecipitate) would be to keep it readily available for cases of life-threatening PPH in order to bypass logistic constraints in supply of fresh frozen plasma, like transport and thawing, and in case of hypofibrinogenemia demonstrated by laboratory testing [60, 77, 83, 84]. A very important practical issue is that in coagulopathic patients with hyperfibrinolysis, antifibrinolytic drugs must be administered before any effort to restore fibrinogen plasma level is undertaken. Also, infusion of starch-based colloids can influence laboratory testing of fibrinogen. If starch solutions have been administered, the threshold for fibrinogen administration in PPH should be raised from 1.5 g/l to 2 g/l [60].

Recombinant Human Factor VII

Recombinant human factor VII (rhFVII) was originally developed for patients with classic hemophilia and inhibitory antibody hemophilia. Physiologically, factor VII is activated by tissue factor and activates factors IX and X to factor IXa. Binding of factor VIIa to tissue factor initiates the cascade that leads to activation of prothrombin to form thrombin, which converts fibrinogen into fibrin, building the clot. In higher doses, FVIIa or rhFVIIa directly activates factor X on the surface of activated platelets, bypassing factor VIII and IX, creating what has been termed a "thrombin burst", which generates large quantities of fibrin at the site of injury. The presumed potential of rhVIIa to reduce blood loss in off-label use to control otherwise uncontrollable bleeding because of its unique mechanism of action [85] has sparked much expectation. However, a recent Cochrane meta-analysis [86] of therapeutic use of rhFVII, including 11 studies in 2,732 patients with ongoing bleeding, showed no significant effect on mortality and control of bleeding. In the setting of PPH, case series and reports have been encouraging [87–89]. For this type of publication, a substantial publication bias must always be assumed, and no controlled trials have been published. One randomized trial has been completed in France, but to our knowledge, no study results are available (clinicaltrials.gov identifier: NCT00370877). The German medical council has raised concerns about the increase in thromboembolic complications [90], but a Cochrane analysis [86] showed no overall increase in adverse thromboembolic events in prophylactic or therapeutic use of rhFVII. However, in the subgroup of patients older than 65, an increase in thromboembolic complication was observed. It is not clear how these safety data can be expanded to PPH, as the procoagulatory state of a parturient might infer an increased risk for thromboembolic complications. Currently, most experts, including an expert panel set up by the manufacturer of rhFVII, advocate the use of rhFVII only in very select situations [60, 84, 91–93].

- rhFVII cannot be a substitute for adequate medical or surgical treatment. In any cases, prior to its use, a definitive diagnosis of the cause of PPH must be established. Practically all cases, except uterine atony without retained fetal tissue, must be treated surgically and are not suitable for rhFVII use. For PPH from uterine atony, after uterotonic agents and uterine massage have been appropriately used, advanced interventions, such as balloon tamponade, B-Lynch suture or radiological embolization of uterine arteries should be considered (the latter, however, is usually not a suitable option for massive, ongoing PPH) [10].
- Before considering rhFVII, acidosis and hypothermia must be corrected, plasma levels of calcium, fibrinogen and platelets must have been restored, as failure to do so will impair or prevent the efficacy of rhFVII. Also, with ongoing arterial bleeding, rhFVII treatment is prone to fail.

If these points have been addressed timely and vigorously, bleeding will have stopped in most cases before the use of rhVII. If not, rhFVII may be used off-label as an attempt to avoid hysterectomy. The recommended dose is 90 mcg/kg bodyweight. If bleeding continues after 10–20 minutes, a second dose can be used. If bleeding continues despite two doses of rhFVII and normothermia/sufficient calcium and fibrinogen plasma levels and platelet count, hysterectomy should not be delayed.

A suggested second indication for rhFVII is immediate unavailability or shortage of blood products. However, in such cases, immediate hysterectomy instead of attempting rhFVII appears more appropriate. It must be pointed out that the availability of rhFVII is by no means a substitute for an adequate infrastructure and logistics, nor should its administration delay any lifesaving intervention [94]. In countries that dispose of a registry, all cases should be entered. Finally, in contrast to, e. g., tranexamic acid, rhFVII is extremely expensive, making it quiet impossible to use outside of resource rich countries, i. e., where 99 % of the fatalities occur.

Other Aspects: Cell Salvage and Point-Of-Care Coagulation Monitoring

Childbirth has traditionally been seen as a contraindication for transfusion of autologous blood collected from the site of operation, especially during Cesarean section, because of concerns about amniotic fluid, fetal squames or phospholipid embolization, further adding to coagulation abnormalities. However, these concerns have been overcome, especially with the use of leukocyte depletion filters. Cell salvage for obstetrics has been endorsed by major obstetric anesthesia societies and the Royal College of Obstetricians and Gynecologists (UK), following laboratory investigations that demonstrated removal of amniotic fluid components and fetal cell detritus and several case series publications. About one third of UK delivery units dispose of cell salvage technology and most of them have added it to PPH protocols [95]. The peripartum use of cell salvage technology has recently been thoroughly reviewed [96]. The main drawbacks for use in PPH are logistic constraints, owing to the unpredicted onset of most cases of PPH. Only in high-risk elective Cesarean sections, e. g., with diagnosed placenta percreta is its routine use feasible, and in our department cell salvage is set up for such cases. Depending on local structures, disposables for a cell salvage machine are cost efficient after 1–2 units of spared packed RBCs [97]. For these cases, leukocyte depletion filters should be available.

With increased attention to hyperfibrinolysis and hypofibrinogenemia, their prognostic value, and recommended interventions to treat these conditions, point-of-care (POC) monitoring of coagulation, e. g., with thromboelastograhy (TEG) or rotation thromboelastometry (ROTEM) and the related FIBTEM, seems to provide useful and timely parameters [98]. A problem in evaluating monitoring methods is that they may be helpful for the assessment of a specific parameter, but they are not therapeutic. They can only be as good as the treatment they prompt – in the worst case they may be harmful. As pointed out earlier, conclusive evidence for most interventions that can be guided by POC coagulation monitoring is lacking. However, provided efficacy of antifibrinolytic drugs and fibrinogen, POC coagulation monitoring can be a valuable tool for goal-directed hemostatic resuscitation. As for cell salvage, however, logistic restraints exist. If a delivery unit is not adjacent to a central operating unit, TEG or ROTEM will be unlikely to be available. However, as platelet count is an important obstetric parameter (e. g., for HELLP diagnostics), many delivery units will be equipped with a POC test for platelet count, which can be very useful in massive PPH.

Conclusion

PPH is the leading cause of maternal morbidity and mortality worldwide. Although global efforts have helped to reduce maternal mortality worldwide, the rate of PPH in developed countries is increasing; nonetheless, 99 % of cases occur in developing countries. Continuing attention has to be paid to further pursue the millennium development goal of a reduction of maternal mortality by three quarters between 1990 and 2015.

Risk profiling can help to identify patients at risk for bleeding, with history of PPH, anomalous insertion of the placenta, and coagulopathy being the most prominent risk factors. Patients with a high risk of PPH should deliver in a specialized center. However, many, if not most cases of PPH will not be predicted, and thus they will occur outside of an optimal setting.

Although several pharmacological interventions have been proposed and will probably prove to be useful in high resource countries, focus should be placed on development, training and quality control of local PPH and mass transfusion protocols that reflect local infrastructure. This approach can substantially help to prevent and manage severe PPH. The main factor determining poor outcome is failure to perform elementary steps, such as delayed diagnosis, staff activation and underresuscitation in case of massive PPH. Many, if not most cases of maternal death due to PPH are considered preventable in resource rich countries, which refers to use of basic measures, not to advanced medical treatment of coagulopathy. Among the proposed pharmacological interventions, uterotonics are the mainstay of therapy. Goals of resuscitation should be adequate fluid therapy and early administration of blood products, ideally according to a mass transfusion protocol. A major priority in anesthesiology management is the maintenance of a basic framework that is needed for coagulation, including normocalcemia, prevention or correction of acidosis, normothermia and platelet count. Use of antifibrinolytics, such as tranexamic acid, and early substitution of fibrinogen to levels > 1.5 g/l, are currently being investigated in larger trials and have the potential for broad application. rhFVII, in contrast, will probably play a minor role for use only in specific situations. Cell salvage and POC coagulation monitoring are recommendable, but logistically difficult to establish. Wherever future trends will go, successful treatment of PPH will remain an interdisciplinary task.

References

1. Berg CJ, Harper MA, Atkinson SM et al (2005) Preventability of pregnancy-related deaths: results of a state-wide review. Obstet Gynecol 106:1228–1234
2. Lewis G (2007) The Confidential Enquiry into Maternal and Child Health (CEMACH). Saving Mothers' Lives: reviewing maternal deaths to make motherhood safer – 2003–2005. The seventh report on confidential enquiries into maternal deaths in the United Kingdom. Available at: http://www.publichealth.hscni.net/sites/default/files/Saving%20Mothers'%20Lives%202003-05%20.pdf. Accessed October 2012
3. Knight M, Callaghan WM, Berg C et al (2009) Trends in postpartum hemorrhage in high resource countries: a review and recommendations from the International Postpartum Hemorrhage Collaborative Group. BMC Pregnancy Childbirth 9:55
4. Thaler I, Manor D, Itskovitz J et al (1990) Changes in uterine blood flow during human pregnancy. Am J Obstet Gynecol 162:121–125
5. Sloan NL, Durocher J, Aldrich T et al (2010) What measured blood loss tells us about postpartum bleeding: a systematic review. BJOG 117:788–800
6. Stafford I, Dildy GA, Clark SL et al (2008) Visually estimated and calculated blood loss in vaginal and cesarean delivery. Am J Obstet Gynecol 199:519.e1–519.e7
7. Gahres EE, Albert SN, Dodek SM (1962) Intrapartum blood loss measured with Cr 51-tagged erythrocytes. Obstet Gynecol 19:455–462
8. Carroli G, Cuesta C, Abalos E et al (2008) Epidemiology of postpartum haemorrhage: a systematic review. Best Pract Res Clin Obstet Gynaecol 22:999–1012

9. Biguzzi E, Franchi F, Ambrogi F et al (2012) Risk factors for postpartum hemorrhage in a cohort of 6011 Italian women. Thromb Res 129:e1–e7
10. Clark SL, Hankins GDV (2012) Preventing maternal death: 10 clinical diamonds. Obstet Gynecol 119:360–364
11. Rudra A, Chatterjee S, Sengupta S et al (2010) Management of obstetric hemorrhage. Middle East J Anesthesiol 20:499–507
12. Nielson EC, Varner MW, Scott JR (1991) The outcome of pregnancies complicated by bleeding during the second trimester. Surg Gynecol Obstet 173:371–374
13. Justus Hofmeyr G, Say L, Metin Gülmezoglu A (2005) Systematic Review: WHO systematic review of maternal mortality and morbidity: the prevalence of uterine rupture. BJOG 112:1221–1228
14. Guise JM (2004) Systematic review of the incidence and consequences of uterine rupture in women with previous caesarean section. BMJ 329:19–25
15. Farinelli CK, Hameed AB (2012) Cardiopulmonary resuscitation in pregnancy. Cardiol Clin 30:453–461
16. Mercier FJ, Van de Velde M (2008) Major obstetric hemorrhage. Anesthesiol Clin 26:53–66
17. Khan KS, Wojdyla D, Say L et al (2006) WHO analysis of causes of maternal death: a systematic review. Lancet 367:1066–1074
18. Wen SW, Huang L, Liston R et al (2005) Severe maternal morbidity in Canada, 1991–2001. CMAJ 173:759–764
19. Waterstone M, Bewley S, Wolfe C (2001) Incidence and predictors of severe obstetric morbidity: case-control study. BMJ 322:1089–1093
20. Hogan MC, Foreman KJ, Naghavi M et al (2010) Maternal mortality for 181 countries, 1980–2008: a systematic analysis of progress towards Millennium Development Goal 5. Lancet 375:1609–1623
21. Creanga AA, Berg CJ, Syverson C et al (2012) Race, ethnicity, and nativity differentials in pregnancy-related mortality in the United States: 1993–2006. Obstet Gynecol 120:261–268
22. Lutomski JE, Byrne BM, Devane D et al (2012) Increasing trends in atonic postpartum haemorrhage in Ireland: an 11-year population-based cohort study. BJOG 119:306–314
23. Bateman BT, Berman MF, Riley LE et al (2010) The epidemiology of postpartum hemorrhage in a large, nationwide sample of deliveries. Anesth Analg 110:1368–1373
24. Berg CJ, Callaghan WM, Syverson C et al (2010) Pregnancy-related mortality in the United States, 1998 to 2005. Obstet Gynecol 116:1302–1309
25. Schutte JM, Steegers EAP, Schuitemaker NWE et al (2010) Rise in maternal mortality in the Netherlands. BJOG 117:399–406
26. Rath W, Surbek D, Kainer F et al (2008) Diagnosis and Therapy of Peripartum Hemorrhage. Leitlinie der Deutschen Gesellschaft für Gynäkologie und Geburtshilfe (DGGG). Available at: http://www.dggg.de/fileadmin/public_docs/Leitlinien/3-3-5-peripartale-blutungen-2010.pdf. Accessed October 2012
27. Gayat E, Resche-Rigon M, Morel O et al (2011) Predictive factors of advanced interventional procedures in a multicentre severe postpartum haemorrhage study. Intensive Care Med 37:1816–1825
28. Naef 3rd RW, Chauhan SP, Chevalier SP et al (1994) Prediction of hemorrhage at cesarean delivery. Obstet Gynecol 83:923–926
29. Prata N, Hamza S, Bell S et al (2011) Inability to predict postpartum hemorrhage: insights from Egyptian intervention data. BMC Pregnancy Childbirth 11:97
30. Begley CM, Gyte GML, Devane D et al (2011) Active versus expectant management for women in the third stage of labour. Cochrane Database Syst Rev CD007412
31. Leduc D, Senikas V, Lalonde AB et al (2009) Active management of the third stage of labour: prevention and treatment of postpartum hemorrhage. J Obstet Gynaecol Can 31:980–993
32. Rogers J, Wood J, McCandlish R et al (1998) Active versus expectant management of third stage of labour: the Hinchingbrooke randomised controlled trial. Lancet 351:693–699

33. B-Lynch C, Keith LG, Lalonde AB, Karoshi M (2006) A Textbook of Postpartum Hemorrhage: A Comprehensive Guide to Evaluation, Management and Surgical Intervention. Sapiens Publishing, Duncow
34. Leong BSH, Chua GSW (2011) Quality of resuscitation in hospitals. Singapore Med J 52:616–619
35. Drife J (1997) Management of primary postpartum haemorrhage. BJOG 104:275–277
36. Sihler KC, Napolitano LM (2010) Complications of massive transfusion. Chest 137:209–220
37. Crofts JF, Ellis D, Draycott TJ et al (2007) Change in knowledge of midwives and obstetricians following obstetric emergency training: a randomised controlled trial of local hospital, simulation centre and teamwork training. BJOG 114:1534–1541
38. Merién AER, van de Ven J, Mol BW et al (2010) Multidisciplinary team training in a simulation setting for acute obstetric emergencies: a systematic review. Obstet Gynecol 115:1021–1031
39. Rizvi F, Mackey R, Barrett T et al (2004) Successful reduction of massive postpartum haemorrhage by use of guidelines and staff education. BJOG 111:495–498
40. Siassakos D, Crofts JF, Winter C et al (2009) The active components of effective training in obstetric emergencies. BJOG 116:1028–1032
41. Su LL, Chong YS (2012) Massive obstetric haemorrhage with disseminated intravascular coagulopathy. Best Pract Res Clin Obstet Gynaecol 26:77–90
42. Vercauteren M, Palit S, Soetens F et al (2009) Anaesthesiological considerations on tocolytic and uterotonic therapy in obstetrics. Acta Anaesthesiol Scand 53:701–709
43. Magalhaes JKRS, Carvalho JCA, Parkes RK et al (2009) Oxytocin pretreatment decreases oxytocin-induced myometrial contractions in pregnant rats in a concentration-dependent but not time-dependent manner. Reprod Sci 16:501–508
44. Dyer RA, Butwick AJ, Carvalho B (2011) Oxytocin for labour and caesarean delivery: implications for the anaesthesiologist. Curr Opin Anaesthesiol 24:255–261
45. Gogarten W, Van Aken H, Kessler P et al (2009) Durchfuehrung von Analgesie- und Anaesthesieverfahren in der Geburtshilfe. 2. Überarbeitete Empfehlungen der Deutschen Gesellschaft für Anästhesiologie und Intensivmedizin. Anaesth Intensivmed 50:S502–S507
46. Thomas TA, Cooper GM (2002) Maternal deaths from anaesthesia: An extract from Why mothers die 1997–1999, the Confidential Enquiries into Maternal Deaths in the United Kingdom. Br J Anaesth 89:499–508
47. Langesæter E, Rosseland LA, Stubhaug A (2011) Haemodynamic effects of oxytocin in women with severe preeclampsia. Int J Obstet Anesth 20:26–29
48. Sweeney G, Holbrook AM, Levine M et al (1990) Pharmacokinetics of carbetocin, a long-acting oxytocin analogue, in nonpregnant women. Curr Therapeutic Res 47:528–540
49. Rydén G, Sjöholm I (1969) Half-life of oxytocin in blood of pregnant and non-pregnant women. Acta Endocrinol 61:425–431
50. Su LL, Chong YS, Samuel M (2012) Carbetocin for preventing postpartum haemorrhage. Cochrane Database Syst Rev CD005457
51. Gohil JT, Tripathi B (2011) A study to compare the efficacy of misoprostol, oxytocin, methyl-ergometrine and ergometrine-oxytocin in reducing blood loss in active management of 3rd stage of labor. J Obstet Gynaecol India 61:408–412
52. Gibbins KJ, Albright CM, Rouse DJ (2013) Postpartum hemorrhage in the developed world: whither misoprostol? Am J Obstet Gynecol (in press)
53. Borgman MA, Spinella PC, Perkins JG et al (2007) The ratio of blood products transfused affects mortality in patients receiving massive transfusions at a combat support hospital. J Trauma 63:805–813
54. Cotton BA, Au BK, Nunez TC et al (2009) Predefined massive transfusion protocols are associated with a reduction in organ failure and postinjury complications. J Trauma Acute Care Surg 66:41–49
55. Onwuemene O, Green D, Keith L (2012) Postpartum hemorrhage management in 2012: Predicting the future. Int J Gynecol Obst 119:3–5

56. Pacheco LD, Saade GR, Gei AF et al (2011) Cutting-edge advances in the medical management of obstetrical hemorrhage. Am J Obstet Gynecol 205:526–532
57. Gutierrez MC, Goodnough LT, Druzin M et al (2012) Postpartum hemorrhage treated with a massive transfusion protocol at a tertiary obstetric center: a retrospective study. Int J Obstet Anesth 21:230–235
58. Snegovskikh D, Clebone A, Norwitz E (2011) Anesthetic management of patients with placenta accreta and resuscitation strategies for associated massive hemorrhage. Curr Opin Anaesthesiol 24:274–281
59. Callum JL, Rizoli S (2012) Plasma transfusion for patients with severe hemorrhage: what is the evidence? Transfusion 52(Suppl 1):30S–37S
60. Gogarten W (2011) Postpartum hemorrhage-an update. Anasthesiol Intensivmed Notfallmed Schmerzther 46:508–514
61. Cerneca F, Ricci G, Simeone R et al (1997) Coagulation and fibrinolysis changes in normal pregnancy: Increased levels of procoagulants and reduced levels of inhibitors during pregnancy induce a hypercoagulable state, combined with a reactive fibrinolysis. Eur J Obstet Gynecol Reprod Biol 73:31–36
62. Macphail S, Talks K (2004) Massive post-partum haemorrhage and management of disseminated intravascular coagulation. Curr Opin Obstet Gynecol 14:123–131
63. Pötzsch B, Ivaskevicius V (2011) Haemostasis management of massive bleeding. Hämostaseologie 31:15–20
64. Rugeri L, Levrat A, David JS et al (2007) Diagnosis of early coagulation abnormalities in trauma patients by rotation thrombelastography. J Thromb Haemost 5:289–295
65. Brenner B (2004) Haemostatic changes in pregnancy. Thromb Res 114:409–414
66. Epiney M, Boehlen F, Boulvain M et al (2005) D-dimer levels during delivery and the postpartum. J Thromb Haemost 3:268–271
67. Shakur H, Roberts I, Bautista R et al (2010) CRASH-2 trial collaborators. Effects of tranexamic acid on death, vascular occlusive events, and blood transfusion in trauma patients with significant haemorrhage (CRASH-2): a randomised, placebo-controlled trial. Lancet 376:23–32
68. Ker K, Edwards P, Perel P, Shakur H, Roberts I (2012) Effect of tranexamic acid on surgical bleeding: systematic review and cumulative meta-analysis. BMJ 344:e3054
69. Rossaint R, Bouillon B, Cerny V et al (2010) Management of bleeding following major trauma: an updated European guideline. Crit Care 14:R52
70. Novikova N, Hofmeyr GJ (2007) Tranexamic acid for preventing postpartum haemorrhage. Cochrane Database Syst Rev CD007872
71. Gungorduk K, Yıldırım G, Asıcıoğlu O et al (2011) Efficacy of intravenous tranexamic acid in reducing blood loss after elective cesarean section: a prospective, randomized, double-blind, placebo-controlled study. Am J Perinatol 28:233–240
72. Movafegh A, Eslamian L, Dorabadi A (2011) Effect of intravenous tranexamic acid administration on blood loss during and after cesarean delivery. BJOG 115:224–226
73. Ferrer P, Roberts I, Sydenham E et al (2009) Anti-fibrinolytic agents in post partum haemorrhage: a systematic review. BMC Pregnancy Childbirth 9:29
74. Ducloy-Bouthors A-S, Jude B, Duhamel A et al (2011) High-dose tranexamic acid reduces blood loss in postpartum haemorrhage. Crit Care 15:R117
75. Fergusson DA, Hébert PC, Mazer CD et al (2008) A comparison of aprotinin and lysine analogues in high-risk cardiac surgery. N Engl J Med 358:2319–2331
76. Peitsidis P, Kadir RA (2011) Antifibrinolytic therapy with tranexamic acid in pregnancy and postpartum. Expert Opin Pharmacother 12:503–516
77. Lier H, Rath W (2011) Current interdisciplinary recommendations for the management of severe postpartum hemorrhage (PPH). Geburtshilfe und Frauenheilkunde 71:577–588
78. (2009) WHO Guidelines for the Management of Postpartum Hemorrhage and Retained Placenta. WHO Press, Geneva
79. Charbit B, Mandelbrot L, Samain E et al (2007) The decrease of fibrinogen is an early predictor of the severity of postpartum hemorrhage. J Thromb Haemost 5:266–273

80. Kratz A, Ferraro M, Sluss PM et al (2004) Laboratory reference values. N Engl J Med 351:1548–1564
81. Mercier FJ, Bonnet MP (2010) Use of clotting factors and other prohemostatic drugs for obstetric hemorrhage. Curr Opin Anaesthesiol 23:310–316
82. Cortet M, Deneux-Tharaux C, Dupont C et al (2012) Association between fibrinogen level and severity of postpartum haemorrhage: secondary analysis of a prospective trial. Br J Anaesth 108:984–989
83. Bell SF, Rayment R, Collins PW et al (2010) The use of fibrinogen concentrate to correct hypofibrinogenaemia rapidly during obstetric haemorrhage. Int J Obstet Anesth 19:218–223
84. Ahonen J, Stefanovic V, Lassila R (2010) Management of post-partum haemorrhage. Acta Anaesthesiol Scand 54:1164–1178
85. Wood AJJ, Mannucci PM (1998) Hemostatic drugs. N Engl J Med 339:245–253
86. Lin Y, Stanworth S, Birchall J et al (2011) Recombinant factor VIIa for the prevention and treatment of bleeding in patients without haemophilia. Cochrane Database Syst Rev CD005011
87. Ahonen J, Jokela R, Korttila K (2007) An open non-randomized study of recombinant activated factor VII in major postpartum haemorrhage. Acta Anaesth Scand 51:929–936
88. Boehlen F, Morales MA, Fontana P et al (2004) Prolonged treatment of massive postpartum haemorrhage with recombinant factor VIIa: case report and review of the literature. BJOG 111:284–287
89. Segal S, Shemesh IY, Blumental R et al (2004) The use of recombinant factor VIIa in severe postpartum hemorrhage. Acta Obstet Gynecol Scand 83:771–772
90. Bundesärztekammer, [German Medical Association] (2009) Cross-sectional guidelines for therapy with blood components and plasma derivatives. Available at: https://www.iakh.de/tl_files/iakh/public/richtlinien/Querschnittsleitlinie_4._Auflage_-_englisch_05.01.2011%20copy.pdf. Accessed October 2012
91. McLintock C, James AH (2011) Obstetric hemorrhage. J Thromb Haemost 9:1441–1451
92. Van De Velde M (2008) Massive obstetric hemorrhage due to abnormal placentation: uterotonic drugs, cell salvage and activated recombinant factor seven. Acta Anaesthesiol Belg 59:197–200
93. Welsh A, Mclintock C, Gatt S et al (2008) Guidelines for the use of recombinant activated factor VII in massive obstetric haemorrhage. Aust NZ J Obstet Gynaecol 48:12–16
94. Vincent JL, Rossaint R, Riou B et al (2006) Recommendations on the use of recombinant activated factor VII as an adjunctive treatment for massive bleeding – a European perspective. Crit Care 10:R120
95. Teig M, Harkness M, Catling S et al (2007) Survey of cell salvage use in obstetrics in the UK. Int J Obstet Anesth 16(Suppl 1):30
96. Tevet A, Grisaru-Granovsky S, Samueloff A et al (2012) Peripartum use of cell salvage: a university practice audit and literature review. Arch Gynecol Obstet 285:281–284
97. Allam J, Cox M, Yentis SM (2008) Cell salvage in obstetrics. Int J Obstet Anesth 17:37–45
98. Huissoud C, Carrabin N, Audibert F et al (2009) Bedside assessment of fibrinogen level in postpartum haemorrhage by thrombelastometry. BJOG 116:1097–1102

Event Medicine: An Evolving Subspecialty of Emergency Medicine

P. E. Pepe and S. Nichols

Introduction

Despite recent declines in world economies and augmented threats of disasters and terrorism, mass gatherings, both planned and unanticipated incidents, have become increasingly common events worldwide [1–15]. From sporting and entertainment productions to large convocations and political demonstrations, situations that bring many thousands of persons together in very close proximity have evolved into escalating challenges for event organizers, local governments and a host of other involved entities [13].

In addition to the challenges of on-site structural integrity, evacuation safety concerns, general security considerations, and a litany of other legal, technical and logistical risk factors, there are also evolving catalogs of medical and health concerns as well [1–7]. Beside the fact that many of the numerous medical conditions that arise during mass gatherings were going to occur whether or not the persons involved were at the event or elsewhere, the circumstances of the event itself may also increase the likelihood a medical emergency.

Clearly, the larger the number of attendees at a given location the larger the number of incidental emergencies that will occur at that site, but depending on the situational logistics, the environmental circumstances, the crowds themselves and the potential barriers to rapid access and treatment, those numbers can be dramati-

P. E. Pepe (✉)
The Section of EMS, Homeland Security and Disaster Medicine, Departments of Surgery/Emergency Medicine, Internal Medicine, Pediatrics and School of Public Health, the University of Texas Southwestern Medical Center, 5323 Harry Hines Boulevard, Mail Code 8579, Dallas, TX 75390-8579, USA
E-mail: Paul.Pepe@UTSW.edu

S. Nichols
Sequel Tour Solutions, 30200 Telegraph Road, Suite 400, Bingham Farms, MI 48025, USA

J.-L. Vincent (Ed.), *Annual Update in Intensive Care and Emergency Medicine 2013*,
DOI 10.1007/978-3-642-35109-9_3, © Springer-Verlag Berlin Heidelberg 2013

cally amplified. Not only could these circumstantial factors precipitate or exacerbate an underlying problem, but they can also generate a new illness or injury in an otherwise healthy individual, or they may also delay time-dependent emergency care. In fact, in most cases, it is the nature of the gathering that will likely increase the risk and precipitate acute illness or injury [8–10].

There are numerous factors that can affect human health, most notably environmental issues (heat, cold, humidity, sunlight, weather, geography, insects), amplified by long waits and lengthy exposure under those conditions [8–10]. In addition, there are injuries and illnesses associated with the availability of alcohol as well as drug intoxication or food-related ailments. Experience has also provided the medical community and event organizers with historic concerns over structural collapses, crowd crush and stampedes. There are also exacerbations of underlying conditions due to situational stresses and the risk of the activity itself leading to either the audience or principals (e. g., performers, athletes, drivers, pilots) being injured.

In addition, one must be prepared for the risks of the site being the nidus for sudden disasters (fires, vehicle/aircraft/boating crashes, tornadoes, lightning strikes) or intentional malfeasance (bombings, shootings, gassings). It is important to take note of all of these medical possibilities because responsible organizers must attempt to best prepare for their occurrence as well as the possible magnitude of these numerous threats [13]. More importantly, it is important to appreciate these risks in order to prevent them in the first place.

Be it heightened and improved security techniques, pro-active public education of attendees, enhanced on-site resources or better logistical and strategic planning, the evolving practice of event medicine requires a new set of competencies for the medical provider [14]. These special knowledge skills involve prospective and well-coordinated communications and planning with event organizers, local public safety systems, media, hospitals, site supervisors and a myriad of other agencies and entities. It also requires longstanding experience in helping to organize these events.

Over the last two decades, there has been a growing number of publications in the medical literature about the health threats and the emergency care provided in mass gatherings as well as the factors that will be more likely to precipitate them [1–10]. The purpose of this particular discussion, however, is to provide an additional perspective on event medicine as a new and rapidly-evolving specialty in the house of medicine. In addition, it will attempt to address an academic (training) roadmap for developing these competencies and also advance a rationale for routinely integrating this type of specialized medical support into organizations responsible for mass gatherings and large-scale events, both public and private [14].

The Evolution of the Need for Event Medicine Practice

The Spectrum of Events

Large-scale assemblies of many thousands of persons have become commonplace events and almost daily occurrences in some communities. In many urban settings, professional football, basketball, polo and racing contests are held several days a week. In addition, many communities hold festivals, community celebrations, parades, and large-scale entertainment concerts throughout the year. In other circumstances, large-scale events may occur over several days (e. g., Hajj pilgrimage, political conventions, economic summits), even over weeks (e. g., summer Olympic games).

Some special events may involve many tens of thousands of persons in a single evening's appearance that will only occur once at a given location, such as a U2 rock concert or a large scale papal visit (Fig. 1). Others may routinely involve 20,000 persons nearly every night (e. g., professional baseball or basketball games). In other circumstances, it may involve a one-time celebration with hundreds of

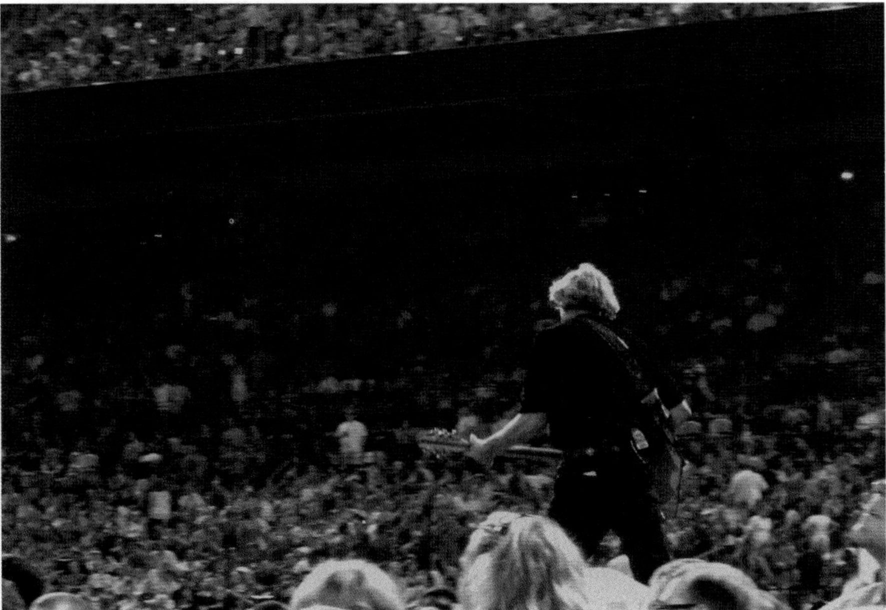

Fig. 1 The enormous volume of persons arriving at some mass gatherings can predict the occurrence of dozens of emergencies just by sheer chance let alone situational factors such as ambient temperature, limited access to water, excessive alcohol consumption, and long waits to get into the venue. In additional to behavioral and environmental factors, event medicine practice is challenged by the variable logistics of mass gatherings

thousands of attendees, such as a National Basketball Association (NBA) or Fédération Internationale de Football Association (FIFA) cup championship parade or celebration. It could also be a single afternoon competition, but with a week or two of lead-up events, such as a Superbowl game.

In turn, these mass gatherings will occur in a myriad of venues ranging from a large stadium, medium-sized arena or racetrack to an outdoor park, hillside field, city streets, private estates, lakesides, seashores and many other locations. Moreover, they occur in a variety of societies on different continents and variable climates. Some may take place at high noon and others in the dark of night.

The Unique Medical Challenges of Mass Gathering Events

Collateral impact may include tremendous traffic congestion and detours, absences from employment and numerous other effects on the local economy [3, 5, 10]. These collateral consequences may include a positive impact, such as enhanced hotel and restaurant profits, also generating tax revenues for the local governments. These effects can also have a negative impact, however, such as scarcity of available accommodation, eateries, ground transportation and other services required by visitors and local residents alike. In some venues, this may even result in an absence of basic supplies, such as water and food. In addition, service providers may even inflate prices in the opportunistic spirit of supply and demand. Furthermore, if local emergency teams and responders are pre-occupied or distracted by the mass gathering event, routine healthcare resources may also be compromised. Therefore, mass gatherings routinely affect the local infrastructure and can create competition for services for the local residents in the affected community, including access to emergency healthcare services. Other factors, such as traffic or venue location, may also inhibit access and egress of emergency vehicles to and from the site should a major catastrophe occur during the event [13].

Another special challenge is the actual configuration of the venue. In the stadium or arena setting, thousands of audience members usually are stacked vertically over many rows making access with equipment difficult and evacuation of the potential patient even more difficult. Even if patients are ambulatory, numerous stairs and steps may be extraordinarily difficult for the ill or injured patient and/or may worsen the condition. Those rows are also cramped areas for delivery of medical care and, without adjacent evacuation, other audience members may be blocking access and egress. In contrast, such as a papal visit, a victory parade or a NASCAR motor speedway, participants are spread across many acres/hectares of land with few landmarks to assist in identifying their exact location, thus delaying their care [15].

At the other end of the spectrum is the need to sequester, provide security and maintain unique discretion in the case of the celebrity, entertainer, political figure or star athlete. This would be another factor that may delay medical care or inhibit optimal response and treatment. Lastly, the proprietary or public relations interests and pressures of the event may result in the principal performer or pivotal member of the tour/production to refuse/defer care when they are in the midst of an evolving emergency. This type of dilemma further poses an extraordinary challenge for the care healthcare provider when the possible myocardial infarction or abdominal catastrophe can be seen as a medical-legal risk, let alone a possible life-threatening danger for the patient.

The Spectrum of Potential Patients

From the point of view of event organizers, there are roughly four or five groups of 'clients' for whom they may need to ensure prompt medical care. This ranges from the principals, their immediate and extended production team, local site staff and the public in attendance, and the involved community at large.

The Special Circumstances of the Principals

The first group of considerations for possible medical attention in event medicine includes the principal(s) and perhaps their immediate family members. This could be the Queen of England, President of Mexico or the Pope. It also could be the lead members of a rock group or athletic celebrities. Their safety and medical care is often less of a challenge in the traditional sense. Many are in great health and have the resources and time to maintain outstanding exercise and training habits. Nevertheless, from time to time, they may also experience routine illnesses/injuries (viral syndromes, allergies, headaches, gastrointestinal illness, trips and falls).

Being transients of sorts, constantly traveling from city to city, they will not have consistency in healthcare delivery or even know their care providers should a medical problem arise. Unless they bring along their own physicians or utilize a team of physicians/medical care providers (e.g., the White House Medical Unit), this can create uncertainty in terms of the quality of care or expertise provided. This concern becomes further augmented when global travel is involved. Local health risks (malaria, water quality, food sources) are further compounded by the quality or lack of healthcare facilities, practitioners and even medication. It is also accentuated by the need for the principal to appear in spite of illness or injury.

Even in familiar urban centers with sophisticated trauma centers, organizers may not always know the optimal place to take their traveling event staff, let alone their central figures. Particularly when discretion is desired to avoid unwanted publicity and maintain security, this question becomes even more pressing.

Production Support Staff

The second group of concern is the immediate support staff of production, tour and team manager and their ancillary staff who routinely accompanying the principal(s). For major rock groups, for example, this can vary from several dozens to several hundreds of personnel. In this example, this tier, which does not even include the local crews that help to build and take down the stage, will span across the group's own management staff, back-up singers/musicians, wardrobe, stage crews and sound personnel to the tour's production team, security personnel, stage managers and a host of others. For a head of state, it may also include an accompanying press corps. For a team, it may include coaches, publicists and a myriad of others.

Experience has shown that the accompanying staff members, by sheer numbers, comprise the most likely group to need medical attention (with the exception of athletes), particularly considering their own transiency circumstances and the same considerations faced by the principals, not only the accompanying travel issues, but the separation from consistencies in healthcare providers. Also tour and local staff may be involved in construction, carpentry and heavy lifting of many mobile objects at variable heights involving sound systems, lighting works, large video screens and the skeletal ('steel') for those stage assets. The nature of this continuous process of building and deconstructing these sets creates an increased risk for injury, both mild and serious alike.

Experience has also demonstrated the absolute need for basic cardiopulmonary resuscitation (CPR), choking techniques and rapid access to automated external defibrillators (AEDs) for those support personnel. It has also demonstrated a spectrum of medical needs for this group, ranging from rapid transport to a trauma center to simple medication refills. Accordingly, it requires prospective knowledge and collaboration with local emergency medical service (EMS) agencies and prospective knowledge and collaboration with the appropriate healthcare facilities and physician experts [14, 16]. Such tactics are routine procedures for the United States' President's travel as well as other heads of state. For similar security and privacy reasons, such prospective planning would seem appropriate for other types of principals and staff as well.

In essence, medical care, just for the tours, teams, production staff, will require several aspects of medical expertise that range from clinical emergency care and training skills (especially CPR and AED training) to preoperative injury management, EMS system oversight skills, tactical medicine, travel and global health expertise, executive medicine and an extended network of EMS system and similarly-skilled physician contacts worldwide.

Local Staff

The third major grouping of personnel that may require medical care are the local staff, including stage hands, equipment movers, security, ushers, vendors and others related to the local venue. Many of these personnel may face the same environmental challenges as the audience as well as some of the same injury threats as the production staff. Often they are employees or sub-contractors of the venue (e. g., arena or stadium) management or the tour itself. This group may involve local police and EMS crews and fire marshal staff as well as federal agents, volunteers and transportation companies or agencies. To some extent, from the organizers and event medicine physician's point of view, this is a cross-over group in terms of direct responsibility (as it generally is for the first two groups).

Audience and Public at Large

The major grouping of persons at risk for medical conditions is, of course, the audience and participants in a mass gathering. Organizers have a vested interest in this group as well as the local staff because any bad publicity stemming from the event could have a significant future public relations impact. Part of the success of a sports franchise or an entertainment tour is that it is considered a safe and enjoyable experience for all involved.

There are now volumes of data that provide not only tabulations of previous demands for medical needs, but also predictive models as well [8–10]. Moreover, previous data have also identified those major predictors to be rather obvious, including the size of the crowd, the nature of the event itself, the climate and length of exposure to elements as well as the availability of alcoholic beverages [8–10]. Clearly an indoor, climate controlled event would have less volume of medical care needs than a summer's day noon-time sports championship victory parade in direct sunlight with extreme humidity. In such a sample circumstance, like many of the other mass gathering events, numerous factors are at play. With crowds diminishing the breeze and air circulation as well as the ability to move about compounded by direct sunlight, the risks for heat illness and exacerbation of other conditions increases exponentially, especially when spectators arrive in the early morning to seize the best positions along the scheduled parade route. Without easy access to water and being reluctant to lose the prized parade route positions, those gatherings can become easy victims for health concerns. Moreover, in the extremely noise-ridden environment, a call for help would be muffled. Worse yet, mobile phone calls for help would likely be inaudible. Even if heard, trying to identify the patient's location in that large crowd of 100,000 plus persons would be difficult at best, even if the street and nearby block location is known.

Such circumstances would be best served by prevention, including alternate timing of the event, vast supplies of water and pro-active public education in terms of what to wear, how to maintain hydration, avoiding the use of alcohol and the employment of a buddy system in which everyone knows ahead of time where the closest public safety official is stationed. In essence, key aspects of event medicine include prospective planning, public education and the supply of resources, such as water, to pre-empt medical emergencies. Public education might also include pre-event concern for those with risk from high ozone levels or considerations of the use of earplugs, sunscreen, insect repellent and numerous other useful adjuncts.

In most western communities, one could expect one true emergency per 10,000 population in a 24 hour period, just at baseline. For an event stretching over several hours involving tens of thousands, several emergencies should occur. Add alcohol, humidity, heat or other factors, and these numbers can be amplified. The problem again is a bystander or friend being able to rapidly contact officials, the responders locating the patient and accessing them readily in the crowds as well as the logistics of the stadium seating or distances at the outdoors track.

Several analysts in mass gathering medicine have estimated the need for one medical care responder team (such as two emergency medical technicians or two paramedics) for every 5,000 to 10,000 attendees with that number rising to one per thousand (or more) depending on the event, climate and logistics [1–15]. This, of course, would be considered separate from dedicated personnel assigned to the production team and principals. Therefore, EMS is a major focus of event medicine and oversight of EMS is a major component of those who practice event medicine.

Accordingly, the question arises as to whether or not the quality of these persons will suffice and meet the standard of care expected in the community served. In many circumstances, private ambulance services may be engaged to spare the local EMS agencies from this additional burden and to curb costs. However, their day-to-day experience may not match the skill level of the municipal public safety responder crews (i. e., 9-1-1, 9-9-9, 1-1-2, responders) and, in addition, their response in a true emergency may not be as well-integrated with the usual EMS-trauma system and day-to-day coordination with the optimal receiving facilities. Therefore, an expert knowledge of EMS systems, EMS personnel and the local contacts (e. g., jurisdictional EMS medical directors) in each venue would be an important aspect of event medicine [14].

Unplanned Events

Enhancing Preparedness Skills for Local Disasters

From time to time, event medicine may become an unplanned function, such as an earthquake or hurricane evacuation, in which tens of thousands are moved to a distant location without their usual support systems, medications or healthcare access. This could also be unexpected volatile civil riot, a political rally turned violent or some other unanticipated events, such as the 'rave' festival that deteriorates with unanticipated levels of drug and alcohol abuse, further exacerbated by heat and humidity. Event medicine doctors and EMS personnel can play a major role in these events by knowing how to rapidly set up on-site 'facilities' as often provided at mass gatherings (e. g., regattas, marathons, festivals). By treating, observing and releasing patients on-site as needed these personnel can help to protect local emergency departments (EDs), let alone render more immediate care.

To some extent, these unexpected incidents can be treated similar to a sudden mass casualty incident. In turn, mass casualty incidents and disaster management experience can be another important skill of the event medicine practitioner as well as routine integration into the local EMS and public health system [17]. In fact, event medicine could be applied to the unexpected public health emergency, such as the sudden need for mass medical care organization or vaccinations in a pandemic or even a nuclear detonation. In fact, event medicine planning and skills have some significant overlap with disaster management and thus large-scale events can be used as an excellent way to help prepare communities for such catastrophes [18, 19].

The Evolving Specialty of Event Medicine

Already an Academic Pursuit in Many Institutions

Event medicine is already becoming a formal function of many institutions and particularly departments of emergency medicine in several medical schools who provide routine services for their local arenas, EMS systems, and professional sports organizations.

Whereas the typical personnel for these functions may be local EMS-based physicians, it is clear that major organizations could readily engage experts who not only understand emergency medical care, tactical medicine, executive medicine, environmental medicine, travel medicine and global health, but also mass casualty incident/disaster management, public health threats and have an extensive network of EMS systems and physicians worldwide [13, 14, 16–20].

In our own organizations, we have begun to train persons in a specialized training apprenticeship over a two-year period that generally follows completion of a traditional emergency medicine residency program. In that apprenticeship, the trainees are not only involved routinely in event medicine deployments, but they are also exposed and deployed to major disasters. They are also integrated into law enforcement tactical teams, are exposed to security details for executives, and are also further exposed to global and travel medicine training [20]. In appropriate circumstance, they are assigned to a more formal apprenticeship involving entertainment tours or assignments to professional sports teams.

Conclusion

Mass gatherings, both planned and unanticipated incidents, have become increasingly common events worldwide. The major events are sporting and entertainment productions that bring many thousands of persons together in very close proximity. In addition to the challenges of on-site safety concerns, general security and numerous logistical risk factors, there are also medical care concerns as well. Event medicine planning involves consideration for the principals (entertainers, athletes, political and religious leaders), production and support staff and the public at large among others. In addition to the fact that many of the numerous medical conditions that arise during mass gatherings were going to occur whether or not the persons involved were at the event or elsewhere, the circumstances of the event itself may also increase the likelihood a medical emergency. It is clear that, today, major event organizers should readily engage experts who not only understand emergency medical care, tactical medicine, executive medicine, environmental medicine, travel medicine and global health, but also mass casualty incident/disaster management, public health threats and have an extensive network of EMS systems and physicians worldwide.

References

1. Sanders AB, Criss E, Stecki P, Meislin HW, Raife J, Allen D (1986) An analysis of medical care at mass gatherings. Ann Emerg Med 15:515–519
2. De Lorenzo RA (1997) Mass gathering medicine: A review. Prehosp Disast Med 12:68–72
3. Zeitz KM, Zeitz CJ, Schneider D, Jarret D (2002) Mass gathering events: retrospective analysis of presentations over seven years at an agricultural and horticultural show. Prehosp Disast Med 17:147–150
4. Michael JA, Barbera JA (1197) Mass gathering medical care: a twenty-five year review. Prehosp Disaster Med 12:305–312
5. Milsten AM, Maguire BJ, Bissell RA, Seaman KG (2002) Mass-gathering medical care: a review of the literature. Prehosp Disast Med 17:151–162
6. McConnell J, Memish Z (2010) The Lancet Conference on mass gatherings medicine. Lancet Infect Dis 10:818–819
7. Memish Z, Alrabeeah AA (2011) Jeddah declaration on mass gatherings health. Lancet Infect Dis 11:342–343
8. Arbon P, Bridgewater FH, Smith C (2001) Mass gathering medicine: a predictive model for patient presentation and transport rates. Prehosp Disast Med 16:150–158
9. Arbon P (2004) The development of conceptual models for mass-gathering health. Prehosp Disast Med 19:208–212
10. Milsten AM, Seaman KG, Liu P, Bissell RA, Maguire BJ (2003) Variables influencing medical usage rates, injury patterns, and levels of care for mass gatherings. Prehosp Disast Med 18:334–346
11. Morimura N, Takahashi K, Katsumi A et al (2007) Mass gathering medicine for the First East Asian Football Championship and the 24th European/South American Cup in Japan. Eur J Emerg Med 14:115–117
12. Zeitz K, Kadow-Griffin C, Zeitz C (2005) Injury occurrences at a mass gathering event. J Emerg Primary Health Care 3: (article 990098)
13. Yancey AH, Jaslow D (2002) Mass gathering medical care. In: Kuehl (ed) Prehospital Systems and Medical Oversight, 3rd edn. Kendall Hunt Publishing, Dubuque, pp 894–913
14. Pepe PE, Copass MK, Fowler RL, Racht EM (2009) Medical direction of emergency medical services systems. In: Cone DC, Fowler R, O'Connor RE (eds) Emergency Medical Services: Clinical Practice and Systems Oversight, Textbook of the National Association of EMS Physicians. Kendall-Hunt Publications, Dubuque, pp 22–52
15. Ombudsman Victoria (1993) The Ombudsman Victoria Report of the investigation into alleged failure of state and local authorities to ensure adequate provision of public transport

and environmental health standards at the "Guns N Roses" Concert at Calder Park Raceway. Govt Printer, Melbourne

16. EMS State of Science (2012) U.S. Metropolitan Municipalities Medical Directors Consortium. Available at: GatheringofEagles.US. Accessed 2nd September 2012
17. Pepe PE, Anderson E (2001) Multiple casualty incident plans: Ten golden rules for prehospital management. Dallas Med J 14:462–468
18. Eastman AL, Rinnert KJ, Nemeth IR, Fowler RL, Minei JP (2007) Alternate site surge capacity in times of public health disaster maintains trauma center and emergency department integrity: Hurricane Katrina. J Trauma 63:253–257
19. North CS, King RV, Polatin P et al (2008) Psychiatric illness among transported hurricane evacuees: acute phase findings in a large receiving shelter site. Psych Annals 38:104–113
20. Metzger JC, Eastman AL, Benitez FL, Pepe PE (2009) The life-saving potential of specialized on-scene medical support for urban tactical operations. Prehosp Emerg Care 13:528–531

Part II

Infections

Update on *Clostridium difficile*

M. Bassetti, D. Pecori, and E. Righi

Introduction

Clostridium difficile represents one of the main causes of infectious diarrhea due to a bacterial strain in the hospital setting. *C. difficile* is a common nosocomial pathogen, particularly among intensive care unit (ICU) patients, whose clinical characteristics often include important risk factors for *C. difficile* infection, such as severe underlying disease and treatment with antimicrobials. Prolonged ICU stay has been identified among the risk factors for *C. difficile* infection [1]. Furthermore, *C. difficile*-associated disease may cause fulminant colitis requiring admission to the ICU [2]. Rates of *C. difficile* infection have risen rapidly over the past decade, along with a trend to increased rates of complications, nosocomial outbreaks, difficult-to-treat recurrent infection, and all-cause mortality within 30 days of *C. difficile* infection [2, 3]. The severity of *C. difficile*-associated disease reflects the emergence of isolates with increased pathogenicity, replicative capacity, and antibiotic resistance. Furthermore, the appearance of *C. difficile* as a community-acquired disease, and the increasing use of immunosuppressive therapies in elderly and debilitated patients has contributed to the spread of *C. difficile*-associated disease. Associated complications include toxic megacolon, bowel perforation, and septic shock. Patients with complicated *C. difficile*-associated disease

M. Bassetti (✉)
Clinica Malattie Infettive, Azienda Ospedaliera Universitaria Santa Maria della Misericordia, Piazzale Santa Maria della Misericordia 15, 33100 Udine Italy
E-mail: mattba@tin.it

D. Pecori
Clinica Malattie Infettive, Azienda Ospedaliera Universitaria Santa Maria della Misericordia, Piazzale Santa Maria della Misericordia 15, 33100 Udine Italy

E. Righi
Clinica Malattie Infettive, Azienda Ospedaliera Universitaria Santa Maria della Misericordia, Piazzale Santa Maria della Misericordia 15, 33100 Udine Italy

J.-L. Vincent (Ed.), *Annual Update in Intensive Care and Emergency Medicine 2013*,
DOI 10.1007/978-3-642-35109-9_4,

display mortality rates of up to 38 %, correlated with significantly prolonged hospitalization especially in the ICU [4].

An increase in treatment failure with metronidazole and challenges related to *C. difficile*-associated disease relapses are other new features of *C. difficile* infection [5]. Although controversial, some authors also report an increased incidence in populations previously considered at low risk [6, 7].

Reduction in antibiotic use, development of infection control committees, and prevention of infection transmission through prompt isolation of infected patients, hand hygiene, and cleaning procedures remain key factors in reducing the incidence of *C. difficile*-associated disease in the critical care setting [8].

The Changing Epidemiology of *C. difficile*

In European hospitals, the number of cases of *C. difficile*-associated disease has increased each year since 2000, and in North America a greater than 3-fold increase in *C. difficile* infection rates during the 5-year period from 2000–2004 has been registered, especially in the elderly [3, 9, 10]. Recent published data in the US report 336,600 hospitalizations related to *C. difficile*-associated disease in 2009, corresponding to 1 in 100 of all hospital stays. In the critical care setting, Lawrence et al. reported an incidence of 0.4–100 cases of infection per 1,000 patient-days per 1,000 admissions, but rates may be higher in outbreak settings and have regional variation [11]. Although elderly hospitalized patients are the main group at risk for developing *C. difficile*-associated disease, recent evidence showed an increased incidence of *C. difficile* infection in populations with no previous antibiotic therapy and low risk groups, such as children [6].

In 2005, molecular analysis identified a new strain of *C. difficile* defined as BI/NAP1/027 (by restriction endonuclease analysis, pulse-field gel electrophoresis, and PCR ribotyping, respectively) responsible for large outbreaks in North America and Europe capable of *in vitro* production of higher levels of toxins A and B [12, 13]. The epidemic, toxin-gene variant ribotype 027 strain is associated with accelerated kinetics *in vitro* and toxin synthesis during stationary growth phases, and mutation in the negative regulator gene (*tcdC*) for production of the binary toxin CDT involved in actin-specific ADP ribosyl transferase activity leading to cytoskeleton disorganization [14, 15]. Furthermore, *C. difficile* ribotype 027 is capable of *in vitro* replication in the presence of non-chloride cleaning agents and displays resistance to fluoroquinolones (MIC > 32 mg/l) [16, 17].

Although only sub-inhibitory concentrations of metronidazole, vancomycin, and linezolid induced toxin production, fluoroquinolones and cephalosporins have been shown to promote ribotype 027 spore germination, cell growth and toxins [18, 19]. Of note, the same *in vitro* model showed that neither piperacillin-tazobactam nor tigecycline induced *C. difficile* toxin production [19]. Finally, ribotype 027 strains with reduced susceptibility to metronidazole have also been found to be transmitted between patients, but their clinical significance in terms of response to antibiotic treatment remains unclear and is still under investigation [20].

Ribotype 027 infections are mostly described in hospitalized patients, but there is recent evidence of community-acquired cases, especially in the community surrounding a hospital in which other cases were diagnosed. A recent study by Wilcox et al. [13] showed an increase in incidence, severity, recurrence, complications and mortality related to *C. difficile*-associated disease with a correlation to ribotype 027 in patients above 65 years. Control of the epidemic *C. difficile* ribotype 027 correlated with a 61 % reduction in cases of *C. difficile* infection between 2007–2010 [21].

Pathogenesis of and Risk Factors for *C. difficile* Infection

C. difficile, a Gram-positive, spore-forming, anaerobic rod can colonize the gut if the normal intestinal flora is altered or absent. Often, asymptomatic colonization is seen in the fecal flora of new-born infants and elderly patients [22]. *C. difficile*-associated disease is a toxin-mediated intestinal disease with highly variable clinical manifestations, ranging from mild diarrhea to severe syndromes, including toxic megacolon, bowel perforation, sepsis, septic shock, and death [23]. Abdominal pain, fever, leukocytosis, and presence of mucus in the stool are the commonest clinical manifestations associated with symptomatic *C. difficile* infection, although they are reported in less than half of patients [24]. Melena or extraintestinal manifestations, such as bacteremia, abscesses, or osteomyelitis are rare [25, 26].

C. difficile is implicated as the causative organism in up to 25 % and 50–75 % of patients who develop antibiotic-associated diarrhea and antibiotic-associated colitis, respectively [4, 27]. Other risk factors associated with *C. difficile*-associated disease are summarized in Table 1 [8, 10, 28–36]. Even though some cases are not associated with previous antibiotic exposure, this remains the principal risk factor for the development of *C. difficile*-associated disease, occurring typically 2 to 3 months before infection [37]. Although all antibiotics can potentially be associated with the development of *C. difficile*-associated disease, some carry a higher risk than others, including clindamycin, cephalosporins and, more recently, fluoroquinolones [38].

Antibiotics play an important role in the development of *C. difficile*-associated disease by disrupting the normal microbiota in the gut and favoring the multiplication and colonization of *C. difficile*. Susceptibility to *C. difficile*-associated disease in patients treated with antibiotics persists for a variable period after the administration of the last dose depending on the molecule administered, i. e., longer time for clindamycin compared to cephalosporins [39, 40]. Hospitalization may expose the patient to a highly-resistant spore contaminated environment, along with the risk of health care workers' sub-optimal hand hygiene. Older patients show greater mortality associated with *C. difficile*-associated disease and more recurrent disease because of their inability to mount a specific serum IgG immune response when exposed to the toxins [41]. Patient exposure to the spores of the microorganism

Table 1 Risk factors associated with *C. difficile*-associated disease in the hospital setting

Risk Factor	Reference
Age ≥ 65 years	[28, 29]
Immunocompromised state (e. g., immunosuppressive drugs, HIV infection, antineoplastic agents)	[29, 30, 31]
Multiple antimicrobials during the previous 3 months	[10, 32, 33]
Severe underlying illness	[28, 29]
Gastrointestinal surgery	[28]
ICU stay	[28]
Multiple antibacterial exposure within 3 months	[28]
Gastrointestinal stimulants and stool softeners	[28, 29]
Reduced health-care worker hand hygiene	[34]
Inadequate environmental disinfection	[8, 34]
Overcrowding and rapid turnover in hospital beds	[34]
Prolonged hospitalization (> 20 days)	[35]
Shared toilet facilities among patients	[34]
Inadequate isolation measures for infected patients	[8, 34]
Emergence of epidemic strains	[36]

HIV: human immunodeficiency virus

occurs mainly through contact with the hospital environment or health care workers. Nevertheless, Best et al. demonstrated the possibility of airborne spread of *C. difficile* spores from patients with symptomatic *C. difficile*-associated disease, recovering *C. difficile* from air sampled at heights up to 25 cm above the toilet seat following flushing a toilet [42].

Following spore germination, the replicating vegetative cells can adhere and penetrate the enterocytes via flagella and proteolytic enzymes, and adhere to the cells through adhesins to colonize the gut. Then, cytotoxic enzymes A and B, the main *C. difficile* virulence factors, cause colonic mucosa cytoskeleton disorganization with inflammatory cytokine production, fluid accumulation and destruction of the intestinal epithelium. As mentioned, the binary toxin produced by *C. difficile* BI/NAP1/027 can increase toxin A and B toxicity and lead to more severe disease [43].

Severe Forms of *C. difficile*-associated Disease

Symptoms of *C. difficile*-associated disease range from a mild self-limited diarrhea to life-threatening colitis. About 30 % of patients with *C. difficile*-associated disease are febrile, and 50 % have leukocytosis. A white blood cell (WBC) count >20,000/μl may herald a patient at risk for rapid progression to fulminant colitis with systemic inflammatory response syndrome (SIRS) and shock. It is important to recognize that presentation of fulminant *C. difficile*-associated disease colitis may be atypical, especially if the patient is immunosuppressed or elderly, and may not necessarily be associated with antibiotic usage [44].

Pseudomembranous colitis and toxic megacolon are pathognomonic of severe *C. difficile*-associated disease. However, pseudomembranes are present in only 50 % of patients with *C. difficile* colitis. Fulminant disease is a potential complication of *C. difficile*-associated disease and colectomy in this group can be life-saving [45]. Unfortunately, hospital mortality in this group of patients ranges from 35 % to 57 % [46]. Although diarrhea is the hallmark of symptomatic *C. difficile*-associated disease, severe abdominal pain and lack of diarrhea could indicate that the patient has ileus with toxic megacolon. High mortality in fulminant colitis is largely the result of lack of timely recognition, for this reason the intensivist should evaluate and manage patients with *C. difficile*-associated disease in order to identify fulminant disease in a timely manner so that colectomy and its timing can be optimized.

There are no validated methods to identify patients at risk for poor outcomes due to *C. difficile* infection, but some factors include advanced age, acute renal insufficiency, WBC count >20,000/μl, immunosuppression, hypoalbuminemia, and at least one organ system failure [46].

Recurrences of *C. difficile*-associated Disease: A Challenging Issue

High rates of *C. difficile*-associated disease recurrence probably represents one of the most challenging aspects of *C. difficile* management. Up to 30 % of patients may experience a second event within 60 days (usually in the first two weeks) from discontinuation of successful treatment with standard therapies, i. e., metronidazole or vancomycin. Recurrence appears to be related to a combination of factors: Failure to re-establish the colonic microflora, persistence of *C. difficile* spores in the intestine, and sub-optimal host immune response to the infecting organism and its toxins. Risk factors for recurrent episodes include: Immunocompromise, exposure to antibacterial agents that disrupt the normal colonic microflora, previous episode of *C. difficile* infection, renal impairment, older age (≥65 years), severe underlying disease, prolonged hospitalization, and ICU stay. Factors that are common in patients hospitalized in ICU, such as the lack of restoration of enteric microbiota, the persistence of *C. difficile* spores within the gut, and deficient host immune response all appear to be related to the chance of recurrence. Furthermore, hospitalized patients who are colonized by the bacteria or experience acute or recurrent infection may represent a reservoir of infection for other patients who share the same environment. Usually, clinical severity does not change significantly between primary events and recurrences; a second cycle of treatment with metronidazole or vancomycin can be efficacious in this scenario, but the therapy remains suboptimal and 40 to 60 % of patients will have one or more relapses [47].

Diagnosis and Therapy of *C. difficile*-associated Disease

The diagnosis of *C. difficile* infection consists of clinical history (i. e., antimicrobial use or/and other risk factors) and presence of diarrhea in combination with laboratory tests. Diagnostic laboratory protocols measure *in vivo C. difficile* toxin production, which is responsible for *C. difficile*-associated disease. Since a rapid and accurate microbiological diagnosis is key, diagnostic algorithms that can provide high sensitivity, rapid turnaround time, and ease of performance are mandatory [48]. Although availability of a rapid diagnostic algorithm for *C. difficile*-associated disease would reduce unnecessary antibiotic treatment and speed implementation of infection control precautions, pre-emptive antibiotic therapy is often started empirically by clinicians.

The detection of toxin A/B from fecal samples by immunoenzymatic methods has been the cornerstone of laboratory *C. difficile* infection diagnosis for over two decades. However, its sensitivity and specificity are suboptimal when used as a standalone assay and it relies on the prevalence of *C. difficile* toxins in stool [49]. Thus, a two-step diagnostic algorithm using a rapid test for both toxin A and B by immunoassay methods followed, in selected cases, by stool culture including isolate toxin testing is performed. Troublesome specimens should always be sent to reference laboratories for culture cytotoxicity neutralization assay (CCNA) confirmatory testing. Other tests include rapid antigen detection of a cell wall-associated enzyme, glutamate dehydrogenase (GDH), as a screening test to rule out negative specimens and test the positive ones for toxin production [50]. Recently, last generation polymerase chain reaction (PCR)-based commercial kits and ribotyping have become available for *C. difficile*-associated disease outbreak monitoring and epidemiological surveys [51, 52].

In addition to microbiological tests, computed tomography (CT) scanning can be useful for recognizing more severe forms of disease detecting colonic mural thickening, intramural gas, and pleural effusion. Laboratory tests showing high WBC counts, low albumin level, and immunosuppression have also been correlated with severe *C. difficile*-associated disease [53].

Treatment of *C. difficile* infection can be challenging. When possible, any antibiotic treatment should be discontinued to allow restoration of the intestinal flora [54]. Often this option is not possible in critically ill patients: In this case, therapy goals are to eradicate the infection despite continuation of concomitant therapy, and to minimize the incidence of recurrence. Metronidazole and vancomycin represent the mainstay for *C. difficile*-associated disease treatment. In a prospective, randomized, double-blind, placebo-controlled trial comparing vancomycin and metronidazole for the treatment of mild and severe *C. difficile*-associated disease [55], metronidazole or vancomycin resulted in clinical cure in 90 % and 98 % of mild forms, respectively; in severe *C. difficile*-associated disease, clinical cure was reached for 76 % and 97 % patients treated with metronidazole or vancomycin, respectively ($p=0.02$). Thus, a superior efficacy of vancomycin was demonstrated for severe cases and the authors recommended it as first-line treatment for severe *C. difficile*-associated disease. Study of *C. difficile*-associated disease recurrences showed no inferiority for metronidazole compared to vancomycin [56]. Thus, vancomycin should be considered as treatment for a first *C. difficile* infection recurrence only in the presence of markers of severe disease (i. e., pseudomembranous colitis, hypotension, rising serum creatinine level) [54]. Conversely, further recurrences should be treated with tapered and/or pulsed vancomycin therapy [54]. Although different tapering schemes have been proposed, this approach has not been validated in comparative studies. Treatment indication and doses are shown in Table 2.

Tigecycline, a glycylcycline derivative of minocycline, also achieves fecal concentrations above the minimum inhibitory concentration (MIC) for *C. difficile*. Tigecycline is not licensed for treatment of *C. difficile*-associated disease and there are no randomized trials but only case reports showing its potential efficacy; thus, it is currently only recommended in cases in which other standard options have failed.

Other antimicrobial treatments include rifaximin, proposed as a rescue option in the treatment of second and later recurrences although high levels of resistance have emerged; ramoplanin, a new lipoglycodepsipeptide, that showed similar results when compared to vancomycin in terms of *C. difficile*-associated disease cure and relapse rates with no emergence of resistance; nitazoxanide, a nitrothiazolide compound with good antimicrobial activity against helminthic and protozoal parasites is still being studied [57, 58]. Fidaxomicin, a macrocyclic antibiotic with good *in vitro* activity against clinical isolates of *C. difficile* (including NAP1/BI/027 strains), has also shown promising results in clinical trials and superiority in recurrence cure rates compared to vancomycin [59]. Furthermore, in individuals taking concomitant antibiotics for other concurrent infections, fidaxomicin was superior to vancomycin in achieving clinical cure (90 % vs. 79.4 %, respectively; $p=0.04$) [60].

Non-antibiotic treatments include toxin-binding agents such as tolevamer, which also neutralizes toxins produced by the NAP1/BI/027 strain, has shown good results on *C. difficile*-associated disease recurrences but lower cure rates when compared with vancomycin and metronidazole, and has a potential place in the treatment of recurrent conditions as supplemental therapy [61]. Treatment with intravenous immunoglobulin (IVIG) to neutralize toxin A by IgG anti-toxin A antibodies has been utilized off-label to treat both refractory and fulminant *C. difficile* infection despite the lack of large randomized controlled trials and few reports of successful treatment in recurrent or severe *C. difficile*-associated disease [62]. Because alterations in the intestinal flora play a critical role in *C. difficile*-associated disease pathogenesis, the use of probiotics (especially *Saccharomyces boulardii* and *Lactobacilli*) is also being studied for treatment of *C. difficile* infection, although the evidence in the literature is not yet sufficient to recommend their

Table 2 Treatment options in *Clostridium difficile* infection in ICU patients

First episode	
Non-severe disease	Stop causative antibiotics if possible Metronidazole 500 mg tid orally for 10–14 days (if oral therapy is possible) Metronidazole 500 mg tid intravenously for 10–14 days (if oral therapy is impossible)
Severe disease	Vancomycin 125 mg qid orally for 10–14 days (if oral therapy is possible) Metronidazole 500 mg tid intravenously for 10 days + intra-colonic vancomycin 500 mg in 100 ml of normal saline every 4–12 h and/or vancomycin 500 mg qid by nasogastric tube (if oral therapy is impossible) Fidaxomicin 200 mg bid orally
First recurrence	Treat as the first episode, according to severity of the disease. Fidaxomicin 200 mg bid orally
Second recurrence	
If oral therapy is possible	Fidaxomicin 200 mg bid orally for 10–14 days Vancomycin 125 mg qid orally for 14 days Consider tapering after initial 14 days therapy: 125 mg bid for 7 days, then 125 mg qid for 7 days, then 125 mg once every 2 days for 8 days (4 doses) and lastly 125 mg once every 3 days for 15 days (5 doses) Consider rifaximin 200–400 mg bid for 10–14 days after vancomycin Consider Saccharomyces boulardii 500 mg bid for 21–28 days
If oral therapy is impossible	Metronidazole 500 mg tid intravenously for 10–14 days + retention enema of vancomycin 500 mg in 100 ml of normal saline every 4–12 and/or vancomycin 500 mg qid by nasogastric tube
Third and later recurrences	Eliminate risk factors Consider tigecycline Consider intravenous immunoglobulin (IVIG) and monoclonal antibodies (ongoing trials) Consider "fecal transplantation"

routine use [63]. Finally, vaccination against *C. difficile* with a toxoid vaccine has proved protective against recurrent *C. difficile*-associated disease [64], and intestinal microbiota transplantation (fecal bacteriotherapy) seems very promising [65].

Conclusion

C. difficile-associated disease diagnosis and treatment is challenging and recurrences are frequent, contributing to its difficult management. A key measure for treating *C. difficile* infection includes discontinuation of antibiotic therapy to allow restoration of the intestinal flora, although this approach is not often applicable in critically ill patients. New therapies aim to eradicate the infection even in the presence of antimicrobial therapy, and to reduce the incidence of recurrence. Metronidazole has shown a poorer response when compared to vancomycin in severe forms of *C. difficile*-associated disease. Oral metronidazole is usually recommended for initial treatment of non-severe *C. difficile*-associated disease. Fidaxomicin may be promising in those patients who cannot tolerate vancomycin, although additional data are needed. New compounds are also under investigation. Nevertheless, infection control measures, awareness of the multiple risk factors along with consideration of possible nosocomial transmission within the ICU, and correct antimicrobial management to limit antibiotic use are key factors to reduce the incidence of *C. difficile*-associated disease in the ICU.

References

1. Cho SM, Lee JJ, Yoon HJ (2012) Clinical risk factors for Clostridium difficile-associated diseases. Braz J Infect Dis 16:256–261
2. Riddle DJ, Dubberke ER (2009) Clostridium difficile infection in the intensive care unit. Infect Dis Clin North Am 23:727–743
3. Tan ET, Robertson CA, Brynildsen S, Bresnitz E, Tan C, McDonald C (2007) Clostridium difficile-associated disease in New Jersey hospitals, 2000–2004 Emerg Infect Dis 13:498–500
4. Owens RC (2006) Clostridium difficile-associated disease: an emerging threat to patient safety: insights from the Society of Infectious Diseases Pharmacists. Pharmacotherapy 26:299–311
5. Musher DM, Aslam S, Logan N et al (2005) Relatively poor outcome after treatment of Clostridium difficile colitis with metronidazole. Clin Infect Dis 40:1586–1590
6. Kim J, Smathers SA, Prasad P, Leckerman KH, Coffin S, Zaoutis T (2008) Epidemiological features of Clostridium difficile-associated disease among inpatients at children's hospitals in the United States, 2001–2006. Pediatrics 122:1266–1270
7. Rouphael NG, O'Donnell JA, Bhatnagar J et al (2008) Clostridium difficile-associated diarrhea: an emerging threat to pregnant women. Am J Obstet Gynecol 198(635):e631–e636
8. Musher DM, Aslam S (2008) Treatment of Clostridium difficile colitis in the critical care setting. Crit Care Clin 24:279–291
9. Kuijper EJ, Barbut F, Brazier JS et al (2008) Update of Clostridium difficile infection due to PCR ribotype 027 in Europe, 2008. Euro Surveill 13:1–7
10. Freeman J, Bauer MP, Baines SD et al (2010) The changing epidemiology of Clostridium difficile infections. Clin Microbiol Rev 23:529–549
11. Lawrence SJ, Puzniak LA, Shadel BN, Gillespie KN, Kollef MH, Mundy LM (2007) Clostridium difficile in the intensive care unit: epidemiology, costs, and colonization pressure. Infect Control Hosp Epidemiol 28:123–130
12. McDonald LC, Killgore GE, Thompson A et al (2005) An epidemic, toxin gene-variant strain of Clostridium difficile. N Engl J Med 353:2433–2441
13. Wilcox MH, Shetty N, Fawley WN et al (2012) Changing epidemiology of Clostridium difficile infection following the introduction of a national ribotyping-based surveillance scheme in England. Clin Infect Dis 55:1056–1063
14. Geric B, Johnson S, Gerding DN, Grabnar M, Rupnik M (2003) Frequency of binary toxin genes among Clostridium difficile strains that do not produce large clostridial toxins. J Clin Microbiol 41:5227–5232

15. Freeman J, Baines SD, Saxton K, Wilcox MH (2007) Effect of metronidazole on growth and toxin production by epidemic Clostridium difficile PCR ribotypes 001 and 027 in a human gut model. J Antimicrob Chemother 60:83–91
16. Akerlund T, Persson I, Unemo M et al (2008) Increased sporulation rate of epidemic Clostridium difficile Type 027/NAP1. J Clin Microbiol 46:1530–1533
17. Spigaglia P, Barbanti F, Mastrantonio P et al (2008) Fluoroquinolone resistance in Clostridium difficile isolates from a prospective study of C. difficile infections in Europe. J Med Microbiol 57:784–789
18. Gerber M, Walch C, Loffler B, Tischendorf K, Reischl U, Ackermann G (2008) Effect of sub-MIC concentrations of metronidazole, vancomycin, clindamycin and linezolid on toxin gene transcription and production in Clostridium difficile. J Med Microbiol 57:776–783
19. Baines SD, Freeman J, Wilcox MH (2005) Effects of piperacillin/tazobactam on Clostridium difficile growth and toxin production in a human gut model. J Antimicrob Chemother 55:974–982
20. Kuijper EJ, Wilcox MH (2008) Decreased effectiveness of metronidazole for the treatment of Clostridium difficile infection? Clin Infect Dis 47:63–65
21. Health Protection Agency. Results of the mandatory Clostridium difficile reporting scheme. Available at: http://www.hpa.org.uk/web/HPAweb&HPAwebStandard/HPAweb_C/119573 3750761 Assessed September 2012
22. Ferraris L, Butel MJ, Campeotto F, Vodovar M, Roze JC, Aires J (2012) Clostridia in premature neonates' gut: incidence, antibiotic susceptibility, and perinatal determinants influencing colonization. PLoS One 7:e30594
23. Rupnik M, Wilcox MH, Gerding DN (2009) Clostridium difficile infection: new developments in epidemiology and pathogenesis. Nat Rev Microbiol 7:526–536
24. Kelly CP, Pothoulakis C, LaMont JT (1994) Clostridium difficile colitis. N Engl J Med 330:257–262
25. Wolf LE, Gorbach SL, Granowitz EV (1998) Extraintestinal Clostridium difficile: 10 years' experience at a tertiary-care hospital. Mayo Clin Proc 73:943–947
26. Pron B, Merckx J, Touzet P et al (1995) Chronic septic arthritis and osteomyelitis in a prosthetic knee joint due to Clostridium difficile. Eur J Clin Microbiol Infect Dis 14:599–601
27. Bartlett JG (2002) Clinical practice. Antibiotic-associated diarrhea. N Engl J Med 346:334–339
28. Bignardi GE (1998) Risk factors for Clostridium difficile infection. J Hosp Infect 40:1–15
29. Kuijper EJ, Coignard B, Tull P (2006) Emergence of Clostridium difficile-associated disease in North America and Europe. Clin Microbiol Infect 12(Suppl 6):2–18
30. Collini PJ, Bauer M, Kuijper E, Dockrell DH (2012) Clostridium difficile infection in HIV-seropositive individuals and transplant recipients. J Infect 64:131–147
31. Barbut F, Corthier G, Charpak Y et al (1996) Prevalence and pathogenicity of Clostridium difficile in hospitalized patients. A French multicenter study. Arch Intern Med 156:1449–1454
32. Bilgrami S, Feingold JM, Dorsky D et al (1999) Incidence and outcome of Clostridium difficile infection following autologous peripheral blood stem cell transplantation. Bone Marrow Transplant 23:1039–1042
33. Nuila F, Cadle RM, Logan N, Musher DM (2008) Antibiotic stewardship and Clostridium difficile-associated disease. Infect Control Hosp Epidemiol 29:1096–1097
34. Loo VG, Libman MD, Miller MA et al (2004) Clostridium difficile: a formidable foe. CMAJ 171:47–48
35. Gerding DN, Olson MM, Peterson LR et al (1986) Clostridium difficile-associated diarrhea and colitis in adults. A prospective case-controlled epidemiologic study. Arch Intern Med 146:95–100
36. van den Hof S, van der Kooi T, van den Berg R, Kuijper EJ, Notermans DW (2006) Clostridium difficile PCR ribotype 027 outbreaks in the Netherlands: recent surveillance data indicate that outbreaks are not easily controlled but interhospital transmission is limited. Euro Surveill 11:E060126 060122

37. Dial S, Kezouh A, Dascal A, Barkun A, Suissa S (2008) Patterns of antibiotic use and risk of hospital admission because of Clostridium difficile infection. CMAJ 179:767–772
38. Johnson S, Samore MH, Farrow KA et al (1999) Epidemics of diarrhea caused by a clindamycin-resistant strain of Clostridium difficile in four hospitals. N Engl J Med 341:1645–1651
39. Merrigan MM, Sambol SP, Johnson S, Gerding DN (2003) Prevention of fatal Clostridium difficile-associated disease during continuous administration of clindamycin in hamsters. J Infect Dis 188:1922–1927
40. Merrigan M, Sambol S, Johnson S, Gerding DN (2003) Susceptibility of hamsters to human pathogenic Clostridium difficile strain B1 following clindamycin, ampicillin or ceftriaxone administration. Anaerobe 9:91–95
41. Kyne L, Warny M, Qamar A, Kelly CP (2001) Association between antibody response to toxin A and protection against recurrent Clostridium difficile diarrhoea. Lancet 357:189–193
42. Best EL, Fawley WN, Parnell P, Wilcox MH (2010) The potential for airborne dispersal of Clostridium difficile from symptomatic patients. Clin Infect Dis 50:1450–1457
43. Barbut F, Decre D, Lalande V et al (2005) Clinical features of Clostridium difficile-associated diarrhoea due to binary toxin (actin-specific ADP-ribosyltransferase)-producing strains. J Med Microbiol 54:181–185
44. Berman L, Carling T, Fitzgerald TN et al (2008) Defining surgical therapy for pseudomembranous colitis with toxic megacolon. J Clin Gastroenterol 42:476–480
45. Sailhamer EA, Carson K, Chang Y et al (2009) Fulminant Clostridium difficile colitis: patterns of care and predictors of mortality. Arch Surg 144:433–439
46. Bobo LD, Dubberke ER, Kollef M (2011) Clostridium difficile in the ICU: the struggle continues. Chest 140:1643–1653
47. Johnson S, Adelmann A, Clabots CR, Peterson LR, Gerding DN (1989) Recurrences of Clostridium difficile diarrhea not caused by the original infecting organism. J Infect Dis 159:340–343
48. Fenner L, Widmer AF, Goy G, Rudin S, Frei R (2008) Rapid and reliable diagnostic algorithm for detection of Clostridium difficile. J Clin Microbiol 46:328–330
49. Planche T, Aghaizu A, Holliman R et al (2008) Diagnosis of Clostridium difficile infection by toxin detection kits: a systematic review. Lancet Infect Dis 8:777–784
50. Tenover FC, Novak-Weekley S, Woods CW et al (2010) Impact of strain type on detection of toxigenic Clostridium difficile: comparison of molecular diagnostic and enzyme immunoassay approaches. J Clin Microbiol 48:3719–3724
51. Peterson LR, Manson RU, Paule SM et al (2007) Detection of toxigenic Clostridium difficile in stool samples by real-time polymerase chain reaction for the diagnosis of C. difficile-associated diarrhea. Clin Infect Dis 45:1152–1160
52. Pancholi P, Kelly C, Raczkowski M, Balada-Llasat JM (2012) Detection of toxigenic Clostridium difficile: comparison of the cell culture neutralization, Xpert C. difficile, Xpert C. difficile/Epi, and Illumigene C. difficile assays. J Clin Microbiol 50:1331–1335
53. Valiquette L, Pepin J, Do XV et al (2009) Prediction of complicated Clostridium difficile infection by pleural effusion and increased wall thickness on computed tomography. Clin Infect Dis 49:554–560
54. Bauer MP, Kuijper EJ, van Dissel JT (2009) European Society of Clinical Microbiology and Infectious Diseases (ESCMID): treatment guidance document for Clostridium difficile infection (CDI). Clin Microbiol Infect 15:1067–1079
55. Zar FA, Bakkanagari SR, Moorthi KM, Davis MB (2007) A comparison of vancomycin and metronidazole for the treatment of Clostridium difficile-associated diarrhea, stratified by disease severity. Clin Infect Dis 45:302–307
56. Pepin J, Routhier S, Gagnon S, Brazeau I (2006) Management and outcomes of a first recurrence of Clostridium difficile-associated disease in Quebec, Canada. Clin Infect Dis 42:758–764
57. Garey KW, Ghantoji SS, Shah DN et al (2011) A randomized, double-blind, placebo-controlled pilot study to assess the ability of rifaximin to prevent recurrent diarrhoea in patients with Clostridium difficile infection. J Antimicrob Chemother 66:2850–2855

58. Musher DM, Logan N, Hamill RJ et al (2006) Nitazoxanide for the treatment of Clostridium difficile colitis. Clin Infect Dis 43:421–427
59. Whitman CB, Czosnowski QA (2012) Fidaxomicin for the treatment of Clostridium difficile infections. Ann Pharmacother 46:219–228
60. Louie TJ, Miller MA, Mullane KM et al (2011) Fidaxomicin versus vancomycin for Clostridium difficile infection. N Engl J Med 364:422–431
61. Weiss K (2009) Toxin-binding treatment for Clostridium difficile: a review including reports of studies with tolevamer. Int J Antimicrob Agent 33:4–7
62. Abougergi MS, Kwon JH (2011) Intravenous immunoglobulin for the treatment of Clostridium difficile infection: a review. Dig Dis Sci 56:19–26
63. Pillai A, Nelson R (2008) Probiotics for treatment of Clostridium difficile-associated colitis in adults. Cochrane Database Syst Rev CD004611
64. Leav BA, Blair B, Leney M et al (2010) Serum anti-toxin B antibody correlates with protection from recurrent Clostridium difficile infection (CDI). Vaccine 28:965–969
65. Gough E, Shaikh H, Manges AR (2011) Systematic review of intestinal microbiota transplantation (fecal bacteriotherapy) for recurrent Clostridium difficile infection. Clin Infect Dis 53:994–1002

Invasive Pulmonary Aspergillosis in Critically Ill Patients

S. Blot, D. Koulenti, and G. Dimopoulos

Introduction

Aspergillus is a ubiquitous fungus that can cause a wide spectrum of diseases including allergy, superficial infection related to (surgical) trauma, and invasive disease [1]. More than 180 species of *Aspergillus* have been described but *A. fumigatus* is most likely to cause disease as it is responsible for about 90 % of cases of invasive aspergillosis. The mechanism of infection is represented by aerosolized conidia by which these organisms spread in the environment and cause pulmonary infection after inhalation. Growth into angio-invasive filamentous forms results in local pulmonary inflammation, invasion, and eventually hematogenous spread to distal organs [1]. As such, nearly every organ can be affected by *Aspergillus* species, albeit that sinopulmonary involvement is most common. Over the past three decades, major advances in healthcare have led to an unwelcome increase in invasive pulmonary aspergillosis largely because of the increasing size of the population at risk [2]. This population includes recipients of hematopoietic stem cell transplants and solid organ transplants, patients with hematological malignancies, patients infected with human immunodeficiency virus (HIV) developing acquired immunodeficiency syndrome (AIDS), and patients receiving immunosuppressive treatment. Furthermore, the use of high-grade supportive care in

S. Blot (✉)
Dept. of Internal Medicine, Ghent University, Ghent, Belgium
E-mail: stijn.blot@UGent.be

D. Koulenti
Dept. of Critical Care Medicine, Attikon University Hospital, University of Athens Medical School, Athens, Greece

G. Dimopoulos
Dept. of Critical Care Medicine, Attikon University Hospital, University of Athens Medical School, Athens, Greece

J.-L. Vincent (Ed.), *Annual Update in Intensive Care and Emergency Medicine 2013*,
DOI 10.1007/978-3-642-35109-9_5, © Springer-Verlag Berlin Heidelberg 2013

severe and life-threatening diseases, specifically in intensive care units (ICUs), has improved survival, but has created a demographic shift in hospital and ICU populations with more debilitated patients at risk for secondary invasive opportunistic infections, such as invasive pulmonary aspergillosis.

Risk Factors for Invasive Pulmonary Aspergillosis

Classic Host Factors

In 2002, the European Organization for the Research and Treatment of Cancer/Mycosis Study Group (EORTC/MSG) defined a set of host factors for the diagnosis of invasive fungal disease [3]. These host factors were revised in 2008 [4] and represent a status of profound immunosuppression. They include: A recent history of severe neutropenia (< 500 neutrophils/mm^3) for at least 10 days; receipt of an allogeneic stem cell transplant; prolonged use of corticosteroids (minimum dose of 0.3 mg/kg/day of prednisone equivalent for > 3 weeks); treatment with other recognized T cell immunosuppressants (e. g., cyclosporine, TNF-α blockers, specific monoclonal antibodies, or nucleoside analogs) during the past three months; and inherited severe immunodeficiency.

It is clear that the spectrum of immunosuppression is broader that that covered by the host factors. For example, a patient infected with HIV who has developed AIDS does not match the EORTC/MSG host factors. It has to be mentioned, however, that the EORTC/MSG criteria for diagnosing invasive fungal disease are primarily developed to select patients with a high likelihood of disease for the purpose of clinical trials, not for daily practice. In ICU settings 30 to 70 % of the cases of invasive aspergillosis arise in the absence of classic host factors [5, 6]. Within the group of ICU patients with classic host factors, chronic obstructive pulmonary disease (COPD) is the most common underlying condition (about 35 %), followed by solid organ transplant [7].

Chronic Obstructive Pulmonary Disease

COPD as such is not considered a host factor by the EORTC/MSG. However, in more severe cases these patients receive corticosteroids for prolonged periods, which puts them into the high-risk category as defined by the EORTC/MSG. Based on the results of several reports, COPD is now broadly recognized as a major risk factor for invasive pulmonary aspergillosis [8]. This risk may be easily overlooked as many COPD patients are chronically colonized with *Aspergillus* species. In a large series of patients with COPD, an average of 16 patients per 1000 admissions were colonized in the respiratory tract with *Aspergillus* species [9]. Probable invasive pulmonary aspergillosis was diagnosed in 22 % of these patients. This data indicate that in case of COPD-associated critical illness, *Aspergillus*-positive respiratory tract samples should not be discarded. COPD patients with GOLD stage III or IV are, in particular, considered to have a substantial risk for invasive pulmonary aspergillosis [8]. Clinical features for invasive pulmonary aspergillosis in COPD patients are, however, non-specific [10]. A thorough diagnostic work-out in patients presenting with *Aspergillus*-positive cultures is advocated.

Additional Risk Factors

A broad range of risk factors has been described. Unfortunately most of these risk factors simply reflect a high index of critical illness. For example, nearly all patients in the ICU with invasive pulmonary aspergillosis are receiving mechanical ventilation, and have high APACHE II and sequential organ failure assessment (SOFA) scores. Such non-specific risk factors do not really speed-up recognition or diagnosis of invasive pulmonary aspergillosis. In a retrospective series, Meersseman et al. [5] found that 7 % of the patients had liver failure. Indeed, it has been demonstrated that decompensated liver disease is an acquired immune deficiency state that may put patients at risk for infection with opportunistic pathogens such as *Aspergillus* [11, 12].

Hartemink et al. suggested that apparently immunocompetent patients with sepsis and associated organ failure might become at risk during the anti-inflammatory phase following the phase of hyperinflammation in severe sepsis [13]. This compensatory anti-inflammatory phase is supposed to be characterized by a status of relative immune paralysis due to neutrophil deactivation, which puts patients at risk for opportunistic infection. Indeed, in a large cohort of ICU patients with invasive pulmonary aspergillosis, approximately half of the patients were admitted to the ICU with signs of sepsis [14]. However, the diagnosis of invasive pulmonary aspergillosis was generally made within the first week of ICU stay, thus not supporting the higher risk of invasive pulmonary aspergillosis in a post-sepsis period.

Meersseman et al. categorized risk factors for invasive aspergillosis among ICU patients into high-, intermediate-, and low-risk [15]. The high-risk category essentially matches the classic host factors. The intermediate category includes prolonged treatment with corticosteroids, COPD, autologous bone marrow transplant, liver cirrhosis with prolonged ICU stay (> 7 days), solid organ cancer, HIV infection, lung transplant, and systemic diseases requiring immunosuppressive therapy. The low-risk category includes patients with major burn injury, solid organ transplants (other than lung), steroid treatment with a duration of < 8 days, prolonged ICU stay (> 21 days), malnutrition, and post-cardiac surgery status. It should be mentioned that the low-risk category in particular involves a large number of patients who will never develop invasive fungal disease. As already mentioned, the discriminative value of such risk factors is low.

As an iatrogenic risk factor, construction or demolition works in the hospital or its environment should be mentioned. In a systematic review of *Aspergillus* outbreaks in hospital settings, it was found that construction or demolition works were considered to be the probable or possible source of the problem in 49% of outbreaks [16].

Diagnosis of Invasive Pulmonary Aspergillosis

The EORTC/MSG Diagnostic Criteria for Invasive Pulmonary Aspergillosis

According to the revised EORTC/MSG definitions for invasive fungal disease, invasive pulmonary aspergillosis is categorized into three major categories reflecting the diagnostic degree of certainty: Proven, probable, and possible invasive fungal disease [4]. A proven diagnosis requires histopathologic evidence of fungal invasion. A diagnosis of probable invasive pulmonary aspergillosis is based on the presence of host factors, clinical features, and positive mycology. Host factors reflect profound immunodeficiency such as neutropenia or treatment with immunosuppressive agents. Clinical features for invasive pulmonary aspergillosis include medical imaging on computed tomography (CT) scan demonstrating suggestive signs of fungal invasion: Dense, well circumscribed lesions, with or without a halo-sign, air crescent sign, or cavity. Mycological criteria include either a direct test (cytology, direct microscopy, or culture) on any respiratory tract aspirate, or galactomannan antigen detection on bronchoalveolar lavage (BAL) fluid or serum. A diagnosis of possible invasive pulmonary aspergillosis is made in the presence of host factors and clinical features, but in the absence of mycological criteria.

The Limited Value of the EORTC/MSG Diagnostic Criteria in the ICU

The diagnostic criteria defined by the EORTC/MSG have been shown to be useful in research and clinical practice in patients with classic host factors [17, 18]. In mechanically ventilated critically ill patients, however, diagnosing invasive pulmonary aspergillosis according to this strict classification is problematic for a number of reasons. First, open lung biopsy may be contraindicated because of coagulation disorders; as such, a diagnosis of proven invasive pulmonary aspergillosis is rare. Second, current definitions of probable or possible invasive pulmonary aspergillosis have been validated only in immunocompromised patients. This is a serious drawback as invasive pulmonary aspergillosis may develop in the absence of predisposing host factors [5, 19]. Third, radiological findings in mechanically ventilated patients are non-specific in the majority of cases [19] in contrast to the very strict definitions of radiological lesions in the EORTC/MSG criteria [4]. Moreover, these lesions need to be documented by CT scan, which is not always feasible in critically ill patients with hemodynamic or respiratory instability. Finally, the value of galactomannan antigen detection in serum is questionable in non-neutropenic patients as circulating neutrophils are capable of clearing the antigen.

"Putative Invasive Pulmonary Aspergillosis": A New Diagnostic Category for Invasive Aspergillosis in ICU Patients

The lack of specific criteria for diagnosing invasive pulmonary aspergillosis in critically ill patients hampers timely initiation of appropriate antifungal therapy. One of the clinical dilemmas in the ICU is the clinical relevance of *Aspergillus*-positive respiratory tract aspirates. Depending on the case-mix in the unit, this is observed in about 1–2 % of mechanically ventilated critically ill patients [6, 19, 20]. The relevance of *Aspergillus*-positive endotracheal aspirates was investigated by Vandewoude et al. who developed a clinical diagnostic algorithm to discriminate *Aspergillus* respiratory colonization from invasive pulmonary aspergillosis [19]. The algorithm considers an *Aspergillus*-positive endotracheal aspirate culture to represent probable invasive pulmonary aspergillosis in the presence of compatible signs, abnormal thoracic medical imaging, and either host factors or BAL fluid positive for *Aspergillus* on direct microscopy and culture (Box 1). In a cohort of 172 ICU patients with *Aspergillus*-positive endotracheal aspirate cultures, 83 were judged to have invasive pulmonary aspergillosis (48.3 %). Histopathology data were available in 26 patients, 19 in the invasive pulmonary aspergillosis group and 9 in the colonization group. In all 26 cases, the diagnosis as based upon the clinical algorithm was confirmed. Yet, because of the low number of histopathology-controlled cases and the single-center design, external validation in a larger cohort was deemed mandatory. This clinical algorithm was recently validated in a multicenter observational study that included 524 ICU patients with *Aspergillus*-positive respiratory tact aspirates [7]. The diagnostic accuracy of this algorithm was evaluated using 115 patients with histopathologic data, considered the gold standard. The algorithm had a specificity of 61 % and a sensitivity of 92 %. The positive and negative predictive values were 61 % and 92 %, respectively. In the total cohort (n = 524), 15 % of the patients had proven invasive pulmonary aspergillosis. According to the EORTC/MSG criteria, only 6 % patients had probable aspergillosis and 79 % of the patients were not classifiable. The algorithm judged 38 % of patients to have putative invasive pulmonary aspergillosis and 47 % to have *Aspergillus* colonization. As such, in a cohort of 524 patients with positive *Aspergillus* cultures, the algorithm diagnosed invasive pulmonary aspergillosis in 32 % more cases than did the EORTC/MSG criteria. Therefore, the algorithm probably encompasses a larger proportion of the true burden of invasive pulmonary aspergillosis in the ICU.

Box 1

Diagnostic criteria for putative invasive pulmonary aspergillosis in critically ill patients [19]. A diagnosis of putative invasive pulmonary aspergillosis requires that all criteria are fulfilled (1 + 2 + 3 + either 4a or 4b).

1. ***Aspergillus*-positive respiratory tract specimen culture**
2. **Compatible signs and symptoms** (one of the following)

- Fever refractory to at least three days of appropriate antibiotic therapy
- Recrudescent fever after a period of defervescence of at least 48 h while still on antibiotics and without other apparent cause
- Pleuritic chest pain
- Pleuritic rub
- Dyspnea
- Hemoptysis
- Worsening respiratory insufficiency in spite of appropriate antibiotic therapy and ventilatory support

3. **Abnormal medical imaging** by portable chest X-ray or CT scan of the lungs
4. **Either 4a or 4b**

 4a. **Host risk factors** (one of the following conditions)

 - Neutropenia (absolute neutrophil count less then 500/mm^3) preceding or at the time of ICU admission
 - Underlying hematological or oncological malignancy treated with cytotoxic agents
 - Glucocorticoid treatment (prednisone or equivalent, >20 mg/day)
 - Congenital or acquired immunodeficiency

 4b. **Semiquantitative *Aspergillus*-positive culture of bronchoalveolar lavage fluid** (+ or ++), without bacterial growth together with a positive cytological smear showing branching hyphae

Galactomannan Antigen Detection in BAL Fluid

Although there remains some debate about the optimal cut-off for the optical density index, the value of galactomannan antigen detection in serum and BAL fluid has been established in neutropenic patients [21, 22]. Currently, a cut-off of 0.5 is used by the US Food and Drug Administration (FDA), whereas a level of 0.7 is generally used in Europe [23, 24]. In non-neutropenic patients, however, the value of galactomannan detection in serum is limited because circulating neutrophils are capable of clearing the antigen. Meersseman et al. evaluated the value of galactomannan detection in BAL fluid in 72 pathology-controlled non-neutropenic ICU patients with an overt risk profile for aspergillosis, as evidenced by thoracic CT scan, underlying and acute conditions [25]. Using a cut-off index of 0.5, the sensitivity and specificity of galactomannan detection in BAL fluid were 88 % and 87 %, respectively. The inclusion of a thoracic CT scan, however, somewhat limits the application of this approach in daily practice. Nevertheless, galactomannan antigen detection in BAL fluid seems to be the best option to diagnose invasive pulmonary aspergillosis in non-neutropenic critically ill patients, in the absence of *Aspergillus*-positive cultures. In case of *Aspergillus*-positive respiratory tract aspirates, additional galactomannan detection on BAL fluid could strengthen the diagnostic certainty of the clinical algorithm used to discriminate *Aspergillus* colonization from invasive disease. This approach, however, needs to be evaluated in a prospective study. It should be mentioned that some antibiotics that are commonly used in ICUs, such as piperacillin-tazobactam, represent an extraneous source of galactomannan resulting in loss of clinical specificity of this diagnostic test [24].

(1,3)-Beta-D-glucan

There has been an emergence of clinical data pertaining to the diagnostic utility of the cell wall component, (1-3)-beta-D-glucan, in serum [24]. (1-3)-Beta-D-glucan is present in the cell wall of most fungal species. The molecule is ubiquitous in the environment and is used as a marker of fungal biomass. The presence of (1-3)-beta-D-glucan in fungal species other than *Aspergillus* means that its role in establishing a specific diagnosis of invasive aspergillosis is not straightforward. False-positive results have been documented in hemodialysis, cardiopulmonary bypass, treatment with immunoglobulin preparations, and exposure to glucan containing gauze (e. g., following major surgery). As these factors are very common in ICU patients, it seems that the value of (1-3)-beta-D-glucan detection lies merely in its high negative predictive value.

Incidence of Invasive Pulmonary Aspergillosis in the ICU

Because of the problematic diagnosis, reliable estimates of the incidence of invasive pulmonary aspergillosis are lacking. Approximately 1 to 2 % of mechanically ventilated patients have *Aspergillus*-positive endotracheal aspirate cultures [19, 20, 26]. In the studies by Vandewoude et al. and Garnacho-Montero et al. a prevalence of invasive pulmonary aspergillosis of 1 % was found [19, 20], whereas Bassetti et al. described a prevalence of just 0.2 % [26]. An important study addressing the epidemiology of invasive aspergillosis in a medical ICU was published by Meersseman et al. [5]. The EORTC/MSG diagnostic criteria were applied in this retrospective study. One-hundred and twenty-seven patients out of 1850 admissions (6.9 %) hospitalized between 2000 and 2003 had microbiological or histopathological evidence of *Aspergillus* during their ICU stay. It is clear that the occurrence rate of invasive pulmonary aspergillosis can vary widely among ICUs. In addition to the already-mentioned problems with diagnosis, differences in case-mix can be responsible for the observed variation in epidemiology. Logically, units with a large number of patients at risk (e. g., COPD, solid organ transplants) will experience higher rates of invasive pulmonary aspergillosis.

Therapeutic Issues

Effective management of invasive pulmonary aspergillosis depends on early initiation of appropriate antifungal agents; delay in treatment initiation is associated with increased mortality. Therefore, the treatment of invasive pulmonary aspergillosis must be initiated upon suspicion of a diagnosis, without need for definitive proof, and should be prolonged beyond resolution of the infection and of any reversible predisposing underlying disease. In the rapidly progressive form of the disease, antifungal agents should be given intravenously. The antifungal agents that are active against *Aspergillus* spp. are: (a) from the class of triazoles: itraconazole, voriconazole and posaconazole; (b) amphotericin B; and (c) echinocandins. In a large prospective surveillance study (PATH Alliance) of invasive fungal infections, which was conducted in North America between 2004 and 2008, voriconazole was the main antifungal agent used for invasive aspergillosis (45.5 %) [27].

Itraconazole has activity against *Aspergillus*, but resistant strains of *A. fumigatus* have already been described [28]. Itraconazole is attractive for long-term therapy because of its oral formulation. Voriconazole provides higher response rates and better survival than amphotericin B in the treatment of probable or proven invasive aspergillosis and is recommended as first-choice treatment [29, 30]. *A. terreus* however, is resistant to amphotericin B both *in vitro* and in animal models, but remains susceptible to itraconazole and voriconazole. Posaconazole has been shown to have significant efficacy against *Aspergillus* as prophylaxis, treatment or salvage therapy for invasive aspergillosis [31]. The use of triazoles may be hampered by drug-related hepatotoxicity and hazardous drug interactions.

Echinocandins (anidulafungin, caspofungin, micafungin) have *in vitro* and in *vivo* activity against *Aspergillus* spp. exerting their antifungal activity by inhibition of biosynthesis of 1,3-beta-glucan in the fungal cell wall. However, only caspofungin has been shown to be effective in patients with proven or probable invasive aspergillosis who are refractory to or intolerant of conventional antifungal treatment, and there are limited data on the use of anidulafungin and micafungin [32]. A recent multicenter, prospective, non-comparative, observational study that assessed the effectiveness and safety of caspofungin in adult hematological patients concluded that 79 % of the patients had complete or partial response on the last day of caspofungin therapy and that the drug was generally well tolerated (non-serious drug-related adverse reactions in 1.7 %) [33].

The management of invasive aspergillosis in critically ill patients is associated with difficulties regarding bioavailability and toxicity. Voriconazole, as already mentioned, is the treatment of choice, but the intravenous form has considerable drug interactions (e. g., reduced clearance of intravenous midazolam) and renal and liver toxicity because of the solvent vehicle [34]. The oral form, however, carries the risk of inadequate absorption and subtherapeutic levels, and no clinical data are available for the bioavailability of oral voriconazole in critically ill patients. The results of the first randomized trial that aimed to evaluate whether routine therapeutic drug monitoring of voriconazole could reduce adverse events or improve treatment response in invasive fungal infections were recently published. The study concluded that routine therapeutic drug monitoring of voriconazole may reduce the rates of drug discontinuation due to adverse events, and may also improve the response to treatment [35].

Posaconazole, although effective, is only available for oral administration, so it is less relevant for critically ill patients [31]. Echinocandins are well tolerated, but clinical trials in critically ill patients are lacking. The severity of critical illness combined with invasive aspergillosis should not justify the risk of insufficient treatment by oral solutions, so intravenous voriconazole or liposomal amphotericin B should be the treatment options. Combination therapy may be considered in breakthrough invasive aspergillosis or in refractory disease, although clear evidence is lacking. Simultaneous inhibition of cell membrane and fungal cell wall biosynthesis, achieved with use of voriconazole and caspofungin, results in a synergistic interaction against *Aspergillus*. Synergy has also been observed *in vitro* between echinocandins and azoles in most, but not all, combinations assessed. The combination of voriconazole and caspofungin was associated with an improved 3-month survival compared with voriconazole alone [36]. Two studies have described clinical experience with caspofungin in combination with liposomal amphotericin B in the management of invasive aspergillosis [37, 38]; in 60 % of these patients, a favorable antifungal response was seen when combination therapy was used. The combination was more successful as a primary therapy than as salvage therapy. Trends toward a higher proportion of favorable responses were observed among patients with pulmonary disease, compared with those with extrapulmonary disease and among neutropenic patients compared with non-neutropenic patients. A recent meta-analysis of studies (1 randomized controlled trial and 7 cohort studies) that assessed the efficacy of combinations of antifungal agents in the treatment of invasive aspergillosis and reported on clinical outcomes concluded that the cumulative evidence is conflicting and of moderate strength [39]. Well-designed, large-scale randomized controlled trials are needed in order to determine the usefulness of antifungal combinations.

Outcome in Invasive Pulmonary Aspergillosis

Despite the availability of potent antifungal agents, mortality rates in patients with invasive pulmonary aspergillosis remain devastatingly high. In general, mortality rates in ICU patients with invasive aspergillosis vary between 70 % and 95 % [5, 6, 20, 40, 41]. In a matched-cohort study, the attributable mortality for invasive aspergillosis was estimated to be 19 % [41]. The high mortality can – at least in part – be attributed to the difficult and, therefore, delayed diagnosis. In non-ICU patients, Nivoix et al. demonstrated that diagnosis at an earlier stage of the disease and with prompt initiation of an appropriate antifungal agent, was associated with significantly better survival [18]. Compared to classic risk groups, ICU patients experience a much more severe course of the disease, with nearly all deaths occurring within the first week after the first culture positive for *Aspergillus* [19]. It can be questioned whether a more prompt initiation of antifungal therapy would contribute to better survival rates in these patients. Recent data from the *Asp*ICU project indicated that delay in the initiation of antifungal therapy was not associated with worse outcome in univariate or multivariate analysis [14]. In a subset of 278 patients with invasive pulmonary aspergillosis, delay in antifungal therapy was only one day in non-survivors (interquartile range 0 to 3 days) vs. two days among survivors (interquartile range 0 to 4 days). This reflects the high degree of accuracy with which clinicians responded to the first positive culture. With currently available diagnostic approaches, it is hardly possible to improve this figure.

In addition to its grim prognosis, invasive pulmonary aspergillosis has an important health-economic burden. Compared with control subjects matched for severity of disease (APACHE II score) and length of ICU stay prior to the infection, patients with invasive aspergillosis had an added length of ICU stay of 12 days, and an added length of mechanical ventilation of 9 days [41]. The economic impact of aspergillosis was investigated by Tong et al., using a large-scale epidemiologic study [42]. Overall, the length of hospitalization was 7.9 vs. 17.7 days in non-aspergillosis and aspergillosis patients, respectively and the mean total hospital charges were approximately $44,000 vs. $97,000. Attention should be given to the fact that in this study patients were compared within the same diagnosis-related group (DRG), but without correction for disease severity and length of stay. Nevertheless, it is obvious that aspergillosis adds substantially to hospital costs.

Conclusion

Invasive pulmonary aspergillosis generally occurs in patients with failing immune function. In addition to profound immunosuppression as reflected by classic host factors, invasive pulmonary aspergillosis can also occur in any patient with a high index of disease severity and associated organ failure. The incidence of invasive pulmonary aspergillosis is hard to estimate because of problems with diagnosis. When lung biopsy is contraindicated because of coagulation disorders or respiratory problems and medical imaging is blurred by mechanical ventilation, the best option is to invest in galactomannan antigen detection on BAL fluid. When the patient presents with *Aspergillus*-positive respiratory tract cultures, a clinical algorithm may lead to a diagnosis of putative invasive pulmonary aspergillosis, a recently established diagnostic category. Despite prompt initiation of adequate antifungal agents, mortality associated with invasive pulmonary aspergillosis in critically ill patients remains unacceptably high. Future research should focus on faster diagnostic techniques and/or the identification of a risk profile that justifies antifungal prophylaxis.

References

1. Marr KA, Patterson T, Denning D (2002) Aspergillosis. Pathogenesis, clinical manifestations, and therapy. Infect Dis Clin North Am 16:875–894
2. Vandewoude K, Vogelaers D, Blot S (2006) Aspergillosis in the ICU – the new 21st century problem. Med Mycol 44(Suppl 1):71–76
3. Ascioglu S, Rex JH, de Pauw B et al (2002) Defining opportunistic invasive fungal infections in immunocompromised patients with cancer and hematopoietic stem cell transplants: an international consensus. Clin Infect Dis 34:7–14
4. De Pauw B, Walsh TJ, Donnelly JP et al (2008) Revised definitions of invasive fungal disease from the European Organization for Research and Treatment of Cancer/Invasive Fungal Infections Cooperative Group and the National Institute of Allergy and Infectious Diseases Mycoses Study Group (EORTC/MSG) Consensus Group. Clin Infect Dis 46:1813–1821
5. Meersseman W, Vandecasteele SJ, Wilmer A, Verbeken E, Peetermans WE, Van Wijngaerden E (2004) Invasive aspergillosis in critically ill patients without malignancy. Am J Respir Crit Care Med 170:621–625
6. Vandewoude K, Blot S, Benoit D, Depuydt P, Vogelaers D, Colardyn F (2004) Invasive aspergillosis in critically ill patients: analysis of risk factors for acquisition and mortality. Acta Clin Belg 59:251–257
7. Blot SI, Taccone FS, Van den Abeele AM et al (2012) A clinical algorithm to diagnose invasive pulmonary aspergillosis in critically ill patients. Am J Respir Crit Care Med 186:56–64
8. Bulpa P, Dive A, Sibille Y (2007) Invasive pulmonary aspergillosis in patients with chronic obstructive pulmonary disease. Eur Respir J 30:782–800
9. Guinea J, Torres-Narbona M, Gijon P et al (2010) Pulmonary aspergillosis in patients with chronic obstructive pulmonary disease: incidence, risk factors, and outcome. Clin Microbiol Infect 16:870–877
10. He H, Ding L, Li F, Zhan Q (2011) Clinical features of invasive bronchial-pulmonary aspergillosis in critically ill patients with chronic obstructive respiratory diseases: a prospective study. Crit Care 15:R5
11. Li D, Chen L, Ding X, Tao R, Zhang YX, Wang JF (2008) Hospital-acquired invasive pulmonary aspergillosis in patients with hepatic failure. BMC Gastroenterol 8:32
12. Prodanovic H, Cracco C, Massard J et al (2007) Invasive pulmonary aspergillosis in patients with decompensated cirrhosis: case series. BMC Gastroenterol 7:2
13. Hartemink KJ, Paul MA, Spijkstra JJ, Girbes AR, Polderman KH (2003) Immunoparalysis as a cause for invasive aspergillosis? Intensive Care Med 29:2068–2071
14. Blot S, Rello J, Dimopoulos G, Vandewoude K, Vogelaers D (2012) Risk factors and outcome in patients critically ill patients with invasive pulmonary aspergillosis. Abstracts of

the Interscience Conference on Antimicrobial Agents and Chemotherapy American Society for Microbiology, San Francisco, 2012, K-951 (abst)

15. Meersseman W, Lagrou K, Maertens J, Van Wijngaerden E (2007) Invasive aspergillosis in the intensive care unit. Clin Infect Dis 45:205–216
16. Vonberg RP, Gastmeier P (2006) Nosocomial aspergillosis in outbreak settings. J Hosp Infect 63:246–254
17. Maertens J, Theunissen K, Verbeken E et al (2004) Prospective clinical evaluation of lower cut-offs for galactomannan detection in adult neutropenic cancer patients and haematological stem cell transplant recipients. Br J Haematol 126:852–860
18. Nivoix Y, Velten M, Letscher-Bru V et al (2008) Factors associated with overall and attributable mortality in invasive aspergillosis. Clin Infect Dis 47:1176–1184
19. Vandewoude KH, Blot SI, Depuydt P et al (2006) Clinical relevance of Aspergillus isolation from respiratory tract samples in critically ill patients. Crit Care 10:R31
20. Garnacho-Montero J, Amaya-Villar R, Ortiz-Leyba C et al (2005) Isolation of Aspergillus spp. from the respiratory tract in critically ill patients: risk factors, clinical presentation and outcome. Crit Care 9:R191–R199
21. Maertens J, Maertens V, Theunissen K et al (2009) Bronchoalveolar lavage fluid galactomannan for the diagnosis of invasive pulmonary aspergillosis in patients with hematologic diseases. Clin Infect Dis 49:1688–1693
22. Maertens J, Verhaegen J, Lagrou K, Van Eldere J, Boogaerts M (2001) Screening for circulating galactomannan as a noninvasive diagnostic tool for invasive aspergillosis in prolonged neutropenic patients and stem cell transplantation recipients: a prospective validation. Blood 97:1604–1610
23. Herbrecht R, Letscher-Bru V, Oprea C et al (2002) Aspergillus galactomannan detection in the diagnosis of invasive aspergillosis in cancer patients. J Clin Oncol 20:1898–1906
24. Hope WW, Walsh TJ, Denning DW (2005) Laboratory diagnosis of invasive aspergillosis. Lancet Infect Dis 5:609–622
25. Meersseman W, Lagrou K, Maertens J et al (2008) Galactomannan in bronchoalveolar lavage fluid: a tool for diagnosing aspergillosis in intensive care unit patients. Am J Respir Crit Care Med 177:27–34
26. Bassetti M, Mikulska M, Repetto E et al (2010) Invasive pulmonary aspergillosis in intensive care units: is it a real problem? J Hosp Infect 74:186–187
27. Azie N, Neofytos D, Pfaller M et al (2012) The PATH (Prospective Antifungal Therapy) Alliance(R) registry and invasive fungal infections: update 2012. Diagn Microbiol Infect Dis 73:293–300
28. Denning DW, Venkateswarlu K, Oakley KL et al (1997) Itraconazole resistance in Aspergillus fumigatus. Antimicrob Agents Chemother 41:1364–1368
29. Herbrecht R, Denning DW, Patterson TF et al (2002) Voriconazole versus amphotericin B for primary therapy of invasive aspergillosis. N Engl J Med 347:408–415
30. Walsh TJ, Anaissie EJ, Denning DW et al (2008) Treatment of aspergillosis: clinical practice guidelines of the Infectious Diseases Society of America. Clin Infect Dis 46:327–360
31. Walsh TJ, Raad I, Patterson TF et al (2007) Treatment of invasive aspergillosis with posaconazole in patients who are refractory to or intolerant of conventional therapy: an externally controlled trial. Clin Infect Dis 44:2–12
32. Maertens J, Raad I, Petrikkos G et al (2004) Efficacy and safety of caspofungin for treatment of invasive aspergillosis in patients refractory to or intolerant of conventional antifungal therapy. Clin Infect Dis 39:1563–1571
33. Jarque I, Tormo M, Bello JL et al (2012) Caspofungin for the treatment of invasive fungal disease in hematological patients (ProCAS Study). Med Mycol (in press)
34. von Mach MA, Burhenne J, Weilemann LS (2006) Accumulation of the solvent vehicle sulphobutylether beta cyclodextrin sodium in critically ill patients treated with intravenous voriconazole under renal replacement therapy. BMC Clin Pharmacol 6:6

35. Park WB, Kim NH, Kim KH et al (2012) The effect of therapeutic drug monitoring on safety and efficacy of voriconazole in invasive fungal infections: A randomized controlled trial. Clin Infect Dis 55:1080–1087
36. Singh N, Limaye AP, Forrest G et al (2006) Combination of voriconazole and caspofungin as primary therapy for invasive aspergillosis in solid organ transplant recipients: a prospective, multicenter, observational study. Transplantation 81:320–326
37. Aliff TB, Maslak PG, Jurcic JG et al (2003) Refractory Aspergillus pneumonia in patients with acute leukemia: successful therapy with combination caspofungin and liposomal amphotericin. Cancer 97:1025–1032
38. Kontoyiannis DP, Hachem R, Lewis RE et al (2003) Efficacy and toxicity of caspofungin in combination with liposomal amphotericin B as primary or salvage treatment of invasive aspergillosis in patients with hematologic malignancies. Cancer 98:292–299
39. Garbati MA, Alasmari FA, Al-Tannir MA, Tleyjeh IM (2012) The role of combination antifungal therapy in the treatment of invasive aspergillosis: a systematic review. Int J Infect Dis 16:e76–81
40. Janssen JJ, Strack van Schijndel RJ et al (1996) Outcome of ICU treatment in invasive aspergillosis. Intensive Care Med 22:1315–1322
41. Vandewoude KH, Blot SI, Benoit D, Colardyn F, Vogelaers D (2004) Invasive aspergillosis in critically ill patients: attributable mortality and excesses in length of ICU stay and ventilator dependence. J Hosp Infect 56:269–276
42. Tong KB, Lau CJ, Murtagh K, Layton AJ, Seifeldin R (2009) The economic impact of aspergillosis: analysis of hospital expenditures across patient subgroups. Int J Infect Dis 13:24–36

Procalcitonin Use to Identify the Infected Heart Failure Patient

R. Choudhary and A. S. Maisel

Introduction

Pulmonary infections substantially increase the risk of mortality in patients with heart failure [1]. Commonly seen in the 65–75 year age group, heart failure complicated by ongoing infection (often leading to sepsis) puts a considerable burden on the healthcare system [2]. Improper and untimely management of such patients has driven up healthcare costs significantly. That being the case, patients with heart failure and superimposed infection (especially pneumonia) often present with overlapping symptoms and signs, making it difficult to distinguish using conventional tools, such as radiographic imaging and blood testing. Studies have shown that patients with preexisting heart failure often experience a worsening of their symptoms due to superimposed infection [3, 4]. Pulmonary infections such as pneumonia have been shown to suppress myocardial function, initiate inflammatory hormone release and worsen heart failure [4].

Procalcitonin (PCT) has been recognized as an excellent marker reflecting the presence and severity of a relevant bacterial infection [5–7]. With documented superiority to conventional markers such as C-reactive protein (CRP) or white blood cell (WBC) count, which lack diagnostic accuracy and are sometimes misleading, PCT has a significant role in facilitating early diagnosis and management of relevant bacterial infection thus lowering the associated morbidity and mortality [7, 8]. Although there is robust evidence supporting use of PCT in detecting bacterial infection, its utility in the setting of acute heart failure patients with pulmonary infection remains uncharted. Recently published results from the Biomarkers in the Assessment of Congestive Heart Failure (BACH) trial have shown that PCT

R. Choudhary (✉)
Capital Health Regional Medical Center, 750 Brunswick Ave, Trenton, NJ 08638, USA
E-mail: dr.rajivc@gmail.com

A. S. Maisel
Veterans Affairs San Diego Healthcare System, 3350 La Jolla Drive, San Diego, CA 92122, USA

J.-L. Vincent (Ed.), *Annual Update in Intensive Care and Emergency Medicine 2013*,
DOI 10.1007/978-3-642-35109-9_6,

cannot only aid in identifying patients with bacterial infection, but can also guide antibiotic use in patients with acute heart failure and superimposed infection [9]. In this chapter we will provide a brief synopsis into the growing utility of PCT to guide treatment in the infected heart failure patient.

Burden of Concomitant Infection in Heart Failure

Heart failure is a growing epidemic affecting millions worldwide and remains one of the leading causes of death [10]. Within the spectrum of heart failure, acute heart failure is an entity that comprises new onset or *de novo* heart failure as well as worsening of preexisting heart failure or acute decompensated heart failure (ADHF) [11]. The prevalence of acute heart failure in the general population can be approximated at 10 %, with an almost > 50 % re-admission rate by 4–6 months. A high in-patient mortality rate of 8 % and short-term mortality rate after discharge of 13 % necessitate effective tailoring of current approaches to improve early diagnosis and risk stratification [12]. The elevated risk of mortality in patients with acute heart failure is associated with the presence of lower respiratory tract infections, such as pneumonia, acute bronchitis, and acute exacerbation of chronic obstructive pulmonary disease (COPD) [13, 14]. The prevalence of acute heart failure and concomitant infection is higher in the elderly age group and is associated with increased risk of mortality and higher re-admission rates [15]. In a population based cohort study of 33,736 patients evaluating the association between preexisting heart failure and 30-day mortality in patients with first time hospitalization for pneumonia revealed that those with a preadmission history of heart failure had a higher risk of mortality from pneumonia (24.4 %) compared to those without (14.4 %) [3]. Furthermore, those in the age group 65–79 years carried an elevated risk of mortality. Factors such as severity of New York Heart Association (NYHA) functional class compounded with improper use of medications significantly contributed to the elevated risk of mortality. Thus, with a currently aging population, strategies to effectively reduce re-admission rates and lower mortality are crucial in order to curb the growing epidemic.

Pathophysiology of Worsening Heart Failure in the Infected Patient

The mechanisms leading to increased mortality in acute heart failure patients with infection can be partly explained by the onset of several changes affecting the optimal functioning of the heart. In addition, causative organisms have been shown to compromise cardiac function by binding host cell-wall receptors, enabling bacterial uptake especially in cardiomyocytes, resulting in decreased cardiac contractility [16]. Acute bacterial infection can also lead to arterial stiffness contributing to an elevated left ventricular afterload pressure; hypoxemia associated with pneumonia can cause an increase in right ventricular afterload [15, 17]. Furthermore, the systemic response to infection in terms of tachycardia can also result in increasing myocardial oxygen demand due to reduced diastolic filling and poor coronary perfusion pressure. The release of pro-inflammatory cytokines can further worsen heart failure by activating compensatory pathways to increase intravascular volume [15–17]. Finally, the continuous ongoing hemodynamic changes in intravascular volume and pressure and the activation of the inflammatory cascade can lead to disruption of coronary plaques resulting in acute coronary syndrome [17, 18].

Procalcitonin Structure and Expression

PCT belongs to the calcitonin superfamily of peptides and is encoded by the CALC 1 gene located on the short arm of chromosome 11 [19–21]. In infective states, the release of bacterial endotoxin results in a ubiquitous expression of CALC 1 gene [21, 22]. It has been suggested that the presence of microbial infection-specific response elements within the CALC 1 gene promoter overrides tissue specific selective expression pattern leading to an overwhelming response to infective stimuli [20, 23]. As a result, systematic proteolytic cleavage and enzymatic degradation result in the release of PCT into the circulation. Containing a 116 amino acid structure and a relatively low molecular weight of 12.8 kDa, PCT levels have been shown to significantly correlate with ongoing infection. In addition, PCT release is mediated by pro-inflammatory cytokines such as tumor necrosis factor (TNF)-α, interleukin (IL)-1β and IL-6, suggesting that both infective and inflammatory stimuli can trigger PCT release [12, 20, 21]. In healthy individuals, post-translational processing of PCT is mostly restricted to neuroendocrine C-cells of the thyroid resulting in the production of biologically active mature calcitonin [17, 24].

In infective states, PCT mRNA upregulation is seen in multiple tissues throughout the body, especially in parenchymal cells of liver, lung, adipose tissue and peripheral mononuclear cells (monocytes and macrophages) but not leukocytes [22, 23]. Nijsten et al. demonstrated that *in vivo* induction of PCT in direct response to administration of TNF-α and IL-6 resulted in increased expression in liver. Moreover, PCT release occurred 12 hours earlier than other acute phase reactant proteins, such as CRP and serum amyloid A [8].

Utility of Procalcitonin in the Infected Heart Failure Patient

A majority of patients with acute heart failure present initially through the emergency department. Most of them present with a universal symptom of dyspnea, which can be difficult to distinguish from underlying non-cardiogenic dyspnea,

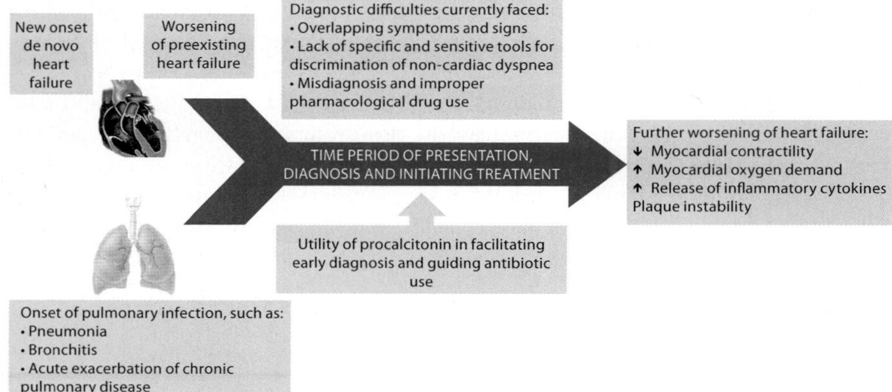

Fig. 1 Proposed outline of the current disparity in the diagnosis and treatment of heart failure patients with bacterial infection. Patients with new-onset and/or worsening preexisting heart failure often present with underlying pulmonary infection which leads to further worsening of heart failure leading to adverse outcomes and even death as outlined at the end of the arrow. The blue arrow represents the time line necessitating effective diagnostic and treatment strategies. On top of the arrow lies the current problem faced, hindering early diagnosis and treatment. Below the arrow lies the proposed solution by incorporating procalcitonin to guide diagnosis and antibiotic use

such as superimposed pneumonia, leading to missed diagnosis and poor outcomes in these patients [17, 25]. The differential diagnosis of dyspnea is challenging. Conventional tools, such as blood tests reporting elevated leukocytes and chest x-rays, have poor specificity, moreover, imaging studies are negative in 20 % of patients with pneumonia [25]. Figure 1 offers a schematic representation of the timeline requiring early action and appropriate treatment in order to prevent further worsening of heart failure and improve patient outcomes.

A recently published study by Maisel et al. demonstrated that PCT levels not only improved diagnostic accuracy in predicting pneumonia in patients with acute heart failure but also proved successful in discriminating non-cardiac dyspnea from cardiac dyspnea [9]. PCT levels added to the diagnostic value of chest x-ray, increasing the area under the curve (AUC) to 0.86 from 0.79 for diagnosing pneumonia. PCT was also found to be more accurate in predicting pneumonia than an elevated WBC count. Multivariate analysis revealed that PCT independently added to overall diagnostic accuracy in predicting pneumonia [9]. Patients with pneumonia were shown to have PCT levels ranging from 0.07–0.58 ng/ml, and in those patients without pneumonia, PCT levels were 0.05–0.12 ng/ml. In a Kaplan-Meier plot of PCT quintiles, patients in the first quintile, with PCT levels < 0.05 ng/ml, had a 92 % survival rate at 90-days, whereas those in the fifth quintile, with PCT levels > 0.21 ng/ml, had a lower, 80.5 % survival rate [9]. The study also highlighted the potential use of PCT levels in guiding antibiotic use in patients with acute heart failure. In patients with PCT levels > 0.21 ng/ml, lack of antibiotic use resulted in worse survival, whereas patients had an elevated risk of mortality when treated with antibiotics if PCT levels were <0.05 ng/ml [9]. In this study, antibiotic treatment was not randomized, highlighting the point that those who were more ill were possibly more likely to receive antibiotics, thus explaining the observed difference in risk of mortality [9]. Despite its limitations, the results shed valuable light into the potential utility of PCT in acute heart failure patients with concomitant infection. To our knowledge, this was the first study of its kind delving into the infected acute heart failure patient.

Natriuretic Peptide and Procalcitonin Guided Treatment

Natriuretic peptides, such as brain natriuretic peptide (BNP), are considered benchmark biomarkers in the diagnosis and prognosis of patients with heart failure. Secreted from the ventricles in direct response to myocyte stretch due to pressure and volume overload, BNP levels are highly sensitive (93 %) and specific (77 %) in diagnosing heart failure using a cut-off of 100 pg/ml. [26] Furthermore, BNP levels carry a high negative predictive value (98 %). Mueller et al. demonstrated that rapid measurement of BNP in heart failure patients with obstructive pulmonary disease was not only helpful in distinguishing between pulmonary dyspnea and cardiac dyspnea but was also able to demonstrate a relative decrease in length of hospital stay and lower cost of treatment [26].

As demonstrated by Maisel et al. BNP used in conjunction with PCT levels may further help to accurately identify patients with heart failure and provide sufficient data on superimposed pulmonary infection, thus enabling a judicious use of pharmacological therapy [9]. A BNP level >400 ng/ml and PCT >0.21 ng/ml accurately identified all patients with acute heart failure and pneumonia whereas those with BNP <100 ng/ml but PCT still >0.21 ng/ml identified those with only pneumonia and no acute heart failure. Similarly, other biomarkers, such as mid-regional proANP (atrial natriuretic peptide) or N-terminal (NT)-proBNP, used in conjunction with PCT may provide valuable diagnostic information in acute heart failure patients with underlying pulmonary disease [9].

Future of Procalcitonin in Heart Failure

With the aforementioned burden of acute heart failure and concomitant pulmonary infections, to reduce growing healthcare costs, effective treatment strategies are required to manage and treat such patients in a timely manner. This would not only improve overall patient outcomes by providing a more accurate diagnosis, but also lower the rates of misdiagnosis and overuse of drugs in the acute setting.

The planned future study, IMPACT (Improved Management of heart failure with ProcAlCiTonin), aims to determine whether PCT-guided antibiotic therapy improves survival in patients with acute heart failure.

Conclusion

The presence of concomitant infection in patients with acute heart failure is associated with high mortality rates, mainly because of misdiagnosis and ineffective treatment due to overlapping symptoms and signs in such patients. Putative markers, such as PCT, are an excellent surrogate of ongoing infection and inflammation providing valuable information regarding the presence of disease and allowing a better and more accurate diagnosis of underlying pulmonary infection in the setting of acute heart failure. PCT adds substantial value to clinical history, physical examination and laboratory testing and should be used in conjunction with additional tests in order to achieve maximum diagnostic accuracy. The prognostic utility of PCT in guiding antibiotic use in infected heart failure patients is promising and must be explored further. Although the area remains relatively new, evaluating PCT in combination with other biomarkers for diagnosis and guiding antibiotic use in heart failure patients is warranted.

References

1. McMurray JJV, Adamopoulos S, Anker SD et al (2012) ESC Guidelines for the diagnosis and treatment of acute and chronic heart failure 2012. The task force for the diagnosis and treatment of Acute and Chronic Heart Failure 2012 of the European Society of Cardiology Developed in collaboration with the Heart Failure Association (HFA) of the ESC. Eur J Heart Fail 33:1787–1847
2. Corrales-Medina VF, Musher DM, Wells GA et al (2012) Cardiac Complications in Patients With Community-Acquired Pneumonia-Incidence, Timing, Risk-Factors, and Association With Short-Term Mortality. Circulation 125:773–781
3. Thomsen RW, Kasatpibal N, Riis A et al (2008) The impact of pre-existing heart failure on pneumonia prognosis: Population based cohort study. J Gen Intern Med 23:1407–1413
4. Musher DM, Rueda AM, Kaka AS, Mapara SM (2007) The association between pneumococcal pneumonia and acute cardiac events. Clin Infect Dis 45:158–165
5. Assicot M, Gendrel D, Carsin H et al (1993) High serum procalcitonin concentrations in patients with sepsis and infection. Lancet 341:515–518
6. Meisner M, Heide A, Schmidt J (2006) Correlation of procalcitonin and C-reactive protein to inflammation, complications, and outcome during the intensive care unit course of multiple-trauma patients. Crit Care 10:R1
7. Christ-Crain M, Stolz D, Bingisser R et al (2006) Procalcitonin guidance of antibiotic therapy in community-acquired pneumonia: a randomized trial. Am J Respir Crit Care Med 174:84–93
8. Nijsten M, Olinga P, Hauw TT et al (2000) Procalcitonin behaves as a fast responding acute phase protein in vivo and in vitro. Crit Care Med 28:458–461
9. Maisel A, Neath SX, Landsberg J et al (2012) Use of procalcitonin for the diagnosis of pneumonia in patients presenting with a chief complaint of dyspnea: results from the BACH (Biomarkers in Acute Heart Failure) trial. Eur J Heart Fail 14:278–286
10. Roger VL, Go AS, Lloyd-Jones DM et al (2011) Heart disease and stroke statistics-2011 update A report from the American Heart Association. Circulation 123:e18–e209
11. Weintraub NL, Collins SP, Pang PS et al (2010) Acute heart failure syndromes: emergency department presentation, treatment, and disposition: Current approaches and future aims. Circulation 122:1975–1996

12. Follath F, Delgado JF, Yilmaz MB et al (2011) Clinical presentation, management and outcomes in the Acute Heart Failure Global Survey of Standard Treatment (ALARM-HF). Intensive Care Med 37:619–626
13. Arnaudis B, Lairez O, Escamilla R et al (2011) Impact of chronic obstructive pulmonary disease severity on symptoms and prognosis in patients with systolic heart failure. Clin Res Cardiol 101:717–726
14. Perry TW, Pugh MJV, Waterer GW et al (2011) Incidence of cardiovascular events following hospital admission for pneumonia. Am J Med 124:244–251
15. Corrales-Medina VF, Suh KN, Rose G et al (2011) Cardiac complications in patients with community-acquired pneumonia: A systematic review and meta-analysis of observational studies. PLoS Med 8:e1001048
16. Fillon S, Soulis K, Rajasekaran S et al (2006) Platelet-activating factor receptor and innate immunity: Uptake of gram-positive bacterial cell wall into host cells and cell-specific pathophysiology. J Immunol 177:6182–6191
17. Christ-Crain M, Muller B (2007) Biomarkers in respiratory tract infections: diagnostic guides to antibiotic prescription, prognostic markers and mediators. Eur Respir J 30:556–573
18. Muller F, Christ-Crain M, Bregenzer T et al (2010) Procalcitonin levels predict bacteremia in patients with community-acquired pneumonia. Chest 138:121–129
19. Russworm S, Wiederhold M, Oberhoffer M et al (1999) Molecular Aspects and Natural Source of Procalcitonin. Clin Chem Lab Med 37:789–797
20. Ittner L, Born W, Rau B et al (2002) Circulating procalcitonin and cleavage products in septicemia compared with medullary thyroid carcinoma. Eur J Endocrinol 147:727–731
21. Meisner M (2007) Pathobiochemistry and clinical use of procalcitonin. Clin Chim Acta 323:17–29
22. Carrol ED, Thomson APJ, Hart CA (2002) Procalcitonin as a marker of sepsis. Int J Antimicrob Agents 20:1–9
23. Linscheid P, Seboek D, Schaer DJ et al (2004) Expression and secretion of procalcitonin and calcitonin gene-related peptide by adherent monocytes and by macrophage-activated adipocytes. Crit Care Med 32:1715–1721
24. Jin M, Khan AI (2009) Procalcitonin: Uses in the clinical laboratory for the diagnosis of sepsis. Lab Med 41:173–177
25. Choudhary R, Gopal D, Kipper B et al (2012) Cardiorenal biomarkers in acute heart failure. J Geriatr Cardiol 9:E1–E13
26. Mueller C, Laule-Kilian K, Frana B et al (2006) Use of B-type natriuretic peptide in the management of acute dyspnea in patients with pulmonary disease. Am Heart J 151:471–477

Part III

Antimicrobials

Systematic Surveillance Cultures as an Aid for Selecting Appropriate Initial Antimicrobial Therapy

P. Depuydt, G. Claeys, and J. Decruyenaere

Introduction

Microbial surveillance aims to monitor the emergence and spread of selected pathogens. With the dramatic increases in acquired antibiotic resistance in many bacterial pathogens, jeopardizing effective treatment of severe infection, surveillance for multidrug resistant (MDR) strains has become a matter of priority [1–3]. Microbial surveillance can be applied on different scales and with different resolutions, depending on the goal it serves. To identify new infectious hazards and update guidelines for empirical treatment of major infections, signals and patterns must be deduced from the systematic registration of key diagnostic cultures, such as blood cultures. A similar form of surveillance based on diagnostic cultures is essential to guide hospital hygiene programs and develop antibiotic formularies in individual hospitals or healthcare facilities. On a much more detailed and specific level, surveillance refers to the search for presence of MDR bacteria in the individual patient; this information is mainly used to guide barrier precautions to limit horizontal spread of these strains. Patient-level surveillance not only encompasses cultures obtained upon clinical suspicion of infection, but is usually complemented by surveillance cultures, cultures taken from patients regardless of suspected infection aimed only at the detection of colonizers, especially of antibiotic resistant organisms. However, whether systematically obtaining surveillance cultures is a

P. Depuydt (✉)
Department of Intensive Care, Ghent University Hospital, De Pintelaan 185, 9000 Ghent, Belgium
E-mail: pieter.depuydt@ugent.be

G. Claeys
Laboratory of Medical Microbiology, Ghent University Hospital, De Pintelaan 185, 9000 Ghent, Belgium

J. Decruyenaere
Department of Intensive Care, Ghent University Hospital, De Pintelaan 185, 9000 Ghent, Belgium

J.-L. Vincent (Ed.), *Annual Update in Intensive Care and Emergency Medicine 2013*,
DOI 10.1007/978-3-642-35109-9_7,

necessary and cost-effective part of a hospital infection control program, and whether it should be used routinely or only in the context of an outbreak is still a matter of discussion [4, 5]. Nevertheless, surveillance cultures may find an application as a tool to support antibiotic decision making, which is the subject of the current review.

How to Use Microbiological Culture Results to Select Antibiotic Therapy for Nosocomial Infection?

In severe infections, such as pneumonia, bloodstream infection or infection complicated by septic shock, it has been repeatedly shown that providing appropriate antibiotic therapy as soon as infection is clinically apparent improves outcome [6–8]. Essentially, initial antibiotic therapy must be chosen empirically; the increasing prevalence of MDR strains in nosocomial infection, more pronounced in the intensive care unit (ICU) than elsewhere in the hospital, increases the risk for an inappropriate empirical choice. To lower this risk as much as possible, broad spectrum antibiotics, often in combination schemes, are recommended for ICU-acquired infection [9, 10]. However, undifferentiated and prolonged use of broad spectrum antibiotics is, itself, the strongest driver for antibiotic resistance, and additional strategies are required to limit the risk of running into uncontrolled escalation [11]. Microbiological identification and susceptibility testing of causative pathogens has a central role in the rationalization of antibiotic therapy, as it allows the antimicrobial spectrum of the treatment to be matched as closely as possible to the pathogen's susceptibility profile, reducing unnecessary selection pressure. Microbiological results become available for guiding antibiotic choices 2 or 3 days after the suspicion of infection and a period of empirical treatment [12]. This two-stage approach, called "de-escalation", is currently advocated as the preferred strategy to achieve a compromise between high odds for appropriate antimicrobial therapy and limiting ecologic selection pressure [13]. However, it has long been acknowledged that pathogenesis of nosocomial infection includes disruption of normal flora and overgrowth by nosocomial pathogens, which then become invasive [14, 15]. Analysis of the effects of selective oropharyngeal and gut decontamination from a recent multicenter study suggested that ICU-acquired bacteremia originated from prior intestinal and respiratory colonization in 45 % and 33 % of episodes, respectively [16]. This observation opens up a window of opportunity to try to detect these pathogens prior to infection by means of surveillance cultures. Anticipating the likely microbial etiology when infection becomes clinically apparent, surveillance cultures results could be used to modify empirical antibiotic therapy accordingly, with better odds for selection of an appropriate drug. In this approach, microbiological data are used to target antibiotic therapy upfront instead of at a second stage.

Can We Predict the Microbial Etiology of Nosocomial Infection by Knowledge of Colonizing Pathogens?

While the concept of colonization preceding nosocomial infection is scientifically robust, it must be detectable in the individual patient in order to be clinically useful for antibiotic guidance. This issue has been addressed in several studies, most of which considered the relationship between microbial etiology of ventilator-associated pneumonia (VAP) and prior cultures from the same patient (Table 1) [17–32]. In a pilot study, Delclaux et al. sampled the lower airways in 50 patients with acute respiratory distress syndrome (ARDS) every 2–3 days and found that 66 % of microbiologically confirmed VAP episodes were preceded by colonization with the same pathogen [17]. Hayon et al. retrospectively compared the microbial etiology of 125 episodes of VAP with 5,576 previously collected cultures, including 732 surveillance cultures [18]. In only 31 % of episodes could all causative pathogens identified in bronchoalveolar lavage (BAL) fluid be identified in previous cultures. Since surveillance cultures were not taken on a regular basis, the time interval between the diagnostic BAL and the last available culture was variable. When the authors only considered cultures from samples taken less than 72 h before clinical suspicion of VAP, concordance between BAL and prior cultures rose to 56 %. In a retrospective study focusing on cardiac surgery patients, only 1 out of 28 episodes of VAP had its pathogen predicted by surveillance cultures [19]. In this study, sampling frequency was low, resulting in a median interval between VAP onset and last culture of 4.5 days, and only 10 episodes of VAP were caused by a typically nosocomial pathogen. Sanders et al. compared 281 diagnostic cultures (endotracheal aspirate [ETA] or BAL) of patients with VAP with ETA obtained 1 to 3 days earlier; 37 % of diagnostic cultures showed pathogens that were not predicted by prior cultures [20]. A much higher concordance between surveillance cultures and diagnostic BAL cultures for suspected VAP was observed by Michel et al. [21]. Endotracheal surveillance cultures were prospectively sampled twice weekly in all intubated patients: 80 % of VAP episodes were caused by pathogens that were identified in earlier surveillance cultures. In a retrospective study in 112 patients with bacteremia of respiratory origin, 70 % of MDR pathogens were identical to those found in previous respiratory surveillance cultures, sampled thrice weekly [22]. Including surveillance cultures sampled from other sites (rectal [stool], oral and urinary) increased sensitivity to 88 %. This percentage was largely confirmed in a subsequent prospective study in the same center [23], in which 69 % and 96 %, respectively, of MDR pathogens causing VAP were found in respiratory or all (including oral, rectal, urinary) surveillance cultures. In a prospective series of 924 episodes of VAP, the presence of methicillin-resistant *Staphylococcus aureus* (MRSA) in nares, oropharynx or tracheal surveillance cultures taken on admission and then weekly had a sensitivity of 70 % for finding the same pathogen in diagnostic cultures [24]. Furthermore, a number of smaller studies have shown that endotracheal surveillance cultures, sampled once or twice weekly, had sensitivities of 60–80 % to predict VAP etiology [25–33].

Table 1 Prediction of microbial etiology of ventilator-associated pneumonia (VAP) by prior surveillance cultures

Author, year [ref]	Number of VAP episodes	Sampling frequency (type of sampling)	Surveillance culture pathogen predictive of VAP etiology (sensitivity)	Surveillance culture pathogen misleading for VAP etiology (1-specificity)
Delclaux, 1997 [17]	24	/2–3d (blind PSB)	66 %	8 %
Bertrand, 2001 [25]	184	/7d (N, R, ETA)	56 % (*Pseudomonas aeruginosa* only)	–
Hayon, 2002 [18]	125	/7d (N,R) (MRSA, acinetobacter only) only clinical ETA	33 %	26 %
Bouza, 2003 [19]	28	/7d (OP, R, ETA)	<5 %	–
Michel, 2006 [21]	41	/3d (ETA)	83 %	5 %
Depuydt, 2006 [22]	112	/2–3d (ETA) /7d (OP, R, U)	70 % (ETA) 88 % (all SC)	15 % (ETA) 46 % (all SC)
Berdal, 2007 [26]	112	/2–3d (OP, ETA)	95 %	27 %
Bagnulo, 2007 [27]	118	/3d (ETA)	60 %	11 %
Depuydt, 2008 [23]	199	/2–3d (ETA) /7d (OP, R, U)	69 % (ETA) 82 % (all SC)	4 % (ETA) 9 % (all SC)
Sanders, 2008 [20]	281	Not specified	57 %	37 %
Papadomichelakis, 2008 [29]	31	/3d (ETA) /7d (R)	82 %	21 %
Boots, 2008 [28]	58	/2–3d (blind mini-BAL)	84 %	50 %
Jung, 2009 [31]	90	/7d (ETA)	72 %	9 %
Joseph, 2010 [32]	36	/3d (ETA)	61 %	9 %
Chan, 2012 [24]	388	/7d (N, OP, ETA) (MRSA only)	70 % (MRSA only)	8 % (MRSA only)
Brusselaers, 2012 [30]	70	/2–3d (ETA)	83 %	4 %

BAL: bronchoalveolar lavage; ETA: endotracheal aspirate; MRSA: methicillin-resistant *Staphylococcus aureus*; N: nasal swab; OP: oropharyngeal culture; PSB: protected specimen brush; R: rectal swab; SC: surveillance culture; U: urinary culture

Few studies have investigated the use of surveillance cultures to predict microbial etiology of nosocomial infections other than VAP. In a retrospective analysis of 157 episodes of bloodstream infection caused by MDR Gram-negative bacteria, 75 % of pathogens causing bacteremia could be detected in a prior surveillance culture; here, surveillance cultures were routinely sampled from multiple sites and using a strict protocol, including thrice weekly obtained oral swabs, urine and ETA, complemented with rectal swabs on admission and then once weekly [34]. The sensitivity of perianal and rectal surveillance cultures to predict MDR Gram-negative bacteria found in clinical cultures was evaluated in a prospective trial: these surveillance cultures, obtained once weekly, had a sensitivity of 78 % [35].

In summary, these data validate the concept that nosocomial infection is preceded by colonization by the causative pathogen in the majority of cases, and that this process can be documented by surveillance cultures. This is best shown for the development of VAP and the prediction of its microbial cause by prior endotracheal aspirates. Although the sensitivities of endotracheal surveillance cultures for prediction of the microbial etiology of VAP were variable across studies, higher values were found in those studies that adopted a formal protocol for obtaining surveillance cultures and that applied a more intense and frequent sampling regimen. Based upon the available data, twice a week appears to be a minimal sampling frequency required to achieve a sensitivity of 60 % or higher.

Use of Surveillance Cultures to Modify Initial Antibiotic Choices

Surveillance cultures may be used to modify empirical antibiotic prescriptions in two ways. First, initial therapy may cover a larger spectrum or include distinct antibiotic classes compared to general empirical schemes, when surveillance cultures show colonization with MDR strains. An example of this process is the use of a fluoroquinolone or trimethoprim-sulfamethoxazole in the presence of *Stenotrophomonas maltophilia* or the use of colistin for multidrug-resistant *Pseudomonas aeruginosa*, as these drugs are rarely included in empirical schemes [23, 30]. As the specificity of surveillance cultures to predict the etiology of infection was above 80 % in most studies (Table 1), only a limited number of cases thus receive unnecessary antibiotic expansion. Second, when MDR are absent from surveillance cultures, this information may be used to prescribe an antibiotic with a smaller spectrum than empirically advocated, or to avoid combination therapy. Evidently, this relies on a high negative predictive value of surveillance cultures, as failing to provide appropriate therapy may have direct adverse consequences on patient outcome. As the sensitivity of surveillance cultures is limited to 60–70 % in most series, mere absence of MDR strains in surveillance cultures does not necessarily justify the choice of a small antimicrobial spectrum. Preferably, surveillance culture results should be incorporated in a decision tree together with other risk factors for MDR infection and considering local prevalence of MDR strains. Using such an approach, negative surveillance cultures can bring the likelihood of involvement of certain MDR pathogens below a threshold at which empirical coverage of these pathogens can be safely withheld [36]. As an example, Harris et al. found that negative nasal surveillance cultures for MRSA reduced the likelihood of finding

MRSA in a clinical culture to 2.4 % if clinical risk factors for MRSA infection were present, and to 1.6 % when absent [37].

There are no controlled trials directly comparing surveillance culture-guided initial antibiotic therapy with strictly empirical therapy. In three observational studies, however, the authors tried to estimate the benefit of surveillance culture-guided therapy by comparing actual initial antibiotic prescription based on regular surveillance cultures to a hypothetical empirical therapy as recommended by guidelines [21–23]. Among the guidelines used as comparators, Michel et al. considered the 1996 American Thoracic Society-Infectious Diseases Society of America (ATS-IDSA) guidelines [21] and Depuydt et al. the 2008 updated ATS-IDSA guidelines [23]. In all studies, actual antibiotic choices were appropriate in more infection episodes than would have been the case if antibiotics had been prescribed empirically; in addition, initial prescriptions were more limited in antimicrobial spectrum and used fewer antibiotic combinations than did empirical schemes. These calculations, however, provide only indirect proof of benefits of surveillance-guided antibiotic prescription over empirical prescription tailored upon local MDR prevalence. Proving superiority of one strategy over the other will require an interventional, preferably randomized trial. When randomizing individual patients to a surveillance or an empirical strategy, a problem of contamination may arise because blinding for the presence of MDR pathogens cannot be done for ethical reasons. This contamination occurs when surveillance cultures showing an MDR pathogen in a patient randomized to the surveillance group influences empirical prescription in a patient from the control group. To avoid this bias, both strategies could be compared by a study using a cluster randomization, or with a before-after design. Apart from comparing rates of appropriate initial antibiotic therapy, it remains to be assessed whether the reduction in antibiotic exposure achieved through a surveillance-guided strategy is more substantial than through a de-escalation strategy.

Can Surveillance Cultures Be Used to Improve Early Diagnosis of VAP?

Whereas early appropriate treatment of VAP is essential for a good outcome, early diagnosis of VAP, based upon a constellation of clinical symptoms and radiographic signs, is imprecise. Adding microbiological data increases accuracy [38] but demands extra time for processing and culturing of samples. Incorporating available microbiological data obtained by regular endotracheal surveillance cultures, Jung et al. increased the accuracy of the clinico-radiological diagnosis of VAP (quantified by the clinical pulmonary infection score) [39]. Recently, interest in endotracheal surveillance cultures has been further boosted by the observation that endotracheal colonization by pathogens may proceed to VAP through an intermediate stage of increasing respiratory symptoms, in parallel with increasing density of pathogens in the lower airways. For these conditions, and for suspected lower respiratory tract infections not meeting full criteria of VAP, the clinical syndrome of ventilator-associated tracheobronchitis (VAT) has been proposed [40]. The relevance of VAT has been confirmed by observational studies showing adverse outcome associated with VAT [41, 42], and by an interventional trial which randomized patients with VAT to receive antibiotic therapy or undergo watchful waiting [43]. The definition of VAT consisted of the combination of fever or leukocytosis, purulent sputum and presence of $> 10^6$ colony forming unit pathogens in ETA in the absence of infiltrates on chest X-ray; importantly, ETAs were sampled as surveillance cultures once weekly and cultured quantitatively. Patients who received antibiotic therapy developed VAP less frequently and had better outcome as reflected by an increase in ventilator-free days and a marginally significant reduction in ICU mortality. This suggests that regular endotracheal surveillance cultures may contribute to early diagnosis of VAT or incipient VAP and trigger early, targeted antibiotic therapy with beneficial effects on outcome. In addition, as this antibiotic therapy is guided by microbiological culture results, less excess selective pressure may be exerted as compared to a standard approach using a clinically based de-escalation therapy. However, larger studies are required before this strategy can be advocated for wider implementation, as it may carry a risk of overtreating patients. Pending more definitive evidence, serial endotracheal surveillance cultures with quantification of pathogens may help to identify the turning point between colonization and infection and the earliest opportunity to intervene with antibiotic therapy.

Microbiological Considerations of Surveillance Cultures

Sampling, processing and interpreting microbiological cultures is different when the goal is diagnosis or surveillance. Diagnostic cultures should identify the cause of infection, and thus preferably come from deep in the affected organ, with precautions to minimize contamination from non-sterile body sites or fluids. In contrast, surveillance cultures aim to detect the presence of potential pathogens, including those that colonize rather than infect the patient at the time of study. As pathogens may differ in their preferential niches for colonization, the body site chosen for surveillance cultures should depend upon the type of pathogen that is targeted. For MRSA, sampling multiple sites may be necessary to obtain good sensitivity; these should include perineal [44, 45] as well as throat swabs [46] and nasal swabs. To detect extended-spectrum beta-lactamase (ESBL)-producing enterobacteriaceae, stool samples may give the best yield, though firm evidence is lacking [35, 47]. On the other hand, as has been discussed above, ETA may be the preferred type of surveillance culture regardless of the pathogen if one aims to guide empirical therapy for VAP.

Because of the complex microflora of colonizing sites, such as the oropharynx or rectum, identification of potential pathogens can be challenging and resource consuming. Selective media with or without added antibiotics may increase the sensitivity for detecting certain high-risk pathogens, which may be otherwise obscured by growth of other bacteria. However, the microbiologist may choose not to report pathogens present in small quantities to the attending clinician to avoid overtreatment. As there is a strong link between increasing density of pathogen colonization with loss of microbial diversity on the one hand and development of infection on the other, semi-quantification, differentiating between low, moderate and heavy growth, or even quantitative cultures provide additional valuable information to the clinician for antibiotic decision-making. However, in other situations, even low numbers are important as they may rapidly increase in number under antibiotic pressure, or give rise to infection at later stages of the hospitalization. Close communication between the attending ICU physician and the microbiologist is essential for judicious guiding of antibiotic therapy by surveillance cultures.

Limitations and Costs of Surveillance Cultures

In all studies on surveillance cultures, a variable though substantial number of nosocomial infections were caused by pathogens that went undetected by surveillance cultures. From the limited data available, it appears that colonization of the respiratory tract is more dynamic than that of the gastrointestinal tract, in which colonization by MDR pathogens may be prolonged [48]. In some cases, the time window between the first appearance of a pathogen in the lower airways and subsequent infection may be too short to be captured by surveillance cultures, which may particularly be the case for highly virulent pathogens, such as *P. aeruginosa* [49]. In addition, biofilm present on endotracheal tubes may act as a source of respiratory infection by MDR pathogens and remain hidden to surveillance by oropharyngeal and endotracheal sampling. In a preliminary study, biofilm found in endotracheal tubes following extubation harbored pathogens that were not detected in surveillance cultures in 24 % of cases, including MRSA and ESBL-producing enterobacteriaceae [50].

The cost and workload associated with a surveillance culture-guided strategy is substantial and probably the most important barrier for promoting the use of systematic surveillance cultures on a wider scale. Apart from potential, but unproven, improvements in patient outcome, the expected benefits will be mostly indirect and result from antibiotic rationalization. A better benefit-cost ratio may be obtained in high risk settings, such as ICUs with high resistance rates [29] or prolonged patient care with high exposure to antibiotics, such as for example burn units [30]. The decision whether to adopt systematic surveillance as a tool for antibiotic decision-making will depend upon the prevalence and diversity of MDR strains in the local ecology, and the need to curtail empirical prescription of broad spectrum drugs. On the other hand, new developments in microbiological techniques, such as rapid identification with mass-spectrography or rapid susceptibility testing, and increasing automation in the microbiology laboratory will shorten the turn-around time of microbiological results, and thus likely reduce the benefit of systematic surveillance cultures. When embarking on a program of surveillance cultures to steer initial therapy, a critical cost-benefit analysis, measuring appropriateness and consumption of early antibiotic therapy before and after the intervention is advisable.

Conclusion

Systematic surveillance cultures show moderate to good prediction for microbial etiology of ICU-acquired infection. This is best documented for VAP, where 50–80 % of the causative pathogens could be identified in prior endotracheal surveillance cultures. Studies that adopted a formal surveillance culture protocol and used a regular sampling schedule of twice a week found higher sensitivities than studies without a protocol or with a lower sampling frequency. In several studies, surveillance cultures have been used to guide initial antibiotic therapy by targeting its spectrum at colonizing pathogens, resulting in high rates of appropriate therapy. Negative surveillance cultures may help to decrease the likelihood that infection is caused by MDR pathogens and thus contribute to antibiotic downsizing. In addition, endotracheal surveillance cultures may help to establish the early diagnosis of VAP. As yet, no interventional studies have compared surveillance culture-guided to empirical antibiotic prescription. Whether the use of systematic surveillance cultures to guide initial antibiotic therapy is cost-effective is currently unknown.

References

1. Bax R, Bywater R, Cornaglia G et al (2001) Surveillance of antimicrobial resistance: what, how and whither. Clin Microbiol Infect 7:316–325
2. Critchley IA, Karlowski JA (2004) Optimal use of antibiotic resistance surveillance systems. Clin Microbiol Infect 10:502–511
3. O'Brien T, Stelling J (2011) Integrated multilevel surveillance of the World's infecting microbes and their resistance to antimicrobial agents. Clin Microbiol Rev 2:281–285
4. Harris AD, McGregor JC, Furuno JP (2006) What infection control interventions should be undertaken to control multidrug-resistant Gram-negative bacteria? Clin Infect Dis 43:S57–S61
5. Aboelela SW, Saiman L, Stone P, Lowy F, Quiros D, Larson E (2006) Effectiveness of barrier precautions and surveillance cultures to control transmission of multidrug-resistant organisms: a systematic review of the literature. Am J Infect Control 34:484–494
6. Kollef MH, Sherman G, Ward S, Fraser VJ (1999) Inadequate antimicrobial treatment of infections: a risk factor for hospital mortality among critically ill patients. Chest 115:462–474
7. Iregui M, Ward S, Sherman G, Fraser VJ, Kollef MH (2002) Clinical importance of delays in the initiation of appropriate antibiotic treatment for ventilator-associated pneumonia. Chest 122:262–268
8. Kuti EL, Patel AA, Coleman CI (2008) Impact of inappropriate antibiotic therapy on mortality in patients with ventilator-associated pneumonia and blood stream infection: A meta-analysis. J Crit Care 23:91–100
9. Ferrer R, Artigas A, Suarez D et al (2009) Effectiveness of treatments for severe sepsis: a prospective, multicenter, observational study. Am J Respir Crit Care Med 180:861–866

10. Kumar A, Zarychanski R, Light B et al (2010) Early combination antibiotic therapy yields improved survival compared with monotherapy in septic shock: A propensity-matched analysis. Crit Care Med 38:1773–1785
11. Geissler A, Gerbeaux P, Granier I, Blanc P, Facon K, Durand-Gasselin J (2003) Rational use of antibiotics in the intensive care unit: impact on microbial resistance and costs. Intensive Care Med 29:49–54
12. Joffe AR, Muscedere J, Marshall JC, Su YH, Heyland DK (2008) The safety of targeted antibiotic therapy for ventilator-associated pneumonia: A multicenter observational study. J Crit Care 23:82–90
13. Niederman MS (2006) De-escalation therapy in ventilator-associated pneumonia. Curr Opin Crit Care 12:452–457
14. Atherton ST, White DJ (1978) Stomach as source of bacteria colonizing respiratory tract during artificial ventilation. Lancet 2:968–969
15. Le Frock JL, Ellis CA, Weinstein L (1979) The relation between aerobic fecal and oropharyngeal microflora in hospitalized patients. Am J Med Sci 277:701–706
16. Oostdijk E, de Smet A, Kesecioglu J, Bonten MJM (2011) The role of intestinal colonization with Gram-negative bacteria as a source for intensive care unit-acquired bacteremia. Crit Care Med 39:961–966
17. Delclaux C, Roupie E, Blot F, Brochard L, Lemaire F, Brun-Buisson C (1997) Lower respiratory tract colonization and infection during severe acute respiratory distress syndrome – Incidence and diagnosis. Am J Respir Crit Care Med 156:1092–1098
18. Hayon J, Figliolini C, Combes A et al (2002) Role of serial routine microbiologic culture results in the initial management of ventilator-associated pneumonia. Am J Respir Crit Care Med 165:41–46
19. Bouza E, Perez A, Munoz P et al (2003) Ventilator-associated pneumonia after heart surgery: a prospective analysis and the value of surveillance. Crit Care Med 31:1964–1970
20. Sanders K, Adhikari N, Friedrich J, Day A, Jiang X, Heyland D (2008) Previous cultures are not clinically useful for guiding empiric antibiotics in suspected ventilator-associated pneumonia: secondary analysis from a randomized trial. J Crit Care 23:58–63
21. Michel F, Franceschini B, Berger P et al (2005) Early antibiotic treatment for BAL-confirmed ventilator-associated pneumonia: a role for routine endotracheal aspirate cultures. Chest 127:589–597
22. Depuydt P, Blot S, Benoit D et al (2006) Antimicrobial resistance in nosocomial bloodstream infection associated with pneumonia and the value of systematic surveillance cultures in an adult intensive care unit. Crit Care Med 34:653–659
23. Depuydt P, Benoit D, Vogelaers D et al (2008) Systematic surveillance cultures as a tool to predict involvement of multidrug antibiotic resistant bacteria in ventilator-associated pneumonia. Intensive Care Med 34:675–682
24. Chan J, Dellit T, Choudhuri J et al (2012) Active surveillance cultures of methicillin-resistant Staphylococcus aureus as a tool to predict methicillin-resistant S. aureus ventilator-associated pneumonia. Crit Care Med 40:1437–1442
25. Bertrand X, Thouverez M, Talon D et al (2001) Endemicity, molecular diversity and colonization routes of Pseudomonas aeruginosa in intensive care units. Intensive Care Med 27:1263–1268
26. Berdal JE, Bjornholt J, Blomfeldt A, Smith-Erichsen N, Bukholm G (2007) Patterns and dynamics of airway colonisation in mechanically-ventilated patients. Clin Microbiol Infect 13:476–480
27. Bagnulo H, Godino M, Galiana A, Bertulo M, Pedreira W (2007) Are routine endotracheal aspirates predictive of the etiology of ventilator-associated pneumonia? Crit Care 11:P87
28. Boots RJ, Phillips GE, George N, Faogali JL (2008) Surveillance culture utility and safety using low-volume blind bronchoalveolar lavage in the diagnosis of ventilator-associated pneumonia. Respirology 13:87–96
29. Papadomichelakis E, Kontopidou F, Antoniadou A et al (2007) Screening for resistant gram-negative micro-organisms to guide empiric therapy of subsequent infection. Intensive Care Med 34:2169–2175

30. Brusselaers N, Logie D, Vogelaers D, Monstrey S, Blot S (2012) Burns, inhalation injury and ventilator-associated pneumonia: Value of routine surveillance cultures. Burns 38:364–370
31. Jung B, Sebbane M, Chanques G et al (2009) Previous endotracheal aspirate allows guiding the initial treatment of ventilator-associated pneumonia. Intensive Care Med 35:101–107
32. Joseph N, Sistla S, Dutta T, Badhe AS, Parija SC (2010) Ventilator-associated pneumonia: role of colonizers and value of routine endotracheal aspirate cultures. Int J Infect Dis 14:E723–E729
33. Lampati L, Maggioni E, Langer M et al (2009) Can routine surveillance samples from tracheal aspirate predict bacterial flora in cases of ventilator-associated pneumonia? Minerva Anestesiol 75:555–562
34. Blot S, Depuydt P, Vogelaers D et al (2005) Colonization status and appropriate antibiotic therapy for nosocomial bacteremia caused by antibiotic-resistant gram-negative bacteria in an intensive care unit. Infect Control Hosp Epidem 26:575–579
35. Snyder G, D'Agata G (2011) Diagnostic accuracy of surveillance cultures to detect gastrointestinal colonization with multidrug-resistant gram-negative bacteria. Am J Infect Control 40:474–476
36. Baba H, Nimmo R, Allworth A et al (2011) The role of surveillance cultures in the prediction of susceptibility patterns of Gram-negative bacilli in the intensive care unit. Eur J Clin Microbiol Infect Dis 30:739–744
37. Harris A, Furuno J, Roghmann M et al (2010) Targeted surveillance of Methicillin-Resistant *Staphylococcus aureus* and its potential use to guide empiric antibiotic therapy. Antimicrob Ag Chemother 54:3143–3148
38. Klompas M (2007) Does this patient have ventilator-associated pneumonia? JAMA 297:1583–1593
39. Jung B, Embriaco N, Roux F et al (2010) Microbiological data, but not procalcitonin improve the accuracy of the clinical pulmonary Infection score. Intensive Care Med 36:790–798
40. Craven D, Chroneou A, Zias N, Hjalmarson KI (2009) Ventilator-associated tracheobronchitis: the impact of targeted antibiotic therapy on patient outcomes. Chest 135:521–528
41. Nseir S, Di Pompeo C, Pronnier P et al (2002) Nosocomial tracheobronchitis in mechanically ventilated patients: incidence. aetiology and outcome. Eur Respir J 20:1483–1489
42. Dallas J, Skrupky L, Abebe N, Boyle WA, Kollef MH (2011) Ventilator-associated tracheobronchitis in a mixed surgical and medical ICU population. Chest 139:513–518
43. Nseir S, Favory R, Jozefowicz E et al (2008) Antimicrobial treatment for ventilator-associated tracheobronchitis: a randomized, controlled, multicenter study. Crit Care 12:R62
44. Matheson A, Christie P, Stari T et al (2012) Nasal swab screening for Methicillin-Resistant Staphylococcus aureus-how well does it perform? A Cross-sectional study. Infect Control Hosp Epidem 33:803–808
45. Lautenbach E, Nachamkin I, Hu BF et al (2009) Surveillance cultures for detection of methicillin-resistant Staphylococcus aureus: diagnostic yield of anatomic sites and comparison of provider- and patient-collected samples. Infection Control Hosp Epidem 30:380–382
46. Batra R, Eziefula C, Wyncoll D, Edgeworth J (2008) Throat and rectal swabs may have an important role in MRSA screening of critically ill patients. Intensive Care Med 34:1703–1706
47. Reddy P, Malczynski M, Obias A et al (2007) Screening for extended-spectrum beta-lactamase producing Enterobacteriaceae among high-risk patients and rates of subsequent bacteremia. Clin Infect Dis 45:846–852
48. O'Fallon E, Gautam S, D'Agata E (2009) Colonization with multidrug-resistant Gram-negative Bacteria: Prolonged duration and frequent cocolonization. Clin Infect Dis 48:1375–1381
49. Yang K, Zhuo H, Guglielmo J, Wiener-Kronisch J (2009) Multidrug-resistant Pseudomonas aeruginosa ventilator-associated pneumonia: the role of endotracheal aspirate surveillance cultures. Ann Pharmacother 43:28–35
50. De Bus L, Boelens J, Claeys G et al (2011) Endotracheal tube biofilm: a hidden reservoir for multidrug-resistant pathogens? Intensive Care Med 37:S199 (abst)

Colistin: An Old Antibiotic as a Last, Invaluable Resort

R. Imberti, M. Regazzi, and G. A. Iotti

Introduction

The last few years have been characterized by the emergence of certain Gram-negative bacteria, especially *Acinetobacter baumannii, Pseudomonas aeruginosa* and *Klebsiella pneumoniae*, which are resistant to almost all currently available antibiotics, except colistin. This fact has prompted a resurgence of interest in colistin, an 'old' antibiotic introduced in 1959 with notable *in vitro* activity against *P. aeruginosa* [1], which was abandoned in the 1970s after the introduction of the aminoglycosides. Colistin is mainly employed in critically ill patients and in individuals with cystic fibrosis. This chapter focuses predominantly on the use of colistin in critically ill patients.

Colistin is a complex antibiotic from several aspects, including taxonomy, pharmaceutical forms, product content in vials (reported as international units [IU] or mg), and dose regimen, thus creating some confusion among clinicians. This confusion is responsible, at least in part, for potentially harmful mistakes and toxicity of colistin.

Colistin (also known as polymyxin E) consists of a complex mixture of polymyxins, the two main ones being colistin A (polymyxin E_1) and colistin B (polymyxin E_2) [2]. Colistin is a bactericidal antibiotic which has concentration-dependent killing and a modest post-antibiotic effect [3]. It binds to the lipopolysaccharides of the outer membrane of Gram-negative bacteria and induces cell death by displac-

R. Imberti (✉)
Direzione Scientifica, Fondazione IRCCS Policlinico S. Matteo, Pavia, Italy
E-mail: r.imberti@smatteo.pv.it

M. Regazzi
Laboratory of Clinical Pharmacokinetics, Fondazione IRCCS Policlinico S. Matteo, Pavia, Italy

G. A. Iotti
Department of Anesthesiology and Critical Care Medicine, Fondazione IRCCS Policlinico S. Matteo, Pavia, Italy

J.-L. Vincent (Ed.), *Annual Update in Intensive Care and Emergency Medicine 2013*,
DOI 10.1007/978-3-642-35109-9_8, © Springer-Verlag Berlin Heidelberg 2013

ing calcium and magnesium. Three pharmaceutical forms of colistin exist: Colistin methanesulfonate (CMS, also known as colistimethate and colistin sulphomethate), colistin sulfate, and colistin base. In the past the terms were used interchangeably in the literature, and even in recent articles it is sometimes not known whether the dose stated refers to CMS or colistin base. Colistin is generally administered systemically (parenterally) as CMS. CMS, which is inactive, is converted to colistin (the active form with antimicrobial activity) both *in vitro* and *in vivo* by hydrolysis of methane sulphonate radicals [4, 5]. CMS is a polyanion, whereas colistin is a polycation. In many countries, CMS is approved for intramuscular (i.m.) use only, and intravenous (i.v.), nebulized and intraventricular use of the drug is off-label.

Pharmacokinetics and Pharmacodynamics

In the past, colistin concentrations in biological fluids and tissues were evaluated by microbiological assays which did not discriminate between CMS and colistin. Moreover, during the incubation period of the microbiological assay, CMS is converted to colistin, resulting in measured concentrations of CMS and colistin that do not reliably reflect their concentration in fluids and tissues. High performance liquid chromatography and mass spectrometry based methods, which enable CMS and colistin to be measured separately and quantified accurately, were introduced only a few years ago [6–8]. In the last decade, the pharmacokinetics of colistin (the active form) and CMS have been studied in animals and critically ill patients using these analytical methods (for a comprehensive review, see Bergen et al. [9]).

Studies in animals have shown that colistin has a very extensive tubular reabsorption and its clearance is mainly via non-renal pathways, whereas CMS undergoes tubular secretion and renal clearance (Fig. 1, [5]). The very high concentration of colistin in urine after systemic CMS administration is very likely due to conversion of CMS within the urinary tract [9].

A few studies performed in critically ill patients with multi-drug resistant (MDR) Gram-negative infections have evaluated the pharmacokinetics of colistin after i.v.

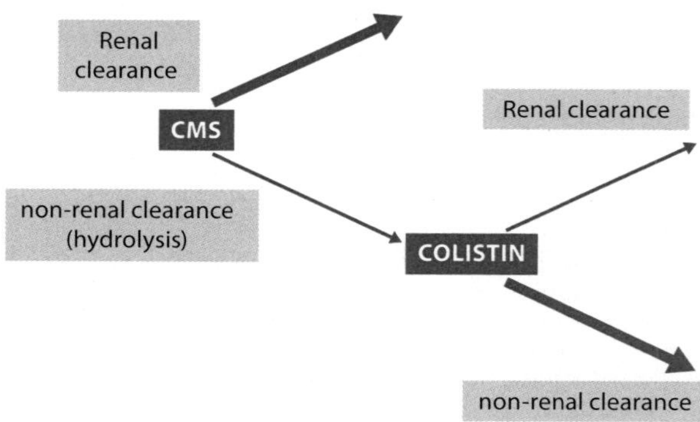

Fig. 1 Schematic representation of the disposition of colistin methanesulfonate (CMS) and the colistin generated from it in the body following i.v. administration of CMS. From [5] with permission

administration of CMS. Imberti et al. [10] showed that with 2 million IU (174 mg) of i.v. CMS every 8 h, the maximum steady state plasma concentration (Cmax,ss) of colistin was 2.21 ± 1.08 mcg/ml (mean ± SD) and the apparent terminal half-life was 5.9 ± 2.6 h (Fig. 2, [10]). Given that the minimum inhibitory concentration (MIC) of colistin is 2 mcg/ml, the Cmax,ss/MIC ratio and AUC_{0-24}/MIC ratio were 1.1 ± 0.5 and 17.3 ± 9.3, respectively. In another study [11], in which patients were treated with 2.8 million IU (approx. 244 mg) of CMS, the Cmax,ss of colistin was 2.93 ± 1.24 mcg/ml and the apparent half-life 7.4 ± 1.7 h. In both studies, two to three hours after CMS administration, plasma colistin concentrations were below the MIC breakpoint of 2 mcg/ml in most patients, indicating that the concentrations of colistin were suboptimal. Plachouras et al. [12], studied CMS and colistin in a population pharmacokinetic analysis. The dose of CMS was 3 million IU (approx. 240 mg) every 8 h. The predicted Cmax values in plasma were 0.60 mcg/ml and 2.3 mcg/ml for the first dose and at steady state, respectively, indicating that patients were exposed to very low plasma colistin concentrations for 2–3 days before reaching steady state, suggesting the need for a loading dose. Also in this study, a large proportion of patients had plasma concentrations below the MIC breakpoint of 2 mcg/ml. Garonzik et al. [13] investigated the pharmacokinetics of CMS and colistin in 105 critically ill patients with a large range of renal function (creatinine clearance 3–169 ml/min/1.72 m^2); some patients were on renal replacement therapy (RRT). These authors showed that with decreasing renal function a larger fraction of CMS was converted to colistin, whereas the clearance of formed colistin decreased. On the basis of their findings, Garonzik et al. [13] developed equations suggesting the loading dose and maintenance dose necessary for various categories of patients (not on RRT, receiving intermittent or continuous RRT) to achieve a given colistin average concentration at steady state (Css,avg) during the dosing interval.

The pharmacodynamic parameters best predicting the efficacy of colistin have not yet been established in humans. However, *in vitro* and *in vivo* animal studies have suggested that the AUC/MIC ratio of total and unbound colistin is the index that best predicts antibacterial activity against *P. aeruginosa* [14, 15].

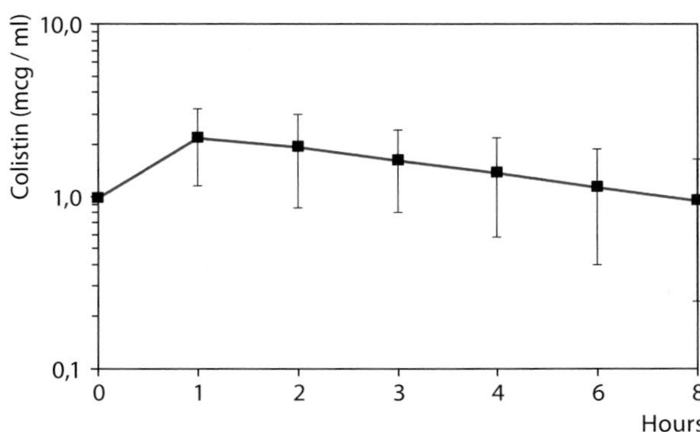

Fig. 2 Plasma concentration of colistin at steady-state following i.v. administration of CMS (2 million IU (174 mg)). From [10] with permission

Lung Tissue Concentration of Colistin After Intravenous Administration of Colistin Methanesulfonate

The efficacy of an antibiotic therapy depends on the susceptibility of the infecting bacteria and the concentration of antibiotic achieved in the target organs. There is concern that after i.v. CMS administration, colistin penetrates poorly into the lungs. Some studies from the 1970s showed that after a single i.v. injection, both free and bound forms of colistin were present in lung tissue, with the concentration of the bound form being considerably higher than that of the free form [16]. Kunin and Bugg [17] showed that after multiple i.v. administration in rabbits, CMS accumulated in lungs in the bound form, and, more recently [18], colistin was detected in mouse lung homogenates. Colistin is positively charged and could, therefore, bind to negatively charged elements of the alveolar basement membrane, making lung tissue binding of colistin plausible. However, the validity of these findings has been questioned by some authors mainly based on the fact that microbiological assays were used in the studies.

Lu et al. [19] reported that colistin was undetectable in lung tissue after i.v. infusion of CMS. We recently showed that colistin was undetectable in bronchoalveolar lavage (BAL) after i.v. administration of CMS (174 mg/8 h) [10]. Although our finding is consistent with that of Lu et al. [19], we drew different conclusions, believing that the correct interpretation of the results lies in the tissue binding of colistin.

Although the issue of lung tissue binding by colistin has very important clinical implications, conclusive information on this issue is still lacking. Several studies in humans showing that i.v. CMS is effective in the treatment of pneumonia caused by MDR Gram-negative bacteria indicate that colistin does indeed penetrate into lung tissue.

Clinical Studies in Ventilator-associated Pneumonia (VAP) and Pneumonia

Although pharmacokinetic studies suggest that the current dosage regimens of i.v. CMS are suboptimal, and despite the possible inadequate diffusion of colistin into the lungs, clinical studies have shown that CMS is effective in the treatment of serious infections caused by MDR Gram-negative bacteria [20–23]. These studies (prospective and retrospective), which compared the effects of i.v. CMS given for the treatment of colistin-only susceptible Gram-negative bacteria with the effects of other antimicrobial agents active on analogous strains, showed that there were no differences in mortality or clinical cure rates. According to a preliminary report of a recent study, administration of high-dose CMS in 28 episodes of blood stream infection and VAP resulted in clinical cure in 82.1 % of cases [23].

Administration of i.v. CMS has also been found to be effective and safe in children and neonates [24–26].

Nebulized Colistin

In order to be active, nebulized CMS must be converted into colistin within the lungs before leaving the respiratory tract by systemic absorption, expectoration or swallowing [27]. A fraction of the CMS dose is absorbed and is then partially converted into colistin within the systemic circulation. Another fraction of the CMS dose is converted into colistin within the lungs and is then partially absorbed within the systemic circulation [27].

Animal studies have shown that direct administration of colistin to the lungs (intranasally or nebulized) was superior to i.v. administration in the treatment of experimental pneumonia caused by *P. aeruginosa* [18, 19]. In humans, the efficacy and safety of nebulized colistin (given as CMS) for the treatment of VAP or nosocomial pneumonia have been investigated in a few, mainly uncontrolled, small clinical trials in adults, children and neonates [28–31]. One retrospective study [29] compared i.v. CMS plus nebulized CMS to i.v. CMS alone in 121 critically ill patients with VAP. Clinical cure was obtained in 79.5 % of patients receiving i.v. CMS plus nebulized CMS and in 60.5 % in patients who received i.v. CMS only ($p = 0.025$). A randomized controlled study performed in 100 adults with VAP caused by Gram-negative bacteria [30] compared the efficacy of systemic antibiotics (mainly carbapenems and CMS) plus nebulized CMS with that of systemic antibiotics without nebulized CMS. Although the microbiological cure rate was significantly higher in patients who received nebulized CMS as adjunctive therapy, a beneficial effect on the clinical cure rate was not demonstrated [30].

The dose of nebulized CMS reported in the literature ranges between 1.5 and 6 million IU/day (approximately 130–520 mg/day) in adults, but the optimal dose is not known. Athanassa et al. [32] reported that the administration of nebulized CMS at a dose of 80 mg/8 h (1 million IU/8 h) to critically ill patients with ventilator-associated tracheobronchitis resulted in a median concentration of colistin in epithelial lining fluid that was above the MIC of all isolated pathogens at 1 and 4 hours post-nebulization, but which declined at 8 hours. The ratio of serum colistin concentration to epithelial lining fluid colistin concentration was 0.17 ($IQ_{25–75}$ 0.13–0.26), with a median serum concentration of 1.2 mcg/ml at 1 hour. These findings suggest that it is probably better to administer higher doses of nebulized CMS and that after treatment with nebulized CMS the serum concentrations of colistin are not negligible. This consideration should be kept in mind when i.v. and nebulized CMS are administered in combination.

There are no relevant clinical studies comparing nebulized CMS with systemic CMS. Nebulized CMS results in lung concentrations which are unattainable by i.v. administration. Monotherapy with nebulized CSM is probably devoid of serious systemic adverse events, but drug lung deposition decreases with loss of aeration and colistin may not reach lung segments with pneumonia [19], a problem shared by all types of nebulized antibiotics. Monotherapy with nebulized CMS is inappropriate when pneumonia is associated with bacteremia.

Combination Therapy

In vitro studies have shown that colistin acts synergistically with other antibiotics (for a comprehensive review see Petrosillo et al. [33]). The antibiotics most frequently combined with colistin are rifampicin and carbapenems. *In vitro* synergy with rifampicin against *P. aeruginosa* and *A. baumannii* was demonstrated in all the studies performed [34–39]. In a mouse model of pneumonia caused by MDR *P. aeruginosa*, maximum synergism was obtained with colistin plus rifampicin [18].

A few clinical studies have investigated colistin (given as CMS) combination therapy. Some of these were non-comparative studies [33]. The comparative studies performed in critically ill patients are scant and present great variability with regards to populations of patients studied, sites of infection, pathogens and definitions of outcome; furthermore, the number of patients included was often low [33]. A recent study performed in 258 patients (86 % of whom were hospitalized in an ICU) infected by *A. baumannii, P. aeruginosa* and *K. pneumoniae* showed that colistin combination therapy was not superior to colistin alone [40]. In contrast, another study which examined 125 patients with bloodstream infections caused by *K. pneumoniae* carbapenemase (KPC)-producing *K. pneumoniae* found that post-antibiogram therapy with a combination of colistin, tigecycline, and meropenem was associated with lower mortality [41]. However, both of these studies have the important limitation of being retrospective. Only large randomized, controlled trials comparing the efficacy and safety of colistin monotherapy vs. colistin combination therapy would be able to resolve the existing uncertainty.

Since i.v. CMS monotherapy results in suboptimal plasma concentrations of colistin even at high doses (see the pharmacokinetics/pharmacodynamics section) and may lead to the emergence of resistance, it is of paramount importance to investigate combination therapy (e. g., i.v. CMS plus another systemic antibiotic, or CMS administered via two different routes).

Minimum Inhibitory Concentrations and Resistance

Different susceptibility breakpoints have been introduced by various organizations. These breakpoints have been obtained with colistin sulfate, the active drug, whereas CMS should not be used for susceptibility testing. According to the European Committee on Antimicrobial Susceptibility Testing (EUCAST) and the US Clinical and Laboratory Standards Institution (CLSI) the susceptibility breakpoint for *A. baumannii* and *K. pneumoniae* is 2 mcg/ml, whereas that for *P. aeruginosa* is 2 mcg/ml according to the CLSI and 4 mcg/ml according to the EUCAST. However, strains of *P. aeruginosa* and *A. baumannii* with a MIC $\leq$ 1 mcg/ml have been reported in several published clinical studies.

Resistance to colistin is not very common and in the period from 2006 to 2009 generally remained stable among the clinical isolates examined [9]. This might be due, in part, to the fact that colistin-resistant bacteria present downregulation of several proteins (outer membrane proteins, chaperones, protein biosynthesis factors, metabolic enzymes), which reduce the microbes' biological fitness and induce phenotype instability [42]. Resistance to colistin is likely due to the increasing use of CMS and colistin heteroresistance to colistin (defined as the presence of colistin-resistant subpopulations in an isolate that is susceptible based upon MIC). Combination therapy might reduce the risk of the emergence of resistance to colistin.

Toxicity

Colistin can be nephrotoxic and neurotoxic. Neurotoxicity has been described after systemic or intraventricular/intrathecal administration of colistin [43]. Manifestations include seizures, aseptic meningitis, hypotonia, neuromuscular blockade with respiratory paralysis, and cauda equina. Neurotoxicity is rare and does not appear to be a major issue in critically ill patients, but this aspect might be underestimated in sedated and mechanically ventilated patients.

Nephrotoxicity is the most common and threatening adverse reaction during CMS/colistin treatment. The frequency of some degree of nephrotoxicity reported in the literature is extremely variable, ranging between 0 and 53 % [43]. The dose of CMS, different definitions of nephrotoxicity, inclusion/exclusion of patients with pre-colistin nephrotoxicity, underlying pathology, and concomitant administration of other potentially nephrotoxic drugs may account for this marked variability. The risk of nephrotoxicity is correlated to the total CMS dose and the duration of CMS therapy [44]. Dose adjustment according to renal function, daily serum creatinine monitoring and careful management of volemia can help to reduce the risk of nephrotoxicity.

Independent of its frequency, nephrotoxicity is a real problem of CMS/colistin therapy, but should not deter the use of this antibiotic, when appropriate. Since no studies have demonstrated that higher doses produce better clinical outcomes, it is our opinion that attempts to reach very high plasma colistin concentrations should not be pursued.

Dose Regimen for Intravenous CMS

When calculating doses, CMS should not be confused with colistin base (1 mg colistin base = 2.4 mg of CMS). The vial concentration of CMS is often reported in IU and not in mg, thus adding a further source of potential confusion. One million

IU of CMS corresponds to approximately 80 mg CMS, but this value, if not reported in the summary of product characteristics, must be verified with the manufacturer. Solutions of CMS must be prepared just before administration.

The optimal dosage regimen is not known. The daily doses reported in the literature vary considerably. The daily dose used in the past was generally lower than that used nowadays, and the daily dose suggested in some summary of product characteristics is still low. Given the lack of comparative clinical studies, we cannot recommend a dose regimen for CMS, but a possible one could be 3–3.5 mg/kg/8 h. In obese patients it is reasonable to refer to the ideal body weight rather than the real one [45]. A loading dose might be beneficial in order to reduce the time taken to reach the steady state concentration [12, 23].

Although colistin is mainly cleared by non-renal mechanisms, since CMS accumulates in patients with renal impairment, its dose must be adjusted in such patients. Garonzik et al. [13] describe equations which can be applied to patients with renal impairment and those on intermittent or continuous RRT.

Central Nervous System Infections

MDR Gram-negative bacteria can cause infections of the central nervous system (CNS; meningitis, ventriculitis, abscesses), which generally occur when patients stay in hospital and are submitted to neurosurgical or otorhinological procedures or have head trauma. Such infections are a therapeutic challenge, and treatment relies on colistin (administered as CMS). CSM and colistin hardly cross the blood-cerebrospinal fluid (CSF) or blood-brain barrier in animals or humans, even if the meninges are inflamed [46, 47], and CMS must, therefore, be administered into the cerebral ventricles or via the intrathecal route. Guidelines published by the Infectious Diseases Society of America (IDSA) suggest that the intraventricular dosage of colistin (presumably CMS) should be 10 mg [48], but the dosages of intraventricular/intrathecal CMS reported in the literature range between 1.6–40 mg, as a single dose or in divided doses [49]. A recent study [50] in which the pharmacokinetics of colistin were evaluated after intraventricular administration of CMS showed that when CMS was administered at doses of $\geq$ 5.2 mg/day, the measured CSF concentrations of colistin were continuously greater than the MIC of 2 mcg/ml, and measured values of C_{trough} (the minimum CSF colistin concentration) ranged between 2.0 and 9.7 mcg/ml (Fig. 3 [50]), which are concentrations that could never be achieved by systemic administration. In contrast, concentrations of colistin were frequently $<$ 2 mcg/ml when the dose of CMS administered was 2.6 mg/day. Although the terminal half-life of drugs is generally longer in the CSF than in plasma, the terminal half-life of colistin in the CSF was comparable to that reported in plasma. Critical factors which were identified or presumed to influence the concentration of colistin in CSF were the rate of transformation of CMS to colistin, the elimination of colistin and CMS through the external efflux

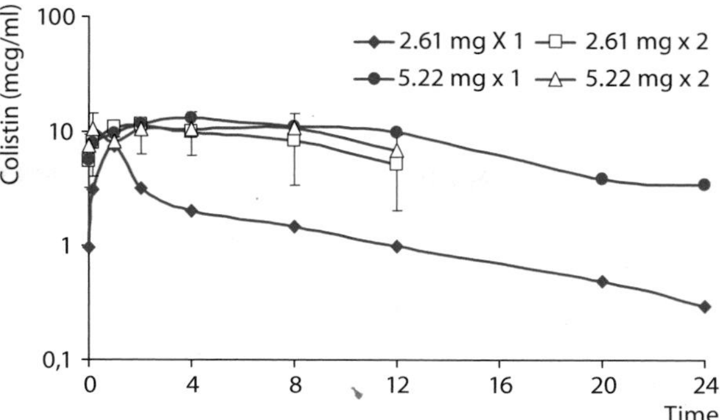

Fig. 3 Concentration-time profiles of colistin at steady-state after intraventricular administration of colistin methanesulfonate (CMS) at different dosage regimens. From [50] with permission

of CSF, the variable amount of spontaneously drained CSF, and the non-uniform time of closure of the external ventricular drainage. For the reasons reported above, Imberti et al. [50] concluded that the daily dose of 10 mg suggested by the IDSA was more prudent.

Clinical studies have shown that intraventricular administration of CMS is effective and safe in the treatment of CNS infections caused by MDR Gram-negative bacteria susceptible only to colistin [49, 50].

Conclusion

Given the current development pipeline, it can be expected that no new antibiotics active against MDR-resistant Gram-negative bacteria will become available in the next few years. Clinicians must be familiar with the use of CMS, to maximize efficacy, minimize the development of resistance and avoid toxicity. In critically ill, adult patients, the i.v. administration of the usual doses of CSM results in apparently suboptimal concentrations in plasma and BAL fluid. Higher doses of CMS given in an attempt to maximize the plasma colistin concentrations may be beneficial, but the efficacy of these regimens has not been investigated and this strategy should not be pursued to the point of causing renal toxicity. There are insufficient clinical data to support the use of nebulized CMS as monotherapy for the treatment of pneumonia. Aerosol therapy as an adjunct to systemic treatment appears promising. Combination therapy (e. g., i.v. CMS plus another antibiotic) could exploit the synergistic bactericidal effects of the two antimicrobial agents, allowing administration of the usual doses of CMS and reducing the risk of renal toxicity, but also in this field, data from sound comparative clinical trials are lacking. For CNS infections, a CMS daily dose of 10 mg administered intraventricularly seems appropriate.

References

1. Duncan IB (1974) Susceptibility of 1,500 isolates of Pseudomonas aeruginosa to gentamicin, carbenicillin, colistin, and polymixin B. Antimicrob Agents Chemother 5:9–15
2. Li J, Nation RL, Milne RW, Turnidge J, Coulthard K (2005) Evaluation of colistin as an agent against multi-resistant Gram-negative bacteria. Int J Antimicrob Agents 25:11–25
3. Li J, Turnidge J, Milne R, Nation RL, Coulthard K (2001) In vitro pharmacodynamic properties of colistin and colistin methanesulphonate against Pseudomonas aeruginosa isolates from patients with cystic fibrosis. Antimicrob Agents Chemother 45:781–785
4. Bergen PJ, Li J, Rayner CR, Nation RL (2006) Colistin methanesulphonate is an inactive prodrug of colistin against Pseudomonas aeruginosa. Antimicrob Agents Chemother 50:1953–1958
5. Li J, Nation RL, Turnidge JD et al (2006) Colistin: the re-emerging antibiotic for multidrug-resistant Gram-negative bacterial infections. Lancet Infect Dis 6:589–601
6. Li J, Milne RW, Nation RL, Turnidge J, Coulthard K, Johnson DW (2001) A simple method for the assay of colistin in human plasma, using pre-column derivatization with 9-fluorenylmethyl chloroformate in solid-phase extraction cartridges and reversed-phase high-performance liquid chromatography. J Chromatogr B Biomed Sci Appl 761:167–175
7. Li J, Milne RW, Nation RL, Turnidge J, Coulthard K, Valentine J (2002) Simple method for assaying colistin methanesulphonate in plasma and urine using high-performance liquid chromatography. Antimicrob Agents Chemother 46:3304–3307
8. Gobin P, Lemaître F, Marchand S, Couet W, Olivier JC (2010) Assay of colistin and colistin methanesulfonate in plasma and urine by liquid chromatography-tandem mass spectrometry. Antimicrob Agents Chemother 54:1941–1948
9. Bergen PJ, Landersdorfer CB, Zhang J et al (2012) Pharmacokinetics and pharmacodynamics of "old" polymyxins: what is new? Diagn Microbiol Infect Dis 74:213–223
10. Imberti R, Cusato M, Villani P et al (2010) Steady-state pharmacokinetics and bronchoalveolar lavage concentration of colistin in critically ill patients after intravenous colistin methanesulphonate administration. Chest 138:1333–1339
11. Markou N, Markantonis SL, Dimitrakis E et al (2008) Colistin serum concentration after intravenous administration in critically ill patients with serious multidrug-resistant, gram-negative bacilli infections: a prospective, open-label, uncontrolled study. Clin Ther 30:143–151
12. Plachouras D, Karvanen M, Friberg LE et al (2009) Population pharmacokinetic analysis of colistin methanesulfonate and colistin after intravenous administration in critically ill patients with infections caused by gram-negative bacteria. Antimicrob Agents Chemother 53:3430–3436
13. Garonzik SM, Li J, Thamlikitkul V et al (2011) Population pharmacokinetics of colistin methanesulfonate and formed colistin in critically ill patients from a multicenter study provide dosing suggestions for various categories of patients. Antimicrob Agents Chemother 55:3284–3294
14. Dudhani RV, Turnidge JD, Coulthard K et al (2010) Elucidation of pharmacokinetic/pharmacodynamic determinant of colistin activity against *Pseudomonas aeruginosa* in murine thigh and lung infection model. Antimicrob Agents Chemother 54:1117–1124
15. Dudhani RV, Turnidge JD, Nation RL, Li J (2010) fAUC/MIC is the most predictive pharmacokinetic/pharmacodynamic index of colistin against Acinetobacter baumannii in murine thigh and lung infection models. J Antimicrob Chemother 65:1984–1990
16. Ziv G, Nouws JFM, van Ginneken CAM (1982) The pharmacokinetics and tissue levels of polymyxin B, colistin and gentamicin in calves. J Vet Pharmacol Therap 5:45–58
17. Kunin CM, Bugg A (1971) Binding of polymyxin antibiotics to tissues. The major determinant of distribution and persistence in the body. J Infect Dis 124:394–400
18. Aoki N, Tateda K, Kikuchi Y et al (2009) Efficacy of colistin combination therapy in a mouse model of pneumonia caused by multidrug-resistant Pseudomonas aeruginosa. J Antimicrob Chemother 63:534–542

19. Lu Q, Girardi C, Zhang M et al (2010) Nebulized and intravenous colistin in experimental pneumonia caused by Pseudomonas aeruginosa. Intensive Care Med 36:1147–1155
20. Reina R, Estenssoro E, Saenz G et al (2005) Safety and efficacy of colistin in *Acinetobacter* and *Pseudomonas* infections: a prospective cohort study. Intensive Care Med 31:1058–1065
21. Kallel H, Hergafi L, Bahloul M et al (2007) Safety and efficacy of colistin compared with imipenem in the treatment of ventilator-associated pneumonia: a matched case-control study. Intensive Care Med 33:1162–1167
22. Michalopoulos AS, Tsiodras S, Rellos K, Mentzelopoulos S, Falagas ME (2005) Colistin treatment in patients with ICU-acquired infections caused by multiresistant Gram-negative bacteria: the renaissance of an old antibiotic. Clin Microbiol Infect 11:115–121
23. Dalfino L, Puntillo F, Mosca A et al (2012) High-dose, extended-interval colistin administration in critically ill patients: is this the right dosing strategy? A preliminary study. Clin Infect Dis 54:1720–1726
24. Iosifidis E, Antachopoulos C, Ioannidou M et al (2010) Colistin administration to pediatric and neonatal patients. Eur J Pediatr 169:867–874
25. Celebi S, Hacimustafaoglu M, Koksal N, Ozkan H, Cetinkaya M (2010) Colistimethate sodium therapy for multidrug-resistant isolates in pediatric patients. Pediatr Int 52:410–414
26. Jajoo M, Kumar V, Jain M, Kumari S, Manchanda V (2011) Intravenous colistin administration in neonates. Pediatr Infect Dis J 30:218–221
27. Marchand S, Gobin P, Brillault J et al (2010) Aerosol therapy with colistin methanesulfonate: a biopharmaceutical issue illustrated in rats. Antimicrob Agents Chemother 54:3702–3707
28. Michalopoulos A, Fotakis D, Virtzili S et al (2008) Aerosolized colistin as adjunctive treatment of ventilator-associated pneumonia due to multidrug-resistant Gram-negative bacteria: a prospective study. Respir Med 102:407–412
29. Korbila IP, Michalopoulos A, Rafailidis PI, Nikita D, Samonis G, Falagas ME (2010) Inhaled colistin as adjunctive therapy to intravenous colistin for the treatment of microbiologically documented ventilator-associated pneumonia: a comparative cohort study. Clin Microbiol Infect 16:1230–1236
30. Rattanaumpawan P, Lorsutthitham J, Ungprasert P, Angkasekwinai N, Thamlikitkul V (2010) Randomized controlled trial of nebulized colistimethate sodium as adjunctive therapy of ventilator-associated pneumonia caused by Gram-negative bacteria. J Antimicrob Chemother 65:2645–2649
31. Nakwan N, Wannaro J, Thongmak T et al (2011) Safety in treatment of ventilator-associated pneumonia due to extensive drug-resistant Acinetobacter baumannii with aerosolized colistin in neonates: a preliminary report. Pediatr Pulmonol 46:60–66
32. Athanassa ZE, Markantonis SL, Fousteri MZ et al (2012) Pharmacokinetics of inhaled colistimethate sodium (CMS) in mechanically ventilated critically ill patients. Intensive Care Med 38:1779–1786
33. Petrosillo N, Ioannidou E, Falagas ME (2008) Colistin monotherapy vs. combination therapy: evidence from microbiological, animal and clinical studies. Clin Microbiol Infect 14:816–827
34. Tascini C, Gemignani G, Ferranti S et al (2004) Microbiological activity and clinical efficacy of a colistin and rifampin combination in multidrug-resistant Pseudomonas aeruginosa infections. J Chemother 16:282–287
35. Giamarellos-Bourboulis EJ, Sambatakou H, Galani I, Giamarellou H (2003) In vitro interaction of colistin and rifampin on multidrug-resistant Pseudomonas aeruginosa. J Chemother 15:235–238
36. Timurkaynak F, Can F, Azap OK, Demirbilek M, Arslan H, Karaman SO (2006) In vitro activities of non-traditional antimicrobials alone or in combination against multidrug-resistant strains of Pseudomonas aeruginosa and Acinetobacter baumannii isolated from intensive care units. Int J Antimicrob Agents 27:224–228
37. Li J, Nation RL, Owen RJ, Wong S, Spelman D, Franklin C (2007) Antibiograms of multidrug-resistant clinical Acinetobacter baumannii: promising therapeutic options for treatment of infection with colistin-resistant strains. Clin Infect Dis 45:594–598

38. Song JY, Kee SY, Hwang IS et al (2007) In vitro activities of carbapenem/sulbactam combination, colistin, colistin/rifampicin combination and tigecycline against carbapenem-resistant Acinetobacter baumannii. J Antimicrob Chemother 60:317–322
39. Bergen PJ, Forrest A, Bulitta JB et al (2011) Clinically relevant plasma concentrations of colistin in combination with imipenem enhance pharmacodynamic activity against multidrug-resistant Pseudomonas aeruginosa at multiple inocula. Antimicrob Agents Chemother 55:5134–5142
40. Falagas ME, Rafailidis PI, Ioannidou E et al (2010) Colistin therapy for microbiologically documented multidrug-resistant Gram-negative bacterial infections: a retrospective cohort study of 258 patients. Int J Antimicrob Agents 35:194–199
41. Tumbarello M, Viale P, Viscoli C et al (2012) Predictors of mortality in bloodstream infections caused by Klebsiella pneumoniae carbapenemase-producing K. pneumoniae: Importance of combination therapy. Clin Infect Dis 55:943–950
42. Fernández-Reyes M, Rodríguez-Falcón M, Chiva C, Pachón J, Andreu D, Rivas L (2009) The cost of resistance to colistin in Acinetobacter baumannii: a proteomic perspective. Proteomics 9:1632–1645
43. Spapen H, Jacobs R, Van Gorp V, Troubleyn J, Honoré PM (2011) Renal and neurological side effects of colistin in critically ill patients. Ann Intensive Care 1:14
44. Hartzell JD, Neff R, Ake J et al (2009) Nephrotoxicity associated with intravenous colistin (colistimethate sodium) treatment at a tertiary care medical center. Clin Infect Dis 48:1724–1728
45. Deryke CA, Crawford AJ, Uddin N, Wallace MR (2010) Colistin dosing and nephrotoxicity in a large community teaching hospital. Antimicrob Agents Chemother 54:4503–4505
46. Antachopoulos C, Karvanen M, Iosifidis E et al (2010) Serum and cerebrospinal fluid levels of colistin in pediatric patients. Antimicrob Agents Chemother 54:3985–3987
47. Markantonis SL, Markou N, Fousteri M et al (2009) Penetration of colistin into cerebrospinal fluid. Antimicrob Agents Chemother 53:4907–4910
48. Tunkel AR, Hartman BJ, Kaplan SL et al (2004) Practice guidelines for the management of bacterial meningitis. Clin Infect Dis 39:1267–1284
49. Falagas ME, Bliziotis IA, Tam VH (2007) Intraventricular or intrathecal use of polymyxins in patients with Gram-negative meningitis: a systematic review of the available evidence. Int J Antimicrob Agents 29:9–25
50. Imberti R, Cusato M, Accetta G et al (2012) Pharmacokinetics of colistin in cerebrospinal fluid after intraventricular administration of colistin methanesulfonate. Antimicrob Agents Chemother 56:4416–4421

Optimizing β-Lactam Antibiotic Therapy in the Critically Ill: Moving Towards Patient-tailored Antibiotic Therapy

M. Carlier, V. Stove, and J. J. De Waele

Introduction

Infection is an extremely important problem in critical care medicine. In a recent point prevalence study, 71 % of over 13,000 patients admitted to intensive care units (ICUs) around the world received antibiotic therapy [1]. Sepsis alone is the leading cause of mortality in non-cardiac ICUs with up to 30 % of patients dying within one month of diagnosis [1, 2]; and the incidence of severe sepsis is increasing at a rate of around 10 % per year [3]. Adequate antibiotic therapy is one of the mainstays in the treatment of sepsis, and several studies have demonstrated that delayed and inappropriate treatment is associated with increased mortality. Timely administration and appropriateness of the spectrum of antibiotic therapy have, therefore, been massively promoted in sepsis guidelines, such as the Surviving Sepsis Campaign and comparable initiatives [4].

More than 70 years after their introduction into clinical practice, β-lactam antibiotics remain the mainstay of treatment for many bacterial infections, because of their large antibacterial spectrum and limited intrinsic toxicity. This class of antibiotic comprises drugs, such as penicillins, carbapenems and cephalosporins, with new agents still being developed.

M. Carlier
Department of Clinical Chemistry, Microbiology and Immunology & Department of Critical Care Medicine, Ghent University, De Pintelaan 185, 9000, Ghent, Belgium

V. Stove
Department of Clinical Chemistry, Microbiology and Immunology & Department of Critical Care Medicine, Ghent University, De Pintelaan 185, 9000, Ghent, Belgium

J. J. De Waele (✉)
Department of Critical Care Medicine, Ghent University, De Pintelaan 185, 9000, Ghent, Belgium
E-mail: Jan.DeWaele@UGent.be

J.-L. Vincent (Ed.), *Annual Update in Intensive Care and Emergency Medicine 2013*,
DOI 10.1007/978-3-642-35109-9_9, © Springer-Verlag Berlin Heidelberg 2013

Despite the clinical experience with β-lactam antibiotics and high clinical cure rates for non-critically ill patients, mortality in patients with severe sepsis is still around 30 %, despite apparently appropriate and timely antibiotic therapy [2]. In recent years, very few new antibiotics have become available, and the same is to be expected in the near future. With increasing rates of antimicrobial resistance, rational use of antibiotics has been advocated, with shorter courses of antibiotic therapy, as well as de-escalation strategies to avoid antibiotic selection pressure. Optimized use of antibiotics to improve outcome and reduce antibiotic resistance is, therefore, the next challenge.

The aim of this chapter is to explore why β-lactam antibiotic therapy may fail in some critically ill patients, to demonstrate the need for optimized β-lactam antibiotic therapy and to describe the methods to achieve this goal. We will address the potential advantages and risks of extended and continuous infusions of β-lactams, including the practical application of this approach. Finally, we will plea for an even more sophisticated method of optimization: Patient-tailored antibiotic therapy.

Why Antibiotic Therapy in Critically Ill Patients is Different: A Question of Pharmacokinetics

Pharmacokinetics (PK) is the study of the movement of drugs into, through and out of the body. Antibiotic dosing regimens are usually determined in healthy adults with normal physiology or non-critically ill patients. Volume of distribution (Vd) and clearance are the key determinants, and the pathophysiological changes observed in critically ill patients appear to have profound effects on both factors [5–7]. Other factors include changes in protein binding and vascular permeability.

Changes in Volume of Distribution

The Vd is a constant factor that relates the plasma concentration (Cp) to the dose (Eq. 1) [8].

$$\text{Dose} = \text{Cp} \times \text{Vd} \tag{1}$$

β-lactam antibiotics are hydrophilic drugs and therefore distribute mainly in the systemic circulation. Therefore, these drugs have a small Vd, usually consistent with the volume of extracellular body water (approximately 0.1–0.6 l/kg) and high concentrations are achieved in plasma [9]. Critically ill patients often have a larger Vd compared to healthy adults, which is also very variable [5]. This increase might be related to the pathology (sepsis, hypoalbuminemia, burns), might be pre-existing (obesity, chronic renal and heart failure) or might be a consequence of clinical interventions [6].

Changes in Clearance

Clearance is defined as the volume of plasma cleared of drug per unit of time. For drugs eliminated by first order kinetics, clearance is the factor that relates the rate of drug elimination to its plasma concentration, Cp (Eq. 2) [8].

$$\text{Rate of drug elimination} = \text{Clearance} \times \text{Cp} \tag{2}$$

β-lactam clearance in severe sepsis is largely dependent on the function of different organ systems, such as the cardiovascular system and the kidneys. Although in the case of a severe infection, myocardial depression may cause decreased organ perfusion as a part of multiple organ dysfunction syndrome, and lead to a reduction in clearance [10], a hyperdynamic circulation may have the opposite effect.

Augmented renal clearance is a phenomenon in which renal elimination of circulating waste matter is enhanced, and has been defined as a creatinine clearance of 130 ml/min/1.73 m^2 or higher [11]. Critically ill patients are at risk of developing augmented renal clearance, because of their pathophysiological disturbances as well as the treatment they receive. The hyperdynamic circulation, characterized by a high cardiac output and low systemic vascular resistance (SVR) results in an augmented blood flow to the major organs, including the kidneys, which enhances kidney function and subsequent elimination of renally cleared antibiotics [12]. Recognizing this augmented renal clearance is important, because this elevated clearance may lead to therapeutic failure and selection of drug resistant strains [13]. The cited incidence of augmented renal clearance varies between 30 and 85 % depending on the studied population and the cut-off used for assessment of augmented renal clearance [14–16].

Changes in Protein Binding

Many drugs, including β-lactam antibiotics bind to proteins. This has many implications, since only the unbound drug is able to distribute into the tissues and bind to its target. This property is especially relevant for highly bound compounds, since small changes in protein binding may result in a large increase in pharmacologically active drug. Although hypoalbuminemia in this context may seem advantageous, this also means that the drug is eliminated faster from the body, and that the antibiotic may 'leak' at an enhanced rate from the circulation. Although protein binding is variable for most β-lactam antibiotics, some express high protein binding, such as flucloxacillin and ertapenem [17]. In the SAFE (Saline vs. Albumin Fluid Evaluation) study, the incidence of hypoalbuminemia (defined as serum albumin levels <25 g/l) was about 40–50 % [18]. The effect of hypoalbuminemia has been insufficiently studied, but is likely to have considerable consequences for moderately to highly protein bound antibiotics.

In summary, all of the pathophysiological changes described above result in a highly variable pharmacokinetic profile, which is also unpredictable. In critically ill patients, standard dosing may lead to under- or overdosing in a considerable number of patients.

Pharmacodynamic Characteristics of β-Lactam Antibiotics

In addition to the PK properties of a drug, the pharmacodynamics (PD) is equally important. PD describes the relationship between the concentration of a drug and its clinical effect. β-lactam antibiotics exhibit a time-dependent killing pattern, meaning that the percentage time above the minimal inhibitory concentration (fT > MIC) of the microorganism is considered the best determinant of efficacy of these antibiotics [19]. Studies have shown that, depending on the antibiotic, 40 to 70 % fT > MIC is necessary to treat infections. To maximize the effect of β-lactam antibiotics, it may be necessary to increase the fT > MIC to 100 % or even to maintain the concentration four to five times the MIC for the entire dosage duration [20]. Further increasing the concentration does not lead to a higher efficacy. The carbapenems are an exception to this rule. The minimum fT > MIC for maximum killing is not known in humans, but bactericidal activity in animal models has suggested that the maximal bactericidal activity is a fT > MIC of 40–50 % [21].

Using the current dosing schemes, these targets are often not reached in critically ill patients. Roberts et al. demonstrated that bolus infusion results in low target attainment (even targets as low as fT > MIC of 50 %) in the majority of (simulated) patients [22, 23]. For meropenem, intermittent bolus dosing resulted in median trough levels of 0 mg/l both in plasma and interstitium [23]. Higher targets are even more difficult to reach. Taccone et al. reported that the target attainment (fT > 4 × MIC between 40 and 70 %, depending on the antibiotic) ranged from 16 to 75 % [24].

From the available evidence it is clear that intermittent bolus dosing rarely results in plasma and tissue concentrations that are deemed necessary for treating severe infections.

How Extended and Continuous β-Lactam Infusions Can Optimize Antibiotic Therapy

Prolonged infusion is intended to optimize the pharmacodynamic profile of β-lactam antibiotics. When the dose is administered as an intermittent infusion, the obtained maximum concentration of the antibiotic (Cmax) is much higher than the concentration needed for maximum killing, as typical MIC values of sensitive microorganisms are < 16 mg/l. Soon after administration of the drug is stopped, the concentration declines quickly, as there is only elimination. However, when the dose is administered as an extended infusion over a period of multiple hours, the Cmax is not as high, as both infusion and elimination occur at the same time, but

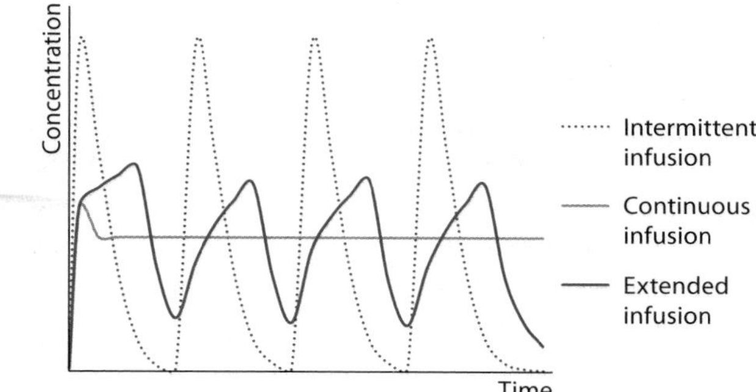

Fig. 1 Pharmacokinetic profiles for the different modes of infusion

still sufficient to maintain adequate concentrations. After the infusion phase, only elimination occurs. When the dose is administered as a constant infusion, there is no elimination phase. The amount of drug leaving the body should equal the amount of drug entering the body, so a constant plasma concentration is obtained. The three modes of infusion are illustrated in Fig. 1.

The available literature agrees that prolonged administration results in a better pharmacokinetic profile in critically ill patients than does intermittent infusion when using the same dose [25–27]. Many studies have demonstrated that prolonged infusion can be as effective (based on PK/PD) as intermittent dosing while using a lower total dose, and thus be associated with reduced costs [28–32]. Recently we showed that an extended 3 hour infusion increased the fT > MIC from 58 to 98 % for piperacillin and from 50 to 81 % for meropenem; higher targets were only reached in a minority of patients [33].

Available Clinical Evidence for Prolonged Infusion

A number of studies have been performed to determine whether the improved PK profile by the use of prolonged infusion translates into better clinical outcomes. Roberts et al. demonstrated that continuous administration of ceftriaxone in septic patients was associated with an improved clinical outcome [34]. Another study evaluating outcomes for 40 septic critically ill patients treated with piperacillin also favored the continuous infusion of piperacillin as it significantly reduced the severity of illness [30]. Moreover, Lorente et al. reported a greater clinical cure of ventilator-associated-pneumonia (VAP) by continuous infusion compared with intermittent infusion when the MIC of the infecting microorganism was 8–16 mg/l in patients without renal failure [35].

A recent, large, prospective study of 240 patients compared continuous infusion of meropenem with intermittent administration (infusions over 30 minutes). The authors found a similar clinical cure rate at the end of therapy, but a higher microbiological success rate in the continuous infusion group. Moreover, the group receiving meropenem as a continuous infusion also had a shorter meropenem-related

ICU stay, a shorter duration of antibiotic therapy and a lower total dose [36]. One comment that can be made on the design of this study is the high dose administered (2 g every 8 hours for intermittent infusion and 4 g as a continuous infusion). Only one study found a mortality advantage for continuous infusion [29].

Other studies did not find improved outcomes when prolonged infusion was used as a mode of administration. In fact, a recent meta-analysis found no clinical advantage for prolonged infusion of β-lactams [37]. The reasons for this finding are probably numerous. First, there are few methodologically sound studies with adequate sample size. Moreover, the improved PK profile when using prolonged infusion logically only results in improved target attainment when the patient is infected with a more resistant microorganism (MIC at least 8 mg/l). Finally, even with the use of prolonged infusion of a standard dose, considerable inter-patient variability still exists, which means that some patients still do not attain minimum targets, while for others, toxicity may occur.

Practical Issues and Considerations When Using Extended or Continuous Infusion

Stability and Compatibility

Not all β-lactam antibiotics are stable for 24 hours at 25 °C. When considering prolonged infusion, each hospital should make sure the antibiotic is sufficiently stable, because stability may vary depending on the solvent and additives used for dissolving the antibiotic. Viaene et al. found meropenem to be stable for maximum 5 hours at room temperature [38], whereas others found it to be stable for longer periods of time [27]. Some antibiotics are stable for more than 24 hours, such as piperacillin/tazobactam [39]; others degrade very quickly, for example, the antibiotic combination, amoxicillin/clavulanic acid. Prolonged infusion of amoxicillin/clavulanic acid would not even be possible, as clavulanic acid seems to be stable for only 30 minutes [40].

Moreover, many β-lactam antibiotics have been shown to be incompatible with other drugs. This does not impose great difficulties in the ICU, because most patients have multiple lumen central venous catheters, but may be a problem in other hospital wards.

Method of Administration

A problem that is often neglected when using extended infusion is the volume of the dead space in the infusion line which can result in incomplete administration of the dose. This effect may have important consequences, especially when a small volume of administration (e. g., 50–100 ml) is chosen. Claus et al. showed that when a volume of 50 ml was used, 40 % of the prescribed antibiotic dose remained in the infusion line when this was not cleared after the administration of the drug [41]. Solutions to this problem include increasing the volume, which may contribute to fluid overload, or using syringe pumps, which may not be universally available [41].

Importance of a Loading Dose

To immediately achieve therapeutic concentrations it is necessary to administer a loading dose. A commonly used approach is to administer a loading dose equal to the first dose administered as an intermittent infusion, immediately followed by continuous or extended infusion [42]. If this loading dose is not administered, the patient is likely to be underdosed.

Toxicity

Many clinicians state that administering β-lactam antibiotics as an extended or continuous infusion is safe, as extremely high values for Cmax are avoided because of the long infusion phase, but extended infusion results in a different PK profile, with higher trough concentrations, for which no solid toxicological research has ever been performed. This seems especially relevant in patients with decreased elimination, in whom there is a risk of accumulation of the drug and resulting toxicity.

For conventional dosing, dose adaptation is also recommended for most β-lactam antibiotics. However, research has shown that even when the antibiotic dosage – using conventional intermittent dosing – was adapted according to kidney function, this was not always sufficient to avoid side effects [43], and it is unlikely that this effect is absent in extended or continuous infusion. The same holds true for patients receiving renal replacement therapy (RRT); a study assessing the variability of antibiotic concentrations in critically ill patients receiving continuous RRT (CRRT) reported excessive trough concentrations for some patients [44].

Underdosing

Although extended and continuous infusion increases exposure of the microorganism to an antibiotic, this may be inadequate in patients in whom the antibiotic is rapidly eliminated. Case reports have shown that some patients require up to 8 or 12 g meropenem to reach adequate serum levels [45]. In these patients, extending the infusion alone did not result in the predefined PK targets being reached and increasing the dose may be necessary in some patients, most likely those who have augmented renal clearance.

Moreover, if there were a saturable, rate limiting transport or elimination mechanism for the antibiotic, the drug would be eliminated continuously at a maximum rate. This effect may result in persistently low concentrations, especially when using continuous infusion as opposed to intermittent or extended infusion where, because of the high peak concentration, effective concentrations can be maintained for some time [46].

PK Modeling and Therapeutic Drug Monitoring to Facilitate Patient-tailored Antibiotic Therapy: An Attempt at Personalized Dosing

Considering the wide variability in antibiotic concentrations in critically ill patients, individually tailored antibiotic therapy is becoming a necessity. At this moment, PK/PD modeling, and antibiotic therapeutic drug monitoring (TDM) are being explored to achieve this. These are the three components of antibiotic optimization, together with prolonged infusion strategies (Fig. 2).

When optimizing β-lactam antibiotic treatment, one must also take into account the susceptibility characteristics of the microorganism. When the MIC of the microorganism is low, lower antibiotic concentrations may be sufficient; conversely, with high MICs (e. g., *Pseudomonas aeruginosa*), (much) higher levels are needed. When starting empirical antibiotic therapy, one must cover a wide range of microorganisms, whilst aiming for the highest PK target. Modeling could be very useful for this purpose: It allows calculation of the optimal starting dose using data from a population pharmacokinetic model in critically ill patients. When the causative microorganism is identified and its susceptibility to the antibiotic determined, lower dosages of the antibiotic may still maintain full efficacy by aiming

Strategy	Extended and continuous infusion	Pharmacokinetic modeling	Therapeutic drug monitoring
Objective	Enhancement of PK/PD profile	Estimation of optimal empirical dose	Patient-tailored antibiotic therapy
Limitations	Drug instability Incompatibility with other drugs Need for special equipment Variable and unpredictable PK	Complex Risk of overdosing Models only predict part of the variability	Expensive Long turnaround time Antibiotic degradation in biological sample Laboratory expertise

Fig. 2 Components of antibiotic optimization. PK: pharmacokinetics; PD: pharmacodynamics

for the optimal PK target (e. g., fT > 1–4 MIC) while avoiding toxicity and decreasing cost. This requires TDM, but has multiple advantages. This combination of PK modeling and TDM allows patient-tailored antibiotic therapy [47]. TDM is indispensable in this context, as no biological variable can predict antibiotic concentrations. Unfortunately, TDM of β-lactam antibiotics is currently challenging with long turnaround times, expensive equipment, logistical problems related to the instability of the samples and the need for well-trained personnel [48]. Efforts to overcome these limitations are urgently needed. We have recently developed a method to determine concentrations of seven β-lactam antibiotics in plasma with a short turnaround time (only 4.5 minutes runtime per sample), which is a step in the right direction for TDM [49].

Conclusion

In the heterogeneous population of an ICU setting, correct antibiotic dosing is problematic because of PK changes in critically ill patients, which are highly variable and unpredictable. This effect may lead to inadequate concentrations in a considerable number of patients. Prolonged infusion optimizes the PK profile by extending the time above the MIC, and several studies have reported improved outcomes, although others did not. However, this entails some practical issues, such as stability and compatibility issues and the need for syringe pumps. Moreover, even with the use of prolonged infusion, the large PK variability between patients still exists, and blind dosing may still lead to under- or overdosing in some patients. TDM allows for individualized dosing, adapted to the physiology of the patient and the MIC of the infecting microorganism, to ensure maximum efficiency and minimal toxicity.

Acknowledgement: Mieke Carlier is funded by a fellowship from the Research Foundation Flanders

References

1. Vincent JL, Rello J, Marshall J et al (2009) International study of the prevalence and outcomes of infection in intensive care units. JAMA 302:2323–2329
2. Rivers E, Nguyen B, Havstad S et al (2001) Early goal-directed therapy in the treatment of severe sepsis and septic shock. N Engl J Med 345:1368–1377
3. Martin GS, Mannino DM, Eaton S, Moss M (2003) The epidemiology of sepsis in the United States from 1979 through 2000. N Engl J Med 348:1546–1554
4. Leibovici L, Shraga I, Drucker M, Konigsberger H, Samra Z, Pitlik SD (1998) The benefit of appropriate empirical antibiotic treatment in patients with bloodstream infection. J Intern Med 244:379–386
5. Roberts JA, Lipman J (2009) Pharmacokinetic issues for antibiotics in the critically ill patient. Crit Care Med 37:840–851

6. Ulldemolins M, Rello J (2011) The relevance of drug volume of distribution in antibiotic dosing. Curr Pharm Biotechnol 12:1996–2001
7. Roberts DM (2011) The relevance of drug clearance to antibiotic dosing in critically ill patients. Curr Pharm Biotechnol 12:2002–2014
8. Hedaya MA (2007) Drug pharmacokinetics following a single IV administration. In: Basic Pharmacokinetics. CRC Press, Boca Raton, pp 23–38
9. Sinnollareddy MG, Roberts MS, Lipman J, Roberts JA (2012) Beta-lactam pharmacokinetics and pharmacodynamics in critically ill patients and strategies for dose optimization: A structured review. Clin Exp Pharmacol Physiol 39:489–496
10. Marshall JC (2001) Inflammation, coagulopathy, and the pathogenesis of multiple organ dysfunction syndrome. Crit Care Med 29:S99–S106
11. Udy AA, Roberts JA, Boots RJ, Paterson DL, Lipman J (2010) Augmented renal clearance implications for antibacterial dosing in the critically ill. Clin Pharmacokinet 49:1–16
12. Di Giantomasso D, May CN, Bellomo R (2003) Vital organ blood flow during hyperdynamic sepsis. Chest 124:1053–1059
13. Udy A, Roberts JA, Boots RJ, Lipman J (2009) You only find what you look for: the importance of high creatinine clearance in the critically ill. Anaesth Intensive Care 37:11–13
14. Fuster-Lluch O, Geronimo-Pardo M, Peyro-Garcia R, Lizan-Garcia M (2008) Glomerular hyperfiltration and albuminuria in critically ill patients. Anaesth Intensive Care 36:674–680
15. Udy A, Boots R, Senthuran S et al (2010) Augmented creatinine clearance in traumatic brain injury. Anesth Analg 111:1505–1510
16. Conil JM, Georges B, Lavit M et al (2007) Pharmacokinetics of ceftazidime and cefepime in burn patients: The importance of age and creatinine clearance. Int J Clin Pharmacol Ther 45:529–538
17. Ulldemolins M, Roberts JA, Rello J, Paterson DL, Lipman J (2011) The effects of hypoalbuminaemia on optimizing antibacterial dosing in critically ill patients. Clin Pharmacokinet 50:99–110
18. Finfer S, Bellomo R, McEvoy S et al (2006) Effect of baseline serum albumin concentration on outcome of resuscitation with albumin or saline in patients in intensive care units: analysis of data from the saline versus albumin fluid evaluation (SAFE) study. BMJ 333:1044–1046
19. Turnidge JD (1998) The pharmacodynamics of beta-lactams. Clin Infect Dis 27:10–22
20. Vogelman B, Craig WA (1986) Kinetics of antimicrobial activity. J Pediatr 108:835–840
21. Ong CT, Tessier PR, Li C, Nightingale CH, Nicolau DP (2007) Comparative in vivo efficacy of meropenem, imipenem, and cefepime against Pseudomonas aeruginosa expressing MexA-MexB-OprM efflux pumps. Diagn Microbiol Infect Dis 57:153–161
22. Roberts JA, Kirkpatrick CMJ, Roberts MS, Dalley AJ, Lipman J (2010) First-dose and steady-state population pharmacokinetics and pharmacodynamics of piperacillin by continuous or intermittent dosing in critically ill patients with sepsis. Int J Antimicrob Agents 35:156–163
23. Roberts JA, Kirkpatrick CMJ, Roberts MS, Robertson TA, Dalley AJ, Lipman J (2009) Meropenem dosing in critically ill patients with sepsis and without renal dysfunction: intermittent bolus versus continuous administration? Monte Carlo dosing simulations and subcutaneous tissue distribution. J Antimicrob Chemother 64:142–150
24. Taccone FS, Laterre PF, Dugernier T et al (2010) Insufficient beta-lactam concentrations in the early phase of severe sepsis and septic shock. Crit Care 14:R126
25. Buijk S, Gyssens IC, Mouton JW, Van Vliet A, Verbrugh HA, Bruining HA (2002) Pharmacokinetics of ceftazidime in serum and peritoneal exudate during continuous versus intermittent administration to patients with severe intra-abdominal infections. J Antimicrob Chemother 49:121–128
26. Georges B, Conil JM, Cougot P et al (2005) Cefepime in critically ill patients: continuous infusion vs. an intermittent dosing regimen. Int J Clin Pharmacol Ther 43:360–369
27. Langgartner J, Vasold A, Glueck T, Reng M, Kees F (2008) Pharmacokinetics of meropenem during intermittent and continuous intravenous application in patients treated by continuous renal replacement therapy. Intensive Care Med 34:1091–1096

28. Thalhammer F, Traunmuller F, El Menyawi I et al (1999) Continuous infusion versus intermittent administration of meropenem in critically ill patients. J Antimicrob Chemother 43:523–527
29. Angus BJ, Smith MD, Suputtamongkol Y et al (2000) Pharmacokinetic-pharmacodynamic evaluation of ceftazidime continuous infusion vs intermittent bolus injection in septicaemic melioidosis. Br J Clin Pharmacol 50:183–191
30. Rafati MR, Rouini MR, Mojtahedzadeh M et al (2006) Clinical efficacy of continuous infusion of piperacillin compared with intermittent dosing in septic critically ill patients. Int J Antimicrob Agents 28:122–127
31. Langgartner J, Lehn N, Glueck T, Herzig H, Kees F (2007) Comparison of the pharmacokinetics of piperacillin and sulbactam during intermittent and continuous intravenous infusion. Chemotherapy 53:370–377
32. Roberts JA, Roberts MS, Robertson TA, Dalley AJ, Lipman J (2009) Piperacillin penetration into tissue of critically ill patients with sepsis-Bolus versus continuous administration? Crit Care Med 37:926–933
33. De Waele J, Carlier M, Hoste E et al (2011) Extended infusion of meropenem and piperacillin in critically ill patients: A pharmacokinetic/pharmacodynamic analysis. Crit Care Med 39:198
34. Roberts JA, Boots R, Rickard CM et al (2007) Is continuous infusion ceftriaxone better than once-a-day dosing in intensive care? A randomized controlled pilot study. J Antimicrob Chemother 59:285–291
35. Lorente L, Jimenez A, Martin MM, Iribarren JL, Jose Jimenez J, Mora ML (2009) Clinical cure of ventilator-associated pneumonia treated with piperacillin/tazobactam administered by continuous or intermittent infusion. Int J Antimicrob Agents 33:464–468
36. Chytra I, Stepan M, Benes J et al (2012) Clinical and microbiological efficacy of continuous versus intermittent application of meropenem in critically ill patients: a randomized open-label controlled trial. Crit Care 16:R113
37. Tamma PD, Putcha N, Suh YD, Van Arendonk KJ, Rinke ML (2011) Does prolonged beta-lactam infusions improve clinical outcomes compared to intermittent infusions? A meta-analysis and systematic review of randomized, controlled trials. BMC Infect Dis 11:181
38. Viaene E, Chanteux H, Servais H, Mingeot-Leclercq MP, Tulkens PM (2002) Comparative stability studies of antipseudomonal beta-lactams for potential administration through portable elastomeric pumps (home therapy for cystic fibrosis patients) and motor-operated syringes (intensive care units). Antimicrob Agents Chemother 46:2327–2332
39. Mathew M, Gupta VD, Bethea C (1994) Stability of piperacillin sodium in the presence of tazobactam sodium in 5% dextrose and normal saline injections. J Clin Pharm Ther 19:397–399
40. Wildfeuer A, Rader K (1996) Stability of beta-lactamase inhibitors and beta-lactam antibiotics in parenteral dosage forms and in body fluids and tissue homogenates: A comparative study of sulbactam, clavulanic acid, ampicillin and amoxycillin. Int J Antimicrob Agents 6:S31–S34 (Reprinted from Arzneim Forsch, vol 41, pg 70, 1991)
41. Claus B, Buyle F, Robays H, Vogelaers D (2010) Importance of infusion volume and pump characteristics in extended administration of beta-lactam antibiotics. Antimicrob Agents Chemother 54:4950
42. Van Herendael B, Jeurissen A, Tulkens PM et al (2012) Continuous infusion of antibiotics in the critically ill: The new holy grail for beta-lactams and vancomycin? Ann Intensive Care 2:22
43. Lemaire-Hurtel AS, Gras-Champel V, Hary L, Masmoudi K, Massy Z, Andréjak M (2009) Recommended dosage adaptation based on renal function is not always sufficient to avoid betalactam antibiotics side effects. Nephrol Ther 5:144–148
44. Roberts DM, Roberts JA, Roberts MS et al (2012) Variability of antibiotic concentrations in critically ill patients receiving continuous renal replacement therapy: A multicenter pharmacokinetic study. Crit Care Med 40:1523–1528

45. Tröger U, Drust A, Martens-Lobenhoffer J, Tanev I, Braun-Dullaeus RC, Bode-Böger SM (2012) Decreased meropenem levels in Intensive Care Unit patients with augmented renal clearance: benefit of therapeutic drug monitoring. Int J Antimicrob Agents 40:370–372
46. Mouton JW, Vinks A (1996) Is continuous infusion of beta-lactam antibiotics worthwhile? Efficacy and pharmacokinetic considerations. J Antimicrob Chemother 38:5–15
47. Roberts JA (2011) Using PK/PD to optimize antibiotic dosing for critically ill patients. Curr Pharm Biotechnol 12:2070–2079
48. Roberts JA, Hope WW, Lipman J (2010) Therapeutic drug monitoring of beta-lactams for critically ill patients: unwarranted or essential? Int J Antimicrob Agents 35:419–420
49. Carlier M, Stove V, Roberts JA, Van de Velde E, De Waele JJ, Verstraete AG (2012) Quantification of seven b-lactam antibiotics and two b-lactamase inhibitors in human plasma using a validated UPLC-MS/MS method. Int J Antimicrob Agents 40:416–422

Antibiotic Adsorption on CRRT Membranes: Impact on Antibiotic Dosing

P. M. Honoré, R. Jacobs, and H. D. Spapen

Introduction

Continuous renal replacement therapy (CRRT) is increasingly used in hemodynamically compromised or unstable patients with severe sepsis and septic shock. Adequate antimicrobial treatment is imperative and directly correlated with outcome in these patients. However, the pharmacokinetic behavior of most antibiotic agents during CRRT has not been investigated in depth. Antibiotics may be eliminated from the circulation by convection but also by adhering to the dialysis membrane itself, which may result in subtherapeutic plasma levels. In this context, the emergence of highly adsorptive dialysis membranes, such as the AN69 surface treated (AN69 ST) and the polymethylmetacrilate (PMMA) membranes among others, raises important questions related to antimicrobial therapy. Currently available data on highly adsorptive membranes relate to chronic hemodialysis in which such membranes have been used for more than a decade to capture small proteins, such as β2-microglobulin, in order to reduce dialysis-associated amyloidosis [1–3]. CRRT employing membranes with enhanced adsorption capacity is not yet widely used in critically ill patients, which explains why pharmacokinetic data have mostly been obtained with 'classic' membranes (e. g., AN69, polyethersulfone, polysulphone) [4, 5]. Current guidelines allow reasonably correct matching of antibiotic

P. M. Honoré (✉)
Intensive Care Departement, University Hospital, Vrije Universiteit Brussel,
1090-Brussels, Belgium
E-mail: Patrick.Honore@uzbrussel.be

R. Jacobs
Intensive Care Departement, University Hospital, Vrije Universiteit Brussel,
1090-Brussels, Belgium

H. D. Spapen
Intensive Care Departement, University Hospital, Vrije Universiteit Brussel,
1090-Brussels, Belgium

J.-L. Vincent (Ed.), *Annual Update in Intensive Care and Emergency Medicine 2013*,
DOI 10.1007/978-3-642-35109-9_10, © Springer-Verlag Berlin Heidelberg 2013

dosing to clearance by conventional membranes, but neglect any potential impact of excessive antibiotic adsorption when highly adsorptive membranes are used [6, 7]. Classic and novel dialysis membranes may indeed have widely different adsorption capacities. This difference has been demonstrated for large cytokines (e. g., high mobility group box [HMGB]-1 protein) and is certainly anticipated to occur for antibiotics [8]. Several landmark *in vitro* studies, although mostly assessing conventional membranes, have also elegantly highlighted a key role of adsorption in antibiotic elimination during CRRT [9, 10].

We reviewed the existing literature regarding adsorption of antibiotics during CRRT to answer the following questions: To what extent are antibiotics adsorbed by conventional and highly adsorptive membranes? Does a difference in adsorption exist between antibiotic classes? Is dose adaptation necessary if adsorption is documented? Antibiotics that undergo significant membrane adsorption are discussed. Eventually, we propose guidelines for dose adaptation of these antibiotics in ICU patients. Future pharmacokinetic studies of antibiotic adsorption are imperative to optimize and refine these preliminary viewpoints.

Aminoglycosides

Preliminary studies showed significant adsorption of tobramycin on polyacrylonitrile (PAN) membranes as well as a concentration dependent adsorption on AN69 membranes [6, 10]. Adsorption of gentamicin on PAN membranes was thought to contribute to the shorter serum half-life and reduced peak concentration of the drug [11]. Investigators from Hong Kong extensively explored amikacin pharmacokinetics. Using 'older' membrane types, in particular AN69, they measured adsorption time, membrane effects, pH, and amikacin concentration. In addition, they investigated the impact of circulating amikacin concentration, membrane surface area, and repeated amikacin dosing on adsorption [12, 13]. They found that *in vitro* membrane adsorption of amikacin was significant, rapid, and dose-related [12, 13]. Adsorption was not reversed by a subsequent decrease in amikacin concentration and depended on filter material, with adsorption on AN69 filters exceeding that on polyamide filters [12]. The observed adsorption was irreversible and de-adsorption never occurred [12]. The amount of amikacin fixed by the membrane was shown to be nearly 900 mg after administration of an excess dose of 2,000 mg for a prolonged period [13]. This magnitude of adsorption will undoubtedly affect therapeutic serum peak amikacin levels. Dose adaptation is thus imperative, the impact of which will become even more important when highly adsorptive membranes are introduced. Consequently, recent suggestions to administer an amikacin loading dose of at least 25 mg [14] to 30 mg [15] in septic shock patients treated with CRRT must already be revised, because they were based on calculations for classical AN69 membranes. The half-life of amikacin was found to be shorter, approximating 24 hours, even in patients receiving CRRT [15]. This is partly explained by the high AN69 membrane sieving coefficient (around 0.9) for amikacin [15] but mainly depends on cumulative membrane adsorption at higher (especially the recently suggested) loading doses [13–15]. The Hong Kong investigators confirmed that this was an antibiotic class effect. A cumulative amikacin dose approaching 1,000 mg was irreversibly bound to the AN69 membrane leaving the latter still incompletely saturated [13]. The same investigators recently demonstrated that aminoglycosides, in particular netilmicin, were also well-absorbed by polyamide membranes [16]. A Japanese study looking at arbekacin and other aminoglycoside behavior during PMMA membrane-based CRRT in critically ill patients also found significant membrane adsorption and suggested higher loading doses should be used [17].

In conclusion, the pharmacokinetics (PK) of aminoglycosides, which are extensively used in ICU patients (e. g., amikacin), need to be reconsidered, particularly when CRRT using highly adsorptive membranes is performed. Primarily, a correct loading dose should be determined to insure adequate bactericidal treatment (Table 1). Thereafter, close drug monitoring is required given the high amount of irreversibly membrane-bound drug at accumulating doses.

Colistin

Colistin is a polypeptide antibiotic composed mainly of polymyxin E_1 and E_2. It is administered parenterally as the prodrug, colistimethate sodium, a fraction of which is hydrolyzed *in vivo* to colistin [18]. Colistin causes rapid bacterial killing in a concentration-dependent manner. Due to its nephrotoxic and, to a lesser extent neurotoxic [18, 19], potential, colistin was progressively supplanted by less toxic antibiotics with a comparable or broader antibacterial spectrum. However, the worldwide resurgence of infections due to multidrug-resistant Gram-negative bacilli has renewed interest in this antimicrobial [19]. Recent experience in patients undergoing CRRT demonstrated a dramatic reduction in the adverse effects of colistin, which permitted significant dose increments resulting in higher peak levels and improved therapeutic efficacy [18, 19]. CRRT elimination of colistin has been recognized for several years, yet the mechanism(s) underlying its removal remained unknown [20]. Very recently, a role of adsorption in the elimination process of colistin was highlighted [21], although still considered to be of relatively minor importance. However, the impact of adsorption was probably underestimated in this study, because CRRT was performed using classic AN69 membranes. With the novel AN69 ST membrane, we convincingly showed that adsorption was by far the major mechanism of elimination (Honoré et al., unpublished data). Comparing the conventional AN69 membrane with its AN69 ST counterpart, colistin adsorption increased from 20 to 80 % [21] (Honoré et al., unpublished data). Quantitative colistin elimination by these new membranes needs to be explored but indirect measurements show that it may be situated between 500 and 1,000 mg as cumulative doses seem to become irreversibly membrane-adsorbed (Honoré et al., unpublished data). These findings, as well as new and upcoming pharmacodynamic

Table 1 Impact on antibiotic dosing of elimination mechanism and degree of membrane adsorption during conventional and highly-adsorptive-membrane continuous renal replacement therapy (H-A-M CRRT)

Antibiotic	Elimination	Dose adsorbed within 24 h	Current dose in CRRT	Class effect	Dose suggested during H-A-M CRRT*
Amino-glycosides (amikacin)	Mainly convection (SC = 0.9) H-A-M CRRT adsorption might reach 50 %	As high as 1,000 mg No saturation Irreversible binding	30 mg/kg loading dose Monitoring serum levels	Yes (tobramycin, netilmycin, arbekacin)	Initially 40 to 45 mg/kg/d
Colistin	Up to 90 % adsorption	Between 5 & 10 MIU No saturation	9 MIU loading dose, then 4.5 MIU bid	No	9 MIU loading dose, then 4.5 MIU tid
Vancomycin	Mainly convection (SC = 0.75) Adsorption might reach 20 %	Up to 1/3 of loading dose (± 350–400 mg) No saturation	20 mg/kg loading dose, then 30 mg/kg/d Monitoring serum levels	Yes (daptomycin)	25 mg/kg loading dose, then 40 mg/kg/d Monitoring serum levels
Teicoplanin	Limited convection (SC = 0.15) Mainly adsorption (90–95 %)	Up to 25 % of loading dose (± 200–250 mg) Saturation unknown	10 mg/kg loading dose bid, repeated 3 times, then 10 mg/kg/d Monitoring serum levels	No	12 mg/kg loading dose bid repeated 3 times, then 12 mg/kg/d Monitoring serum levels
Levofloxacin	Mainly convection (SC = 0.8) Saturation present (SatC = 0.75)	Up to 30 % of loading dose (± 250–300 mg) Saturation present	750 mg loading dose, then 500 mg bid	Highly possible but not yet shown	1,000 mg loading dose, then 500 mg/d tid

* hypothetical dose, needs to be confirmed

SC: sieving coefficient; SatC: saturation coefficient; MIU: million international units; bid: twice daily; tid: three times a day

insights, will obviously prompt reconsideration of colistin dosage. The currently accepted colistin dose of 3 million IU tid should be increased, at least up to 4 million IU qid. The most recently published guidelines suggest that colistin be administered as a loading dose of 9 million IU followed by 4.5 million IU bd [22], with adaptations of the daily dose according to glomerular filtration rate (GFR). No dose reduction is needed during CRRT (using 'old' membrane types) but, once again, this must be validated when highly adsorptive membranes are used.

In conclusion, CRRT permits higher colistin dosing and may enhance the therapeutic effect of the drug without increasing side-effects. However, colistin is significantly adsorbed by membranes with enhanced adsorption to the point that daily doses should be substantially increased (Table 1).

Glycopeptides

Vancomycin

Studies on adsorption of vancomycin to dialysis membranes are scarce. Still, experimental proof exists that commonly used filters are able to irreversibly fix vancomycin. Tian et al. studied the vancomycin adsorption capacity of AN69, polyamide, and polysulfone membranes in an *in vitro* hemofiltration model [7]. Vancomycin (36 mg) was added to a known volume of a blood-crystalloid mixture (target concentration 50 mg/l) and pumped through a closed circuit. Adsorption, calculated from the fall in concentration over 120 min, to the 0.6-m PAN filters was significantly greater (10.08 ± 2.26 mg) than to the 0.6-m polyamide (5.20 ± 1.82 mg) or 0.7-m polysulfone (4.80 ± 2.40 mg) filters. Cumulative adsorption was not changed after reducing vancomycin serum concentration by dilution with 500 ml lactated Ringer's solution. These findings suggest that the degree of vancomycin adsorption depends on filter material and occurs mainly when the AN69 membrane is used. Theoretically, AN69 might irreversibly fix almost one third of the initial dose. If proven *in vivo*, loading and maintenance doses of vancomycin will have to be adapted accordingly. Because we routinely apply CRRT using the AN69 ST hemofilter, we were able to identify retrospectively that daily vancomycin maintenance doses close to 3,000 mg were needed during the first 3 treatment days [23]. Choi and co-workers demonstrated that, within the first hour after changing the membrane, a striking decline in vancomycin trough concentration occurred, which necessitated a considerable increase in the continuous infusion dose [24].

In conclusion, experimental data suggest substantial vancomycin adsorption during CRRT, and especially when using AN69 membranes. These preliminary data need to be confirmed by clinical trials. Meanwhile, clinicians working with highly adsorptive membranes, such as AN69 ST, are advised to carefully monitor vancomycin trough levels, especially after a filter change [23].

Teicoplanin

Shiraishi and co-workers recently found that teicoplanin was adsorbed by PMMA membranes [25]. Teicoplanin (50 mg/l) was circulated throughout the beaker in an *in vitro* hemodiafiltration circuit, mimicking maximum plasma concentrations of the drug after administration of a standard dose. Teicoplanin concentrations in the plasma surrogate and ultrafiltrate were determined by high performance liquid chromatography. Teicoplanin was predominantly adsorbed on PMMA membranes but not ultrafiltrated [25]. In the same experiment, the researchers also detected significant adsorption of the drug on PAN membranes. In an *in vivo* study this time, teicoplanin was strongly eliminated during CRRT when AN69 membranes were used [26]. In this experiment, elimination through convection was almost negligible (sieving coefficient of teicoplanin was 0.15 as compared to 0.9 for amikacin [27]) and thus teicoplanin was predominantly adsorbed, confirming the *in vitro* data [25, 26].

In conclusion, preliminary data indicate significant membrane adsorption of teicoplanin in spite of its poor convection rate. Teicoplanin doses should be adapted and given more frequently in order to keep trough levels at an optimal range between 15 and 25 mg/l [28].

Daptomycin

Other glycopeptides such as daptomycin may also be significantly adsorbed onto PAN membranes but *in vitro* data are very preliminary [29] and need to be confirmed in large studies *in vivo*.

Quinolones

The Hong Kong investigator group observed significant *in vitro* adsorption of levofloxacin during CRRT with conventional AN69 membranes [9, 30]. Approximately one third of a 100 mg dose was captured by the membrane. Recent investigations elicited substantial 'extra-renal' elimination of ciprofloxacin [31, 32]. Although not specifically assessed and thus not proven, it is plausible that this important extra-renal elimination of ciprofloxacin could be attributed in part to an adsorption process, especially when AN69 membranes are used. Ciprofloxacin has a sieving coefficient exceeding 0.8. Thus, in case of significant adsorption, lower serum concentrations are expected. Because both bactericidal effect and risk of developing resistance during quinolone treatment depend on high peak concentrations, it is evident that important dose adaptations must be anticipated during CRRT [9, 30]. This was illustrated in a case report describing a patient undergoing CRRT in whom ciprofloxacin dose could be increased to 800 mg bid without side-effects [33]. However, more data are needed to support these preliminary experimental and clinical findings.

In conclusion, within the group of quinolones, levofloxacin is highly membrane adsorbed. Data for ciprofloxacin are not yet available but indirect evidence suggests a similar, though not quantified, adsorption. Globally, lower peak concentrations are to be expected, which compromise the efficacy of these drugs and enhance the risk of bacterial resistance.

Significant dose adaptations of quinolones must be anticipated during CRRT. Additional studies are eagerly awaited to better delimit the role of adsorption, in particular when using highly adsorptive membranes.

Conclusion

For decades, adsorption has been overlooked as a potential mechanism for antibiotic elimination during CRRT. Only recently, several key investigations have convincingly demonstrated that, at least for some antibiotics, membrane adsorption plays an important role in eliminating active drug from the circulation. This effect is clinically relevant since it may mean that significant antibiotic dose adaptation is needed in critically ill patients undergoing CRRT. Moreover, the expanding use of highly adsorptive membranes will accentuate this adsorptive 'loss' and dramatically change current guidelines for antibiotic dosing during CRRT [34]. Information regarding membrane adsorption of antibiotics is still scarce, mostly derived from *in vitro* studies, limited to certain antibiotic classes (aminoglycosides, colistin, glycopeptides, and quinolones), and virtually non-existent with regard to the use of novel membranes with much higher adsorption capacity than those that are currently employed. Adequate antibiotic treatment is a cornerstone of treatment for severe sepsis and septic shock. Because many septic patients will require CRRT, more studies are urgently needed to better define the optimal dose regimens for all relevant antibiotic classes.

References

1. Chanard J, Lavaud S, Randoux C, Rieu P (2003) New insights in dialysis membrane biocompatibility: relevance of adsorption properties and heparin binding. Nephrol Dial Transplant 18:252–257
2. Randoux C, Gillery P, Georges N, Lavaud S, Chanard J (2001) Filtration of native and glycated beta2-microglobulin by charged and neutral dialysis membranes. Kidney Int 60:1571–1577
3. Hoenich NA, Stamp S (2000) Clinical performance of a new high-flux synthetic membrane. Am J Kidney Dis 36:345–352
4. Susla GM (2009) The impact of continuous renal replacement therapy on drug therapy. Clin Pharmacol Ther 86:562–565
5. Heintz BH, Matzke GR, Dager WE (2009) Antimicrobial dosing concepts and recommendations for critically ill adult patients receiving continuous renal replacement therapy or intermittent hemodialysis. Pharmacotherapy 29:562–577
6. Kronfol NO, Lau AH, Barakat MM (1987) Aminoglycoside binding to polyacrylonitrile hemofilter membranes during continuous hemofiltration. ASAIO Trans 33:300–303
7. Tian Q, Gomersall CD, Leung PP et al (2008) The adsorption of vancomycin by polyacrylonitrile, polyamide, and polysulfone hemofilters. Artif Organs 32:81–84

8. Yumoto M, Nishida O, Moriyama K et al (2011) *In vitro* evaluation of high mobility group box 1 protein removal with various membranes for continuous hemofiltration. Ther Apher Dial 15:385–393
9. Choi G, Gomersall CD, Lipman J et al (2004) The effect of adsorption, filter material and point of dilution on antibiotic elimination by haemofiltration: an *in vitro* study of levofloxacin. Int J Antimicrob Agents 24:468–472
10. Cigarran-Guldris S, Brier ME, Golper TA (1991) Tobramycin clearance during simulated continuous arteriovenous hemodialysis. Contrib Nephrol 93:120–123
11. Kraft D, Lode H (1979) Elimination of ampicillin and gentamicin by hemofiltration. Klin Wochenschr 57:195–196
12. Tian Q, Gomersall CD, Ip M et al (2008) Adsorption of amikacin, a significant mechanism of elimination by hemofiltration. Antimicrob Agents Chemother 52:1009–1013
13. Tian Q, Gomersall CD, Ip M, Joynt GM (2011) Effect of preexposure to aminoglycosides on *in vitro* adsorption of amikacin by polyacrylonitrile hemofilters. Antimicrob Agents Chemother 55:3641–3642
14. Taccone FS, De Backer D, Laterre PF et al (2011) Pharmacokinetics of a loadingdose of amikacin in septic patients undergoing continuous renal replacement therapy. Int J Antimicrob Agents 37:531–535
15. Gálvez R, Luengo C, Cornejo R et al (2011) Higher than recommended amikacin loading doses achieve pharmacokinetic targets without associated toxicity. Int J Antimicrob Agents 38:146–151
16. Lam PKN, Tian Q, Ip M, Gomersall CD (2010) *In vitro* adsorption of gentamicin and netilmicin by polyacrylonitrile and polyamide hemofiltration filters. Antimicrob Agents Chemother 54:963–965
17. Ikawa K, Morikawa N, Suyama H, Ikeda K, Yamanoue T (2009) Pharmacokinetics and pharmacodynamics of once-daily arbekacin during continuous venovenous hemodiafiltration in critically ill patients. J Infect Chemother 15:420–423
18. Spapen HD, Jacobs R, Van Gorp V, Troubleyn J, Honoré PM (2011) Renal and neurological side effects of colistin in critically ill patients. Ann Intensive Care 25:14
19. Spapen HD, Honoré PM, Gregoire N et al (2011) Convulsions and apnoea in a patient infected with New Delhi metallo-β-lactamase-1 Escherichia coli treated with colistin. J Infect 63:468–470
20. Marchand S, Frat JP, Petitpas F et al (2010) Removal of colistin during intermittent haemodialysis in two critically ill patients. J Antimicrob Chemother 65:1836–1837
21. Markou N, Fousteri M, Markantonis SL et al (2012) Colistin pharmacokinetics in intensive care unit patients on continuous venovenous haemodiafiltration: an observational study. J Antimicrob Chemother 67:2459–2462
22. Dalfino L, Puntillo F, Mosca A et al (2012) High-dose, extended-interval colistin administration in critically ill patients: is this the right dosing strategy? A preliminary study. Clin Infect Dis 54:1720–1726
23. Honoré PM, Jacobs R, Joannes-Boyau O et al (2013) Newly designed CRRT membranes for sepsis and SIRS: a pragmatic approach for bedside intensivists summarizing the more recent advances. A systematic structured review. ASAIO Journal (in press)
24. Choi G, Gomersall CD, Tian Q, Joynt GM, Freebairn R, Lipman J (2009) Principles of antibacterial dosing in continuous renal replacement therapy. Crit Care Med 37:2268–2282
25. Shiraishi Y, Okajima M, Sai Y, Miyamoto K, Inaba H (2012) Elimination of teicoplanin by adsorption to the filter membrane during haemodiafiltration: screening experiments for linezolid, teicoplanin and vancomycin followed by *in vitro* haemodiafiltration models for teicoplanin. Anaesth Intensive Care 40:442–449
26. Bellmann R, Falkensammer G, Seger C, Weiler S, Kountchev J, Joannidis M (2010) Teicoplanin pharmacokinetics in critically ill patients on continuous veno-venous hemofiltration. Int J Clin Pharmacol Ther 48:243–249
27. Armendariz E, Chelluri L, Ptachcinski R (1990) Pharmacokinetics of amikacin during continuous veno-venous hemofiltration. Crit Care Med 18:675–676

28. Meyer B, Traunmüller F, Hamwi A et al (2004) Pharmacokinetics of teicoplanin during continuous hemofiltration with a new and a 24-h used highly permeable membrane: rationale for therapeutic drug monitoring-guided dosage. Int J Clin Pharmacol Ther 42:556–560
29. Wagner CC, Steiner I, Zeitlinger M (2009) Daptomycin elimination by CVVH in vitro: evaluation of factors influencing sieving and membrane adsorption. Int J Clin Pharmacol Ther 47:178–186
30. Tian Q, Gomersall CD, Wong A et al (2006) Effect of drug concentration on adsorption of levofloxacin by polyacrylonitrile haemofilters. Int J Antimicrob Agents 28:147–150
31. Malone RS, Fish DN, Abraham E, Teitelbaum I (2001) Pharmacokinetics of levofloxacin and ciprofloxacin during continuous renal replacement therapy in critically ill patients. Antimicrob Agents Chemother 45:2949–2954
32. Bellmann R, Egger P, Gritsch W et al (2002) Pharmacokinetics of ciprofloxacin in patients with acute renal failure undergoing continuous venovenous haemofiltration: influence of concomitant liver cirrhosis. Acta Med Austriaca 29:112–116
33. Utrup TR, Mueller EW, Healy DP, Callcut RA, Peterson JD, Hurford WE (2010) High-dose ciprofloxacin for serious gram-negative infection in an obese, critically ill patient receiving continuous venovenous hemodiafiltration. Ann Pharmacother 44:1660–1664
34. Honoré PM, Jacobs R, Boer W et al (2012) New insights regarding rationale, therapeutic target and dose of hemofiltration and hybrid therapies in septic AKI. Blood Purif 33:44–51

Part IV

Sepsis Mechanisms and Therapies

Hyperinflammation and Mediators of Immune Suppression in Critical Illness

A. C. Morris, A. J. Simpson, and T. S. Walsh

Introduction

Critical illness, constituting an acute illness or injury resulting in organ dysfunction and failure, is associated with a profound, systemic activation of the immune system and inflammation-mediated organ damage [1]. However, critically ill patients also suffer a high rate of nosocomial infection with secondary sepsis being a common cause of death [2]. This high prevalence of secondary infections argues for the influence of an immune suppression that may, at first glance, appear paradoxical in light of the pro-inflammatory nature of many critical illnesses. Although immune cell hypo-function has been noted in clinical and experimental critical illnesses, the mediators of these effects remain poorly defined. This review will present the recent evidence accumulating for the role of pro-inflammatory mediators in driving immune dysfunction, and how this insight may, in part, explain the apparent paradox of immune suppression occurring in a patient with manifestations of hyperinflammation [3].

A. C. Morris
Center for Inflammation Research, University of Edinburgh, Queen's Medical Research Institute, 47 Little France Crescent, Edinburgh EH16 4TJ, Scotland, UK

A. J. Simpson
Institute of Cellular Medicine, Newcastle University, Newcastle upon Tyne, NE2 4HH, England, UK

T. S. Walsh (✉)
Center for Inflammation Research, University of Edinburgh, Queen's Medical Research Institute, 47 Little France Crescent, Edinburgh EH16 4TJ, Scotland, UK
E-mail: Timothy.walsh@ed.ac.uk

J.-L. Vincent (Ed.), *Annual Update in Intensive Care and Emergency Medicine 2013*,
DOI 10.1007/978-3-642-35109-9_11, © Springer-Verlag Berlin Heidelberg 2013

Nosocomial Infection in Intensive Care

Estimates of the prevalence of nosocomial infection among general medical and surgical patients range from 4–6 % [4]. In striking contrast, among patients requiring organ support in intensive care units (ICU), the prevalence rises to 25–40 % [2, 5]. These latter rates are similar to those found in frank neutropenia [6]. Although attributing direct mortality to nosocomial infection remains problematic, one infection alone, ventilator associated pneumonia (VAP), has an estimated mortality of 20–30 % [7]. This high prevalence of nosocomial infection, combined with the frequency of otherwise commensal organisms among the infecting organisms [5] suggests a profound degree of immune suppression.

Systemic Inflammation and Immune Suppression in Critical Illness

Critical illness is frequently associated with a systemic inflammatory response syndrome (SIRS), characterized by physiological manifestations of inflammation (altered temperature, leukocytosis or bone marrow suppression, tachycardia and tachypnea). This inflammatory response is accompanied by biochemical and immunological evidence of immune system activation [1, 8, 9], and can be precipitated by both sterile and infective insults. Despite disparate initiating events, the stereotyped SIRS response arises from final common pathways, with the release of endogenous inflammatory mediators including tumor necrosis factor (TNF)-α, interleukins (IL)-1, 6, and 8, and complement activation [1, 8–10].

Prompted by the failures of therapies aimed at neutralizing these pro-inflammatory mediators, the concept of a counter-regulatory but equally maladaptive anti-inflammatory response known as the "compensatory anti-inflammatory response syndrome" (CARS) was proposed [11]. The general concept has been of SIRS-CARS being a biphasic process with inflammation being followed by immune hypoactivity and recovery occurring as the immune hypofunction resolved [12]. However, whilst the biphasic SIRS-CARS continuum provided an interesting theoretical framework, it lacks experimental demonstration and does not fit with the clinical picture seen amongst critically ill patients in the ICU. Clinically, many patients show signs of persisting inflammation, and immune-mediated organ damage while simultaneously remaining highly susceptible to secondary infections, suggesting the term complex immune dysfunction syndrome (CIDS).

Immune hypoactivity has now been demonstrated in virtually all immune cell types, including innate actors such as neutrophils [13, 14], monocytes [15], tissue macrophages [16] and dendritic cells [17], as well as in the adaptive immune system in T cells [18], B cells [19] and natural killer (NK) cells [20] (Table 1 [12, 13, 15, 16, 18–28]). However, it is undoubtedly true that critical illness is associated with a profound degree of immune activation and systemic inflammation [1].

Table 1 Immune defects and immunosuppressive responses identified in patients and animal models of critical illness

Cell type	Finding	References
Neutrophils	Impaired phagocytosis, reactive oxygen species production, transmigration	[13, 24, 32, 36, 38]
Monocytes	Reduced production of tumor necrosis factor in response to LPS	[15, 21, 23, 24]
Macrophages	Reduced production of tumor necrosis factor in response to LPS	[16]
T lymphocytes	Decreased proliferative response, increased apoptosis, increased proportion of regulatory T cells	[12, 18, 19, 22, 50]
B lymphocytes	Impaired antigen-specific responses	[19]
Natural killer cells	Reduced cytokine responses to LPS	[20]
Dendritic cells	Decreased antigen presentation	[19, 50]

LPS: lipopolysaccharide

One possible reason for the variable and apparently contradictory findings of immune cell function from different reports may be the time point at which the measurement is made. In animal models, in which pre-morbid sampling is feasible and there is certainty over time and severity of onset, most studies indicate a rapid pro-inflammatory response with immune cell activation/hyperactivity with later onset of hypoactivity [12]. In human studies, monocyte deactivation is largely reported to occur several days after admission to intensive care [21], as are T cell impairments [22]; however, this is not universally the case and apparently 'early onset' immune suppression is noted in some reports [23, 24]. In these latter cases, it is possible that the early 'hyperactive' phase may well have been missed in the pre-ICU period. What is also clear is that the 'immune status' (i. e., hyper- or hypo-active) may depend on which aspect of cellular function is examined, with increasing evidence that both pro- and anti-inflammatory mediators may be elevated at the same time [29].

Neutrophils: Exemplars of the Hyper-/hypo-inflammatory Duality

Of the immune cells discussed above, one type in particular appears to exemplify this apparent dualistic state by demonstrating features of both activation and dysfunction simultaneously – the neutrophil. Organ dysfunction in critically ill patients is, to a considerable degree, driven by neutrophils [30]. These key immune cells tend to display surface markers of 'activation', notably elevated levels of

CD11b and CD64 and diminished CD16 in critical illness [31], although one study has also demonstrated diminished inducibility of these receptors [32]. Neutrophils from critically ill patients demonstrate enhanced release of proteolytic enzymes such as human neutrophil elastase (HNE) in response to *ex-vivo* lipopolysaccharide (LPS) [33] with elevated levels also being seen in patient plasma [34]. Similar findings are made when examining other neutrophil granule contents, such as myeloperoxidase (MPO) [35]. Despite their accumulation and damage of organs, neutrophils from critically ill patients display impaired transmigration and chemotaxis [25].

In recent work by our group we have demonstrated that, in patients with the severe nosocomial infection, VAP, neutrophils exhibit profound impairment of phagocytic ability and production of reactive oxygens species (ROS) [13]. However, the same neutrophils also expressed enhanced surface markers of 'activation' (elevated CD11b, CD64, decreased CD16) and induced greater inflammation in alveolar cells [13], while the patients had higher levels of plasma HNE and MPO. This dualistic dysfunction was not restricted to the plasma compartment, as alveolar neutrophils demonstrated a similar impairment in phagocytosis [13], and alveolar fluid had high levels of alveolar inflammatory cytokines [36] and the neutrophil-derived enzymes, HNE and matrix metalloproteinases (MMP) 8 and 9 [37]. This apparently paradoxical super-position of both pro-inflammatory activation and failure of key anti-microbial functions within the same cell type was illuminated by the finding that dysfunction was driven by an excess of the pro-inflammatory complement split product, C5a [13].

C5a Is a Key Mediator of Neutrophil Dysfunction

C5a is an anaphylotoxin derived from complement C5, and is released in large quantities in a variety of diseases that can precipitate critical illness including sepsis, major trauma, pancreatitis and major surgery. C5a has a range of deleterious effects when released in large quantities, including activating the coagulation system via tissue factor and stimulating the production of inflammatory cytokines, such as high mobility group box protein (HMGB)-1 [38]. C5a is also directly chemoattractive to neutrophils as well as stimulating the release of ROS and lytic enzymes, such as HNE [26]. These effects have been implicated in sepsis-associated organ damage and outcomes [39]. C5a was demonstrated to be a key mediator of neutrophil dysfunction in animal models of sepsis [27], and more recently in humans with critical illness [13, 14].

C5a has a very short plasma half-life (2–3 min), and is predominantly removed by binding to its major receptor, CD88, which is then internalized by CD88-bearing cells [40]. This can make determining C5a levels and cellular exposure difficult. However, the key finding that CD88 downregulation relates to complement exposure and correlates with neutrophil function [13, 14] allows determination of C5a mediated dysfunction in humans.

Having identified C5a as a key mediator of neutrophil dysfunction, the question arises of clinical relevance and time course. In the study of patients with suspected VAP [13] the samples were taken at the time of clinical suspicion, typically 8 days after admission to ICU and, therefore, it was not possible to determine whether C5a-mediated dysfunction preceded, or was a consequence of, nosocomial infection. In addition, although immune depression is suggested to be a late phenomenon in critical illness [12], C5a release occurs early [41]. If this hypothesis is correct, dysfunction should occur similarly early.

The correlation between CD88 and impaired phagocytosis, the hallmark of C5a-mediated neutrophil dysfunction in humans, was also found in samples taken earlier in the course of ICU admission [14], importantly before any ICU-acquired infection had occurred. Indeed, neutrophil CD88 was below levels seen in healthy volunteers in the majority of patients at study admission (i. e., <48 hours after ICU admission), with counts tending to fall further during admission suggesting ongoing complement activation. This observation was backed up by the finding of increasing C3a (a proxy measure of C5a release) among patients with neutrophil dysfunction, in contrast to static or falling levels among those without dysfunction. These findings are suggestive of ongoing complement activation in the patients with neutrophil dysfunction/low CD88.

Patients with C5a-mediated neutrophil dysfunction had a considerably higher risk of nosocomial infection (relative risk [RR] 5.4, 95 % confidence interval [CI] 1.4–21.0) than patients without dysfunction. Time-series analysis showed a significant difference between the two groups, with the dysfunction group showing a steady increase in infections over their stay whilst those without dysfunction remained relatively resistant to infection even if they remained in the ICU for some time [14].

A mechanism by which C5a impairs phagocytosis by neutrophils has recently been elucidated [13, 14]. Following ligation of CD88, the intracellular signaling system PI3 K is activated. The delta isoform then proceeds to impair activation of the small GTPase RhoA, which in turn inhibits the actin polymerization required for phagocytosis. These defects have been demonstrated in *ex vivo* C5a treated neutrophils and in those extracted from critically ill patients. Intriguingly, elevated intracellular levels of cAMP, which can arise from excessive beta-agonist stimulation, also impair phagocytosis via the same mechanism [42] although the actions of C5a are independent of cAMP [13]. Importantly, the growth factor/cytokine, granulocyte-macrophage colony-stimulating factor (GM-CSF), is able to restore RhoA activity and thus rescue phagocytic ability in neutrophils [13, 14]. This effect provides a new potential therapeutic angle and is currently being tested in a clinical trial (ClinicalTrials.gov identifier NCT01653665).

Additional Pro-inflammatory Drivers of Dysfunction

In addition to C5a, other classically 'pro-inflammatory' molecules have been shown to drive neutrophil dysfunction. Formylated peptides, such as fMLP, are found in bacterial cell walls as well as those of mitochondria. The fMLP receptor acts via the same G-coupled protein isoforms as the C5a receptor, namely the $G_{\alpha i2}$ subunit and *in vitro* can induce a similar defect in phagocytosis [13]. The recent finding of formylated peptides derived from the release of mitochondria following major trauma [43] suggests another way in which a precipitant of critical illness can induce both immune activation and hypoactivity simultaneously.

In patients with alcoholic hepatitis, another well-established cause of systemic immune activation that bears some comparison to sepsis, Mookerjee and colleagues demonstrated defects in neutrophil phagocytosis and ROS production [44]. These defects predicted the subsequent occurrence of nosocomial infections, and could be reproduced in neutrophils from healthy volunteers by application of patient plasma or directly with LPS, and blocked by extracting LPS or inhibiting the LPS receptor, CD14. LPS hyporesponsiveness in monocytes, termed monocyte deactivation, is a well-characterized component of immune suppression in sepsis [15]. As LPS can itself induce a state of deactivation in monocytes, this could induce additional immunosuppressive effects. LPS is commonly found in plasma and other body fluids from critically ill patients, even in the absence of Gram-negative infection. Indeed extracorporeal LPS absorption with polymyxin hemoperfusion has shown early promise in human sepsis [45].

Additional mediators of immune dysfunction are likely to be identified over the next few years. The alveolar space of patients with VAP demonstrates high levels of pro-inflammatory molecules [36, 37] and bronchoalveolar lavage (BAL) fluid from these patients can induce a defect in phagocytic and bactericidal functions of healthy donor neutrophils [13]. The nature of this pulmonary inhibitor is currently undetermined, although it acts in a C5a independent fashion [13].

The co-existence of immune dysfunction and inflammatory disease is not restricted to sepsis and similar precipitants of critical illness. In human immunodeficiency virus (HIV), infection activation of complement has been associated with increased C5a, reduced neutrophil CD88 and impaired neutrophil function [46]. In other diseases with a major inflammatory component, including Crohn's disease, chronic renal impairment and congestive cardiac failure, immune dysfunction is common [47, 48].

Sepsis and SIRS result not only in immune activation but also in activation of a number of other neuro-humoral systems, with the catecholamines being key mediators of the frequently seen tachycardia and hyperdynamic circulation. Exogenous catecholamines and adrenergic drugs are regularly administered to patients to reverse vasodilatation, and later stage reductions in cardiac output. Acting via beta-receptors, these hormones and drugs can impair functions of neutrophils [13] and T cells [48]. Although these effects have not been definitively demonstrated in human sepsis, it is highly likely that part of the immune suppression seen is beta-adrenergic mediated. This may explain the reductions in nosocomial infections seen in burns patients treated with propranolol [49] and some of the benefit of beta-blockers in animal models of sepsis [50].

The Influence of Multiple Immune Dysfunctions

Whilst there is growing evidence of the role of pro-inflammatory molecules directly mediating immune dysfunction, it is undoubtedly the case that a significant amount of immune failure arises from inappropriate or overly exuberant counter-regulatory anti-inflammatory responses to the primary immune activation. Elevated levels of regulatory T-cells, which inhibit T-cell proliferation, are found in sepsis and major trauma [22] and are associated with poor outcomes. Recent work has identified elevated levels of myeloid derived suppressor cells, dendritic cells and B-cells [28], although the influence of these specific findings on patient outcomes remains to be fully determined.

Immune cell dysfunctions do not occur in isolation. Our group has recently demonstrated concurrent dysfunctions of monocytes, neutrophils and T-cells in a cohort of critically ill patients [51]. Whilst 11 % of patients demonstrated no immune dysfunction, 23 % had dysfunction of 1 cell type, 45 % dysfunction of two cell types and 21 % had dysfunction across all three cell types examined. This cumulative burden of immune dysfunction was associated with a progressive increase in the risk of developing nosocomial infection, ranging from 0 % amongst patients with no dysfunction to 75 % of those with all three [51]. It is likely that the effects of immune cell dysfunction are not simply additive, but synergistic.

The field of immune failure in critical illness is relatively new, with much still to be determined. Key questions that remain include the time course of dysfunction, especially the recovery phase and whether recovery is a pre-requisite for over-all recovery from critical illness and successful discharge from hospital. Further work is required to clarify the relative contributions of different mediators of immune cell dysfunction, with this knowledge hopefully illuminating new therapeutic avenues. It can be hoped that better characterization of markers of immune failure will allow effective trials of targeted immunostimulatory and immunomodulatory therapies, and this must remain a key focus for this field.

The picture emerging from recent work on immune failure in critical illness is coming closer to describing the picture seen clinically, of systemic inflammation and inflammation-mediated organ failure coupled with significant vulnerability to nosocomial infection and death from sepsis. In a manner that can be considered analogous to disseminated intravascular coagulopathy (DIC), demonstrating both thrombosis and coagulopathy, we see a complex state of both pro and anti-inflammatory actions simultaneously and sometimes even in the same cell type.

Conclusion

Immune failure is key to understanding the pathophysiology of critical illness, and can be considered another organ failure. Some of this is failure is driven by molecules which also drive the inflammatory response (e. g., C5a, LPS, fMLP), which may explain the duality of inflammation and immune suppression, immune mediated organ failures, and susceptibility to nosocomial infection/death from sepsis. The classical conceptions of SIRS and CARS fail to adequately describe the situation at an immune cellular level. We suggest that these concepts should be refined to reflect the reality of an immune failure in which collateral host damage occurs simultaneously with markedly impaired anti-microbial defenses. The mixture of novel 'pro-inflammatory' molecules driving cellular failure, alongside over-zealous counter-regulatory processes is perhaps best described as a 'complex immune dysfunction syndrome'.

References

1. Adibconquy M, Cavaillon J (2007) Stress molecules in sepsis and systemic inflammatory response syndrome. FEBS Lett 581:3723–3733
2. Vincent JL, Bihari DJ, Suter P et al (1995) The prevalence of nosocomial infection in intensive care units in Europe. Results of the European Prevalence of Infection in Intensive Care (EPIC) Study. EPIC International Advisory Committee. JAMA 274:639–644
3. Ward PA (2011) Immunosuppression in sepsis. JAMA 306:2618–2619
4. Pellizzer G, Mantoan P, Timillero L et al (2008) Prevalence and risk factors for nosocomial infections in hospitals of the Veneto region, north-eastern Italy. Infection 36:112–119
5. Vincent JL, Rello J, Marshall J et al (2009) International study of the prevalence and outcomes of infection in intensive care units. JAMA 302:2323–2329
6. The GIMEMA Investigators (1991) Prevention of bacterial infection in neutropenic patients with hematologic malignancies. A randomized, multicenter trial comparing norfloxacin with ciprofloxacin. Ann Intern Med 115:7–12
7. Chastre J, Fagon J (2002) Ventilator-associated pneumonia. Am J Respr Crit Care Med 165:867–903
8. Sakamoto Y, Mashiko K, Matsumoto H, Hara Y, Kutsukata N, Yokota H (2010) Systemic inflammatory response syndrome score at admission predicts injury severity, organ damage and serum neutrophil elastase production in trauma patients. J Nihon Med Sch 77:138–144
9. Miyaoka K, Iwase M, Suzuki R et al (2005) Clinical evaluation of circulating interleukin-6 and interleukin-10 levels after surgery-induced inflammation. J Surg Res 125:144–150
10. Bianchi ME (2007) DAMPs, PAMPs and alarmins: all we need to know about danger. J Leuk Biol 81:1–5
11. Bone RC (1996) Sir Isaac Newton, sepsis, SIRS, and CARS. Crit Care Med 24:1125–1128
12. Hotchkiss RS, Karl IE (2003) The pathophysiology and treatment of sepsis. N Engl J Med 348:138–150
13. Morris AC, Kefala K, Wilkinson TS et al (2009) C5a mediates peripheral blood neutrophil dysfunction in critically ill patients. Am J Respir Crit Care Med 180:19–28
14. Morris AC, Brittan M, Wilkinson TS et al (2011) C5a-mediated neutrophil phagocytic dysfunction is RhoA-dependent and predicts nosocomial infection in critically ill patients. Blood 117:5178–5188
15. Döcke W, Randow F, Syrbe U et al (1997) Monocyte deactivation in septic patients: restoration by IFN-gamma treatment. Nat Med 3:678–681
16. Flohé SB, Agrawal H, Flohé S, Rani M, Bangen JM, Schade FU (2008) Diversity of interferon gamma and granulocyte-macrophage colony-stimulating factor in restoring immune dysfunction of dendritic cells and macrophages during polymicrobial sepsis. Mol Med 14:247–256

17. Yanagawa Y, Onoe K (2007) Enhanced IL-10 production by TLR4- and TLR2-primed dendritic cells upon TLR restimulation. J Immunol 178:6173–6180
18. Heidecke CD, Hensler T, Weighardt H et al (1999) Selective defects of T lymphocyte function in patients with lethal intraabdominal infection. Am J Surg 178:288–292
19. Mohr A, Polz J, Martin EM (2012) Sepsis leads to a reduced antigen-specific primary antibody response. Eur J Immunol 42:341–352
20. Souza-Fonseca-Guimaraes F, Parlato M, Fitting C, Cavaillon JM, Adib-Conquy M (2012) NK cell tolerance to TLR agonists mediated by regulatory T cells after polymicrobial sepsis. J Immunol 15:5850–5858
21. Meisel C, Schefold JC, Pschowski R et al (2009) Granulocyte-macrophage colony-stimulating factor to reverse sepsis-associated immunosuppression: A double-blind, randomized, placebo-controlled multicenter trial. Am J Respir Crit Care Med 180:640–648
22. Venet F, Chung CS, Monneret G et al (2008) Regulatory T cell populations in sepsis and trauma. J Leuk Biol 83:523–535
23. Lukaszewicz AC, Grienay M, Resche-Rigon M et al (2009) Monocytic HLA-DR expression in intensive care patients: interest for prognosis and secondary infection prediction. Crit Care Med 37:2746–2752
24. Danikas DD, Karakantza M, Theodorou GL, Sakellaropoulos GC, Gogos CA (2008) Prognostic value of phagocytic activity of neutrophils and monocytes in sepsis. Correlation to CD64 and CD14 antigen expression. Clin Exp Immunol 154:87–97
25. Arraes SM, Freitas MS, da Silva SV et al (2006) Impaired neutrophil chemotaxis in sepsis associates with GRK expression and inhibition of actin assembly and tyrosine phosphorylation. Blood 108:2906–2913
26. Ward PA (2004) The dark side of C5a in sepsis. Nat Rev Immunol 4:133–142
27. Huber-Lang M, Younkin EM, Sarma JV et al (2002) Complement-induced impairment of innate immunity during sepsis. J Immunol 169:3223–3231
28. Boomer JS, To K, Chang KC et al (2011) Immunosuppression in patients who die of sepsis and multiple organ failure. JAMA 21:2594–2605
29. Osuchowski MF, Welch K, Siddiqui J, Remick DG (2006) Circulating cytokine/inhibitor profiles reshape the understanding of the SIRS/CARS continuum in sepsis and predict mortality. J Immunol 177:1967–1974
30. Brown KA, Brain SD, Pearson JD, Edgeworth JD, Lewis SM, Treacher DF (2006) Neutrophils in development of multiple organ failure in sepsis. Lancet 368:157–169
31. Muller Kobold A, Tulleken JE, Zijlstra JG et al (2000) Leukocyte activation in sepsis; correlations with disease state and mortality. Intensive Care Med 26:883–892
32. Rosenbloom AJ, Pinsky MR, Napolitano C et al (1999) Suppression of cytokine-mediated beta2-integrin activation on circulating neutrophils in critically ill patients. J Leuk Biol 66:83–89
33. Ertel W, Jarrar D, Jochum M et al (1994) Enhanced release of elastase is not concomitant with increased secretion of granulocyte-activating cytokines in whole blood from patients with sepsis. Arch Surg 129:90–97
34. Nuijens JH, Abbink JJ, Wachtfogel YT et al (1992) Plasma elastase alpha 1-antitrypsin and lactoferrin in sepsis: evidence for neutrophils as mediators in fatal sepsis. J Lab Clin Med 119:159–168
35. Kothari N, Keshari RS, Bogra J et al (2011) Increased myeloperoxidase enzyme activity in plasma is an indicator of inflammation and onset of sepsis. J Crit Care 26:435.e1– 435.e7
36. Morris AC, Kefala K, Wilkinson TS et al (2010) Diagnostic importance of pulmonary interleukin-1 beta and interleukin-8 in ventilator-associated pneumonia. Thorax 65:201–207
37. Wilkinson TS, Morris AC, Kefala K et al (2013) Ventilator-associated pneumonia is characterized by excessive release of neutrophil proteases in the lung. Chest (in press)
38. Rittirsch D, Flierl M, Ward P (2008) Harmful molecular mechanisms in sepsis. Nat Rev Immunol 8:776–787

39. Gardinali M, Padalino P, Vesconi S et al (1992) Complement activation and polymorphonuclear neutrophil leukocyte elastase in sepsis. Correlation with severity of disease. Arch Surg 127:1219–1224
40. Oppermann M, Götze O (1994) Plasma clearance of the human C5a anaphylatoxin by binding to leucocyte C5a receptors. Immunology 82:516–521
41. Fosse E, Pillgram-Larsen J, Svennevig JL et al (1998) Complement activation in injured patients occurs immediately and is dependent on the severity of the trauma. Injury 29:509–514
42. Kamanova J, Kofronova O, Masin J et al (2008) Adenylate cyclase toxin subverts phagocyte function by RhoA inhibition and unproductive ruffling. J Immunol 181:5587–5597
43. Zhang Q, Raoof M, Chen Y et al (2010) Circulating mitochondrial DAMPs cause inflammatory responses to injury. Nature 464:104–107
44. Mookerjee R, Stadlbauer V, Lidder S et al (2007) Neutrophil dysfunction in alcoholic hepatitis superimposed on cirrhosis is reversible and predicts the outcome. Hepatology 46:831–840
45. Cruz DN, Antonelli M, Fumagalli R et al (2009) Early use of polymyxin B hemoperfusion in abdominal septic shock. JAMA 301:2445–2452
46. Meddows-Taylor S, Pendle S, Tiemessen CT (2001) Altered expression of CD88 and associated impairment of complement 5a-induced neutrophil responses in human immunodeficiency virus type 1-infected patients with and without pulmonary tuberculosis. J Infect Dis 15:662–665
47. Korzenik JR (2007) Is Crohn's disease due to defective immunity? Gut 56:2–5
48. Maisel AS (1994) Beneficial effects of metoprolol treatment in congestive heart failure. Reversal of sympathetic-induced alterations of immunologic function. Circulation 90:1774–1780
49. Jeschke MG, Norbury WB, Finnerty CC, Branski LK, Herndon DN (2007) Propranolol does not increase inflammation, sepsis, or infectious episodes in severely burned children. J Trauma 62:676–681
50. Ackland GL, Yao ST, Rudiger A et al (2010) Cardioprotection, attenuated systemic inflammation, and survival benefit of beta1-adrenoceptor blockade in severe sepsis in rats. Crit Care Med 38:388–394
51. Morris AC (2011) Unravelling the paradox, how inflammation leads to immuno-suppression and secondary infection. Journal of the Intensive Care Society 12:56–57 (abst)

Immunoglobulins in Sepsis: Which Patients will Benefit the Most?

Z. Molnár, A. Nierhaus, and F. Esen

Introduction

After decades of research, septic shock and related multiple organ dysfunction still remain the leading causes of mortality on our intensive care units (ICUs) worldwide [1]. Although in a recent large multicenter clinical trial the mortality was only 24.2 % [2], data from large international registries reveal a figure of around 50 % [1]. Searching for further treatment modalities for patients suffering from septic shock is, therefore, warranted. In addition to early stabilization of vital functions and antibiotic treatment, modulation of the immune system and the host response may be an important therapeutic approach. It has been shown that serum immunoglobulin concentrations are low during severe infection [3], and patients in septic shock with low IgG and IgM levels have higher mortality rates compared to those with normal immunoglobulin levels [4]. Polyclonal intravenous immunoglobulins (IVIGs) have been used in critical care for decades. These agents can modulate the host immune response in many ways. Several studies and meta-analyses on the use of polyclonal immunoglobulins as adjunctive therapy for sepsis have been published [5–7]. The results of each meta-analysis were very similar, showing that the reduction in mortality was greater with an IgM-enriched IVIG preparation (IgM preparation) compared to standard IVIG preparations containing

Z. Molnár
Department of Anesthesiology and Intensive Care, University of Szeged, 6. Semmelweis St, 6725 Szeged, Hungary

A. Nierhaus
Department of Critical Care, University Medical Center Hamburg-Eppendorf, Martinistr. 52, 20246 Hamburg, Germany

F. Esen (✉)
Department of Anesthesiology and Intensive Care, Medical Faculty of İstanbul, University of İstanbul, Capa Klinikleri, 34093 İstanbul, Turkey
E-mail: fesen@hisarhospital.com

J.-L. Vincent (Ed.), *Annual Update in Intensive Care and Emergency Medicine 2013*,
DOI 10.1007/978-3-642-35109-9_12,

almost only IgG (IgG preparations). A recent summary on *in vivo* and *in vitro* evidence nicely showed the superiority of the IgM preparation as compared to IgG preparations [8]. However, there are several open questions, such as the optimal timing of administration, the appropriate dose of IgM, the target population, and the relatively high cost, which limit its use [9].

The aims of this current chapter are to provide an overview on the rationale of IgM supplementation in severe sepsis and septic shock and to give the authors' opinion on the target patient population who may benefit most from this treatment.

Rationale for IgM Supplementation in Sepsis

Based on the differences in the amino acid sequences in the constant region of the heavy chains, immunoglobulins can be divided into five different classes: IgG, IgM, IgA, IgD and IgE. Each immunoglobulin class differs markedly from the others in its physical and biological properties. IgM is the first class of antibody to be produced in the immune response. It is a larger molecule compared to IgG, and is present in the serum in concentrations 8–10 times lower than those of IgG. Moreover, the half-life of the smaller IgG molecule is four times longer than that of the large IgM molecule. Studies of mice deficient in secreted IgM have provided unexpected insights into its role in several diverse processes, from B cell survival to atherosclerosis, as well as in autoimmunity and protection against infection. IgM has stronger phagocytosis promoting activity as compared to IgG, which has been known for more than 50 years [10]. Among the various distinct properties that underlie the functions of IgM, two stand out: Its polyreactivity and its ability to facilitate the removal of apoptotic cells. In addition, new B cell-targeted therapies for the treatment of autoimmunity have been shown to cause a reduction in serum IgM, potentially disrupting the functions of this immunoregulatory molecule and increasing susceptibility to infection [11]. Another important effect of IgM is to protect from the endotoxin burst after successful antibiotic treatment [12]. The principal modes of action of IgM with respect to its antibacterial activity are summarized in Fig. 1.

Since the first publication of successful IVIG treatment of a child with idiopathic thrombocytopenic purpura in 1981, IVIG has been shown to be effective in several autoimmune and systemic inflammatory conditions, mainly in hematology and neurology [13, 14]. For IgM substitution, an intravenous IgM preparation (Pentaglobin, Biotest, Germany) was developed and introduced into clinical use in 1985 with a relative composition of 76 % IgG, 12 % IgA and 12 % IgM.

The intravenous IgM preparation was first investigated in 1991, in a homogeneous (medical) septic patient population [15]. Sixty-nine patients in septic shock with high endotoxin levels were randomized to receive IgM-preparation or placebo. The study was discontinued after an interim analysis of data, because the difference between the mortality rates (4 % vs. 32 %) was statistically significant in favor of the IgM group. Another prospective, randomized controlled study in a

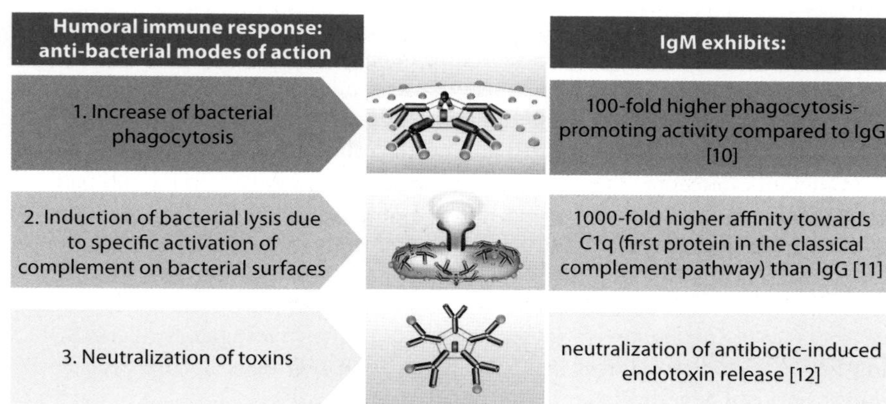
Humoral immune response:
anti-bacterial modes of action
IgM exhibits:
1. Increase of bacterial phagocytosis
100-fold higher phagocytosis-promoting activity compared to IgG [10]
2. Induction of bacterial lysis due to specific activation of complement on bacterial surfaces
1000-fold higher affinity towards C1q (first protein in the classical complement pathway) than IgG [11]
3. Neutralization of toxins
neutralization of antibiotic-induced endotoxin release [12]

Fig. 1 The role of IgM in the humoral immune response

mixed medical and surgical patient population evaluated the effect of IgM treatment on the progression of organ function and sepsis [16]. Serial measurements of procalcitonin (PCT) levels, APACHE II and sequential organ failure assessment (SOFA) scores were monitored over 8 days. PCT levels showed a statistically significant decrease in the treatment group ($p < 0.001$) but improvement in SOFA and APACHE II scores could not be demonstrated. Septic shock incidence (38 % vs. 57 %) and 28-day mortality rates (23.8 % vs. 33.3 %) were lower in the IgM-treated group but did not reach significance. Interpretation of these results is difficult because of the small sample size. In a similar study including 68 patients with septic shock, a significant mortality reduction (22 % vs. 40 %) in the IgM-treatment arm was reported [17]. Patients in the intervention group had higher APACHE II scores as compared to controls (21.27 ± 7.23 vs. 10.5 ± 4.6), which may serve as an explanation for the difference in mortality between these two studies. Rodríguez et al. [18] assessed the impact on outcome of adjuvant therapy with a high-dose IgM preparation in critically ill patients who underwent surgery for intra-abdominal sepsis. In this multicenter, prospective trial, 56 patients with severe sepsis and septic shock of intra-abdominal origin were randomized within 24 hours after the onset of symptoms. The administration of Pentaglobin in addition to antibiotic therapy was associated with a 20 % mortality reduction in the intent-to-treat analysis. The lack of significant difference in the mortality rate between the two groups may be attributable to the small sample size. In the subset of patients who received adequate antibiotic therapy, a significant reduction in mortality for the IgM-treated group was found, with reductions in the relative and absolute risk of death of 74 and 25 %, respectively.

More recently, Hentrich et al. [19] investigated the role of intravenous Pentaglobin in neutropenic patients with severe sepsis and septic shock. In the largest trial on the use of polyclonal immunoglobulin ($n = 211$), they failed to document any benefit of IVIG therapy based on 28-day mortality rate. The main criticism of this clinical investigation is that most of the patients were low grade septic patients showing none or one organ failure with a relatively low mortality suggesting that these patients are not a target population for IVIG treatment.

The results from two large prospective randomized controlled studies on the effects of IgG treatment in septic patients (Score-based Immunoglobulin Treatment in Sepsis [SBITS] study) [20] and post-cardiac surgery patients with severe systemic inflammatory response syndrome (ESSICS study) [21] have recently been published by the same group. The SBITS study revealed no reduction in mortality with administration of IgG in the total study population or in subgroups. Given the statistical power, the study does not nourish hope for IVIG therapy in septic patients. These results were further supported by the second study on post-cardiac surgery patients with severe sepsis [21]. The investigators of the SBITS and ESSICS studies claimed that this failure with IgG does not necessarily exclude a survival benefit shown by IgM preparations.

The strongest recommendation for IgG and IgM treatment in sepsis is based on four meta-analyses published over the last 10 years [5–7, 22]. In the latest meta-analysis performed by the Cochrane group and published in 2010, 84 studies were screened, of which 42 were excluded. Of the remaining 42 trials, polyclonal IgG preparations were administered to adults in 10 trials (n = 1,430) and 7 trials used the IgM preparation (n = 528). The meta-analysis showed significant reductions in mortality compared to placebo or no intervention, with a relative risk reduction in the IgM-treated group vs. placebo (RR = 0.66, 95 % CI 0.51–0.85).

These data represent current clinical evidence regarding the rationale for IgM treatment in sepsis. Regarding guidelines, the Surviving Sepsis Campaign [23] did not mention IgM treatment in adults, whereas the German sepsis guideline gives a "C" degree recommendation that IgM preparations may be considered in severe sepsis and septic shock, but not IgG preparations [24].

Who Would Benefit the Most From IgM at What Point in Time?

Most sepsis trials recruit patients based simply on the American College of Chest Physicians/Society of Critical Care Medicine (ACCP/SCCM) consensus definitions [25], but whether this is the best approach has been a subject of debate in recent years. Can we regard septic shock due to peritonitis after surgery as identical to that caused by pneumonia? Is there an exact diagnostic measure to capture the moment when systemic inflammatory response syndrome (SIRS), infection, sepsis, severe sepsis or septic shock occurs? According to a recent study, there is a significant difference in the PCT value between medical and surgical patients fulfilling the same consensus criteria, SIRS: 0.33 (0.13–1) vs. 5.70 (2.65–8.35), septic shock: 8.4 (3.63–76) vs. 34 (7.1–76) ng/ml [26]. It was also reported that there was a significant difference between the best cut-off values to differentiate between survivors and non-survivors in medical vs. surgical patients: 1 ng/ml (80 % sensitivity, 94 % specificity) and 6 ng/ml (76 % sensitivity, 72.7 % specificity), respectively. The same consensus criteria were fulfilled in both patient groups with a completely different inflammatory response and outcome. Therefore, one cannot regard sepsis as a homogeneous disease. This uncertainty may have led to inhomogeneous groups of patients in several clinical trials with selection bias, sampling error, and eventually failure to produce significant results [27, 28]. This effect may also explain why disease severity and mortality rates tend to be higher in registries or databases (i. e., in reality) than in clinical trials [1].

If the indication to administer IgM was based simply on the above mentioned consensus criteria of 'septic shock', it would lead to a multitude of patients receiving IVIG (most of them unnecessarily), which would impose great financial strains on many ICUs. There are studies which used a more complex severity scoring system instead of the consensus criteria, one of which is the SBITS study [20]. Unfortunately, although it is the largest prospective randomized immunoglobulin study to date (n=653), the drug investigated was an IgG preparation and not an IgM preparation. Another limitation of the results is that the study was performed in the early 1990 s (published years later in 2007), and many therapeutic and diagnostic concepts have changed fundamentally since then, making the results difficult to apply to current practice.

Inflammatory markers, such as PCT [16, 29], or immunoglobulin levels [4] have also been suggested or investigated as biologically plausible indicators of those patients who may benefit from IgM treatment. PCT is a reliable sepsis marker and prognostic factor, and may also have use in differentiating between etiologies [26]; thus it may have useful additional value in patient selection. Unfortunately, PCT-assisted or guided IgM treatment has not been investigated yet. Although it has been reported that patients with low immunoglobulin levels had higher mortality rates than patients with normal concentrations [4], the results of this study are difficult to apply in everyday practice for several reasons. The study was performed on 21 patients only, with 12 in the hypo-IgG and 9 in the normal IgG group. Furthermore, it is difficult to know whether the low IgG was related to a pre-existing condition, and we know nothing about the kinetics of immunoglobulin levels in acute illness; therefore, interpreting a single admission value remains difficult.

Regarding the timing of IgM treatment, a recent retrospective study found that survivors received treatment with the IgM preparation significantly earlier (23 vs. 62 h) [30]. In the study by Rodríguez et al. [18] patients also received the IgM preparation within 24 hours after surgery.

Despite the controversies regarding the indications for IgM treatment in sepsis, IgM has been used for more than two decades in several countries and hundreds of ICUs without clear evidence or guidelines. Therefore, we tried to develop a consensus, using published data and unpublished own audits and adapting our own clinical practice and experience of more than 10 years of IgM use, in order to give a recommendation on who would, in our view, benefit the most from IgM treatment (Table 1 [18, 19, 28]). The first element of this concept is severity. Rather than using any of the consensus criteria or severity scores, we suggest to consider treatment once early resuscitation/stabilization is finished, antibiotic treatment has been started, but the patient is not improving clinically, i. e., vasopressor require-

Table 1 Suggested target patients for treatment with IgM-enriched preparations

Requirements	Comments and Concepts	Reference
Severity	Persistence of septic shock or severe sepsis with > 2 organ dysfunctions after initial resuscitation/treatment	Heintrich et al. [19] Expert opinion
Timing	As early as possible. Best effects are expected if treatment is initiated within the first 8 h of sepsis.	Berlot et al. [28]
	Late start of treatment (48 h) is not recommended.	Expert opinion
Target groups/subgroups with the highest benefit probability	Abdominal infections in surgical patients (peritonitis) presumably Gram-negative bacterial infections	Rodriguez et al. [18]
	Meningococcal sepsis Toxic shock syndrome Overwhelming post splenectomy infection Necrotizing fasciitis	Expert opinion
Dosage (80 kg)	50 ml/h for the first 6 h (15 g), followed by 15 ml/h for 72 h (54 g), daily re-evaluation	Expert opinion
Exclusion criteria	Standing DNR order or limitation of therapy, incurable metastatic malignant disease, neutropenia due to hematological malignancies and according to SPC	Expert opinion

DNR: do-not-resuscitate; SPC: summary of product characteristics

ments are still increasing or cannot be reduced, and there are still at least two failing organs [19]. The second issue is timing. IgM should be started as early as possible to help the initial fight against infection [28], and we do not recommend its use after 48 hours, as by that time there are too many confounding factors, hence benefit is not expected. The third issue is the etiology of sepsis. We do not believe that "all sepsis is the same", therefore we have listed five target groups that are most likely to benefit. There is some evidence that in peritonitis after surgery due to Gram-negative infections, mortality can be dramatically reduced by early IgM treatment [18]. The other four conditions are the most common reasons for fulminant sepsis; hence, we suggest early administration of IgM. We also suggest dosages and which patients who should be excluded as candidates for the treatment.

Conclusion

The positive results of clinical trials published so far suggest that IgM-preparations have a definite role in sepsis treatment, and many reviews and meta-analyses have been published over the years addressing the beneficial effects of IVIGs.

However, which subgroup of patients with sepsis will benefit most remains to be shown. Without more evidence and based on the best of our knowledge and clinical experience, it seems reasonable to assume that the early administration of IgM in sufficiently sick patients will result in the greatest benefit.

Acknowledgement: The authors would like to thank Professor Giorgio Berlot, PD Dr. Henning Ebelt and Professor Massimo Girardis for sharing their results and experience with us, without which this article could not have been completed.

References

1. Martin G, Brunkhorst FM, Janes JM et al (2009) The international PROGRESS registry of patients with severe sepsis: drotrecogin alfa (activated) use and patient outcomes. Crit Care 13:R103
2. Ranieri VM, Thompson BT, Barie PS et al (2012) Drotrecogin alfa (activated) in adults with septic shock. N Engl J Med 366:2055–2064
3. Werdan K (2001) Pathophysiology of septic shock and multiple organ dysfunction syndrome and various therapeutic approaches with special emphasis on immunoglobulins. Ther Apher 5:115–122
4. Taccone FS, Stordeur P, De Backer D, Creteur J, Vincent JL (2009) γ-globulin levels in patients with community-acquired septic shock. Shock 32:379–385
5. Alejandria MM, Lansang MA, Dans LF, Mantaring JB (2002) Intravenous immunoglobulin for treating sepsis and septic shock. Cochrane Database Syst Rev CD0011090
6. Kreymann KG, de Heer G, Nierhaus A, Kluge S (2007) Use of polyclonal immunoglobulins as adjunctive therapy for sepsis or septic shock. Crit Care Med 35:2677–2685
7. Laupland KB, Kirkpatrick AW, Delaney A (2007) Polyclonal intravenous immunoglobulin for the treatment of severe sepsis and septic shock in critically ill adults: a systematic review and meta-analysis. Crit Care Med 35:2686–2692
8. Esen F, Tugrul S (2009) IgM enriched immunoglobulins in sepsis. In: Vincent JL (ed) Yearbook of Intensive Care and Emergency Medicine. Springer-Verlag, Berlin, pp 102–110
9. Neugebauer EAM (2007) To use or not to use? Polyclonal intravenous immunoglobulins for the treatment of sepsis and septic shock. Crit Care Med 35:2855
10. Cohen S, Porter RB (1964) Structure and biological activity of immunoglobulins. Adv Immunol 27:287–349
11. Ehrenstein MR, Notley CA (2010) The importance of natural IgM: scavenger, protector and regulator. Nat Rev Immunol 10:778–786
12. Oesser S, Schulze C, Seifert J (1999) Protective capacity of a IgM/IgA-enriched polyclonal immunoglobulin-G preparation in endotoxemia. Res Exp Med (Berl) 198:325–339
13. Imbach P, Barandun S, d'Apuzzo V et al (1981) High-dose intravenous gammaglobulin for idiopathic thrombocytopenic purpura in childhood. Lancet 1:1228–1231
14. Harvey III RD (2005) The patient: emerging clinical applications of intravenous immunoglobulins. Pharmacotherapy 25:85S–93S
15. Schedel I, Dreikhausen U, Nentwig B et al (1991) Treatment of gram-negative septic shock with an immunoglobulin preparation: A prospective, randomised clinical trial. Crit Care Med 19:1104–1113
16. Tugrul S, Ozcan PE, Akinci O et al (2002) The effects of IgM-enriched immunoglobulin preparations in patients with severe sepsis. Crit Care 6:357–362
17. Karatzas S, Boutzouka E, Venetsanou K et al (2002) The effect of IgM-enriched immunoglobulin preparations in patients with severe sepsis: another point of view. Crit Care 6:543–544

18. Rodríguez A, Rello J, Neira J et al (2005) Effects of high dose of intravenous immunoglobulin and antibiotics on survival for severe sepsis undergoing surgery. Shock 23:298–304
19. Hentrich M, Fehnle K, Ostermann H et al (2006) IgMA-enriched immunoglobulin in neutropenic patients with sepsis syndrome and septic shock: A randomized, controlled, multiple-center trial. Crit Care Med 34:1319–1325
20. Werdan K, Pilz G, Bujdoso O et al (2007) Score-based immunoglobulin G therapy of patients with sepsis: the SBITS study. Crit Care Med 35:2693–2701
21. Werdan K, Pilz G, Müller-Werdan U et al (2008) Immunoglobulin G treatment of postcardiac surgery patients with score-identified severe systemic inflammatory response syndrome – the ESSICS study. Crit Care Med 36:716–723
22. Alejandria MM, Lansang MAD, Dans LF, Mantaring III JB (2010) Intravenous immunoglobulin for treating sepsis, severe sepsis and septic shock (update 2010). Cochrane Database Syst Rev (2):CD001090
23. Dellinger RP, Levy MM, Carlet JM et al (2008) Surviving Sepsis Campaign: International guidelines for management of severe sepsis and septic shock: 2008. Intensive Care Med 34:17–60
24. Reinhart K, Brunkhorst FM, Bone H-G et al (2010) Prevention, diagnosis, therapy and follow-up care of sepsis: 1st revision of S-2k guidelines of the German Sepsis Society (Deutsche Sepsis-Gesellschaft e.V. (DSG)) and the German Interdisciplinary Association of Intensive Care and Emergency Medicine (Deutsche Interdisziplinäre Vereinigung für Intensiv- und Notfallmedizin (DIVI)). GMS German Medical Science 8:1612–3174
25. American College of Chest Physicians – Society of Critical Care Medicine (1992) Consensus Conference: Definitions for sepsis and organ failure and guidelines for the use of innovative therapies in sepsis. Crit Care Med 20:864–875
26. Clec'h C, Fosse JP, Karoubi P et al (2006) Differential diagnostic value of procalcitonin in surgical and medical patients with septic shock. Crit Care Med 34:102–107
27. Cohen J (1999) The "failure" of clinical trials in sepsis. Curr Opin Crit Care 330:339–340
28. Vincent JL (2010) We should abandon randomized controlled trials in the intensive care unit. Crit Care Med 38(Suppl):S534–S538
29. Molnar Z, Fogas J (2012) Timing IgM treatment in sepsis: is procalcitonin the answer? In: Vincent JL (ed) Annual Update in Intensive Care and Emergency Medicine 2012. Springer-Verlag, Berlin, pp 109–115
30. Berlot G, Vassallo MC, Busetto N et al (2012) Relationship between the timing of administration of IgM and IgA enriched immunoglobulins in patients with severe sepsis and septic shock and the outcome: A retrospective analysis. J Crit Care 27:167–171

Macrophage Migration Inhibitory Factor in Critical Illness: Dr. Jekyll and Mr. Hyde?

C. Stoppe, J. Bernhagen, and S. Rex

Introduction

In critically ill patients, sepsis and its sequelae belong to the leading causes of death world-wide. During the last decades, the incidence of sepsis has been constantly increasing [1, 2]. Apart from the administration of antibiotics, treatment of sepsis still comprises mainly supportive strategies (including fluid resuscitation and administration of vasopressors). Several promising pharmacotherapeutic approaches failed to show beneficial effects, such as the inhibition of tumor necrosis factor (TNF)-α, the modulation of relative adrenal insufficiency and the administration of activated protein C [3–5].

Interestingly, neutralization of macrophage migration inhibitory factor (MIF) activity belongs to the rare therapies that have been shown to effectively reduce mortality from septic shock in an animal model [6, 7]. In contrast, increasing evidence suggests that MIF might paradoxically exhibit beneficial and protective effects in the setting of ischemia-reperfusion injury, but also in certain infectious diseases [8–11]. Given the central role of MIF within the innate immune response, pathogenesis of sepsis and ischemia-reperfusion injury, it is tempting to speculate

C. Stoppe (✉)
Institute of Biochemistry and Molecular Cell Biology, RWTH Aachen University, Pauwelsstraße 30, 52074 Aachen, Germany
E-mail: christian.stoppe@gmail.com

J. Bernhagen
Institute of Biochemistry and Molecular Cell Biology, RWTH Aachen University, Pauwelsstraße 30, 52074 Aachen, Germany

S. Rex
Department of Anesthesiology, University Hospitals Gasthuisberg, KU Leuven, Herestraat 49, 3000 Leuven, Belgium

J.-L. Vincent (Ed.), *Annual Update in Intensive Care and Emergency Medicine 2013*,
DOI 10.1007/978-3-642-35109-9_13,

that, in future, modulating MIF release may represent a fascinating pharmacological approach for various pathological conditions in which inflammatory pathways are critically involved.

Macrophage Migration Inhibitory Factor: Its Functional Role Within the Immune System

The innate immune system belongs to the first line of defense mechanisms against microbial infections and is immediately activated when a pathogenic stimulus passes the host's natural defense barriers [12]. The initial detection of invasive pathogens is carried out by sentinel cells of the innate immune system, which are located in tissues with direct environmental contact. Binding of pathogen-associated molecular patterns (PAMPs) to pattern recognition receptors, such as Toll-like receptors (TLR), activates signal transduction pathways and transcription of various immune genes, resulting in the release of immuno-regulatory molecules [12], amongst which cytokines represent the most powerful effector molecules.

Cytokines play a pivotal role in orchestrating the cellular and humoral immune response to infectious stimuli. Animals in which genes encoding cytokines or cytokine receptors are mutated or deleted show an increased susceptibility to infection [13]. In contrast, the uncontrolled release of pro-inflammatory mediators might result in a life-threatening overwhelming inflammatory response that is known to be associated with severe complications and fatal outcome in patients with sepsis and septic shock [14].

MIF was one of the first inflammatory mediators to be discovered about half a century ago by David, who described its cytokine-like characteristics [15]. He demonstrated inhibitory effects of MIF on random cell migration *in vitro* – hence the name "macrophage migration inhibitory factor". It took until 1993, for MIF to be 're-discovered' as a cytokine released from the pituitary gland after exposure to endotoxins (lipopolysaccharide, LPS), serving to regulate the neuro-inflammatory response to infectious stimuli [16]. Subsequently, animal studies demonstrated that immunoneutralization of MIF protected mice from endotoxin shock and revealed that MIF counter-regulates the immunosuppressive and protective effects of glucocorticoids [16, 17]. These observations resulted in the suggestion that the severity of endotoxin shock is at least partially determined by the balance between (anti-inflammatory) glucocorticoids and circulating (pro-inflammatory) MIF levels. MIF thus was a previously unrecognized endogenous antagonist of the anti-inflammatory action of glucocorticoids. Under the assumption that MIF might represent an important cross-link between the endocrine and immune system, several studies emerged investigating the role of MIF within the inflammatory response [13]. These studies revealed that the pro-inflammatory effects of MIF are mediated by signal transduction initiated on binding to the major histocompatibility complex, class-II invariant chain, CD74 [18] (Fig. 1).

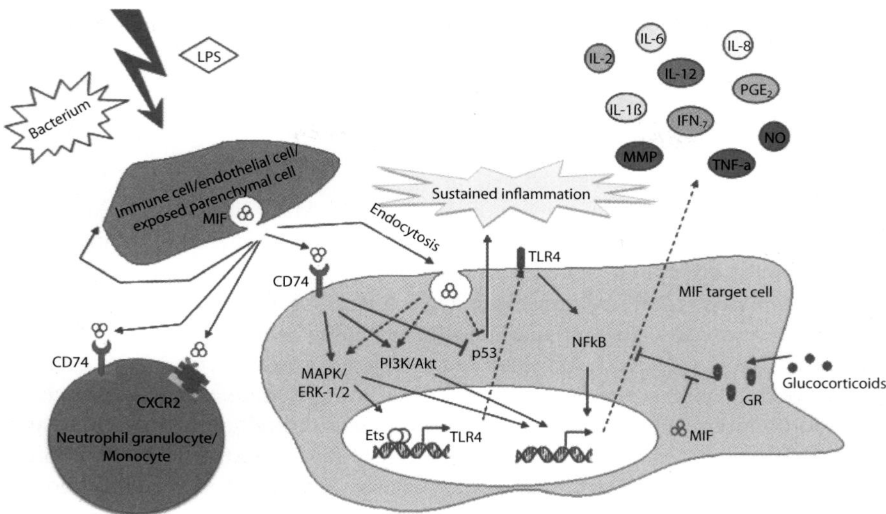

Fig. 1 Schematic illustration of macrophage migration inhibitory factor (MIF) secretion after an initial pathogen stimulus. MIF binds to the CD74-receptor (classical receptor mediated pathway) or undergoes endocytosis (non-classical endocytic pathway) and leads to the activation of different pro-inflammatory pathways with the release of various cytokines, inhibition of glucocorticoid induced anti-inflammatory effects and inhibition of apoptosis. Moreover, MIF promotes leukocyte recruitment to the inflammatory site (probably mostly neutrophils through the G-protein coupled chemokine receptor 2 [CXCR2] and monocytes through CXCR2 and CXCR2/CD74 complexes). For further explanations, see text. LPS: lipopolysaccharide; Ets: transcription factor E-twenty six; TLR4: Toll-like receptor 4; MAPK: mitogen-activated protein kinase; MMP: matrix metalloproteinases; ERK: extracellular signal-regulated kinase; PI3K: phosphatidylinositol 3-kinase; Akt: protein B kinase; IL: interleukin; TNF: tumor necrosis factor; NO: nitric oxide; MMP: matrix metalloproteinase; PG: prostaglandin; GR: glucocorticoid receptor

MIF not only interacts with CD74, but also has high affinity interactions with the chemokine receptors, CXCR2 and CXCR4. MIF-mediated activation of CXCR2 and CXCR4 exhibits chemokine-like functions and has been identified to regulate leukocyte recruitment into infectious and inflammatory sites. In addition, MIF has been shown to be critically involved in the inflammatory pathogenesis of experimental atherosclerosis [19]. Whether MIF, in addition to interacting with CD74, CXCR2 and CXCR4, also binds to a specific cognate MIF-receptor remains unknown.

Studies have demonstrated that MIF regulates the production and release of TNF-α, interleukin (IL)-1β, IL-2, IL-6, IL-8, IL-12, interferon (IFN)-γ [13, 20–22], nitric oxide (NO) [13], matrix metalloproteinase [23] and prostaglandin E_2 (PGE_2) [24]. As a proof of principle, the genetic deletion of MIF results in a significantly reduced release of inflammatory mediators, such as TNF-α, IL-1β and PGE_2, from macrophages [20, 24]. MIF is, therefore, considered to be one of the most important upstream regulators of the innate immune reaction.

The fact that MIF is stored in preformed vesicles in the cytosol in various cell types (macrophages, dendritic cells, B- and T-cells) [13] and rapidly released upon pathogen stimulus [19], further underlines MIF's unique role within the inflammatory response. In particular, the cytosolic storage of MIF profoundly distinguishes MIF from other inflammatory cytokines that require transcriptional activation and mRNA translation before release [25].

MIF has several distinctive functional properties. MIF regulates the expression of TLR4, thereby facilitating the sensing of pathogens [26]. Furthermore, MIF controls cell cycling, cell growth and apoptosis by activation of 'pro-survival kinases', such as extracellular signal-regulated kinase-1/2 (ERK1/2) [27] as well as by regulation of the c-Jun activation domain binding protein (JAB) 1/COP9 signalosome subunit (CSN) 5, and the tumor suppressor protein, p53 [13]. ERK1/2 represents a specific subset of the mammalian mitogen-activated protein kinases (MAPK) family, which are ubiquitously expressed intracellular signaling kinases critically involved in the regulation of cell cycling by activating transcription factors and/or some downstream protein kinases. The c-Jun N-terminal kinases (JNK) modulate various cellular functions, including proliferation, differentiation and apoptosis. Recently, Lue and colleagues [28] reported that rapid stimulation of the JNK signaling pathway is mediated through CXCR4 and co-dependent on CD74 in T cells and fibroblasts. Given the fact that MIF blocks JNK-mediated apoptosis [10], Lue and colleagues suggest that MIF can promote inflammatory response in a JNK-dependent manner [28].

Elevated MIF levels inhibit accumulation of p53 in the cytoplasm of macrophages, promoting an enhanced survival of monocytes/macrophages and a sustained pro-inflammatory action by the increased production of TNF-α, IL-1β and PGE_2 [23], allowing more efficient eradication of pathogens. On the other hand, if unbalanced, these effects might soon become harmful and contribute to the development of shock [20, 23]. In fact, immuno-neutralization or genetic deletion of MIF is known to protect mice from both endotoxin and exotoxin shock [16, 23].

MIF in Infectious and Acute Inflammatory Diseases

Circulating values of MIF in healthy persons range between 2 to 10 ng/ml and follow a circadian rhythm that mimics the rhythm of plasma cortisol and peaks at approximately 8 a.m. [29]. In contrast, circulating MIF levels are elevated in patients with sepsis and septic shock due to massive release from immune cells during the inflammatory response, reaching median concentrations up to 18 ng/ml (6.6–154.4 ng/ml) and differing significantly from healthy controls [6, 13]. Upon the recognition of pathogens, MIF is secreted from monocytes, macrophages, dendritic cells, T- and B-cells, neutrophils, eosinophils, basophils or mast cells, but is also expressed in tissues with environmental contact, such as the lungs and the gastrointestinal tract [13].

The first reports indicating a pivotal role of MIF within the pathophysiology of sepsis go back to investigations in 1993 when Bernhagen and colleagues observed major MIF release after stimulation with LPS in an animal model [6, 16]. Calandra et al. also reported an overwhelming increase in circulating MIF levels in patients with severe sepsis and septic shock [6]. Beishuizen et al. confirmed these data and found significantly higher MIF values in non-survivors compared to survivors from septic shock [30]. Moreover, elevated MIF values were described to predict worsening of outcome [20] and mortality in septic shock [7]. Gando and colleagues [31] found high circulating MIF levels in septic patients with disseminated intravascular coagulation (DIC) that were correlated with soluble fibrin levels. MIF might, therefore, be crucially involved in thrombotic processes in septic patients with DIC.

MIF is known to exhibit antioxidant properties [11, 32], comparable to thioredoxin-1 (Trx). Elevated plasma levels of Trx and MIF have been shown to correlate in septic patients and have been suggested to contribute to redox homeostasis and to counteract oxidative stress [33].

Considering central nervous system (CNS) infections, MIF has been shown to be markedly increased in patients with meningococcal disease [34], in whom MIF values correlated with illness severity, and were extremely elevated in patients with shock. Levels of MIF were significantly increased in the cerebrospinal fluid (CSF) from patients with meningitis and encephalitis. Likewise, Østergaard and Benfield observed an association between elevated MIF levels and severity of illness in patients with cerebral infections [35]. Recently, Renner and colleagues suggested that MIF gene polymorphisms might affect the occurrence, severity and outcome of children with meningococcal disease [36].

Moreover, elevated MIF levels have been reported in patients with acute pancreatitis and pancreatic necrosis. Of note, MIF values within 24 hours after the onset of pain were found to be an independent predictor for the development of pancreatic necrosis [37].

In urinary tract infections, Otukesh and colleagues [38] attempted to differentiate upper and lower urinary tract involvement in children. Interestingly, the MIF/creatinine ratio was significantly lower in patients with acute cystitis compared to those with pyelonephritis, which may reflect infiltration of kidneys by immune cells [38].

MIF has also been shown to play a key role in the inflammatory response in acute respiratory distress syndrome (ARDS). Within the lungs, MIF is constitutively expressed by alveolar macrophages, the bronchial epithelium, and the alveolar capillary endothelium. Patients with ARDS exhibit significantly higher MIF levels in bronchoalveolar (BAL) fluid compared to healthy control patients [21]. Likewise, elevated MIF levels were found in BAL fluid in a model of LPS-induced lung injury. Immunoneutralization of MIF reduces the secretion of TNF and IL-8 and decreases neutrophil accumulation, suggesting that MIF can control neutrophil infiltration in the lungs and promote the pulmonary inflammatory response in ARDS [39].

Given the cumulating evidence indicating a pivotal role for MIF in the pathophysiology of infection and sepsis, MIF is emerging as a promising target for therapies modulating the inflammatory response in patients with sepsis and septic shock. Of note, MIF levels were found to remain elevated over a time span of several days in septic patients. This facet might provide a wide window for therapeutic administration of anti-MIF antibodies and is in apparent contrast to previous futile strategies that aimed to inhibit TNF-α and IL-1 in septic patients [3]. It can be speculated that – owing to the different kinetic characteristics of the various cytokines, with a rapid decrease in TNF-α and IL-1 – treatments aimed at antagonizing cytokines were applied too late, as circulating levels of TNF-α and IL-1 had already returned to baseline values. Interestingly, Calandra et al. demonstrated that anti-MIF treatment protected mice from lethal peritonitis even if administered up to 8 hours after cecal ligation and puncture [6].

Notwithstanding, it has to be acknowledged that recently reported findings paradoxically suggest a potentially beneficial role of MIF in certain conditions and time windows. Pollak et al. demonstrated increased susceptibility to bacterial superinfection after MIF neutralization in a murine model of peritonitis [40]. Yende and colleagues demonstrated that polymorphisms associated with higher MIF gene expression are associated with a survival benefit in patients with community acquired pneumonia [41]. These intriguing findings preclude widespread generalization of the above-reported findings in septic patients and indicate that the ambiguous role of MIF values has to be interpreted cautiously within the context of different clinical settings.

The Value of MIF as a Biomarker in SIRS and Sepsis

Various studies have demonstrated that circulating MIF levels correlate with the severity of illness and predict clinical outcome in septic patients (see above) [13, 21, 30–36]. Several investigators have specifically addressed the question as to whether determinations of MIF levels might be able to differentiate between non-infectious and infectious origins of inflammatory disease. Lehmann et al. found postoperative MIF release to be significantly increased but comparable in patients with infectious and non-infectious inflammation [42]. In contrast, in patients undergoing cardiac surgery with the use of cardiopulmonary bypass (CPB), de Mendonça-Filho and colleagues demonstrated that postoperative MIF values were increased and significantly higher in patients who developed septic complications with microbiological proven infection [43].

Kofoed and colleagues [44] found that circulating MIF values fairly predicted culture-proven bacteremia, but had only limited diagnostic power to discriminate between bacterial and non-bacterial causes of sepsis when compared to procalcitonin (PCT) and C-reactive protein (CRP). Of note, the predictive value could be significantly increased by the combination of different markers [44]. In patients with severe burn injury, Grieb and colleagues reported that combined determination of MIF and PCT was useful for discriminating between post-burn inflammation in survivors and systemic inflammatory response syndrome (SIRS) or sepsis with lethal outcome [45].

Although previous studies have repeatedly reported that MIF is critically involved in the development of organ dysfunction and associated with bad outcome in the critically ill patient, the diagnostic value of MIF is still controversial. The reasons might be due to the heterogeneous patient populations included in the various trials and to the large variance in inflammatory responses. The controversy can also be attributed to the fact that MIF exerts ambiguous and contradicting effects. Whether perioperative determination of MIF may provide helpful information, therefore, has to be clarified in larger and preferably multicenter studies.

MIF in Myocardial Ischemia-Reperfusion Injury

Within the myocardium, MIF has also been shown to be induced by endotoxins, to initiate the release of various pro-inflammatory cytokines, to induce apoptosis of cardiomyocytes and to promote cardiac dysfunction in sepsis and endotoxemia. Inhibition of MIF's pro-inflammatory activities resulted in an improvement of cardiomyocyte survival and myocardial function [46]. One study also suggested that during myocardial ischemia-reperfusion injury, MIF exacerbates ischemic tissue damage [47].

However, an increasing body of evidence has revealed various protective mechanisms of MIF in the setting of myocardial ischemia-reperfusion injury (Table 1, Fig. 2) [9–11, 13, 18, 34, 45, 48, 49]: First, MIF release from stores within cardiomyocytes activates adenosine monophosphate-activated protein kinase (AMPK) in an autocrine/paracrine manner [9]. The activation of AMPK exerts cardioprotective effects by activating anaerobic glycolysis in the ischemic heart, initiating glucose transporter-4 translocation, increasing glucose uptake and resulting in reduced myocardial damage and apoptosis. Second, the release of endogenous MIF from cardiomyocytes is known to inhibit the activation of the JNK pathway [10]. The JNK pathway regulates essential processes such as inflammation, cell differentiation and apoptosis and thus promotes myocardial damage in ischemia-reperfusion injury. In fact, animal studies with MIF-knockout mouse hearts showed increased myocardial necrosis and apoptosis when compared to MIF wild-type mice [10]. Third, MIF is known to promote neovascularization during hypoxia [50], which may be of particular interest in patients with myocardial infarction or undergoing cardiac surgery. Herein, myocardial tissue regularly suffers from oxygen undersupply, which may be compensated for by promoting neovascularization. Fourth, MIF protects against oxidative stress resulting from ischemia-reperfusion injury in myocardial infarction owing to its intrinsic thiolprotein oxidoreductase activity [32].

Stoppe et al. recently reported possible cardioprotective effects of MIF in cardiac surgical patients [8]. Cardiac surgery with the use of CPB provokes myocardial ischemia-reperfusion injury, which contributes to perioperative inflammation and morbidity/mortality. Interestingly, MIF levels reached peak values at admis-

Table 1 Overview of macrophage migration inhibitory factor (MIF)-dependent mechanisms that provide protective effects during myocardial ischemia and reperfusion injury

Pathophysiological condition	MIF activity	Net effect	References
Acute myocardial infarction	Increased MIF levels	Unknown	[48]
Resuscitation after out of hospital cardiac arrest	Increased MIF levels after ROSC with early decrease	Unknown	[49]
Cardiac surgery	Perioperative increase with early decrease after termination of surgery	MIF levels after termination of surgery: – inverse correlation with SOFA/SAPS – direct correlation with cardiac power index	[18]
		MIF levels in the later post-operative time course: Associated with worse out-come and organ dysfunction	[45]
Ischemia/reperfusion – experimental data	Elevated MIF levels (after hypoxia or ischemia)	Reduction in oxidative stress	[11, 34]
		AMPK activation Inhibition of JNK-mediated apoptosis Neovascularization and angiogenesis ERK1/2-activation	[9] [10] [49] [13]
	Significantly reduced (MIF knockout) stress	Reduced infarct size, reduced apoptosis	

ERK: extracellular signal-regulated kinase; JNK: c-Jun N-terminal kinases; AMPK: adenosine monophosphate-activated protein kinase; SOFA: sequential organ failure assessment; ROSC: return of spontaneous circulation

sion to the ICU. The circulating MIF levels decreased throughout the observation period and reached preoperative values already 4 h after admission to the ICU. Interestingly, postoperative MIF values were inversely correlated with simplified acute physiology score (SAPS) II and sequential organ failure assessment (SOFA) score during the early postoperative stay. Moreover, MIF values on postoperative day 1 were related to the calculated cardiac power index and correlated inversely with troponin T levels [8].

The primary trigger of perioperative MIF release in cardiac surgery remains speculative and is assumed to result from ischemia-reperfusion or inflammation. Further studies are warranted that specifically investigate the perioperative modulation of MIF by various effectors.

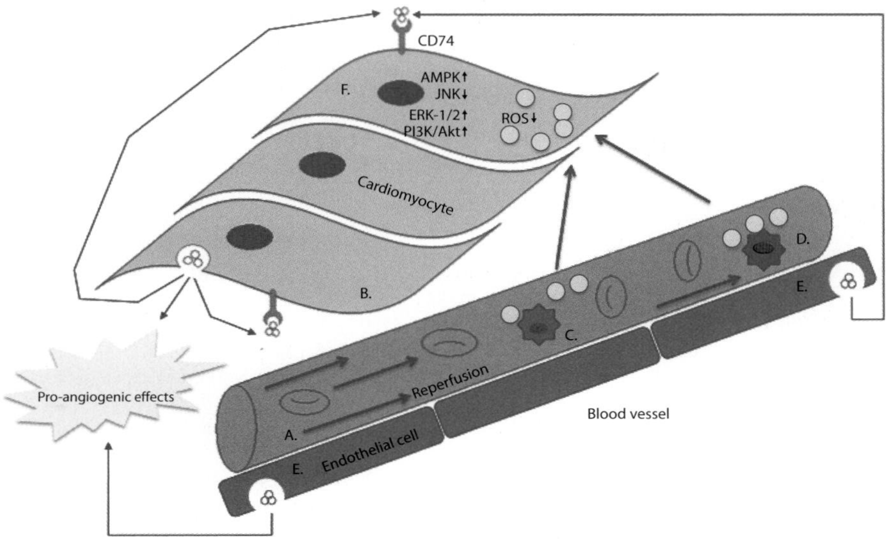

Fig. 2 Macrophage migration inhibitory factor (MIF) in ischemia-reperfusion injury. Potential cardioprotective mechanisms of MIF. Ischemia with subsequent reperfusion (*A*) leads to excessive release of MIF from cardiomyocytes (*B*) and endothelial cells (*E*) and results in massive release of reactive oxygen species (ROS, light blue circles) from neutrophils (*C*) and other immune cells (*D*). The potential cardioprotective mechanisms of MIF are summarized in *F*. For further explanations, see text. ERK: extracellular signal-regulated kinase; PI3 K: phosphatidylinositol 3-kinase; Akt: protein B kinase; JNK: c-Jun N-terminal kinases; AMPK: adenosine monophosphate-activated protein kinase

Conclusion

MIF acts as a key upstream player within the inflammatory response and has several biological functions, such as control of cell growth and arrest, sensing of pathogenic stimuli, leukocyte recruitment into inflammatory foci, inhibition of glucocorticoid induced immunosuppression and prevention of immune cell apoptosis. Yet, overall, the functional role of MIF in inflammation and infection seems double-edged: On the one hand, the pro-inflammatory effects of MIF are essential for an effective host defense. On the other hand, an unbalanced MIF release may be associated with organ dysfunction and various other deleterious effects. Recent findings regarding cardioprotection by MIF in the setting of myocardial ischemia-reperfusion injury add further complexity.

Further research has to focus primarily on a more comprehensive understanding of the ambivalent and possibly time-dependent effects of MIF and on potential ways to modulate MIF release in various pathological settings in which inflammatory pathways are critically involved.

Acknowledgments: Without naming them individually, we are very thankful to numerous friends and colleagues with whom we have shared our research on MIF and who have helped us with valuable comments over many years. Furthermore, we are indebted to the technical assistance of M. Coeuru for designing the figures.

References

1. Vincent JL, Sakr Y, Sprung CL et al (2006) Sepsis in European intensive care units: results of the SOAP study. Crit Care Med 34:344–353
2. Martin GS, Mannino DM, Eaton S, Moss M (2003) The epidemiology of sepsis in the United States from 1979 through 2000. N Engl J Med 348:1546–1554
3. Abraham E (1999) Why immunomodulatory therapies have not worked in sepsis. Intensive Care Med 25:556–566
4. Sprung CL, Annane D, Keh D et al (2008) Hydrocortisone therapy for patients with septic shock. N Engl J Med 358:111–124
5. Ranieri VM, Thompson BT, Barie PS et al (2012) Drotrecogin alfa (activated) in adults with septic shock. N Engl J Med 366:2055–2064
6. Calandra T, Echtenacher B, Roy DL et al (2000) Protection from septic shock by neutralization of macrophage migration inhibitory factor. Nat Med 6:164–170
7. Al-Abed Y, Dabideen D, Aljabari B et al (2005) ISO-1 binding to the tautomerase active site of MIF inhibits its pro-inflammatory activity and increases survival in severe sepsis. J Biol Chem 280:36541–36544
8. Stoppe C, Grieb G, Rossaint R et al (2012) High postoperative blood levels of macrophage migration inhibitory factor are associated with less organ dysfunction in patients after cardiac surgery. Mol Med 18:843–850
9. Miller EJ, Li J, Leng L et al (2008) Macrophage migration inhibitory factor stimulates AMP-activated proteinkinase in the ischaemic heart. Nature 451:578–582
10. Qi D, Hu X, Wu X, Merk M, Leng L, Bucala R, Young LH (2009) Cardiac macrophage migration inhibitory factor inhibits JNK pathway activation and injury during ischemia/reperfusion. J Clin Invest 119:3807–3816
11. Koga K, Kenessey A, Powell SR, Sison CP, Miller EJ, Ojamaa K (2010) Macrophage migration inhibitory factor provides cardioprotection during ischemia/reperfusion by reducing oxidative stress. Antioxid Redox Signal 14:1191–1202
12. Janeway Jr CA, Medzhitov R (2002) Innate immune recognition. Ann Rev Immunol 20:197–216
13. Calandra T, Roger T (2003) Macrophage migration inhibitory factor: a regulator of innate immunity. Nat Rev Immunol 3:791–800
14. Calandra T, Bochud PY, Heumann D (2002) Cytokines in septic shock. Curr Clin Top Infect Dis 22:1–23
15. David JR (1966) Delayed hypersensitivity in vitro: its mediation by cell-free substances formed by lymphoid cell-antigen interaction. Proc Natl Acad Sci USA 56:72–77
16. Bernhagen J, Calandra T, Mitchell RA et al (1993) MIF is a pituitary-derived cytokine that potentiates lethal endotoxaemia. Nature 365:756–759
17. Calandra T, Bernhagen J, Metz CN et al (1995) MIF as a glucocorticoid-induced modulator of cytokine production. Nature 377:68–71
18. Leng L, Metz CN, Fang Y et al (2003) MIF signal transduction initiated by binding to CD74. J Exp Med 197:1467–1476
19. Bernhagen J, Krohn R, Lue H et al (2007) MIF is a noncognate ligand of CXC chemokine receptors in inflammatory and atherogenic cell recruitment. Nat Med 13:587–596
20. Calandra T, Bernhagen J, Mitchell RA, Bucala R (1994) The macrophage is an important and previously unrecognized source of macrophage migration inhibitory factor. J Exp Med 179:1895–1902

21. Bozza FA, Gomes RN, Japiassu AM et al (2003) Macrophage migration inhibitory factor levels correlate with fatal outcome in sepsis. Shock 22:309–313
22. Donnelly SC, Haslett C, Reid PT et al (1997) Regulatory role for macrophage migration inhibitory factor in acute respiratory distress syndrome. Nat Med 3:320–323
23. Onodera S, Kaneda K, Mizue Y, Koyama Y, Fujinaga M, Nishihira J (2000) Macrophage migration inhibitory factor up-regulates expression of matrix metalloproteinases in synovial fibroblasts of rheumatoid arthritis. J Biol Chem 275:444–450
24. Mitchell RA, Liao H, Chesney J et al (2002) Macrophage migration inhibitory factor (MIF) sustains macrophage proinflammatory function by inhibiting p53: regulatory role in the innate immune response. Proc Natl Acad Sci USA 99:345–350
25. Fingerle-Rowson G, Koch P, Bikoff R et al (2003) Regulation of macrophage migration inhibitory factor expression by glucocorticoids in vivo. Am J Pathol 162:47–56
26. Roger T, David J, Glauser MP, Calandra T (2001) MIF regulates innate immune responses through modulation of Toll-like receptor 4. Nature 414:920–924
27. Mitchell RA, Metz CN, Peng T, Bucala R (1999) Sustained mitogen-activated protein kinase (MAPK) and cytoplasmic phopholipase A2 activation by macrophage migration inhibitory factor (MIF). J Biol Chem 274:18100–18106
28. Lue H, Dewor M, Leng L, Bucala R, Bernhagen J (2011) Activation of the JNK signalling pathway by macrophage migration inhibitory factor (MIF) and dependence on CXCR4 and CD74. Cell Signal 23:135–144
29. Petrovsky N, Socha L, Silva D, Grossman AB, Metz C, Bucala R (2003) Macrophage migration inhibitory factor exhibits a pronounced circadian rhythm relevant to its role as a glucocorticoid counter-regulator. Immunol Cell Biol 81:137–143
30. Beishuizen A, Thijs LG, Haanen C, Vermes I (2001) Macrophage migration inhibitory factor and hypothalamo-pituitary-adrenal function during critical illness. J Clin Endocrinol Metab 86:2811–2816
31. Gando S, Sawamura A, Hayakawa M, Hoshino H, Kubota N, Nishihira J (2007) High macrophage migration inhibitory factor levels in disseminated intravascular coagulation patients with systemic inflammation. Inflammation 30:118–124
32. Thiele M, Bernhagen J (2005) Link between macrophage migration inhibitory factor and cellular redox regulation. Antioxid Redox Signal 7:1234–1248
33. Leaver SK, Maccallum NS, Pingle V et al (2010) Increased plasma thioredoxin levels in patients with sepsis: positive association with macrophage migration inhibitory factor. Intensive Care Med 36:336–341
34. Sprong T, Pickkers P, Geurts-Moespot A et al (2007) Macrophage migration inhibitory factor (MIF) in meningococcal septic shock and experimental human endotoxemia. Shock 27:482–487
35. Østergaard C, Benfield T (2009) Macrophage migration inhibitory factor in cerebrospinal fluid from patients with central nervous system infection. Crit Care 13:R101
36. Renner P, Roger T, Bochud PY et al (2012) A functional microsatellite of the macrophage migration inhibitory factor gene associated with meningococcal disease. FASEB J 26:907–916
37. Rahman SH, Menon KV, Holmfield JH, McMahon MJ, Guillou JP (2007) Serum macrophage migration inhibitory factor is an early marker of pancreatic necrosis in acute pancreatitis. Ann Surg 245:282–289
38. Otukesh H, Fereshtehnejad SM, Hoseini R et al (2009) Urine macrophage migration inhibitory factor (MIF) in children with urinary tract infection: a possible predictor of acute pyelonephritis. Pediatric Nephrology 24:105–111
39. Makita H, Nishimura M, Miyamoto K et al (1998) Effect of anti-macrophage migration inhibitory factor antibody on lipopolysaccharide-induced pulmonary neutrophil accumulation. Am J Respir Crit Care Med 158:573–579
40. Pollak N, Sterns T, Echtenacher B, Mannel DN (2005) Improved resistance to bacterial superinfection in mice by treatment with macrophage migration inhibitory factor. Infect Immun 73:64884–64892

41. Yende S, Angus DC, Kong L et al (2009) The influence of macrophage migration inhibitory factor gene polymorphisms on outcome from community-acquired pneumonia. FASEB J 23:2403–2411
42. Lehmann LE, Novender U, Schroeder S et al (2001) Plasma levels of macrophage migration inhibitory factor are elevated in patients with severe sepsis. Intensive Care Med 27:1412–1415
43. de Mendonca-Filho HT, Gomes RV, de Almeida Campos LA et al (2004) Circulating levels of macrophage migration inhibitory factor are associated with mild pulmonary dysfunction after cardiopulmonary bypass. Shock 22:533–537
44. Kofoed K, Andersen O, Kronborg G et al (2007) Use of plasma C-reactive protein, procalcitonin, neutrophils, macrophage migration inhibitory factor, soluble urokinase-type plasminogen activator receptor, and soluble triggering receptor expressed on myeloid cells-1 in combination to diagnose infections: a prospective study. Crit Care 11:R38
45. Grieb G, Simons D, Piatkowski A, Bernhagen J, Steffens GC, Pallua N (2009) Macrophage migration inhibitory factor-A potential diagnostic tool in severe burn injuries? Burns 36:335–342
46. Chagnon F, Metz CN, Bucala R, Lesur O (2005) Endotoxin-induced myocardial dysfunction: Effects of macrophage migration inhibitory factor neutralization. Circ Res 96:1095–1102
47. Gao XM, Liu Y, White D et al (2011) Deletion of macrophage migration inhibitory factor protects the heart from severe ischemia-reperfusion injury: a predominant role of anti-inflammation. J Mol Cell Cardiol 50:991–999
48. Yu CM, Lai KW, Chen YX, Huang XR, Lan HY (2003) Expression of macrophage migration inhibitory factor in acute ischemic myocardial injury. J Histochem Cytochem 51:625–631
49. Stoppe C, Fries M, Rossaint R et al (2012) Blood levels of macrophage migration inhibitory factor after successful resuscitation from cardiac arrest. PLoS One 7:e33512
50. Amin MA, Volpert OV, Woods JM, Kumar P, Harlow LA, Koch AE (2003) Migration inhibitory factor mediates angiogenesis via mitogen-activated protein kinase and phosphatidylinositol kinase. Circ Res 93:321–329

Part V

Adjunct Therapies

Standardized Reporting, Registration, and a Multicenter, Multispecies Approach to Preclinical (Animal) Trials

M. C. Reade and E. Kirkman

Introduction

Opinions on the ethics of using animal models of human disease to test novel pharmacological and other therapies are diverse [1]. We make no comment on whether animal experimentation as a concept is 'ethical', other than to note that animal (or 'preclinical') models of disease are currently considered mandatory in drug development, and only proceed if approved by institutional ethics boards which balance cost (to the animal) and benefit. The only rational approach to this situation is to make the most efficient use of this resource. This notion is codified in the internationally accepted principle of the "3Rs": Replacement, reduction, and refinement (Table 1) [2].

Preclinical and clinical trials of pharmaceuticals aim to test efficacy, safety, and ultimately net benefit when applied by practitioners. As researchers involved in assessing drugs that show early promise for the treatment of patients with trauma, using animal models and clinical phase II and III trials in humans, we are struck by the different conceptual frameworks of these two experimental paradigms. There are good historical reasons underpinning many of these differences. However, the science and practice of clinical trials in humans, particularly those relevant to critical care medicine, has developed remarkably over the last few decades [3]. Like others [4], we note the common failure to translate promising animal-derived data into successful clinical trials. In this chapter, we explore whether elements of the modern approach to clinical trials could usefully be ap-

M. C. Reade (✉)
Joint Health Command, Australian Defence Force, c/- Level 9, University of Queensland Health Sciences Building, Royal Brisbane & Women's Hospital, Queensland 4029, Australia
E-mail: michael.reade@defence.gov.au

E. Kirkman
Defence Science and Technology Laboratory, Porton Down, Salisbury SP4 0JQ, United Kingdom

J.-L. Vincent (Ed.), *Annual Update in Intensive Care and Emergency Medicine 2013*, 167
DOI 10.1007/978-3-642-35109-9_14, © Springer-Verlag Berlin Heidelberg 2013

Table 1 The "3Rs" guiding use of animal models of human disease

Replacement	The first question to be asked of any proposed animal experimentation: Can the research question be answered using another technique (such as pharmacokinetic modeling) such that the animal experiments can be *replaced*. If not possible, the following two principles must be applied.
Reduction	The number of animals used for the experiments must be *reduced* to the minimum needed to answer the research question. The caveat to this principle is that studying too few animals to answer the question risks invalidating the results, meaning the lives of the animals used would be wasted.
Refinement	The pain, suffering or harm felt by the animals must be minimized by *refinement* of the experimental technique wherever possible.

plied to preclinical research, in order to promote greater efficiency, transparency, and less wasted effort. Specifically, we propose the formation of networks of preclinical trialists that could perform multicenter, multispecies evaluations of promising new therapies that would act as a bridge between preclinical and clinical research. We explicitly do not address the use of animals for teaching, antibody or tissue production, studies attempting to produce transgenic or gene-knockout disease models, studies attempting to understand pathogenic mechanisms, and toxicology studies.

Current Paradigms of Clinical and Preclinical Research

Clinical Trials in Critical Care Medicine

Most of the interventions applied by intensivists have never been subjected to a formal clinical trial, as their effects are immediately apparent. Examples include vasopressors for shock, oxygen for hypoxemia, and funnel-web spider antivenom, which was licensed for use after experience in only two patients [5]. However, the incremental gain that can be expected of most additions to 'common sense' interventions is low. Large samples are needed to detect small effects, a realization that has led critical care medicine to embrace the notion of the multicenter clinical trial. Although some contend that the multicenter clinical trial paradigm is inappropriate for the heterogeneous group of patients with life-threatening illness [6], the many problems of single-center studies (such as lack of applicability to more diverse populations, lack of blinding, unequal allocation of resources to treatment groups, and lack of *a priori* analysis plans) [7] argue against a return to the days when limited evidence was over-extrapolated into practice. The numerous instances of benefit in single-center trials contradicted when interventions were tested more widely (such as tight glycemic control [8], high-dose hemofiltration [9] and corticosteroids for acute respiratory distress syndrome [ARDS] [10]), also argue for the necessity of large scale multicenter effectiveness trials.

A critical concept in modern clinical trial research is the distinction between small *efficacy* trials and large multicenter *effectiveness* trials. Efficacy trials test an intervention implemented in a controlled manner in a carefully selected population: The ability to produce an effect. All subjects receive either the intervention or its comparator, and are best analyzed according to the intervention received. In contrast, effectiveness trials test the policy of applying an intervention, accepting that in practice it might be applied to some 'wrong' subjects within the trial, not well applied, and that subjects may cross over from the intervention to control groups for a variety of informative reasons. Effectiveness trials must be analyzed according to intention to treat, thereby accounting for the many possible reasons why an intervention may not work when applied to a population. Efficacy trials are not pilot studies for effectiveness trials; rather, they are essential preludes that inform the design and viability of such pilot studies.

Preclinical (Animal) Trials Relevant to Critical Care Medicine

Preclinical experiments of potential therapeutic agents serve two purposes: To investigate pathophysiological/pathogenic and pharmacologic mechanisms, and to assess the balance of risk and benefit prior to experimental use in humans. Mechanistic studies can be exploratory research [11], which looks for patterns in data without testing a pre-specified hypothesis, or can test the hypothesis that a drug works in a particular way. There is no direct analogy to human pharmacology clinical trials, and we offer no critique of these processes. However, animal trials of therapeutics can also test the hypothesis that a drug (or other intervention) is of benefit in a particular condition. This is confirmatory research. Whilst directly analogous to a human clinical trial, we note the methods adopted in these two experimental paradigms can be quite different.

Drawing on the experience of misleading single center clinical trials, few intensivists would now accept as sufficient evidence the result of a study performed by single-center advocates of an intervention performed in an unblinded, non-randomized manner in a small (and potentially iteratively-derived) sample from a population sharing few features in common with that postulated to be eligible for the drug treatment in question. Perhaps curiously to clinicians schooled in evidence-based medicine, these features typify most preclinical studies – a situation that is recognized in leading journals as unacceptable [12].

Numerous studies have highlighted methodological deficiencies in animal trial research, summarized in Table 2. For example, a recent systematic review of 271 papers published between 1999–2005 reporting *in vivo* research on rodents or non-human primates [13] found that only 12 % reported using some form of randomization and that only 14 % determining outcome using a qualitative score reported assessor blinding. Animal studies without randomization and blinding are five times more likely to report a positive effect [14]. Others have found similar evidence of poor quality (judged by the standards of human trials): Of 133 publi-

Table 2 Features of clinical and preclinical trial research relevant to critical care medicine

Clinical	Preclinical
Randomized	Often non-randomized
Investigators blinded to treatment allocation	Investigators unblinded to treatment allocation
Outcome assessment frequently made by blinded non-investigators	Outcome assessment routinely made by unblinded investigators
Multicenter	Single center
Heterogeneous population that is similar to the population in which the drug would be applied	Homogenous population that is dissimilar in many respects to the analogous human population (e. g., animals are routinely young, of one sex, and without comorbidity)
Outcome measures increasingly assessed at a time point relevant to the patient, such as 90-day mortality	Outcome measures assessed a few hours after treatment
Mortality is a common endpoint	Mortality is uncommonly an endpoint. Most animals in critical care studies are euthanized at the end of the experiment
Experimental therapy applied in the context of all other elements of 'best practice'	Experimental therapy often (though not always) applied as a single therapy
Sample size calculated from pilot data on variability, prospectively informing an understanding of the power of the trial to find a difference between samples (if one is present) with a certain statistical significance	Sample size is rarely prospectively calculated. Sometimes an iterative approach to sample size is adopted, in which trends to significant differences between groups are 'pursued' with additional subjects

cations in a veterinary journal between 1992–1993, 30 % had weaknesses in design, 45 % in analysis, and 26 % had conclusions inconsistent with the analysis [15].

Despite accepted desirability of presenting sample size calculations in animal trials [11], of 271 reports of animal studies identified for review, none reported how the number of animals required to be studied had been determined [13]. This raises suspicion that the number chosen reflects tradition, feasibility, or an iterative approach whereby more and more animals are studied until any effect reaches statistical significance. This is acceptable in exploratory research, but not in hypothesis-testing. It risks wastage of animals, either studying more than are required to be reasonably certain of an effect, or because too few are studied, making lack of an observed effect meaningless [12]. Adding extra animals increases the chance of type I error (concluding a difference when none is present). Ideally, animal study sample sizes should be calculated in the same way as in human studies – with pilot trials used to determine likely effect size and variability [11]. Once the variability is known, the number of animals needed to be fairly sure (e. g., 80 % sure) of showing an effect of a certain size with a particular certainly can be calculated. Few animal studies pre-specify their primary outcome [12]. Instead, various endpoints are often subjected to statistical tests, usually without adjustment for multiple comparisons and so with a higher than reported type I error [15].

Numerous decisions must be made in animal trials that can influence the generalizability of results. It is sometimes desirable to start with simple models to elucidate basic mechanisms. Often these simple models are not designed to closely replicate clinical reality, but rather to address specific aspects of a condition or treatment. This can be an essential step in understanding a more complex clinical situation, or interpreting the outcome of complex models. For example, the evidence for hypotensive resuscitation in trauma is dominated by trials (both human and animal) of short times to hemorrhage control, but many guidelines to not acknowledge this and leave timelines open ended. Porton Down Defence Science and Technology Laboratory therefore compared the pathophysiological problems associated with hypotensive resuscitation (at one extreme) and traditional Advanced Trauma Life Support aggressive fluid resuscitation (at the other) after combined hypovolemic shock and blast injury [16]. Bleeding was simulated by withdrawing blood from the arterial cannula, avoiding the risk of rebleeding. Although this did not replicate clinical reality, the purpose of the study was to compare the systemic pathophysiology of both approaches, rather than to advocate one approach over the other. Once such mechanisms had been elucidated, a model more closely representing clinical reality was used to compare what had become standard care (hypotensive resuscitation) with an approach ("novel hybrid resuscitation") based on hypotheses derived from the mechanistic studies [17].

It is important that the limitations of these 'simple' studies are acknowledged and respected, and that more complex trials (involving animal models or clinical studies) are not leap-frogged when new treatments are brought into practice. Regrettably, this is sometimes forgotten. Many animal models replicate disease but not the intercurrent standard treatments received by most patients: For example, drugs in animal trials of cardiac arrest are usually given earlier than is possible in clinical practice, and delay in therapy is an important predictor of efficacy [18]. Fluid resuscitation in a rat sepsis model reduced mortality from 74 % to 14 % [19], yet many animal models of sepsis do not involve fluid resuscitation; even when they do, monitoring is rarely as sophisticated as in human intensive care [20]. The severity of an experimental insult is often chosen to optimize the effect of an intervention, rather than to replicate the human condition, yet baseline risk of death is a prime determinant of efficacy. For example, a review of animal sepsis models found a control group mortality of 88 %, compared to 39 % in humans [21]. Animal experiments are usually performed using young animals of one sex, yet age [22] and sex [23] are clear determinants of lethality of septic insults in animals. Animals rarely have any comorbidity, despite the influence of comorbidity on response to acute physiological stress [24]. The method of producing the model of the human clinical state can vary widely: For example, sepsis models can use intravenous endotoxin, cecal ligation and puncture, or the intravenous administration of exogenous live bacteria.

Choice of species is a crucial decision in animal trials. The systems biology of some species can produce a misleading conclusion if applied more generally: For example, the ability of mice to enter naturally a state of torpor probably explained the ability of hydrogen sulfide to protect against ischemia, an effect which could not be reproduced in other species without this natural ability [25]. The US Food and Drug Administration (FDA) mandates toxicology testing of new pharmaceuticals in at least two mammalian species [26], commonly a rodent (usually rat) and non-rodent (initially dog; later sheep or pig) model [27].

Most preclinical trial programs do not adopt a systematic or between-laboratory coordinated approach to these issues. The result is different models with apparently divergent results. For example, a recent review of the preclinical evidence for hemostatic dressings [28] found variations in rate of bleeding at the time of application, choice of vessels, method of laceration, duration of hemorrhage before application, resuscitation regimen after application, and application with or without prior vascular control. This made for a confusing picture, with the only possible conclusion being that different dressings appeared most effective in different circumstances.

Systematic Review and Meta-analysis in Animal Research

Some of the problems highlighted above might be overcome by well-conduced meta-analyses that could integrate knowledge derived from many different models. However, the number of meta-analyses of animal data is around 10% of that for clinical trials in humans [29]. There are numerous reasons for this disparity. Animal studies are particularly prone to publication bias [30, 31]. The threshold to test a therapy in animals is lower than in humans, and the expense involved is generally less. Therefore, animal experiments have a greater chance of producing a 'negative' result. Negative animal trials of experimental compounds unlikely to be tested again are more difficult to publish than negative but anticipated human trials.

Any meta-analysis is only as valid as its constituent studies. Most of the animal studies identified in a systematic comparison of animal and human trial results [32] would not have been suitable for inclusion in a meta-analysis if randomization, allocation concealment and blinded assessment of outcome were mandatory criteria.

An Historical Perspective: Why Have These Two Systems Evolved So Differently?

Trial Design

There are numerous possible explanations for these differences in approach to human and animal trials. It is entirely reasonable to construct early animal experiments as small efficacy trials. There is no point testing a drug in a variety of species and experimental conditions if it has no effect in the hypothesized optimal model. Animals comprising this model can be bred to be near-identical or genetically identical, reducing the imperative to use randomization to control for unobserved confounding. In small-scale projects, the scientist conducting the experiment commonly also assesses outcome. Lack of blinding is a problem if outcomes are not entirely objective. Sometimes a scientist wishes to screen a number of variations of a drug therapy; it makes sense to do this in a limited number of animals, and progress only the most promising to more extensive study. However, hypothesis-testing experiments often closely follow exploratory mechanistic or early efficacy research, making it easy to muddle the two concepts and not prespecify primary outcomes or planned analyses in the 'definitive' preclinical trial.

Model Selection

Animal experiments rightly aim to demonstrate the effect of an intervention if one is present. This may be easier in an animal model with a higher than clinically applicable mortality, such as one without intercurrent treatments, such as fluids or antibiotics, or one with an overwhelming septic insult. It is usually not possible for technical or logistic reasons to apply the full spectrum of intensive care interventions to animal models over the days to weeks common in clinical intensive care. Animal species are often selected on the basis of familiarity and precedent in published literature: if a drug for a particular condition has been successfully translated from a rat model to a human therapy, it seems reasonable to test other drugs for that condition in rats. Animals must be treated humanely, meaning any noxious stimuli must be performed under anesthesia – which may alter physiological responses. All these are valid justifications to make little change to the manner in which early efficacy studies are conducted in animals.

There does, however, seem to be a large evidence gap between small animal experiments conducted in tightly regulated conditions, and the translation into expensive human clinical trials. Infrequently, this is because the animal model has been simplified so much that it is no longer representative of clinical mechanisms: For example, modeling the lactic acidemia of shock by infusion of hydrochloric acid. More commonly, though, we sense the problem is in the more subtle aspects of trial design. Many promising drugs fail to cross the preclinical/clinical divide, a problem that the US Institute of Medicine identified as one of the two major problems facing clinical research [33].

Drugs Failing to Cross the Preclinical/Clinical Divide

Most drugs showing sufficient promise in preclinical models to be tested in humans fail to enter practice [34]. Perel et al. [32] systematically reviewed the animal evidence underpinning six clinical interventions for which there was unequivocal clinical trial evidence of a treatment effect (either benefit or harm). Five of the six interventions chosen (corticosteroids for traumatic brain injury, antifibrinolytics in hemorrhage, thrombolysis in acute ischemic stroke, tirilazad in acute ischemic stroke, and antenatal corticosteroids to prevent neonatal respiratory distress syndrome) were relevant to critical care medicine. In general, the standard of experimental design and reporting was poor. In three examples (thrombolysis, antenatal corticosteroids and tirilazad), results of the animal experiments, when taken together, agreed with the subsequent human clinical trial. However, 17 reports of animal studies of corticosteroids for head injury and 18 reports of animal studies of tirilazad for acute stroke showed net benefit, whereas subsequent definitive clinical trials showed net harm. Eight reports of animal studies of antifibrinolytics in hemorrhage did not demonstrate efficacy, in contrast to a subsequent large clinical trial. There are numerous prominent examples of medications showing promise in preclinical studies but failing in large human effectiveness trials [20]. Some models fail to cross the divide between animal species, such as hydrogen sulfide as protection for ischemia [25].

Failing to cross the preclinical/clinical divide comes at considerable cost. Sometimes (fortunately rarely) this is to the trial participants themselves, such as the life-threatening cytokine storm precipitated in a phase I trial of a CD28 monoclonal antibody [35], or less dramatically the higher mortality associated with the higher doses of tumor necrosis factor antibody fragment dimer in patients with septic shock [36]. More commonly, the cost is financial, with the lost opportunity being the development of other drugs that may have been more successful. There would clearly be substantial benefit if the gap between preclinical and clinical studies could be bridged.

Strategies to Improve

We are not the first to identify the problems listed and to suggest possible solutions. A US Department of Defense-sponsored workshop in 2000 brought together 38 research groups working on novel therapies for hemorrhagic shock [37]. In principle, agreement to standardize many potential confounding factors was reached, including the physiologic state of the animal (temperature, caging density, feeding and hydration status, etc.), experimental procedures (anesthesia, rate of bleeding, duration of hypotension prior to resuscitation, etc.), resuscitation protocol (type of fluid used as control, rate and volume of fluid), time of endpoint assessment, selection of surrogate and explanatory endpoints (cardiovascular dynamics, indices of organ perfusion, blood loss, markers of inflammation, etc.), and outcomes (mortality, organ failure, etc.). Regrettably, no consensus emerged from the meeting, nor has any developed since.

We believe a number of developments would increase the proportion of drugs crossing the preclinical/clinical divide, many of which draw from the lessons learnt and the improvements made in human clinical trials over the last 20 years:

Table 3 Features of the reporting of clinical and preclinical research relevant to critical care medicine

Clinical	Preclinical
Primary data available to regulatory authorities	Primary data rarely publically available
Requirement for prospective trial registration	No trial register exists
Increasing trend for publication of an *a priori* statistical analysis plan	No requirement for pre-specified analyses
Publication bias is present, but variable	Publication bias is common
Frequently subjected to systematic review and aggregate meta-analysis	Uncommonly subjected to systematic review
Increasingly subjected to planned individual patient data meta-analysis	Only one individual animal data meta-analysis of a critical care preclinical study has ever been published [38]

Improving the Reporting of Animal Experiments

Preclinical studies are generally reported quite differently to modern clinical trials (Table 3) [38]. Just as implementation of the CONSORT guidelines [39] improved the reporting of human clinical trials, the 2010 Animal Research: Reporting In Vivo Experiments (ARRIVE) guidelines [40] aim for the same effect in preclinical research. Developed in consultation with the major research funding bodies in the United Kingdom, these are a checklist of 20 pieces of information essential to the understanding of how an experiment was performed, its biological relevance, and the reliability and validity of its findings. The GOLD checklist for animal experiments [41] has similar goals. Neither standard has emerged as dominant, though the major UK research funding organizations mandate use of the ARRIVE guidelines in the programs they fund.

Facilitating Unbiased Systematic Reviews and Meta-analysis in Animal Research Using a Trial Registry

In 2004, the International Committee of Medical Journal Editors identified publication bias against 'negative' clinical trials in humans as a major problem, in response mandating pre-registration in a clinical trial registry as a requirement for publication [42]. The system is not perfect: Of registered trials completed before 2007, only 46 % had been published at the time of a 2009 systematic review [43]. Compulsory notification of trial results is gathering momentum: Since 2008, studies falling under US Food and Drug Administration Amendments Act legislation must report their results in a trial registry, although presently the minority have done so [44].

While the benefits of compulsory registration and reporting of preclinical trial results is acknowledged, institutional support for analogous mandatory requirements is at an earlier stage. The Collaborative Approach to Meta-Analysis and Review of Animal Data in Experimental Studies (CAMARADES) group [31], focused mainly on neurological disease, has advocated a standardized approach to meta-analysis, and hosts a repository of animal trial data to which investigators are invited to contribute. There is not, however, any requirement for preclinical trial registration or mandatory reporting, such as is the case for human studies. Any trial performed but not registered or reported is lost forever – an untenable waste of resources – and so we advocate for an international preclinical trials registry that would facilitate the reporting of negative as well as positive results. Consolidation of available evidence should facilitate better understanding of the risks and benefits of progressing to human studies, especially if meta-analyses can be performed using individual subject rather than aggregate data.

Multicenter, Multispecies Animal Effectiveness Trials to Follow Single-Center Efficacy Studies

Meta-analysis of small or poor-quality center studies can be misleading – as was the case in the meta-analysis of human albumin resuscitation trials [45], and also the discordant results of meta-analyses of trials of stress-ulcer prophylaxis [46]. Critical care physicians, in particular, have come to rely on multicenter trials to test the effectiveness of broad application of a new intervention. We believe that many interventions could be usefully assessed in multicenter, multispecies clinical trials as a final step before progressing to human studies. This approach would have a number of beneficial effects:

a) It would take account of possible species-specific or strain-specific effects that have in the past led to misleading results [25], leading to greater external validity;
b) The larger numbers of animals involved would allow assessment of the effects of sex, age and comorbidity;
c) It would allow assessment of a novel intervention by investigators less driven to find a beneficial effect of a particular approach;
d) It would ideally assess animals across a spectrum of baseline risk, with the intention of quantifying interaction of risk and therapy with outcome;
e) It would allow sufficient power to identify subtle effect sizes too small to be detected convincingly in smaller studies;
f) It would increase confidence that the results had been checked by data monitors independent of the site investigators, and properly analyzed by independent statisticians according to a pre-specified plan;
g) It should increase the attractiveness of a research program to funding agencies aiming to more effectively coordinate the use of grant money; and
h) It should increase the ability to publish the results, in much the same way as large human effectiveness studies generate great interest in advance of publication.

Protocols for such multicenter, multispecies trials would ideally incorporate, where possible, the features of multicenter human trial design known to increase validity: Randomization (using block and stratified techniques where appropriate); blinding to allocation during the course of the experiment and in the assessment of results; standardized (or at least clinically representative) intercurrent therapy; data monitoring by an independent committee that can recommend modification or discontinuation of the trial; sample size calculations based on pilot data; and *a priori* registration of analysis plans. Prospective registration of protocols and analysis plans would be encouraged or mandated. If possible, endpoints that reflect clinical utility (such as mortality) should be preferred over surrogates, with the caveat that surrogate endpoints can be an effective strategy to reduce animal suffering at earlier stages. A steering committee would design the study and take overall responsibility for publishing its results. Results would be published according to accepted guidelines, and there would be an implicit commitment by investigators to submit their data to individual subject data meta-analysis.

Overcoming Barriers to Multicenter, Multispecies Research

If the merits of a multicenter, multispecies approach to late phase preclinical studies seem so clear, it is useful to hypothesize why very few investigators have adopted this approach. It can be difficult to replicate the same model in different centers. This was identified as a major problem in the Multicenter Animal Spinal Cord Injury Study [4], but one that could be overcome by experience and training [47]. This problem would also be overcome if each center tested the intervention using its own model, adding to external validity. Preclinical investigators generally receive less academic or institutional credit for collaborative work in comparison to human clinical trialists, at least in developed trial networks such as the ANZICS Clinical Trials Group. Aiming to develop national research infrastructure, funding mechanisms tend to prioritize national over international research efforts. There is less precedent in preclinical research for the acceptance of ethics reviews performed in other institutions or countries. There are, at present, few trial coordinating centers capable of data management, monitoring, and reporting preclinical studies. However, these were all problems that faced critical care trialists 20 years ago; all have been overcome, to the benefit of the research endeavor.

Early Steps Towards Multicenter, Multispecies Research

We are not the first group to recognize the potential for translating clinical trial approaches back into preclinical testing. In toxicology, European Registration, Evaluation, Authorization and Restriction of Chemicals (REACH) legislation [48] aims to minimize animal testing and maximize collaboration by forming Substance Information Exchange Forums for investigators dealing with the same substance. Dirnagl and Fisher [49] and Bath et al. [50] recently suggested multicenter and multispecies preclinical trials of novel ischemic stroke therapies. A positive step towards an active collaboration directly relevant to trauma was recently announced in the field of traumatic brain injury: The five US center Operation Brain Trauma Therapy consortium [4], funded in large part by the US military in response to the current military epidemic of blast-induced traumatic brain injury (TBI). Their planned approach involves a number of steps:

1. Putative therapies will be screened in rodents across a spectrum of established TBI models;
2. Agreed objective outcomes (such as lesion volume and cognitive outcomes) will be assessed;
3. Promising therapies will be tested in more complex models that more closely represent clinical reality: for example, TBI + hemorrhagic shock or inflammation, and also across a spectrum of disease severity; and lastly
4. The most promising approaches will be tested in a common porcine TBI model in a number of centers. The most promising of all will proceed to human clinical trials.

Various drug candidates have already been identified and prioritized on the basis of understandings of mechanism of action. Centers will use their own preclinical models, rather than imperfectly attempting to recreate those of others. By studying models with varying severities of illness, drugs will hopefully be identified for particular indications. This military-funded collaboration is, to our knowledge, the first of its type in a field relevant to critical care medicine, and is hopefully the first step for preclinical research on a trail blazed by the founders of the critical care trials groups around 20 years ago.

Conclusion

In this chapter, in order to illustrate opportunities for improvement, we have highlighted a number of examples in which preclinical animal models have provided incomplete information. We feel it necessary to point out that this should not be misinterpreted by those wishing to advance a particular ethical view that animal research is not warranted or does not achieve its stated objectives. If anything, we argue for adding an extra step in preclinical research, rather than its diminution. However, we also argue that animal research must be done as efficiently and effectively as possible. While there is still a place for single center unblinded exploratory and mechanistic research, we feel that adding the extra step of a multicenter, multispecies trial, along with trial registration and proper design and reporting of preclinical studies, should make the use of animals more justified by increasing their benefit.

We have outlined many of the features of the modern approach to human clinical trials that we feel could be usefully applied to the advanced preclinical assessment of novel therapeutics in order to reduce the number of drugs that look promising in animal studies but fail translation into humans. Like the Operation Brain Trauma Therapy consortium, we are in a fortunate position as investigators of novel therapies relevant to combat casualty care. Under the auspices of The Technical Cooperation Program (http://www.acq.osd.mil/ttcp/) and in collaboration with New Zealand, Canadian and United States partners, we plan coordinated preclinical studies of interventions such as putative 'pharmacological' resuscitation fluids, clotting factor concentrates and replacements, and novel therapies for TBI. While military-sponsored research groups such as ours are taking advantage of existing collaborative structures, we see little reason why this approach should not receive the support of the broader critical care research community.

Acknowledgement: We are grateful to Professor Rinaldo Bellomo both for planting the notion of multicenter, multispecies preclinical trials, and for driving the development of the ANZICS Clinical Trials Group, an effective demonstration of the value of multicenter collaborative research in critical care medicine.

References

1. Weatherall D (2007) Animal research: the debate continues. Lancet 369:1147–1148
2. Russell WMS, Burch RL (1959) The principles of humane experimental technique. Methuen & Co. Ltd, London
3. Angus DC, Mira JP, Vincent JL (2010) Improving clinical trials in the critically ill. Crit Care Med 38:527–532
4. Kochanek PM, Bramlett H, Dietrich WD et al (2011) A novel multicenter preclinical drug screening and biomarker consortium for experimental traumatic brain injury: operation brain trauma therapy. JTrauma 71:S15–S24
5. Fisher MM, Raftos J, McGuinness RT et al (1981) Funnel-web spider (Atrax robustus) antivenom. 2. Early clinical experience. Med J Aust 2:525–526
6. Vincent JL (2010) We should abandon randomized controlled trials in the intensive care unit. Crit Care Med 38:S534–S538
7. Bellomo R, Warrillow SJ, Reade MC (2009) Why we should be wary of single-center trials. Crit Care Med 37:3114–3119
8. Finfer S, Chittock DR, Su SY et al (2009) Intensive versus conventional glucose control in critically ill patients. N Engl J Med 360:1283–1297
9. Bellomo R, Cass A, Cole L et al (2009) Intensity of continuous renal-replacement therapy in critically ill patients. N Engl J Med 361:1627–1638
10. Steinberg KP, Hudson LD, Goodman RB et al (2006) Efficacy and safety of corticosteroids for persistent acute respiratory distress syndrome. N Engl J Med 354:1671–1684
11. Festing MF, Altman DG (2002) Guidelines for the design and statistical analysis of experiments using laboratory animals. ILAR J 43:244–258
12. Macleod M (2011) Why animal research needs to improve. Nature 477:511
13. Kilkenny C, Parsons N, Kadyszewski E et al (2009) Survey of the quality of experimental design, statistical analysis and reporting of research using animals. PLoS One 4:e7824
14. Bebarta V, Luyten D, Heard K (2003) Emergency medicine animal research: does use of randomization and blinding affect the results? Acad Emerg Med 10:684–687

15. McCance I (1995) Assessment of statistical procedures used in papers in the Australian Veterinary Journal. Aust Vet J 72:322–328
16. Garner J, Watts S, Parry C, Bird J, Cooper G, Kirkman E (2010) Prolonged permissive hypotensive resuscitation is associated with poor outcome in primary blast injury with controlled hemorrhage. Ann Surg 251:1131–1139
17. Kirkman E, Watts S, Cooper G (2011) Blast injury research models. Philos Trans R Soc Lond B Biol Sci 366:144–159
18. Reynolds JC, Rittenberger JC, Menegazzi JJ (2007) Drug administration in animal studies of cardiac arrest does not reflect human clinical experience. Resuscitation 74:13–26
19. Smith III EF, Slivjak MJ, Egan JW, Gagnon R, Arleth AJ, Esser KM (1993) Fluid resuscitation improves survival of endotoxemic or septicemic rats: possible contribution of tumor necrosis factor. Pharmacology 46:254–267
20. Dyson A, Singer M (2009) Animal models of sepsis: why does preclinical efficacy fail to translate to the clinical setting? Crit Care Med 37:S30–S37
21. Eichacker PQ, Parent C, Kalil A et al (2002) Risk and the efficacy of antiinflammatory agents: retrospective and confirmatory studies of sepsis. Am J Respir Crit Care Med 166:1197–1205
22. Turnbull IR, Wlzorek JJ, Osborne D, Hotchkiss RS, Coopersmith CM, Buchman TG (2003) Effects of age on mortality and antibiotic efficacy in cecal ligation and puncture. Shock 19:310–313
23. Kadioglu A, Cuppone AM, Trappetti C et al (2011) Sex-based differences in susceptibility to respiratory and systemic pneumococcal disease in mice. J Infect Dis 204:1971–1979
24. Reade MC, Milbrandt EB, Angus DC (2007) The impact of chronic disease on response to infection: more than just reduced physiological reserve? In: Vincent JL (ed) Yearbook of Intensive Care and Emergency Medicine. Springer, Heidelberg, pp 197–207
25. Haouzi P (2011) Murine models in critical care research. Crit Care Med 39:2290–2293
26. Center for Drug Evaluation and Research (1996) Guidance for industry: single dose acute toxicity testing for pharmaceuticals. Available at http://www.fda.gov/downloads/Drugs/.../Guidances/ucm079270.pdf. Accessed Oct 2012
27. Zbinden G (1993) The concept of multispecies testing in industrial toxicology. Regul Toxicol Pharmacol 17:85–94
28. Pusateri AE, Holcomb JB, Kheirabadi BS, Alam HB, Wade CE, Ryan KL (2006) Making sense of the preclinical literature on advanced hemostatic products. J Trauma 60:674–682
29. Sandercock P, Roberts I (2002) Systematic reviews of animal experiments. Lancet 360:586
30. Korevaar DA, Hooft L, ter Riet G (2011) Systematic reviews and meta-analyses of preclinical studies: publication bias in laboratory animal experiments. Lab Anim 45:225–230
31. Sena ES, van der Worp HB, Bath PM, Howells DW, Macleod MR (2010) Publication bias in reports of animal stroke studies leads to major overstatement of efficacy. PLoS Biol 8:e1000344
32. Perel P, Roberts I, Sena E et al (2007) Comparison of treatment effects between animal experiments and clinical trials: systematic review. BMJ 334:197
33. Sung NS, Crowley Jr WF, Genel M et al (2003) Central challenges facing the national clinical research enterprise. JAMA 289:1278–1287
34. Kimmelman J, London AJ (2011) Predicting harms and benefits in translational trials: ethics, evidence, and uncertainty. PLoS Med 8:e1001010
35. Eastwood D, Findlay L, Poole S et al (2010) Monoclonal antibody TGN1412 trial failure explained by species differences in CD28 expression on CD4+ effector memory T-cells. Br J Pharmacol 161:512–526
36. Fisher CJ Jr, Agosti JM, Opal SM et al (1996) Treatment of septic shock with the tumor necrosis factor receptor: Fc fusion protein. The Soluble TNF Receptor Sepsis Study Group. N Engl J Med 334:1697–1702
37. Majde JA (2003) Animal models for hemorrhage and resuscitation research. J Trauma 54:S100–S105

38. Bath PM, Gray LJ, Bath AJ, Buchan A, Miyata T, Green AR (2009) Effects of NXY-059 in experimental stroke: an individual animal meta-analysis. Br J Pharmacol 157:1157–1171
39. Moher D, Hopewell S, Schulz KF et al (2010) CONSORT 2010 Explanation and Elaboration: Updated guidelines for reporting parallel group randomised trials. J Clin Epidemiol 63:e1–e37
40. Kilkenny C, Browne WJ, Cuthill IC, Emerson M, Altman DG (2010) Improving bioscience research reporting: the ARRIVE guidelines for reporting animal research. PLoS Biol 8:e1000412
41. Hooijmans CR, Leenaars M, Ritskes-Hoitinga M (2010) A gold standard publication checklist to improve the quality of animal studies, to fully integrate the Three Rs, and to make systematic reviews more feasible. Altern Lab Anim 38:167–182
42. DeAngelis C, Drazen JM, Frizelle FA et al (2004) Clinical trial registration: a statement from the International Committee of Medical Journal Editors. Med J Aust 181:293–294
43. Ross JS, Mulvey GK, Hines EM, Nissen SE, Krumholz HM (2009) Trial publication after registration in ClinicalTrials.Gov: a cross-sectional analysis. PLoS Med 6:e1000144
44. Prayle AP, Hurley MN, Smyth AR (2012) Compliance with mandatory reporting of clinical trial results on ClinicalTrials.gov: cross sectional study. BMJ 344:d7373
45. Cochrane Injuries Group Albumin Reviewers (1998) Human albumin administration in critically ill patients: systematic review of randomised controlled trials. BMJ 317:235–240
46. Cook DJ, Reeve BK, Guyatt GH et al (1996) Stress ulcer prophylaxis in critically ill patients. Resolving discordant meta-analyses. JAMA 275:308–314
47. Basso DM, Beattie MS, Bresnahan JC et al (1996) MASCIS evaluation of open field locomotor scores: effects of experience and teamwork on reliability. Multicenter Animal Spinal Cord Injury Study. JNeurotrauma 13:343–359
48. Regulation (EC) No1907/2006 of the European Parliament and of the Council of 18 December 2006, concerning the Registration, Evaluation, Authorisation and Restriction of Chemicals (REACH), establishing a European Agency, amending Directive 1999/45/EC and Repealing Council Regulation (EEC) No 793/93 and Commission Regulation (EC) No1488/94 as well as Council Directive 76/769/EEC and Commission Directives 91/155/EEC, 93.67/EEC, 93/105/EC and 2000/21/EC. Available at http://eur-lex.europa.eu/LexUriServ/LexUriServ.do?uri=OJ:L:2007:136:0003:0280:en:PDF. Accessed Oct 2012
49. Dirnagl U, Fisher M (2012) International, multicenter randomized preclinical trials in translational stroke research: it's time to act. J Cereb Blood Flow Metab 32:933–935
50. Bath PM, Macleod MR, Green AR (2009) Emulating multicentre clinical stroke trials: a new paradigm for studying novel interventions in experimental models of stroke. Int J Stroke 4:471–479

Vitamin D and the Critically Ill Patient: An Update for the Intensivist

A. Krishnan, P. Nair, and B. Venkatesh

Introduction

The prime role of vitamin D has always been thought to be the maintenance of calcium and phosphate homeostasis, thereby maintaining adequate bone mineralization and good cardiac and skeletal muscle function. Over the past decade, accumulating molecular and biochemical data, along with clinical and observational studies in different groups of patients seem to suggest that this hormone exerts a significantly wider range of 'pleiotropic' effects (Table 1) [1–5] on different organ systems in the body. The discovery that most tissues and cells in the body have vitamin D receptors and that several possess the 1-α hydroxylase enzyme, has provided novel insights into the additional non-skeletal or pleiotropic actions of this vitamin. Consequently perturbations in vitamin D status have been implicated in a variety of non-musculoskeletal disease states. For example, deficiency of calcitriol (the physiologically active form of vitamin D) has been shown to correlate with the development of a number of autoimmune diseases, such as type 1 diabetes mellitus, multiple sclerosis, rheumatoid arthritis, systemic lupus erythematosus and inflammatory bowel disease [6]. Moreover association with adverse outcomes in association with hypovitaminosis D has been reported in cardiac transplant recipients [7] and in the general population [8, 9].

A. Krishnan
Department of Intensive Care, Princess Alexandra Hospital, Brisbane, Australia

P. Nair
Department of Intensive Care, St. Vincent's Hospital, Sydney, NSW, Australia

B. Venkatesh (✉)
Department of Intensive Care, Princess Alexandra and Wesley Hospitals, University of Queensland, Australia
E-mail: bala_venkatesh@health.qld.gov.au

J.-L. Vincent (Ed.), *Annual Update in Intensive Care and Emergency Medicine 2013*,
DOI 10.1007/978-3-642-35109-9_15, © Springer-Verlag Berlin Heidelberg 2013

Table 1 Pleiotropic effects of vitamin D

Organ system	Pleiotropic Effects
Anti-infective	Induces cathelicidin antimicrobial peptide (*camp*) and defensin β2 (*defβ*) genes [1], thereby improving innate immunity. Stimulates release of neutrophil lipocalin (NGAL) which is a bacteriostatic agent [2].
Anti-inflammatory and immunomodulatory	Decreases TNF-α production from macrophages by decreasing nuclear factor-kappa B (NF-κβ) [3]. Inhibits lipopolysaccharide stimulated expression of pro-inflammatory cytokines including intercellular adhesion molecule (ICAM-1), platelet endothelial adhesion molecule (PECAM)-1, and interleukin (IL)-6 on human umbilical vein cords [4].
Cardiovascular	Anti-inflammatory, anti-atherosclerotic, and direct cardioprotective effects, hypertension control by inhibition of renin release, improved outcomes by parathyroid hormone suppression [5].

These significant extra-skeletal effects have resulted in suggestions that hypovitaminosis D may be an "invisible accomplice" to morbidity and mortality in the intensive care unit (ICU), resulting in the conduct of a number of studies in these patients [10]. Several observational studies have found an association between hyopvitaminosis D and adverse outcomes in the critically ill, raising suggestions that these patients should receive routine vitamin D supplementation.

Given the burgeoning volume of literature on vitamin D and critical illness, we felt an update is timely for the intensivist. In this review, we will briefly review the physiology, clarify the terminology and definitions of vitamin D deficiency, examine the differences in metabolism of vitamin D in ICU patients when compared with the general population, the current evidence on the role of this hormone in the critically ill, and the problems with sample collection and interpretation of laboratory results. We will finally critically appraise whether routine supplementation is justified in the ICU and the directions for future research.

Forms of Vitamin D

Vitamin D exists in multiple forms: The two main forms are vitamin D2 (ergocalciferol) and vitamin D3 (cholecalciferol). Vitamin D1 is a combination of ergosterol and lumisterol (1:1) and as it is a mixture of compounds rather than a pure vitamin D product, the term D1 is no longer used. Ergocalciferol is found in plants, yeast, and invertebrates but not produced by vertebrates. The precursor of ergocalciferol is ergosterol. Only D3 is produced in the human body. D2 is not produced by vertebrates as they lack the precursor ergosterol. For physiological replacement, vitamin D3 is thought to be 87 % more potent than vitamin D2.

Physiology

Cholecalciferol is largely produced from 7-dehydrocholesterol in the skin by the effects of ultraviolet B light. Choleciferol in turn binds to D-binding protein (DBP) and is transported to the liver. Successive hydroxylation steps then occur: The first step occurs in the liver to 25(OH)D3 (also known as calcidiol) and the second hydroxylation to 1α,25$(OH)_2$D3 (also known as calcitriol) by the action of 1α-hydroxylase enzyme takes place in the proximal renal tubular cells. 1α,25$(OH)_2$D3 is the active form and binds to the vitamin D receptor (VDR) resulting in transcriptional regulation of target genes. The VDR is present widely in different cells of the body including intestine, renal tubular cells, as well as endocrine glands like parathyroid and pancreas, and immune cells [11]. Around 88 % of 25(OH)D3 is bound to DBP and most of the remainder to albumin, with only 0.03 % remaining free in the plasma. Renal 1α-hydroxylase enzyme is very tightly regulated by parathyroid hormone (PTH), serum calcium levels and fibroblast growth factor (FGF) 23. In addition to the kidney, there are several other tissues in the body that express the CYP27B1 gene that codes for the 1α-hydroxylase enzyme [12]. Extra-renal 1α-hydroxylase is not activated by hypocalcemia or by PTH, but by tissue-specific stimuli [12] such as lipopolysaccharide (LPS) [13] and Th1 cytokines [14]. The role of the extra-renal 1α-hydroxylase enzyme is unclear, but autocrine production of 1α,25$(OH)_2$D3 may play a very important role in the pleiotropic effects of this hormone.

Definitions of Vitamin D Deficiency

It is unclear what levels of vitamin D are needed to meet physiologic requirements of the individual. There is no universally accepted definition of what constitutes vitamin D deficiency [15]. Even though 1α,25$(OH)_2$D3 is the active moiety and is responsible for the physiological effects, 25(OH)D3 levels are used to assess vitamin D status because the half-life of 25(OH)D3 is 2–3 weeks, whereas that of 1α,25$(OH)_2$D3, is only a few hours. Moreover calcitriol produced at the tissue level cannot be assessed in the serum.

Vitamin D sufficiency is defined by serum 25(OH)D3 level $>$75 nmol/l, a level that has been shown to suppress PTH secretion [16]. Serum 25(OH)D3 levels between 50–75 nmol/l are defined as insufficiency and $<$50 nmol/l as deficiency. Serum concentrations between 25–50 nmol/l are defined as mild deficiency, 10–25 nmol/l as moderate deficiency and $<$10 nmol/l as severe deficiency. PTH secretion and subsequent renal 1α-hydroxylase activation usually maintain serum levels of 1α,25$(OH)_2$D3 until 25(OH)D3 levels decrease $<$10 nmol/l. The currently recommended target serum level for 25-OH D by the Institute of Medicine report is 50–125 nmol/l. The recommended daily requirement of 600–800 IU/day may not be sufficient in critically ill patients to achieve adequate serum vitamin D levels [17]. This has led to a higher recommended dose to prevent vitamin D deficiency for the at risk population with a ceiling dose of up to 10,000 IU/day [18].

Vitamin D Assay Considerations and Caveats for Interpreting a Random Measurement in the Critically Ill

Serum 25(OH)D3 levels vary significantly depending on the method used to estimate them. The most common method used to estimate 25(OH)D3 levels is the radioimmunoassay [19]. Other methods include chromatographic separation followed by direct detection, e. g., high-performance liquid chromatography (HPLC). Most of these tests are referenced against isotope dilution liquid chromatography-tandem mass spectroscopy as gold standard (LC-MS) [20]. A recently published study showed excellent concordance between two LC-MS assays but other automated assays, except DiaSorin RIA, showed significant inaccuracies, especially when measuring low levels of 25(OH)D3 [21]. Consequently, the Diasorin RIA is now considered the gold standard. Many smaller centers do not have access to LC-MS and hence most laboratories need to be aware of the limitations of the assay method used to estimate 25(OH)D3 levels.

In critically ill patients, there are a number of caveats when interpreting serum vitamin D levels. A recent study in patients undergoing cardiopulmonary bypass (CPB) showed that levels of both 25(OH)D3 and 1α,25$(OH)_2$D3 decreased by around 30 % when measurements were performed in close proximity to fluid loading [22]. Levels of both of these compounds returned to normal over the ensuing four days when the effects of fluid loading had abated. This effect is likely to have significant implications in critically ill patients with severe sepsis or trauma who receive large volumes of fluid for resuscitation. Another uncertain aspect is the validity of a single measurement in assessing a patient's vitamin D status. Venkatesh et al. demonstrated that there is marked plasma hour to hour variability in 25(OH)D3 levels in critically ill patients, thus questioning the validity of a single measurement [23]. Of the fourteen patients studied, 50 % showed significant cross-over between groups (of deficiency, insufficiency and sufficiency) due to significant hour to hour variability in levels. It is unclear whether repeated measurements over a few days need to be made to determine the vitamin D status of the patient.

Factors Contributing to Vitamin D Deficiency in the Critically Ill Population

A number of factors may act in tandem to cause vitamin D deficiency in ICU patients. The prevalence of vitamin D deficiency in the community is about 50 %.

Consequently a large number of patients are deficient on admission to the ICU. Moreover, critically ill patients have significantly reduced exposure to UVB light due to chronic illness, reduced vitamin D intake and altered metabolism of the hormone by chronic disease or medications [19]. Furthermore, the calcium-PTH-vitamin D axis may be affected in critically ill patients in whom levels of circulatory cytokines are very high. Interleukin-6 (IL-6) and tumor necrosis factor-alpha (TNF-α) have been shown to suppress PTH release in patients with chronic renal failure [24]. However, the effect of inflammation on $1\alpha,25(OH)_2D3$ levels has not been conclusively established. A recent study in cardiac surgical patients who underwent CPB, a model of inflammation, demonstrated that $1\alpha,25(OH)_2D3$ levels increased significantly above baseline around 4 days after CPB [22].

It is also possible that $1\alpha,25(OH)_2D3$ levels may be significantly blunted either by poor tissue production in critical illness or PTH resistance [25]. Bjorkman et al. demonstrated attenuated parathyroid function despite low 25(OH)D3 levels in immobilized patients [26]. This effect may also contribute to decreased $1\alpha,25(OH)_2D3$ production. Levels of DBP, a Gc globulin, decrease after injury or trauma and appear to predict morbidity and mortality in some studies [27, 28]. Endocytosis in the proximal tubular of the filtered 25(OH)D3 bound to DBP is essential for its activation to$1\alpha,25(OH)_2D3$ [29]. However, decrease in DBP is unlikely to have a significant impact on 25(OH)D3 levels or its activation to $1\alpha,25(OH)_2D3$ for two major reasons: After the initial drop in an acute illness, DBP levels rebound [30]; more importantly, most of the DBP in the body is not bound to vitamin D and, therefore, levels have to drop considerably before impacting on 25(OH)D3 levels in a clinically significant manner [31].

Summary of Current Literature on Serum Vitamin D Status and Outcomes in the Critically Ill Population

Over the past decade, a number of studies have not only demonstrated vitamin D deficiency in ICU patients but many of them have also shown an association with morbidity and mortality in these patients. Several have also reported a high prevalence of vitamin D insufficiency/deficiency ranging from 38 % to 100 % in critically ill patients. The reported prevalence is close to 50 % higher than in patients in general medical wards. Mean 25-OH D levels, in all except one study, ranged from 10 to 40 nmol/l, within the very deficient to insufficient range. A number of studies have demonstrated an association between vitamin D deficiency/insufficiency and illness severity, ICU length of stay, ventilator requirement, infection rates, blood culture positivity, and hospital mortality. These are summarized in Table 2 [32–47].

Table 2 Summary of vitamin D studies in adult and pediatric ICU patients

Author	Ref	Year	N	Type of study	Outcome
Flynn et al.	[34]	2012	66 adult, surgical	Prospective, observational	25(OH)D3 levels < 50 nmol/l associated with greater length of hospital stay, risk of infection and organ dysfunction
Braun et al.	[35]	2012	1,325 adult	Retrospective observational	Low 25(OH)D3 levels at time of ICU admission is a predictor of all-cause mortality
Higgins et al.	[36]	2012	196 adult	Prospective	25(OH)D3 levels reduced during ICU stay. Low levels associated with longer time to ICU discharge and a trend to increased risk of infection
Morandi et al.	[37]	2012	120 adult medical	Prospective	25(OH)D3 levels measured early during critical illness are not important determinants of delirium risk.
Arnson et al.	[38]	2012	130 adult medical	Prospective observational	Patients with 25(OH)D3 levels > 50 nmol/l survived longer than those without. No difference in 60-day outcomes.
Matthews et al.	[39]	2012	258, adult surgical	Prospective observational	Patients with moderate and severe 25(OH)D3 deficiency had increased mortality, length of ICU stay and ICU treatment cost compared to those patients with normal or mildly deficient status
McNally et al.	[40]	2012	326 pediatric	Prospective cohort	25(OH)D3 levels < 50 nmol/l in 69 % of population. Associated with increased catecholamine administration, longer PICU length of stay and greater severity of illness.
Madden et al.	[41]	2012	511 pediatric	Prospective cohort	High rate of vitamin D deficiency, associated with higher severity scores on admission
Braun et al.	[33]	2011	2,399 adult	Retrospective, observational	25(OH)D3 deficiency before admission predicts short- and long-term all cause mortality and blood culture positivity
Venkatram et al.	[42]	2011	932 adult medical	Retrospective, observational	Higher hospital mortality for vitamin D deficient but not insufficient patients.

Table 2 *Continued*

Author	Ref	Year	N	Type of study	Outcome
Cecchi et al.	[43]	2011	170 adult	Prospective, observational	25(OH)D3 levels significantly lower in septic patients compared to those with trauma. No relationship between vitamin D levels and outcome
McKinney et al.	[44]	2011	136 adult	Retrospective observational	Over one-third of patients deficient in 25(OH)D3. Deficiency associated with increased length of ICU stay and greater risk of death
Lucidarme et al.	[45]	2010	134 adult	Prospective, observational	25(OH)D3 low in 79 % of population. No mortality association with severity of deficiency
Lee et al.	[46]	2009	42 adult	Prospective, observational	Worsening mortality with reducing 25(OH)D3 levels, seven patients with undetectable 25(OH)D3 levels with three deaths (all had cancer)
Jeng et al.	[32]	2009	49 adult vs. 21 controls	Prospective, observation	25(OH)D3 levels significantly lower in critically ill patients when compared with controls and correlated positively with LL-37 levels in septic patients
Van den Berghe et al.	[47]	2003	22 adult	Prospective, observational	Severe deficiency of 25(OH)D3 and 1α,25(OH)$_2$D3 in critically ill patients on ICU admission when compared to controls. No improvement with administration of standard doses of 25(OH)D3 but cytokine levels decrease

All these studies are observational, with three of the largest ones being retrospective. It has been hypothesized that with a normal circulating vitamin D level, individual target tissues are possibly able to increase local formation of 1,25-dihydroxy D to meet tissue demand during critical illness but this mechanism fails during states of deficiency resulting in worsening existing organ dysfunction in critically ill patients, leading to poor outcomes; i. e., the observed association between increased mortality and vitamin D deficiency in the general population may be magnified during critical illnesses, translating into excess morbidity and mortality [10] (Fig. 1). The causal relationship between low 25(OH)D3 levels and outcomes has not been proven in any of the above studies, but becomes relevant in light of the increasing volume of evidence.

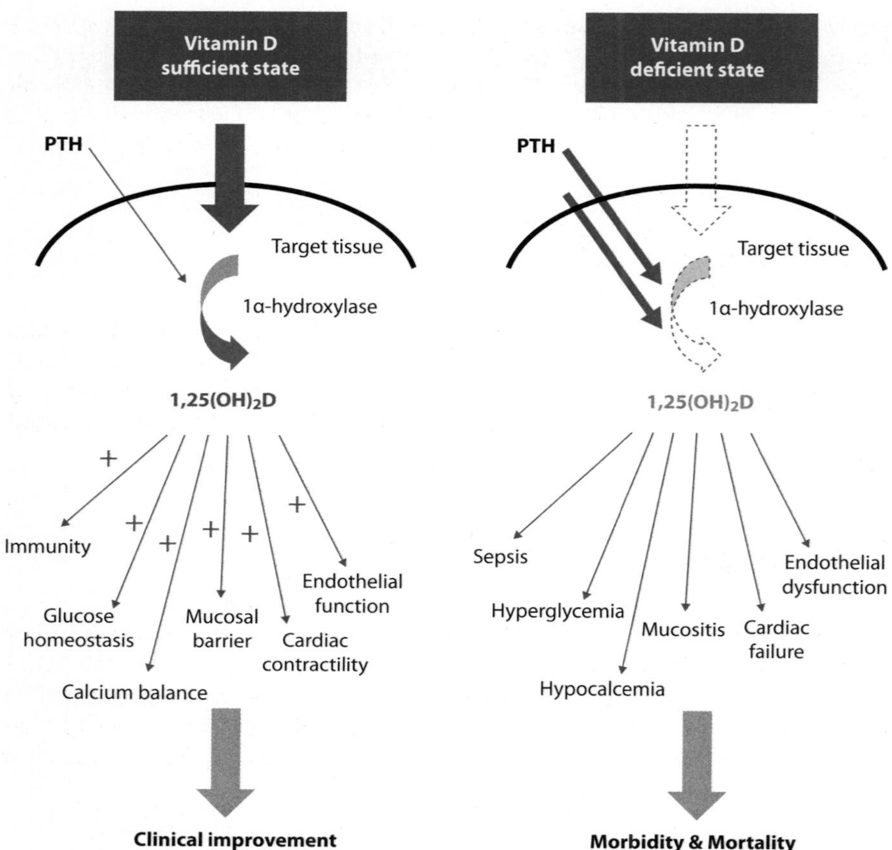

Fig. 1 Potential pathophysiological basis for hypovitaminosis D-induced organ dysfunction. From [10] with permission

Potential Clinical Manifestations of Vitamin D Deficiency in the Critically Ill Patient

Potential consequences of vitamin D deficiency may include altered immune responses and predisposition to infection, impaired cardiovascular function and myopathy.

Infection and Immunity

Cathelicidin (LL-37) is an antimicrobial peptide, the synthesis of which is critically dependent on 1,25(OH)D3 levels. It is important for innate immunity and expressed at airway, bladder and gastrointestinal epithelial surfaces. Jeng at al. have shown a positive correlation between 25(OH)D3 levels and circulating LL-37 levels [32]. A recent study has shown that the vitamin D status of umbilical cord blood impacts on innate immune response in the newborn [48]. Braun et al. [33] have shown that patients with 25(OH)D3 deficiency have greater blood culture positivity.

Cardiac Function

The VDR is expressed widely in the cardiovascular system including on vascular smooth muscle, endothelium and cardiomyocytes. Vitamin D has been shown to decrease plasma renin activity [49], and to correlate inversely with incidence of coronary artery calcification [50]. Low levels of 25(OH)D3 have been associated with poor prognosis in heart failure patients [51].

Skeletal Muscle Function

The association of 25(OH)D3 deficiency and muscle weakness is very clear with symptoms responding well to vitamin D supplementation [52]. Low 25(OH)D3 levels may also caused diminished muscle strength to increased PTH secretion [53]. This may have implications in the ICU, especially in chronic patients who may experience difficulties with mobilization or weaning from mechanical ventilation.

Vitamin D Supplementation in ICU Patients

Despite all the recent evidence that has linked hypovitaminosis D to adverse outcomes in ICU patients, there are only four interventional trials with sample sizes that are too small to draw any inferences regarding outcome benefit [47, 54–56] (Table 3).

Patients with very low levels of 25(OH)D3 tend to show a much more pronounced increment in levels to administration of supplemental vitamin D [15]. In critically ill patients with altered pharmacokinetics, multiple organ dysfunction, gastrointestinal malfunction, and varying degrees of vitamin D deficiency, the dose response to supplementation is unpredictable, unless it is administered parenterally.

Although vitamin D has an excellent risk profile, reports of hypercalcemia, hypercalciuria, vascular calcification and acute renal failure exist, particularly in the setting of unrecognized underlying hyperparathyroidism or the presence of granulomatous disease [57].

Table 3 Trials of vitamin D supplementation in the ICU

Author	Ref	Year	N	Intervention	Outcome
Amrein et al.	[54]	2011	25	High-dose 540,000 U PO Prospective, double-blind	Normalization of 25(OH)D3 levels, no complications like hypercalcemia or hypercalciuria
Mata-Garandos et al.	[55]	2010	33	3 groups – control, 1.5 mg cholecalciferol, 2 mcg i.v. calcitriol Observational	Normalization of 25(OH)D3 levels in those receiving cholecalciferol, no change in the other two groups
Ingels et al.	[56]	2010	24	Cholecalciferol i.v. loading 8,000 U followed by 600 IU daily	Normalization of 25(OH)D3 levels, transient increase in LL-37 levels when compared to placebo
Van den Berghe et al.	[47]	2003	22	Cholecalciferol i.v. 200 IU vs. 500 IU	No correction of 25(OH)D3 levels in either group, cytokine levels suppressed in patients that received the higher dose

Vitamin D as a Pleiotropic Agent in the ICU: Is it Ready for Prime Time?

While the flood of information on the putative benefits of vitamin D continues to flow in, there are still unanswered questions that need resolution before routine supplementation can be recommended in ICU patients.

1. What is the optimal level of vitamin D that is required for pleiotropic benefits?
2. Does a single measurement reflect a patient's vitamin D status and if not, what time points should be used for sampling?
3. What is the relationship between plasma and tissue vitamin D activity?
4. Is serum vitamin D purely a marker of disease severity or is there a biological role?
5. Does vitamin D supplementation improve organ function and mortality in critically ill patients?

As we seek and find more answers to the above questions, vitamin D may well evolve as a cheap and effective agent that could modify the course of a wide range of ICU conditions or fall by the wayside as yet another drug that promised much but delivered little.

References

1. Wang TT, Nestel FP, Bourdeau V et al (2004) Cutting edge: 1,25-dihydroxyvitamin D3 is a direct inducer of antimicrobial peptide gene expression. J Immunol 173:2909–2912
2. Goetz DH, Holmes MA, Borregaard N, Bluhm ME, Raymond KN, Strong RK (2002) The neutrophil lipocalin NGAL is a bacteriostatic agent that interferes with siderophore-mediated iron acquisition. Mol Cell 10:1033–1043
3. Talmor Y, Bernheim J, Klein O, Green J, Rashid G (2008) Calcitriol blunts pro-atherosclerotic parameters through NF-κβ and p38 in vitro. Eur J Clin Invest 38:548–554
4. Cohen-Lahav M, Douvdevani A, Chaimovitz C, Shany S (2007) The anti-inflammatory activity of 1,25-dihydroxyvitamin D3 in macrophages. J Steroid Biochem Mol Biol 103:558–562
5. Pilz S, Tomaschitz A, Marz W et al (2011) Vitamin D, cardiovascular disease and mortality. Clin Endocrinol (Oxf) 75:575–584
6. Szodoray P, Nakken B, Gaal J et al (2008) The complex role of vitamin D in autoimmune diseases. Scand J Immunol 68:261–269
7. Zittermann A, Schleithoff SS, Gotting C et al (2009) Calcitriol deficiency and 1-year mortality in cardiac transplant recipients. Transplantation 87:118–124
8. Melamed ML, Michos ED, Post W, Astor B (2008) 25-hydroxyvitamin D levels and the risk of mortality in the general population. Arch Intern Med 168:1629–1637
9. Holick MF (2006) High prevalence of vitamin d inadequacy and implications for health. Mayo Clin Proc 81:353–373
10. Lee P, Nair P, Eisman JA, Center JR (2009) Vitamin D deficiency in the intensive care unit: an invisible accomplice to morbidity and mortality? Intensive Care Med 35:2028–2032
11. Haussler MR, Jurutka PW, Mizwicki M, Norman AW (2011) Vitamin D receptor (VDR)-mediated actions of 1α,25(OH)2vitamin D3: Genomic and non-genomic mechanisms. Best Prac Res Clin Endocrinol Metab 25:543–559
12. Adams JS, Hewison M (2012) Extrarenal expression of the 25-hydroxyvitamin D-1-hydroxylase. Arch Biochem Biophys 523:95–102
13. Reichel H, Koeffler HP, Barbers R, Norman AW (1987) Regulation of 1,25-dihydroxyvitamin D3 production by cultured macrophages from normal human donors and from patients with pulmonary sarcoidosis. J Clin Endocrinol Metab 65:1201–1209
14. Adams JS, Singer FR, Gacad MA et al (1985) Isolation and structural identification of 1,25-dihyrdoxyvitamin D produced by cultured alveolar macrophages in sarcoidosis. J Clin Endocrinl Metab 60:960–966
15. Heaney RP (2011) Assessing vitamin D status. Curr Opin Clin Nutr Metab Care 14:440–444
16. Durazo-Arvizu RA, Dawson-Hughes B, Sempos CT et al (2010) Three-phase model harmonizes estimates of the maximal suppression of parathyroid hormone by 25-hydroxyvitamin D in persons 65 years of age and older. J Nutr 140:595–599
17. Ross AC, Taylor CL, Yaktine AL et al (2011) Dietary reference intakes for calcium and vitamin D. In: Del Valle HB (ed) Institute of Medicine: Dietary Reference Intakes for Calcium and Vitamin D. National Academies Press, Washington
18. Hollick MF, Binkley NC, Bischoff-Ferrari HA et al (2001) Evaluation, treatment, and prevention of vitamin D deficiency: an endocrine society clinical practice guideline. J Clin endocrinol Metab 96:1911–1930
19. Pittas AG, Laskowski U, Kos L, Saltzman E (2012) The role of vitamin D in adults requiring nutrition therapy. J Parent Enteral Nutr 34:70–78
20. Tai SS, Bedner M, Phinney KW (2010) Development of a candidate reference measurement procedure for the determination of 25-hydroxyvitamin D3 and 25-hydroxyvitamin D2 in human serum using isotope-dilution liquid chromatography-tandem mass spectrometry. Anal Chem 82:1942–1948

21. Farrell CJL, Martin S, McWhinney B, Straub I, Williams P, Herrmann M (2012) State-of-the-art vitamin D assays: a comparison of automated immunoassays with liquid chromatography-tandem mass spectrometry methods. Clin Chem 58:531–542
22. Krishnan A, Ochola J, Mundy J et al (2010) Acute fluid shifts influence the assessment of vitamin D status in critically ill patients. Crit Care 14:R216
23. Venkatesh B, Davidson B, Robinson K, Pascoe R, Appleton C, Jones M (2012) Do random estimations of vitamin D3 and parathyroid hormone reflect the 24-hour profile in the critically ill? Intensive Care Med 38:177–179
24. Feroze U, Molnar MZ, Dukkipati R, Kovesdy CP, Kalantar-Zadeh K (2011) Insights into nutritional and inflammatory aspects of low parathyroid hormone in dialysis patients. J Ren Nutr 21:100–104
25. Lee P (2011) Vitamin D metabolism and deficiency in critical illness. Best Prac Res Clin Endocrinol Metab 25:769–781
26. Bjorkman MP, Sorva AJ, Risteli J, Tilvis RS (2009) Low parathyroid hormone levels in bedridden geriatric patients with vitamin D deficiency. J Am Geriatr Soc 57:1045–1050
27. Dahl B, Schiodt FV, Ott P et al (2003) Plasma concentration of Gc-globulin is associated with organ dysfunction and sepsis after injury. Crit Care Med 31:152–156
28. Meier U, Gressner O, Lammert F, Fressner AM (2006) Gc globulin: roles in response to injury. Clin Chem 52:1247–1253
29. Nykjaer A, Dragun D, Walther D et al (1999) An endocytic pathway essential for renal uptake and activation of the steroid 25(OH) vitamin D3. Cell 96:507–515
30. Dahl B, Schiodt FV, Rudolph S, Ott P, Kiaer T, Heslet L (2001) Trauma stimulates the synthesis of Gc-globulin. Intensive Care Med 27:394–399
31. Chun RF (2012) New perspectives on the vitamin D binding protein. Cell Biochem Funct 30:445–456
32. Jeng L, Yamshchikov AV, Judd SE et al (2009) Alterations in vitamin D status and anti-microbial peptide levels in patients in the intensive care unit with sepsis. J Transl Med 7:28
33. Braun A, Chang D, Mahadevappa K et al (2011) Association of low serum 25-hydroxyvitamin D levels and mortality in the critically ill. Crit Care Med 39:671–677
34. Flynn L, Zimmerman LH, McNorton K et al (2012) Effects of vitamin D deficiency in critically ill surgical patients. Am J Surg 203:379–382
35. Braun AB, Gibbons FK, Litonjua AA, Giovannucci E, Christopher KB (2012) Low serum 25-hydroxyvitamin D at critical are initiation is associated with increased mortality. Crit Care Med 40:63–72
36. Higgins DM, Wischmeyer PE, Queensland KM, Sillau SH, Sufit AJ, Heyland DK (2012) Relationship of vitamin D deficiency to clinical outcomes in critically ill patients. J Parenter Enteral Nut 36:713–720
37. Morandi A, Narnett N, Miller RR 3rd, Pandharipande PP, Ely EW, Ware LB (2013) Vitamin D and delirium in critically ill patients: a preliminary investigation. J Crit Care (in press)
38. Arnson Y, Gringauz I, Itzhaky D, Amital H (2012) Vitamin D deficiency is associated with poor outcomes and increased mortality in severely ill patients. QJM 105:633–639
39. Matthews RL, Ahmed Y, Wilson KL et al (2012) Worsening severity of vitamin D deficiency is associated with increased length, surgical intensive care unit cost, and mortality rate in surgical intensive care unit patients. Am J Surg 204:37–43
40. McNally JD, Menon K, Chakraborty P et al (2012) The association of vitamin D status with pediatric critical illness. Pediatrics 130:429–436
41. Madden K, Feldman HA, Smith EM et al (2012) Vitamin D deficiency in critically ill children. Pediatrics 130:421–428
42. Venkatram S, Chilimuri S, Adrish M, Salako A, Patel M, Diaz-Fuentes G (2011) Vitamin D deficiency is associated with mortality in the medical intensive care unit. Crit Care 15:R292
43. Cecchi A, Bonizzoli M, Douar S et al (2011) Vitamin D deficiency in septic patients at ICU admission is not a mortality predictor. Minerva Anestesiol 77:1184–1189
44. McKinney JD, Bailey BA, Garrett LH, Peiris P, Manning T, Peiris AN (2011) Relationship between vitamin D status and ICU outcomes in veterans. J Am Med Dir Assoc 12:208–211

45. Lucidarme O, Messai E, Mazzoni T, Arcade M, du Cheyron D (2010) Incidence and risk factors of vitamin D deficiency in critically ill patients: results from a prospective observational study. Intensive Care Med 36:1609–1611
46. Lee P, Eisman JA, Center JR (2009) Vitamin d deficiency in critically ill patients. N Engl J Med 360:1912–1914
47. Van den Berghe G, Van Roosbroeck D, Vanhove P et al (2003) Bone turnover in prolonged critical illness: effect of vitamin D. J Clin Endocrinol Metab 88:4623–4632
48. Walker VP, Zhang X, Rastegar I et al (2011) Cord blood vitamin D status impacts innate immune response. J Clin Endocrinol Metab 96:1835–1843
49. Resnick LM, Muller FB, Laragh JH (1986) Calcium-regulating hormones in essential hypertension: relation to plasma rennin activity and sodium metabolism. Ann Intern Med 105:649–654
50. Watson KE, Abrolat ML, Malone LL et al (1997) Active serum vitamin D levels are inversely correlated with coronary calcification. Circulation 96:2755–1760
51. Liu LC, Voors AA, van Veldhuisen D et al (2011) Vitamin D status and outcomes in heart failure patients. Eur J Heart Fail 13:619–625
52. Haroon M, Fitzgerald O (2012) Vitamin D deficiency: Subclinical and clinical consequences on musculoskeletal health. Curr Rheumatol Rep 14:286–293
53. Visser M, Deeg DJ, Lips P et al (2003) Low vitamin D and high parathyroid hormone levels as determinants of loss of muscle strength and muscle mass (sarcopenia): the Longitudinal Aging Study Amsterdam. J Clin Endocrinol Metab 88:5766–5772
54. Amrein K, Sourij H, Wagner G et al (2011) Short-term effects of high-dose oral vitamin D3 in critically ill vitamin D deficient patients: a randomized, double-blind placebo-controlled pilot study. Crit Care 15:R104
55. Mata-Garandos J, Vargas-Vasserot J, Ferreiro-Vera C, de Castro L, Guerrero Pavon R, Quesada Gomez J (2010) Evaluation of vitamin D endocrine system (VDES) status and response to treatment of patients in intensive care units (ICUs) using an on-line SPE-LC-MS/MS method. J Ster Biochem Mol Biol 121:452–455
56. Ingels C, Van Cromphaut S, Wouters P et al (2010) Effect of restoration of 25OHD3 status in prolonged critical illness on serum innate immunity parameters LL-37 and sCD163. Crit Care 14(Suppl 1):590 (abst)
57. Bischoff-Ferrari HA, Shao A, Dawson-Hughes B, Hathcock J, Giovannucci E, Willett WC (2010) Benefit-risk assessment of vitamin D supplementation. Osteoporos Int 21:1121–1132

Part VI

Hemodynamic Optimization

Autonomic Dysfunction Is the Motor of Chronic Critical Illness

A. Toner, J. Whittle, and G. L. Ackland

Introduction

Many of the insults that lead to critical illness, such as sepsis, trauma and major surgery, either cause, or are perhaps the consequence of, profound alterations in autonomic nervous system control. Several cardinal features of chronic critical illness – regardless of the etiology – support the assertion that autonomic dysfunction is a core mechanism underlying the development and perpetuation of multiorgan failure. By reconsidering the spectrum that autonomic dysfunction encompasses, we explore the pivotal and multi-faceted impact exerted by aberrant autonomic control in chronic critical illness.

Established Autonomic Dysfunction Is Common in Patients Who Develop Critical Illness

Unequivocally, the majority of patients in the intensive care unit (ICU) exhibit established, predisposing features of chronic disease prior to requiring critical care [1]. Established autonomic dysfunction is highly prevalent in patients with com-

A. Toner
Department of Anesthesia and Intensive Care Medicine, St. George's Hospital, Blackshaw Road, London SW17 8QT, UK

J. Whittle
Department of Anesthesia, Pain Management and Critical Care, University College London, London NW1 2BU, UK

G. L. Ackland (✉)
Academy of Medical Sciences/Health Foundation Clinician Scientist, Wolfson Institute for Biomedical Research, Department of Medicine, University College London, London WC1E 6BT, UK
E-mail: g.ackland@ucl.ac.uk

J.-L. Vincent (Ed.), *Annual Update in Intensive Care and Emergency Medicine 2013*,
DOI 10.1007/978-3-642-35109-9_16, © Springer-Verlag Berlin Heidelberg 2013

mon medical comorbidities [2]. In addition, many critically ill patients manifest previously unsuspected, subclinical pathology. For example, autonomic abnormalities can be detected in pre-disease states, such as pre-hypertension [3]. Although various techniques have been used to detect alterations in autonomic control in a wide range of diseases, chiefly concentrating on the autonomic modulation of heart rate (heart rate variability) and the arterial baroreflex, the lack of population norms, variable acquisition and analysis techniques, and lack of long term follow-up limit comparability across studies [4].

Autonomic Dysfunction Is a Ubiquitous Feature at the Onset of Critical Illness

Irrespective of baseline autonomic function, experimental and clinical studies have demonstrated rapid and profound alterations in autonomic function following a range of apparently disparate pathologies leading to critical illness. Activation of the sympathetic nervous system is central to a coordinated cardiorespiratory, metabolic and immune response to infection and tissue injury. Indeed, early survival following endotoxemic shock is critically dependent upon the maintenance of an elevated sympathetic drive. Expression of heat shock protein (HSP)-70 prevents circulatory collapse via inhibition of inducible nitric oxide synthase (iNOS) gene expression in the rostral ventrolateral medulla, the crucial brainstem substrate that generates increased sympathetic activity [5]. Acute hyperadrenergic stimulation is characterized by a several fold increase in the levels of circulating catecholamines and rapid, parallel reductions in heart rate variability [6], most elegantly demonstrated by infusing endotoxin in healthy volunteers [7]. The speed with which these dysautonomic changes occur partly reflects rapid changes in afferent information conveyed to autonomic control centers.

Consistent with this idea, experimental data derived from laboratory models of critical illness show that afferent neural sensors are pivotal in shaping autonomic control during early sepsis. For example, in addition to sensing levels in blood oxygen, carbon dioxide and hydrogen ions, the carotid body chemoreceptors detect circulating inflammatory mediators that enhance hypoxic sensitivity [8]. These laboratory data explain, at least in part, the appearance of the ubiquitous features of tachycardia and tachypnea at the onset of critical illness, which frequently occur in the absence of hypoxia and/or acidosis, both key triggers of increased peripheral chemosensitivity. Acute transection of the carotid sinus nerve, which conveys both circulating biologic information transduced by the carotid body chemosensitive cells and blood pressure changes to brainstem control centers, increases mortality in experimental endotoxemia [9], through undefined mechanisms. The loss of chemoreflex and/or baroreflex responses in critically ill septic patients is associated with higher mortality [10]. Whether this reflects an intrinsic failure of autonomic control, as suggested by post-mortem data from septic patients [11], or the unavoidable consequences of modern critical care treatment remains unclear. Several common clinical interventions, including sedation [12] and neuromuscular blockade [13], markedly reduce, if not ablate, the carotid chemoreflex, and also profoundly alter baroreflex control [14]. The unavoidable, 'off-target' effects of immobilization and anxiety also contribute to this dysautonomic phenotype. Enforced bed-rest in healthy volunteers results in a reduction in heart rate variability after less than 24 hours, particularly in the high frequency range that reflects parasympathetic modulation of the heart [15]. Similarly, acute psychological stress reduces baroreflex sensitivity, whilst increasing heart rate and blood pressure; β-adrenergic blockade enhances baroreflex sensitivity during acute psychological stress [16]. Remarkably, experimental models of bed-rest also demonstrate a mechanistic interaction between dysautonomia and anhedonia [17], relevant to the negative prognostic impact of depression on outcome of critical illness [18]. These data suggest that the potential benefit of early physical, occupational and/or behavioral therapy [19] could be mediated through partial preservation or restoration of autonomic control.

Persistence of Autonomic Dysfunction in Established Critical Illness

The rapid development, or unmasking, of autonomic dysfunction early in critical illness leads to more sinister pathologic derangement (Fig. 1). Using just two examples, namely cardiac dysfunction and immune paralysis, the persistence of autonomic dysfunction at both cellular and integrative physiologic levels helps explain the irreversible cycle of multiorgan dysfunction that typifies the frequent failure to successfully capitalize on the ability of the modern critical care facility to prevent early mortality.

Autonomic Dysfunction Drives Cardiac Injury and Failure

The functional disconnection between the autonomic nervous system and the heart during critical illness has been described as "cardiac uncoupling" [20]. Several consequences of cardiac uncoupling ensue in critical illness. Myocardial cell injury can be induced by excessive sympathetic activity, through the accumulation of intracellular calcium triggering myocardial necrosis [21]. A prothrombotic state and metabolic dysregulation [22], induced by sympathetic activation, may also contribute. Acute psychological stress alone triggers coagulation and endothelial cell activation (reviewed in detail elsewhere [22]), an effect abolished by non-specific β-blockade. Thus, autonomic dysfunction-induced injury is likely to contribute to the elevated troponin levels seen frequently in critically ill patients [23]. This mechanism may underpin the association between autonomic dysfunction and poorer clinical outcomes.

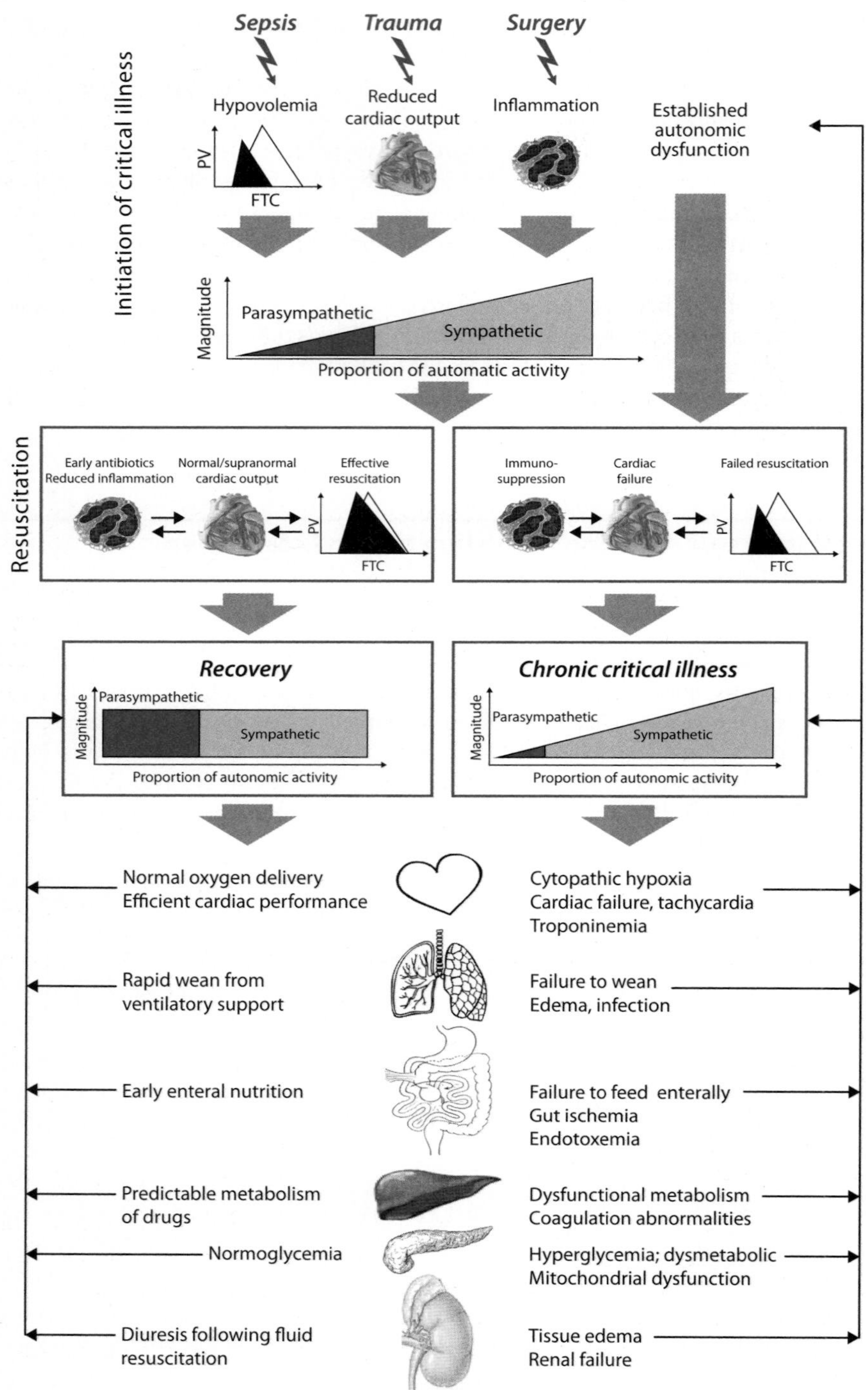

Initiation of critical illness
Sepsis
Trauma
Surgery
Hypovolemia
Reduced cardiac output
Inflammation
Established autonomic dysfunction
PV
FTC
Magnitude
Parasympathetic
Sympathetic
Proportion of automatic activity
Resuscitation
Early antibiotics Reduced inflammation
Normal/supranormal cardiac output
Effective resuscitation
Immuno-suppression
Cardiac failure
Failed resuscitation
Recovery
Chronic critical illness
Proportion of autonomic activity
Normal oxygen delivery
Efficient cardiac performance
Cytopathic hypoxia
Cardiac failure, tachycardia
Troponinemia
Rapid wean from ventilatory support
Failure to wean
Edema, infection
Early enteral nutrition
Failure to feed enterally
Gut ischemia
Endotoxemia
Predictable metabolism of drugs
Dysfunctional metabolism
Coagulation abnormalities
Normoglycemia
Hyperglycemia; dysmetabolic
Mitochondrial dysfunction
Diuresis following fluid resuscitation
Tissue edema
Renal failure

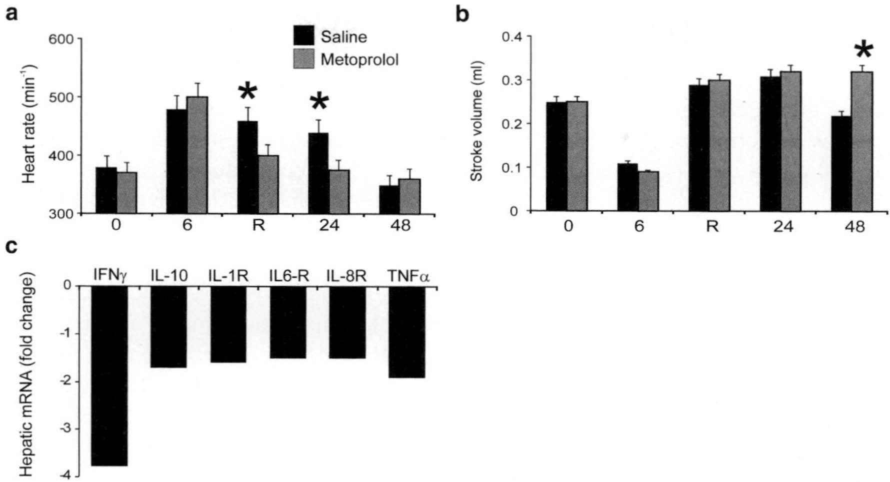

Fig. 2 β-blockade is beneficial in polymicrobial sepsis. **a** Reduction in heart rate following metoprolol treatment commenced 6 h after fecal peritonitis in adult rats. R denotes immediate period following fluid resuscitation, which was commenced 6 h after the onset of sepsis (n = 6 rats/group). **b** Improvement in stroke volume (measured by transthoracic echocardiography) following sustained metoprolol treatment for 2 days, commenced 6 h after fecal peritonitis in adult rats. **c** Hepatic genes associated with inflammation were downregulated by metoprolol pretreatment for 2 days before endotoxin administration in adult rats. Negative fold-change compared to saline treated rats. IFN: interferon; IL: interleukin; R: receptor; TNF: tumor necrosis factor. Asterisk denotes $p \leq 0.05$; all data mean ± SD. (Data from [28])

◀ **Fig. 1** Autonomic dysfunction is the motor for chronic critical illness: Concept. Failure to adequately hemodynamically resuscitate patients after major trauma, surgery or sepsis leads to persistent sympathetic activation, and parasympathetic withdrawal, thereby establishing autonomic dysfunction and fuelling multiple-organ dysfunction of varying severity. Pre-existing autonomic dysfunction, prior to (or as the result of) the insult, predisposes patients to irreversible autonomic dysfunction and deterioration in pre-existing organ dysfunction. Adequate resuscitation limits the impact of sympathetic activation, restores autonomic control and facilitates more rapid recovery from the initiating insult. For brevity, effects on musculoskeletal and cognitive impairment have been omitted. PV: peak velocity (cardiac contractility); FTC: corrected flow time, as measured by esophageal Doppler cardiac output monitor

In the absence of direct myocardial injury, prolonged sympathetic activation results in β-adrenoreceptor downregulation and desensitization – the process of uncoupling receptors from their downstream signaling effectors [24]. Various inflammatory mediators also directly impair cardiac receptor signaling [25]. This desensitization has been demonstrated in critical illness; several investigators have shown that an impaired cardio-metabolic physiologic response to exogenous β-adrenoreceptor stimulation is associated with increased mortality [26]. Interestingly, attenuation of increased sympathetic drive during sepsis using cardioselective β-blockers (Fig. 2) and α_2-agonists [27] may prevent these deleterious developments, although extra-cardiac mechanisms that indirectly reduce cardiac inflammation may also contribute [28]. The preservation of parasympathetic function, which is otherwise rapidly reduced at the onset of critical illness, also limits organ injury through a range of mechanisms. In addition to enabling more efficient cardiac performance [29] through under-appreciated synchrony with sympathetic activation (chiefly by increasing diastolic filling time and reducing cardiac work), intact vagal innervation limits cardiac (and extra-cardiac) inflammation [30] and enables neural reflexes to reduce myocardial injury [31]. Inter-organ crosstalk mediated neurally by the parasympathetic autonomic nervous system limits myocardial loss following coronary ischemia-reperfusion injury [31]. Distant organ injury, produced experimentally by bilateral occlusion of the femoral arteries, dramatically attenuates myocardial damage following transient coronary artery ligation, and is dependent on intact vagal innervations [31].

In summary, the combination of sympathetic activation and loss of parasympathetic cardiac modulation promotes a state of induced heart failure. The consequent inability to mount appropriate, integrated cardiovascular responses to subsequent infectious and other iatrogenic challenges is likely to play a key role in the failure to recover from critical illness. For example, cardiac failure is an important mechanism underlying the failure to wean successfully from ventilatory support [32]; failed planned or unplanned extubation is associated with marked clinical deterioration and increased morbidity and mortality.

Autonomic Dysfunction Results in Immune Paralysis

Since the initial bidirectional link between autonomic and immune systems was made by focusing on cytokine activation of the hypothalamic-adrenal axis, an abundance of experimental data has emerged demonstrating that corticosteroid-independent and parasympathetic mechanisms mediate stress-induced immunodepression. Neuro-anatomical studies have demonstrated extensive sympathetic innervation of the thymus, spleen, lymph nodes and bone marrow [33], in addition to parasympathetic innervation [30]. *In vitro* studies have shown that sympathetic and parasympathetic neurotransmitters can modulate all aspects of the immune response, including cytokine production, lymphocyte proliferation, and antibody secretion [34]. Although apparently anatomically unconnected, cardiac dysfunction and monocyte deactivation share pivotal mechanistic links in the pathogenesis of chronic critical illness through the development of autonomic dysfunction. Paralleling concomitant impaired myocardial performance [35], lymphocytes exposed to tumor necrosis factor (TNF)-α [36] or obtained from septic patients [37] exhibit impaired production of cyclic adenosine monophosphate (c-AMP) following β-adrenergic receptor stimulation, the levels of which help determine the balance between cellular activation and suppression.

Regardless of the precipitating causes of critical illness, several clinical studies have demonstrated that monocytic deactivation, which is characterized by reduced

HLA-DR expression, diminished antigen-presentation and bactericidal killing, is associated with a substantially increased risk of infection and higher mortality [38]. This inability of monocytes to provide immunosurveillance at such a key juncture, when critically ill patients are most susceptible to endogenous danger molecules and exogenous sources of infection, represents a crucial mechanism in conferring increased, sustained risk of failing to recover. In monocytes, catecholamines rapidly inhibit endotoxin-induced TNF-α production while increasing the release of the anti-inflammatory cytokine, interleukin (IL)-10 [39]. Similarly, $CD14^+$ monocytes from patients with septic shock demonstrate β-adrenergic desensitization following catecholamine stimulation [40], an effect recapitulated by *ex vivo* incubation of monocytes from healthy volunteers with lipopolysaccharide (LPS) and isoproterenol. The rapid production of anti-inflammatory cytokines, such as IL-10, results in spontaneous sepsis/pneumonia within 3 days of experimentally induced stroke, the mortality from which is reduced by administering propranolol [39]. Attenuation of sympatho-excitation, either through α_2-agonists administered into the central nervous system (CNS) [27], or peripheral β-blockade [28, 41], reduces mortality in sepsis. Restoration of vagal tone, loss of which would remove the α_7-nicotinic anti-inflammatory component from the neuroimmune arsenal [42], may contribute.

Deficient host immunity may not be the only contributor to the susceptibility of the chronically critically ill patient to recurrent infections. Host-pathogen interactions are shaped by adrenergic mechanisms that may be central to this phenomenon. The pro- and anti-inflammatory phenotype conferred by α- and β-adrenoreceptors alters depending on the presence of bacteria [43], with established sympathetic nervous system activation predisposing to accumulation of bacteria in tissue and an increased likelihood of secondary sepsis. Endogenous and exogenous catecholamines administered at therapeutically relevant levels stimulate bacterial growth and increase virulence of bacteria. Promotion of bacterial growth occurs via formation of direct complexes with the ferric iron within transferrin and lactoferrin, enabling bacterial sequestration of the normally inaccessible, but nutritionally key, host iron [44].

Therapeutic Precedents for Reversing Autonomic Dysfunction in Critical Illness

Modulation of autonomic control has either been directly explored, or inadvertently altered, in a chronic disease that bears many parallels to the syndrome of chronic critical illness (Fig. 3). As with many forms of chronic critical illness, autonomic dysregulation is recognized as a core feature of chronic heart failure, which is also characterized by increased sympathetic drive, high levels of circulating catecholamines and cortisol, accompanied by the withdrawal of parasympathetic activity [45]. Elevated plasma levels of pro-inflammatory cytokines [46], and deficient immunity [47] are also common features of chronic heart failure.

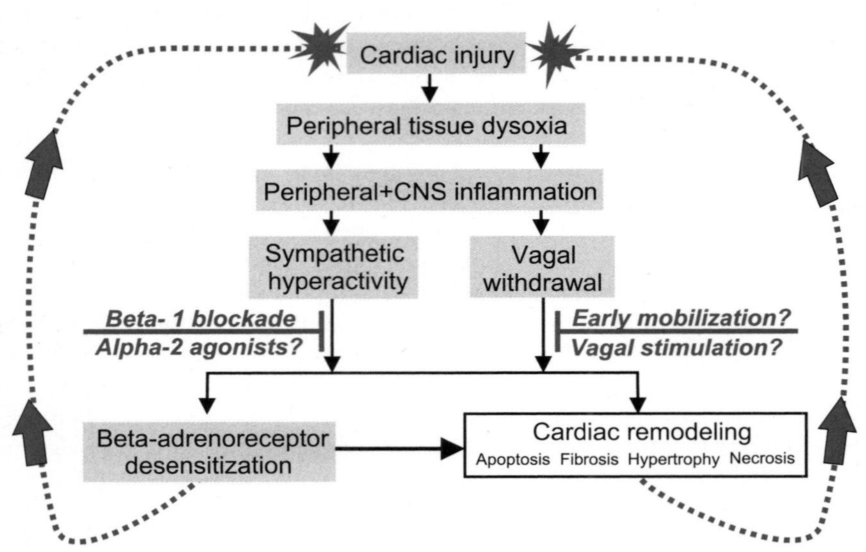

Fig. 3 Pathophysiologic parallels between chronic heart failure and established critical illness. Heart failure is a syndrome of multiorgan dysfunction driven by cardiac injury, tissue dysoxia, inflammation, autonomic dysfunction and consequent β-adrenoreceptor desensitization, generating a vicious pathophysiologic cycle which can be broken by sympatholysis and/or restoration of parasympathetic drive. Carefully titrated β_1-blockade improves outcome in heart failure; clinical trials exploring restoration of vagal tone in heart failure are currently in process

Importantly, cardiac failure can no longer be considered as a syndrome exclusive to the periphery, since neurohumoral activation is driven by concomitant changes in the central nervous system. A range of evidence-based, beneficial clinical treatments including angiotensin-converting enzyme (ACE)-inhibition and β-blockade are mechanistically bound together by autonomic modulation. Extensive clinical trials in heart failure [45] and proof-of-principle studies in human septic patients [48] have demonstrated the (arguably) counterintuitive finding that sympatholytics preserve, or improve, left ventricular performance. Laboratory interventions targeted at the CNS, chiefly aimed at reducing the adverse peripheral effects of sympatho-excitation, achieve superior clinical results in experimental heart failure. Compared to conventional peripheral delivery, chronic administration of ACE inhibitors and β_1 adrenoreceptor blockers directly into the CNS is more effective in reducing left ventricular remodeling, improving baroreceptor regulation of sympathetic nerve activity and reducing plasma levels of pro-inflammatory cytokines [49]. Clinical interventions using β-blockade in heart failure confer beneficial effects beyond improving cardiac performance and restoring autonomic balance; β blockade has also been shown to restore humoral immunity [47] and reduce plasma levels of pro-inflammatory cytokines [46]. Similarly, reductions in, or loss of, vagal activity is a predictor of high mortality in chronic heart failure [45]. Importantly, restoring parasympathetic modulation via electrical stimulation of the vagus nerve improves cardiac function, heart rate variability and baroreflex sensitivity, as well as attenuating excessive neurohormonal and inflammatory activation in experimental heart failure induced in different species [50]. Clinical trials are now in progress.

Conclusion

Established chronic critical illness presents a massive therapeutic challenge that requires novel approaches. Far from representing another biomarker of critical illness, autonomic dysfunction drives fundamental mechanisms that demonstrate it must be regarded as a mediator of an apparently impenetrable pathophysiologic cycle of multiorgan dysfunction. Greater understanding is required of the integrative, neurophysiologic and cellular mechanisms through which autonomic dysfunction impedes recovery, particularly using models of human injury and inflammation. Exploitation of innate mechanisms, such as remote preconditioning, and recognizing clinical interventions that may inadvertently do harm are important approaches to consider. Modulating autonomic dysfunction, through a variety of therapeutic avenues and radical – though rational – approaches, offers several exciting opportunities to minimize, or reverse, the devastating long-term consequences of chronic critical illness.

Acknowledgments: Supported by Academy of Medical Sciences/Health Foundation Clinician Scientist scheme (GLA), National Institute for Health Research Central and East London Clinical Research Network (GLA), Centre for Anaesthesia, Critical Care and Pain Management, University College London (JW), and HCA International Perioperative Medicine fellowships (AT, JW). This work was undertaken at University College London Hospitals NHS Trust/University College London who received a proportion of funding from the Department of Health UK NIHR Biomedical Research Centre funding scheme.

References

1. Angus DC, Linde-Zwirble WT, Lidicker J, Clermont G, Carcillo J, Pinsky MR (2001) Epidemiology of severe sepsis in the United States: analysis of incidence, outcome, and associated costs of care. Crit Care Med 29:1303–1310
2. Phillips JK (2012) Autonomic dysfunction in heart failure and renal disease. Front Physiol 3:219
3. Davis JT, Rao F, Naqshbandi D et al (2012) Autonomic and hemodynamic origins of prehypertension: central role of heredity. J Am Coll Cardiol 59:2206–2216
4. Seely AJ, Macklem PT (2004) Complex systems and the technology of variability analysis. Crit Care 8:R367–R384
5. Chan JY, Ou CC, Wang LL, Chan SH (2004) Heat shock protein 70 confers cardiovascular protection during endotoxemia via inhibition of nuclear factor-kappaB activation and inducible nitric oxide synthase expression in the rostral ventrolateral medulla. Circulation 110:3560–3566

6. de Montmollin E, Aboab J, Mansart A, Annane D (2009) Bench-to-bedside review: Beta-adrenergic modulation in sepsis. Crit Care 13:230
7. Godin PJ, Fleisher LA, Eidsath A et al (1996) Experimental human endotoxemia increases cardiac regularity: results from a prospective, randomized, crossover trial. Crit Care Med 24:1117–1124
8. Ackland GL, Kasymov V, Gourine AV (2007) Physiological and pathophysiological roles of extracellular ATP in chemosensory control of breathing. Biochem Soc Trans 35:1264–1268
9. Tang GJ, Kou YR, Lin YS (1998) Peripheral neural modulation of endotoxin-induced hyperventilation. Crit Care Med 26:1558–1563
10. Schmidt H, Muller-Werdan U, Hoffmann T et al (2005) Autonomic dysfunction predicts mortality in patients with multiple organ dysfunction syndrome of different age groups. Crit Care Med 33:1994–2002
11. Sharshar T, Gray F, Lorin de la Grandmaison G et al (2003) Apoptosis of neurons in cardiovascular autonomic centres triggered by inducible nitric oxide synthase after death from septic shock. Lancet 362:1799–1805
12. Akada S, Fagerlund MJ, Lindahl SG, Sakamoto A, Prabhakar NR, Eriksson LI (2008) Pronounced depression by propofol on carotid body response to CO2 and K+-induced carotid body activation. Respir Physiol Neurobiol 160:284–288
13. Eriksson LI, Sato M, Severinghaus JW (1993) Effect of a vecuronium-induced partial neuromuscular block on hypoxic ventilatory response. Anesthesiology 78:693–699
14. Ebert TJ (2005) Sympathetic and hemodynamic effects of moderate and deep sedation with propofol in humans. Anesthesiology 103:20–24
15. Hughson RL, Yamamoto Y, Maillet A et al (1994) Altered autonomic regulation of cardiac function during head-up tilt after 28-day head-down bed-rest with counter-measures. Clin Physiol 14:291–304
16. Truijen J, Davis SC, Stok WJ et al (2011) Baroreflex sensitivity is higher during acute psychological stress in healthy subjects under beta-adrenergic blockade. Clin Sci 120:161–167
17. Moffitt JA, Grippo AJ, Beltz TG, Johnson AK (2008) Hindlimb unloading elicits anhedonia and sympathovagal imbalance. J Appl Physiol 105:1049–1059
18. Desai SV, Law TJ, Needham DM (2011) Long-term complications of critical care. Crit Care Med 39:371–379
19. Schweickert WD, Pohlman MC, Pohlman AS et al (2009) Early physical and occupational therapy in mechanically ventilated, critically ill patients: a randomised controlled trial. Lancet 373:1874–1882
20. Norris PR, Ozdas A, Cao H et al (2006) Cardiac uncoupling and heart rate variability stratify ICU patients by mortality: a study of 2088 trauma patients. Ann Surg 243:804–812
21. Ellison GM, Torella D, Karakikes I et al (2007) Acute beta-adrenergic overload produces myocyte damage through calcium leakage from the ryanodine receptor 2 but spares cardiac stem cells. J Biol Chem 282:11397–11409
22. Barnes SJ, Ackland GL (2010) Beta-adrenoreceptor modulation of metabolic, endocrine and immunologic function during critical illness. Endocr Metab Immune Disord Drug Targets 10:292–300
23. Landesberg G, Vesselov Y, Einav S, Goodman S, Sprung CL, Weissman C (2005) Myocardial ischemia, cardiac troponin, and long-term survival of high-cardiac risk critically ill intensive care unit patients. Crit Care Med 33:1281–1287
24. DeWire SM, Ahn S, Lefkowitz RJ, Shenoy SK (2007) Beta-arrestins and cell signaling. Annu Rev Physiol 69:483–510
25. Coggins M, Rosenzweig A (2012) The fire within: cardiac inflammatory signaling in health and disease. Circ Res 110:116–125
26. Collin S, Sennoun N, Levy B (2008) Cardiovascular and metabolic responses to catecholamine and sepsis prognosis: a ubiquitous phenomenon? Crit Care 12:118
27. Hofer S, Steppan J, Wagner T et al (2009) Central sympatholytics prolong survival in experimental sepsis. Crit Care 13:R11

28. Ackland GL, Yao ST, Rudiger A et al (2010) Cardioprotection, attenuated systemic inflammation, and survival benefit of beta1-adrenoceptor blockade in severe sepsis in rats. Crit Care Med 38:388–394
29. Paton JF, Nalivaiko E, Boscan P, Pickering AE (2006) Reflexly evoked coactivation of cardiac vagal and sympathetic motor outflows: observations and functional implications. Clin Exp Pharmacol Physiol 33:1245–1250
30. Rosas-Ballina M, Tracey KJ (2009) The neurology of the immune system: neural reflexes regulate immunity. Neuron 64:28–32
31. Mastitskaya S, Marina N, Gourine A et al (2012) Cardioprotection evoked by remote ischaemic preconditioning is critically dependent on the activity of vagal pre-ganglionic neurones. Cardiovasc Res 95:487–494
32. Heunks LM, van der Hoeven JG (2010) Clinical review: the ABC of weaning failure – a structured approach. Crit Care 14:245
33. Nance DM, Sanders VM (2007) Autonomic innervation and regulation of the immune system (1987–2007). Brain, Behav Immun 21:736–745
34. Tracey KJ (2010) Understanding immunity requires more than immunology. Nat Immunol 11:561–564
35. Silverman HJ, Penaranda R, Orens JB, Lee NH (1993) Impaired beta-adrenergic receptor stimulation of cyclic adenosine monophosphate in human septic shock: association with myocardial hyporesponsiveness to catecholamines. Crit Care Med 21:31–39
36. Singh M, Notterman DA, Metakis L (1993) Tumor necrosis factor produces homologous desensitization of lymphocyte beta 2-adrenergic responses. Circ Shock 39:275–278
37. Bernardin G, Kisoka RL, Delporte C, Robberecht P, Vincent JL (2003) Impairment of beta-adrenergic signaling in healthy peripheral blood mononuclear cells exposed to serum from patients with septic shock: involvement of the inhibitory pathway of adenylyl cyclase stimulation. Shock 19:108–112
38. Monneret G, Lepape A, Venet F (2011) A dynamic view of mHLA-DR expression in management of severe septic patients. Crit Care 15:198
39. Meisel C, Meisel A (2011) Suppressing immunosuppression after stroke. N Engl J Med 365:2134–2136
40. Link A, Selejan S, Maack C, Lenz M, Bohm M (2008) Phosphodiesterase 4 inhibition but not beta-adrenergic stimulation suppresses tumor necrosis factor-alpha release in peripheral blood mononuclear cells in septic shock. Crit Care 12:R159
41. Suzuki T, Morisaki H, Serita R et al (2005) Infusion of the beta-adrenergic blocker esmolol attenuates myocardial dysfunction in septic rats. Crit Care Med 33:2294–2301
42. Rosas-Ballina M, Olofsson PS, Ochani M et al (2011) Acetylcholine-synthesizing T cells relay neural signals in a vagus nerve circuit. Science 334:98–101
43. Straub RH, Linde HJ, Mannel DN, Scholmerich J, Falk W (2000) A bacteria-induced switch of sympathetic effector mechanisms augments local inhibition of TNF-alpha and IL-6 secretion in the spleen. FASEB J 14:1380–1388
44. Lyte M, Freestone PP, Neal CP et al (2003) Stimulation of Staphylococcus epidermidis growth and biofilm formation by catecholamine inotropes. Lancet 361:130–135
45. Schwartz PJ, De Ferrari GM (2011) Sympathetic-parasympathetic interaction in health and disease: abnormalities and relevance in heart failure. Heart Fail Rev 16:101–107
46. Gage JR, Fonarow G, Hamilton M, Widawski M, Martinez-Maza O, Vredevoe DL (2004) Beta blocker and angiotensin-converting enzyme inhibitor therapy is associated with decreased Th1/Th2 cytokine ratios and inflammatory cytokine production in patients with chronic heart failure. Neuroimmunomodulation 11:173–180
47. Maisel AS (1994) Beneficial effects of metoprolol treatment in congestive heart failure. Reversal of sympathetic-induced alterations of immunologic function. Circulation 90:1774–1780
48. Gore DC, Wolfe RR (2006) Hemodynamic and metabolic effects of selective beta1 adrenergic blockade during sepsis. Surgery 139:686–694
49. Felder RB, Yu Y, Zhang ZH, Wei SG (2009) Pharmacological treatment for heart failure: a view from the brain. Clin Pharmacol Ther 86:216–220
50. Schwartz PJ, De Ferrari GM (2009) Vagal stimulation for heart failure: background and first in-man study. Heart Rhythm 6:S76–S81

Hemodynamic Adaptation to Hypoxia in Neonatal Critical Care

H. A. van Elteren, C. Ince, and I. K. M. Reiss

Introduction

Hypoxia is a condition that is not only observed in critically ill patients admitted to the intensive care unit (ICU): Approximately 140 million people live in a high altitude environment and face chronic hypoxia [1], and every human being has experienced extreme hypoxic conditions *in utero*. The fetus can survive and grow under these conditions because of decreased metabolic demands and altered cardiovascular circulation. Naturally, if oxygen delivery (DO_2) does not meet oxygen consumption (VO_2), the fetus will suffer and will eventually require critical care. For this condition, the term dysoxia is appropriate, as it describes the condition in which the need for oxygen to sustain cellular respiration (mitochondrial oxygen requirement for fueling oxidative phosphorylation to produce ATP needed for the energy requirements of cells to live and function) exceeds that being supplied by the microcirculation [2]. It can be argued that the holy grail of critical medicine is the identification of dysoxia and its adequate treatment. In neonatal intensive care, this quest is confounded by the changing metabolic requirements of the neonate as its growth progresses.

H. A. van Elteren
Department of Pediatrics, Division of Neonatology, Erasmus Medical Center-Sophia Children's Hospital, University Medical Center, Rotterdam, The Netherlands

C. Ince
Department of Intensive Care Adults, Erasmus Medical Center, University Medical Center, Rotterdam, The Netherlands

I. K. M. Reiss (✉)
Department of Pediatrics, Division of Neonatology, Erasmus Medical Center-Sophia Children's Hospital, University Medical Center, Rotterdam, The Netherlands
i.reiss@erasmusmc.nl

J.-L. Vincent (Ed.), *Annual Update in Intensive Care and Emergency Medicine 2013*, 211
DOI 10.1007/978-3-642-35109-9_17, © Springer-Verlag Berlin Heidelberg 2013

Both intra- and extra-uterine adaptation mechanisms are known to come into play to avoid hypoxia and cellular dysfunction. Although these mechanisms are protective, they can potentially be pathological, as there are limitations to these defense mechanisms. These mechanisms can further be confounded by treatment modalities that may themselves cause harm. For example, after birth, diseases associated with maladaptation, such as patent ductus arteriosus (PDA) and persistent pulmonary hypertension of the newborn (PPHN), are often treated with excessive amounts of oxygen. However, it has become clear that hyperoxia itself can cause damage by the formation of reactive oxygen species (ROS). Although ROS have prominent signaling properties important in both normal and patho-physiological states of vasodilation [3], ROS can also cause membrane lipid peroxidation and DNA fragmentation [4]. In neonates, there is direct and indirect evidence that ROS play a role in a variety of conditions, including bronchopulmonary dysplasia (BPD), retinopathy of prematurity, periventricular leukomalacia (PVL) and necrotizing enterocolitis (NEC) [5]. As technology has advanced, treatment of newborns as young as 22 weeks gestational age has been realized. Unfortunately, this trend has also seen an increase in the incidence of maladaptation in newborns. The understanding of oxygen transport and handling pathways in the developing fetus, as well as methods of monitoring and treating such a developing condition, is the challenge facing the neonatologist today.

In this review, we will discuss cardiovascular adaptation and maladaptation to hypoxia in fetal and postnatal life and its consequences for further development. We will briefly discuss monitoring techniques to identify the presence of hemodynamic mechanisms associated with (mal)adaptation to hypoxia.

Antenatal Adaptation to Hypoxia

Oxygen transfer to the fetus is mainly regulated by uterine artery blood flow [6]. In intrauterine life, the human fetus is subject to a hypoxic environment. Extrapolations from animal studies suggest that under normal conditions, human fetal PaO_2 is between 2.5 and 3.5 kPa [7]. Low partial pressure of oxygen also implies that fetal tissues are more susceptible to a state of oxygen insufficiency. Several maternal and environmental conditions can impede the process of oxygen delivery. The following three forms of antenatal hypoxia have been suggested: (1) Pre-placental hypoxia, in which both the mother and her fetus become hypoxic (high-altitude, cyanotic maternal heart disease); (2) utero-placental hypoxia, in which maternal oxygenation is normal, but the utero-placental circulation is impaired (pre-eclampsia, placental insufficiency); and (3) post-placental hypoxia, in which only the fetus is hypoxic due to fetal disease [8]. Most of the data regarding the effects of hypoxia have been acquired from animal studies in which different techniques have been used to mimic chronic hypoxia. However, it is unclear whether these models of chronic hypoxemia result in the same adaptive mechanisms as occur in hypoxemic neonates.

In normal fetal life, metabolism and VO_2 are decreased compared to extrauterine life. Many physiological functions are reduced, including respiratory effort, gastrointestinal digestion and absorption and renal tubular re-absorption. There is also no need to maintain thermoregulation because the thermal environment is maintained by the mother. These changes result in reduced tissue VO_2. From an evolutionary perspective, it is assumed that the hypoxic environment is important for development, as it protects the fetus from oxidative damage [9]. The hypoxic environment is also critical for lung development, as the hypoxic environment stabilizes hypoxia inducible factor (HIF). HIF is a family of transcription factors that play a central role in cellular adaptation to insufficient oxygen. Under normoxic conditions (cellular O_2 concentration $>5\%$), HIF proteins are degraded. The expression of HIF-1 proteins and the level of HIF-1 DNA binding activity increases exponentially from an oxygen fraction from 5% O_2 to 0.5% O_2 [10]. HIF-1 is activated during fetal development, and it is also active during the normal homeostasis of most tissues. In the human lung at 8 to 13 weeks of gestation, HIF-1α expression is mainly restricted to branching epithelium, whereas HIF-2α appears to be present in the vascular structures of the lung parenchyma [11]. Mouse models have identified the different functions of HIF subunits. HIF-1α knockout mice suffer from severe cardiovascular defects and die *in utero*, whereas HIF-2α knockout mice suffer from postnatal respiratory distress due to insufficient surfactant production and slow heart rate [12].

HIF-1 target genes include those encoding vascular endothelial growth factor (VEGF), erythropoietin, glucose transporters, and glycolytic enzymes [13]. Enhanced erythropoiesis results in higher hematocrit and hemoglobin concentrations in cord blood. The proportion of fetal hemoglobin (HbF) in cord blood is generally increased at high altitudes compared to equivalent populations at sea-level [14]. The affinity of fetal hemoglobin for oxygen is substantially greater than that of adult hemoglobin. The P50 value for HbF (i. e., the partial pressure of oxygen at which the protein is 50 % saturated) is roughly 19 mm Hg, whereas adult hemoglobin has a value of approximately 26.8 mm Hg [15]. This phenomenon is a result of decreased binding of 2,3-diphosphoglycerate (2,3-DPG) to HbF. The increase in HbF concentrations results in higher oxygen saturation at the same partial pressure of oxygen. HbF cells are also more compliant than adult hemoglobin cells, making it easier for them to enter the capillaries of the microcirculation [16].

The fetal heart has an improved protection mechanism to prevent hypoxia-induced cell death compared to the adult heart. This resistance has been attributed to the enhanced capacity of the immature heart for glycolysis and protection against oxidative stress [17, 18]. Increased adrenergic activity and elevated plasma concentration of catecholamines results in positive chronotropic and inotropic stimulation of the heart leading to an increase in cardiac output [19]. There is also an altered distribution in cardiac output. Hypoxic stress in the ovine fetus increases umbilical venous return through the ductus venosus and the preferential streaming of this blood through the foramen ovale, facilitating the delivery of the most highly oxygenated blood to the upper body and thus to the heart and brain

[20]. Blood flow to the gastrointestinal, renal and peripheral vascular beds decreases [21].

Studies in both animal and human fetuses show an increase in oxygen extraction when DO_2 is diminished [22, 23]. The fetus is also capable of switching metabolic rate depending on oxygen levels. In response to hypoxia, the fetus can reduce its oxygen demands or it can increase its metabolic demands to prevent hyperoxia [24]. These adaptation mechanisms can maintain conditions until a 50% fall in placental blood flow occurs. Hereafter, a decrease in fetal movement is required to reduce VO_2 [25]. Obstetricians consider this to be a risk factor for adverse pregnancy outcome.

Antenatal Maladaptation to Hypoxia

If fetal adaptation mechanisms are insufficient, chronic hypoxia leads to altered cardiac and pulmonary development. Lung development can be divided into the following five stages based on histological appearance: Embryonic (1–7 wk gestation); pseudoglandular (5–17 wk gestation); canalicular (16–26 wk gestation); saccular (24–38 wk gestation); and alveolar stage (36 wk gestation onward) [26]. By 17 weeks of gestation, all preacinar pulmonary and bronchial arteries are formed. Thereafter, there is an increase in lung capillaries. In response to hypoxia, pulmonary vascular remodeling occurs. This remodeling is characterized by the combination of hypertrophy and hyperplasia of the cells within each layer of the vessel wall. There is increased smooth muscle proliferation and muscularization of the normally muscle-free peripheral arteries. The intima is infiltrated with fibroblasts, and the adventitia shows increased production of extracellular matrix with deposition of collagen and elastin [27]. These changes result in thickening of the blood vessel wall, increased pulmonary vascular resistance (PVR), and reduced compliance. Vascular remodeling can occur at any stage of fetal lung development and also occurs in the postnatal period [28]. Compared to adults, these vascular changes are greater and occur more rapidly in newborns [29]. This results in more severe pulmonary hypertension and generally lower oxygen saturation levels. The intracellular mechanisms underlying vascular remodeling are complex and have recently been discussed in excellent reviews [28, 30]. Unfortunately, vascular remodeling can only be observed by histopathological examination and cannot be predicted on antenatal ultrasound.

In normal cardiac development, at 8 weeks of gestation, the heart is developed to a completely looped 4-chamber organ [31]. Hemodynamic characteristics, such as ventricular volume, stroke volume, and cardiac output, increase with gestational age, whereas ejection fraction decreases as gestation advances. The combined cardiovascular output in human fetuses, estimated by the Doppler technique, steadily increases from 50 ml/min at 18 weeks to 1,200 ml/min (approximately 400 ml/kg/min) at term. Normal fetal cardiovascular physiology is characterized by ventricular volumes that are larger on the right and ejection fractions that are greater for the left ventricle. This results in similar left and right ventricular stroke volume and cardiac output [32].

In chronic hypoxia, fetal cardiac development is impaired in both structure and function [33]. Animal studies have shown that chronic hypoxia in the first trimester causes ventricle septum defects, myocardial thinning, cardiomyocyte hypertrophy, ventricle dilation and detachment of the epicardium [34–36]. This phenomenon leads to a lower heart rate, decreased cardiac output and lowered contractility [37, 38]. Developmental changes to chronic hypoxia are not restricted to cardiovascular tissue. Changes in other fetal tissues are beyond the scope of this paper.

Postnatal Hemodynamics and Maladaptation

The fetal circulation is characterized by a high PVR, and this resistance is accompanied by a constant state of pulmonary hypertension. Of the blood pumped out by the right ventricle, approximately 10 % enters the lung via pulmonary arteries; the majority enters the aorta via the ductus arteriosus [39]. As a result of the low vascular resistance of the placenta, the high vascular resistance of the fluid-filled fetal lungs, and the presence of the fetal channels, the fetal circulation functions as a parallel circuit with right-to-left shunting of relatively oxygenated blood through the foramen ovale and less-saturated blood across the ductus arteriosus. At birth, an impressive fall in PVR and an increase in systemic vascular resistance (SVR) results in the transition from fetal to an adult circulation, including the closure of the foramen ovale and ductus arteriosus. Various mechanical factors and vasoactive agent signaling pathways contribute to the decrease in PVR. Of these factors, the endothelium-derived nitric oxide pathway (EDNO), prostacyclin (PGI_2) and endothelin-1 (ET-1) pathways seem to have the greatest clinical importance. A newborn infant prior to the 37th week of gestation is considered to be preterm. The use of antenatal corticosteroids and exogenous surfactant therapy made it possible to treat premature infants as young as 22 weeks of gestation. Cardiovascular physiology in preterm newborns is altered compared to adults, and hemodynamic values differ between the broad ranges of prematurity. Reference values for gestational age are shown in Table 1 [40]. The preterm newborn has a limited ability to respond to changes in determinants of the cardiac output, due to fewer mitochondria and energy stores. Consequently, the preterm infant heart is less able to respond to stresses that occur in the postnatal period, such as increased peripheral vascular resistance with resultant increased afterload. Large ductus arteriosus and high mean airway pressure can further impede systemic blood flow during a period when the preterm infant is particularly vulnerable to blood flow changes and hypoxia.

Chronic hypoxia has a major influence on postnatal adaptation and *vice versa*. Most data in humans on this subject were gathered from comparison of high-altitude vs. sea-level newborns. At birth, mean pulmonary artery pressure (PAP) is equal in newborns born at high altitude and at sea level, with values of 60 mm Hg.

Table 1 Reference values for heart rate and blood pressure in premature infants [40]. Data are presented as means and 95 % confidence intervals

Gestational age (weeks)	Heart rate (beats/minute)	Mean blood pressure (mm Hg)	Systolic blood pressure (mm Hg)	Diastolic blood pressure (mm Hg)
<24	160 (120–190)	27 (20–37)	35 (25–45)	23 (15–30)
24–28	157 (115–185)	31 (23–40)	40 (30–50)	26 (17–34)
28–32	150 (110–180)	36 (28–45)	45 (35–55)	30 (22–40)
32–37	136 (90–175)	42 (33–50)	55 (45–65)	35 (28–43)
37–40	130 (70–170)	45 (36–55)	60 (55–75)	40 (32–47)

Within 72 hours, PAP decreases and remains at values of 12 mm Hg through further life. At high altitude, there is a persistent high PAP with values of 55 mm Hg after 72 hours of birth and 28 mm Hg during adolescence and adulthood [41]. As a result, there is persistent right ventricle hypertrophy with a similar decreasing pattern as in PAP [42]. These factors contribute to a persistent fetal circulation including a prolonged right-left shunt over the ductus arteriosus, a 30–40-fold higher incidence of persistent ductus arteriosus and persistence of an anatomically patent foramen ovale in 44 % of children at the age of 6 months [43–45]. Most striking is the estimation of a 100-fold increase of PPHN in infants born in hypoxic conditions [46].

Persistent Pulmonary Hypertension of the Newborn

PPHN must be distinguished from pulmonary hypertension in children or adults. In children, congenital heart disease or idiopathic pulmonary hypertension accounts for the majority of cases [47], while in adults, chronic obstructive pulmonary disease (COPD), left heart disease and connective tissue disease are more frequent causes of pulmonary hypertension.

PPHN due to maladaptation is different than other forms of PPHN. PPHN generally can be divided into the following three groups: (1) Those with abnormally constricted pulmonary vasculature due to lung parenchymal diseases, such as meconium aspiration syndrome, respiratory distress syndrome (RDS), or pneumonia; (2) those with hypoplastic vasculature, as observed in congenital diaphragmatic hernia; and (3) those with lungs of normal parenchyma but remodeled pulmonary vasculature [48]. This last group suffers from what is known as idiopathic PPHN, but antenatal vascular remodeling almost certainly plays a major role in the etiology. Understanding the regulation of the perinatal pulmonary circulation has helped the development of new treatments for PPHN. Inhaled NO has proven its value in newborns, decreasing the need for extracorporeal membrane oxygenation (ECMO) [49]. Other potential treatment options currently being studied in neonates include inhibition of cGMP degradation by PDE5 with sildenafil, inhibition of cAMP degradation with milrinone, and inhibition of ET-1 with bosentan [50–52]. However, as only small randomized controlled trials have been performed in newborns, their clinical value remains uncertain.

Consequences of Maladaptation to Hypoxia

Exposure to chronic hypoxia and persistent fetal circulation leads to increased mortality and morbidity in newborns and children [53, 54]. Epidemiological studies have indicated that high-altitude pregnancies increase the risk of intrauterine growth restriction (IUGR) and low birth weight. Infants born small for gestational age are at higher risk for prematurity, asphyxia, necrotizing enterocolitis and bronchopulmonary dysplasia and thus have increased morbidity and mortality rates [55, 56]. In adult life, small for gestational age infants also have a more than 1.5-fold increased risk of cardiovascular disease compared to age- and gender-matched controls who were born appropriate for gestational age [57].

Reaching a situation of normoxia can reverse the cellular and structural changes in the pulmonary vasculature. In pulmonary hypertensive rats, 6 weeks of normoxia resulted in reversal of vessel wall thickness and vascular smooth muscle cell infiltration in preacinar arteries [58]. However, right ventricle systolic pressure shows incomplete reversal. Sartori et al. demonstrated that survivors of perinatal pulmonary hypertension had a significantly greater increase in PAP at high altitude compared to healthy controls [59]. These findings suggest that a transient perinatal insult to the pulmonary circulation leaves a persistent and potentially fatal imprint, which predisposes patients to a pathological response when activated in adult life.

Oxygen: Treatment or Trouble?

As technology has helped to treat newborns as young as 22 weeks gestational age, the use of oxygen therapy has become more and more standard as the perception that dysoxia is prevalent and can be corrected by administering oxygen via respiration gained acceptance. As gestational age decreases, the incidence of maladaptation and specific neonatal disorders, such as PPHN, persistent ductus arteriosus and RDS, increases [60]. However, as knowledge of oxygen therapy has increased over time, it has become clear that administration of high fractions of oxygen also has serious side effects. Excessive oxygen administration results in increased mitochondrial production of ROS, as well as reactive nitrogen species (RNS), which cause membrane and DNA fragmentation [61]. Under normal physiological conditions, O_2 and NO form hydrogen peroxide (H_2O_2), which is a stable cell-signaling molecule in vascular homeostasis [3]. In the situation of increased ROS availability, however, ROS and NO can form the highly reactive peroxynitrite ($ONOO^-$). This oxidant and others have the potential to produce vasoconstriction, cytotoxicity, and damage to surfactant proteins and lipids. The premature infant is especially susceptible to ROS- and RNS-induced damage for two major reasons. First, increases in antioxidant capacity occur in the latter part of gestation in preparation for the transition to extra-uterine life and, in early stages, this capacity is undeveloped. Adequate concentrations of antioxidants, such as catalase, glutathione peroxidase and superoxide dismutase, may therefore be absent at birth [62]. Second, the ability to increase synthesis of antioxidants in response to hyperoxia or other oxidant challenges is relatively impaired [4].

ROS are directly responsible for DNA damage and thus carcinogenesis [63]. A higher target of oxygen saturation increases the incidence of severe retinopathy of prematurity and BPD in extreme preterm infants [64, 65]. Resuscitation in the delivery room with 100 % oxygen even increases mortality rates [66, 67]. In later life, ROS is responsible for cell aging [68, 69], carcinogenesis and childhood leukemia [70, 71]. Conversely, higher targets of oxygen saturation reduce mortality in extreme preterm infants [64, 72]. These data indicate that there is a clear balance between 'drug action' and side-effects in oxygen therapy. In standard critical care, tissue oxygenation and oxygen availability at the microvascular level is not routinely measured. We hypothesize that gaining such insight into the oxygen transport pathways at the level of the microcirculation for the critically ill neonatal patient can result in an improved monitoring environment, leading to treatment strategies aimed at optimizing tissue oxygenation and resolving dysoxia. Such a strategy would result in a more rational use of oxygen therapy, thereby restricting its harmful side effects.

Monitoring of Maladaptation in the Newborn

In (premature) newborns, hemodynamic monitoring remains complicated compared to adults; methods should be accurate along the entire spectrum of gestational age and birth-weight, useful in neonates with extra- and intra-cardiac shunting, validated against one of the 'gold standards' and most of all be practical and non-invasive [73]. However, many measuring techniques are impractical, due to the lack of appropriately sized materials, and the risks of use outweigh the potential benefits.

The following three key components in the physiology of DO_2 to the tissues can be identified: Uptake of oxygen in the lung, transport and delivery of oxygen from the lung to the tissues, and oxygen uptake and utilization by the tissues [74]. Recent innovations in hemodynamic monitoring have helped neonatal and pediatric intensivists to visualize tissue perfusion and oxygenation in a non-invasive manner. These techniques have allowed evaluation of cardiac output, systemic vascular resistance, organ blood flow distribution and tissue DO_2 at the bedside. However, lack of validation and reference values complicates clinical use [73].

Adaptation is not limited to DO_2 or tissue oxygen extraction. Techniques need to be combined to allow monitoring of changes in neonatal adaptation. This approach has not yet been attempted in neonatal critical care. The identification of whether tissues suffer from dysoxia, i. e., the condition where oxygen availability is inadequate to meet the mitochondrial needs of the parenchymal cells to sustain oxidative phosphorylation, can be regarded as a 'holy grail' in this respect.

Tissue perfusion has been measured in newborns during the adaptation phase mainly using orthogonal polarization spectral (OPS) imaging and its successor, sidestream dark field (SDF) imaging. SDF imaging uses a light guide, which is surrounded by green light (530 nm) emitting diodes (LED). The light penetrates the tissue, illuminates the microcirculation, and is absorbed by hemoglobin of the erythrocytes. The flowing red blood cells perfusing the microvessels are visualized. Quantitative assessments of microvascular variables are possible using specialized software off-line. Different variables can be measured, including vascular density (FCD), heterogeneity of perfusion and microvascular blood flow. A disadvantage of the OPS/SDF imaging techniques is that the resolution is limited due to the use of analog video cameras and the fact that the technology does not allow instant on-line bedside quantification of images [75]. These shortcomings may have been resolved by the recent introduction of a computer-controlled high resolution imaging sensor-based device based on incident dark field imaging [76], which holds promise in this respect [75].

The FCD in the skin of premature infants decreases significantly over the first month of life. A correlation has been found with decreases in hemoglobin concentration [77]. It has been supposed that higher FCD in the first week of postnatal life may be related to higher cardiac output in the first week. The microcirculation has been measured in newborns with severe respiratory failure directly after birth. ECMO treatment did not improve the microcirculation after 24 hours. Interestingly, the use of inhaled NO did have this effect, which highlights the role of NO in adaptation [78, 79].

Tissue oxygenation has been measured in newborns during the adaptation phase using near-infrared spectroscopy (NIRS). NIRS is based on the transparency of biological tissue to light in the near-infrared part of the spectrum (700–1,000 nm) and its subsequent absorption by oxygenated hemoglobin (O_2Hb) and deoxygenated hemoglobin (HHb) in the blood vessels that are within the near-infrared light beam. Absorption changes in near-infrared light can later be converted into concentration changes of O_2Hb and HHb. NIRS has mainly been used for cerebral oxygen saturation [80–82]. However, small numbers and great inter-patient variability gave limited information concerning normal ranges during the first weeks of life.

Conclusion

Chronic hypoxia has major influences on fetal development and physiology in newborns. There are several adaptation mechanisms to protect against hypoxia.

Maladaptation has been related to neonatal disorders and cardiovascular disease in adult life. Combining imaging techniques is necessary for an optimal view of adaptation. Better understanding of pathophysiological pathways in maladaptation can help clinicians find the optimal treatment for hypoxia.

References

1. Moore LG, Charles SM, Julian CG (2011) Humans at high altitude: hypoxia and fetal growth. Respir Physiol Neurobiol 178:181–190
2. Ince C, Sinaasappel M (1999) Microcirculatory oxygenation and shunting in sepsis and shock. Crit Care Med 27:1369–1377
3. Widlansky ME, Gutterman DD (2011) Regulation of endothelial function by mitochondrial reactive oxygen species. Antioxid Redox Signal 15:1517–1530
4. Davis JM, Auten RL (2010) Maturation of the antioxidant system and the effects on preterm birth. Semin Fetal Neonatal Med 15:191–195
5. Lee JW, Davis JM (2011) Future applications of antioxidants in premature infants. Curr Opin Pediatr 23:161–166
6. Julian CG, Wilson MJ, Lopez M et al (2009) Augmented uterine artery blood flow and oxygen delivery protect Andeans from altitude-associated reductions in fetal growth. Am J Physiol Regul Integr Comp Physiol 296:1564–1575
7. Mitchell JA, Van Kainen BR (1992) Effects of alcohol on intrauterine oxygen tension in the rat. Alcohol Clin Exp Res 16:308–310
8. Kingdom JC, Kaufmann P (1997) Oxygen and placental villous development: origins of fetal hypoxia. Placenta 18:613–621
9. Hutter D, Kingdom J, Jaeggi E (2010) Causes and mechanisms of intrauterine hypoxia and its impact on the fetal cardiovascular system: a review. Int J Pediatr 401323
10. Jiang BH, Semenza GL, Bauer C, Marti HH (1996) Hypoxia-inducible factor 1 levels vary exponentially over a physiologically relevant range of O2 tension. Am J Physiol 271:1172–1180
11. Groenman F, Rutter M, Caniggia I, Tibboel D, Post M (2007) Hypoxia-inducible factors in the first trimester human lung. J Histochem Cytochem 55:355–363
12. Compernolle V, Brusselmans K, Acker T et al (2002) Loss of HIF-2alpha and inhibition of VEGF impair fetal lung maturation, whereas treatment with VEGF prevents fatal respiratory distress in premature mice. Nat Med 8:702–710
13. Semenza GL, Agani F, Iyer N et al (1999) Regulation of cardiovascular development and physiology by hypoxia-inducible factor 1. Ann NY Acad Sci 874:262–268
14. Ballew C, Haas JD (1986) Hematologic evidence of fetal hypoxia among newborn infants at high altitude in Bolivia. Am J Obstet Gynecol 155:166–169
15. Prystowsky H, Hellegers A, Cotter J, Bruns P (1959) Fetal blood studies. XII. On the relationship between the position of the oxygen dissociation curve of human fetal blood and adult-fetal hemoglobin. Am J Obstet Gynecol 77:585–588
16. Linderkamp O, Guntner M, Hiltl W, Vargas VM (1986) Erythrocyte deformability in the fetus, preterm, and term neonate. Pediatr Res 20:93–96
17. Ascuitto RJ, Ross-Ascuitto NT (1996) Substrate metabolism in the developing heart. Semin Perinatol 20:542–563
18. Druyan S, Cahaner A, Ashwell CM (2007) The expression patterns of hypoxia-inducing factor subunit alpha-1, heme oxygenase, hypoxia upregulated protein 1, and cardiac troponin T during development of the chicken heart. Poult Sci 86:2384–2389
19. Ostadal B, Kolar F (2007) Cardiac adaptation to chronic high-altitude hypoxia: beneficial and adverse effects. Respir Physiol Neurobiol 158:224–236
20. Richardson BS, Bocking AD (1998) Metabolic and circulatory adaptations to chronic hypoxia in the fetus. Comp Biochem Physiol A Mol Integr Physiol 119:717–723

21. Rurak DW, Richardson BS, Patrick JE, Carmichael L, Homan J (1990) Blood flow and oxygen delivery to fetal organs and tissues during sustained hypoxemia. Am J Physiol 258:1116–1122
22. Bocking AD, White SE, Homan J, Richardson BS (1992) Oxygen consumption is maintained in fetal sheep during prolonged hypoxaemia. J Dev Physiol 17:169–174
23. Postigo L, Heredia G, Illsley NP et al (2009) Where the O2 goes to: preservation of human fetal oxygen delivery and consumption at high altitude. J Physiol 587:693–708
24. Singer D, Muhlfeld C (2007) Perinatal adaptation in mammals: the impact of metabolic rate. Comp Biochem Physiol A Mol Integr Physiol 148:780–784
25. Boddy K, Dawes GS, Fisher R, Pinter S, Robinson JS (1974) Foetal respiratory movements, electrocortical and cardiovascular responses to hypoxaemia and hypercapnia in sheep. J Physiol 243:599–618
26. Hislop A (2005) Developmental biology of the pulmonary circulation. Paediatr Respir Rev 6:35–43
27. Stenmark KR, Fagan KA, Frid MG (2006) Hypoxia-induced pulmonary vascular remodeling: cellular and molecular mechanisms. Circ Res 99:675–691
28. Gao Y, Raj JU (2010) Regulation of the pulmonary circulation in the fetus and newborn. Physiol Rev 90:1291–1335
29. Stenmark KR, Aldashev AA, Orton EC et al (1991) Cellular adaptation during chronic neonatal hypoxic pulmonary hypertension. Am J Physiol 261:97–104
30. Sylvester JT, Shimoda LA, Aaronson PI, Ward JP (2012) Hypoxic pulmonary vasoconstriction. Physiol Rev 92:367–520
31. Manner J (2000) Cardiac looping in the chick embryo: a morphological review with special reference to terminological and biomechanical aspects of the looping process. Anat Rec 259:248–262
32. Hamill N, Yeo L, Romero R et al (2011) Fetal cardiac ventricular volume, cardiac output, and ejection fraction determined with 4-dimensional ultrasound using spatiotemporal image correlation and virtual organ computer-aided analysis. Am J Obstet Gynecol 205:1–10
33. Patterson AJ, Zhang L (2010) Hypoxia and fetal heart development. Curr Mol Med 10:653–666
34. Ream M, Ray AM, Chandra R, Chikaraishi DM (2008) Early fetal hypoxia leads to growth restriction and myocardial thinning. Am J Physiol Regul Integr Comp Physiol 295:583–595
35. Clemmer TP, Telford IR (1966) Abnormal development of the rat heart during prenatal hypoxic stress. Proc Soc Exp Biol Med 121:800–803
36. Sharma SK, Lucitti JL, Nordman C, Tinney JP, Tobita K, Keller BB (2006) Impact of hypoxia on early chick embryo growth and cardiovascular function. Pediatr Res 59:116–120
37. Kamitomo M, Onishi J, Gutierrez I, Stiffel VM, Gilbert RD (2002) Effects of long-term hypoxia and development on cardiac contractile proteins in fetal and adult sheep. J Soc Gynecol Investig 9:335–341
38. Gilbert RD (1998) Fetal myocardial responses to long-term hypoxemia. Comp Biochem Physiol A Mol Integr Physiol 119:669–674
39. Rasanen J, Wood DC, Weiner S, Ludomirski A, Huhta JC (1996) Role of the pulmonary circulation in the distribution of human fetal cardiac output during the second half of pregnancy. Circulation 94:1068–1073
40. Pejovic B, Peco-Antic A, Marinkovic-Eric J (2007) Blood pressure in non-critically ill preterm and full-term neonates. Pediatr Nephrol 22:249–257
41. Sime F, Banchero N, Penaloza D, Gamboa R, Cruz J, Marticorena E (1963) Pulmonary hypertension in children born and living at high altitudes. Am J Cardiol 11:143–149
42. Aparicio Otero O, Romero Gutierrez F, Harris P, Anand I (1991) Echocardiography shows persistent thickness of the wall of the right ventricle in infants at high altitude. Cardioscience 2:63–69
43. Gamboa R, Marticorena E (1971) Pulmonary arterial pressure in newborn infants in high altitude. Arch Inst Biol Andina 4:55–66

44. Penaloza D, Arias-Stella J, Sime F, Recavarren S, Marticorena E (1964) The heart and pulmonary circulation in children at high altitudes: Physiological, anatomical, and clinical observations. Pediatrics 34:568–582
45. Niermeyer S (2003) Cardiopulmonary transition in the high altitude infant. High Alt Med Biol 4:225–239
46. Walsh-Sukys MC, Tyson JE, Wright LL et al (2000) Persistent pulmonary hypertension of the newborn in the era before nitric oxide: practice variation and outcomes. Pediatrics 105:14–20
47. Haworth SG, Hislop AA (2009) Treatment and survival in children with pulmonary arterial hypertension: the UK Pulmonary Hypertension Service for Children 2001–2006. Heart 95:312–317
48. Steinhorn RH (2010) Neonatal pulmonary hypertension. Pediatr Crit Care Med 11:79–84
49. Hoffman GM, Ross GA, Day SE, Rice TB, Nelin LD (1997) Inhaled nitric oxide reduces the utilization of extracorporeal membrane oxygenation in persistent pulmonary hypertension of the newborn. Crit Care Med 25:352–359
50. Baquero H, Soliz A, Neira F, Venegas ME, Sola A (2006) Oral sildenafil in infants with persistent pulmonary hypertension of the newborn: a pilot randomized blinded study. Pediatrics 117:1077–1083
51. Bassler D, Kreutzer K, McNamara P, Kirpalani H (2010) Milrinone for persistent pulmonary hypertension of the newborn. Cochrane Database Syst Rev CD007802
52. Mohamed WA, Ismail M (2012) A randomized, double-blind, placebo-controlled, prospective study of bosentan for the treatment of persistent pulmonary hypertension of the newborn. J Perinatol 32:608–613
53. Julian CG, Wilson MJ, Moore LG (2009) Evolutionary adaptation to high altitude: a view from in utero. Am J Hum Biol 21:614–622
54. Lozano JM (2001) Epidemiology of hypoxaemia in children with acute lower respiratory infection. Int J Tuberc Lung Dis 5:496–504
55. Zeitlin J, El Ayoubi M, Jarreau PH et al (2010) Impact of fetal growth restriction on mortality and morbidity in a very preterm birth cohort. J Pediatr 157:733–739
56. Malloy MH (2007) Size for gestational age at birth: impact on risk for sudden infant death and other causes of death, USA 2002. Arch Dis Child Fetal Neonatal Ed 92:473–478
57. Kaijser M, Bonamy AK, Akre O et al (2008) Perinatal risk factors for ischemic heart disease: disentangling the roles of birth weight and preterm birth. Circulation 117:405–410
58. Sluiter I, van Heijst A, Haasdijk R et al (2012) Reversal of pulmonary vascular remodeling in pulmonary hypertensive rats. Exp Mol Pathol 93:66–73
59. Sartori C, Allemann Y, Trueb L, Delabays A, Nicod P, Scherrer U (1999) Augmented vasoreactivity in adult life associated with perinatal vascular insult. Lancet 353:2205–2207
60. Koch J, Hensley G, Roy L, Brown S, Ramaciotti C, Rosenfeld CR (2006) Prevalence of spontaneous closure of the ductus arteriosus in neonates at a birth weight of 1000 grams or less. Pediatrics 117:1113–1121
61. Freeman BA, Crapo JD (1981) Hyperoxia increases oxygen radical production in rat lungs and lung mitochondria. J Biol Chem 256:10986–10992
62. Georgeson GD, Szony BJ, Streitman K et al (2002) Antioxidant enzyme activities are decreased in preterm infants and in neonates born via caesarean section. Eur J Obstet Gynecol Reprod Biol 103:136–139
63. Aust AE, Eveleigh JF (1999) Mechanisms of DNA oxidation. Proc Soc Exp Biol Med 222:246–252
64. Carlo WA, Finer NN, Walsh MC et al (2010) Target ranges of oxygen saturation in extremely preterm infants. N Engl J Med 362:1959–1969
65. Saugstad OD, Aune D (2011) In search of the optimal oxygen saturation for extremely low birth weight infants: a systematic review and meta-analysis. Neonatology 100:1–8
66. Vento M, Saugstad OD (2011) Oxygen supplementation in the delivery room: updated information. J Pediatr 158:e5–e7

67. Saugstad OD, Speer CP, Halliday HL (2011) Oxygen saturation in immature babies: revisited with updated recommendations. Neonatology 100:217–218
68. Sastre J, Pallardo FV, Vina J (2000) Mitochondrial oxidative stress plays a key role in aging and apoptosis. IUBMB Life 49:427–435
69. Sastre J, Pallardo FV, Garcia de la Asuncion J, Vina J (2000) Mitochondria, oxidative stress and aging. Free Radic Res 32:189–198
70. Spector LG, Klebanoff MA, Feusner JH, Georgieff MK, Ross JA (2005) Childhood cancer following neonatal oxygen supplementation. J Pediatr 147:27–31
71. Naumburg E, Bellocco R, Cnattingius S, Jonzon A, Ekbom A (2002) Supplementary oxygen and risk of childhood lymphatic leukaemia. Acta Paediatr 91:1328–1333
72. Stenson B, Brocklehurst P, Tarnow-Mordi W, trial UKBI, Australian BIIt, New Zealand BIIt (2011) Increased 36-week survival with high oxygen saturation target in extremely preterm infants. N Engl J Med 364:1680–1682
73. Soleymani S, Borzage M, Seri I (2010) Hemodynamic monitoring in neonates: advances and challenges. J Perinatol 30:38–45
74. Top AP, Tasker RC, Ince C (2011) The microcirculation of the critically ill pediatric patient. Crit Care 15:213
75. Bezemer R, Bartels SA, Bakker J, Ince C (2012) Clinical review: Clinical imaging of the sublingual microcirculation in the critically ill – where do we stand? Crit Care 16:224
76. Sherman H, Klausner S, Cook WA (1971) Incident dark-field illumination: a new method for microcirculatory study. Angiology 22:295–303
77. Kroth J, Weidlich K, Hiedl S, Nussbaum C, Christ F, Genzel-Boroviczeny O (2008) Functional vessel density in the first month of life in preterm neonates. Pediatr Res 64:567–571
78. Top AP, Buijs EA, Schouwenberg PH, van Dijk M, Tibboel D, Ince C (2012) The Microcirculation is unchanged in neonates with severe respiratory failure after the initiation of ECMO Treatment. Crit Care Res Pract 2012:372956
79. Top AP, Ince C, Schouwenberg PH, Tibboel D (2011) Inhaled nitric oxide improves systemic microcirculation in infants with hypoxemic respiratory failure. Pediatr Crit Care Med 12:e271–e274
80. McNeill S, Gatenby JC, McElroy S, Engelhardt B (2011) Normal cerebral, renal and abdominal regional oxygen saturations using near-infrared spectroscopy in preterm infants. J Perinatol 31:51–57
81. Wijbenga RG, Lemmers PM, van Bel F (2011) Cerebral oxygenation during the first days of life in preterm and term neonates: differences between different brain regions. Pediatr Res 70:389–394
82. van Bel F, Lemmers P, Naulaers G (2008) Monitoring neonatal regional cerebral oxygen saturation in clinical practice: value and pitfalls. Neonatology 94:237–244

Ventriculo-arterial Decoupling in Acutely Altered Hemodynamic States

F. Guarracino, R. Baldassarri, and M. R. Pinsky

Introduction

The dynamic interaction between the heart and the systemic circulation allows the cardiovascular system to be efficient in providing adequate cardiac output and arterial pressures necessary for sufficient organ perfusion [1]. The cardiovascular system provides adequate pressure and flow to the peripheral organs in different physiological (rest and exercise) and pathological conditions because of the continuous modulation of the arterial system compliance, stiffness and resistance with respect to left ventricular (LV) systolic performance [2]. Cardiac output is the final result of this dynamic modulation. Because LV stroke volume depends on myocardial contractility and loading conditions (preload and afterload), both cardiac and arterial dysfunction can lead to acute hemodynamic decompensation and shock. According to the underlying pathophysiological mechanisms, altered hemodynamic profiles can be classified as primarily reflecting cardiogenic, hypovolemic, obstructive or distributive shock.

Low cardiac output resulting in systemic hypoperfusion requires prompt and adequate treatment to restore cardiovascular function and prevent organ hypoperfusion. Current clinical guidelines recommend resuscitation with intravascular fluid infusions supplemented with selective use of inotropes and vasopressors to

F. Guarracino (✉)
Department of Cardiothoracic Anesthesia and Intensive Care Medicine, Azienda Ospedaliero Universitaria Pisana, Via Paradisa, 2, 56123 Pisa, Italy
E-mail: fabiodoc64@hotmail.com

R. Baldassarri
Department of Cardiothoracic Anesthesia and Intensive Care Medicine, Azienda Ospedaliero Universitaria Pisana, Via Paradisa, 2, 56123 Pisa, Italy

M. R. Pinsky
Department of Critical Care Medicine, University of Pittsburgh, 606 Scaife Hall, 3550 Terrace Street, Pittsburgh, PA 15261, USA

J.-L. Vincent (Ed.), *Annual Update in Intensive Care and Emergency Medicine 2013*, DOI 10.1007/978-3-642-35109-9_18, © Springer-Verlag Berlin Heidelberg and BioMed Central Ltd. 2013

reverse shock in critically ill patients [3, 4]. However, the treatment of acute hemodynamic impairment should be tailored based on the etiological mechanism of the cardiovascular dysfunction. Herein lies a major problem with present guidelines: They cannot distinguish the underlying causes of impaired LV stroke volume leading to impaired cardiac output.

Ventriculo-arterial Coupling

The concept that the cardiovascular system works better when the heart and the arterial system are coupled has been well demonstrated [5, 6]. When the heart pumps blood into the vascular tree at a rate and volume that matches the capability of the arterial system to receive it, both cardiovascular performance and its associated cardiac energetics are optimal [7, 8]. A contractility or arterial tone that is too high or too low decouples these processes and can lead to cardiac failure independent of myocardial ischemia or the toxic effects of sepsis and related systemic disease processes. This optimization means that the LV workload and the arterial system optimally match when the left ventricle ejects the blood into the arterial system and is quantified by ventriculo-arterial (V-A) coupling analysis. This process is optimized without excessive changes in LV pressure, and the mechanical energy of LV ejection is completely transferred from the ventricle to the arterial system [9, 10]. The role of V-A coupling in the management of critically ill patients with severe hemodynamic instability and shock is becoming increasingly clear.

V-A coupling can be defined as the ratio of the arterial elastance (Ea) to the ventricular elastance (Ees). This ratio was first proposed by Suga [11] as a method to evaluate the mechanical efficiency of the cardiovascular system and the interaction between cardiac performance and vascular function. The Ea/Ees ratio has been consistently demonstrated to be a reliable and effective measure of cardiovascular performance [9, 11, 12]. Burkhoff and Sagawa, and successively many other investigators, have demonstrated that when the Ea/Es is near unity, the efficiency of the system is optimal. In this case, the left ventricle provides an adequate stroke volume with the lowest possible energetic consumption [13, 14]. Thus, V-A coupling is an effective index of the mechanical performance of the left ventricle and of the dynamic modulation of the cardiovascular system. In addition, the Ea/Ees reflects cardiac energetics. The balance between myocardial oxygen consumption and the mechanical energy required to perform this work appears to be optimal when the heart and the peripheral vascular system are coupled.

The area of the LV pressure-volume (P-V) loop (Fig. 1) during a single cardiac cycle represents the total mechanical energy of the heart during that beat and has a linear correlation with myocardial oxygen consumption [15]. The energetic efficiency of the cardiovascular system is optimal when all the pulsating energy of the heart is transmitted to the arterial system [12]. Effective understanding of V-A coupling requires an appropriate understanding of the concepts of the determinants,

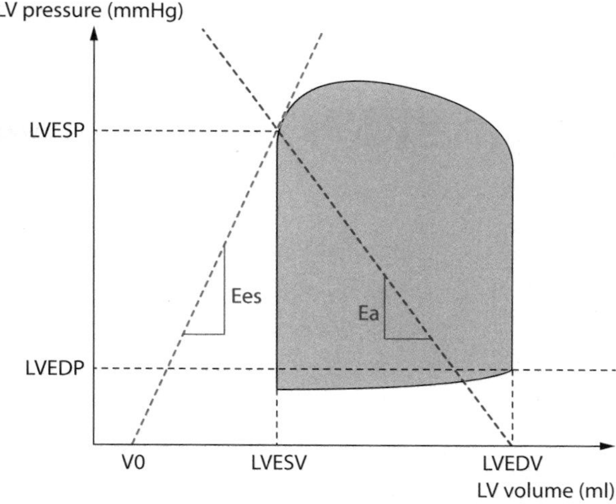

Fig. 1 The left ventricular (LV) P-V loop. The P-V loop area is highlighted in blue. The slopes of LV elastance (Ees) and arterial elastance (Ea) are shown. ESV: end-systolic volume; ESP: end-systolic pressure; EDV: end-diastolic volume; EDP: end-systolic pressure

Ea and Ees. And the effective use of these concepts requires an understanding as to how they may be derived at the bedside in critically ill patients.

Left Ventricular Elastance (Ees)

When the left ventricle ejects, arterial pressure increases and the LV stroke volume is transferred into the aorta. As LV volume decreases to its end-systolic minimum, the actual end-systolic volume (ESV) is a function of not only intrinsic cardiac contractility, but also arterial pressure. For the same LV end-diastolic volume (EDV) and intrinsic cardiac contractility, if arterial pressure at end-systole were less, then LVESV would also be lower and LV stroke volume greater. Similarly, increasing arterial pressure has the opposite effect to increasing LVESV and decreasing stroke volume. Importantly, the resultant potential end-systolic pressure-volume points possible as arterial pressure is independently varied describe a tight linear relationship called the end-systolic pressure-volume relationship (ESPVR). The slope of the ESPVR is the LV elastance (Ees) (Fig. 1) and is determined for the intrinsic contractility of the heart. The steeper the slope, the greater the contractility [16]. Ees (mm Hg/ml) is a useful, load independent index of myocardial contractility and LV inotropic efficiency (end-systolic LV stiffness) [17]. Although myocardial contractility is the main determinant of LV systolic function, biochemical properties of the LV myocytes (stiffness, compliance, fibrosis, etc.), cardiac myocyte contraction synchrony and geometric remodeling of the LV chamber can also significantly influence LV performance [18]. Therefore, Ees should be considered as an integrated measure of LV systolic performance derived from the complex association between the inotropic efficiency and the functional, structural and geometric characteristics of the left ventricle [19].

Arterial Elastance (Ea)

Ea (mm Hg/ml) is the expression of the total afterload imposed on the left ventricle and represents the complex association of different arterial properties including wall stiffness, compliance and outflow resistance. Thus, the total arterial compliance, impedance and the systolic and diastolic time interval are significant components of the arterial load [11]. Graphically, Ea can be described as the slope of the line running from the LVEDV to the LV end-systolic pressure (ESP) on the P-V loop (Fig. 1). Operationally, Ea can be defined as the capability of the arterial vessels to increase pressure when LV stroke volume increases.

A-V Coupling Measurement

According to the seminal studies of Frank and Starling, Grossman and colleagues, and subsequently other investigators, LV contractile function can be evaluated by the relationship between the ESP and the ESV [20, 21]. After the experimental investigations of Suga and Sugawa on isolated canine hearts, the assessment of V-A coupling in humans has been less successful because of the invasive techniques needed to acquire these measures. Because of the recognized importance of V-A coupling in the management of critically ill patients, much effort has been put into achieving non-invasive measurement approaches [22]. Despite several proposed non-invasive approaches to evaluate Ea/Ees, only the modified single beat method developed by Chen et al. has been validated against the invasive measurement of Ees [23]. The single beat method is based on the assumption that be-

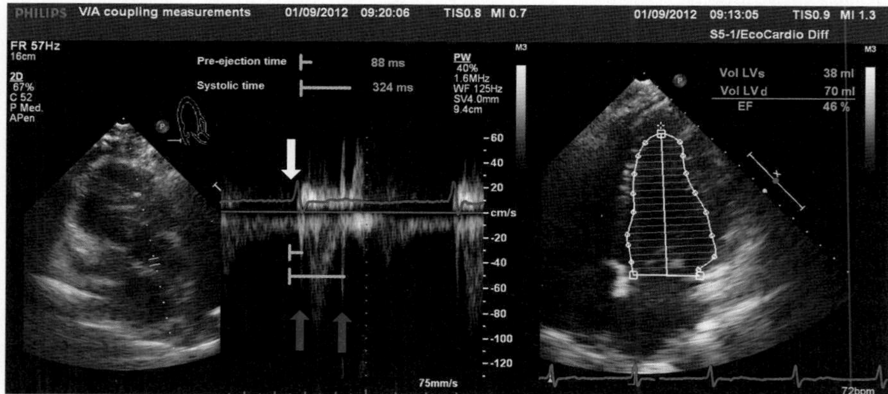

Fig. 2 Echocardiographic measurements of left ventricular (LV) time intervals (*left*) and LV ejection fraction (EF, *right*). The white arrow indicates the beginning of the QRS complex, the dark blue arrows indicate the aortic valve opening and closure. The light blue lines show the time interval measurements

cause the time-variation of LV elastance is not influenced by loading conditions or heart rate (HR), the evaluation of the P-V loop can be obtained by a single heart beat [24]. The non-invasive method developed by Chen et al. utilizes echocardiographic measures of LV end-diastolic and end-systolic areas. Chen et al. demonstrated that this method could be used for obtaining the single-beat measure of Ees (Ees[SB]), through the measure of LV ejection fraction (LVEF), stroke volume, pre-ejection time and systolic time interval (Fig. 2) when coupled with systolic and diastolic arterial pressure measurements [23].

Ea is calculated as ESP/stroke volume. From the rearrangement of this equation, Ea is proportional to the sum of HR, arterial resistance and [(ESP – mean arterial pressure[MAP])/stroke volume]. Since end-systolic arterial pressure occurs slightly after peak systolic pressure is achieved, Ea can be calculated as 0.9 × systolic arterial pressure/stroke volume, where 0.9 × systolic arterial pressure equals LVESP [23, 25].

Since all these measures can be readily made at the bedside, it is possible to assess V-A coupling in critically ill patients.

Ventriculo-arterial Decoupling in Altered Hemodynamic States

Although the occurrence of V-A decoupling is generally associated with pathological states, in some physiological conditions, such as during exercise or with increased age, a mismatch between LV performance and arterial system function can occur.

According to the physiological changes occurring during exercise, the cardiovascular system modulates its performance to provide adequate pressure and flow to peripheral organs in the presence of increased metabolic demand. Because the Ea/Ees is normally coupled in healthy humans at rest, during exercise Ees increases more than Ea; consequently, the ratio of Ea to Ees decreases [26]. Because LV performance and, therefore, Ees normally increases during exercise, Ea can increase, decrease or be unchanged. The Ea modifications impact Ea/Ees in conditions of increased LV work. Ea generally increases in elderly people as a consequence of the structural changes in the arterial properties (compliance, stiffness, pulse wave). The mismatch between Ea and Ees during exercise can be blunted in elderly people because of a reduction in the cardiovascular reserve. Furthermore, cardiovascular diseases (hypertension, coronary artery disease, diabetes mellitus), which have an impact on V-A coupling, frequently occur in elderly patients.

Cardiovascular impairment leading to acute systemic hypotension and shock can occur in many different clinical scenarios. Cardiovascular dysfunction is generally characterized by an altered Ea/Ees due to either the decrease in Ees or to the significant increase in Ea. Operationally, the system becomes uncoupled when the ratio of arterial to ventricular elastance is > 1 (Ea/Ees > 1), while an Ea increase is the consequence of an increase of the arterial load.

Ventriculo-arterial Decoupling Due to Decreased Ees

According to the hemodynamic profile of the underlying pathology, an Ees decrease indicates an impairment in myocardial contractility, resulting in reduction of LV performance. Although myocardial ischemia and acute myocardial infarction are the most common causes of LV contractile dysfunction, other pathologies, such as myocarditis and severe cardiomyopathy (dilative and hypertrophic), can be characterized by myocardial depression and diminished Ees [27, 28]. The acute decompensation of LV function can lead to severe hemodynamic impairment and shock.

Acute Heart Failure

Acute failure of LV systolic function is characterized by the inability of the heart to provide an adequate stroke volume to match the metabolic demands of the body. Acute systolic cardiac dysfunction results in both a low ejection fraction and increased filling pressures in the attempt to maintain a sufficient stroke volume. For this reason, the LV ESPVR is shifted downward and rightward, and Ees decreases. At the same time, Ea significantly increases because of increased sympathetic tone as the normal response of the autonomic nervous system to compensate for the reduced LV stroke volume. Thus, one sees tachycardia and increased arterial tone [2]. Hence, the cardiovascular system is generally uncoupled in acute heart failure, and Ea/Ees increases up to three or four fold [29]. Therefore, the treatment of acute heart failure is usually to decrease Ea by calcium channel blockers, beta-blockers and other vasodilating agents, whereas Ees is increased by inotrope infusions. Traditionally, the management of acute heart failure is based on inotropic agents aimed to improve myocardial contractility and to restore organ perfusion [30]. The inotropic agents commonly employed in the treatment of acute heart failure (catecholamines and phosphodiesterase III inhibitors) induce well-described adverse effects, such as increased myocardial oxygen consumption, arrhythmias and increased mortality [12]. In recent years, the therapeutic use of the novel calcium sensitizer, levosimendan, has been progressively emphasized because of its inotropic and vasodilator properties [31, 32]. Because of its intrinsic performance, levosimendan impacts both Ea and Ees and improves V-A coupling [12]. Moderate systemic arterial hypotension can be induced by levosimendan, which then requires the administration of low doses of norepinephrine. The association between the inotropic and vasopressor action seems to improve cardiovascular performance by matching Ea and Ees.

Cardiac Surgery

Cardiogenic shock is the most severe clinical manifestation of perioperative acute heart failure after cardiac surgery and leads to systemic hypoperfusion and organ dysfunction that generally requires either pharmacological or mechanical support. The acute reduction in Ees, from many different causes that range from inadequate myocardial protection to myocardial stunning, is usually the main reason for the uncoupled Ea/Ees ratio.

Treatment with inodilator drugs in post-cardiotomy acute heart failure has been demonstrated to be effective in restoring V-A coupling and improving LV performance [33, 34].

Tachycardia

Tachycardia induced by stress conditions and during exercise is generally well tolerated by healthy people. Indeed, the increase in HR is a compensatory mechanism that enhances myocardial contractility and LV performance [2]. This force-frequency relationship has beneficial effects on cardiac performance, which contribute to maintain the efficiency of the cardiovascular system and provide optimal V-A coupling. The intrinsic mechanism underlying the force-frequency relationship is most likely the dynamic balance of the intracellular Ca_2^+ concentration [35]. In acute heart failure patients, baseline LV V-A uncoupling can be significantly worsened by tachycardia because the normal force-frequency relationship is impaired.

Acute Systemic Hypotension

Several different etiological mechanisms can cause hypotension, but systemic arterial hypotension is generally the first and often life-threatening symptom of acute cardiovascular dysfunction. Either heart failure or circulatory impairment can lead to systemic arterial hypotension and hemodynamic decompensation. Because peripheral organ perfusion strictly depends on the MAP, systemic arterial hypotension should be promptly reversed. According to recommended treatments, fluid resuscitation is generally the first therapeutic approach [3, 4]. Indeed, the hemodynamic response to fluid administration depends on either the increase in stroke volume consequent to fluid resuscitation or on other factors, including arterial tone [1, 36]. MAP is the product of the interaction between LV stroke volume and arterial system function expressed by the Ea. Recently, we proposed a bedside method to evaluate the dynamic arterial elastance (Eadyn) to determine which patients are responders to fluid resuscitation [37]. In mechanically ventilated patients, Eadyn corresponds to the ratio of pulse pressure variation (PPV) to stroke volume variation (SVV) during a single positive pressure breath. The bedside evaluation of the Eadyn should allow either functional assessment of arterial tone or of fluid responsiveness in severely hypotensive patients. Further investigations are required because of both the limitations of the published studies and the small populations enrolled, but the predictive value of Eadyn suggests a useful application in clinical practice.

Although MAP is the main determinant of organ perfusion, it can also be influenced by flow distribution and tissue oxygenation. Despite the restoration of a normal MAP, patients with cardiovascular dysfunction can suffer from decreased organ oxygenation and perfusion [38]. In this context, a sufficient MAP should be maintained in hemodynamically instable patients to prevent any further tissue injury [3].

Ventriculo-arterial Decoupling Due To Increased Ea

Acute Systemic Hypertension

Increased arterial pressure represents the most common cause of pressure overload of the left ventricle and plays a key role in the evolution of ventricular hypertrophy, dysfunction and failure. Hypertensive crisis is characterized by a sudden increase in blood pressure associated with or followed by signs of impairment in target organs, such as heart, kidney and brain. Most patients arriving at the emergency department with elevated blood pressure and acute pulmonary edema have a normal LVEF, suggesting that acute heart failure in these situations is due to diastolic dysfunction [39]. However, LV systolic dysfunction has also been reported in association with uncontrolled systemic hypertension, which may be responsible for the development of acute heart failure and pulmonary edema [40]. In these situations, the acute LV decompensation dramatically improves with rapid blood pressure normalization.

The mechanism by which a hypertensive crisis may cause acute and severe LV systolic dysfunction, even causing acute pulmonary edema, consists of acute V-A uncoupling because of an abrupt and exaggerated increase in Ea. Such afterload mismatch leads to an exhaustion of the preload reserve of the left ventricle [40]. The rapid reduction in elevated blood pressure by aggressive treatment usually induces a regression of myocardial dysfunction by restoring Ea and, therefore, a coupling of the Ea/Ees ratio. Thus, consideration of the pathophysiological role of V-A decoupling allows the true pathogenic mechanism of acute heart failure in a patient with normal LV systolic function to be determined.

Ventriculo-arterial Decoupling in Septic Shock

The hemodynamic profile of septic shock is primarily characterized by generalized vasodilatation resulting in severe hypotension with systemic hypoperfusion [41]. The occurrence of myocardial depression and eventual cardiac dysfunction has been largely recognized in patients with septic shock, although the pathogenetic mechanisms of the myocardial injury are not yet completely understood [42, 43].

In most of the patients with septic shock, cardiovascular efficiency is impaired, and the Ea/Ees becomes uncoupled ($Ea/Ees > 1$). The hemodynamic profile is characterized by both the significant increase in Ea and the decrease in Ees. Because the increase in Ea is generally induced by pharmacological vasoconstriction (norepinephrine) and the consequent increase in arterial tone, a decrease in Ees generally depends on the reduction in myocardial contractility. Whatever the underlying mechanism, when A-V uncoupling occurs in septic shock, the cardiac energetics are unfavorable and are often sacrificed to maintain tissue perfusion. Despite the severe hemodynamic dysfunction, Ea/Ees can be normally coupled in patients with septic shock (Ea/Ees = 1). In these cases, the proper interaction between LV performance and arterial system function can depend on both a normal cardiac function and on a proper therapeutic approach with fluid administration, inotropes and vasoconstrictors.

According to international guidelines, management of septic shock requires either fluid resuscitation or the employment of vasopressors (norepinephrine) to maintain an adequate cardiac output and tissue perfusion [4]. The use of inotropes is recommended when cardiac dysfunction and an increase in filling pressures occur. Recently, the use of levosimendan has been suggested for the treatment of myocardial dysfunction associated with septic shock [44, 45].

Right Ventricular Dysfunction and V-A Coupling

The cardiovascular system can be acutely decompensated by right ventricular (RV) failure with consequent severe hemodynamic instability and systemic hypoperfusion [46]. The RV dysfunction can be due to intrinsic mechanisms that occur in myocardial infarction or can be secondary to an increase in the RV afterload caused by pulmonary hypertension. Despite the underlying etiological mechanisms, RV uncoupling can occur [47].

Because the right ventricle contributes to the efficiency of the cardiovascular system through right V-A coupling, the assessment of the Ea/Ees of the right side of the circulation can play a role in the management of critically ill patients [48]. RV V-A coupling expresses the optimal interaction between RV performance and function of the pulmonary vascular system. When Ees decreases (RV acute myocardial infarction, septic shock) or Ea increases (pulmonary hypertension, acute respiratory distress syndrome [ARDS]), the right side of the cardiovascular apparatus becomes uncoupled.

Although evaluation of RV elastance requires invasive techniques with significant limitations for clinical practice, non-invasive models to assess the RV Ea/Ees have recently been proposed. Pulmonary artery catheterization and cardiac magnetic resonance may be useful in determining RV V-A coupling [48, 49].

Conclusion

Although the management of shock patients has traditionally been based on advanced hemodynamic monitoring, the role of echocardiography in the evaluation of patients with acute hemodynamic decompensation has been progressively expanding in the last decades.

The management of critically ill patients with acutely altered hemodynamic states can benefit from the assessment of V-A coupling. Since the introduction of echocardiographic methods to assess cardiovascular function, the bedside evaluation of the Ea/Ees has become available and reliable.

The diagnostic function of echocardiographic assessment is enhanced by its capability to contribute to an evaluation of the Ea/Ees ratio and, therefore, V-A coupling in patients with acute hemodynamic impairment. The assessment of cardiovascular function by evaluation of the Ea/Ees ratio can offer an adjunctive perspective for understanding the pathophysiology of altered hemodynamic profiles, and for guiding therapeutic strategies and testing the effectiveness of treatments. However, this concept still needs to be tested in large trials.

References

1. Pinsky MR (2000) Both perfusion pressure and flow are essential for adequate resuscitation. Sepsis 4:143–146
2. Chantler PD, Lakatta EG (2012) Arterial-ventricular coupling with aging and disease. Front Physio 3:90
3. Antonelli M, Levy M, Andrews PJ et al (2007) Hemodynamic monitoring in shock and implications for management. International Consensus Conference. Intensive Care Med 33:575–590
4. Dellinger RP, Levy MM, Carlet JM et al (2008) Surviving sepsis campaign: international guidelines for management of severe sepsis and septic shock. Intensive Care Med 34:17–60
5. Binkley PF, Van Fossen DB, Nunziala E, Unverferth DV, Leier CV (1990) Influence of positive inotropic therapy on pulsatile hydraulic load and ventricular-vascular coupling in congestive heart failure. J Am Coll Cardiol 15:1127–1135
6. Elzinga G, Westerhof N (1991) Matching between ventricle and arterial load. Circ Res 68:1495–1500
7. Kass DA, Kelly RP (1992) Ventriculo-arterial coupling: concepts, assumptions, and applications. Ann Biomed Eng 20:41–62
8. Starling MR (1993) Left ventricular–arterial coupling relations in the normal human heart. Am Heart J 125:1659–1666
9. Sunagawa K, Maughan WL, Burkhoff D, Sagawa K (1983) Left ventricular interaction with arterial load studied in isolated canine ventricle. Am J Physiol 245:H773–H780
10. Kelly RP, Ting CT, Yang TM et al (1992) Effective arterial elastance as index of arterial vascular load in humans. Circulation 86:513–521
11. Suga H (1969) Time course of left ventricular pressure-volume relationship under various end-diastolic volume. Jap Heart J 10:509–515
12. Guarracino F, Cariello C, Danella A et al (2007) Effect of levosimendan on ventriculo-arterial coupling in patients with ischemic cardiomyopathy. Acta Anaesthesiol Scand 51:1217–1224
13. Sunagawa K, Maughan WL, Sagawa K (1985) Optimal arterial resistance for the maximal stroke work studied in isolated canine left ventricle. Circ Res 56:586–595
14. Burkhoff D, Sagawa K (1986) Ventricular efficiency predicted by an analytical model. Am J Physiol 250:1021–1027
15. Hayash K, Shigemi K, Shishido T, Sugimachr M, Sunagawa K (2000) Single-beat Estimation of Ventricular End-systolic Elastance-effective Arterial Elastance as an Index of Ventricular Mechanoenergetic Performance. Anesthesiology 92:1769–1776

16. Blaudszun G, Morel DR (2011) Relevance of the volume-axis intercept, V0, compared with the slope of end-systolic pressure–volume relationship in response to large variations in inotropy and afterload in rats. Exp Physiol 96:1179–1195
17. Sagawa K, Suga H, Shoukas AA, Bakalar KM (1977) End-systolic pressure/volume ratio: a new index of ventricular contractility. Am J Cardiol 40:748–753
18. Borlaug BA, Kass DA (2008) Ventricular-vascular interaction in heart failure. Heart Fail Clin 4:23–36
19. Kass DA (2002) Age-related changes in ventricular-arterial coupling: pathophysiologic implications. Heart Fail Rev 7:51–62
20. Grossman W, Braunwald E, Mann T, McLaurin LP, Green LH (1977) Contractile state of the left ventricle in man as evaluated from end-systolic pressure-volume relations. Circulation 56:845–852
21. Sagawa K (1981) The end-systolic pressure-volume relation of the ventricle: definition modifications and clinical use. Circulation 63:1223–1227
22. Senzaki H, Chen CH, Kass DA (1996) Single-beat estimation of end-systolic pressure-volume relation in humans: a new method with the potential for noninvasive application. Circulation 94:2497–2506
23. Chen CH, Fetics B, Nevo E et al (2001) Noninvasive single-beat determination of left ventricular end-systolic elastance in humans. J Am Coll Cardiol 38:2028–2034
24. Shishido T, Hayashi K, Shigemi K, Sato T, Sugimachi M, Sunagawa K (2000) Single-beat estimation of end-systolic elastance using bilinearly approximated time-varying elastance curve. Circulation 102:1983–1989
25. Zanon F, Aggio S, Baracca E et al (2009) Ventricular-arterial coupling in patients with heart failure treated with cardiac resynchronization therapy: may we predict the long-term clinical response? Eur J Echocardiogr 10:106–111
26. Najjar SS, Schulman SP, Gerstenblith G et al (2004) Age and gender affect ventricular-vascular coupling during aerobic exercise. J Am Coll Cardiol 44:611–617
27. Widyastuti Y, Stenseth R, Berg KS, Pleym H, Wahba A, Videm V (2012) Preoperative and intraoperative prediction of risk of cardiac dysfunction following open heart surgery. Eur J Anaesthesiol 29:143–151
28. Buja LM (2005) Myocardial ischemia and reperfusion injury. Cardiovasc Pathol 14:170–175
29. Fox JM, Maurer MS (2005) Ventriculo-vascular coupling in systolic and diastolic heart failure. Curr Heart Fail Rep 2:204–211
30. Majure DT, Teerlink JR (2011) Update on the management of acute decompensated heart failure. Curr Treat Options Cardiovasc Med 13:570–585
31. Toller WG, Stranz C, Nieminen MS (2006) Levosimendan, a new inotropic and vasodilator agent. Anaesthesiology 104:556–569
32. Landoni G, Mizzi A, Biondi-Zoccai G et al (2010) Levosimendan reduces mortality in critically ill patients. A meta-analysis of randomized controlled studies. Minerva Anestesiol 76:276–286
33. De Santis V, Vitale D, Tritapepe L (2010) Levosimendan and cardiac surgery. J Cardiothorac Vasc Anesth 24:210
34. Toller W, Algotsson L, Guarracino F et al (2013) Perioperative use of levosimendan: Best practice in operative settings. J Cardiothorac Vasc Anesth (in press)
35. Masutani S, Cheng HJ, Tachibana H, Little WC, Cheng CP (2011) Levosimendan restores the positive force-frequency relation in heart failure. Am J Physiol Heart Circ Physiol 301:H488–H496
36. Monge García MI, Gil Cano A, Gracia Romero M (2011) Dynamic arterial elastance to predict arterial pressure response to volume loading in preload-dependent patients. Crit Care 15:R15
37. Pinsky MR (2002) Functional hemodynamic monitoring: applied physiology at the bedside. In: Vincent JL (ed) Yearbook of Intensive Care and Emergency Medicine. Springer, Heidelberg, pp 534–551

38. Lamia B, Chemla D, Richard C, Teboul JL (2005) Clinical review: interpretation of arterial pressure wave in shock states. Crit Care 9:601–606
39. Little WC (2001) Hypertensive pulmonary oedema is due to diastolic dysfunction. Eur Heart J 22:1961–1964
40. Ross J (1997) On variations in the cardiac hypertrophic response to pressure overload. Circulation 95:1349–1351
41. Vieillard-Baron A (2011) Septic cardiomyopathy. Ann Intensive Care 1:6
42. Hunter JD, Doddi M (2010) Sepsis and the heart. Br J Anaesth 104:3–11
43. Young JD (2004) The heart and circulation in severe sepsis. Br J Anaesth 93:114–120
44. De BD, Taccone FS, Radermacher P (2007) Levosimendan in septic shock: another piece in the puzzle, but many pieces are still lacking. Intensive Care Med 33:403–405
45. Pinto BB, Rehberg S, Ertmer C, Westphal M (2008) Role of levosimendan in sepsis and septic shock. Curr Opin Anaesthesiol 21:168–177
46. Price LC, Wort SJ, Finney SJ, Marino PS, Brett SJ (2010) Pulmonary vascular and right ventricular dysfunction in adult critical care: current and emerging options for management: a systematic literature review. Crit Care 14:R169
47. Kevin LG, Barnard M (2007) Right ventricular failure. Contin Educ Anaesth Crit Care Pain 7:89–94
48. Grignola JC, Ginés F, Bia D, Armentano R (2007) Improved right ventricular–vascular coupling during active pulmonary hypertension. Int J Cardiol 115:171–182
49. Sanz J, García-Alvarez A, Fernández-Friera L et al (2012) Right ventriculo-arterial coupling in pulmonary hypertension: a magnetic resonance study. Heart 98:238–243

New Pharmacological Strategy in Acute Heart Failure: Vasodilators vs. Inotropes

L. Lemasle, E. Gayat, and A. Mebazaa

Introduction

Acute heart failure is a major public health issue. Acute heart failure is common, especially among the elderly and is a major cause of hospitalization, including to the intensive care unit (ICU), and of mortality. Based on the Framingham cohort, the incidence of heart failure after 65 years old is approaching the figure of 10 per 10,000 residents and life expectancy after 40 years old in subjects with heart failure is reduced 5-fold compared with the general population [1, 2]. The prevalence of chronic heart failure is 1 to 2 % in the adult population and 6 to 10 % in people over 65 years old and is increasing [3, 4].

Similar to the increasing incidence of chronic heart failure, the number of hospitalizations for acute heart failure has tripled over the last thirty years and now represents 5 % of hospital admissions. It is the first cause of hospitalization in patients over 65 years. Acute heart failure represents half of the spending on heart failure, care of which consumes 2 % of national health expenditure [5].

Acute heart failure is one of the earliest described diseases. Indeed, its clinical symptoms are well known by any physician (dyspnea, liver pain, crackles on auscultation). However, its epidemiology has only recently become an area of interest [6]. During the last forty years, the definition of acute heart failure remained un-

L. Lemasle
Department of Anesthesiology and Intensive Care Medicine, Hôpitaux Universitaires Saint Louis Lariboisière, Université Paris Diderot, 2 rue Ambroise Paré, 75010 Paris, France

E. Gayat
Department of Anesthesiology and Intensive Care Medicine, Hôpitaux Universitaires Saint Louis Lariboisière, Université Paris Diderot, 2 rue Ambroise Paré, 75010 Paris, France

A. Mebazaa (✉)
Department of Anesthesiology and Intensive Care Medicine, Hôpitaux Universitaires Saint Louis Lariboisière, Université Paris Diderot, 2 rue Ambroise Paré, 75010 Paris, France
E-mail: alexandre.mebazaa@lrb.aphp.fr

J.-L. Vincent (Ed.), *Annual Update in Intensive Care and Emergency Medicine 2013*,
DOI 10.1007/978-3-642-35109-9_19,

Box 1 Definitions of acute heart failure syndromes

Acute decomposed heart failure	Signs and symptoms of acute heart failure that are mild do not fulfill the criteria for cardiogenic shock, pulmonary edema or hypertensive crisis.
Pulmonary edema	Patients present with severe respiratory distress, tachypnea, and orthopnea with rales over the lung fields. Arterial oxygen saturation is usually 90 % on room air prior to treatment with oxygen
Hypertensive heart failure	Signs and symptoms of heart failure accompanied by high blood pressure and usually relatively preserved LV systolic function, with a chest radiograph compatible with acute pulmonary edema. There is evidence of increased sympathetic tone with tachycardia and vasoconstriction.
Cardiogenic shock	Defined as evidence of tissue hypoperfusion induced by heart failure after adequate correction of preload. There are no diagnostic hemodynamic parameters. However, typically, cardiogenic shock is characterized by reduced systolic blood pressure and absent or low urine output.
Isolated right heart failure	Characterized by a low output syndrome in the absence of pulmonary congestion with increased jugular venous pressure, with or without hepatomegaly, and low LV filling pressures.
High output failure	Characterized by high cardiac output usually with rapid heart rate, with warm peripheries, pulmonary congestion and sometimes low blood pressure, as in septic shock.

clear and included various conditions ranging from acute pulmonary edema during a hypertensive crisis to cardiogenic shock following a myocardial infarction. The word heart in "acute heart failure" has misled generations who thought that acute heart failure was always related to systolic dysfunction. Recent epidemiological studies have shown that acute heart failure is, in fact, not a disease but a syndrome [7–9]. The European Society of Cardiology (ESC) and the European Society of Intensive Care Medicine (ESICM) have further classified acute heart failure patients into six categories (Box 1) [10, 11], forming the basis for the new concept of acute heart failure syndromes. These definitions should now be used in our daily practice and in future studies on acute heart failure.

In Europe, there has been a substantial and continuous decrease in acute heart failure as the underlying cause of death in the past twenty years, similar to what had already been described in other cardiovascular diseases [12] (Fig. 1). There has been an accompanying increase in age at death from acute heart failure in both men and women. These results are encouraging and may be related to a better management of acute heart failure over the past twenty years. The European guidelines on the management of acute heart failure may have had beneficial effects [12].

The syndrome of acute heart failure is due either to decompensated chronic heart failure or to the occurrence of heart failure on a healthy heart (*de novo*), as in myocardial infarction. It is important to differentiate chronic decompensated heart

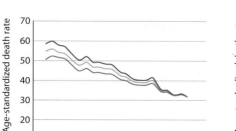

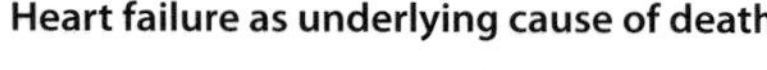

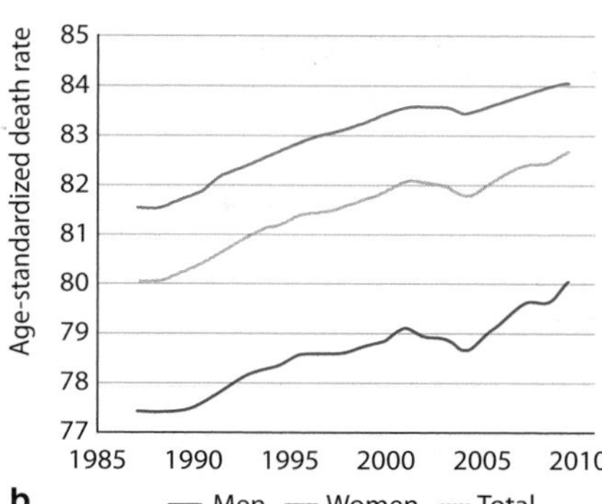

Fig. 1 Heart failure as an underlying cause of death in Europe. **a** Age-standardized death rates and **b** mean age at death from heart failure. Data represent the total population of the seven studied European countries (adapted from [12] with permission)

failure and acute heart failure on a healthy heart because the physiological response will be much more pronounced in the case of *de novo* acute heart failure. In addition, acute heart failure in a healthy heart will occur in a patient who is not taking long-term cardiovascular drugs (so few drug interactions with drugs administered during the acute epidose). In *de novo* acute heart failure, the overall blood volume is normal or low compared with decompensated chronic heart failure, in which it is normal or high.

The goals in the treatment of acute heart failure are first to improve the condition as rapidly as possible in order to ensure short- and long-term survival. The episode of acute heart failure and the drugs used should ideally not reduce the survival of these patients. The optimal agent for the treatment of acute heart failure would be one that would decrease ventricular filling pressures, improve clinical symptoms and renal function, preserve myocardial tissue, reduce plasma concentrations of neurohormones, and would not create arrhythmia or symptomatic hypotension. In fact, at present, no agent has all these characteristics.

Although the treatment of chronic heart failure has evolved over the past twenty years that of acute heart failure has been limited. However, in recent years, a better understanding of pathophysiological mechanisms has enabled a reflection on the available treatments [14].

Why More Vasodilator?

Among the available drugs for acute heart failure, vasodilators are very close to the ideal drug but are still underused.

Physiopathologic Evidence

Nitrates act directly on smooth muscle by releasing nitric oxide (NO) from the parent molecule. Whatever the dose, nitrates are associated with constant venodilation, but arterial vasodilatation increases progressively with increased plasma nitrate concentration [15]. This vasodilatation is associated with decreased preload and afterload and coronary vasodilatation. The final consequences of these hemodynamic modifications is decreased blood pressure and left ventricular filling pressure [16]. Vasodilators should be tried as a first-line therapy in acute heart failure when blood pressure is high: Hypertensive acute heart failure and decompensated chronic heart failure with an elevated systolic blood pressure. Recent data suggest an improvement in survival associated with the use of vasodilating drugs in acute heart failure [13]. These results are based on the analysis of an international observational study, which included more than 5,000 patients admitted for acute heart

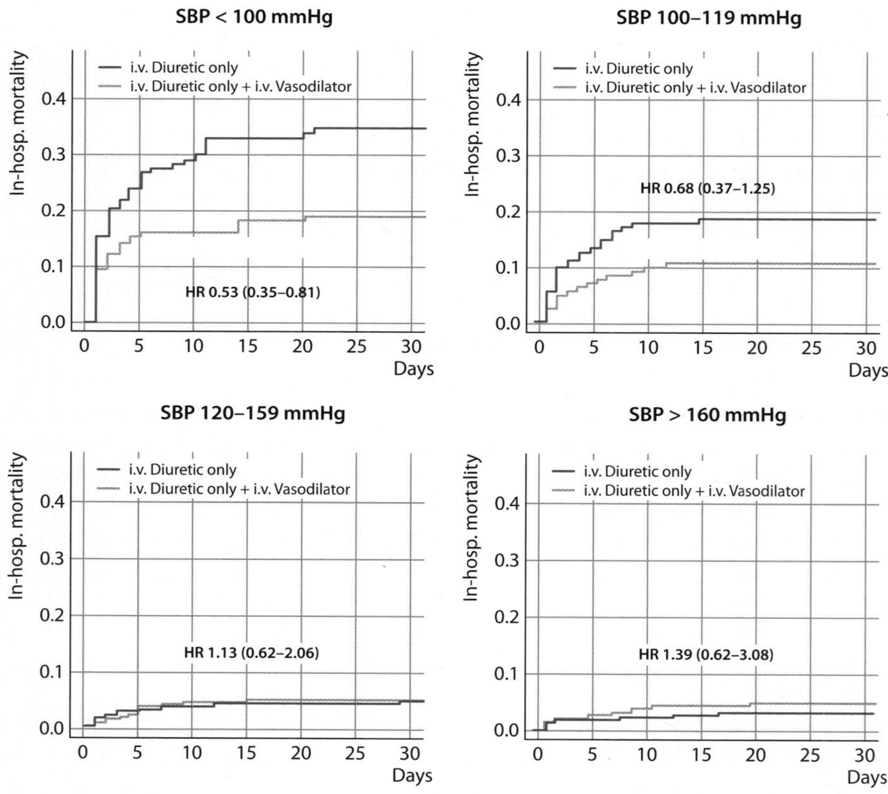

Fig. 2 Effects of intravenous (i.v.) vasodilators on in-hospital mortality of patients with various levels of systolic blood pressure (adapted from [13] with permission). SBP: systolic blood pressure; HR: hazard ratio

failure. The aim of this study was to identify the risks and benefits of intravenous (i.v.) drugs in patients hospitalized with acute decompensated heart failure. The acute heart failure global survey of standard treatment (ALARM-HF) reviewed in-hospital treatments in eight countries. In terms of in-hospital survival, a vasodilator in combination with a diuretic performed better than treatment with only a diuretic. Although other evidence of beneficial effect of nitrates on short term outcome is needed, the ALARM-HF study indicates that nitrates are safe in acute heart failure patients with normal blood pressure at admission.

Intravenous nitrates and sodium nitroprusside are currently recommended in acute heart failure patients with SBP > 110 mm Hg and may be used with caution in patients with SBP between 90 and 110 mm Hg (class of recommendation I, level of evidence B [10, 11]). Moreover, nitrates can be administered by sublingual pulverization, especially in an emergency or by i.v. administration. Continuous infusion doses must be adapted according to the drug. During congestive heart failure, recommended doses are usually 1 to 8 mg/h for nitroglycerin. Recent data show that nitrates can be used in patients with acute heart failure with systolic blood pressure close to 100 mm Hg (Fig. 2). They are contraindicated in cardiogenic shock.

In all cases, effects on dyspnea and blood pressure should be monitored closely. Of note, adverse effects of nitrates are usually dose-dependent and consist of headache, flush, tachycardia and palpitations, and hypotension. These effects are reversed by withdrawal of the drug.

Finally, the venodilation effect of nitrates leads to decreased central venous pressure and thus limits organ congestion, which constitutes one major determinant of organ dysfunction, particularly kidney dysfunction, in acute heart failure.

Is Nitrate the Only Efficient Vasodilator?

Neseritide, a recombinant form of human B-type natriuretic peptide (BNP) is a powerful vasodilator, which has been used for acute dyspnea due to pulmonary edema. However, a recent trial, the Acute Study of Clinical Effectiveness of Nesiritide in Decompensated Heart Failure (ASCEND-HF), showed no beneficial effect compared to standard of care [17]. Thus, for now, there is no strong evidence to support use of vasodilator other than nitrates in acute heart failure.

Association with Diuretics

Diuretics are frequently used in acute heart failure patients, although the rationale of their use is not supported by high-level evidence. There is evidence to suggest that indications for high doses of diuretics should be limited and that diuretics should be used at lower doses than in the past. In hypertensive acute heart failure, the leading cause of pulmonary edema in France and around the world, there is no prior hypervolemia. Diuretic therapy when given at high doses (>1 mg/kg) can quickly exceed its goal and cause hypovolemia. It is preferable to focus on the use of vasodilators if the aim is to quickly improve symptoms in acute heart failure patients. Similarly, decompensated chronic heart failure does not necessarily mean 'associated' hypervolemia. In contrast, for a patient in decompensated chronic heart failure, with dyspnea and clear signs of hypervolemia, including dilated jugular veins in a sitting position, diuretics are indicated, but at lower doses than before, e. g., bolus of i.v. furosemide 40 mg, with a maximum of 100 mg i.v. in the 6 first hours and 240 mg maximum in the first 24 hours. It has been shown that the initial dose of diuretics should not exceed 80 mg [18]. Yilmaz et al. [18] studied the impact of diuretic dosing on mortality in acute heart failure using a propensity-matched analysis on data from the ALARM-HF study. A post-hoc analysis was performed to determine if there was an interaction between i.v. bolus diuretic dosing and outcomes. Patients were classified as receiving high- or low-dose i.v. furosemide if their total initial 24 h dose was above or below 1 mg/kg, respectively. The conclusion of this study was that initial i.v. doses of diuretics were not associated, *per se*, with increased in-hospital mortality. However, high dose diuretics are harmful in patients with comorbidities, such as diabetes or previous kidney dysfunction.

In summary, nitrates are indicated as first line therapy, together with non-invasive ventilation, in acute heart failure, especially in patients with high blood pressure and high left ventricular filling pressure. Diuretics should be started at a dose <1 mg/kg with monitoring of cardiac output and dyspnea less than two hours later. Table 1 reports dose, indication and potential side effects of vasodilators in acute heart failure according to the ESC guidelines.

Table 1 Indications and dosing of intravenous vasodilators in acute heart failure (HF) according to the ESC guidelines [10, 11]

Vasodilator	Indication	Dosing	Main side-effects	Other
Nitro-glycerin	Pulmonary congestion/edema BP > 90 mm Hg	Start 10–20 mcg/min, increase up to 200 mcg/min	Hypotension, headache	Tolerance on continuous use
Isosorbide dinitrate	Pulmonary congestion/edema BP > 90 mm Hg	Start with 1 mg/h, increase up to 10 mg/h	Hypotension, headache	Tolerance on continuous use
Nitroprusside	Hypertensive HF congestion/edema BP > 90 mm Hg	Start with 0.3 mcg/min and increase up to 5 mcg/kg/min	Hypotension, isocyanate toxicity	Light sensitive
Nesiritide	Hypertensive HF congestion/edema BP > 90 mm Hg	Bolus 2 mcg/kg + infusion 0.015–0.003 mcg/kg/min	Hypotension	

Why Less Inotrope?

The use of inotropes in acute heart failure is very controversial. Increasing evidence indicates detrimental effects on survival, regardless of the severity of the acute heart failure [19, 20]. Inotropes such as dobutamine (beta-1 adrenergic agonist) are a 'classical' treatment for acute heart failure. However, epidemiological studies have shown that they are indicated in less than 10% of patients [21]. The use of inotropic agents should be exceptional and motivated only by the presence of signs of hypoperfusion (e. g., oliguria, mottling) with or without hypotension and with or without pulmonary edema refractory to diuretics and vasodilators.

The ideal inotropic agent should improve contractility of the left ventricle and right ventricle without increasing heart rate, increasing the pre- or post-load, or increasing oxygen consumption. It should also have beneficial effects on diastolic function, maintaining adequate diastolic coronary perfusion and cardiac output. Finally, it should have a rapid onset of action and a short half-life. Such an agent does not exist.

Inotropes should be used with care because they cause an increase in the cellular concentration of calcium and myocardial oxygen consumption [22]. The two main side effects are rhythm disorders and myocardial ischemia. Inotropes are not useful in acute heart failure with a high systolic blood pressure and are not indicated as first line in acute heart failure with a normal blood pressure [23]. Inotropes which are used for their short-term hemodynamic benefits have been frequently shown to have little or no effect on clinical outcomes. Indeed, despite their expected beneficial effect on cardiac output and/or blood pressure, all inotropes and vasopressors may carry the risk of increased myocardial ischemia and arrhythmias, leading to a detrimental effect on short-term outcomes [19]. However, data are limited, and the interpretation of findings is often skewed by the fact that positive inotropes are administered to patients with the most severe acute heart failure who already carry a high risk of death.

For example, the Outcomes of a Prospective Trial of Intravenous Milrinone for Exacerbations of Chronic Heart Failure (OPTIME-CHF) study showed no benefit of milrinone administered to 949 patients hospitalized for acute heart failure; an increase in arrhythmias was observed and coronary patients had a poorer prognosis [24]. A retrospective analysis of over 65,000 records of file ADHERE also showed that inotropes were associated with excess mortality compared to conventional treatment [21]. Moreover, analysis of the Acute Decompensated Heart Failure National Registry (ALARM-HF) database revealed a deleterious effect of inotropes on survival in acute heart failure [13]. In this study, the authors demonstrated that the use of an i.v. positive inotropic agent was associated with an increased risk of in-hospital death (Fig. 3). Based on these results, conclusions could be drawn about three categories of agents: (1) epinephrine and norepinephrine markedly worsened the risk of in-hospital death; (2) dopamine and dobutamine moderately worsened the risk of in-hospital death; (3) levosimendan had no or a slight beneficial effect on the risk of in-hospital death [13].

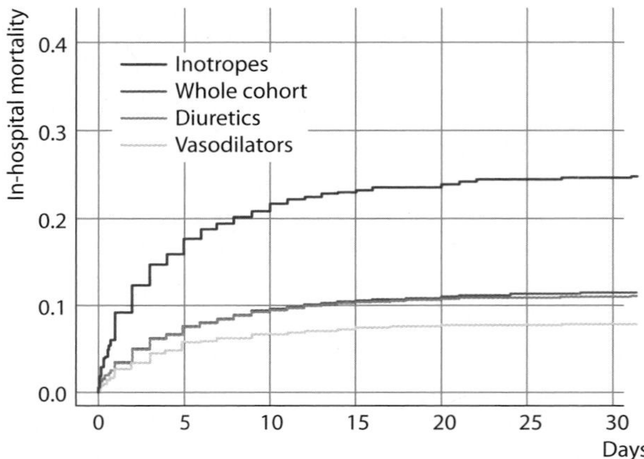

Fig. 3 Effects of the main intravenous drugs administered during the first 48 h to patients with acute heart failure on in-hospital mortality. Whole cohort (n = 4,953), diuretics (n = 4,167), vasodilators (mostly nitrates, n = 1,930), inotropes and/or vasopressors (n = 1,617) (adapted from [13] with permission)

Dobutamine is a positive inotropic agent for which uncertainty exists concerning its effect on mortality. A systematic review and meta-analysis of randomized controlled trials about dobutamine for patients with severe heart failure was published in 2012 [25]. Fourteen studies, with 673 participants were included: Dobutamine was not associated with improved mortality in patients with acute heart failure, and there was a trend towards an increase in mortality with use of dobutamine compared with placebo or standard care, although this did not reach statistical significance.

Levosimendan is a pyridazinone-dinitrile derivative that increases troponin C affinity for Ca^{2+} and stabilizes the conformation of troponin C. Levosimendan has positive inotropic properties without impairing ventricular relaxation or inducing cystolic Ca^{2+} overload, owing to improvement in sensitivity of the contractile apparatus to intracellular Ca^{2+}. These inodilatory properties lead to a dramatic increase in cardiac output with a concomitant reduction in cardiac filling pressures in failing hearts. Despite the fact that it does not seem to induce ventricular arrhythmias and prolongation of the QT interval, levosimendan augments heart rate and increases the incidence of atrial fibrillation especially in case of high bolus or prolonged administration (> 48 h).

According to recent ESC guidelines [10, 11], levosimendan is recommended as a second-line treatment in acute heart failure (recommendation level IIB, level of evidence B). Levosimendan may be administered as a bolus dose (3–12 mg/kg) over 10 min followed by a continuous infusion (0.05–0.2 mg/kg/min for 24 h). The infusion rate may be increased once stability is confirmed. In patients with systolic blood pressure < 100 mm Hg, the infusion should be started without a bolus dose to avoid hypotension.

Finally, cardiac myosin activators are recently discovered small molecules that directly stimulate the activity of cardiac myosin motor protein resulting in improvement of cardiac contractility without alterations of intracellular calcium concentration. Administration of a cardiac myosin activator in healthy volunteers caused an increase in stroke volume and cardiac contractility without affecting myocardial oxygen consumption. These promising results should be evaluated in

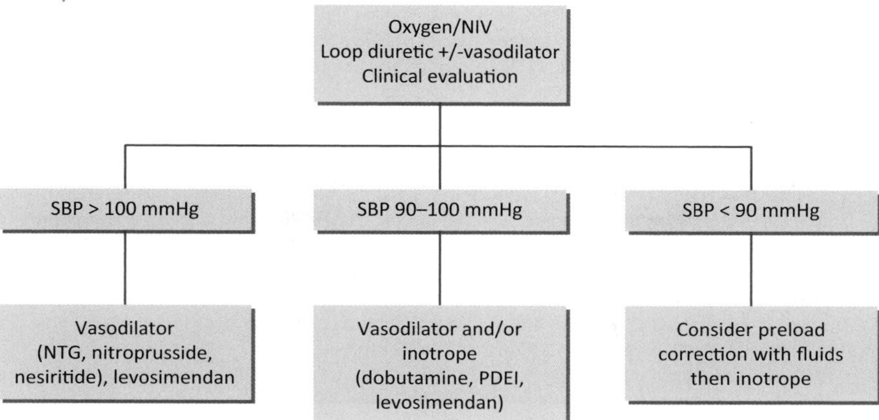

Fig. 4 Proposed algorithm for the use of intravenous drugs in acute heart failure according to the ESC guidelines [10, 11]. NIV: non-invasive ventilation; SBP: systolic blood pressure; NTG: nitroglycerin; PDEI: phosphodiesterase inhibitor

large scale randomized trials involving patients with acute heart failure and impaired cardiac contractility [26].

Conclusion

New evidence to guide the management of acute heart failure has emerged recently. Epidemiological studies based on large registers have helped clarify the definition of acute heart failure syndromes. Compared to chronic heart failure, very few studies of high level evidence have been conducted in the setting of acute heart failure. However, there is sufficient evidence to recommend using more vasodilators associated with lower doses of diuretics. Inotropes should be considered only in cases of acute heart failure associated with organ hypoperfusion and, among the available inotropes, dobutamine seems to be associated with an important rate of adverse events. Figure 4 is a proposed algorithm for management which summarizes the respective places of the different i.v. drugs in the management of patients with acute heart failure.

References

1. Lloyd-Jones D, Adams R, Carnethon M et al (2009) Heart disease and stroke statistics – 2009 update: a report from the American Heart Association Statistics Committee and Stroke Statistics Subcommittee. Circulation 119:480–486
2. Lloyd-Jones DM, Larson MG, Leip EP et al (2002) Lifetime risk for developing congestive heart failure: the Framingham Heart Study. Circulation 106:3068–3072

3. Roger VL, Weston SA, Redfield MM et al (2004) Trends in heart failure incidence and survival in a community-based population. JAMA 292:344–350
4. McMurray JJ, Pfeffer MA (2005) Heart failure. Lancet 365:1877–1889
5. Dar O, Cowie MR (2008) Acute heart failure in the intensive care unit: epidemiology. Crit Care Med 36(1 Suppl):S3–S8
6. Gheorghiade M, Mebazaa A (2005) Introduction to acute heart failure syndromes. Am J Cardiol 96:1G–4G
7. Adams Jr KF, Fonarow GC, Emerman CL et al (2005) Characteristics and outcomes of patients hospitalized for heart failure in the United States: rationale, design, and preliminary observations from the first 100,000 cases in the Acute Decompensated Heart Failure National Registry (ADHERE). Am Heart J 149:209–216
8. Cleland JG, Swedberg K, Follath F et al (2003) The EuroHeart Failure survey programme – a survey on the quality of care among patients with heart failure in Europe. Part 1: patient characteristics and diagnosis. Eur Heart J 24:442–463
9. Zannad F, Mebazaa A, Juilliere Y et al (2006) Clinical profile, contemporary management and one-year mortality in patients with severe acute heart failure syndromes: The EFICA study. Eur J Heart Fail 8:697–705
10. Nieminen MS, Bohm M, Cowie MR et al (2005) Executive summary of the guidelines on the diagnosis and treatment of acute heart failure: the Task Force on Acute Heart Failure of the European Society of Cardiology. Eur Heart J 26:384–416
11. McMurray JJ, Adamopoulos S, Anker SD et al (2012) ESC Guidelines for the diagnosis and treatment of acute and chronic heart failure 2012: The Task Force for the Diagnosis and Treatment of Acute and Chronic Heart Failure 2012 of the European Society of Cardiology. Developed in collaboration with the Heart Failure Association (HFA) of the ESC. Eur Heart J 33:1787–1847
12. Laribi S, Aouba A, Nikolaou M et al (2012) Trends in death attributed to heart failure over the past two decades in Europe. Eur J Heart Fail 14:234–239
13. Mebazaa A, Parissis J, Porcher R et al (2011) Short-term survival by treatment among patients hospitalized with acute heart failure: the global ALARM-HF registry using propensity scoring methods. Intensive Care Med 37:290–301
14. Cotter G, Moshkovitz Y, Milovanov O et al (2002) Acute heart failure: a novel approach to its pathogenesis and treatment. Eur J Heart Fail 4:227–234
15. Imhof PR, Ott B, Frankhauser P, Chu LC, Hodler J (1980) Difference in nitroglycerin dose-response in the venous and arterial beds. Eur J Clin Pharmacol 18:455–460
16. Publication Committee for the VMAC Investigators (2002) Intravenous nesiritide vs nitroglycerin for treatment of decompensated congestive heart failure: a randomized controlled trial. JAMA 287:1531–1540
17. O'Connor CM, Starling RC, Hernandez AF et al (2011) Effect of nesiritide in patients with acute decompensated heart failure. N Engl J Med 365:32–43
18. Yilmaz MB, Gayat E, Salem R et al (2011) Impact of diuretic dosing on mortality in acute heart failure using a propensity-matched analysis. Eur J Heart Fail 13:1244–1252
19. Thackray S, Easthaugh J, Freemantle N, Cleland JG (2002) The effectiveness and relative effectiveness of intravenous inotropic drugs acting through the adrenergic pathway in patients with heart failure – a meta-regression analysis. Eur J Heart Fail 4:515–529
20. Felker GM, O'Connor CM (2001) Inotropic therapy for heart failure: an evidence-based approach. Am Heart J 142:393–401
21. Abraham WT, Adams KF, Fonarow GC et al (2005) In-hospital mortality in patients with acute decompensated heart failure requiring intravenous vasoactive medications: an analysis from the Acute Decompensated Heart Failure National Registry (ADHERE). J Am Coll Cardiol 46:57–64
22. Katz AM (1986) Potential deleterious effects of inotropic agents in the therapy of chronic heart failure. Circulation 73(III):184–190
23. Petersen JW, Felker GM (2008) Inotropes in the management of acute heart failure. Crit Care Med 36(1 Suppl):S106–S111

24. Cuffe MS, Califf RM, Adams Jr KF et al (2002) Short-term intravenous milrinone for acute exacerbation of chronic heart failure: a randomized controlled trial. JAMA 287:1541–1547
25. Tacon CL, McCaffrey J, Delaney A (2012) Dobutamine for patients with severe heart failure: a systematic review and meta-analysis of randomised controlled trials. Intensive Care Med 38:359–367
26. Parissis JT, Rafouli-Stergiou P, Stasinos V, Psarogiannakopoulos P, Mebazaa A (2010) Inotropes in cardiac patients: update 2011. Curr Opin Crit Care 16:432–441

Goal Directed Therapy: A Review

M. Gruenewald and B. Bein

Introduction

The issue of hemodynamic optimization has attracted increasing interest over the last two decades, following publication of several studies that have suggested beneficial effects of so called "goal-directed therapy" on patient outcomes. Whereas in the past large volumes of crystalloids were administered in order to replace an ambiguous 'third space loss' [1], delivering an individually adapted amount of fluids based on advanced hemodynamic monitoring should now be considered standard of care [2]. The main goal of this individually tailored therapy is an optimal oxygen supply to the vital organs in critical situations, such as high-risk surgery, critical illness or post-cardiac arrest syndrome. Oxygen delivery (DO_2) depends on oxygen transport capacity, which in turn is determined by the hemoglobin concentration, its saturation with oxygen and cardiac output. Consequently, therapy is based on optimization of cardiac function with its key determinants preload, contractility and afterload. Current concepts include the use of fluids, inotropes and vasopressors. With respect to fluids, it is crucial to avoid additional harm to our patients, e. g., by fluid overload. Furthermore, the concept of "one fits all" is most probably wrong and health care professionals should define specific therapeutic goals in order to meet the individual needs of our patients [3]. Therefore, a patient's medical history and comorbidities as well as the type of surgical procedure are important aspects that must be considered.

M. Gruenewald (✉)
Department of Anesthesiology and Intensive Care Medicine, University Hospital Schleswig-Holstein (UKSH), Campus Kiel, Schwanenweg 21, 24105 Kiel, Germany
E-mail: matthias.gruenewald@uksh.de

B. Bein
Department of Anesthesiology and Intensive Care Medicine, University Hospital Schleswig-Holstein (UKSH), Campus Kiel, Schwanenweg 21, 24105 Kiel, Germany

J.-L. Vincent (Ed.), *Annual Update in Intensive Care and Emergency Medicine 2013*,
DOI 10.1007/978-3-642-35109-9_20,

The present chapter aims to provide a comprehensive review of the development of goal-directed fluid therapy, discuss the current evidence and provide an outlook on future concepts.

Where We Come From

For a long time, the administration of intravenous fluids was based on empirical values and simple calculations such as the "4-2-1 rule" [4]. This is not surprising because only clinical evaluation and static filling pressures were available for estimation of fluid needs. The importance of fluid therapy on patient outcome remained rather unclear. Large volumes of crystalloids were administered to replace the suggested volume deficit caused by preoperative fasting, blood and urine loss, perspiration and a so called "third space loss" [1]. This mysterious third spacing was the rationale for liberal fluid administration, since it was suggested that large amounts of fluid were lost into this third space.

'Liberal' vs. 'Restrictive' Infusion Regimes

The 'liberal' fluid strategy aimed to administer a large amount of fluids in order to preserve intravascular volume and achieve a sufficient organ perfusion. In daily clinical practice, patients were treated with large amounts of unbalanced crystalloids both in anesthesiology and in the intensive care unit (ICU). Liberal intraoperative fluid therapy often resulted in fluid overload with extensive weight gain and deleterious effects on patient outcome [5, 6].

In contrast, a 'restrictive' fluid therapy aims to limit the amount of fluid administered in order to protect organs, e. g., the bowel, from swelling due to interstitial edema. However, this strategy may also cause complications such as renal failure and possibly result in a prolonged hospital stay [7].

As such, the terms 'liberal' and 'restrictive' are impractical as they are not clearly defined and may be associated with varying amounts of fluid administered. A nice review comparing 'liberal' vs. 'restrictive' fluid therapy highlights this inconsistency in the underlying definitions [8].

The Pulmonary Artery Catheter

With the introduction of the pulmonary artery catheter (PAC) by William Swan and Jeremy Ganz in the 1970s, hemodynamic status could be evaluated at the bedside. It was not until 1988, however, that Shoemaker et al. first reported benefits of using supranormal values obtained with the PAC as therapeutic goals for high-risk surgery patients [9]. In this study, however, a standardized algorithm for guidance to reach these goals was not defined. A few years later, however, one of the first controlled studies using such an algorithm was performed and reported fewer intra- and postoperative complications in vascular surgery patients if hemodynamic optimization based on PAC values was performed before surgery [10]. The study showed that 26 % of patients only required fluids whereas another 37 % additionally required inotropes for optimization of their hemodynamic status.

So far, the largest trial examining the impact of goal-directed optimization was performed between 1990 and 1999 in 19 Canadian hospitals [11]. A total of 1,994 patients were randomized into two groups. Patients in the intervention group were equipped with a PAC and the following goals were defined: Hematocrit $\geq 27\,\%$; mean arterial pressure (MAP) ≥ 70 mm Hg; heart rate < 120 bpm; DO_2 550–600 ml/min/m^2; cardiac output 3.5–4.5 l/min; pulmonary artery occlusion pressure (PAOP) ≥ 18 mm Hg. The control group was treated with standard care and not equipped with a PAC. Interestingly, the investigators observed no difference between groups with regard to complications (except for lung embolism, which occurred significantly more often in the catheter group), length of hospital stay or one-year mortality. Although these results were at first disappointing, this study nevertheless contributed a fundamental insight into the feasibility of goal-directed therapy and raised an important discussion about the right goals. Interestingly, in about one third of all patients in the intervention group the predefined goals were not reached.

Minimal Invasive Cardiac Output Monitoring

With the increased use of the PAC, a wide range of complications was reported. Also, insertion of a PAC is sometimes difficult and time-consuming. These aforementioned shortcomings led to the development of less invasive hemodynamic monitoring devices.

The trans-cardiopulmonary thermodilution technique allows determination of cardiac output without catheterization of the right heart. The technique only needs a central venous line and a specific thermistor-tipped arterial catheter, most often placed in the femoral artery. Trans-cardiopulmonary thermodilution yields new variables that reflect cardiac filling, such as the global end-diastolic volume index (GEDVI), or pulmonary edema, such as the extra vascular lung water index (EVLWI). Integration of these variables into a goal-directed protocol in cardiac surgery resulted in a decreased use of catecholamines as well as a shorter duration on the ventilator and a shorter ICU stay [12]. In addition to trans-cardiopulmonary thermodilution, the PiCCO device allows for continuous determination of cardiac output by pulse contour analysis after calibration of the underlying algorithm by thermodilution [13, 14]. Subsequently, other pulse contour based monitors were introduced into the market, which also enable continuous cardiac output monitoring beat-to-beat after calibration by a reference method (most often indicator dilution technique). In addition to determination of cardiac output, pulse contour analysis allows for evaluation of the heart-lung interaction during mechanical ventilation. An increased variation in stroke volume over a predefined time frame indicates fluid responsiveness [15], an essential component in goal-directed therapy. Recently, advanced pulse contour algorithms, based on demographic data and empirical datasets that do not require calibration by a reference technique allow a more simple application by connecting to a standard radial arterial line. Therefore, the beneficial effects of goal-directed therapy have become available for patients who do not require invasive monitoring with a femoral line [16]. Nonetheless, these techniques still suffer from significant bias during clinical situations with changing vascular resistance that do not permit their ubiquitous use [17, 18].

Esophageal Doppler

Another technique, esophageal Doppler, has also been proposed for guidance of fluid optimization. Sinclair et al. used Doppler-derived variables for goal-directed fluid therapy in patients undergoing hip surgery and reported faster recovery of patients in the intervention group [19]. Others used the esophageal Doppler for fluid optimization in patients undergoing abdominal surgery and reported comparable benefits [20]. Even though esophageal Doppler is a minimally invasive technique, its use for continuous evaluation is hampered by the lack of stability of the signal during surgical manipulation or movement.

Where We Are

The increasing interest in perioperative goal-directed therapy has changed anesthesiologists' attitudes towards fluid administration and optimization of cardiac output. Modern perioperative concepts are changing and no longer restricted to the immediate period during surgery. To date we understand that fluid management may influence long term outcomes. We are gaining more and more insight into the choice of adequate goals, timing of therapy and selection of patients who benefit most. At present, monitoring devices are readily available, yielding various variables (Table 1) that may be integrated into goal-directed therapy protocols.

The concept of extensive preoperative fasting ("nil by mouth after midnight") has been discouraged in the modern perioperative management of patients. It has been shown that fasting of 6 hours for solid food and 2 hours for fluids is safe and associated with positive effects on outcome [21]. However, up to 50 % of our patients will still respond with a significant increase in stroke volume and cardiac output after adequate volume administration and may, therefore, benefit from fluid therapy [22]. The main goal of optimization is to provide adequate DO_2 to vital organs and prevent hypoperfusion and hypoxia. Given an adequate hemoglobin concentration and sufficient oxygenation, cardiac output is the main determinant of DO_2. Therefore, goal-directed therapy is often based on optimization of stroke volume, which in turn is dependent on preload, contractility and afterload as reflected in the Frank-Starling curve. Preload itself does not imply preload (or fluid) responsiveness as individual fluid responsiveness depends on the dynamic characteristics of cardiac contractility and compliance. As outlined above, the dynamic variables obtained from heart-lung interactions during mechanical ventilation indicate fluid responsiveness and may be used to guide fluid administration. These variables can be either obtained from pulse contour analysis (pulse pressure variation [PPV], stroke volume variation [SVV]), esophageal Doppler (variation of velocity time integral (ΔVTI)) or even non-invasively by the plethysmographic signal (pleth variability index [PVI]). Unfortunately, these variables only work reliably during controlled mechanical ventilation and are further influenced by tidal volume [23], intra-abdominal hypertension [24] and vasoactive medication [25]. Therefore, volumetric variables obtained from trans-cardiopulmonary thermodilution (such as the GEDVI) or approaches such as the passive leg raising maneuver are clinically important measures of fluid responsiveness.

Table 1 Variables for determination of oxygen delivery

<table>
<tr><td colspan="7">Oxygen Delivery</td></tr>
<tr><td colspan="7">DO_2</td></tr>
<tr><td colspan="5">Cardiac Output</td><td>Transport Capacity</td><td>Oxygenation</td></tr>
<tr><td colspan="5">CO/CI</td><td rowspan="10">Hb/Hct</td><td rowspan="10">SaO_2
PaO_2</td></tr>
<tr><td colspan="4">Stroke Volume</td><td rowspan="2">Heart Rate</td></tr>
<tr><td colspan="4">SV/SVI</td></tr>
<tr><td colspan="2">Preload</td><td>Contractility</td><td>Afterload</td><td rowspan="7">bpm</td></tr>
<tr><td>Preload</td><td>Volume Responsiveness</td><td></td><td></td></tr>
<tr><td>GEDVI</td><td>SVV</td><td>dP/dtmax</td><td>SVR/SVRI</td></tr>
<tr><td>LVEDV</td><td>PPV/SPV</td><td>CPI</td><td rowspan="4"></td></tr>
<tr><td>FTc</td><td>PVI</td><td>CFI/GEF</td></tr>
<tr><td>CVP</td><td>ΔVpeak</td><td>LVEF</td></tr>
<tr><td>PAOP</td><td>GEDVI</td><td>LVSWI</td></tr>
</table>

DO_2: oxygen delivery (mlO_2/min); CO/CI: cardiac output/index (l/min; l/min/m^2); Hb: hemoglobin (g/dl); Hct: hematocrit (%); SaO_2: arterial saturation of oxygen (%); PaO_2: partial pressure of arterial oxygen (mmHg); GEDVI: global end-diastolic volume index (ml/m^2); LVEDV: left ventricular end-diastolic volume (ml); FTc: flowtime corrected for heart rate (ms); CVP: central venous pressure (mmHg); PAOP: pulmonary arterial occlusion pressure (mmHg); SVV: stroke volume variation (%); PPV: pulse pressure variation (%); SPV: systolic pressure variation (%); PVI: pleth variability index; ΔVpeak: variation of peak flow velocity (%); LVEF: left ventricular ejection fraction (%); CFI: cardiac function index; GEF: global ejection fraction (%); CPI: cardiac power index (W/m^2); dP/dtmax: maximum increase in left ventricular pressure (mmHg/s); LVSWI: left ventricular stroke work index (g/m/m^2); SVR/SVRI: systemic vascular resistance/index (dyn/s/cm^5 [/m^2])

Table 2 Clinical criteria for identification of high-risk patients. (One criterion present yields classification of high risk). Modified from [9]

1.	Severe cardiopulmonary disease with dysfunction (acute myocardial infarction, dilative cardiomyopathy, ejection fraction < 40 %)
2.	Age > 70 years with limited physiologic reserve of one or more vital organs
3.	Sepsis (hemodynamic instability, septic cardiomyopathy)
4.	Respiratory failure ($PaO_2/FiO_2 < 300$, $PaCO_2 > 45$ mm Hg, $FEV_1 < 60$ % of predicted value)
5.	Chronic cirrhosis (Child B or C)
6.	Acute renal failure (urea > 45 mg/dl, creatinine > 3 mg/dl)
7.	Extensive surgery of carcinoma (e. g., esophagectomy, total gastrectomy, surgery > 8 h)
8.	Acute abdominal catastrophe (e. g., pancreatitis, gangrenous bowel, peritonitis)
9.	Major vascular surgery (e. g., aortic surgery)
10.	Severe trauma (life-threatening condition)
11.	Acute bleeding (> 2.5 l of blood, hematocrit < 20 %)

Although it has been shown to be less predictive of fluid responsiveness than other measures, central venous pressure (CVP) is probably still the most frequently used variable to estimate volume status. The interpretation of CVP should be based on its trend over time, on the parallel estimation of stroke volume and also consider transmitted pressures. One of the most important trials regarding goal-directed therapy used the CVP to guide fluid administration [26]. Apart from the controversial discussion regarding the goals of this study, it highlighted the impact of timing of therapy. It is a straightforward concept that the longer an organ suffers from hypoxia, the greater the damage. Kern and Shoemaker showed that goal-directed therapy was beneficial if started early and before organ failure had occurred [27]. Therefore, it is advisable to integrate goal-directed therapy in high-risk surgery with a high possibility of large volume turnover. However, it is not always possible to foresee the invasiveness end extent of a surgical procedure. Goal-directed management may, thus, be started during the procedure or at the beginning of postoperative intensive care in order to reduce complications [28]. Since health care resources are limited, it is reasonable to use costly intensive monitoring devices only in patients who will benefit from them in terms of reduction in lengths of ICU and hospital stay. Goal-directed therapy had most impact when patients in the respective control groups had mortality rates of 20 % or higher [27, 29]. However, identification of high-risk patients is not easy and often not successful [30]. The best approach is probably to consider individual patient comorbidities and the risk of the surgical procedure. Whereas the cardiac risk can for example be assessed by scores, such as the revised cardiac risk index [31], the type of surgery should also be considered [32]. A possible approach, including individual and procedure-related risks may be found in the modified Shoemaker criteria (Table 2) [9].

Table 3 Selection of current meta-analyses on goal-directed therapy (GDT)

Author	Year	Number of studies	Number of patients	Main message	Conclusion
Kern [27]	2002	21	2341	GDT decreases mortality if: Started early Control group mortality > 20 % Difference in DO_2	GDT is beneficial
Poeze [38]	2005	21	4175	GDT decreases mortality in high-risk surgery	GDT is beneficial
Giglio [34]	2009	16	3410	GDT decreases rate of minor and major gastrointestinal complications	GDT is beneficial
Rahbari [39]	2009	9	971	GDT and restrictive volume management decrease morbidity after colorectal resection	GDT and "restriction" is beneficial
Brienza [35]	2009	20	4220	GDT decreases risk of renal impairment in surgical patients	GDT is beneficial
Dalfino [33]	2011	26	4188	GDT decreases incidence of postoperative infections	GDT is beneficial
Gurgel [29]	2011	32	5056	GDT decreases morbidity and mortality in high-risk surgical patients	GDT is beneficial
Hamilton [37]	2011	29	4805	GDT decreases morbidity and mortality in moderate and high-risk surgical patients	GDT is beneficial
Corcoran [36]	2012	23	3861	GDT and restrictive volume management decrease complication rate and length of hospital stay	GDT and "restriction" is beneficial

DO_2: oxygen delivery

There is an increasing number of meta-analyses dealing with individualized goal-directed therapy and evidence is growing that patient outcomes may be improved by this strategy [27, 29, 33–39] (Table 3). The British National Institute for Health and Clinical Excellence has recommended the individualized optimization of intravascular volume in high-risk surgical patients (www.nice.org.uk). As stated above, the impact of goal-directed therapy increases with the risk of the patients [27, 29]. Individualized goal-directed therapy can reduce the number of major complications such as infections (e. g., wound infections, pneumonia) [33], gastrointestinal complications [34], renal complications [35, 36] and shorten length of hospital stay [36]. Another recent meta-analysis based on 29 studies showed that goal-directed therapy improved morbidity and mortality of high-risk surgical patients [37]. However, the authors showed nicely that there is still a need for more studies with higher quality and a multicenter design. Several trials are currently recruiting patients in order to provide more valuable data (clinicaltrials.gov: NCT00766519, NCT01473446 and NCT01458678).

Where We Are Going

Hemodynamic monitoring devices are being developed with ever increasing frequency to reduce invasiveness and complication rates. Advanced monitoring derived from non-invasive plethysmography, non-invasive finger arterial waveform analysis, bioreactance or bioimpedance will potentially become interchangeable with traditional invasive hemodynamic techniques. Clinicians need reliable tools, otherwise therapy based on the measures obtained will not be effective. Moreover, the use of hemodynamic tools without a reasonable protocol will not provide any benefit to the patient [40]. A protocol for goal-directed therapy must consider key issues, such as available monitoring in the respective institution, the individual morbidity of the patient as well as the surgical procedure. A basic concept is presented in Fig. 1.

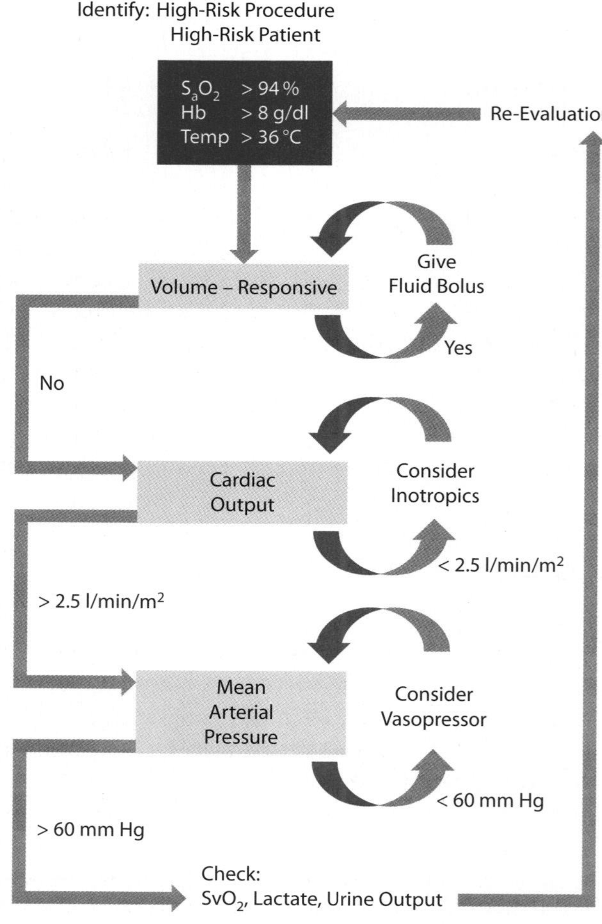

Fig. 1 Suggested protocol for goal-directed therapy

In the future, a well-defined algorithm may be integrated into computer-assisted closed-loop systems as realized in automatic insulin pumps or used for guidance of sedation [41, 42]. Whereas automatic systems may be more precise in monitoring one or more key variables and in regulating the therapeutic interventions necessary to control a system, the complexity of the physiologic model and the disease will not allow these systems to completely replace the clinician. At present, development is focusing on decision support systems that propose a certain action and, thereby, support the caregivers. An up-to-date review regarding this issue in the context of fluid therapy has recently been published [43].

Another promising computer-based option in fluid therapy could be improvement in the detection of hypovolemia using advanced statistical methods such as genetic algorithms [44]. These complex mathematical methods integrate several hemodynamic variables, which may potentially improve the prediction of hypovolemia; however, no data from large scale trials are currently available that prove beneficial effects on outcome.

Conclusion

Perioperative fluid therapy has an important effect on long-term outcome. Individualized goal-directed fluid therapy has attracted considerable interest in recent years. Modern advanced hemodynamic monitoring enables bedside evaluation of fluid status and may be used to guide therapy. Several meta-analyses conclude that the use of goal-directed therapy improves outcomes, when used in high-risk patients and started before organ failure has occurred. New non-invasive devices are being marketed that still need to prove reliability in challenging clinical situations. We need large good quality multicenter studies to gain more knowledge on the impact of goal-directed therapy on outcome. Future concepts may use closed-loop systems as well as integrated mathematical methods to assist the clinician in the challenging perioperative task of hemodynamic optimization.

References

1. Jacob M, Chappell D, Rehm M (2009) The "third space" – fact or fiction? Best Pract Res Clin Anaesthesiol 23:145–157
2. Michard F (2011) The burden of high-risk surgery and the potential benefit of goal-directed strategies. Crit Care 15:447
3. Reuter DA (2012) Pragmatic fluid optimization in high-risk surgery patients: when pragmatism dilutes the benefits. Crit Care 16:106
4. Bailey AG, McNaull PP, Jooste E, Tuchman JB (2010) Perioperative crystalloid and colloid fluid management in children: where are we and how did we get here? Anesth Analg 110:375–390
5. Lowell JA, Schifferdecker C, Driscoll DF, Benotti PN, Bistrian BR (1990) Postoperative fluid overload: not a benign problem. Crit Care Med 18:728–733

6. Holte K, Jensen P, Kehlet H (2003) Physiologic effects of intravenous fluid administration in healthy volunteers. Anesth Analg 96:1504–1509
7. Holte K, Foss NB, Andersen J et al (2007) Liberal or restrictive fluid administration in fast-track colonic surgery: a randomized, double-blind study. Br J Anaesth 99:500–508
8. Bundgaard-Nielsen M, Secher NH, Kehlet H (2009) "Liberal" vs. "restrictive" perioperative fluid therapy – a critical assessment of the evidence. Acta Anaesthesiol Scand 53:843–851
9. Shoemaker WC, Appel PL, Kram HB, Waxman K, Lee TS (1988) Prospective trial of supranormal values of survivors as therapeutic goals in high-risk surgical patients. Chest 94:1176–1186
10. Berlauk JF, Abrams JH, Gilmour IJ, O'Connor SR, Knighton DR, Cerra FB (1991) Preoperative optimization of cardiovascular hemodynamics improves outcome in peripheral vascular surgery. A prospective, randomized clinical trial. Ann Surg 214:289–297
11. Sandham JD, Hull RD, Brant RF et al (2003) A randomized, controlled trial of the use of pulmonary-artery catheters in high-risk surgical patients. N Engl J Med 348:5–14
12. Goepfert MS, Reuter DA, Akyol D, Lamm P, Kilger E, Goetz AE (2007) Goal-directed fluid management reduces vasopressor and catecholamine use in cardiac surgery patients. Intensive Care Med 33:96–103
13. Godje O, Hoke K, Goetz AE et al (2002) Reliability of a new algorithm for continuous cardiac output determination by pulse-contour analysis during hemodynamic instability. Crit Care Med 30:52–58
14. Linton NW, Linton RA (2001) Estimation of changes in cardiac output from the arterial blood pressure waveform in the upper limb. Br J Anaesth 86:486–496
15. Michard F, Teboul JL (2000) Using heart-lung interactions to assess fluid responsiveness during mechanical ventilation. Crit Care 4:282–289
16. Cecconi M, Fasano N, Langiano N et al (2011) Goal-directed haemodynamic therapy during elective total hip arthroplasty under regional anaesthesia. Crit Care 15:R132
17. Bein B, Meybohm P, Cavus E et al (2007) The reliability of pulse contour-derived cardiac output during hemorrhage and after vasopressor administration. Anesth Analg 105:107–113
18. Gruenewald M, Meybohm P, Renner J et al (2011) Effect of norepinephrine dosage and calibration frequency on accuracy of pulse contour-derived cardiac output. Crit Care 15:R22
19. Sinclair S, James S, Singer M (1997) Intraoperative intravascular volume optimisation and length of hospital stay after repair of proximal femoral fracture: randomised controlled trial. BMJ 315:909–912
20. Wakeling HG, McFall MR, Jenkins CS et al (2005) Intraoperative oesophageal Doppler guided fluid management shortens postoperative hospital stay after major bowel surgery. Br J Anaesth 95:634–642
21. Brady M, Kinn S, Stuart P (2003) Preoperative fasting for adults to prevent perioperative complications. Cochrane Database Syst Rev: CD004423
22. Marik PE, Cavallazzi R, Vasu T, Hirani A (2009) Dynamic changes in arterial waveform derived variables and fluid responsiveness in mechanically ventilated patients: a systematic review of the literature. Crit Care Med 37:2642–2647
23. Renner J, Cavus E, Meybohm P et al (2007) Stroke volume variation during hemorrhage and after fluid loading: impact of different tidal volumes. Acta Anaesthesiol Scand 51:538–544
24. Renner J, Gruenewald M, Quaden R et al (2009) Influence of increased intra-abdominal pressure on fluid responsiveness predicted by pulse pressure variation and stroke volume variation in a porcine model. Crit Care Med 37:650–658
25. Renner J, Meybohm P, Hanss R, Gruenewald M, Scholz J, Bein B (2009) Effects of norepinephrine on dynamic variables of fluid responsiveness during hemorrhage and after resuscitation in a pediatric porcine model. Paediatr Anaesth 19:688–694
26. Rivers E, Nguyen B, Havstad S et al (2001) Early goal-directed therapy in the treatment of severe sepsis and septic shock. N Engl J Med 345:1368–1377
27. Kern JW, Shoemaker WC (2002) Meta-analysis of hemodynamic optimization in high-risk patients. Crit Care Med 30:1686–1692

28. Pearse R, Dawson D, Fawcett J, Rhodes A, Grounds RM, Bennett ED (2005) Early goal-directed therapy after major surgery reduces complications and duration of hospital stay. A randomised, controlled trial [ISRCTN38797445]. Crit Care 9:R687–R693
29. Gurgel ST, do Nascimento Jr P (2011) Maintaining tissue perfusion in high-risk surgical patients: a systematic review of randomized clinical trials. Anesth Analg 112:1384–1391
30. Moonesinghe SR, Mythen MG, Grocott MP (2011) High-risk surgery: epidemiology and outcomes. Anesth Analg 112:891–901
31. Lee TH, Marcantonio ER, Mangione CM et al (1999) Derivation and prospective validation of a simple index for prediction of cardiac risk of major noncardiac surgery. Circulation 100:1043–1049
32. Boersma E, Kertai MD, Schouten O et al (2005) Perioperative cardiovascular mortality in noncardiac surgery: validation of the Lee cardiac risk index. Am J Med 118:1134–1141
33. Dalfino L, Giglio MT, Puntillo F, Marucci M, Brienza N (2011) Haemodynamic goal-directed therapy and postoperative infections: earlier is better. A systematic review and meta-analysis. Crit Care 15:R154
34. Giglio MT, Marucci M, Testini M, Brienza N (2009) Goal-directed haemodynamic therapy and gastrointestinal complications in major surgery: a meta-analysis of randomized controlled trials. Br J Anaesth 103:637–646
35. Brienza N, Giglio MT, Marucci M, Fiore T (2009) Does perioperative hemodynamic optimization protect renal function in surgical patients? A meta-analytic study. Crit Care Med 37:2079–2090
36. Corcoran T, Rhodes JE, Clarke S, Myles PS, Ho KM (2012) Perioperative fluid management strategies in major surgery: a stratified meta-analysis. Anesth Analg 114:640–651
37. Hamilton MA, Cecconi M, Rhodes A (2011) A systematic review and meta-analysis on the use of preemptive hemodynamic intervention to improve postoperative outcomes in moderate and high-risk surgical patients. Anesth Analg 112:1392–1402
38. Poeze M, Greve JW, Ramsay G (2005) Meta-analysis of hemodynamic optimization: relationship to methodological quality. Crit Care 9:R771–R779
39. Rahbari NN, Zimmermann JB, Schmidt T, Koch M, Weigand MA, Weitz J (2009) Meta-analysis of standard, restrictive and supplemental fluid administration in colorectal surgery. Br J Surg 96:331–341
40. Takala J, Ruokonen E, Tenhunen JJ, Parviainen I, Jakob SM (2011) Early non-invasive cardiac output monitoring in hemodynamically unstable intensive care patients: a multi-center randomized controlled trial. Crit Care 15:R148
41. Leslie K, Absalom A, Kenny GN (2002) Closed loop control of sedation for colonoscopy using the Bispectral Index. Anaesthesia 57:693–697
42. Liu N, Chazot T, Hamada S et al (2011) Closed-loop coadministration of propofol and remifentanil guided by bispectral index: a randomized multicenter study. Anesth Analg 112:546–557
43. Rinehart J, Liu N, Alexander B, Cannesson M (2012) Review article: closed-loop systems in anesthesia: is there a potential for closed-loop fluid management and hemodynamic optimization? Anesth Analg 114:130–143
44. Bardossy G, Halasz G, Gondos T (2011) The diagnosis of hypovolemia using advanced statistical methods. Comput Biol Med 41:1022–1032

Part VII

The Peripheral Circulation

Clinical Significance of Peripheral Circulation Abnormalities in Critically Ill Patients

A. Lima, M. E. Van Genderen, and J. Bakker

Introduction

The development of therapeutic goals and priorities for the intensive care setting depends on an accurate evaluation of the adequacy of organ perfusion. Clinically, the major causes of poor tissue perfusion can be divided into systemic and regional causes. Although inadequate systemic circulatory function may be directly measured, regional causes of altered tissue perfusion are more difficult to measure and more tenuous in appearance. From an etiological perspective, the most common cause of regional hypoperfusion in critically ill patients is an alteration in peripheral vascular function. A variety of factors contribute to these derangements in the peripheral circulation, and most of these alterations are present in both septic and non-septic shock. These factors are currently attributed to a combination of pathological derangements, including impaired arteriolar vasoregulation and capillary perfusion. These derangements are mainly observed in peripheral vascular beds, such as the skin, muscle, and gastrointestinal tract. Although these vascular beds are functionally and metabolically different organs, at a circulatory level they are remarkably similar. Blood flow in these organs is moderately to strongly influenced by sympathetic vasoconstrictor mechanisms. In this regard, coronary,

A. Lima
Department of Intensive Care Adults, Erasmus MC University Medical Center,
Erasmus University Rotterdam, PO Box 2040, room H602, 3000 CA Rotterdam, the Netherlands

M. E. Van Genderen
Department of Intensive Care Adults, Erasmus MC University Medical Center,
Erasmus University Rotterdam, PO Box 2040, room H602, 3000 CA Rotterdam, the Netherlands

J. Bakker (✉)
Department of Intensive Care Adults, Erasmus MC University Medical Center,
Erasmus University Rotterdam, PO Box 2040, room H602, 3000 CA Rotterdam, the Netherlands
E-mail: jan.bakker@erasmusmc.nl

J.-L. Vincent (Ed.), *Annual Update in Intensive Care and Emergency Medicine 2013*,
DOI 10.1007/978-3-642-35109-9_21,

Table 1 Methods of monitoring the peripheral circulation according to the peripheral vascular bed

Peripheral vascular bed	Method of evaluation	Advantage	Limitations
Skin	Physical examination with capillary refill time on the nail-bed, and visual inspection for mottling (elbow or knee)	Depends only on physical examination; categorical judgment (capillary refill time > 5 s) has substantial overall agreement between trained observers; easily performed at the bedside	Difficult interpretation during central hypothermia
Skin	Body temperature gradient ($dT_{c\text{-}p}$, $dT_{p\text{-}a}$, $T_{skin\text{-}diff}$)	Validated method to estimate dynamic variations in skin blood flow when compared to skin temperature itself	At least two temperature probes required; does not reflect the variations in real time; difficult interpretation during central hypothermia
Skin	PPI	Easily obtained from pulse oximeter; reflects real-time changes in peripheral circulation vasomotor tone	Limited to finger; not accurate during patient motion
Muscle	NIRS	Assessment of oxygenation in all vascular compartments; it can be applied to measuring regional blood flow and oxygen consumption	Requires specific software to display the variables
Gastrointestinal mucosa (sublingual, ileostomy, colostomy)	SDF	Direct visualization of the microcirculation	Observer-related bias; semi-quantitative measure of perfusion; requires specific software to analyze the variables

$dT_{c\text{-}p}$: temperature gradient central-to-peripheral; $dT_{p\text{-}a}$: temperature gradient peripheral-to-ambient; $T_{skin\text{-}diff}$: forearm-to-fingertip skin-temperature gradient; PPI: peripheral perfusion index; NIRS: Near-infrared spectroscopy; SDF: Sidestream darkfield

cerebral, and renal circulations have a high degree of autoregulation with poor sympathetic control. However, skeletal muscle, gastrointestinal, and cutaneous circulations are under predominantly sympathetic control with a poor degree of autoregulation [1]. Observations on the behavior of the peripheral circulation permit the recognition of two broad phases during the development of shock, irrespective of initiating factors. There is an initial period during which compensatory mechanisms predominate. Neurohumoral response-induced vasoconstriction preserves the perfusion to vital organs at the expense of decreased perfusion to the peripheral tissues. Blood flow variations, therefore, follow a similar response pattern in the skin, muscle and gastrointestinal vascular beds, which makes these tissues highly sensitive for detecting occult tissue dysoxia during acute circulatory shock [2–5]. With the progression of circulatory shock and after initiation of appropriate therapy, the active participation of the peripheral circulation in supporting tissue perfusion becomes less striking and ultimately disappears. Some patients enter a phase of stability, and alterations in the peripheral circulation may no longer reflect the acute compensatory mechanisms. Other factors, such as mechanical ventilation, vasopressor, vasodilators, sedatives and opiate use overcome the neurohumoral physiologic response. Nevertheless, this may explain why abnormalities in the peripheral circulation still persist after a patient has reached systemic hemodynamic stability [6, 7]. Although the metabolic functional disturbances that occur in cutaneous, muscle or gastrointestinal tissues following circulatory shock have been studied in detail, most of these studies are limited to comparing one vascular bed to another. To what extent each peripheral vascular bed contributes to tissue hypoperfusion in shock remains to be studied. Multiple clinical studies have shown that circulatory abnormalities in any of these peripheral tissues are independent predictors of tissue hypoperfusion when compared to traditional global variables of resuscitation [8–10]. In light of these observations, interest in monitoring circulation in these peripheral vascular beds as a method of detecting inadequate tissue perfusion has become widespread in the intensive care unit (Table 1). The purpose of this chapter, therefore, is to summarize current knowledge about available techniques to detect abnormalities in peripheral perfusion and oxygenation in critically ill patients. We will focus this review on methods that are readily available for clinical use at the bedside, particularly clinical examination of the peripheral circulation and non-invasive optical monitoring devices.

Clinical Examination of the Peripheral Circulation

Clinical examination of the peripheral circulation allows for rapid and repeated assessment of critically ill patients at the bedside. The peripheral circulation can be easily assessed by performing a careful physical examination that involves touching the skin or measuring capillary refill time. Clinical signs of abnormal skin circulation consist of a cold, pale, clammy, and mottled skin, as well as an increase in capillary refill time. In particular, capillary refill time has been advocated as a measure of abnormal skin perfusion. Pressure is applied to the distal phalanx of the index finger for 15 seconds, which squeezes the blood from the cutaneous tissue. With the patient's hand held above their heart, the health care provider measures the time it takes for blood to return to the tissue after releasing finger pressure (Fig. 1). A delayed return of normal color indicates decreased skin perfusion and is usually related to decreased skin blood flow or derangement of the cutaneous microcirculation. Assessing skin temperature will assist in

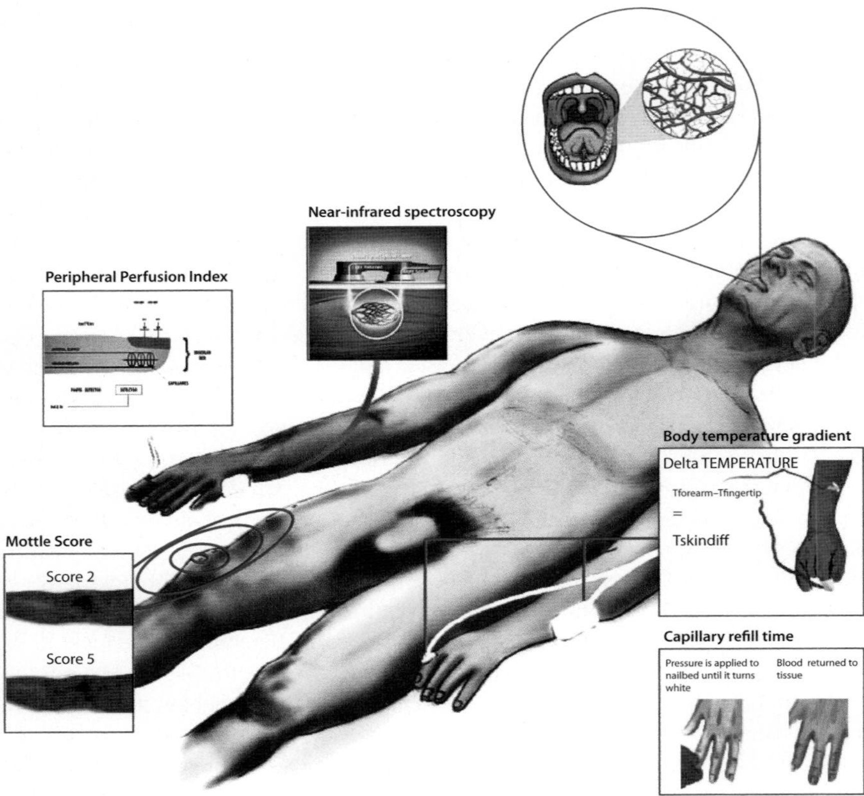

Fig. 1 Monitoring methods of the peripheral circulation for clinical use at the bedside

evaluating the cause of sluggish capillary refill. Assuming normal core temperature, decreased skin blood flow, as a cause of delayed capillary refill time, can be estimated by measuring skin temperature because cold extremities reflect the constriction of cutaneous vessels that ultimately decrease the amount of blood volume within the peripheral vasculature [11]. Warm extremities indicate adequate cutaneous blood flow. A delayed capillary refill time in this condition suggests cutaneous microcirculatory derangement [12]. Over the past 30 years, the definition of a delayed capillary refill time has been debated in the literature. Based on clinical observations, the upper limit of normal for capillary refill time is often considered to be 2 seconds [13]. In pediatric and adult intensive care patients, a capillary refill time <2 seconds was shown to have little predictive value for assessing the adequacy of resuscitation in post-cardiac surgery patients and patients with septic shock [14, 15]. A delayed return of more than 2 seconds seems to be of limited value in critically ill adult patients because the upper limit of normal in a healthy population has been shown to be <4.5 seconds [16]. Applying this upper limit of normality, we have been able to demonstrate that a capillary refill time >5 seconds in patients following initial hemodynamic optimization in the intensive care unit (ICU) was of great value. Using capillary refill time, we were able to discriminate hemodynamically stable patients with more severe organ dysfunction [17]. In addition, patients with a prolonged capillary refill time had significantly higher odds of developing worsening organ failure than patients with a normal capillary refill time. Similar observations have been made during therapeutic hypothermia following cardiac arrest [18]. In this controlled observational study of mild systemic hypothermia, capillary refill time was shorter in survivors at admission and improved even further directly after rewarming, while in non-survivors, a prolonged capillary refill time persisted during the rewarming period. A positive likelihood ratio was calculated after rewarming and indicated that a capillary refill time exceeding 11.5 seconds was obtained at least 1.8–17.0 times more often in non-survivors than survivors. In addition, the authors found that, after rewarming to achieve normal core temperature, the sequential organ failure assessment (SOFA) score was significantly higher in patients with a more prolonged capillary refill time; this was largely attributed to the significantly higher scores for the respiratory, cardiovascular, and renal systems. Importantly, this does not necessarily indicate causality. One concern among physicians about the use of capillary refill time as a clinical assessment tool for evaluating critically ill patients is its suspected lack of reproducibility within and between observers. Despite these current questions that are raised about the reliability of capillary refill time, the subjective assessment of capillary refill time in a heterogeneous population of seriously ill patients has been shown to be reliable among different observers and for repeated measurements. During 1,038 consecutive daily capillary refill time measurements in 173 patients, we observed a substantial overall agreement between trained observers, instructed intensivists, and ICU nurses in determining prolonged capillary refill time (capillary refill time > 5 seconds) with an inter-rater correlation coefficient (ICC) of (0.85 [95% CI 0.82–0.86]) [19]. It can thus be concluded that a capillary refill time with a cut-off of 5 seconds can be of prognostic value in critically ill patients and a clinically better indicator of circulatory shock than the original cut-off of 2 seconds.

Pallor, mottling and cyanosis are key visual indicators of reduced circulation to the skin. Mottling of the skin is easily recognized and is often encountered in critically ill patients. It is defined as a bluish skin discoloration that typically manifests near the elbows or knees and has a distinct patchy pattern. Mottling is the result of heterogeneous small vessel vasoconstriction and is thought to reflect abnormal skin perfusion. To analyze mottling objectively, Ait-Oufella et al. recently developed a clinical scoring system (from 0 to 5) based on the area of mottling from the knees to the periphery [20]. This group reported that a higher mottling score within 6 hours after initial resuscitation, independent of systemic hemodynamics, was a strong predictive factor of 14-day mortality during septic shock. This scoring system is very easy to learn, has good interobserver agreement, and can be used at the bedside.

Although skin temperature has been shown to be an easily accessible parameter for assessing circulatory shock severity, more recent research has demonstrated that body temperature gradients can better reflect changes in cutaneous blood flow for critically ill patients than the absolute skin temperature [21–23]. Body temperature gradients are determined by the temperature difference between two measurement points, such as peripheral-to-ambient, central-to-toe, and forearm-to-fingertip ($T_{skin\text{-}diff}$). Increased vasoconstriction during circulatory shock leads to decreased skin temperature and a diminished ability of the core to regulate its temperature before hypothermia occurs. Consequently, core temperature is maintained at the cost of the periphery to maintain vital organ perfusion, resulting in an increased central-to-peripheral temperature difference when vasoconstriction decreases fingertip blood flow. This concept establishes the central-to-toe temperature difference as an indicator of peripheral perfusion in critically ill patients. A normal temperature gradient of 3 to 7 °C occurs once the patient's hemodynamics have been optimized. Because the effect of the operating room environment on skin and body temperature changes during surgery, especially with the use of cardiopulmonary bypass (CPB), $T_{skin\text{-}diff}$ may be a more reliable measurement because the two skin temperatures are exposed to the same ambient temperature as the fingertip [24, 25]. Experimental studies have suggested $T_{skin\text{-}diff}$ thresholds of 0 °C for initiating vasoconstriction and 4 °C for severe vasoconstriction. In critically ill adult patients, $T_{skin\text{-}diff}$ measurements conducted simultaneously with clinical observation have helped to address the reliability of subjective peripheral perfusion assessment and are able to indicate abnormal peripheral perfusion in the post-resuscitation period [18].

Optical Monitoring

Optical methods directly apply light with different wavelengths to tissue components and use the scattering characteristics of the tissue to assess different tissue-states [26]. At physiologic concentrations, the molecules that absorb most of the light are hemoglobin, myoglobin, cytochrome, melanins, carotenes, and bilirubin. These substances can be quantified and measured in intact tissues using simple optical methods. The assessment of tissue oxygenation is based on the specific absorption spectrum of oxygenated hemoglobin (HbO_2) and deoxygenated hemoglobin (Hb). Commonly used optical methods for peripheral circulation monitoring are pulse oximeter signaling (peripheral perfusion index), near-infrared spectroscopy (NIRS) and sidestream darkfield (SDF) imaging.

Peripheral Perfusion Index

The peripheral perfusion index (PPI) is derived from the photoelectric plethysmographic signal of pulse oximetry and has been used as a non-invasive measure of peripheral circulation in critically ill patients [27–31]. Pulse oximetry is a monitoring technique used in nearly every trauma, critically ill, and surgical patient. The principle of pulse oximetry is based on two light sources with different wavelengths (660 nm and 940 nm) that are emitted through the cutaneous vascular bed of a finger or earlobe. A detector at the far side measures the intensity of the transmitted light at each wavelength, and the oxygen saturation is derived from the ratio between the red light (660 nm) and the infra-red light (940 nm) absorbed. Since other tissues, such as connective tissue, bone, and venous blood, absorb light, pulse oximetry distinguishes the pulsatile component of arterial blood from the non-pulsatile component of other tissues. Thus, the PPI is calculated as the ratio between the pulsatile component (arterial compartment) and the non-pulsatile component (other tissues) of the light reaching the detector of the pulse oximeter and it is calculated independently from the patient's oxygen saturation. Alterations in peripheral perfusion are accompanied by variations in the pulsatile component, and because the non-pulsatile component does not change, the ratio changes. As a result, the value displayed on the monitor reflects changes in peripheral circulation (Fig. 1).

Because the size of the pulsatile portion increases with vasodilation and decreases with vasoconstriction, changes in the PPI reflect changes in peripheral vasomotor tone. This was first demonstrated in a model of axillary plexus-induced vasodilatation; the analgesic effect of this nerve block could be predicted within minutes using the increase in PPI as a measure of concomitant peripheral vasodilatation in patients undergoing hand surgery [27]. Similarly, the PPI was shown to be rapidly reduced following sympathetic response-induced vasoconstriction after the introduction of a nociceptive skin stimulus or an intravenous injection of epinephrine or norepinephrine [30, 31]. Furthermore, in a lower body negative pressure model, the PPI also rapidly decreased following sympathetic activation in healthy volunteers who underwent stepwise decreases in venous return [32]. In a large population of healthy volunteers, the median PPI value was 1.4 % [28]. In critically ill patients, the same value was found to represent a very sensitive cut-off point for determining abnormal peripheral perfusion, as defined by a prolonged capillary refill time and an increased skin temperature difference [28]. The inclusion of PPI into the pulse oximeter signal is a recent advance in the clinical monitoring of the peripheral circulation in critically ill patients. Furthermore, PPI is easily obtained and non-invasive.

Near-Infrared Spectroscopy

NIRS offers a technique for continuous, non-invasive, bedside monitoring of tissue oxygenation. Like pulse oximetry, NIRS uses the principles of light transmission and absorption to non-invasively measure the concentrations of hemoglobin and oxygen saturation (StO_2) in tissues. NIRS has greater tissue penetration than pulse oximetry and provides a global assessment of oxygenation in all vascular compartments (arterial, venous, and capillary). The tissue penetration is directly related to the spacing between illumination and detection fibers. With 25 mm spacing, approximately 95 % of the detected optical signal is from a depth of zero to 23 mm. The variables that are analyzed using NIRS can either be directly calculated or derived from physiological interventions, such as an arterial and venous vascular occlusion test (VOT). Using the VOT, NIRS can be applied to measure regional blood flow and oxygen consumption by following the rate of HbO_2 and Hb changes [33]. In the venous occlusion method, a pneumatic cuff is inflated to a pressure of approximately 50 mm Hg. Such pressure blocks venous occlusion, but does not impede arterial inflow. As a result, venous blood volume and pressure increase. NIRS can reflect this change by an increase in HbO_2, Hb and total hemoglobin (tHb). In an arterial occlusion method, the pneumatic cuff is inflated to a pressure of approximately 30 mm Hg greater than the systolic pressure. This pressure blocks both venous outflow and arterial inflow. Depletion of locally available O_2 is monitored by NIRS as a decrease in HbO_2 and a simultaneous increase in Hb, whereas tHb remains constant. After releasing the occluding cuff, a hyperemic response is observed. Blood volume increases rapidly, which results in an increase in HbO_2 and a quick washout of Hb (Fig. 2).

Nevertheless, the utility of NIRS for managing critically ill patients remains a matter of debate. Publications using NIRS have described profound alterations in microvascular function in patients suffering from different pathophysiological conditions, such as sepsis and traumatic shock [34–38]. In a study by Shapiro et al. [38], the dynamic NIRS variables collected during a VOT were strongly associated with the severity of organ dysfunction and mortality in patients with septic shock. In this study, the StO_2 recovery slope was most sensitive for predicting mortality. This finding is of special interest because there is a lack of agreement on how to standardize a method for performing a VOT [39, 40]. When

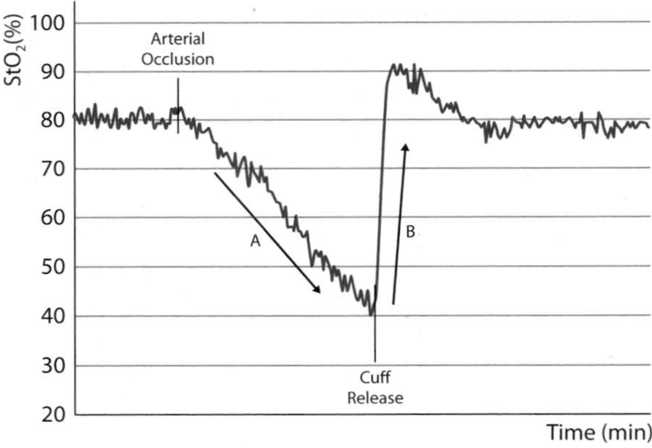

Fig. 2 Tissue muscle oxygen saturation (StO_2) during 3 minutes of arterial occlusion. (*A*) Rate of StO_2 deoxygenation: The velocity at which StO_2 decreases during arterial occlusion, expressed as %/min. Rapid deoxygenation rate corresponds to higher oxygen extraction rates. (*B*) Rate of StO_2 reoxygenation: The velocity at which StO_2 increases from cuff release to the maximal reoxygenation during reactive hyperemia, which reflects mainly microcirculatory vascular reactivity

measured on the thenar eminence, NIRS-derived measurements are influenced by the condition of the peripheral circulation [12]. Nevertheless, when used in conjunction with other peripheral perfusion methods, repeated StO_2 monitoring has the potential to assess the effect of therapeutic interventions on the peripheral microvascular circulation in various shock states. Similarly, Colin et al. [41] investigated StO_2 measurements in three different sites (masseter, deltoid, and thenar) during the first 6 hours of severe sepsis resuscitation and compared these measurements to the central venous oxygen saturation ($ScvO_2$). These authors found that StO_2 values measured on the masseter muscle could better predict $ScvO_2 > 70\%$ than thenar tissue oxygen saturation (area under the curve, 0.80 vs. 0.67; $p = 0.02$). In addition, they showed that StO_2 measured on either the masseter or deltoid muscle was a better predictor of 28-day mortality than StO_2 measured on the thenar eminence. This observation indicates that StO_2 on the masseter muscle may be a more powerful indicator of resuscitation than measurements taken on the thenar eminence.

Although NIRS can potentially be very useful for assessing tissue oxygenation and perfusion, additional studies are still being conducted to clarify its role in the clinical management of ICU patients. The relatively poor precision and the lack of standardization among the different instruments suggest that further technological advances are required before NIRS can be adopted more widely in the clinical setting.

Sidestream Dark Field

SDF imaging techniques have recently been introduced and allow for the direct visualization of the microcirculation. This technology has been incorporated into a small handheld video microscope that can be directly applied to superficial mucosa. One of the most easily accessible sites in humans for peripheral circulation monitoring is the sublingual mucosa, but ileostomies, colostomies, and rectal mucosa can also be investigated. Studies applying orthogonal polarization spectral (OPS) imaging (earlier predecessor of SDF) and SDF have focused on the microcirculation in disease states, as well as during therapy in surgery, emergency medicine, and intensive care medicine [42–44]. OPS imaging and SDF imaging have had an important clinical impact by observing the sublingual microcirculation during sepsis, shock, and resuscitation [42–46] (Fig. 1).

The results from clinical observational studies have shown that sublingual microcirculatory alterations before resuscitation and their lack of improvement after resuscitation have been associated with an increased risk of morbidity and mortality. Trzeciak et al. [44] studied the effects of early goal-directed therapy on indices of sublingual microcirculatory perfusion in early sepsis. These authors demonstrated that early increases in sublingual microcirculatory perfusion were associated with a reduced severity of organ dysfunction. In addition, the investigators found a correlation between sublingual microcirculatory and macrocirculatory parameters during early treatment. This correlation was lost in the latter phases of sepsis, which emphasizes the importance of time in improving peripheral circulation during sepsis therapy. Sublingual microcirculatory alterations have also been reported during the early phase of non-septic shock, such as in severe heart failure and out-of-hospital cardiac arrest patients [18, 45]. Therefore, microcirculatory dysfunction has been associated with morbidity and mortality in a wide array of clinical scenarios. Nevertheless, the overall prevalence of sublingual microcirculatory dysfunction in critically ill patients is still unknown. To address this issue, a large international, multicenter, observational study has been conducted to investigate the prevalence of sublingual microcirculatory alterations in critically ill patients, irrespective of their underlying disease [10]. With more than 500 patients included, this study aims to assess the sublingual microcirculation in critically ill patients located in 40 participating ICUs. The results of this study will provide important insight for future interventional studies.

Clinical Applications in Patient Management

From the above, we can conclude that clinical and hemodynamic parameters must be combined with measures of the peripheral circulation to continuously monitor the critically ill patient and maintain adequate tissue perfusion. Although the mechanisms involved in shock resuscitation are not yet fully understood, it is clear that the persistence of an abnormal peripheral circulation measured in skin, muscle, sublingual or intestinal mucosa is associated with worse patient outcomes. It is likely that interventions specifically aimed at the peripheral vascular bed would have a greater effect on regional perfusion. This concept originated in the 1990s with clinical trials of different types of vasodilators (prostacyclin, N-acetylcysteine) targeting splanchnic perfusion as assessed by gastric tonometry [47]. These studies demonstrated an improvement in gastric perfusion with drug administration, which suggests that successful microcirculatory recruitment had occurred. More recently, some studies have evaluated short-term infusions of nitroglycerine in septic or non-septic shock and demonstrated significant improvements in capillary perfusion [46, 48]. One of these studies was a randomized controlled trial in 70 patients with septic shock and failed to show significant differences in the evolution of the sublingual microcirculation between the control and nitroglycerine-treated groups [46]. Although this study precluded the effectiveness of nitroglycerine on sublingual microvascular flow, the cutaneous circulation, as measured by central-to-toe temperature, significantly improved in the nitroglycerine-treated group compared to the control group. This finding highlights the need to identify the best peripheral vascular bed to target during and after resuscitation therapy for shock. Other less-specific therapeutic approaches have been shown to have positive effects on the peripheral circulation. For instance, Futier et al. [49] recently showed that the administration of a fluid challenge improved peripheral tissue oxygenation in patients undergoing major abdominal surgery. Whether these interventions are capable of resuscitating different peripheral vascular beds remains to be determined. Current studies are underway to determine the effects of these interventions on the peripheral circulation of critically ill patients.

Conclusion

Resuscitation of circulatory shock is aimed at re-establishing adequate tissue perfusion through optimization of traditional end-points, such as mean arterial pressure, cardiac output and its determinants. Therefore, monitoring critically ill patients in the early hours of shock is essential to recognize alterations in these pre-defined end-points and assess whether a patient needs active intervention. Although the initial objective of hemodynamic monitoring is the restoration of these global macrocirculatory variables, abnormalities in the peripheral circulation may still persist and are related to the development of organ failure. When these conditions remain unrecognized, abnormalities in the peripheral circulation may worsen the prognosis for critically ill patients. This scenario has led to a growing interest in non-invasive methods designed to evaluate regional perfusion in peripheral tissues. These methods may be a valuable adjunct to standard global parameters when predicting or diagnosing ongoing tissue hypoperfusion. We propose that global parameters of oxygen transport be complemented by monitoring parameters of the peripheral circulation. This is not a novel idea, as evidenced by the many studies performed on the use of the microcirculation as a marker of the severity of shock. Real-time assessment of the peripheral circulation at the bedside is easily obtained using non-invasive monitoring techniques. Moreover, it is a simple approach that can be rapidly applied throughout the hospital, including the emergency department, operating room, wards and ICU.

References

1. Guyton AC (2000) Local control of blood flow by the tissues, and humoral regulation. In: Guyton AC, Hall JE (eds) Textbook of Medical Physiology. W.B. Saunders Company, Philadelphia, pp 175–182
2. Guzman JA, Dikin MS, Kruse JA (2005) Lingual, splanchnic, and systemic hemodynamic and carbon dioxide tension changes during endotoxic shock and resuscitation. J Appl Physiol 98:108–113
3. Guzman JA, Lacoma FJ, Kruse JA (1998) Relationship between systemic oxygen supply dependency and gastric intramucosal PCO2 during progressive hemorrhage. J Trauma 44:696–700
4. Shepherd AP, Kiel JW (1992) A model of countercurrent shunting of oxygen in the intestinal villus. Am J Physiol 262:H1136–H1142
5. Schlichtig R, Kramer DJ, Pinsky MR (1991) Flow redistribution during progressive hemorrhage is a determinant of critical O2 delivery. J Appl Physiol 70:169–178

6. Chien LC, Lu KJ, Wo CC, Shoemaker WC (2007) Hemodynamic patterns preceding circulatory deterioration and death after trauma. J Trauma 62:928–932
7. Poeze M, Solberg BC, Greve JW, Ramsay G (2005) Monitoring global volume-related hemodynamic or regional variables after initial resuscitation: What is a better predictor of outcome in critically ill septic patients? Crit Care Med 33:2494–2500
8. Lima A, Jansen TC, van Bommel J, Ince C, Bakker J (2009) The prognostic value of the subjective assessment of peripheral perfusion in critically ill patients. Crit Care Med 37:934–938
9. van Genderen ME, van Bommel J, Lima A (2012) Monitoring peripheral perfusion in critically ill patients at the bedside. Curr Opin Crit Care 18:273–279
10. Vellinga NA, Boerma EC, Koopmans M et al (2012) Study design of the microcirculatory shock occurrence in acutely ill patients (microSOAP): an international multicenter observational study of sublingual microcirculatory alterations in intensive care patients. Crit Care Res Pract 2012:121752
11. Lima A, van Genderen ME, Klijn E, Bakker J, van Bommel J (2012) Peripheral vasoconstriction influences thenar oxygen saturation as measured by near-infrared spectroscopy. Intensive Care Med 38:606–611
12. Lima A, van Bommel J, Sikorska K et al (2011) The relation of near-infrared spectroscopy with changes in peripheral circulation in critically ill patients. Crit Care Med 39:1649–1654
13. Champion HR, Sacco WJ, Copes WS et al (1989) A revision of the Trauma Score. J Trauma 29:623–629
14. Bailey JM, Levy JH, Kopel MA, Tobia V, Grabenkort WR (1990) Relationship between clinical evaluation of peripheral perfusion and global hemodynamics in adults after cardiac surgery. Crit Care Med 18:1353–1356
15. Tibby SM, Hatherill M, Murdoch IA (1999) Capillary refill and core-peripheral temperature gap as indicators of haemodynamic status in paediatric intensive care patients. Arch Dis Child 80:163–166
16. Schriger DL, Baraff L (1988) Defining normal capillary refill: variation with age, sex, and temperature. Ann Emerg Med 17:932–935
17. Lima A, Jansen TC, van Bommel J, Ince C, Bakker J (2009) The prognostic value of the subjective assessment of peripheral perfusion in critically ill patients. Crit Care Med 37:934–938
18. van Genderen ME, Lima A, Akkerhuis M, Bakker J, van Bommel J (2012) Persistent peripheral and microcirculatory perfusion alterations after out-of-hospital cardiac arrest are associated with poor survival. Crit Care Med 40:2287–2294
19. Lima A, van Genderen M, Boerstrea T, Bakker J, van Bommel J (2011) Is bedside clinical examination of capillary refill time reproducible in critically ill patients between different observers? A inter-rater variability study. Intensive Care Med 37:S215 (abst)
20. Ait-Oufella H, Lemoinne S, Boelle PY et al (2011) Mottling score predicts survival in septic shock. Intensive Care Med 37:801–807
21. Curley FJ, Smyrnios NA (2003) Routine monitoring of critically ill patients. In: Irwin RS, Cerra FB, Rippe JM (eds) Intensive Care Medicine. Lippincott Williams & Wilkins, Philadelphia, pp 250–270
22. Rubinstein EH, Sessler DI (1990) Skin-surface temperature gradients correlate with fingertip blood flow in humans. Anesthesiology 73:541–545
23. Akata T, Kanna T, Yoshino J et al (2004) Reliability of fingertip skin-surface temperature and its related thermal measures as indices of peripheral perfusion in the clinical setting of the operating theatre. Anaesth Intensive Care 32:519–529
24. House JR, Tipton MJ (2002) Using skin temperature gradients or skin heat flux measurements to determine thresholds of vasoconstriction and vasodilatation. Eur J Appl Physiol 88:141–145
25. Sessler DI (2003) Skin-temperature gradients are a validated measure of fingertip perfusion. Eur J Appl Physiol 89:401–402

26. Flewelling R (2000) Noninvasive optical monitoring. In: Bronzino JD (ed) The Biomedical Engineering Handbook. Springer, Berlin, pp 1–10
27. Galvin EM, Niehof S, Verbrugge SJ et al (2006) Peripheral flow index is a reliable and early indicator of regional block success. Anesth Analg 103:239–243
28. Lima AP, Beelen P, Bakker J (2002) Use of a peripheral perfusion index derived from the pulse oximetry signal as a noninvasive indicator of perfusion. Crit Care Med 30:1210–1213
29. Takeyama M, Matsunaga A, Kakihana Y et al (2011) Impact of skin incision on the pleth variability index. J Clin Monit Comput 25:215–221
30. Mowafi HA, Ismail SA, Shafi MA, Al Ghamdi AA (2009) The efficacy of perfusion index as an indicator for intravascular injection of epinephrine-containing epidural test dose in propofol-anesthetized adults. Anesth Analg 108:549–553
31. Biais M, Cottenceau V, Petit L et al (2011) Impact of norepinephrine on the relationship between pleth variability index and pulse pressure variations in ICU adult patients. Crit Care 15:R168
32. Lima A, van Genderen M, Klijn E et al (2011) P69 Perfusion index as a predictor for central hypovolemia in humans. Crit Care 15(Suppl 1):24 (abst)
33. Lima A, Bakker J (2005) Noninvasive monitoring of peripheral perfusion. Intensive Care Med 31:1316–1326
34. De Blasi RA, Palmisani S, Alampi D et al (2005) Microvascular dysfunction and skeletal muscle oxygenation assessed by phase-modulation near-infrared spectroscopy in patients with septic shock. Intensive Care Med 31:1661–1668
35. Doerschug KC, Delsing AS, Schmidt GA, Haynes WG (2007) Impairments in microvascular reactivity are related to organ failure in human sepsis. Am J Physiol Heart Circ Physiol 293:H1065–H1071
36. Gomez H, Torres A, Polanco P et al (2008) Use of non-invasive NIRS during a vascular occlusion test to assess dynamic tissue O(2) saturation response. Intensive Care Med 34:1600–1607
37. Skarda DE, Mulier KE, Myers DE, Taylor JH, Beilman GJ (2007) Dynamic near-infrared spectroscopy measurements in patients with severe sepsis. Shock 27:348–353
38. Shapiro NI, Arnold R, Sherwin R et al (2011) The association of near-infrared spectroscopy-derived tissue oxygenation measurements with sepsis syndromes, organ dysfunction and mortality in emergency department patients with sepsis. Crit Care 15:R223
39. Mayeur C, Campard S, Richard C, Teboul JL (2011) Comparison of four different vascular occlusion tests for assessing reactive hyperemia using near-infrared spectroscopy. Crit Care Med 39:695–701
40. Damoisel C, Payen D (2011) Vascular occlusion tests: do we need another definition? Crit Care Med 39:2587–2588
41. Colin G, Nardi O, Polito A et al (2012) Masseter tissue oxygen saturation predicts normal central venous oxygen saturation during early goal-directed therapy and predicts mortality in patients with severe sepsis. Crit Care Med 40:435–440
42. Sakr Y, Dubois MJ, De Backer D, Creteur J, Vincent JL (2004) Persistent microcirculatory alterations are associated with organ failure and death in patients with septic shock. Crit Care Med 32:1825–1831
43. Spronk PE, Ince C, Gardien MJ et al (2002) Nitroglycerin in septic shock after intravascular volume resuscitation. Lancet 360:1395–1396
44. Trzeciak S, McCoy JV, Phillip DR et al (2008) Early increases in microcirculatory perfusion during protocol-directed resuscitation are associated with reduced multi-organ failure at 24 h in patients with sepsis. Intensive Care Med 34:2210–2217
45. De Backer D, Creteur J, Dubois MJ, Sakr Y, Vincent JL (2004) Microvascular alterations in patients with acute severe heart failure and cardiogenic shock. Am Heart J 147:91–99
46. Boerma EC, Koopmans M, Konijn A et al (2010) Effects of nitroglycerin on sublingual microcirculatory blood flow in patients with severe sepsis/septic shock after a strict resus-

citation protocol: a double-blind randomized placebo controlled trial. Crit Care Med 38:93–100

47. Buwalda M, Ince C (2002) Opening the microcirculation: can vasodilators be useful in sepsis? Intensive Care Med 28:1208–1217
48. den Uil CA, Caliskan K, Lagrand WK et al (2009) Dose-dependent benefit of nitroglycerin on microcirculation of patients with severe heart failure. Intensive Care Med 35:1893–1899
49. Futier E, Christophe S, Robin E et al (2011) Use of near-infrared spectroscopy during a vascular occlusion test to assess the microcirculatory response during fluid challenge. Crit Care 15:R214

The Microcirculation in Hemorrhagic Shock

A. Harrois, S. Tanaka, and J. Duranteau

Introduction

Hemorrhagic shock is characterized by both macrovascular hemodynamic abnormalities (decreased venous return, decreased cardiac output and systemic hypotension) and alterations of the microcirculation. The microcirculation is a critical component of the cardiovascular system, which regulates flow to the tissues. Several studies have shown a significant decrease in microvascular blood flow in various organs during the acute phase of hemorrhagic shock and resuscitation [1–4]. Persistence of these microvascular alterations is believed to be a contributing factor to the development of organ dysfunction. The pathogenesis of the microvascular alterations involves both vascular and cellular components. In current clinical practice, guidelines for resuscitation are provided by monitoring macrocirculatory variables, such as arterial blood pressure, heart rate, and cardiac output. However, whether these resuscitation procedures are effective in restoring organ microcirculation remains to be elucidated. The purpose of this review is to focus on the mechanisms involved in the development of microvascular alterations in

A. Harrois
Département d'Anesthésie et de Réanimation Chirurgicale, Université Paris-Sud,
Hôpitaux universitaires Paris-Sud, Assistance Publique Hôpitaux de Paris, Hôpital de Bicêtre,
78, rue du Général Leclerc, 94275 Le-Kremlin-Bicêtre Cedex, France

S. Tanaka
Département d'Anesthésie et de Réanimation Chirurgicale, Université Paris-Sud,
Hôpitaux universitaires Paris-Sud, Assistance Publique Hôpitaux de Paris, Hôpital de Bicêtre,
78, rue du Général Leclerc, 94275 Le-Kremlin-Bicêtre Cedex, France

J. Duranteau (✉)
Département d'Anesthésie et de Réanimation Chirurgicale, Université Paris-Sud,
Hôpitaux universitaires Paris-Sud, Assistance Publique Hôpitaux de Paris, Hôpital de Bicêtre,
78, rue du Général Leclerc, 94275 Le-Kremlin-Bicêtre Cedex, France
E-mail: jacques.duranteau@bct.aphp.fr

J.-L. Vincent (Ed.), *Annual Update in Intensive Care and Emergency Medicine 2013*,
DOI 10.1007/978-3-642-35109-9_22,

hemorrhagic shock and to discuss the potential therapeutic implications for resuscitation in hemorrhagic shock.

Cardiovascular Response in Hemorrhagic Shock

In the acute phase of hemorrhage, macrovascular and microvascular responses rapidly act to compensate for the loss of blood volume and to limit tissue hypoxia.

Macrovascular Response

The macrovascular compensatory mechanism involves the autonomic nervous system. Decreases in venous return and arterial pressure lead to unloading of cardiopulmonary and arterial baroreceptors inducing a decrease in the activation of the vasomotor inhibitory center in the brainstem, which leads to activation of the sympathetic center and inhibition of vagal activity (sinoatrial node). The increased activity of the sympathetic nerves produces an increase in heart rate, cardiac contractility and arterial and venous tone with an activation of the renin-angiotensin-aldosterone system. The magnitude of the compensatory vasoconstriction that follows is the net result of the interaction of the effects of norepinephrine (from the peripheral nerves) and epinephrine (from the adrenal medulla) on the peripheral vascular adrenoreceptors, and nonadrenergic mechanisms (i. e., angiotensin and vasopressin). Arterial vasoconstriction rapidly decreases non-vital organ blood flow (musculocutaneous, splanchnic and renal blood flow) to maintain perfusion pressure and blood flow to vital organs (the heart and the brain). It is important to keep in mind that the sympathetic stimulation exerts both arterial and venous α-adrenergic stimulation [5]. Indeed, in addition to its arterial vasoconstricting action, the sympathetic stimulation induces venoconstriction (specially in splanchnic circulation) enhancing a shift of splanchnic blood volume to the systemic circulation [6]. This venous adrenergic stimulation may recruit blood from the venous unstressed volume helping to maintain venous return and cardiac output [6].

Microvascular Response

The microcirculation regulates the distribution of blood flow throughout individual organs to provide adequate oxygen delivery (DO_2) for the oxygen demands of every cell within an organ. In order to achieve this, the microcirculation responds to changes in metabolic demand by limiting blood flow in microvascular units with low oxygen demand and increasing blood flow in microvascular units with high oxygen demand. This microvascular heterogeneity of blood flow is an essential property of normal microcirculatory perfusion to provide adequate DO_2 for the tissue. During hemorrhagic shock, in addition to the macrovascular distribution of arterial blood flow at the expense of non-vital organs, blood flow is redistributed within the capillary networks of each organ according to arteriolar and capillary resistances, rheologic factors and oxygen demand. Increase in arteriolar and capillary resistances associated with unfavorable rheologic factors takes blood flow away from microvascular units with low oxygen demands and non-essential cell functions. The microvascular units where the blood flow is reduced most severely might adjust their function and their energy utilization to prevent hypoxia. This down-regulation of cellular metabolism is called conformance or hibernation [7]. The possible involvement of such a mechanism may limit tissue hypoxia. However, the observed increase in lactate level during the acute phase of hemorrhagic shock indicates the limits of this adaptative metabolic down-regulation.

The microvascular response to the decrease in DO_2 in microvascular units with high oxygen demand involves several compensatory mechanisms to increase oxygen extraction and maintain tissue oxygenation. Two major mechanisms have been proposed to account for the local oxygen delivery regulation: Regulation of arteriolar tone and control of the functional surface area for oxygen exchange.

Regulation of the Arteriolar Tone

Arterioles dilate in response to decreased tissue PO_2 to increase perfusion and DO_2. The arteriolar tone is the net result of the interaction of the autonomic nervous system, vasoactive substances in the blood (catecholamines, angiotensin and vasopressin) and local regulation of arteriolar tone. Local regulation of arteriolar tone is a crucial factor in microvascular regulation to match oxygen supply to oxygen demand. Several mechanisms contribute to the local regulation of arteriolar tone, including response to intraluminal pressure (myogenic response), shear stress on the endothelial cells (shear-dependent response), and tissue metabolite concentrations (metabolic response).

The vascular myogenic response refers to the intrinsic ability of a blood vessel to constrict to an increase in intraluminal pressure or dilate to a decrease in intraluminal pressure. The vasodilation induced by shear stress (nitric oxide [NO]-dependent mechanism) is dependent on endothelial sensing/transduction of the shear induced by blood flow. The proposed mechanosensors on the luminal surface of the endothelium include components of the glycocalyx (glycoproteins and proteoglycans), stretch-activated ion channels, cytoskeletal rearrangements and cell-cell and cell-extracellular matrix connections [8].

The metabolic response allows the vascular tone to adapt to cellular oxygen demand. During hemorrhagic shock, the decrease in DO_2 limits the production of adenosine 5′ triphosphate (ATP) and adenosine 5′ diphosphate (ADP) accumulates because its stock is not completely rephosphorylated with a resulting accumulation of ADP and its degradation products (adenosine 5′ monophosphate [AMP], adenosine). Furthermore, glycolysis is activated with a production of lactate and hydrogen ion. Adenosine, lactate and hydrogen ions are arteriolar vasodilators and contribute to the close link between metabolite production and tissue oxygenation. CO_2 is also a powerful vasodilator, which accumulates when there is an increase in cellular metabolism or reduced clearance of CO_2 during tissue hypoperfusion.

Finally, an increasingly important role in the regulation of the microvascular tone and in the matching of oxygen supply to oxygen demand is being attributed to the red blood cell (RBC) and the hemoglobin molecule. Ellsworth et al. [9, 10] suggest that the RBC behaves as a mobile oxygen-sensor and controls vascular tone by means of release of ATP. ATP is released from erythrocytes in response to mechanical deformation of the membrane, to exposure to low PO_2 associated with a decrease in the hemoglobin oxygen saturation within erythrocytes, and to receptor-mediated activation of erythrocyte membrane-bound ß-adrenergic receptors or prostacyclin receptors. The erythrocyte-derived ATP can then interact with endothelial purinergic receptors, inducing release of vasodilator mediators. This vasodilation is conducted in a retrograde fashion, resulting in increased blood flow (oxygen supply) to areas of increased oxygen demand. Certainly this concept still needs to be confirmed, but it is an attractive track to explain the microvascular response to oxygen demand. Other mechanisms involving the erythrocyte in the regulation of the vascular tone have been proposed. Stamler et al. proposed that the erythrocyte could regulate DO_2 through the transport of NO in a protected form as S-nitrosothiol (SNO) [11, 12]. This vasorelaxant moiety is released by hemoglobin when the hemoglobin oxygen saturation falls in response to an increase in local oxygen demand. Finally, another hypothesis has been proposed in which deoxyhemoglobin would function as a nitrite reductase to transform nitrite (NO_2^-) into NO with resulting vasodilatory action [13, 14]. The possible involvement of other oxygen sensors, such as cytochrome oxidase or NADPH oxidase, is interesting, but requires further work to establish their respective contribution.

Control of Functional Surface Area for Oxygen Exchange

To maintain tissue oxygenation despite the decrease in DO_2, there is an immediate need to extract more oxygen from the incoming blood. Oxygen extraction depends on the incoming blood flow (convective oxygen transport determined mainly by arteriolar tone) and on the functional surface area for oxygen exchange (diffusive oxygen transport) related to the number of RBCs and the number of perfused capillaries. Thus, oxygen extraction is facilitated by a high capillary density which increases the surface area for oxygen exchange and reduces capillary-to-mitochondrial diffusion distances (Fig. 1).

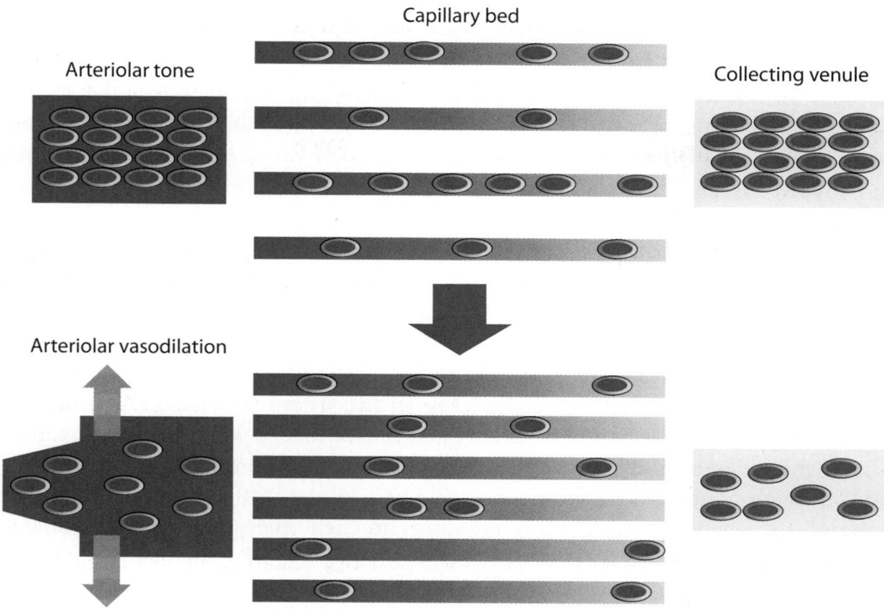

Fig. 1 Schematic representation of the microvascular response to a decrease in oxygen delivery in microvascular units with high oxygen demands

This high capillary density can be achieved by recruiting capillaries (i. e., initiation of RBC flux in previously non-flowing capillaries). However, in some microvascular beds, such as skeletal muscle or myocardium microcirculation, it has been reported that most capillaries may sustain RBC flux at rest and capillary recruitment does not appear to be requisite for the increase in oxygen extraction [15, 16]. So, in these microcirculations, the oxygen extraction is mainly dependent on the distribution of RBC within the previously flowing capillaries. Recruitment is then more a longitudinal recruitment (along the vessel) than a recruitment of new capillaries [16]. Capillary resistance and rheologic factors (blood viscosity and RBC deformability) determine the RBC distribution within the capillary bed [17, 18]. These factors play a crucial role in determining capillary homogeneity and functional capillary density, especially at low flow states [19]. During the acute phase of hemorrhagic shock, the decrease in capillary pressure will cause increased net fluid absorption with fluid shift from the interstitium to the vascular compartment helping to restore blood volume. This effect associated with hemodilution during the resuscitation phase could theoretically decrease blood viscosity and contribute to decrease the heterogeneity of RBC distribution. However, during the late phase of hemorrhagic shock, the inflammatory process can induce fluid leakage with fluid shift to the interstitial compartment resulting in an increase in viscosity and heterogeneity of RBC distribution [20, 21].

Alterations of the Microcirculation in Hemorrhagic Shock

Despite efficient microvascular adaptative mechanisms, when the blood loss is severe enough, alterations of microcirculatory blood flow and tissue oxygenation have been described in various experimental models of hemorrhagic shock. Progressive decrease in cardiac output and oxygen delivery induces a progressive decrease in capillary blood flow, RBC velocities and functional capillary density with an increase in flow heterogeneity [4, 22]. These microvascular alterations are more pronounced in non-vital organ microcirculations (splanchnic, renal and musculocutaneous microcirculations) and in microvascular units with low oxygen demand and non-essential cell functions. Increase in RBC aggregation causing blood flow slowing with intermittent/no flow capillaries and 'plasmatic' capillaries contribute to the increased heterogeneity (Fig. 2) [2]. There is evidence that hemorrhagic shock impairs RBC deformability and causes RBC cellular damage [23, 24]. These microvascular alterations are associated with a decrease in microvascular PO_2 through convective arteriovenous shunting, direct diffusion of oxygen from arterioles to venules lying in close proximity to each other, and functional shunting of disadvantaged microcirculatory units [25, 26].

In septic shock, alteration of microcirculatory blood flow is a major pathophysiological feature. Microvascular density and microvascular blood flow are both reduced in association with an increased heterogeneous perfusion in septic patients [27, 28]. Moreover, the degree of microvascular impairment has a prognostic value since it worsens in non-surviving septic patients compared to those who ultimately overcome their septic episode [29]. Early systemic hemodynamic

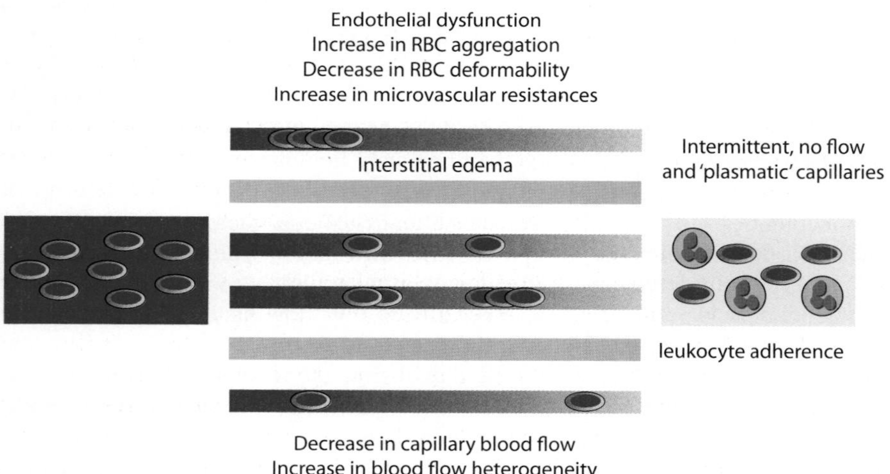

Fig. 2 Illustration of potential mechanisms involved in the development of microvascular alterations in hemorrhagic shock

resuscitation of septic patients may improve the time-course of microcirculatory dysfunction and eventually patient outcome. However, even when systemic hemodynamic alterations seem to be reversed with fluid resuscitation and vasoactive agents, significant alterations in the microcirculation may persist and participate in the development of multiple organ failure. Therefore in septic shock, relationships between macrovascular hemodynamic and microcirculatory changes during resuscitation are complex (global hemodynamics do not necessarily reflect regional microcirculation) with a critical disorder of the microcirculation. Nakajima et al. [30] compared microvascular perfusion in intestinal villi in mouse models of septic shock and hemorrhagic shock. These authors demonstrated that, after one hour at the same level of hypotension (mean arterial pressure [MAP] $\approx$ 40 mm Hg), mucosal perfusion disorders were considerably more pronounced in endotoxin-induced hypotension than in hemorrhagic hypotension. RBC velocity was maintained in hemorrhagic shock but not during endotoxic shock. During the initial phase of hemorrhagic shock, the microvasculature was still able to regulate microvascular perfusion, but during sepsis the regulatory response was impaired. Similar results were achieved by Fang et al. [3], who found that impaired buccal capillary blood flow in septic animals (cecal ligation and perforation) was more severe than that in hemorrhagic animals with the same level of hypotension. In addition, major findings reported by these authors were that the impaired buccal capillary blood flow was similar in both types of shock for the same reduction in cardiac index and that significantly improved global hemodynamics after fluid resuscitation did not effectively improve the buccal capillary blood flow in septic shock, in contrast to the hemorrhagic shock condition during which buccal capillary blood flow was significantly improved. Therefore, microvascular alterations are closely related to macrocirculatory variables (especially cardiac index and DO_2) during hemorrhage and resuscitation [3, 31]. Hence, fluid resuscitation, associated with blood transfusion, is the major therapy to improve the microcirculation in hemorrhagic shock. In this respect, Legrand et al. [26] reported that correcting arterial blood pressure and cardiac index with only fluid resuscitation was not a guarantee for providing sufficient oxygen and correct shock-induced microcirculatory hypoxia. Only transfusion of blood associated with fluid resuscitation was able to improve tissue oxygenation [26]. Blood transfusion has to be considered early during the management of hemorrhagic shock to improve microvascular DO_2 and match oxygen supply to oxygen demand.

Even if a considerable part of the microvascular alterations during hemorrhagic shock are closely related to a decrease in DO_2, other factors could be involved in addition to hemodynamic factors; these include changes in the microvascular endothelium, leukocyte adherence to venules, interstitial and endothelial edema, RBC alterations, and coagulation activation (Fig. 2). During the resuscitation phase of hemorrhagic shock, neutrophil rolling and adherence to postcapillary venules is enhanced with leukocyte plugging and resulting increase in vascular resistances [1]. In addition, generation of reactive oxygen species (ROS) precedes leukocyte adherence following hemorrhagic shock and promotes endothelial dysfunction with an increase in microvascular permeability and tissue edema, which may lead to alterations in oxygen diffusion [32]. Machiedo et al. [24] reported that transfusion of RBCs from trauma/hemorrhagic shock rats into naïve rats led to impaired microcirculatory flow to several important organs, including the lungs, spleen, ileum, and cecum, as well as deleterious systemic hemodynamic effects with reduced cardiac output. The role of these factors tends to increase with the degree of inflammation. Presumably, when the inflammatory response is marked (e. g., severe or sustained hemorrhagic shock, traumatic hemorrhagic shock or associated hypoxemia), sepsis-like microvascular alterations with persistent alterations may be observed despite adequate macrovascular resuscitation and associated with organ dysfunction. This possibility is supported by studies documenting that microcirculatory alterations partly persist after resuscitation despite correction of macrovascular parameters. For example, persistent decreased microcirculatory PO_2 values have been reported despite an adequate macrovascular resuscitation [25, 26].

It should be stressed that observations about alterations of the microcirculation in hemorrhagic shock are mainly derived from experimental models during the acute phase of resuscitation. Thus, assessing microvascular alterations in hemorrhagic shock patients seems urgent.

Implications for Resuscitation of Patients with Hemorrhagic Shock

Objectives of Fluid Resuscitation

In hemorrhagic shock, the therapeutic priority is to stop the bleeding as quickly as possible. A critical element in the resuscitation of patients with hemorrhagic shock is to prevent a potential increase of bleeding by being too aggressive. Indeed, fluid resuscitation may promote coagulopathy by diluting coagulation factors and favoring hypothermia. Moreover, an excessive arterial pressure can favor bleeding by preventing clot formation. Two concepts have emerged in recent years: The concept of 'low volume resuscitation' and that of 'hypotensive resuscitation'. Often these two concepts are merged. Indeed, the fluid resuscitation strategy and the blood pressure target are two associated elements during hemorrhagic shock resuscitation. Several experimental studies have suggested that limited administration of fluids with a low blood-pressure level as an endpoint may decrease bleeding without the associated increased risk of death, if lasting for a short period of time [33, 34]. Recently, Li et al. reported that a target resuscitation pressure of 50–60 mm Hg was the ideal blood pressure for uncontrolled hemorrhagic shock in rats [35]. Ninety minutes of permissive hypotension is the tolerance limit and 120 min of hypotensive resuscitation can cause a significant alteration in mitochondrial function and severe organ damage and should be avoided [35]. Therefore, the initial objective is to control bleeding as soon as possible and to maintain a minimal arterial pressure to limit tissue hypoxia, inflammation and organ dysfunction. European guidelines for the management of the bleeding trauma patient recommend a target systolic blood pressure of 80 to 100 mm Hg in the acute phase of hemorrhagic shock until major bleeding has been stopped [36]. However, the optimal level of blood pressure during resuscitation of patients with hemorrhagic shock is still debated and we need more experimental and clinical studies to evaluate the consequences of hypotensive resuscitation on the microcirculation and tissue oxygenation. It appears crucial to develop bedside devices to assess microcirculatory perfusion or tissue oxygenation to better titrate the hemodynamic resuscitation strategy during hemorrhagic shock.

It is important to remember that restoration of the microcirculation implies not only restoration of blood volume to enhance organ perfusion, but also restoration of the functional capillary density. In this respect, it is crucial to test the influence of the currently used therapies (i. e., fluids, vasopressors and transfusion) on functional capillary density.

Fluid Resuscitation and Vasoactive Agents

Hypertonic saline (HTS) has been proposed as an interesting tool to improve the microcirculation in trauma hemorrhagic shock. It has been reported in experimental studies that resuscitation with HTS improves intestinal perfusion associated with selective arteriolar vasodilation of distal premucosal arterioles (A3), decreases interstitial and endothelial edema and prevents leukocyte adhesion to postcapillary venules and hemorrhagic shock-induced inflammation [1, 37]. However, despite these microvascular beneficial effects, fluid resuscitation with HTS failed to improve outcomes in trauma patients with hemorrhagic shock in recent studies [38, 39]. Moreover, there was a higher mortality rate in patients receiving HTS who did not receive any blood transfusion in the first 24 hours. To explain this effect, the authors evoked the possibility that out-of-hospital administration of HTS could mask the signs of hypovolemia and delay the diagnosis of hemorrhagic shock.

In the context of restoring functional capillary density, a new approach to fluid resuscitation is based on fluid with high viscosity in order to increase plasma viscosity and wall shear stress with NO production causing microcirculatory vasodilation with resulting capillary recruitment. Cabrales et al. suggested that hemorrhagic shock resuscitation (hamster window model) with polyethylene glycol (PEG)-conjugated bovine serum albumin provides early and long-term sustained systemic and microvascular recovery compared to hydroxyethyl starch (HES) [40]. Recently in the same model, Villela et al. reported that increasing blood and plasma viscosities during hemorrhage resuscitation with increased viscosity Ringer's lactate (addition of 0.3 % alginate) significantly improved arteriolar diameter and venular flow and maintained functional capillary density [41]. It is obvious that this concept has to be confirmed but thinking about the rheological properties of fluids could generate new ways of improving the microcirculation.

Vasopressor agents may be transiently required in hemorrhagic shock to maintain tissue perfusion in the presence of life-threatening hypotension, even when fluid expansion is in progress and hypovolemia has not yet been corrected. The microvascular effects of vasopressors in hemorrhagic shock are still under debate. More works will be required to establish the net microvascular effect of vasopressors during resuscitation of hemorrhagic shock patients. It is conceivable that correction of hypotension by vasopressors may improve microvascular perfusion by increasing the driving pressure of capillary beds [42, 43].

Transfusion

As previously mentioned, early administration of RBCs is a priority to maintain arterial DO_2 and to restore effective microcirculation and tissue oxygenation [25, 26]. An increasing body of data suggests that RBC plays a crucial role as an oxygen sensor in the regulation of microvascular tone and in the matching of oxygen supply to oxygen demand. Therefore, blood transfusion may improve microvascular DO_2 not only as an oxygen carrier but also as an oxygen sensor that improves functional capillary density by interfering with local microvascular control [44, 45]. This finding is important because a better understanding of the role of the RBC could change transfusion strategy and influence recommended optimal hemoglobin levels in hemorrhagic shock; moreover, it may be relevant to assess the impact of the quality of transfused RBCs on the microcirculation [46].

Conclusion

In hemorrhagic shock, a considerable part of the microvascular alterations are closely related to macrocirculatory variables (especially DO_2). Other factors could be involved in addition to macrohemodynamic factors. These include changes in the microvascular endothelium, leukocyte adherence to postcapillary venules, interstitial and endothelial edema, RBC deformability alterations, and coagulation activation. Restoration of the microcirculation after hemorrhagic shock has to focus on improvement in the functional capillary density within the organ. In this respect, it is crucial to test the influence of currently used therapies in hemorrhagic shock (i. e., fluids, vasopressors and transfusion) on functional capillary density. It is important to develop bedside devices to assess microcirculatory perfusion and tissue oxygenation to better titrate the hemodynamic resuscitation strategy during hemorrhagic shock. Understanding the impact of currently used therapies in hemorrhagic shock is the first step toward developing interventions that target microcirculatory perfusion.

References

1. Pascual JL, Ferri LE, Seely AJ et al (2002) Hypertonic saline resuscitation of hemorrhagic shock diminishes neutrophil rolling and adherence to endothelium and reduces in vivo vascular leakage. Ann Surg 236:634–642
2. Sordia T, Tatarishvili J, Varazashvili M, McHedlishvili G (2004) Hemorheological disorders in the microcirculation following hemorrhage. Clin Hemorheol Microcirc 30:461–462
3. Fang X, Tang W, Sun S, Huang L, Chang YT, Castillo C, Weil MH (2006) Comparison of buccal microcirculation between septic and hemorrhagic shock. Crit Care Med 34 (Suppl):S447–S453
4. Dubin A, Pozo MO, Ferrara G et al (2009) Systemic and microcirculatory responses to progressive hemorrhage. Intensive Care Med 35:556–564
5. Imai Y, Satoh K, Taira N (1978) Role of the peripheral vasculature in changes in venous return caused by isoproterenol, norepinephrine, and methoxamine in anesthetized dogs. Circ Res 43:553–561
6. Gelman S, Mushlin PS (2004) Catecholamine-induced changes in the splanchnic circulation affecting systemic hemodynamics. Anesthesiology 100:434–439
7. Schumacker PT (1998) Oxygen supply dependency in critical illness: an evolving understanding. Intensive Care Med 24:97–99
8. Dahl KN, Kalinowski A, Pekkan K (2010) Mechanobiology and the microcirculation: cellular, nuclear and fluid mechanics. Microcirculation 17:179–191
9. Ellsworth ML, Ellis CG, Goldman D, Stephenson AH, Dietrich HH, Sprague RS (2009) Erythrocytes: Oxygen sensors and modulators of vascular tone. Physiology 24:107–116
10. Sprague RS, Bowles EA, Achilleus D, Ellsworth ML (2010) Erythrocytes as controllers of perfusion distribution in the microvasculature of skeletal muscle. Acta Physiologica 202:285–292
11. Jia L, Bonaventura C, Bonaventura J, Stamler JS (1996) S-nitrosohaemoglobin: a dynamic activity of blood involved in vascular control. Nature 380:221–226
12. Stamler JS, Jia L, Eu JP et al (1997) Blood flow regulation by S-nitrosohemoglobin in the physiological oxygen gradient. Science 276:2034–2037
13. Cosby K, Partovi KS, Crawford JH et al (2003) Nitrite reduction to nitric oxide by deoxyhemoglobin vasodilates the human circulation. Nat Med 9:1498–1505
14. Gladwin MT, Crawford JH, Patel RP (2004) The biochemistry of nitric oxide, nitrite, and hemoglobin: role in blood flow regulation. Free Radic Biol Med 36:707–717
15. Kindig CA, Richardson TE, Poole DC (2002) Skeletal muscle capillary hemodynamics from rest to contractions: implications for oxygen transfer. J Appl Physiol 92:2513–2520
16. Poole DC, Copp SW, Hirai DM, Musch TI (2011) Dynamics of muscle microcirculatory and blood-myocyte O2 flux during contractions. Acta Physiologica 202:293–310
17. Bateman RM, Sharpe MD, Ellis CG (2003) Bench-to-bedside review: Microvascular dysfunction in sepsis – hemodynamics, oxygen transport, and nitric oxide. Crit Care 7:359
18. Ellis CG, Jagger J, Sharpe M (2005) The microcirculation as a functional system. Crit Care 9(Suppl 4):S3
19. Groom AC, Ellis CG, Wrigley SJ, Potter RF (1995) Capillary network morphology and capillary flow. Int J Microcirc Clin Exp 15:223–230
20. Funk W, Baldinger V (1995) Microcirculatory perfusion during volume therapy. A comparative study using crystalloid or colloid in awake animals. Anesthesiology 82:975–982
21. Hoffmann JN, Vollmar B, Laschke MW, Inthorn D, Schildberg FW, Menger MD (2002) Hydroxyethyl starch (130 kD), but not crystalloid volume support, improves microcirculation during normotensive endotoxemia. Anesthesiology 97:460–470
22. Vajda K, Szabo A, Boros M (2004) Heterogeneous microcirculation in the rat small intestine during hemorrhagic shock: Quantification of the effects of hypertonic-hyperoncotic resuscitation. Eur Surg Res 36:338–344

23. Zaets SB, Berezina TL, Morgan C et al (2003) Effect of trauma-hemorrhagic shock on red blood cell deformability and shape. Shock 19:268–273
24. Machiedo GW, Zaets SB, Berezina TL et al (2009) Trauma-hemorrhagic shock-induced red blood cell damage leads to decreased microcirculatory blood flow. Crit Care Med 37:1000–1010
25. Ince C, Sinaasappel M (1999) Microcirculatory oxygenation and shunting in sepsis and shock. Crit Care Med 27:1369–1377
26. Legrand M, Mik EG, Balestra GM et al (2010) Fluid resuscitation does not improve renal oxygenation during hemorrhagic shock in rats. Anesthesiology 112:119–127
27. De Backer D, Creteur J, Preiser JC, Dubois MJ, Vincent JL (2002) Microvascular blood flow is altered in patients with sepsis. Am J Respir Crit Care Med 166:98–104
28. Trzeciak S, Dellinger RP, Parrillo JE et al (2007) Early microcirculatory perfusion derangements in patients with severe sepsis and septic shock: relationship to hemodynamics, oxygen transport, and survival. Ann Emerg Med 49:88–98
29. Sakr Y, Dubois MJ, De Backer D, Creteur J, Vincent JL (2004) Persistent microcirculatory alterations are associated with organ failure and death in patients with septic shock. Crit Care Med 32:1825–1831
30. Nakajima Y, Baudry N, Duranteau J, Vicaut E (2001) Microcirculation in intestinal villi: a comparison between hemorrhagic and endotoxin shock. Am J Respir Crit Care Med 164:1526–1530
31. van Iterson M, Bezemer R, Heger M, Siegemund M, Ince C (2012) Microcirculation follows macrocirculation in heart and gut in the acute phase of hemorrhagic shock and isovolemic autologous whole blood resuscitation in pigs. Transfusion 52:1552–1559
32. Childs EW, Udobi KF, Wood JG, Hunter FA, Smalley DM, Cheung LY (2002) In vivo visualization of reactive oxidants and leukocyte-endothelial adherence following hemorrhagic shock. Shock 18:423–427
33. Capone AC, Safar P, Stezoski W, Tisherman S, Peitzman AB (1995) Improved outcome with fluid restriction in treatment of uncontrolled hemorrhagic shock. J Am Coll Surg 180:49–56
34. Kowalenko T, Stern S, Dronen S, Wang X (1992) Improved outcome with hypotensive resuscitation of uncontrolled hemorrhagic shock in a swine model. J Trauma 33:349–353
35. Li T, Zhu Y, Hu Y et al (2011) Ideal permissive hypotension to resuscitate uncontrolled hemorrhagic shock and the tolerance time in rats. Anesthesiology 114:111–119
36. Rossaint R, Bouillon B, Cerny V et al (2010) Management of bleeding following major trauma: an updated European guideline. Crit Care 14:R52
37. el Zakaria R, Tsakadze NL, Garrison RN (2006) Hypertonic saline resuscitation improves intestinal microcirculation in a rat model of hemorrhagic shock. Surgery 140:579–587
38. Bulger EM, Jurkovich GJ, Nathens AB et al (2008) Hypertonic resuscitation of hypovolemic shock after blunt trauma: a randomized controlled trial. Arch Surg 143:139–148
39. Bulger EM, May S, Kerby JD et al (2011) Out-of-hospital hypertonic resuscitation after traumatic hypovolemic shock. Ann Surg 253:431–441
40. Cabrales P, Intaglietta M, Tsai AG (2005) Increased plasma viscosity sustains microcirculation after resuscitation from hemorrhagic shock and continuous bleeding. Shock 23:549–555
41. Villela NR, Tsai AG, Cabrales P, Intaglietta M (2011) Improved resuscitation from hemorrhagic shock with Ringer's lactate with increased viscosity in the hamster window chamber model. J Trauma 71:418–424
42. Deruddre S, Cheisson G, Mazoit JX, Vicaut E, Benhamou D, Duranteau J (2007) Renal arterial resistance in septic shock: effects of increasing mean arterial pressure with norepinephrine on the renal resistive index assessed with Doppler ultrasonography. Intensive Care Med 33:1557–1562

43. Georger JF, Hamzaoui O, Chaari A, Maizel J, Richard C, Teboul JL (2010) Restoring arterial pressure with norepinephrine improves muscle tissue oxygenation assessed by near-infrared spectroscopy in severely hypotensive septic patients. Intensive Care Med 36:1882–1889
44. Sakr Y, Chierego M, Piagnerelli M et al (2007) Microvascular response to red blood cell transfusion in patients with severe sepsis. Crit Care Med 35:1639–1644
45. Yuruk K, Almac E, Bezemer R, Goedhart P, de Mol B, Ince C (2011) Blood transfusions recruit the microcirculation during cardiac surgery. Transfusion 51:961–967
46. Raat NJH, Ince C (2007) Oxygenating the microcirculation: the perspective from blood transfusion and blood storage. Vox Sang 93:12–18

Perioperative Monitoring of Tissue Perfusion: New Developments

C. Boer

Introduction

Textbook descriptions of physiological regulation systems in the human body are frequently simplified to enable application of these concepts in clinical practice. An example of a complex control system that has been simplified for clinical monitoring purposes is the maintenance of tissue perfusion. Although tissue perfusion depends on local vasomotor tone, metabolic regulation and cardiac output, perioperative monitoring is in most cases restricted to non-invasive arterial blood pressure measurements in combination with heart rate and oxygen saturation in patients undergoing low risk surgery. The use of more specific indices for tissue perfusion and fluid responsiveness, such as stroke volume, cardiac output, oxygen delivery and consumption, stroke volume variation (SVV) and pulse pressure variation (PPV), is generally restricted to the intensive care setting and high-risk surgical procedures, mainly due to the vulnerability of these specific patient populations.

The limited use of indicators of tissue perfusion and fluid responsiveness in the general surgical population is partly caused by the unavailability of specific minimally invasive monitoring devices. With the recent validation of novel hemodynamic devices that allow online monitoring of stroke volume, cardiac output and PPV we enter a new era of more extensive hemodynamic assessment during low-to-moderate risk surgery.

This chapter first illustrates the relation between arterial blood pressure, microcirculatory perfusion and organ blood flow to underline the limitations of arterial blood pressure as a hemodynamic representative for organ perfusion. Subsequently, the value of hemodynamic indices to guide perioperative vasopressor and fluid management are described, and an overview is presented of available monitoring

C. Boer (✉)
Department of Anesthesiology, Institute for Cardiovascular Research,
VU University Medical Center, De Boelelaan 1117, 1081 HV Amsterdam, the Netherlands
E-mail: c.boer@vumc.nl

J.-L. Vincent (Ed.), *Annual Update in Intensive Care and Emergency Medicine 2013*,
DOI 10.1007/978-3-642-35109-9_23, © Springer-Verlag Berlin Heidelberg 2013

devices that could be implemented for the perioperative use of these indices. Finally, an example is provided to illustrate the applicability and value of dynamic hemodynamic indices in the perioperative setting.

Guidance of Organ Perfusion by Arterial Blood Pressure

During anesthesia, maintenance of organ perfusion pressure by vasoactive substances is routinely guided by arterial blood pressure values. The concept is based on the assumption that the administration of vasopressor agents leads to constriction of arterioles, thereby improving organ perfusion pressure and blood flow. The contrasting effects of phenylephrine administration on arterial blood pressure and cardiac output, which are schematically represented in Fig. 1, however, illustrate the limitations of arterial blood pressure as a guide for the maintenance of organ perfusion. With the administration of two incremental concentrations of phenylephrine, the mean arterial blood pressure (MAP) increases as expected. In parallel, cardiac output unexpectedly decreases, leading to an unwanted reduction in tissue perfusion. This phenomenon was nicely demonstrated by Brassard et al. in healthy volunteers [1]. The reduction in cardiac output after phenylephrine administration is partly ascribed to an increase in venous resistance rather than a reduction in stroke volume, which remains relatively stable under different concentrations of phenylephrine [1, 2]. In contrast, whereas phenylephrine treatment reduced cardiac output in anesthetized patients, this phenomenon was not observed during ephedrine treatment [2, 3], suggesting that the effects of vasopressor agents on arterial blood pressure and cardiac output are not universal.

Although the deviating effects of phenylephrine on MAP and cardiac output are commonly known, this example illustrates that the absence of information with respect to stroke volume and cardiac output during general surgery may prohibit adequate clinical decision making in patients that require optimal tissue perfusion.

The weakness of arterial blood pressure as a representation of tissue perfusion can additionally be demonstrated by data presented by Bellomo and Giantomasso

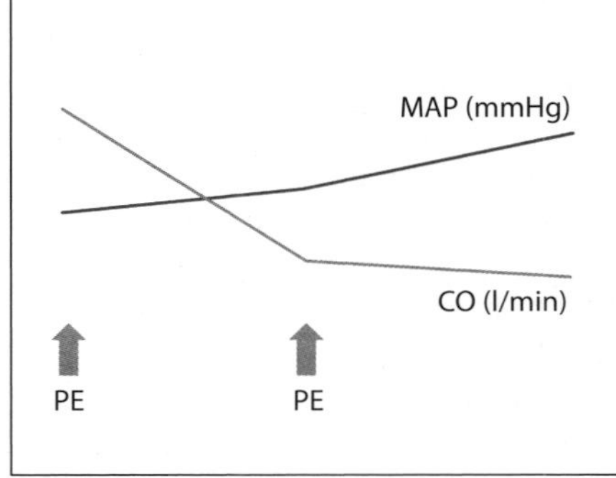

Fig. 1 The administration of two incremental concentrations of phenylephrine (PE) induces an increase in mean arterial pressure (MAP). Despite the increase in arterial blood pressure, phenylephrine administration is associated with a reduction in cardiac output (CO), which is not detected in the absence of adequate hemodynamic monitoring

[4]. They describe that the relation between perfusion pressure and tissue blood flow not only depends on the specific organ system, but that this relation is shifted rightwards in case of cardiac or renal disease. In particular, under disease conditions, a higher perfusion pressure is required to obtain a similar tissue blood flow when compared to healthy conditions [4]. Moreover, the use of vasopressor therapy under different disease conditions was associated with distinct effects on arterial pressure and cardiac output. Again, from this example it can be concluded that the sole measurement of arterial blood pressure is inadequate to reflect the level of tissue perfusion, and should be complemented with additional hemodynamic indices to fully understand the effects of specific interventions on tissue blood flow.

The Relation Between Arterial Blood Pressure and Microcirculatory Perfusion

The microcirculation is involved in the distribution of blood and its nutritive constituents to organs, and is responsible for adequate metabolic exchange in all areas of the human body in rest, and during exercise, surgery or illness. The regulatory mechanisms responsible for maintenance of microcirculatory perfusion are, however, not completely understood. This is further complicated by the technical difficulties associated with clinical evaluation of microcirculatory perfusion during surgery or intensive care.

The simplest representation of the microvascular control system is based on an arterial blood pressure-driven regulation of microcirculatory perfusion. This control system is, among others, complemented by autoregulation mechanisms that involve metabolic, myogenic and endothelial pathways in the microvasculature, all contributing to preservation of flow to vital tissues and organs. However, as these metabolic, myogenic and endothelial processes cannot be monitored online in the clinical setting, arterial blood pressure is frequently the only guidance to monitor tissue perfusion.

There is an ongoing debate as to whether arterial blood pressure changes affect the microcirculatory perfusion such that this leads to changes in tissue perfusion. If true, one might assume that anesthesia or illness influences the relation between arterial blood pressure and microcirculatory perfusion, thereby leading to disturbed tissue perfusion. However, there are several examples in the literature showing that this relation is not linear. Using ketanserin, an antihypertensive drug acting on serotonin, α-1/2-adrenergic and histamine receptors, Elbers et al. showed that the reduction in arterial blood pressure was not paralleled by disturbances in perfused capillary density in normovolemic cardiosurgical patients [5]. Others found that, despite a 20 mm Hg increase in arterial blood pressure by phenylephrine, sublingual medium-sized vessel blood flow was unaffected whereas in small vessels it was even depressed [6].

De Backer et al. described the relationship between system hemodynamics and microcirculatory perfusion as relatively loose, especially within the physiological

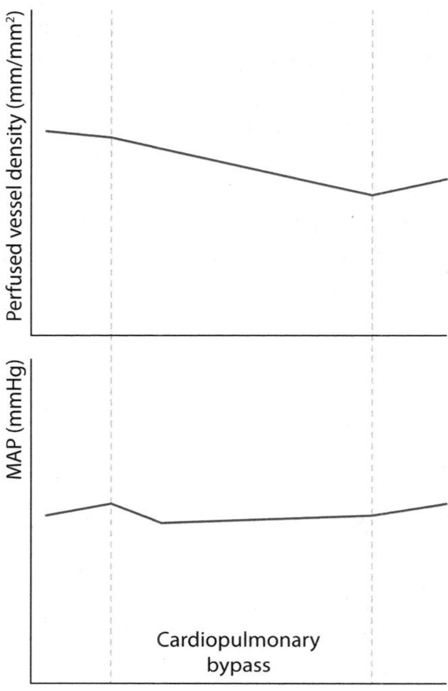

Fig. 2 Changes in the microvascular perfused vessel density (*upper panel*) and mean arterial pressure (MAP; *lower panel*) during cardiopulmonary bypass. The perfused vessel density decreased during bypass, irrespective of the observed restoration of arterial blood pressure

range of cardiac output and arterial blood pressure [7]. Indeed, in patients with septic shock, an increase in blood pressure by vasoactive agents was not beneficial for microcirculatory perfusion for an MAP exceeding 65 mm Hg [8]. In addition, we showed that pulsatile blood flow during cardiopulmonary bypass (CPB) was associated with preservation of microcirculatory perfusion when compared to laminar flow; this effect was irrespective of systemic hemodynamics [9]. From our findings, we concluded that the regulation of microcirculatory perfusion not only depends on the driving force of arterial blood pressure, but additionally involves metabolic, rheological and endothelial factors.

Figure 2 is a simplified representation of the relation between microcirculatory perfusion (upper panel) and MAP (lower panel) as observed in our patients during non-pulsatile CPB [9]. The initiation of CPB was associated with a decrease in microcirculatory perfused vessel density and MAP. Whereas the MAP, which fluctuated around 60 mm Hg, was restored to baseline values throughout the surgical procedure, the microcirculatory perfusion density decreased continuously. These findings further suggest that, in case of relatively normal arterial blood pressure values, volume challenges and vasoactive substances may be relatively ineffective as modulators of microcirculatory perfusion.

However, in cases of severe blood pressure derangement, perfusion of the microcirculation is clearly disturbed as was recently shown by two cases of nitroglycerin-induced hypotension [10]. Nitroglycerin-induced vasodilation resulted in an initial increase in the arteriolar diameter and microcirculatory flow, but was followed by a reduction in the microvessel blood velocity during the hypotensive phase [10]. In a study by Thooft et al., an increase in MAP above 65 mm Hg using vasopressor therapy in patients with septic shock and arterial hypotension was associated with augmentation of the microvascular perfused vessel density [11]. Moreover, Pottecher et al. showed that passive leg raising, which induces a fluid shift and increase in arterial blood pressure, improved sublingual microcirculatory perfusion in preload-responsive severe septic patients [12]. These findings may suggest that volume and pharmacological interventions to correct hypotensive episodes can affect the perfusion of the microcirculation, particularly in fluid-responsive patients or patients with insufficient vasomotor tone. Altogether, under conditions of severe blood pressure derangements and disease, the relation between arterial blood pressure and microcirculatory perfusion may be altered, and is inadequately reflected by arterial blood pressure measurements alone.

Perioperative Use of Dynamic Hemodynamic Indices

Despite the number of literature reports showing that perioperative fluid and inotropic therapy should preferably not only be based on arterial blood pressure, this mind shift is still not adopted in general anesthesia. This may partly be explained by the lack of validated devices for minimally invasive monitoring of indicators of tissue perfusion that can be easily applied in the intraoperative period.

In 2011, two systematic reviews were published that focused on the effects of preemptive hemodynamic monitoring and therapy and maintenance of perioperative tissue perfusion on patient outcome [13, 14]. The review by Hamilton et al. showed that hemodynamic monitoring and therapy based on indices like cardiac output, oxygen delivery (DO_2), stroke volume or PPV, but not MAP or central venous pressure (CVP), was associated with a reduction in mortality and surgical complications. Specific subgroup mortality analyses revealed that cardiac index (CI) or DO_2 were superior to stroke volume as hemodynamic optimization targets. One study was included showing that PPV may alternatively be used to optimize hemodynamic strategies [15]. Interestingly, the review by Hamilton further showed that a combination of fluid therapy with vasopressor administration was superior for the hemodynamic optimization of surgical patients than fluid therapy alone [13].

The second review by Gurgel and do Nascimento showed that perioperative monitoring of cardiac output and oxygen delivery and consumption is of added value in the improvement of outcome in high-risk surgical patients [14]. Both papers demonstrated that preemptive hemodynamic monitoring and therapy may contribute to improved patient outcomes in the surgical setting. However, most studies included in the reviews used CI and oxygen delivery and consumption to guide intraoperative vasopressor or fluid therapy. Until recently, these indices required invasive monitoring, including pulmonary artery catheter measurements or PiCCO technology, which limited the applicability of these indices in the general perioperative setting. With the introduction of Doppler-ultrasound cardiac output monitoring, automated application of arterial pulse wave or pulse oximetry algorithms for the calculation of stroke volume, and non-invasive arterial blood pressure measurement devices it is, however, expected that more and more anesthesiologists will use static and dynamic hemodynamic indices for tissue perfusion in the operating room.

Table 1 gives an overview of hemodynamic monitoring devices that are available for the perioperative setting. Briefly, hemodynamic monitoring is either based on esophageal Doppler-ultrasound (Cardio-Q®), non-invasive Doppler-ultrasound (USCOM®), intra-arterial blood pressure monitoring (PiCCO®, Flotrac®, LiDCO®, ProAQT®), non-invasive bioreactance measurements (NICOM®) or non-invasive continuous arterial blood pressure measurements using a finger cuff (Nexfin®, Finapres®). The applicability of these devices in the postoperative period mainly depends on the invasiveness of the technology, which can be categorized as highly invasive (Cardio-Q, PiCCO), minimally invasive (Flotrac, LiDCO, ProAQT) and non-invasive (USCOM, NICOM, Nexfin, Finapres).

All devices provide information on the effects of vasopressor therapy (stroke volume, cardiac output, CI, systemic vascular resistance [SVR]), whereas SVV and PPV for the evaluation of the fluid responsiveness of a patient are not provided by the Cardio-Q or Finapres. Postoperative monitoring of cardiac output and fluid responsiveness during general ward admission is only possible with non-invasive devices like the USCOM, NICOM, Nexfin and Finapres. The Cardio-Q and USCOM devices assess stroke volume based on Doppler-ultrasound flow measurements, and require additional arterial pressure monitoring. The pressure-based devices use specific algorithms to calculate stroke volume, cardiac output and SVV based on different arterial waveform analysis algorithms; this has been extensively reviewed by Montenij et al [16].

Table 1 Hemodynamic monitoring devices for the perioperative setting.

	Technique	Invasive	Continuous measurements	SV/CO	SVV	PPV	Ward
CardioQ	Doppler	+	+	+	–	–	–
PiCCO	Thermodilution/ arterial line	+	+/–	+	+	+	–
Flotrac/LiDCO/ ProAQT	Arterial line	+	+	+	+	+	–
USCOM	Doppler	–	–	+	+	–	+
NICOM	Bioreactance	–	+	+	+	–	+
Nexfin	Finger cuff	–	+	+	+	+	+
Finapres	Finger cuff	–	+	+	–	–	+

CO: cardiac output; SV: stroke volume; SVV: stroke volume variation; PPV: pulse pressure variation; ward: general surgical ward

The introduction of novel hemodynamic monitoring devices in the general surgical setting allows specific evaluation of organ perfusion parameters and fluid responsiveness by a minimally invasive approach. However, integration of these stand-alone devices with existing anesthesia machines, the absence of large clinical outcome studies in low-to-moderate risk surgical patients and the costs of probes and catheters still limits the applicability of these devices in routine clinical practice.

Non-invasive Monitoring of Dynamic Hemodynamic Indices: An Example

The measurement of dynamic hemodynamic indices based on arterial blood pressure monitoring previously required the presence of an intra-arterial blood pressure catheter. However, the number of patients receiving an intra-arterial line during non-cardiovascular surgical procedures is limited and varies widely among countries. Moreover, there is a tendency to restrict intra-arterial blood pressure measurements to high-risk surgery or patients with multiple comorbidities, mainly due to economical reasons and the risk of complications. The observed reduction in invasive perioperative monitoring conflicts with the increasing interest in measuring static and dynamic indices to monitor the effects of vasopressor therapy and fluid responsiveness in surgical patients.

Alternatively, blood pressure measurements based on non-invasive arterial blood pressure evaluation technologies may be used to derive information on cardiac output and the variation in pulse pressure or stroke volume in low-to-moderate risk surgical patients. In our hospital, we increasingly use Nexfin non-invasive finger arterial blood pressure measurements to gain beat-to-beat information on arterial blood pressure, cardiac output and pulse pressure variation. Nexfin non-invasive arterial blood pressure measurements are based on the volume clamp method that was described by Peňáz and Wesseling [17, 18]. The Nexfin monitor provides beat-to-beat information about the arterial blood pressure and cardiac output using a redesigned finger cuff for better signal to noise ratio [19–21]. We have shown that Nexfin arterial blood pressure measurements reproducibly reflect autonomic function responses in volunteers, and have a high level of agreement with intra-arterial blood pressure measurements in children [22] and adults [19, 20]. Moreover, the calculation of stroke volume and cardiac output based on the Nexfin CO-trek algorithm showed a high level of agreement with invasive cardiac output measurements using a pulmonary artery catheter [21].

Although the clinical value of non-invasive arterial blood pressure measurements in the perioperative setting should be further elaborated, studies in our group showed that the availability of dynamic hemodynamic indices may indeed be of interest for the general anesthesiologist. Figure 3 shows the trends in MAP (upper panel), CI (middle panel) and PPV (lower panel) at baseline, during Trendelenburg positioning and on return to the supine position in an American Society

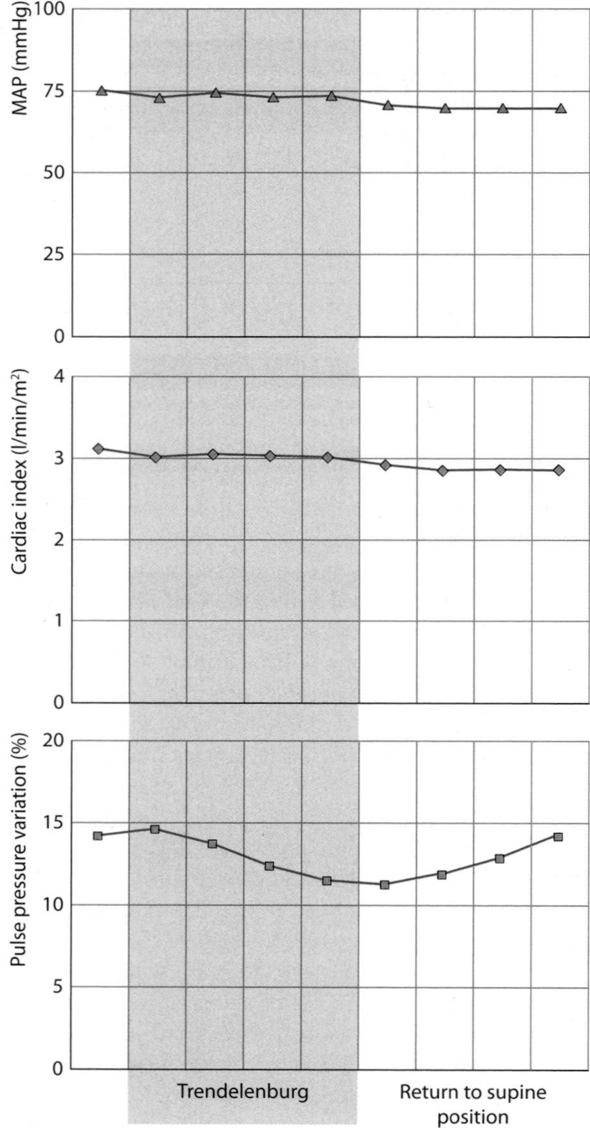

Fig. 3 Changes in mean arterial pressure (*upper panel*), cardiac index (*middle panel*) and pulse pressure variation (*lower panel*) during Trendelenburg positioning in a mechanically ventilated patient

of Anesthesiologists (ASA) II patient who was anesthetized and mechanically ventilated (unpublished data). Measurements were performed before surgical incision, and the patient had no cardiac arrhythmias that might have disturbed PPV measurements, and a closed thorax. To measure PPV, the tidal volume during mechanical ventilation was set to 8 ml/kg. MAP was measured using the CC-Nexfin device (Bmeye BV, Amsterdam, the Netherlands), which additionally provides information on CI and PPV. As shown in Fig. 3, Trendelenburg positioning induced only a small change in MAP and CI, whereas the PPV visibly reduced by 3–4 %. PPV returned to baseline values after repositioning the patient in the supine position. These data are not only supportive for a role of non-invasive arterial blood pressure measurements in relatively healthy patients undergoing surgery, but show that PPV measurements may be of added value in the monitoring of volume changes in the perioperative setting. However, further investigation of these novel indices in the general surgical population is warranted, in particular with respect to the limitations of their applicability [23] and the relation to patient outcome.

Conclusion

Non-invasive or invasive arterial blood pressure measurements are generally used during low-to-moderate risk surgery to guide vasopressor and fluid therapy. However, perioperative arterial blood pressure values provide only limited information with respect to tissue perfusion. In particular, although microvascular organ perfusion is partly pressure-driven, other factors, such as baseline blood pressure, metabolic and endothelial influences and specific disease conditions, may affect the relationship between perfusion pressure and tissue blood flow. Implementation of hemodynamic monitoring devices that enable assessment of stroke volume, cardiac output, SVV and PPV may be additionally used to guide vasopressor and fluid therapy and maintain adequate tissue perfusion. Although there is increasing evidence that minimally invasive monitoring of these indices may be of added value in general surgery, the limitations of these indices and their effects on patient outcome after general surgery should be further evaluated in large clinical trials.

References

1. Brassard P, Seifert T, Wissenberg M, Jensen PM, Hansen CK, Secher NH (2010) Phenylephrine decreases frontal lobe oxygenation at rest but not during moderately intense exercise. J Appl Physiol 108:1472–1478
2. Thiele RH, Nemergut EC, Lynch 3rd C (2011) The physiologic implications of isolated alpha(1) adrenergic stimulation. Anesth Analg 113:284–296
3. Meng L, Cannesson M, Alexander BS et al (2011) Effect of phenylephrine and ephedrine bolus treatment on cerebral oxygenation in anaesthetized patients. Br J Anaesth 107:209–217
4. Bellomo R, Giantomasso DD (2001) Noradrenaline and the kidney: friends or foes? Crit Care 5:294–298
5. Elbers PW, Ozdemir A, van Iterson M, van Dongen EP, Ince C (2009) Microcirculatory imaging in cardiac anesthesia: ketanserin reduces blood pressure but not perfused capillary density. J Cardiothorac Vasc Anesth 23:95–101
6. Maier S, Hasibeder WR, Hengl C et al (2009) Effects of phenylephrine on the sublingual microcirculation during cardiopulmonary bypass. Br J Anaesth 102:485–491

7. De Backer D, Ortiz JA, Salgado D (2010) Coupling microcirculation to systemic hemodynamics. Curr Opin Crit Care 16:250–254
8. Boerma EC, Ince C (2010) The role of vasoactive agents in the resuscitation of microvascular perfusion and tissue oxygenation in critically ill patients. Intensive Care Med 36:2004–2018
9. Koning NJ, Vonk AB, van Barneveld LJ et al (2012) Pulsatile flow during cardiopulmonary bypass preserves postoperative microcirculatory perfusion irrespective of systemic hemodynamics. J Appl Physiol 112:1727–1734
10. Atasever B, Boer C, Lust E, van der Kuil M et al (2011) Quantitative imaging of microcirculatory response during nitroglycerin-induced hypotension. J Cardiothorac Vasc Anesth 25:140–144
11. Thooft A, Favory R, Salgado DR et al (2011) Effects of changes in arterial pressure on organ perfusion during septic shock. Crit Care 15:R222
12. Pottecher J, Deruddre S, Teboul JL et al (2010) Both passive leg raising and intravascular volume expansion improve sublingual microcirculatory perfusion in severe sepsis and septic shock patients. Intensive Care Med 36:1867–1874
13. Hamilton MA, Cecconi M, Rhodes A (2011) A systematic review and meta-analysis on the use of preemptive hemodynamic intervention to improve postoperative outcomes in moderate and high-risk surgical patients. Anesth Analg 112:1392–1402
14. Gurgel ST, do Nascimento Jr P (2011) Maintaining tissue perfusion in high-risk surgical patients: a systematic review of randomized clinical trials. Anesth Analg 112:1384–1391
15. Lopes MR, Oliveira MA, Pereira VO, Lemos IP, Auler Jr JO, Michard F (2007) Goal-directed fluid management based on pulse pressure variation monitoring during high-risk surgery: a pilot randomized controlled trial. Crit Care 11:R100
16. Montenij LJ, de Waal EE, Buhre WF (2011) Arterial waveform analysis in anesthesia and critical care. Curr Opin Anaesthesiol 24:651–656
17. Peñáz J (1954) A portable finger plethysmograph. Scr Med (Brno) 27:213–234
18. Wesseling KH, De Wit B, Van der Hoeven GMA, Van Goudoever J, Settels JJ (1995) Physiocal, calibrating finger vascular physiology for Finapres. Homeostasis 36:67–82
19. Eeftinck Schattenkerk DW, van Lieshout JJ, van den Meiracker AH et al (2009) Nexfin noninvasive continuous blood pressure validated against Riva-Rocci/Korotkoff. Am J Hypertens 22:378–383
20. Martina JR, Westerhof BE, van Goudoever J et al (2012) Noninvasive continuous arterial blood pressure monitoring with Nexfin®. Anesthesiology 116:1092–1103
21. Bogert LW, Wesseling KH, Schraa O et al (2010) Pulse contour cardiac output derived from non-invasive arterial pressure in cardiovascular disease. Anaesthesia 65:1119–1125
22. Garnier RP, van der Spoel AG, Sibarani-Ponsen R, Markhorst DG, Boer C (2012) Level of agreement between Nexfin non-invasive arterial pressure with invasive arterial pressure measurements in children. Br J Anaesth 109:609–615
23. Michard F, Biais M (2012) Rational fluid management: dissecting facts from fiction. Br J Anaesth 108:369–371

Part VIII

Cardiac Arrest

Improving the Local Chain-of-Survival to Improve Survival After Out-of-Hospital Cardiac Arrest

K. Sunde

Introduction

Approximately 275,000 Europeans every year suffer from out-of-hospital cardiac arrest (OHCA) and are treated by the local Emergency Medical Systems (EMS) [1, 2]. Despite evolving evidence based guidelines for cardiopulmonary resuscitation (CPR), survival rates after OHCA have not improved much in the majority of places around the world. However, there is a huge variety in worldwide survival, with some cities having survival rates greater than 20–30 % and some with just a few percent survival [1, 2]. These significant survival differences can partly be explained by different definitions of OHCA [2], but are mainly due to overall quality within the local chain-of-survival [3] (Fig. 1, upper left panel): Early arrest recognition and call for help, early CPR, early defibrillation, and early post-resuscitation care. Whereas CPR and defibrillation have received the most attention and been the major research areas over the present three decades, post-resuscitation care has received more focus just in the last 10 years.

Chain of Survival

Successful survival (defined as a survived patient with a normal to just a slightly reduced neurological function, independent, back to normal life activities and work) is very dependent on well functioning pre- and in-hospital systems of care. A focused, goal-directed treatment strategy throughout the local chain-of-survival is of utmost importance. In other words, all stages influencing outcome for the OHCA patient, such as early recognition, initiation of bystander CPR, activation

K. Sunde (✉)
Surgical Intensive Care Unit Ullevål, Department of Anesthesiology,
Division of Emergencies and Critical Care, Oslo University Hospital, N-0407 Oslo, Norway
E-mail: kjetil.sunde@medisin.uio.no

J.-L. Vincent (Ed.), *Annual Update in Intensive Care and Emergency Medicine 2013*,
DOI 10.1007/978-3-642-35109-9_24, © Springer-Verlag Berlin Heidelberg 2013

of the EMS system, good quality Basic Life Support (BLS), early defibrillation, good quality Advanced Life Support (ALS), and finally, goal-directed, standardized good quality post-resuscitation care including percutaneous coronary intervention (PCI) and therapeutic hypothermia as well as a rehabilitation plan, have to be predefined and optimized within the system.

How is this achievable? First, it is very important to document the current situation and outcomes within the local system. This is possible by documenting Utstein data for OHCA [4], which is a very useful and recommended tool for evaluating and critically assessing the local chain-of-survival. Thereby, areas along the chain-of-survival that are in need of improvement can be identified. The two important and decisive questions that then need to be asked are:

1. Are we happy with the survival rate within our institution?
2. If not, where are the weak links?

The most important step is, therefore, to document and understand that there is a potential for improved survival within the local system. Further, the weak links, partly responsible for this bad outcome, have to be identified and challenged. Efforts to improve the weakest links have to be initiated and strictly implemented.

Formula for Survival

It is well known that adherence to CPR guidelines is suboptimal. This has been shown for several groups, even for health care professionals performing ALS [5, 6]. The development of good clinical guidelines does not insure their use in practice, and implementation of changes takes time [7]. Therefore, improving skill performance is even more important than solely concentrating on the content of the guidelines. It has been suggested that patient outcome is a product of medical science, educational efficiency and local implementation [8]. This has been called the Utstein Formula of Survival (Fig. 1, upper right panel) [8, 9]. Science tells us what to do based on the evidence, education tells us how to teach based on the science, and implementation what to do and how to do it. In other words, it does not help if the level of scientific evidence is high, education is excellent, but local implementation and adoption into clinical practice are low. As a consequence, the survival rate will stay low, although the potential for improved outcome is present. Implementation is the crucial part of changing behavior, and must be focused on and defined if new treatment strategies are to be followed locally. Changing clinical practice is sometimes as difficult as the basic science and clinical trial work that leads to the discovery of beneficial therapies [10]. In an American Heart Association (AHA) Consensus Recommendation from 2011, Neumar et al. summarized the important implementation strategies for improving survival after OHCA in the United States [11]. The lower panel of Figure 1 shows the 71 factors that can impact on the local chain-of-survival and thereby influence the Utstein Formula of Survival.

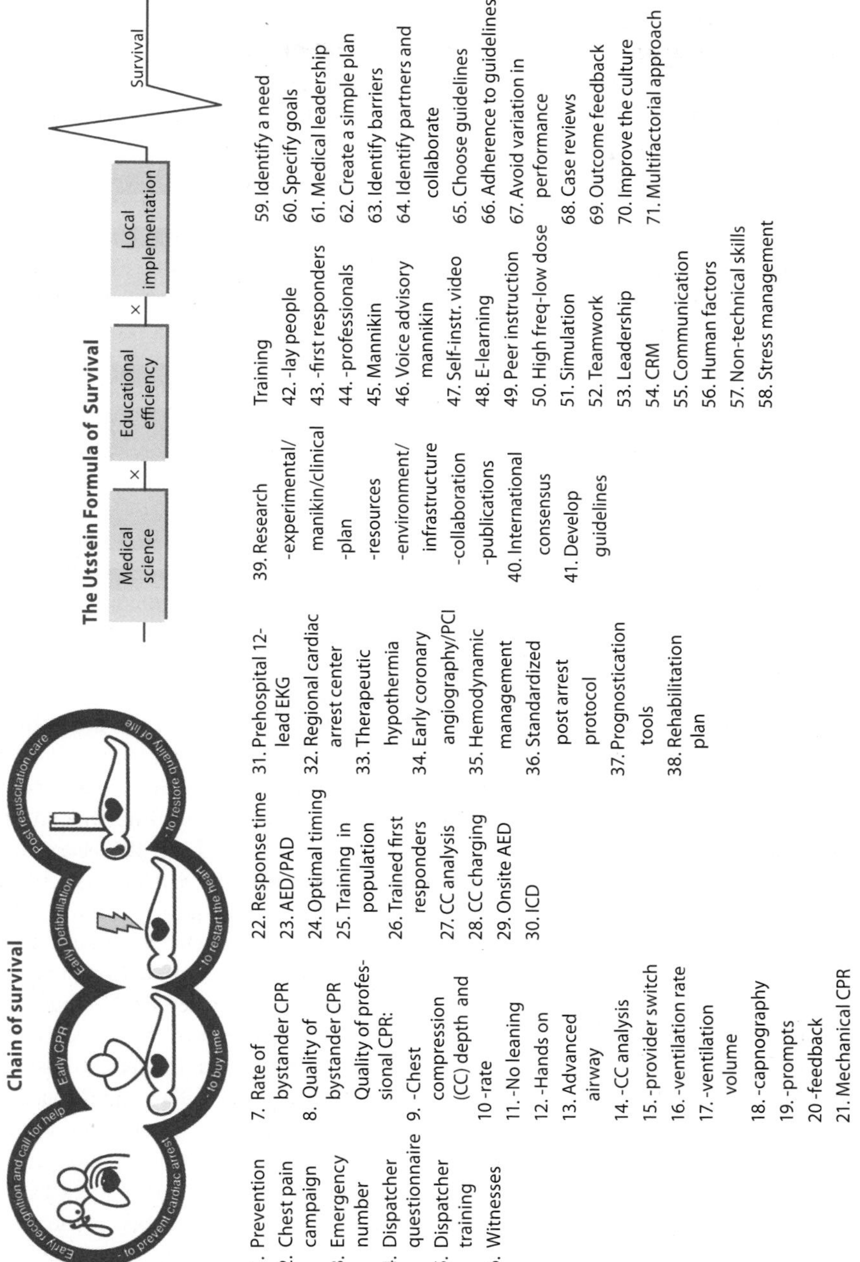

Fig. 1 *Upper left panel*: Chain of survival (with permission from Laerdal Medical); *upper right panel*: Formula of survival (with permission from Laerdal Medical); *lower panel*: Seventy-one factors that impact on the local chain of survival and, thereby, influence the Utstein Formula of survival

The Oslo Experience

In Oslo, Norway, survival to hospital discharge for OHCA was below 10 % for the last 30 years [12–14]. The city of Oslo covers 454 km^2 and has approximately 550,000 inhabitants. Oslo has a one-tiered community-run EMS system. All acute care ambulances are manned with paramedics. On weekdays between 07:30 and 22:00, a physician-manned ambulance staffed by two paramedics and an anesthesiologist functions on the same level as the regular paramedic staffed ambulances. All paramedics are trained to use defibrillators in manual mode. Endotracheal intubation is the standard method for securing the airways, followed by uninterrupted chest compressions with 10–12 interposed ventilations per minute. There are several hospitals taking care of OHCA patients, but the majority of the patients (60–70 %) are admitted to a 24 hour PCI center: Oslo University Hospital Ullevål.

We recently evaluated survival after OHCA in Oslo over a ten-year period, during which some important changes in the local chain-of-survival were implemented at different time periods [15]. During the first period (1996–1998), ambulance personnel provided ALS according to the 1992 Guidelines [16], resulting in poor ALS quality with long periods without vital organ perfusion and few shocks resulting in return of spontaneous circulation (ROSC) (many unsuccessful shocks increasing the time without perfusion) [13]. There was no standardized post-resuscitation care treatment plan at any of the five receiving hospitals in Oslo at that time. Modified 2000 Guidelines [17], with more focus on chest compression quality and three minutes of CPR prior to and between defibrillation, were implemented prior to the second period (2001–2003), based on findings from some local ALS studies [13, 18]. The main aim of these changes was to optimize vital organ perfusion by minimizing interruptions in chest compression, and for the timing of defibrillation to be improved. We thus improved the second and third link in our local chain-of-survival. Paramedics were actively involved in the suggested changes and also in the training campaign. Data from the local studies [13, 18] were actively used in training and implementation.

During this time, we had no standardized in-hospital post-resuscitation care. We had, however, realized that quality of hospital care after cardiac arrest matters [19], and the landmark studies on therapeutic hypothermia after OHCA had just been published [20, 21]. Further, in a study from Norway, we documented that survival to discharge varied between 34 % and 56 % in four different hospital regions [22]. These data were later confirmed in Sweden, US, Japan and recently Germany [23–26]. As a consequence, in 2002/3 we developed a standardized goal-directed post-resuscitation treatment plan with focus on optimizing hemodynamics, treating the cause of arrest early, coronary angiography and subsequent PCI if indicated, therapeutic hypothermia for 24 hours, avoiding hyperglycemia, and early seizure detection and treatment through a protocolized system of care [27]. If coronary angiography and/or PCI were indicated, patients were directly transported from the scene to one of the two hospitals with this capacity (24 hours/day). The post-resuscitation protocols were applied to all patients regardless of initial rhythm or causes if active treatment was desired [27]. At Oslo Ullevål University

Hospital, these radical treatment changes were introduced with a clearly defined implementation strategy and presented at different meetings, in different departments, for nurses and doctors. After two years, we documented an improvement in successful survival from 26 % to 56 % [27], which was sustained in subsequent years [28]. In Table 1, a summary of the treatment plan is presented.

Our local chain-of-survival was thus changed throughout this 10-year period, with a special focus on the weakest links: The first period (1996–1998) had poor

Table 1 Summary of the standard operating procedures for post-resuscitation care at Oslo University Hospital Ullevål 2003–2009. From [15] with permission

Emergency bundle		
Withhold intensive care DNAR order End-stage malignancy	*Coronary angiography* Transport patients without delay to coronary angiography when cardiologist suspects AMI (ST-segment elevation or other symptoms/signs judged to indicate AMI)	*MTH* All comatose patients, when in doubt, cool. Relative contraindications trauma and primary coagulopathy.
Also consider on a patient to patient basis: Small chance of survival (un-witnessed and initial AS/PEA and resuscitated more than 0.5 h) Very advanced age (no absolute age limit)		Start cooling immediately with refrigerated NaCl 0.9 % (30 ml/kg) and ice-packs. Maintain 33 °C for 24 h with surface or invasive automated cooling device. Deep sedation (fentanyl and midazolam or propofol) Intermittent muscle relaxant (only if sedation fails to control shivering) Re-warm 0.5 °C/h (terminate sedation at 36 °C)
Management bundle		
Monitor EKG and pulse oximetry Invasive pressures, arterial line and CVC ($CVSO_2$, SO_2, PO_2, PCO_2, pH, electrolytes, blood sugar) Temperature (bladder) Chest X-ray Echocardiography (consider IABP or dobutamine/epinephrine if pump failure)	*Targets* Pulse 60–100/min MAP> 65 mm Hg (dopamine, norepinephrine) SO_2 > 95–98 %, pCO_2 5–6 kPa $CVSO_2$ > 70 % Urine output > 1 ml/kg/h pH > 7.1, BE > –10 mmol/l Blood sugar 5–8 mmol/l Haemoglobin > 9–10 g/dl	*Prognostication* *Base treatment withdrawal in patients that remain comatose 72 h after re-warming on:* Clinical examination by consultant neurologist (NSE and EEG as deemed necessary) Interdisciplinary consensus to withdraw care

AMI: acute myocardial infarction; BE: base excess; CVC: central venous catheter; $CSVO_2$: central venous oxygen saturation; DNAR: do not attempt resuscitation; EKG: electrocardiogram; EEG: electronencephalography; IABP: intra aortic balloon pump; MTH: mild therapeutic hypothermia; NSE: neuron specific enolase; PEA: pulseless electral activity; SO_2: arterial oxygen saturation. Conversion factors: 1 kPa = 7.5 mm Hg; 1 mmol/l = 18 mg/dl (blood sugar)

ALS quality and poor post-resuscitation care; the second period (2001–2003) had good ALS quality but poor post-resuscitation care; and the third period (2004–2005) had good ALS quality (no additional changes since the 2001–2003 period) and good post-resuscitation care. During these three different time periods, 1,320 patients received ALS for OHCA [15].

Table 2 Demographic characteristics and overall outcome (all causes/all initial rhythms) in the three different time periods. Period 1 (1996–1998) with poor ALS/poor post-arrest care, period 2 (2001–2003) with good ALS/poor post-arrest care and period 3 with good ALS/good post-arrest care. From [15] with permission

	1996–1998	2001–2003	2004–2005	p value
ALS initiated	454	449	417	
Age	65 ± 18	64 ± 18	65 ± 17	0.88
Gender (% male)	329 (72)	323 (72)	293 (70)	0.48
Cardiac etiology	313 (69)	349 (78)	281 (67)	0.76
Location				
Home	226 (50)	291 (65)	224 (54)	0.20
Public	168 (37)	112 (25)	143 (34)	0.34
Other/unknown	60 (13)	46 (10)	50 (12)	0.55
Initial rhythm				
VF/VT	181 (40)	164 (34)	138 (33)	0.039
Asystole	192 (42)	233 (52)	189 (45)	0.33
PEA/other/unknown	81 (18)	52 (12)	90 (22)	0.17
Witnessed arrest	361 (80)	276 (61)	302 (72)	0.022
Bystander CPR	248 (55)	217 (48)	225 (54)	0.84
Response interval[a]	7 ± 4	9 ± 4	9 ± 4	<0.001
ROSC at any time point	135 (30)	153 (34)	149 (36)	0.058
Admitted to ICU[b]	102 (23)	128 (29)	119 (29)	0.040
Discharged	31 (7)	45 (10)	54 (13)	0.002
CPC 1–2[c]	26 (6)	38 (9)	51 (12)	0.001
CPC 3–4	5	4	3	
Discharged (CPC 1–2/admitted ICU)	25 %	30 %	43 %	0.005

All variables given as numbers (percentages in parenthesis) except age and response interval (mean ± SD). p values are obtained from linear by linear associations for trend over time periods for categorical data and from ANOVA for continuous data. ALS: advanced life support; VF: ventricular fibrillation; VT: ventricular tachycardia; PEA: pulseless electrical activity; CPR: cardiopulmonary resuscitation; ROSC: return of spontaneous circulation; ICU: intensive care unit; CPC: cerebral performance category. Response interval: time from call received to ambulance arrival.

[a] Ambulanced witnessed arrests excluded from analysis

[b] Missing information for 8 patients in the second time period

[c] CPC score missing for 3 patients in the second time period

The results showed that there was a significantly improved overall survival to hospital discharge across the three time periods, from 7 % to 10 % and 13 %, respectively, p = 0.001 (Table 2). Survival with favorable neurological outcome (Clinical Performance Category [CPC] 1–2) was also significantly improved (6 %, 9 %, and 12 %, respectively for the different time periods, p = 0.001). OHCA patients with a cardiac cause also had significantly improved survival rates, from 9 % to 12 % and 17 %, respectively (p = 0.003). And, finally, among those patients with the best survival potential, bystander witnessed cardiac arrests with a cardiac cause and initial ventricular fibrillation (VF), survival with a favorable neurological outcome was 14 %, 22 % and 33 %, respectively (p = 0.001). Interestingly, we documented that despite an increase in negative prognostic factors such as more unwitnessed non-VF arrests and increased response intervals, outcome improved two-fold during these 10 years (Table 2) [15].

This survival benefit was achieved through improvements in quality of ALS and post-resuscitation care. ALS training focused on optimizing chest compressions by stressing the importance of adequate force and rate as well as limiting hands-off intervals. Clinical studies also documented that the quality of chest compressions in our EMS improved markedly over the years [29, 30]. Since none of the ALS components, such as drug administration [31, 32], intubation or advanced airway management [31], have been documented to improve survival, optimal compression quality is, in addition to early defibrillation, the most important task during resuscitation [33]. The increase in survival, however, was most prominent for the third time period [15], demonstrating the importance of improved post-resuscitation care. This factor has also been emphasized in recent international guidelines [33] as well as in a recent review paper [34].

Results from Other Systems

Our findings are in agreement with recent studies reporting temporal improvements in survival within different EMS systems [35, 36]. A study from Seattle reported cumulative effects of four EMS program changes with overall survival to hospital discharge improving from 31 % to 45 % during a 30-year period in patients with witnessed VF arrest [35]. The local chain-of-survival was strengthened by focusing on the second and third links with strategies to provide early BLS through telephone assisted CPR and early defibrillation through public access defibrillators and equipping first responders with defibrillators [35]. Similarly, a large-scale population-based study from Japan reported improved survival during an eight year period after implementing changes to the first three links in their local chain-of-survival [36]. By training lay-persons in BLS, introducing telephone-assisted CPR, placing public access defibrillators, and training emergency medical technicians in defibrillation, tracheal intubation and administration of epinephrine, they noted increased neurological intact survival (from 6 % to 16 %) for patients with witnessed VF arrest [36]. Similar improvements have recently been seen after engaging a whole community in OHCA treatment on the Danish island, Bornholm [37].

In Minnesota, the initiative was taken even further. In 2010, Lick et al. published promising results from the "Take Heart America Project" at two sites in Minnesota, where all four previously weak links in their chain-of-survival were changed and improved [38]. The focus was on improving bystander CPR rate (training campaign) and professional ALS performance (compression quality, impedance threshold device, defibrillation strategy) through skilled training, and also improved in-hospital care with the goal of admitting OHCA patients to specialized cardiac arrest centers capable of performing PCI and therapeutic hypothermia. Survival to hospital discharge for all patients after OHCA improved significantly from 8.5 % to 19 % [38]. Finally, a recent study from Stavanger, Norway, showed the survival potential after OHCA, when, in an optimized system, every fourth patient after all cardiac arrests (independent of cause and initial rhythm), and every second patient after initial witnessed VF arrests had good cerebral outcomes [39].

Conclusion

Continuous focus on the importance of a well-functioning chain-of-survival with specific strategies to improve quality of care during ALS and post-resuscitation care results in improved outcomes after OHCA. In order to continuously improve outcomes from cardiac arrest in any EMS system, attention should be paid to all aspects of the chain-of-survival. Resuscitation Outcomes Consortium Investigators in the USA showed in 2008 that the overall outcome for OHCA varied between 3–16 % for EMS systems with median response intervals of 7 minutes [40]. With a response interval of 9 minutes in Oslo, outcomes have moved from mid-range to top-end of this scale by improving the local chain-of-survival. Such system variations may make a huge impact on results from multicenter intervention clinical trials, and institutions should be encouraged to identify and improve weak links in their chain-of-survival to optimize quality of care before randomizing patients. Consensus on science, and future guidelines, are totally dependent on trials of good quality, with treatment of good quality along the chain-of-survival, to obtain the important answers we need with the final goal of getting more neurologically intact survivors back to a meaningful life. Nike's famous phrase should be remembered and used: "Just do it". But, importantly, the implementation strategy has to be predefined and carefully planned!

References

1. Atwood C, Eisenberg MS, Herlitz J, Rea TD (2005) Incidence of EMS-treated out-of-hospital cardiac arrest in Europe. Resuscitation 67:75–80
2. Berdowski J, Berg RA, Tijssen JG, Koster RW (2010) Global incidences of out-of-hospital cardiac arrest and survival rates: Systematic review of 67 prospective studies. Resuscitation 81:1479–1487

3. Cummins RO, Ornato JP, Thies WH, Pepe PE (1991) Improving survival from sudden cardiac arrest: the "chain of survival" concept. A statement for health professionals from the Advanced Cardiac Life Support Subcommittee and the Emergency Cardiac Care Committee, American Heart Association. Circulation 83:1832–1847
4. Jacobs I, Nadkarni V, Bahr J et al (2004) Cardiac arrest and cardiopulmonary resuscitation outcome reports: update and simplification of the Utstein templates for resuscitation registries: a statement for healthcare professionals from a task force of the International Liaison Committee on Resuscitation (American Heart Association, European Resuscitation Council, Australian Resuscitation Council, New Zealand Resuscitation Council, Heart and Stroke Foundation of Canada, InterAmerican Heart Foundation, Resuscitation Councils of Southern Africa). Circulation 110:3385–3397
5. Abella BS, Alvarado JP, Myklebust H et al (2005) Quality of cardiopulmonary resuscitation during in-hospital cardiac arrest. JAMA 293:305–310
6. Wik L, Kramer-Johansen J, Myklebust H et al (2005) Quality of cardiopulmonary resuscitation during out-of-hospital cardiac arrest. JAMA 293:299–304
7. Berdowski J, Schmohl A, Tijssen JG, Koster RW (2009) Time needed for a regional emergency medical system to implement resuscitation Guidelines 2005-The Netherlands experience. Resuscitation 80:1336–1341
8. Chamberlain DA, Hazinski MF (2003) Education in resuscitation. Resuscitation 59:11–43
9. Castrén M (2008) Pre-hospital airway management – time to provide the same standard of care as in the hospital. Acta Anaesthesiol Scand 52:877–878
10. Weinert CR, Mann HJ (2008) The science of implementation: changing the practice of critical care. Curr Opin Crit Care 14:460–465
11. Neumar RW, Barnhart JM, Berg RA et al (2011) Implementation strategies for improving survival after out-of-hospital cardiac arrest in the United States: consensus recommendations from the 2009 American Heart Association Cardiac Arrest Survival Summit. Circulation 123:2898–2910
12. Lund I, Skulberg A (1976) Cardiopulmonary resuscitation by lay people. Lancet 2:702–704
13. Sunde K, Eftestol T, Askenberg C, Steen PA (1999) Quality assessment of defibrillation and advanced life support using data from the medical control module of the defibrillator. Resuscitation 41:237–247
14. Naess AC, Steen PA (2004) Long term survival and costs per life year gained after out-of-hospital cardiac arrest. Resuscitation 60:57–64
15. Lund-Kordahl I, Olasveengen TM, Lorem T, Samdal M, Wik L, Sunde K (2010) Improving outcome after out-of-hospital cardiac arrest by strengthening weak links of the local Chain of Survival; quality of advanced life support and post-resuscitation care. Resuscitation 81:422–426
16. Advanced Life Support Working Party of the European Resuscitation Council (1992) Guidelines for advanced life support. Resuscitation 24:111–121
17. Anonymous (2000) Guidelines for cardiopulmonary resuscitation and emergency cardiovascular care – An international consensus on science. Resuscitation 46:3–437
18. Wik L, Hansen TB, Fylling F et al (2003) Delaying defibrillation to give basic cardiopulmonary resuscitation to patients with out-of-hospital ventricular fibrillation: a randomized trial. JAMA 289:1389–1395
19. Engdahl J, Abrahamsson P, Bång A, Lindqvist J, Karlsson T, Herlitz J (2000) Is hospital care of major importance for outcome after out-of-hospital cardiac arrest? Experience acquired from patients with out-of-hospital cardiac arrest resuscitated by the same Emergency Medical Service and admitted to one of two hospitals over a 16-year period in the municipality of Göteborg. Resuscitation 43:201–211
20. The Hypothermia After Cardiac Arrest (HACA) study group (2002) Mild TH to improve the neurologic outcome after cardiac arrest. N Engl J Med 346:549–556
21. Bernard SA, Gray TW, Buist MD et al (2002) Treatment of comatose survivors of out-of-hospital cardiac arrest with induced hypothermia. N Engl J Med 346:557–563

22. Langhelle A, Tyvold SS, Lexow K, Hapnes S, Sunde K, Steen PA (2003) In-hospital factors associated with improved outcome after out-of-hospital cardiac arrest. A comparison between four regions in Norway. Resuscitation 56:247–263
23. Herlitz J, Engdahl J, Svensson L, Angquist KA, Silfverstolpe J, Holmberg S (2006) Major differences in 1-month survival between hospitals in Sweden among initial survivors of out-of-hospital cardiac arrest. Resuscitation 70:404–409
24. Carr BG, Kahn JM, Merchant RM, Kramer AA, Neumar RW (2009) Inter-hospital variability in post-cardiac arrest mortality. Resuscitation 80:30–34
25. Kajino K, Iwami T, Daya M et al (2010) Impact of transport to critical care medical centers on outcomes after out-of-hospital cardiac arrest. Resuscitation 81:549–554
26. Wnent J, Seewald S, Heringlake M et al (2012) Choice of hospital after out-of-hospital cardiac arrest – a decision with far reaching consequences – a study in a large German city. Crit Care 16:R164
27. Sunde K, Pytte M, Jacobsen D et al (2007) Implementation of a standardised treatment protocol for post resuscitation care after out-of-hospital cardiac arrest. Resuscitation 73:29–39
28. Tømte O, Andersen GØ, Jacobsen D, Drægni T, Auestad B, Sunde K (2011) Strong and weak aspects of an established post-resuscitation treatment protocol-A five-year observational study. Resuscitation 82:1186–1193
29. Olasveengen TM, Wik L, Kramer-Johansen J, Sunde K, Pytte M, Steen PA (2007) Is CPR quality improving? A retrospective study of out-of-hospital cardiac arrest. Resuscitation 75:260–266
30. Olasveengen TM, Vik E, Kuzovlev A, Sunde K (2009) Effect of implementation of new resuscitation guidelines on quality of cardiopulmonary resuscitation and survival. Resuscitation 80:407–411
31. Stiell IG, Wells GA, Field B et al (2004) Advanced Cardiac Life Support in Out-of-Hospital Cardiac Arrest. N Engl J Med 351:647–656
32. Olasveengen TM, Sunde K, Brunborg C, Thowsen J, Steen PA, Wik L (2009) Intravenous drug administration during out-of-hospital cardiac arrest: a randomized trial. JAMA 302:2222–2229
33. Deakin CD, Nolan JP, Soar J et al (2011) European Resuscitation Council Guidelines for Resuscitation 2010 Section 4. Adult advanced life support Resuscitation 81:1305–1352
34. Nolan JP, Lyon RM, Sasson C et al (2012) Advances in the hospital management of patients following an out of hospital cardiac arrest. Heart 98:1201–1206
35. Becker L, Gold LS, Eisenberg M, White L, Hearne T, Rea T (2008) Ventricular fibrillation in King County, Washington: A 30-year perspective. Resuscitation 79:22–27
36. Iwami T, Nichol G, Hiraide A et al (2009) Continuous improvements in "chain of survival" increased survival after out-of-hospital cardiac arrests: a large-scale population-based study. Circulation 119:728–734
37. Møller Nielsen A, Lou Isbye D, Knudsen Lippert F, Rasmussen LS (2012) Engaging a whole community in resuscitation. Resuscitation 83:1067–1071
38. Lick CJ, Aufderheide TP, Niskanen RA et al (2011) Take Heart America: A comprehensive, community-wide, systems-based approach to the treatment of cardiac arrest. Crit Care Med 39:26–33
39. Lindner TW, Søreide E, Nilsen OB, Torunn MW, Lossius HM (2011) Good outcome in every fourth resuscitation attempt is achievable – an Utstein template report from the Stavanger region. Resuscitation 82:1508–1513
40. Nichol G, Thomas E, Callaway CW et al (2008) Regional variation in out-of-hospital cardiac arrest incidence and outcome. JAMA 300:1423–1431

Stent Choice in Patients Undergoing Primary Percutaneous Coronary Intervention

G. Biondi-Zoccai, M. Peruzzi, and G. Frati

Introduction

Acute myocardial infarction (AMI) due to persistent ST-segment elevation or new left bundle branch block represents the most severe form of acute coronary syndrome, and a true medical emergency. Despite its historically ominous prognosis, ongoing developments in the delivery of care, reperfusion techniques, available medical devices and ancillary pharmacologic therapy have brought remarkable improvements in the prognosis of these patients. Indeed, whereas 21-day mortality was 13 % in the placebo arm of the 1986 landmark Gruppo Italiano per lo Studio della Streptochinasi nell'Infarto Miocardico (GISSI) study [1], it can now be as low as 3.5 % at 1 year in patients managed according to state-of-the-art care, such as in the Everolimus-eluting stent vs. bare-metal stent in ST-segment elevation myocardial infarction (EXAMINATION) trial [2].

Despite such major improvements, several questions remain as to the most appropriate combination of devices and drugs to maximize timely reperfusion while minimizing the risk of early or late adverse events.

G. Biondi-Zoccai (✉)
Department of Medico-Surgical Sciences and Biotechnologies, Sapienza University of Rome, Corso della Repubblica 79, 04100 Latina, Italy
E-mail: giuseppe.biondizoccai@uniroma1.it

M. Peruzzi
Department of Medico-Surgical Sciences and Biotechnologies, Sapienza University of Rome, Corso della Repubblica 79, 04100 Latina, Italy

G. Frati
Department of Medico-Surgical Sciences and Biotechnologies, Sapienza University of Rome, Corso della Repubblica 79, 04100 Latina, Italy

J.-L. Vincent (Ed.), *Annual Update in Intensive Care and Emergency Medicine 2013*,
DOI 10.1007/978-3-642-35109-9_25,

Scope of the Problem and Evidence in Favor of Coronary Stents

Percutaneous coronary intervention (PCI) is well established as the most effective and safe reperfusion means in patients with ST-elevation myocardial infarction (STEMI), when this procedure can be performed within 120 minutes from symptom onset and even more so if radial access can be employed [3, 4]. Indeed, in a comprehensive meta-analysis of 23 randomized trials, Keeley et al. [3] showed that percutaneous revascularization was associated with a significantly lower risk of death or major adverse cardiac events in such patients in comparison to fibrin-specific or non-fibrin-specific thrombolytic agents.

Whereas PCI once entailed only, or mainly, percutaneous transluminal coronary angioplasty (PTCA), it is now routinely based on concomitant stent implantation [5]. As demonstrated extensively by Nordmann and colleagues [5], even in patients with STEMI, routine bare-metal stent implantation is associated with a lower 12-month risk of reinfarction (odds ratio = 0.67 [95 % confidence interval 0.45–0.99]) and repeat revascularization (odds ratio = 0.48 [0.39–0.59]).

The introduction of first-generation drug-eluting stents in 2002 revolutionized the care of patients with stable coronary artery disease, and soon the question of the risk-benefit balance of drug-eluting stents in comparison to bare-metal stents even in the setting of STEMI became important. Why is this clinical setting so peculiar and potentially hazardous for drug-eluting devices? Of course, the culprit lesions of patients with STEMI are highly active atherosclerotic plaques with a major potential for recurrent thrombosis and further plaque activation. Moreover, the ubiquitous presence of red and/or white thrombus makes these lesions much more likely than stable coronary lesions to be associated with acute, subacute, late, and very late stent thrombosis. Therefore, routine use of drug-eluting stents in such a prothrombotic milieu in order to minimize the risk of re-stenosis and repeat revascularization has often been challenged as too hazardous.

Comparison Between Bare-Metal and Drug-Eluting Stents

First-generation stents include by convention sirolimus-eluting stents (Cypher, Cordis, Miami, FL, USA) and paclitaxel-eluting stents (Taxus, Boston Scientific, Natick, MA, USA), with the possible addition of zotarolimus-eluting stents (Endeavor, Medtronic, MN, USA). They have proved remarkably effective in selected patients and lesions [6], but their safety, even in uncomplicated patients and lesions, has been repeatedly questioned [7, 8]. Only recently, were Palmerini et al. able to disprove the safety threat potentially posed by drug-eluting stents [9].

A few years after their approval in short and simple lesions of subjects without severe coronary instability, first-generation drug-eluting stents were formally compared with bare-metal stents in patients with STEMI [10]. In their comprehensive patient-level analysis including 11 randomized trials and 6,298 patients focusing only on sirolimus- or paclitaxel-eluting stents, De Luca et al. [10] showed that first-generation drug-eluting stents led to significantly lower 3-year rates of repeat revascularization (hazard ratio = 0.57 [0.50–0.66]) without any statistically significant increase in the risk of all cause death, recurrent myocardial infarction, or overall stent thrombosis in comparison to bare-metal stents. Conversely, drug-eluting stents were associated with a significantly higher risk of very late (> 1 year) stent thrombosis and reinfarction. Thus, although the overall safety and efficacy of such devices can be considered established, long-term safety remains incompletely appraised. Accordingly, duration and intensity of dual antiplatelet therapy in these patients receiving first-generation drug-eluting stents continues to be individualized to minimize bleeding risk while maximizing anti-thrombotic effects [11, 12].

Second-Generation Drug-Eluting Stents

The introduction of second- or new-generation drug-eluting stents has been welcomed as a major development in the management of patients with coronary artery disease, under the premises that these devices may maintain the anti-restenotic effect of first-generation devices while providing a lower risk of thrombosis. Among second-generation devices, we may include biolimus-eluting stents (Biomatrix, Biosensors, Singapore; Nobori, Terumo, Tokyo, Japan), everolimus-eluting stents (Promus or Promus Element, Boston Scientific; Xience, Abbott Vascular, Santa Clara, CA, USA), and second-generation zotarolimus-eluting stents (Resolute, Medtronic, Minneapolis, MN, USA).

A limited number of studies have appraised the risk-benefit balance of these devices in subjects with STEMI, but important data have been provided by the COMPARE [13], RESOLUTE All Comers [14], LEADERS [15], and COMFORTABLE AMI trials [16]. Moreover, the comprehensive review by Palmerini et al., including several trials focusing on such patients, is also crucial for informed decision-making (Table 1) [9].

Specifically, the comparison of the everolimus eluting Xience-V stent with the paclitaxel eluting Taxus Liberté stent trial (COMPARE) demonstrated the superiority of everolimus-eluting stents in comparison to paclitaxel-eluting stents in a large cohort of unselected and real-world patients, including 452 subjects with STEMI [13]. In this specific set of patients, everolimus-eluting stents reduced the risk of death, myocardial infarction and repeat revascularization, but also the risk of stent thrombosis (relative risk = 0.30 [0.12–0.73], p = 0.005).

The RESOLUTE All Comers trial included 2,292 patients with coronary artery disease, and randomized them to second-generation zotarolimus-eluting stents or everolimus-eluting stents [14]. As many as 29 % of these subjects had AMI as an admission diagnosis. Notably, clinical events occurred up to 2 years with a similar frequency in both groups in overall analyses, with the notable exception of definite stent thrombosis, which was less common in patients receiving everolimus-eluting stents (0.3 % vs. 1.2 % at 12 months, p = 0.01). Findings in the AMI subgroup were largely in agreement with those stemming from the overall analysis.

Table 1 Risk* of stent thrombosis with different drug-eluting stents (DES) in comparison to bare-metal stents (modified from [9])

Device	Definite stent thrombosis			Definite or probable stent thrombosis		
	Early	Late (>1 month)	Cumulative at 1 year	Early	Late (>1 month)	Cumulative at 1 year
1st-generation DES						
PES	0.79 (0.49–1.27)	1.09 (0.44–2.48)	0.83 (0.54–1.22)	0.83 (0.50–1.35)	1.25 (0.62–2.61)	0.82 (0.55–1.17)
SES	0.54 (0.30–0.90)	0.50 (0.18–1.25)	0.57 (0.36–0.88)	0.46 (0.26–0.79)	0.51 (0.22–1.09)	0.50 (0.32–0.72)
PC-ZES	0.97 (0.47–2.04)	2.01 (0.50–9.09)	1.09 (0.58–2.13)	1.17 (0.53–2.72)	2.10 (0.60–9.20)	1.13 (0.60–2.11)
2nd-generation DES						
Bio-linx-ZES	3.08 (0.40–78.96)	1.32 (0.16–14.32)	1.71 (0.43–9.27)	0.32 (0.09–0.99)	1.70 (0.33–10.83)	0.53 (0.21–1.26)
EES	0.21 (0.11–0.42)	0.27 (0.08–0.74)	0.23 (0.13–0.41)	0.32 (0.17–0.60)	0.42 (0.17–0.95)	0.34 (0.21–0.53)

*reported as odds ratios (95 % credible intervals), with odds ratios > 1 favoring bare-metal stents. Biolinx-ZES: Biolinx-coated (second-generation) zotarolimus-eluting stent; EES: everolimus-eluting stent; PC-ZES: phosphorylcholine-coated (first-generation) zotarolimus-eluting stent; PES: paclitaxel-eluting stent; SES: sirolimus-eluting stent

The Limus Eluted from A Durable vs. ERodable Stent coating (LEADERS) trial compared biolimus-eluting stents with a bioresorbable polymer vs. sirolimus-eluting stents with a permanent polymer in 1,707 unselected patients with coronary artery disease, 16 % of whom had STEMI [15]. Biolimus-eluting stents were associated with a similar rate of adverse events in comparison to sirolimus-eluting stents, but tended to have a remarkably lower risk of definite stent thrombosis at 2 years (2 % vs. 4 %, p = 0.09).

Finally, the Comparison of Biolimus Eluted From an Erodible Stent Coating With Bare Metal Stents in Acute ST-Elevation Myocardial Infarction (COMFORTABLE AMI) trial included 1,161 patients with STEMI, randomizing them to biolimus-eluting stents or bare-metal stents [16]. As expected, biolimus-eluting stents reduced the risk of the composite end-point of death, recurrent myocardial infarction or repeat revascularization. However, these devices led to an unexpected reduction in the risk of target-vessel reinfarction (hazard ratio = 0.20 [0.06–0.69], p = 0.01) and a strong trend toward fewer stent thromboses (hazard ratio = 0.42 [0.15–1.19], p = 0.10).

Reconciling the Evidence

The comprehensive network meta-analysis by Palmerini and colleagues [9], pooling data from 49 randomized clinical trials and 50,844 patients, offers a unique opportunity to summarize all the evidence regarding the safety and, together with the work from Bangalore et al. [17, 18], the efficacy of drug-eluting stents. Specifically, Palmerini et al. included trials comparing bare-metal stents with everolimus-, paclitaxel-, sirolimus-, and zotarolimus-eluting stents. Moreover, 9 trials focused only on patients with STEMI, whereas many others were real-world pragmatic trials (thus also including such high-risk subjects). Bayesian analyses based on Markov chain Monte Carlo (MCMC) estimation methods enabled the computation of detailed data regarding definite stent thrombosis, and definite/probable stent thrombosis at different time points (early [< 1 month], late [> 1 month], at 1 year, very late [> 1 year], and at 2 years). Analyses showed that, across the board, everolimus-eluting stents were the safest drug-eluting stents available, even when including second-generation devices in the analyses. However, the truly paradigm-shifting finding was that everolimus-eluting stents were associated with a lower rate of stent thrombosis in comparison to bare-metal stents (Table 1), with

Table 2 Pros and cons of different coronary stents in patients undergoing primary percutaneous coronary intervention

Device	Risk of				Ease of use	Cost	Safety with short-term DAPT
	TLR/TVR	MI	Death	ST			
BMSs	+	+/–	+/–	+/–	+	–	+
1st-generation DES							
PES	+/–	+/–	+/–	+/–	+/–	+/–	–
SES	–	+/–	+/–	+/–	+/–	+/–	–
PC–ZES	+/–	+/–	+/–	+/–	+/–	+/–	–
2nd-generation DES							
AES	–	+/–	+/–	+/–	+/–	+	–
BES	–	+/–	–	+/–	+/–	+	–
Biolinx-ZES	–	+/–	+/–	+/–	+/–	+	–
EES	–	–	+/–	–	+/–	+	+/–

+: high; +/–: average; –: low; AES: amphilimus-eluting stent; BES: biolimus-eluting stent; BMS: bare-metal stent; Biolinx-ZES: Biolinx-coated (second-generation) zotarolimus-eluting stent; DAPT: dual antiplatelet therapy; DES: drug-eluting stent; EES: everolimus-eluting stent; MI: myocardial infarction; PC-ZES: phosphorylcholine-coated (first-generation) zotarolimus-eluting stent; PES: paclitaxel-eluting stent; SES: sirolimus-eluting stent; ST: stent thrombosis; TLR: target lesion revascularization; TVR: target vessel revascularization clear statistical evidence of such an unprecedented effect as early as after only 1 month, and as late as after 2 years of follow-up. Despite these apparently surprising results, some pathophysiologic explanations are available. Indeed, a number of important *in vitro* or animal studies have suggested that the polymers (poly n-butyl methacrylate, vinylidene fluoride, and hexafluoropropylene), the drug (everolimus), or their combination may exert beneficial antithrombotic and plaque silencing effects [19–21]. Specifically, Kolandaivelu et al. suggested that the combination of thin-strut design and proprietary polymer coating reduced thrombus deposition in an *in vitro* model of coronary stenting [19]. Conversely, Verheye et al. [20] and Van Dyck and colleagues [21] provided evidence from atherosclerotic animal models that stents coated with everolimus promote macrophage autophagy in atherosclerotic plaques and reduce the extent of peri-strut inflammation.

In keeping with these astonishing results supporting the safety of everolimus-eluting stents and the predictable anti-restenotic efficacy of these devices [17, 18], such drug-eluting stents represent the therapeutic choice with the most favorable risk-benefit balance for patients with STEMI requiring PCI and eligible for dual antiplatelet therapy for at least 3 months (Table 2).

Avenues for Future Research and Practice

Despite the plethora of studies already conducted on coronary stents that have included patients with AMI, several questions remain unanswered. Indeed, the belief that a drug-eluting stent with a totally bioresorbable polymer might be safer than a device with a permanent polymer is shared by many clinicians and researchers [22]. Only dedicated and suitably sized randomized trials and network meta-analyses will be able to address this issue.

The future widespread availability and ensuing adoption of bioresorbable vascular scaffolds may change completely the way we treat patients with coronary artery disease in general and those with STEMI in particular. [23] However, the evidence base in favor or against these hitherto unprecedented devices is even more limited than the evidence base regarding stents with bioresorbable polymers. Accordingly, only time will tell if these scaffolds will be able to become workhorse devices and whether their use will translate into meaningful clinical benefits for real-world patients.

Conclusion

The management of STEMI has changed dramatically during the last few decades thanks to concomitant improvements in medical therapy and developments in mechanical reperfusion [24]. Bare-metal stents and drug-eluting stents are now commonplace in the treatment of culprit and non-culprit lesions of these patients.

Whereas individualization of treatment remains the safest and most effective management strategy, we believe that patients without a high bleeding risk and likely to continue dual antiplatelet therapy for 3 or more months after transradial primary PCI are best served by everolimus-eluting stent implantation and concomitant antiplatelet therapy for 3 or more months with aspirin plus either prasugrel or ticagrelor [12, 25–28]. Combining biolimus-eluting stenting with 6 months or more of dual antiplatelet therapy also appears to be a promising treatment choice.

References

1. Gruppo Italiano per lo Studio della Streptochinasi nell'Infarto Miocardico (GISSI) (1986) Effectiveness of intravenous thrombolytic treatment in acute myocardial infarction. Lancet 1:397–402
2. Sabate M, Cequier A, Iñiguez A, et al (2012) Everolimus-eluting stent versus bare-metal stent in ST-segment elevation myocardial infarction (EXAMINATION): 1 year results of a randomised controlled trial. Lancet 380:1482–1490
3. Keeley EC, Boura JA, Grines CL (2003) Primary angioplasty versus intravenous thrombolytic therapy for acute myocardial infarction: a quantitative review of 23 randomised trials. Lancet 361:13–20
4. Romagnoli E, Biondi-Zoccai G, Sciahbasi A, et al (2012) Radial versus femoral randomized investigation in ST-segment elevation acute coronary syndrome: The RIFLE-STEACS (Radial Versus Femoral Randomized Investigation in ST-Elevation Acute Coronary Syndrome) Study. J Am Coll Cardiol 60:2481–2489
5. Nordmann AJ, Hengstler P, Harr T, Young J, Bucher HC (2004) Clinical outcomes of primary stenting versus balloon angioplasty in patients with myocardial infarction: a meta-analysis of randomized controlled trials. Am J Med 116:253–262
6. Hill RA, Dündar Y, Bakhai A, Dickson R, Walley T (2004) Drug-eluting stents: an early systematic review to inform policy. Eur Heart J 25:902–919
7. Nordmann AJ, Briel M, Bucher HC (2006) Mortality in randomized controlled trials comparing drug-eluting vs. bare metal stents in coronary artery disease: a meta-analysis. Eur Heart J 27:2784–2814
8. Camenzind E, Steg PG, Wijns W (2007) Stent thrombosis late after implantation of first-generation drug-eluting stents: a cause for concern. Circulation 115:1440–1455
9. Palmerini T, Biondi-Zoccai G, Della Riva D et al (2012) Stent thrombosis with drug-eluting and bare-metal stents: evidence from a comprehensive network meta-analysis. Lancet 379:1393–1402
10. De Luca G, Dirksen MT, Spaulding C et al (2012) Drug-eluting vs bare-metal stents in primary angioplasty: a pooled patient-level meta-analysis of randomized trials. Arch Intern Med 172:611–621
11. Biondi-Zoccai GG, Lotrionte M, Agostoni P et al (2006) A systematic review and meta-analysis on the hazards of discontinuing or not adhering to aspirin among 50,279 patients at risk for coronary artery disease. Eur Heart J 27:2667–2674
12. Biondi-Zoccai G, Lotrionte M, Agostoni P et al (2011) Adjusted indirect comparison meta-analysis of prasugrel versus ticagrelor for patients with acute coronary syndromes. Int J Cardiol 150:325–331
13. Kedhi E, Gomes M, Joesoef KS et al (2012) Everolimus-eluting stents and paclitaxel-eluting stents in patients presenting with myocardial infarction: insights from the two-year results of the COMPARE prospective randomised controlled trial. EuroIntervention 7:1376–1385

14. Silber S, Windecker S, Vranckx P, Serruys PW (2011) Unrestricted randomised use of two new generation drug-eluting coronary stents: 2-year patient-related versus stent-related outcomes from the RESOLUTE All Comers trial. Lancet 377:1241–1247
15. Stefanini GG, Kalesan B, Serruys PW et al (2011) Long-term clinical outcomes of biodegradable polymer biolimus-eluting stents versus durable polymer sirolimus-eluting stents in patients with coronary artery disease (LEADERS): 4 year follow-up of a randomised non-inferiority trial. Lancet 378:1940–1948
16. Räber L, Kelbæk H, Ostoijc M et al (2012) Effect of biolimus-eluting stents with biodegradable polymer vs bare-metal stents on cardiovascular events among patients with acute myocardial infarction: the COMFORTABLE AMI randomized trial. JAMA 308:777–787
17. Bangalore S, Kumar S, Fusaro M et al (2012) Short- and long-term outcomes with drug-eluting and bare-metal coronary stents: a mixed-treatment comparison analysis of 117,762 patient-years of follow-up from randomized trials. Circulation 125:2873–2891
18. Bangalore S, Kumar S, Fusaro M et al (2012) Outcomes with various drug eluting or bare metal stents in patients with diabetes mellitus: mixed treatment comparison analysis of 22,844 patient years of follow-up from randomised trials. BMJ 345:e5170
19. Kolandaivelu K, Swaminathan R, Gibson WJ et al (2012) Stent thrombogenicity early in high-risk interventional settings is driven by stent design and deployment and protected by polymer-drug coatings. Circulation 123:1400–1409
20. Verheye S, Martinet W, Kockx MM et al (2007) Selective clearance of macrophages in atherosclerotic plaques by autophagy. J Am Coll Cardiol 49:706–715
21. Van Dyck CJ, Hoymans VY, Bult H, et al (2013) Resolute® and xience V® polymer-based drug-eluting stents compared in an atherosclerotic rabbit double injury model. Catheter Cardiovasc Interv (in press)
22. Meredith IT, Verheye S, Dubois CL et al (2012) Primary endpoint results of the EVOLVE trial: a randomized evaluation of a novel bioabsorbable polymer-coated, everolimus-eluting coronary stent. J Am Coll Cardiol 59:1362–1370
23. Brugaletta S, Heo JH, Garcia-Garcia HM et al (2012) Endothelial-dependent vasomotion in a coronary segment treated by ABSORB everolimus-eluting bioresorbable vascular scaffold system is related to plaque composition at the time of bioresorption of the polymer: indirect finding of vascular reparative therapy? Eur Heart J 33:1325–1333
24. Puymirat E, Simon T, Steg PG et al (2012) Association of changes in clinical characteristics and management with improvement in survival among patients with ST-elevation myocardial infarction. JAMA 308:998–1006
25. Alexopoulos D, Galati A, Xanthopoulou I et al (2012) Ticagrelor versus prasugrel in acute coronary syndrome patients with high on-clopidogrel platelet reactivity following percutaneous coronary intervention: a pharmacodynamic study. J Am Coll Cardiol 60:193–199
26. Montalescot G, Wiviott SD, Braunwald E et al (2009) Prasugrel compared with clopidogrel in patients undergoing percutaneous coronary intervention for ST-elevation myocardial infarction (TRITON-TIMI 38): double-blind, randomised controlled trial. Lancet 373:723–731
27. Cannon CP, Harrington RA, James S et al (2010) Comparison of ticagrelor with clopidogrel in patients with a planned invasive strategy for acute coronary syndromes (PLATO): a randomised double-blind study. Lancet 375:283–293
28. Steg PG, James SK, Atar D, et al (2012) ESC Guidelines for the management of acute myocardial infarction in patients presenting with ST-segment elevation: The Task Force on the management of ST-segment elevation acute myocardial infarction of the European Society of Cardiology (ESC). Eur Heart J 33:2569–2619

Cardiac Index During Therapeutic Hypothermia: Which Target Value Is Optimal?

R. Giraud, N. Siegenthaler, and K. Bendjelid

Introduction

Mild therapeutic hypothermia is now recognized as standard therapy in patients resuscitated from out-of-hospital cardiac arrest (OHCA), and is recommended in comatose patients suffering from cardiac arrest related to ventricular fibrillation (VF) [1]. In these patients, maintaining an adequate tissue oxygen delivery (DO_2) is crucial. However, during hypothermia, clinical signs of hypoperfusion such as cold, clammy skin and delayed capillary refill are not reliable and monitoring devices must, therefore, be used to measure or estimate the cardiac index (CI). However, there are no recommendations regarding the target value of CI in the hypothermic patient. In this article, the authors attempt to provide clinicians with some rationale to guide their therapy for the management of CI in patients treated with mild therapeutic hypothermia.

Mild Therapeutic Hypothermia

Neurologic outcome and survival rates are improved in patients treated with mild therapeutic hypothermia [2, 3]. The reason for the improved survival is probably

R. Giraud
Intensive Care Service, Geneva University Hospitals, 4 Rue Gabrielle Perret-Gentil, CH-1211 Geneva 14, Switzerland

N. Siegenthaler
Intensive Care Service, Geneva University Hospitals, 4 Rue Gabrielle Perret-Gentil, CH-1211 Geneva 14, Switzerland

K. Bendjelid (✉)
Intensive Care Service, Geneva University Hospitals, 4 Rue Gabrielle Perret-Gentil, CH-1211 Geneva 14, Switzerland
E-mail: karim.bendjelid@hcuge.ch

J.-L. Vincent (Ed.), *Annual Update in Intensive Care and Emergency Medicine 2013*,
DOI 10.1007/978-3-642-35109-9_26, © Springer-Verlag Berlin Heidelberg and BioMed Central Ltd. 2013

related to the preservation of cerebral function. During mild therapeutic hypothermia, clinical data demonstrate that heart rate is significantly reduced, an effect that usually improves left ventricular (LV) filling [4]. Whereas CI usually decreases with hypothermia, mild therapeutic hypothermia exerts positive inotropic effects in isolated human and pig myocardium. The phenomenon of increased inotropism during mild therapeutic hypothermia is not associated with increased sarcoplasmic reticulum Ca^{2+}-content or increased Ca^{2+}-transients [5]. Moreover, recent studies using animal species and in humans have provided accumulating evidence suggesting that mild therapeutic hypothermia may also improve cardiac performance [5, 6]. Therefore, the higher survival rates may also be related to positive hemodynamic effects of cooling in patients already suffering from cardiac disease. Furthermore, a study about the hemodynamic effects of mild therapeutic hypothermia in 20 consecutive patients admitted in cardiogenic shock after successful resuscitation from OHCA showed that these patients seemed to benefit from mild therapeutic hypothermia in terms of myocardial performance, catecholamine usage, and survival when compared to a historic control group of matched patients treated without hypothermia [7]. Moreover, animal studies have shown that, in myocardial infarction, hypothermia decreases oxygen consumption and infarct size [8]. The positive inotropic effect of mild therapeutic hypothermia measured by systolic function has also been demonstrated in *in vivo* studies [5, 9] and can be measured echocardiographically by the significant increase in ejection fraction (EF) and the augmented contraction velocity measured by pulse contour analysis. However, as shown by Lewis et al., increasing the heartrate (HR) under hypothermic conditions has a negative impact on LV contractility [9]. Although systolic performance is clearly improved at all temperature steps investigated, pronounced hypothermia may impair diastolic function [10]. However, in the temperature range recommended for mild therapeutic hypothermia in cardiac arrest patients (32–34 °C) [11, 12], diastolic function seems to be preserved [6]. Although mild therapeutic hypothermia may have direct repercussions on the myocardium, a study by Bernard et al. showed no clinically significant effect on cardiac arrhythmias in the hypothermia group [13].

Which CI Target Value Is Optimal in Hypothermic Patients

In order to maintain perfusion pressure and as a result of hypothermia, the systemic vascular resistance (SVR) increases. As a result, mean arterial pressure (MAP) decreases only slightly with mild therapeutic hypothermia despite a significant decrease in CI. This reaction to hypothermia is explained by the vasoconstriction of peripheral arteries and arterioles [14] and the stabilization of MAP reducing the vasopressor dosage. Furthermore, the need for volume in mild therapeutic hypothermia can be explained by the induction of 'cold diuresis' through a combination of increased venous return (vasoconstriction), activation of atrial natriuretic peptide, decreased levels of antidiuretic hormone and renal antidiuretic hormone receptor levels, and tubular dysfunction [15, 16].

There is considerable confusion about the standard of care for critically ill patients undergoing mild therapeutic hypothermia, in particular related to the subject of hemodynamic optimization. For example, for many years it was commonly taught that although the patient's body temperature decreases, CI values should be as normal as those of normothermic patients. However, although a significant decrease in CI may lead to inadequate organ perfusion in normothermic patients, Bergman et al. failed to demonstrate that a low cardiac output caused lower mixed venous oxygen saturation (SvO_2) in patients undergoing mild therapeutic hypothermia [17]. This suggests that, parallel to the drop in CI, oxygen consumption decreases also because of the lower body temperature. In other words, during mild therapeutic hypothermia, the workload for the heart may be lower because of the lower resting energy metabolism required at a lower body temperature [17]. In fact, the overall metabolic rate decreases by approximately 8 % per °C amounting to a decrease of 32 % when the target temperature of 33 °C is reached, thus oxygen consumption and CO_2 production are reduced. This effect holds true for the heart itself, in which the diminished heart rate reduces the metabolic demand even further. In addition, mild therapeutic hypothermia induces coronary vasodilatation and increases myocardial perfusion [18]. This belief is corroborated by the fact that under cardiopulmonary bypass (CPB), a technique performed with moderate systemic hypothermia (28 to 32 °C), blood flow and CI are maintained between 2.2 and 2.4 l/min/m^2, without detrimental effects.

Bohr Effects During Alpha- and Ph-Stat Hypothermia

During hypothermia, SvO_2 measurement depends on the blood gas analysis technique (alpha-stat, pH-stat) used and the impact of the decrease in temperature on the affinity of hemoglobin for oxygen (Bohr Effect). Indeed, whether a pH-stat or alpha-stat strategy is the ideal acid-base management during severe hypothermic circulatory arrest has been the subject of contention. Advocates of pH-stat management (which aims for a partial pressure of CO_2 [PCO_2] of 40 mm Hg and pH of 7.40 at the patient's actual temperature) claim that the resulting higher CO_2 causes cerebral vasodilatation and faster and more homogeneous cooling. They also suggest that the resulting acidotic protocol of this acid-base management facilitates the release of oxygen from hemoglobin, a fact that offsets the hypothermic leftward shift of the oxygen dissociation curve (Bohr Effect). On the other hand, proponents of alpha-stat management, in which there is an alkaline drift during hypothermia, state that this allows cerebral auto-regulation to continue and that cellular transmembrane pH gradients and protein function are maintained. Indeed, when alpha-stat pH management is used, the PCO_2 decreases (and solubility increases); thus a hypothermic patient with a pH of 7.40 and an arterial PCO_2 of 40 mm Hg (measured at 37 °C) will, in reality, have a lower $PaCO_2$ and this will manifest as a relative respiratory alkalosis coupled with decreased cerebral blood flow. In addition, the alkaline pH improves cerebral protection during the ischemic insult. However, there is evidence to suggest that the best technique for acid-base management in patients undergoing deep hypothermic circulatory arrest during cardiac surgery is also dependent upon the age of the patient with better results using alpha-stat in the adult than in the pediatric patient [19].

What Exactly Does SvO_2 Mean During Mild Therapeutic Hypothermia?

Although mild therapeutic hypothermia induces a decrease in both HR and CI, in the majority of cases SvO_2 value remains stable (Fig. 1). However, during this condition there is sometimes an increase in systemic arterial lactate levels and it is unclear whether this is caused by increased anaerobic metabolism. The pathogenesis of this disorder is uncertain, but it appears not to relate to inadequate DO_2 [20]. Therefore, the use of inotropic drugs in order to increase CI to 'normal' values may be futile or even harmful because of its negative impact on LV contractility,

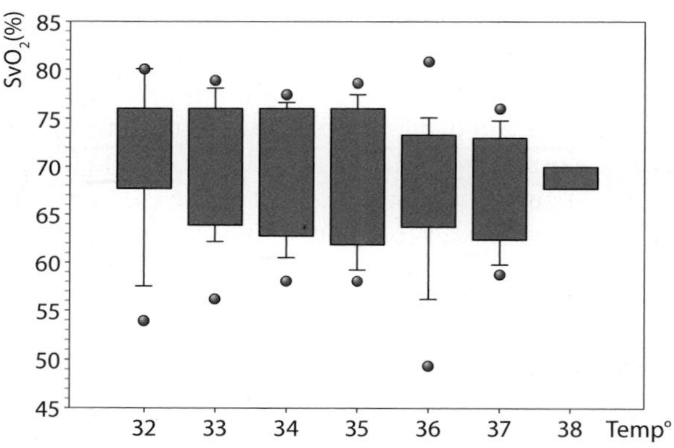

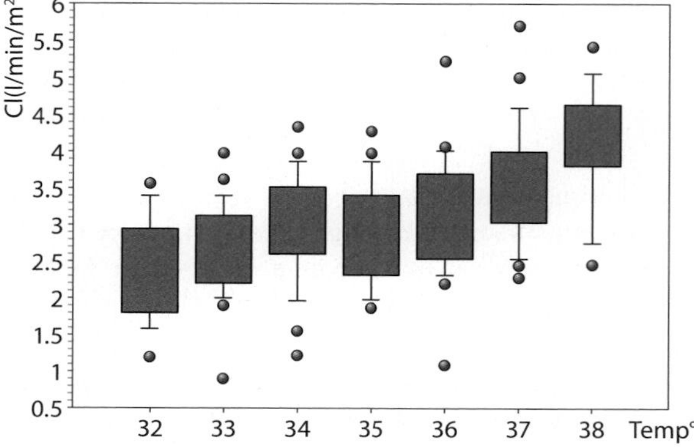

Fig. 1 Effects of temperature level on cardiac index (CI) and mixed venous oxygen saturation (SvO_2) values in 27 patients undergoing mild therapeutic hypothermia (alpha-Stat management. Bendjelid et al., unpublished data). Please note that a continuous decrease in CI is not associated with the same decrease in SvO_2 values

ventricular arrhythmias and increase in oxygen uptake (VO_2). The best indicator of good tissue perfusion in patients undergoing mild therapeutic hypothermia seems to be SvO_2 and not CI. However, another misconception arises from the relatively large differences between SvO_2 values measured in patients undergoing the alpha-stat and the pH-stat acid-base management. Indeed, oxygen extraction is decreased during mild therapeutic hypothermia as the oxyhemoglobin dissociation curve shifts left (Bohr Effect). And, the increased oxygen affinity of hemoglobin during this hypothermic state could also be aggravated by the alkalotic environment (oxyhemoglobin dissociation curve shifts left; Bohr Effect) produced by the alpha-stat method, to the point of developing tissue hypoxia [21]. In this sense, SvO_2 monitoring could be a valuable tool to optimize DO_2 in the hypothermic patient, where the optimal value of SvO_2 is adjusted according to the acid-base management of blood gas measurements.

Conclusion

Although mild therapeutic hypothermia is now recognized as the standard therapy in patients resuscitated from OHCA, optimal target CI values are not clear. However, based on the pathophysiology of the effects of hypothermia, it is possible to find answers regarding the hemodynamic management of these patients. Indeed, it seems futile and even dangerous to try to normalize CI to 'normal' values. However, it does seem appropriate to monitor SvO_2 values and arterial lactate levels in these patients, taking into account the impact of hypothermia and acid-base management on the oxyhemoglobin dissociation curve.

References

1. Arrich J, Holzer M, Herkner H, Mullner M (2009) Hypothermia for neuroprotection in adults after cardiopulmonary resuscitation. Cochrane Database Syst Rev CD004128
2. The Hypothermia after Cardiac Arrest Study Group (2002) Mild therapeutic hypothermia to improve the neurologic outcome after cardiac arrest. N Engl J Med 346:549–556
3. Holzer M, Bernard SA, Hachimi-Idrissi S, Roine RO, Sterz F, Mullner M (2005) Hypothermia for neuroprotection after cardiac arrest: systematic review and individual patient data meta-analysis. Crit Care Med 33:414–418
4. Reil JC, Bohm M (2007) The role of heart rate in the development of cardiovascular disease. Clin Res Cardiol 96:585–592
5. Weisser J, Martin J, Bisping E et al (2001) Influence of mild hypothermia on myocardial contractility and circulatory function. Basic Res Cardiol 96:198–205
6. Jacobshagen C, Pelster T, Pax A et al (2010) Effects of mild hypothermia on hemodynamics in cardiac arrest survivors and isolated failing human myocardium. Clin Res Cardiol 99:267–276
7. Zobel C, Adler C, Kranz A et al (2012) Mild therapeutic hypothermia in cardiogenic shock syndrome. Crit Care Med 40:1715–1723

8. Miki T, Liu GS, Cohen MV, Downey JM (1998) Mild hypothermia reduces infarct size in the beating rabbit heart: a practical intervention for acute myocardial infarction? Basic Res Cardiol 93:372–383
9. Lewis ME, Al-Khalidi AH, Townend JN, Coote J, Bonser RS (2002) The effects of hypothermia on human left ventricular contractile function during cardiac surgery. J Am Coll Cardiol 39:102–108
10. Fischer UM, Cox Jr. CS, Laine GA, Mehlhorn U, Allen SJ (2005) Mild hypothermia impairs left ventricular diastolic but not systolic function. J Invest Surg 18:291–296
11. Neumar RW, Nolan JP, Adrie C et al (2008) Post-cardiac arrest syndrome: epidemiology, pathophysiology, treatment, and prognostication. A consensus statement from the International Liaison Committee on Resuscitation (American Heart Association, Australian and New Zealand Council on Resuscitation, European Resuscitation Council, Heart and Stroke Foundation of Canada, InterAmerican Heart Foundation, Resuscitation Council of Asia, and the Resuscitation Council of Southern Africa); the American Heart Association Emergency Cardiovascular Care Committee; the Council on Cardiovascular Surgery and Anesthesia; the Council on Cardiopulmonary, Perioperative, and Critical Care; the Council on Clinical Cardiology; and the Stroke Council. Circulation 118:2452–2483
12. Nolan JP, Neumar RW, Adrie C et al (2008) Post-cardiac arrest syndrome: epidemiology, pathophysiology, treatment, and prognostication. A Scientific Statement from the International Liaison Committee on Resuscitation; the American Heart Association Emergency Cardiovascular Care Committee; the Council on Cardiovascular Surgery and Anesthesia; the Council on Cardiopulmonary, Perioperative, and Critical Care; the Council on Clinical Cardiology; the Council on Stroke. Resuscitation 79:350–379
13. Bernard SA, Gray TW, Buist MD et al (2002) Treatment of comatose survivors of out-of-hospital cardiac arrest with induced hypothermia. N Engl J Med 346:557–563
14. Reuler JB (1978) Hypothermia: pathophysiology, clinical settings, and management. Ann Intern Med 89:519–527
15. Allen DE, Gellai M (1993) Mechanisms for the diuresis of acute cold exposure: role for vasopressin? Am J Physiol 264:R524–R532
16. Polderman KH, Tjong Tjin Joe R, Peerdeman SM, Vandertop WP, Girbes AR (2002) Effects of therapeutic hypothermia on intracranial pressure and outcome in patients with severe head injury. Intensive Care Med 28:1563–1573
17. Bergman R, Braber A, Adriaanse MA, van Vugt R, Tjan DH, van Zanten AR (2010) Haemodynamic consequences of mild therapeutic hypothermia after cardiac arrest. Eur J Anaesthesiol 27:383–387
18. Frank SM, Satitpunwaycha P, Bruce SR, Herscovitch P, Goldstein DS (2003) Increased myocardial perfusion and sympathoadrenal activation during mild core hypothermia in awake humans. Clin Sci (Lond) 104:503–508
19. Abdul Aziz KA, Meduoye A (2010) Is pH-stat or alpha-stat the best technique to follow in patients undergoing deep hypothermic circulatory arrest? Interact Cardiovasc Thorac Surg 10:271–282
20. Raper RF, Cameron G, Walker D, Bowey CJ (1997) Type B lactic acidosis following cardiopulmonary bypass. Crit Care Med 25:46–51
21. Miyamoto TA, Miyamoto KJ (2000) Is it justified to disregard the Bohr effect during alpha-stat hypothermia? Ann Thorac Surg 69:973–975

Therapeutic Hypothermia: Is It Effective for Non-VF/VT Cardiac Arrest?

C. Sandroni, F. Cavallaro, and M. Antonelli

Introduction

Sudden cardiac death represents a major health problem. In adults, the prevalence of out-of-hospital cardiac arrest (OHCA) attended by the emergency medical services (EMS) ranges from 52 to 112 per 100,000 person-years in developed countries [1], whereas the prevalence of adult in-hospital cardiac arrest (IHCA) ranges from 1 to 5 per 1,000 patient admissions [2].

Mortality from cardiac arrest exceeds 90 % in OHCA [1, 3] and 70 % in most studies on IHCA [4–6]. Patients who have a shockable rhythm, i. e., ventricular fibrillation (VF) or pulseless ventricular tachycardia (VT), on initial electrocardiogram (EKG) have a consistently higher survival than those whose initial cardiac rhythm is non-shockable, i. e., asystole or pulseless electrical activity (PEA).

More than two-thirds of initially resuscitated patients die before hospital discharge [7, 8]. The major causes of hospital mortality are post-resuscitation brain and myocardial dysfunction [9, 10]. Mild therapeutic hypothermia can reduce the severity of post-resuscitation brain injury and improve survival in patients who remain comatose after resuscitation from cardiac arrest. In 2002, two randomized clinical

C. Sandroni (✉)
Department of Anesthesiology and Intensive Care, Catholic University School of Medicine, Largo Agostino Gemelli 8, 00168 Rome, Italy
E-mail: sandroni@rm.unicatt.it

F. Cavallaro
Department of Anesthesiology and Intensive Care, Catholic University School of Medicine, Largo Agostino Gemelli 8, 00168 Rome, Italy

M. Antonelli
Department of Anesthesiology and Intensive Care, Catholic University School of Medicine, Largo Agostino Gemelli 8, 00168 Rome, Italy

J.-L. Vincent (Ed.), *Annual Update in Intensive Care and Emergency Medicine 2013*, DOI 10.1007/978-3-642-35109-9_27, trials showed improved neurological outcome [11, 12] in a total of 350 comatose adults resuscitated from OHCA who were cooled to 32–34 °C for 12–24 hours shortly after recovery of spontaneous circulation. The largest of these trials [12] also showed a significant reduction in mortality within six months in patients treated with mild therapeutic hypothermia. Both these trials included only patients who had VF/VT as the initial rhythm.

Based on these results, subsequently confirmed by a meta-analysis [13], the International Liaison Committee on Resuscitation (ILCOR) recommended in 2003 the use of mild therapeutic hypothermia for all comatose survivors after OHCA due to VF/VT [14]; this recommendation was confirmed in the current 2010 Guidelines for Cardiopulmonary Resuscitation [15]. However, only 25–30 % of OHCA patients have VF/VT as the initial recorded cardiac rhythm [1], and this percentage has decreased in recent years [16, 17], partly because of the advent of implantable cardioverter-defibrillators for the prevention and treatment of patients at risk of lethal arrhythmias [18]. The prevalence of VF/VT rhythms in IHCA does not exceed 25–30 % either [2]. For the remaining 70–75 % of patients who undergo cardiac arrest with non-VF/VT rhythms, indications for receiving therapeutic hypothermia after resuscitation are less clear.

Hypothermia for Non-VF/VT Cardiac Arrest

The evidence on whether use of mild therapeutic hypothermia could improve prognosis in comatose patients resuscitated from non-VF/VT cardiac arrest is sparse. We identified 15 observational studies (Table 1) and 2 randomized trials.

Randomized Clinical Trials

Use of mild therapeutic hypothermia for the treatment of patients resuscitated from non-VF/VT cardiac arrest has been described in two randomized trials, even though neither was specifically designed to assess the benefit of mild therapeutic hypothermia in this patient population. One trial was a feasibility study on a helmet device for inducing hypothermia after resuscitation [19], the other examined the effect of isovolemic high-volume hemofiltration alone or combined with mild therapeutic hypothermia to improve survival after cardiac arrest [20]. These trials included a total of only 44 patients with non-VF/VT rhythms. Within this small subgroup, patients treated with mild therapeutic hypothermia had a higher survival rate at six months than did controls (5/22 vs. 2/22; risk ratio [RR] for mortality 0.85 [0.65–1.11] $p = 0.24$).

Table 1 Characteristics of 15 observational studies including data on use of mild therapeutic hypothermia in patients with non-ventricular fibrillation/ventricular tachycardia (VF/VT) cardiac arrest.

Author [Reference]	Arrest location	Patients	Non-VF/VT		Initiation of hypothermia	Cooling method	Control group	Definition of poor outcome	Length of follow-up
			Total	Cooled					
Holzer 2006 [27]	Mixed (OHCA 67 %)	1,038	534	28	In-hospital	Internal	Concurrent	CPC 3–5	30 days
Oddo 2006 [21]	OHCA	109	23	12	In-hospital	External	Historical	CPC 3–5	Discharge
Heer 2007 [26]	Mixed	76	18	10	In-hospital	Internal	Historical	NA	Discharge
Sunde 2007 [29]	OHCA	119	15	6	In-hospital	Mixed	Historical	CPC 3–5	Discharge
Arrich 2007 [23]	Mixed (OHCA 83 %)	587	197	124	In-hospital	Mixed	Concurrent	CPC 3–5	Discharge
Rittenberger 2008 [38]	Mixed (OHCA 56 %)	241	81	42	In-hospital	Mixed	Concurrent	Discharged to a nursing home	Discharge
Storm 2008 [28]	OHCA	126	49	18	In-hospital	Mixed	Historical	CPC 3–5	Discharge
Don 2009 [24]	OHCA	491	313	122	In-hospital	External	Historical	CPC 2–5	Discharge
Whitfield 2009 [30]	OHCA	123	28	15	Pre/In-hospital	Mixed	Historical	Discharged to a nursing home	Discharge
Gaieski 2009 [39]	OHCA	38	18	9	In-hospital	Mixed	Historical	CPC 3–5	Discharge
Bro-Jeppesen 2009 [25]	OHCA	156	48	27	Pre/In-hospital	Mixed	Historical	CPC 3–5	6 months
Derwall 2009 [37]	OHCA	68	28	13	In-hospital	Mixed	Concurrent	CPC 3–5	14 days
Dumas 2011 [33]	OHCA	1,145	437	261	In-hospital	External	Historical	CPC 3–5	Discharge
Storm 2012 [34]	Mixed (OHCA 73 %)	387	175	87	In-hospital	Mixed	Historical	CPC 1–2	90 days
Lundbye 2012 [35]	Mixed (OHCA 52 %)	100	100	52	In-hospital	Internal	Historical	CPC 3–5	Discharge

OHCA: out-of-hospital cardiac arrest; CPC: Cerebral Performance Category

Observational Studies

A series of observational studies evaluated the effects of mild therapeutic hypothermia in non-VF/VT patients (Table 1). In a retrospective analysis from Oddo et al. [21] of a database on the implementation of mild therapeutic hypothermia in an intensive care unit (ICU), the rates of good neurological outcome (Cerebral Performance Category [CPC] 1–2 [22]) in a small subgroup of patients resuscitated from non-VF/VT arrest and treated with mild therapeutic hypothermia was not significantly better than that of historical controls (2/12 vs. 1/11; p=0.99).

In 2007, the results of the European Resuscitation Council Hypothermia After Cardiac Arrest Registry (HACA-R) were published [23]. This multicenter observational study included data from 19 participating centers on 587 patients resuscitated from cardiac arrest, around 18 % of which had occurred in hospital. The non-FV/VT subgroup included 197 subjects, 124 (63 %) of whom were treated using mild therapeutic hypothermia. The rate of survival to hospital discharge was significantly higher in mild therapeutic hypothermia-treated patients (45/124 (35 %) vs. 14/73 (19 %); p=0.023). The rate of the combined endpoint of death (CPC=5) and poor neurological outcome (CPC 3–4) was also lower – although not significantly – in the mild therapeutic hypothermia group (89/124 [71 %] vs. 59/73 [81 %] p=0.21). In this study, only univariate analysis was performed, so no correction was made for pre- and intra-arrest potential confounders. Another limitation was the risk of selection bias, because the choice of using hypothermia in a given patient was left to the discretion of the treating physician.

In 2009, a large, retrospective study by Don et al. [24] on implementation of mild therapeutic hypothermia in a community hospital during a five year-period was published. The study included a total of 491 patients with OHCA with all rhythms, of whom 313 (74 %) had non-VF/VT cardiac arrest. Patients enrolled after implementation of the therapeutic hypothermia protocol were compared with historical controls. Results showed that whereas in patients with VF/VT the hypothermia period was associated with significantly higher rates of survival to hospital discharge and favorable neurological outcome as compared to the pre-hypothermia period (44/81 [54.3 %] vs. 36/93 [38.7 %]; p=0.04 and 28/81 [34.6 %] vs. 14/93 [15 %]; p=0.01, respectively), there were no significant improvements in patients resuscitated from non-VF/VT rhythms (26/122 [21 %] vs. 37/191 [19 %], p=0.78 and 14/122 [11 %] vs. 17/191 [9 %], p=0.82, respectively). Moreover, results of multivariable analysis showed a slight trend towards a worse outcome for the mild therapeutic hypothermia period in patients with non-VF/VT rhythms (favorable neurological outcome odds ratio [OR] 0.82 [0.41–1.60]; survival to discharge OR 0.92 [0.37–2.32]).

Other smaller observational studies on mild therapeutic hypothermia were carried out between 2006 and 2009 [25–30]. None of these studies was designed to specifically investigate the association between mild therapeutic hypothermia and prognosis of non-VF/VT rhythms. The majority of these studies documented a non-significant trend towards better outcome when mild therapeutic hypothermia was used in patients with non-VF/VT cardiac arrest.

A recent systematic review and meta-analysis by Kim et al. [31] evaluated the two randomized studies reported above and 12 non-randomized studies for a total of 1,336 non-VF/VT patients, 412 (30.8 %) of whom were treated using mild therapeutic hypothermia. The quality of evidence was assessed using the GRADE methodology [32]. The results showed that the quality of evidence in all studies was very low. Most of the studies had substantial risks of bias and 9/12 had a high degree of imprecision, because of their small sample size. Pooled data from the two small randomized studies showed a non-significant trend toward a lower 6-month mortality with mild therapeutic hypothermia (RR 0.85 [0.65–1.11]). Meta-analysis of the 12 observational studies showed a significant reduction in hospital mortality (RR 0.84 [0.78–0.92]) and a non-significant trend towards better neurological outcome (RR for poor neurological outcome 0.95 [0.90–1.01]) after mild therapeutic hypothermia. The authors concluded that mild therapeutic hypothermia was associated with reduced in-hospital mortality for adult patients resuscitated from non-shockable cardiac arrest, but also suggested caution in interpreting the results, given a substantial risks of bias and the low quality of the evidence.

Results of the Most Recent Studies

Three very recent studies that were not included in the systematic review by Kim et al. [31] reported conflicting results on the potential benefit of mild therapeutic hypothermia in patients with non-VF/VT cardiac arrest. A first study by Dumas et al. [33] reported data from a prospective French database including 1,145 OHCA patients, 437 of whom were non-VF/VT patients. The association between mild therapeutic hypothermia and good neurological outcome at discharge (CPC 1 or 2) was quantified by logistic regression analysis. Mild therapeutic hypothermia was induced in 457/708 (65 %) patients with VF/VT and in 261/437 (60 %) with non-VF/VT. After adjustment for confounders, the results showed that whereas mild therapeutic hypothermia was associated with a significantly better neurological outcome at discharge in VF/VT patients, there was a trend towards a worse outcome in non-VF/VT patients (OR 1.90 [1.18–3.06] vs. 0.71 [0.37–1.36]).

Another prospective single-center observational study was conducted by Storm et al. [34] in a university hospital setting with historical controls. The paper enrolled 387 consecutive patients with all rhythms who had been admitted to the ICU after cardiac arrest. Mild therapeutic hypothermia was induced in 201 patients (87 with non-VF/VT), who were compared with 186 historical controls (88 with non-VF/VT). Univariate analysis showed a non-significant trend towards better neurological outcome in non-VF/VT patients treated with mild therapeutic hypothermia (24/87 [27.8 %] vs 16/88 [18 %], $p = 0.17$). On Cox regression analysis, however, the risk for poor neurological outcome at discharge in the two groups was almost identical (hazard ratio [HR] 0.98 [0.53–1.50]). Kaplan-Meier analysis revealed no differences in 90-day survival with or without mild therapeutic hypothermia ($p = 0.82$).

Finally, a recent small single-center observational study by Lundbye et al. [35] compared neurological outcome and survival at hospital discharge in 52 non-VF/VT cardiac arrest patients treated using mild therapeutic hypothermia compared with 48 historical controls who did not receive mild therapeutic hypothermia. In contrast with the previous two studies, the rates of good neurological outcome (15/52 [29 %] vs. 6/48 [13 %]; p = 0.021) and survival to discharge (20/52 [38 %] vs. 9/48 [19 %]; p = 0.03) were significantly higher in patients treated with mild therapeutic hypothermia. These results were confirmed after controlling for confounders using binomial logistic regression (OR 4.35 [1.10–17.24], p = 0.04 and OR 5.65 [1.66–19.23], p = 0.006, respectively).

The Forest plots in Fig. 1a, b summarize the results of 12 observational studies reporting survival to discharge (1,581 patients, Fig. 1a) and of 13 observational studies reporting neurological outcome (1,998 patients, Fig. 1b). Data pooled according to a fixed effect model show a significant reduction in the RR for hospital mortality (0.88 [0.82–0.95]) and a smaller but significant reduction in RR for poor neurological outcome (0.95 [0.90–0.99]) in patients treated using mild therapeutic hypothermia. However, in spite of pooled results favoring treatment, the effect is not consistent, with large studies showing increased RR for poor neurological outcome associated with use of mild therapeutic hypothermia [33] (Fig. 1b).

In comparison with the results of randomized trials in VF/VT patients [36], analysis of the available evidence shows that use of mild therapeutic hypothermia in comatose patients resuscitated from non-VF/VT cardiac arrest is associated with a small effect size, particularly as regards neurological outcome, with several studies [24, 30, 33, 37, 38] suggesting no effect or even a possible harm from mild therapeutic hypothermia. There are many possible explanations for this observation. One explanation could be that patients who undergo a cardiac arrest with non-VF/VT rhythms represent a more heterogeneous population as compared to those with a VF/VT arrest. Sudden death due to VF/VT is usually the result of cardiac causes, such as arrhythmia or acute myocardial ischemia, whereas non-VF/VT rhythms (asystole or PEA) have a wider variety of causes, such as hypoxia, hypovolemia, sepsis, pulmonary thromboembolism, or cardiac tamponade. These causes are often associated with major comorbidities, which could reduce the chances of patient survival after resuscitation, regardless of the protective effect of mild therapeutic hypothermia. Moreover, cardiac arrest from these causes is often preceded by generalized hypoxia or hypoperfusion, which may further worsen cerebral anoxic damage. Finally, since asystole represents the final evolution of all cardiac arrest rhythms, its presence may indicate a long collapse-to-resuscitation interval and/or poor or absent bystander resuscitation, both of which are associated with a high risk of irreversible neurological damage. In some studies, therefore, non-VF/VT patients could have been simply too ill to benefit from mild therapeutic hypothermia.

Heterogeneity observed in study results may also be explained by differences in case mix and in cooling protocols. For example, some studies included only OHCA patients, whereas others included both IHCA and OHCA (see Table 1). Two of the studies that documented lack of benefit from mild therapeutic hypo-

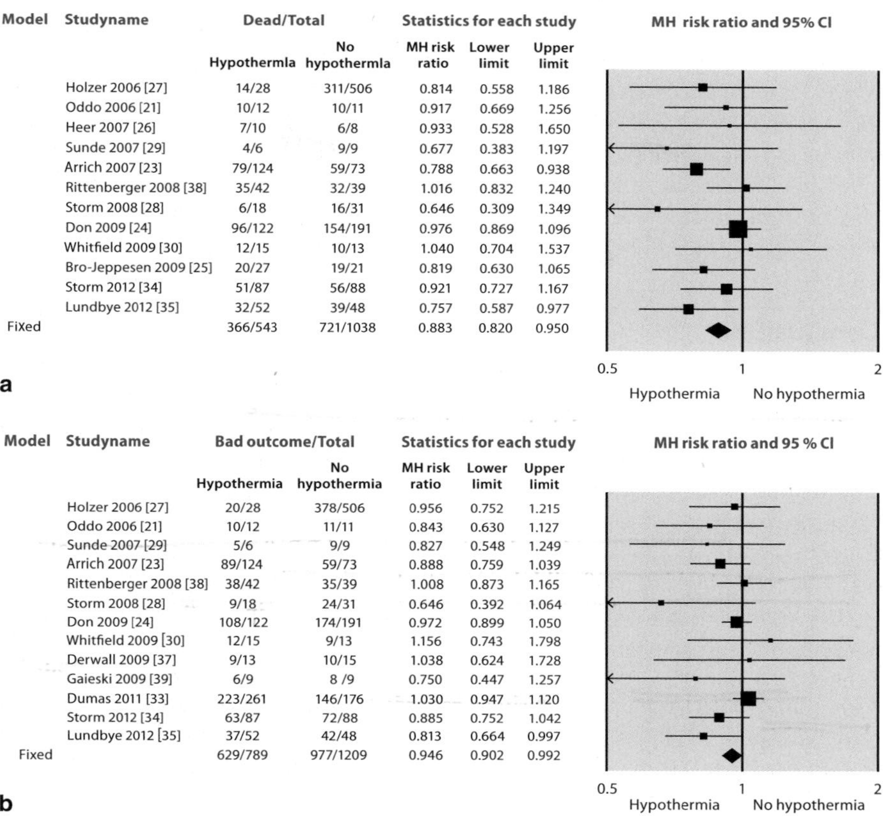

a

Model	Studyname	Dead/Total Hypothermla	Dead/Total No hypothermla	MH risk ratio	Lower limit	Upper limit
	Holzer 2006 [27]	14/28	311/506	0.814	0.558	1.186
	Oddo 2006 [21]	10/12	10/11	0.917	0.669	1.256
	Heer 2007 [26]	7/10	6/8	0.933	0.528	1.650
	Sunde 2007 [29]	4/6	9/9	0.677	0.383	1.197
	Arrich 2007 [23]	79/124	59/73	0.788	0.663	0.938
	Rittenberger 2008 [38]	35/42	32/39	1.016	0.832	1.240
	Storm 2008 [28]	6/18	16/31	0.646	0.309	1.349
	Don 2009 [24]	96/122	154/191	0.976	0.869	1.096
	Whitfield 2009 [30]	12/15	10/13	1.040	0.704	1.537
	Bro-Jeppesen 2009 [25]	20/27	19/21	0.819	0.630	1.065
	Storm 2012 [34]	51/87	56/88	0.921	0.727	1.167
	Lundbye 2012 [35]	32/52	39/48	0.757	0.587	0.977
Fixed		366/543	721/1038	0.883	0.820	0.950

b

Model	Studyname	Bad outcome/Total Hypothermia	Bad outcome/Total No hypothermia	MH risk ratio	Lower limit	Upper limit
	Holzer 2006 [27]	20/28	378/506	0.956	0.752	1.215
	Oddo 2006 [21]	10/12	11/11	0.843	0.630	1.127
	Sunde 2007 [29]	5/6	9/9	0.827	0.548	1.249
	Arrich 2007 [23]	89/124	59/73	0.888	0.759	1.039
	Rittenberger 2008 [38]	38/42	35/39	1.008	0.873	1.165
	Storm 2008 [28]	9/18	24/31	0.646	0.392	1.064
	Don 2009 [24]	108/122	174/191	0.972	0.899	1.050
	Whitfield 2009 [30]	12/15	9/13	1.156	0.743	1.798
	Derwall 2009 [37]	9/13	10/15	1.038	0.624	1.728
	Gaieski 2009 [39]	6/9	8 /9	0.750	0.447	1.257
	Dumas 2011 [33]	223/261	146/176	1.030	0.947	1.120
	Storm 2012 [34]	63/87	72/88	0.885	0.752	1.042
	Lundbye 2012 [35]	37/52	42/48	0.813	0.664	0.997
Fixed		629/789	977/1209	0.946	0.902	0.992

Fig. 1 Forest plot of risk ratio for mortality **a** and poor neurological outcome **b** in observational studies of patients resuscitated from non-VF/VT cardiac arrest. Data were partially reproduced from [31] with Author's permission

thermia used the external surface cooling method, which may require longer times to achieve the target temperature than with intravascular cooling.

Finally, apart from two trials with minimal sample sizes, all the published studies on mild therapeutic hypothermia for non-VF/VT arrest are observational. This makes controlling of confounders extremely difficult to achieve and introduces further sources of bias. Studies in which the control group was represented by concurrent patients not treated using mild therapeutic hypothermia are prone to selection bias, and in those with historical controls, the results may reflect secular trends in patient or disease characteristics or changes in resuscitation practice rather than the effect of the study intervention.

To be correctly addressed, the question as to whether mild therapeutic hypothermia may be beneficial in patients with asystole or PEA as the initial cardiac rhythm will require a purposely designed, high-quality randomized controlled trial. However, in order to demonstrate an increase in survival from 25 % to 30 % with a 0.05 risk of a type-1 error (alpha) and a 0.20 risk of type-II error (beta) using univariate analysis, a minimum of 1,100 patients resuscitated from non-VF/VT would be required. Such a large sample size would be difficult to collect, considering that only about 10 % of patients resuscitated from cardiac arrest of all rhythms survive to hospital admission [8]. Moreover, this trial may even raise ethical issues, since pooled results from observational studies suggest a modest but significant benefit from mild therapeutic hypothermia in non-FV/VT cardiac arrests.

Conclusions

Non-VF/VT are the most common initial cardiac rhythms recorded in both in-hospital and out-of-hospital cardiac arrests. Unfortunately, patients with non-VF/VT rhythms also represent the majority of those who die despite resuscitation, and interventions able to improve the prognosis of this patient category are eagerly awaited. Whereas mild therapeutic hypothermia has been consistently demonstrated to improve outcomes after VF/VT cardiac arrest, its use in patients with non-VF/VT arrest has produced conflicting results. Pooled data from available studies show that the use of mild therapeutic hypothermia for 24 hours in comatose patients resuscitated from non-VF/VT arrest was associated with a 15 % reduction in hospital mortality and with a minimal, albeit significant improvement in neurological outcome at discharge. The quality of evidence supporting these results, however, is very poor, since it is based almost exclusively on observational studies, most of which were not specifically designed to evaluate the benefit of mild therapeutic hypothermia in non-VF/VT patients. Randomized controlled trials of adequate sample size are necessary to address this question.

References

1. Berdowski J, Berg RA, Tijssen JG, Koster RW (2011) Global incidences of out-of-hospital cardiac arrest and survival rates: Systematic review of 67 prospective studies. Resuscitation 81:1479–1487
2. Sandroni C, Nolan J, Cavallaro F, Antonelli M (2007) hospital cardiac arrest: incidence, prognosis and possible measures to improve survival. Intensive Care Med 33:237–245
3. Nichol G, Thomas E, Callaway CW et al (2008) Regional variation in out-of-hospital cardiac arrest incidence and outcome. JAMA 300:1423–1431
4. Nadkarni VM, Larkin GL, Peberdy MA et al (2006) First documented rhythm and clinical outcome from in-hospital cardiac arrest among children and adults. JAMA 295:50–57
5. Peberdy MA, Kaye W, Ornato JP et al (2003) Cardiopulmonary resuscitation of adults in the hospital: a report of 14,720 cardiac arrests from the National Registry of Cardiopulmonary Resuscitation. Resuscitation 58:297–308
6. Sandroni C, Ferro G, Santangelo S et al (2004) hospital cardiac arrest: survival depends mainly on the effectiveness of the emergency response. Resuscitation 62:291–297

7. Nolan JP, Laver SR, Welch CA, Harrison DA, Gupta V, Rowan K (2007) Outcome following admission to UK intensive care units after cardiac arrest: a secondary analysis of the ICNARC Case Mix Programme Database. Anaesthesia 62:1207–1216
8. Stiell IG, Wells GA, Field BJ et al (1999) Improved out-of-hospital cardiac arrest survival through the inexpensive optimization of an existing defibrillation program: OPALS study phase II. Ontario Prehospital Advanced Life Support. JAMA 281:1175–1181
9. Laver S, Farrow C, Turner D, Nolan J (2004) Mode of death after admission to an intensive care unit following cardiac arrest. Intensive Care Med 30:2126–2128
10. Nolan JP, Neumar RW, Adrie C et al (2008) Post-cardiac arrest syndrome: epidemiology, pathophysiology, treatment, and prognostication. A Scientific Statement from the International Liaison Committee on Resuscitation; the American Heart Association Emergency Cardiovascular Care Committee; the Council on Cardiovascular Surgery and Anesthesia; the Council on Cardiopulmonary, Perioperative, and Critical Care; the Council on Clinical Cardiology; the Council on Stroke. Resuscitation 79:350–379
11. Bernard SA, Gray TW, Buist MD et al (2002) Treatment of comatose survivors of out-of-hospital cardiac arrest with induced hypothermia. N Engl J Med 346:557–563
12. The HACA study group (2002) Mild therapeutic hypothermia to improve the neurologic outcome after cardiac arrest. N Engl J Med 346:549–556
13. Holzer M, Bernard SA, Hachimi-Idrissi S, Roine RO, Sterz F, Mullner M (2005) Hypothermia for neuroprotection after cardiac arrest: systematic review and individual patient data meta-analysis. Crit Care Med 33:414–418
14. Nolan JP, Morley PT, Hoek TL, Hickey RW (2003) Therapeutic hypothermia after cardiac arrest. An advisory statement by the Advancement Life support Task Force of the International Liaison committee on Resuscitation. Resuscitation 57:231–235
15. Peberdy MA, Callaway CW, Neumar RW et al (2010) Part 9: post-cardiac arrest care: 2010 American Heart Association Guidelines for Cardiopulmonary Resuscitation and Emergency Cardiovascular Care. Circulation 122:S768–S786
16. Agarwal DA, Hess EP, Atkinson EJ, White RD (2009) Ventricular fibrillation in Rochester, Minnesota: experience over 18 years. Resuscitation 80:1253–1258
17. Cobb LA, Fahrenbruch CE, Olsufka M, Copass MK (2002) Changing incidence of out-of-hospital ventricular fibrillation. JAMA 288:3008–3013
18. Hulleman M, Berdowski J, de Groot JR et al (2012) Implantable cardioverter-defibrillators have reduced the incidence of resuscitation for out-of-hospital cardiac arrest caused by lethal arrhythmias. Circulation 126:815–821
19. Hachimi-Idrissi S, Corne L, Ebinger G, Michotte Y, Huyghens L (2001) Mild hypothermia induced by a helmet device: a clinical feasibility study. Resuscitation 51:275–281
20. Laurent I, Adrie C, Vinsonneau C et al (2005) High-volume hemofiltration after out-of-hospital cardiac arrest: a randomized study. J Am Coll Cardiol 46:432–437
21. Oddo M, Schaller MD, Feihl F, Ribordy V, Liaudet L (2006) From evidence to clinical practice: effective implementation of therapeutic hypothermia to improve patient outcome after cardiac arrest. Crit Care Med 34:1865–1873
22. Brain Resuscitation Clinical Trial I Study Group (1986) A randomized clinical study of cardiopulmonary-cerebral resuscitation: design, methods, and patient characteristics. Brain Resuscitation Clinical Trial I Study Group Am J Emerg Med 4:72–86
23. Arrich J (2007) Clinical application of mild therapeutic hypothermia after cardiac arrest. Crit Care Med 35:1041–1047
24. Don CW, Longstreth Jr WT, Maynard C et al (2009) Active surface cooling protocol to induce mild therapeutic hypothermia after out-of-hospital cardiac arrest: a retrospective before-and-after comparison in a single hospital. Crit Care Med 37:3062–3069
25. Bro-Jeppesen J, Kjaergaard J, Horsted TI et al (2009) The impact of therapeutic hypothermia on neurological function and quality of life after cardiac arrest. Resuscitation 80:171–176
26. Heer C (2007) Hypothermia after cardiac arrest – experiences in routine use on a medical intensive care unit. Intensivmedizin und Notfallmedizin 44:303–307

27. Holzer M, Mullner M, Sterz F et al (2006) Efficacy and safety of endovascular cooling after cardiac arrest: cohort study and Bayesian approach. Stroke 37:1792–1797
28. Storm C, Steffen I, Schefold JC et al (2008) Mild therapeutic hypothermia shortens intensive care unit stay of survivors after out-of-hospital cardiac arrest compared to historical controls. Crit Care 12:R78
29. Sunde K, Pytte M, Jacobsen D et al (2007) Implementation of a standardised treatment protocol for post resuscitation care after out-of-hospital cardiac arrest. Resuscitation 73:29–39
30. Whitfield AM, Coote S, Ernest D (2009) Induced hypothermia after out-of-hospital cardiac arrest: one hospital's experience. Crit Care Resusc 11:97–100
31. Kim YM, Yim HW, Jeong SH, Klem ML, Callaway CW (2012) Does therapeutic hypothermia benefit adult cardiac arrest patients presenting with non-shockable initial rhythms?: A systematic review and meta-analysis of randomized and non-randomized studies. Resuscitation 83:188–196
32. Guyatt GH, Oxman AD, Vist GE et al (2008) GRADE: an emerging consensus on rating quality of evidence and strength of recommendations. BMJ 336:924–926
33. Dumas F, Grimaldi D, Zuber B et al (2011) Is hypothermia after cardiac arrest effective in both shockable and nonshockable patients?: insights from a large registry. Circulation 123:877–886
34. Storm C, Nee J, Roser M, Jorres A, Hasper D (2012) Mild hypothermia treatment in patients resuscitated from non-shockable cardiac arrest. Emerg Med J 29:100–103
35. Lundbye JB, Rai M, Ramu B et al (2012) Therapeutic hypothermia is associated with improved neurologic outcome and survival in cardiac arrest survivors of non-shockable rhythms. Resuscitation 83:202–207
36. Arrich J, Holzer M, Herkner H, Mullner M (2009) Hypothermia for neuroprotection in adults after cardiopulmonary resuscitation. Cochrane Database Syst Rev CD004128
37. Derwall M, Stoppe C, Brucken D, Rossaint R, Fries M (2009) Changes in S-100 protein serum levels in survivors of out-of-hospital cardiac arrest treated with mild therapeutic hypothermia: a prospective, observational study. Crit Care 13:R58
38. Rittenberger JC, Guyette FX, Tisherman SA, DeVita MA, Alvarez RJ, Callaway CW (2008) Outcomes of a hospital-wide plan to improve care of comatose survivors of cardiac arrest. Resuscitation 79:198–204
39. Gaieski DF, Band RA, Abella BS et al (2009) Early goal-directed hemodynamic optimization combined with therapeutic hypothermia in comatose survivors of out-of-hospital cardiac arrest. Resuscitation 80:418–424

Cerebral Oximetry in Cerebral Resuscitation After Cardiac Arrest

A. Ahn, J. Nolan, and S. Parnia

Introduction

Interestingly, despite great medical progress over the past 50 years, survival from cardiac arrest has improved only slightly [1, 2] and long-term neurological, cognitive and functional deficits are common [3]. Pathophysiologically, cardiac arrest represents a state of generalized whole-body ischemia resulting from either a no-flow or a low-flow state that culminates in inadequate organ perfusion and oxygen delivery (DO_2) leading to cellular damage and death [1]. On-going inflammatory responses and cellular damage continue even after return of spontaneous circulation (ROSC), and are confounded by the problem of ischemia-reperfusion injury [1]. As a result of this unique pathological state, first termed "post resuscitation disease" in 1972 [4], even though spontaneous circulation may initially be restored in up to 50 %, many of the early survivors die in the subsequent hours to days because of a combination of neurological dysfunction, cardiac dysfunction, ischemia-reperfusion injury and persistent inflammatory responses [1].

One of the major limitations in current practice is the inability to measure and hence optimize end-organ perfusion in real-time because of the lack of a clear physiological marker to guide the quality of care being delivered with respect to vital organ and in particular brain perfusion. During cardiopulmonary resuscitation (CPR) and in the post-resuscitation period, such a marker could improve outcome

A. Ahn
Resuscitation Research Group, Department of Medicine, Division of Critical Care Medicine, Stony Brook Medical Center, New York, NY, USA

J. Nolan (✉)
Department of Anesthesia and Critical Care, Royal United Hospital, Bath, BA1 3NG, UK
E-mail: jerry.nolan@nhs.net

S. Parnia
Resuscitation Research Group, Department of Medicine, Division of Critical Care Medicine, Stony Brook Medical Center, New York, NY, USA

J.-L. Vincent (Ed.), *Annual Update in Intensive Care and Emergency Medicine 2013*, 337
DOI 10.1007/978-3-642-35109-9_28, © Springer-Verlag Berlin Heidelberg 2013

by ensuring early recognition of poor perfusion. Adjustments in CPR could then improve coronary and cerebral perfusion and ultimately outcome. This review focuses on the potential role of cerebral oximetry as a novel tool that may be used both for prognostication and as a real-time indicator of the balance between oxygen delivery and uptake in brain tissue during CPR and in the post-resuscitation period.

Cerebral Oximetry as a Prognosticator and Real-Time Marker of Cerebral Perfusion During CPR

The use of end tidal carbon dioxide (etCO_2) has been proposed recently as a general marker of effective overall circulation and perfusion as well as ROSC during cardiac arrest [5], but does not indicate the quality of cerebral perfusion or DO_2. In clinical practice, the electroencephalogram (EEG) is often used to assess cerebral ischemia during procedures such as cardiac and neurosurgery [6]. One of the major limitations of EEG technology is that although useful as an indicator of cortical activity, it does not provide a measure of real-time DO_2 and brain tissue perfusion. Technical limitations, such as long preparation times, prevent conventional EEG being used reliably during cardiac arrest. Recently, small portable EEG devices, which use bispectral technology, have also been studied in cardiac arrest, but they are susceptible to movement artifacts and are, therefore, unreliable during resuscitation [7].

Cerebral oximetry works by non-invasively transmitting and detecting harmless near-infrared light through sensors that are placed on the patient's forehead, and is not susceptible to motion artifact. Just as with the commonly used pulse oximetry devices, which measure changes in the oxygen saturation of arterial blood, cerebral oximetry monitors changes in oxygen saturation in the cerebral cortex. This device thus has the potential to provide cerebral oxygen values in real time and, consequently, cerebral perfusion during cardiac arrest and in the post-resuscitation period. Cerebral oximetry relies on near-infrared spectroscopy (NIRS), which is based on the Beer Lambert law. According to this law, the absorption of light through any medium is proportional to: (1) the length the light has to travel; (2) the concentration of molecules with light absorbing properties (chromophores) present in the medium; and (3) the molar extinction coefficient (i. e., the measure of how strongly the molecules (chromophores) absorb light at a given wavelength) [8].

Use of NIRS is possible in biological tissue, because although the tissues themselves are relatively transparent to near-infrared light in the 400–1,000 nm range, specific chromophores present in tissues absorb wavelengths of light in this spectrum [9]. Water and melanin both express low optical absorption, which enables near-infrared light to pass through several centimeters of tissue, including skin, subcutaneous tissue, and bone without being absorbed significantly [10]. The attenuation of light at a given wavelength is caused by light scattering in tissue, which is related to the properties of specific chromophores. NIRS measures the decrease in optical intensity, expressed as the change in optical density per centimeter of tissue [8]. Organometallic molecules, such as hemoglobin, have characteristic infrared absorption spectra that shift with oxygenation and thereby permit the identification of oxygenated and deoxygenated molecules with spectroscopy [11]. In brain tissue, there are three principal chromophores: Oxyhemoglobin, deoxyhemoglobin and oxidized cytochrome aa_3 [8]. NIRS determines the ratio of oxyhemoglobin to deoxyhemoglobin and calculates the cerebral hemoglobin oxygen saturation [12], thus providing an index of changes in regional brain hemoglobin oxygen saturation. Since 70–80 % of blood in the measured areas of brain tissue is venous, these data represent mainly cerebral venous saturation [13].

This technology relies typically on two or more wavelengths of light. The second wavelength is used to eliminate common background absorption, subject pigment variability, or optical path length [8]. A series of equations are then used to create an algorithm that provides data about concentration changes for each specific chromophore. Because the scattering characteristics of mammalian tissues cause light to travel in an elliptical path between the tissue and the detectors, by adjusting the spacing and position of the detectors it is possible to determine the depth of tissue from which light is being measured [8]. Thus, most cerebral oximeters have a second detector, which is positioned on the sensor, to collect data derived from the contributions to the signal from superficial (skin, subcutaneous tissue, and bone) tissue and distinguish this from deep (brain) tissue [8].

Validation Studies of Cerebral Oximetry Using NIRS

Baseline Variables

Although, in principle, different body positions can impact hemodynamic functions and influence systemic and organ perfusion and oxygenation, in healthy subjects head position does not alter readings across a range of oxygenation and ventilation [14, 15]. However, in patients with increased intracranial pressure (ICP), position change may lead to decreased cerebral perfusion pressure (CPP) and DO_2 [13], which should also be considered in cardiac arrest patients. There are no gender specific differences in measurements. In one study of 111 hemodynamically stable patients, it was demonstrated that values obtained from male and female subjects were similar (M 61 ± 12 %; F 61 ± 9 %) and although weight, height, and head size also did not impact on regional cerebral oxygen saturation values, patient age, hemoglobin concentration, and sensor location did alter saturation values [16]. With respect to age and sensor position, whereas there was a statistically significant alteration, the measurements (58–64 %) remained within the normal range (the normal range may vary a little based upon the different manufacturers but lies approximately in the 60–80 % range), making it unlikely that these findings are clinically significant in the context of shock and cardiac arrest, during which values typically decrease to below 40 or even 20 % [17, 18]. Perhaps the most important observation in this study [16] was that at baseline there was some variability with respect to cerebral saturation in a few patients who, although hemodynamically stable, expressed abnormally low readings of 15–20 % (overall range 15–89 %), suggesting that some 'normal' patients may be outliers. Thus, as with any monitoring tool or laboratory reading, some outliers whose results fall outside those of the majority of the population limit any proscribed 'normal' range and, as such, clinical correlation is needed with the use of this technology.

NIRS is not typically influenced by comorbid conditions, including risk factors for cardiovascular disease, such as hypertension, history of myocardial infarction, factor VIIc, factor VIIIc, cholesterol and high-density lipoprotein (HDL)-cholesterol, smoking or diabetes mellitus [19]. Advanced age affects cerebral blood flow in the temporal and temporoparietal regions of the cortex although this is not the usual site for obtaining cerebral oximetry readings [19]. Melanin pigmentation may attenuate NIRS readings in persons with darker skin [20]. Hyperbilirubinemia may directly alter cerebral oximetry readings and interfere with cerebral oxygen saturation in patients with icterus [21, 22], because bilirubin, a heme breakdown product, can act as a chromophore, albeit mostly at wavelengths below those used for NIRS measurements. Conjugated bilirubin, in particular, may also absorb light in the NIRS range, as demonstrated by the use of NIRS in screening for biliary atresia in infants [23].

Although occlusion of the intracranial circulation reduces cerebral saturation substantially, occlusion of the extracranial circulation causes only a mild and non-clinically significant reduction. In one study, baseline levels were 67.4 ± 8.5 % and decreased to 65.6 ± 8.3 % after occlusion of the extracranial circulation [24], whereas in another small study, scalp ischemia led to a reduction in cerebral oxygenation from a mean of 72 ± 6 % to 59 ± 7 % [25].

In one study, NIRS values in healthy subjects were compared with those in 18 subjects who had been dead for an average of 19.8 ± 18.2 hours and had been kept at a temperature of 18 °C. The mean (± SD) cerebral oxygen saturation in the dead subjects was 51.0 ± 26.8 %, whereas in the control group it was 68.4 ± 5.2 %. After removal of the brain at autopsy in five of the dead subjects, the cerebral saturation was 73.4 ± 13.3 % [26]. These findings may reflect some obvious limitations of this technology in the form of venous hyperoxia, where non-functioning or dead tissue no longer extracts oxygen, which leads to abnormally high venous saturation levels [27].

The Effect of Oxygen, Carbon Dioxide, Sedatives and Neuromuscular Blocking Drugs on NIRS

Although cerebral blood flow is affected little by changes in the PaO_2 in the normal range, hypoxemia with SaO_2 below 90 % leads to an increase in cerebral perfusion as measured by transcranial Doppler [28]. Cerebral blood flow and perfusion are also linearly related to $PaCO_2$; cerebral vasodilatation occurs during hypercapnia and vasoconstriction during hypocapnia [29]. NIRS values correlate well with changes in CO_2 values [30, 31]. Regional cerebral saturation measured by NIRS is also affected directly by changes in systemic blood oxygen saturation. Cerebral oximetry values have been shown to decrease following induced hypoxia [32]. The administration of oxygen increases mean cerebral saturation, and this is enhanced by the administration of sedatives, general anesthetics and neuromuscular blocking drugs. In one study, after administering 100% oxygen, cerebral oxygen saturation increased from $62 \pm 9.5\%$ to $67.8 \pm 10.6\%$; giving thiopental, fentanyl and rocuronium increased it further to 80.2 ± 9.7, reflecting increased DO_2 and decreased oxygen consumption [33]. This potential additive or synergistic effect could have a significant impact on preserving neuronal tissue lying at the ischemic threshold following cardiac arrest and in other brain injury states.

The Effect of Low Cardiac Output and Hypothermia on NIRS

NIRS has been validated in both low cardiac output states and hypothermia. Reduced cardiac output decreases systemic DO_2, which leads to increased brain oxygen extraction and lower cerebral oxygen saturation as measured using NIRS [34–36]. Reductions in cardiac output are associated with decreased cerebral oxygen saturation because of increased brain oxygen extraction resulting from reduced brain DO_2. In one study, treatment of patients with normotensive acute heart failure, increased the mean cerebral saturation 34% (20–58) to 50% (19–91) ($p < 0.02$) [35]. Cerebral oximetry values correlate with left ventricular (LV) dysfunction during exercise testing [36]. Hypothermia is another factor that independently affects cerebral metabolism and the balance between oxygen supply and demand leading to increased cerebral oxygen saturation because of reduced cerebral metabolism and oxygen uptake [37]. Cerebral oximetry by NIRS has been used and validated for measuring cerebral oxygen saturation during hypothermia [38–40] and confirmed previous observations.

Application of NIRS During Cardiac Arrest

Cerebral oximetry reflects the balance between regional oxygen supply and demand. Several factors impact the delivery of oxygen to the brain, including hemoglobin concentration, arterial oxygen saturation and cardiac output. Under physiological conditions, oxygen transport to brain tissue is kept constant by compensatory mechanisms involving cerebral blood flow; however, during critical conditions such as cardiac arrest, cerebral compensatory mechanisms are unable to meet oxygen demand, which leads to increased oxygen extraction and decreased cerebral oxygen saturation. NIRS does not rely on pulsatile blood flow, which makes it particularly valuable during the no-flow or low-flow state that occurs in cardiac arrest [41].

Although, NIRS has been used extensively in patients in several different medical specialties including neurology and neurosurgery [42], trauma [43], vascular

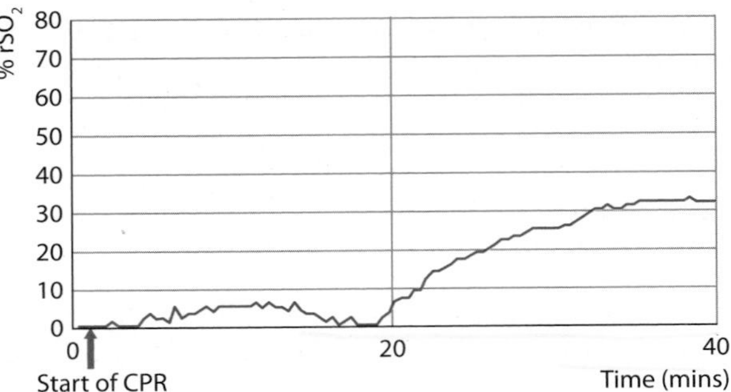

Fig. 1 The impact of cardiopulmonary resuscitation (CPR) on cerebral oximetry values (rSO_2) during cardiac arrest

surgery [44], and cardiac surgery [45], to date, there have been few studies of cerebral oximetry during cardiac arrest. These studies indicate that cerebral saturation may correlate with outcome [17, 18]. In one small study of 16 out-of-hospital cardiac arrests (OHCA), all patients with a mean cerebral oxygen saturation of 17 % or less (lower limit of detection was 15 %) did not survive [17]. Within this group, four patients achieved ROSC and in these patients readings increased transiently to 40–60 % [17]. In another study of 18 OHCA patients admitted to an emergency department, the nine patients who survived for one week achieved a significantly higher median cerebral oxygen saturation on arrival than did non-survivors (63 % vs. 46 % $p=0.003$) [18]. In a recent study, 33 of 132 OHCA patients had a cerebral saturation of 15 % (lowest measurable limit) on emergency department arrival and none survived [46]. In another study, 92 OHCA patients had favorable neurological outcomes; whereas up to 50 % of survivors with regional cerebral saturation values >40 % had a good neurological outcome, none of the patients with a cerebral oxygen saturation ≤ 25 % survived [47].

There have also been multiple case reports describing the use of NIRS in cardiac arrest. Interestingly, in one prolonged cardiac arrest involving an 87-year-old female inpatient with severe aortic stenosis scheduled for aortic valve replacement, continuous measurements correlated with continuous mixed venous oximetry. In this case, regional cerebral saturation decreased rapidly from 70 % to a minimum of approximately 30 %, and increased back to approximately 50 % with CPR. After 25 min of chest compressions, cardiopulmonary bypass (CPB) was commenced and this increased the cerebral oxygen values to pre-cardiac arrest levels [48]. Another recent case report of cardiac arrest during aortic valve surgery demonstrated similar observations [49]. These case reports show that cerebral oximetry has the potential to provide real-time information on cerebral oxygen delivery and consumption during resuscitation.

Although there is clearly very limited experience with this technology during cardiac arrest, data derived from studies so far indicate that it may be a valuable tool for prognostication and real-time monitoring of cerebral perfusion and DO_2 during CPR. Our own early experience with the use of NIRS during in-hospital cardiac arrest has also shown that this condition is typically associated with very low cerebral oxygen saturation values ($\leq$15–20 %); however, with continued CPR these values can be increased (Fig. 1). There was a significant difference in mean

NIRS recordings in patients who achieved ROSC compared with those who did not (35 ± 5 % vs. 18 ± 0.4 %; $p = 0.001$) [50].

Conclusion

Cerebral oximetry using NIRS may prove to be a valuable real-time monitor of the quality of CPR, and in particular cerebral resuscitation. It may also provide data that can contribute to prognostication in individual patients. Further studies are needed to understand the utility of this technology during CPR and in the post-resuscitation period.

References

1. Neumar RW, Nolan JP, Adrie C et al (2008) Post-cardiac arrest syndrome: epidemiology, pathophysiology, treatment, and prognostication. A consensus statement from the International Liaison Committee on Resuscitation (American Heart Association, Australian and New Zealand Council on Resuscitation, European Resuscitation Council, Heart and Stroke Foundation of Canada, InterAmerican Heart Foundation, Resuscitation Council of Asia, and the Resuscitation Council of Southern Africa); the American Heart Association Emergency Cardiovascular Care Committee; the Council on Cardiovascular Surgery and Anesthesia; the Council on Cardiopulmonary, Perioperative, and Critical Care; the Council on Clinical Cardiology; and the Stroke Council. Circulation 118:2452–2483
2. Kudenchuk PJ, Redshaw JD, Stubbs BA et al (2012) Impact of changes in resuscitation practice on survival and neurological outcome after out-of-hospital cardiac arrest resulting from nonshockable arrhythmias. Circulation 125:1787–1794
3. Mateen FJ, Josephs KA, Trenerry MR et al (2011) Long-term cognitive outcomes following out-of-hospital cardiac arrest. Neurology 77:1438–1445
4. Negovsky VA (1972) The second step in resuscitation: the treatment of the "post-resuscitation disease.". Resuscitation 1:1–7
5. Heradstveit BE, Sunde K, Sunde GA, Wentzel-Larsen T, Heltne JK (2012) Factors complicating interpretation of capnography during advanced life support in cardiac arrest – a clinical retrospective study in 575 patients. Resuscitation 83:813–818
6. de Vries JW, Bakker PF, Visser GH, Diephuis JC, van Huffelen AC (1998) Changes in cerebral oxygen uptake and cerebral electrical activity during defibrillation threshold testing. Anesth Analg 87:16–20
7. Fatovich D, Jacobs I, Celenza A, Paech M (2006) An observational study of bispectral index monitoring for out of hospital cardiac arrest. Resuscitation 69:207–212
8. Pollard V, Prough DS (1998) Cerebral oxygenation: Near infrared spectroscopy. In: Tobin MJ (ed) Principles and Practice of Intensive Care Monitoring. McGraw-Hill Professional, New York, pp 1019–1034
9. Jöbsis FF (1977) Noninvasive infrared monitoring of cerebral and myocardial oxygen sufficiency and circulatory parameters. Science 198:1264–1267
10. Boulnois JL (1986) Photophysical processes in recent medical laser developments: a review. Lasers Med Sci:47–66
11. Tamura T, Hazeki O, Takada M, Tamura M (1985) Absorbance profile of red blood cell suspension in vitro and in situ. Adv Exp Med Biol 191:211–217

12. Pollard V, Prough DS, DeMelo AE et al (1996) Validation in volunteers of a near-infrared spectroscope for monitoring brain oxygenation in vivo. Anesth Analg 82:269–277
13. McCormick PW, Stewart M, Ray P et al (1991) Measurement of regional cerebrovascular hemoglobin oxygen saturation in cats using optical spectroscopy. Neurol Res 13:65–70
14. Fuchs G, Schwarz G, Kulier A, Litscher G (2000) The influence of positioning on spectroscopic measurements of brain oxygenation. J Neurosurg Anesthesiol 12:75–80
15. Pollard V, Prough DS, DeMelo AE et al (1996) The influence of carbon dioxide and body position on near-infrared spectroscopic assessment of cerebral hemoglobin oxygen saturation. Anesth Analg 82:278–287
16. Kishi K, Kawaguchi M, Yoshitani K, Nagahata T, Furuya H (2003) Influence of patient variables and sensor location on regional cerebral oxygen saturation measured by INVOS 4100 near-infrared spectrophotometers. J Neurosurg Anesthesiol 15:302–306
17. Newman DH, Callaway CW, Greenwald IB, Freed J (2004) Cerebral oximetry in out-of-hospital cardiac arrest: standard CPR rarely provides detectable hemoglobin-oxygen saturation to the frontal cortex. Resuscitation 63:189–194
18. Müllner M, Sterz F, Binder M, Hirschl MM, Janata K, Laggner AN (1995) Near infrared spectroscopy during and after cardiac arrest – preliminary results. Clin Intensive Care 6:107–111
19. Claus JJ, Breteler MMB, Hasan D et al (1998) Regional cerebral blood flow and cerebrovascular risk factors in the elderly population. Neurobiol Aging 19:57–64
20. Wassenaar EB, Van den Brand JGH (2005) Reliability of near-infrared spectroscopy in people with dark skin pigmentation. J Clin Monit Comput 19:195–199
21. Madsen PL, Skak C, Rasmussen A, Secher NH (2000) Interference of cerebral near-infrared oximetry in patients with icterus. Anesth Analg 90:489–493
22. Song JG, Jeong SM, Shin WJ et al (2011) Laboratory variables associated with low near-infrared cerebral oxygen saturation in icteric patients before liver transplantation surgery. Anesth Analg 112:1347–1352
23. Akiyama T, Yamauchi Y (1994) Use of near infrared reflectance spectroscopy in the screening for biliary atresia. J Pediatr Surg 29:645–647
24. Samra SK, Stanley JC, Zelenock GB, Dorje P (1999) An assessment of contributions made by extracranial tissues during cerebral oximetry. J Neurosurg Anesthesiol 11:1–5
25. Germon TJ, Kane NM, Manara AR, Nelson RJ (1994) Near-infrared spectroscopy in adults: effects of extracranial ischaemia and intracranial hypoxia on estimation of cerebral oxygenation. Br J Anaesth 73:503–506
26. Schwarz G, Litscher G, Kleinert R, Jobstmann R (1996) Cerebral oximetry in dead subjects. J Neurosurg Anesthesiol 8:189–193
27. Rivers EP (1992) Venous hyperoxia after cardiac arrest. Chest 102:1787–1793
28. Gupta AK, Menon DK, Czosnyka M, Smielewski P, Jones JG (1997) Thresholds for hypoxic cerebral vasodilation in volunteers. Anesth Analg 85:817–820
29. Harper AM, Glass HI (1965) Effect of alterations in the arterial carbon dioxide tension on the blood flow through the cerebral cortex at normal and low arterial pressures. J Neurol Neurosurg Psychiat 28:449–452
30. Smielewski P, Kirkpatrick P, Minhas P, Pickard JD, Czosnyka M (1995) Can cerebrovascular reactivity be measured with NIRS? Stroke 26:2285–2292
31. Smielewski P, Czosnyka M, Pickard JD, Kirkpatrick P (1997) Clinical evaluation of near-infrared spectroscopy for testing cerebrovascular reactivity in patients with carotid artery disease. Stroke 28:331–338
32. Henson LC, Calalang C, Temp JA, Ward DS (1998) Accuracy of a cerebral oximeter in healthy volunteers under conditions of isocapnic hypoxia. Anesthesiology 88:58–65
33. Baraka AS, Nawfal M, El-Khatib M, Haroun-Bizri S (2005) Regional cerebral oximetry after oxygen administration. Br J Anaesth 95:720
34. Paquet C, Deschamps A, Denault AY et al (2008) Baseline regional cerebral oxygen saturation correlates with left ventricular systolic and diastolic function. J Cardiothorac Vasc Anesth 22:840–846

35. Madsen PL, Nielsen HB, Christiansen P (2000) Well-being and cerebral oxygen saturation during acute heart failure in humans. Clin Physiol 20:158–164
36. Koike A, Itoh H, Oohara R et al (2004) Cerebral oxygenation during exercise in cardiac patients. Chest 125:182–190
37. Polderman KH (2009) Mechanisms of action, physiological effects, and complications of hypothermia. Crit Care Med 37:S186–S202
38. Rubio A, Hakami L, Münch F et al (2008) Noninvasive control of adequate cerebral oxygenation during low-flow antegrade selective cerebral perfusion on adults and infants in the aortic arch surgery. J Card Surg 23:474–479
39. Leyvi G, Bello R, Wasnick JD, Plestis K (2006) Assessment of cerebral oxygen balance during deep hypothermic circulatory arrest by continuous jugular bulb venous saturation and near-infrared spectroscopy. J Cardiothorac Vasc Anesth 20:826–833
40. Kadoi Y, Kawahara F, Saito S et al (1999) Effects of hypothermic and normothermic cardiopulmonary bypass on brain oxygenation. Ann Thorac Surg 68:34–39
41. Tobias JD (2006) Cerebral oxygenation monitoring: near-infrared spectroscopy. Expert Rev Med Dev 3:235–243
42. Shojima M, Watanabe E, Mayanagi Y (2004) Cerebral blood oxygenation after cerebrospinal fluid removal in hydrocephalus measured by near-infrared spectroscopy. Surg Neurol 62:312–318
43. Gracias VH, Guillamondegui OD, Stiefel MF et al (2004) Cerebral cortical oxygenation: A pilot study. J Trauma 56:469–472
44. Vernieri F, Tibuzzi F, Pasqualetti P et al (2004) Transcranial doppler and near-infrared spectroscopy can evaluate the hemodynamic effect of carotid artery occlusion. Stroke 35:64–70
45. Kurth CD, Steven JL, Montenegro LM et al (2001) Cerebral oxygen saturation before congenital heart surgery. Ann Thorac Surg 72:187–192
46. Ito N, Nanto S, Nagao K, Hatanaka T, Kai T (2010) Regional cerebral oxygen saturation predicts poor neurological outcome in patients with out-of-hospital cardiac arrest. Resuscitation 81:1736–1737
47. Ito N, Shinsuke N, Nagao K, Hatanaka T, Nishiyama K, Tatsuro K (2012) Regional cerebral oxygen saturation on hospital arrival is a potential novel predictor of neurological outcomes at hospital discharge in patients with out-of-hospital cardiac arrest. Resuscitation 83:46–50
48. Paarmann H, Heringlake M, Sier H, Schön J (2010) The association of non-invasive cerebral and mixed venous oxygen saturation during cardiopulmonary resuscitation. Interact Cardiovasc Thorac Surg 11:371–373
49. Mayr NP, Martin K, Kurz J, Tassani P (2011) Monitoring of cerebral oxygen saturation during closed-chest and open-chest CPR. Resuscitation 82:635–636
50. Parnia S, Nasir A, Shah C, Patel R, Mani A, Richman P (2012) A feasibility study evaluating the role of cerebral oximetry in predicting return of spontaneous circulation in cardiac arrest. Resuscitation 83:982–985

Prognostication of Coma After Cardiac Arrest and Therapeutic Hypothermia

M. Oddo

Introduction

Following the introduction of therapeutic hypothermia and the implementation of standardized post-resuscitation care, the number of patients who survive from coma after cardiac arrest has significantly increased [1]. Previous to use of therapeutic hypothermia, clinical neurological examination at 72 hours was considered the gold standard for outcome prognostication of coma after cardiac arrest [2]. However, therapeutic hypothermia and the drugs used to induce therapeutic cooling alter drug elimination and may significantly modify neurological (mainly motor) response [3, 4], thereby rendering clinical examination less reliable and potentially insufficient, when used alone, to adequately predict the prognosis of coma after cardiac arrest. Emerging evidence from independent centers demonstrates that the addition to neurological examination of other prognostic tools – mainly electroencephalography (EEG), somato-sensory evoked potentials (SSEP) and serum neuron-specific enolase (NSE) – significantly improves prognostication of coma after cardiac arrest and therapeutic hypothermia. The implementation of such a multimodal prognostic approach into critical care practice should improve the care of comatose cardiac arrest patients.

M. Oddo (✉)
Department of Critical Care Medicine, CHUV-Lausanne University Hospital
and Faculty of Biology and Medicine, University of Lausanne, Rue du Bugnon 46, BH 08.623,
CH-1011 Lausanne, Switzerland
E-mail: mauro.oddo@chuv.ch

J.-L. Vincent (Ed.), *Annual Update in Intensive Care and Emergency Medicine 2013*, 347
DOI 10.1007/978-3-642-35109-9_29, © Springer-Verlag Berlin Heidelberg 2013

Neurological Examination to Assess Prognosis After Cardiac Arrest and Therapeutic Hypothermia

Clinical examination is an essential step to assess prognosis; however, recent clinical studies have shown that neurological tests may have reduced prognostic accuracy in comatose cardiac arrest patients treated with induced hypothermia.

Motor Response

Bouwes et al., in a recent study including 391 adult comatose patients after cardiac arrest treated with therapeutic hypothermia, found that motor response gave a false outcome prediction in up to 10–15 % of patients (false positive rate of 10 % for poor prognosis, with a 95 % confidence interval [CI] of 6–16) [5]. This study confirmed previous findings from other groups who found that motor response at 72 hours gave a false positive rate of 12 % [4] and up to 24 % [6] for poor prognosis. Importantly, recovery of full motor reaction may take up to 6 days after cardiac arrest and therapeutic hypothermia [3] and sedatives given during therapeutic hypothermia may also be a potential confounder [4].

Brainstem Reflexes

Although of higher predictive value than motor response, the absence of pupillary/corneal reflexes is not uniformly associated with a poor prognosis: some patients may still awake and recover, with a false positive rate of 4–6 % for poor prognosis, according to recent studies [4–7].

EEG to Improve Prognostication After Cardiac Arrest and Therapeutic Hypothermia

Analysis of Dynamic EEG Changes

Previous to the introduction of therapeutic hypothermia, the value of EEG to help with the prognostication of coma after cardiac arrest was already well known [2, 8]. In particular, the analysis of dynamic EEG changes and the dichotomization between a 'reactive' (i. e., a change in the EEG trace upon a painful stimulation) versus a 'non-reactive' EEG background was useful to discriminate between good versus poor prognosis [9].

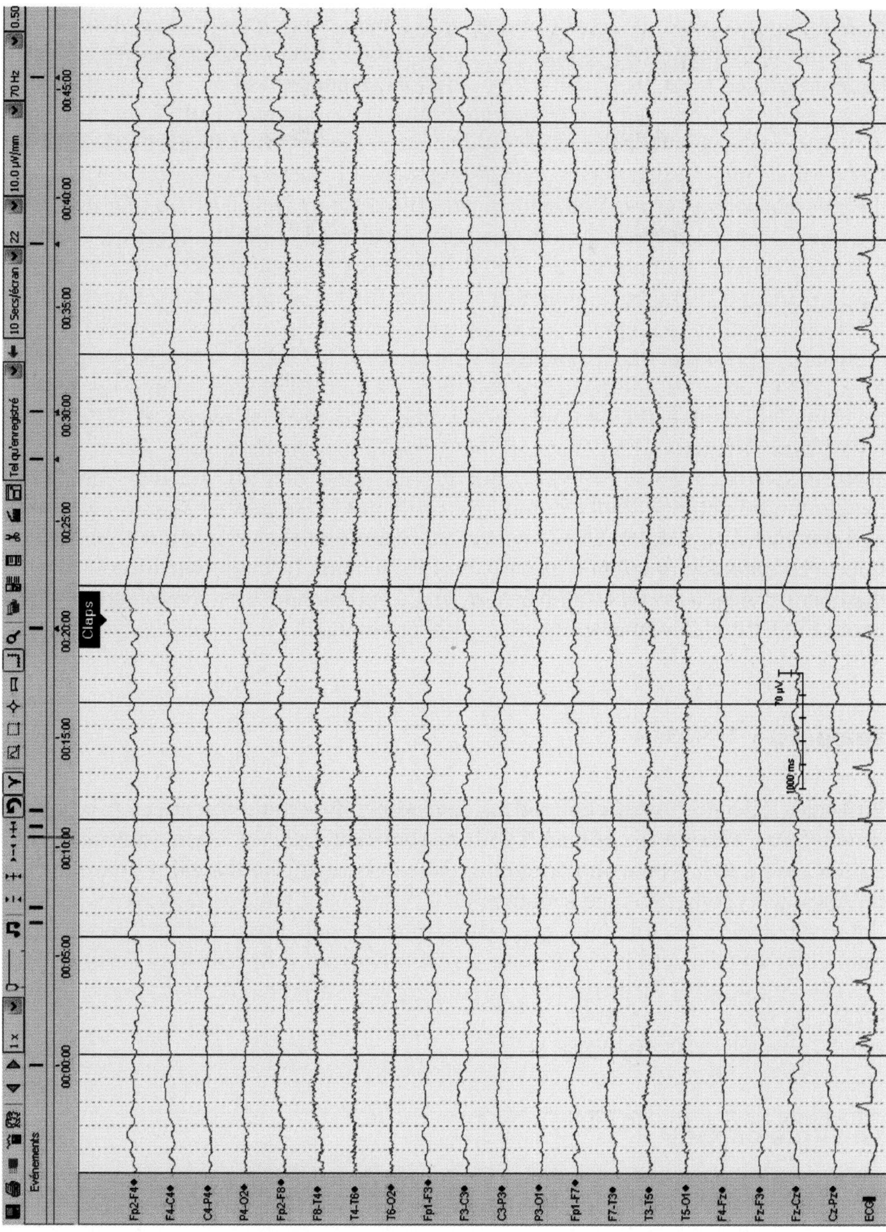

Fig. 1 EEG reactivity. The figure shows the EEG recorded on one illustrative patient during therapeutic hypothermia, 18 hours after cardiac arrest. Illustrated is an example of EEG reactivity: Upon stimulation (claps), the EEG background changes, i. e., increased frequency/reduced amplitude. The patient regained consciousness and had a good recovery

Emerging clinical evidence from several single center prospective studies suggests that EEG may indeed improve coma prognostication after cardiac arrest in patients treated with therapeutic hypothermia. Rundgren et al., in a preliminary study using a simplified amplitude-integrated EEG approach, first demonstrated that the presence of a continuous EEG pattern (as opposed to an EEG showing flat periods and/or spontaneous burst-suppression patterns) during the early hypothermic phase was associated with regain of consciousness [10]. Using the same approach, the same group more recently confirmed these findings in a larger cohort [11]. The additive value of EEG patterns to prognosticate coma after cardiac arrest and therapeutic hypothermia was further confirmed by Fugate et al., who showed that 'malignant' EEG patterns consisting of burst-suppression/generalized suppression were associated with death [7]. Finally, when looking at dynamic EEG changes, the presence of a non-reactive EEG background upon painful stimulation was also strongly associated with poor recovery [6, 7]. On the other hand, a reactive EEG background (Fig. 1) is a positive sign, which is often associated with a good recovery: our group found that all survivors had EEG background reactivity, and the majority of them (74%) had a favorable outcome at 3 months [12]. Adding EEG to standard neurological examination significantly improved outcome prediction as early as 12–24 hours from cardiac arrest – during therapeutic hypothermia – and increased the prediction of good outcome compared to SSEP [12]. Other groups had similar results [13].

Seizures

Post-anoxic seizures/status epilepticus (including myoclonus status epilepticus) are generally considered as malignant EEG patterns and are very often associated with a poor outcome [7, 14–16], particularly when occurring in the early phase during therapeutic hypothermia and sedation [12]. A subset of patients however who have 'late' seizures (i. e., after the rewarming phase) and display other 'good' signs (including EEG reactivity and presence of brainstem reflexes) may survive with a good neurological recovery [17]: these patients warrant aggressive anti-epileptic therapy.

The Role of SSEP

SSEP are usually performed to confirm a bad prognosis of coma after cardiac arrest and therapeutic hypothermia. The predictive value of SSEP for poor prognosis has indeed been confirmed in this setting by several recent studies [5–7]. Except in very rare cases [18], bilateral absence of the N20 component is invariably associated with irreversible coma and poor prognosis [19]. The main limitation of SSEP is when predicting the potential for good recovery in patients who have an N20 component but show coma or impairment of consciousness. For patients in such a 'gray zone' of uncertain prognosis, a multimodal approach (including neurological examination, EEG and NSE) is strongly recommended: In this context, EEG reactivity significantly improves prognostic accuracy, because those patients with a reactive EEG background have a high chance of recovery [6, 12, 17].

Serum Neuron-Specific Enolase

Serum NSE is a marker of the severity of global brain ischemia and at present appears to be the biomarker with the highest prognostic value after cardiac arrest and therapeutic hypothermia [20–22]. Before the therapeutic hypothermia era, serum NSE levels above 33 µg/l 24–72 hours after cardiac arrest were strongly, although not invariably, associated with poor prognosis [2, 5, 23]. Tiainen et al. however showed in a randomized study of patients treated with therapeutic hypothermia versus normothermia that hypothermia may significantly reduce serum NSE levels; the decreasing levels of serum NSE suggest a selective attenuation of delayed neuronal death by therapeutic hypothermia [24]. From a clinical standpoint, this study indicates that applying one single cut-off level may potentially be misleading. This suggestion has indeed been repeatedly shown by all recent studies in which the predictive value of NSE was tested and compared to that of other prognostic tools [25]. Much higher cut-off serum NSE values than 33 µg/l were necessary to reach an false positive rate of 0 % [20, 22, 26], with values as high as 78.9 µg/l needed to predict a poor outcome with a specificity of 100 % [26]. In a cohort of 61 consecutive comatose cardiac arrest patients treated with therapeutic hypothermia, we found 5 subjects who survived (of whom 3 had a full recovery) despite peak serum NSE > 33 µg/l at 48–72 hours [22]. In summary, as for all previous prognostic tools, serum NSE should be integrated into a multimodal prognostic algorithm.

Multimodal Prognostic Algorithm

The implementation of therapeutic hypothermia and of standardized post-resuscitation care has increased the number of patients who survive from acute coma after cardiac arrest and have the potential for good long-term recovery. Among early survivors, some still undergo early death in the intensive care unit (ICU) from post-cardiac arrest syndrome or refractory global brain dysfunction (absent brainstem reflexes, early myoclonus, non-reactive EEG, absent bilateral N20, highly elevated serum NSE levels) and irreversible coma. An increasing number of patients survive the early ICU phase after therapeutic hypothermia, and may eventually awaken and recover. In these patients, neurological examination (particularly motor signs) may not be enough to adequately predict prognosis: Additional prognostic tools – particularly EEG, SSEP and NSE – are of great value to improve early outcome prediction and avoid misleading prognostication (Fig. 2).

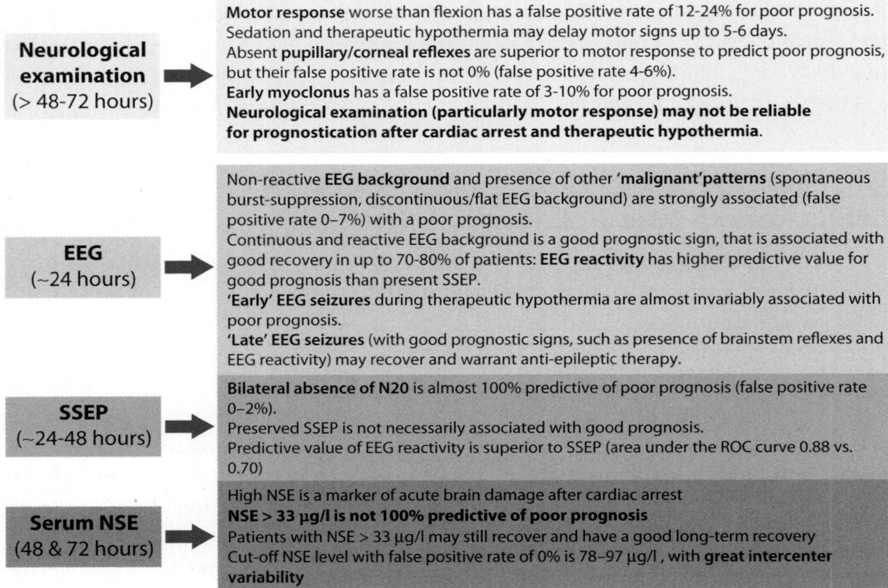

Fig. 2 Multimodal prognostication of coma after cardiac arrest and therapeutic hypothermia. The figure summarizes the timing after cardiac arrest of all available tools to predict recovery from coma. The prognostic performance is expressed as the false-positive rate for poor prognosis. EEG: electroencephalography; SSEP: somato-sensory evoked potentials; ROC: receiver operating characteristic; NSE: neuron-specific enolase

Perspectives and Areas for Future Clinical Investigation

Blood Biomarkers of Acute Cerebral Damage after Cardiac Arrest

Astrocytic soluble 100B protein (S-100B) levels have also been investigated for prognosis after cardiac arrest and studies have shown an association between elevated levels of S-100B in the blood within 24 hours from cardiac arrest and a poor prognosis [25, 27]. S-100B may represent an alternative biomarker to NSE. Preliminary studies have examined the value of other blood biomarkers, including glial fibrillary acidic protein [28], neurofilament H [29] and procalcitonin [28].

Neuroimaging

Diffusion magnetic resonance imaging (MRI) with the use of apparent diffusion coefficient (ADC) maps has been recently used to quantify brain damage after cardiac arrest and therapeutic hypothermia [30–33]. Spatial and temporal differences in ADC may provide insight into mechanisms of hypoxic-ischemic brain injury and, hence, recovery [31, 33]. The ideal time window for prognostication using diffusion MRI is 2–5 days after cardiac arrest: When comparing MRI in this time window to neurological examination at 3 days, diffusion MRI improved the sensitivity for predicting poor outcome by 38 %, while maintaining 100 % specificity [32]. Interestingly, when combining diffusion MRI with serum NSE, ADC-based predictions identified an additional 5 poor outcome patients out of 14 with 48-h NSE levels less than 78.9 µg/l [34], again illustrating the importance of a multimodal approach for the prognostication of comatose cardiac arrest patients.

Auditory Evoked Potentials

The frontal cortex network of auditory discrimination is emerging as a valid tool to assess cognitive function and recovery in humans with neuropsychiatric and neurological diseases [35]. This auditory-frontal cortical deficiency can be objectively measured with the so-called mismatch negativity (MMN). Fischer et al. first reported the value of MMN in comatose cardiac arrest patients not treated with therapeutic hypothermia [36]. When performed after the acute phase, on average at 10 days from cardiac arrest, all patients in whom SSEP or auditory evoked potentials were abolished did not awaken (100 % specificity). More importantly however, all patients in whom MMN was present did wake (100 % specificity); therefore, MMN was superior to SSEP for the prediction of awakening and had the best specificity and positive predictive value for good recovery. Our group recently focused on the prognostic value of automated auditory discrimination and MMN in 30 comatose cardiac arrest patients treated with therapeutic hypothermia in whom evoked potentials were performed at two time points (during and after therapeutic hypothermia). All patients (11/30) who displayed an early improvement in auditory discrimination across the two recordings regained consciousness [37].

Conclusion

Prognostication of coma after cardiac arrest and therapeutic hypothermia requires a multimodal approach. Neurological examination remains the first step: Motor response may be delayed up to 5 days after cardiac arrest because of the therapeutic hypothermia and may not be sufficient to accurately predict prognosis in all patients. The addition of EEG as a second step improves prognostic accuracy; in particular, presence of an early (within 24 hours from cardiac arrest) reactive EEG background is a good sign whereas a non-reactive or burst-suppressed EEG pattern is an ominous sign. Bilateral absence of N20 on SSEP at 24–48 hours is almost invariably associated with a poor prognosis and is helpful to confirm irreversible coma. Serum NSE at 48–72 hours may be useful to assess the severity of acute brain damage; however, the cut-off values for poor prognosis are higher in patients treated with therapeutic hypothermia, thus serum NSE should be used only as a complementary tool and never alone. Diffusion MRI and auditory evoked potentials provide new insight into the mechanisms of hypoxic-ischemic brain injury and may improve the prediction of long-term recovery in comatose survivors of cardiac arrest.

References

1. Peberdy MA, Callaway CW, Neumar RW et al (2010) Part 9: post-cardiac arrest care: 2010 American Heart Association Guidelines for Cardiopulmonary Resuscitation and Emergency Cardiovascular Care. Circulation 122(18 Suppl 3):S768–S786
2. Wijdicks EF, Hijdra A, Young GB, Bassetti CL, Wiebe S (2006) Practice parameter: prediction of outcome in comatose survivors after cardiopulmonary resuscitation (an evidence-based review): report of the Quality Standards Subcommittee of the American Academy of Neurology. Neurology 67:203–210
3. Thenayan AE, Savard M, Sharpe M, Norton L, Young B (2008) Predictors of poor neurologic outcome after induced mild hypothermia following cardiac arrest. Neurology 71:1535–1537
4. Samaniego EA, Mlynash M, Caulfield AF, Eyngorn I, Wijman CA (2011) Sedation confounds outcome prediction in cardiac arrest survivors treated with hypothermia. Neurocrit Care 15:113–119
5. Bouwes A, Binnekade JM, Kuiper MA et al (2012) Prognosis of coma after therapeutic hypothermia: A prospective cohort study. Ann Neurol 71:206–212
6. Rossetti AO, Oddo M, Logroscino G, Kaplan PW (2010) Prognostication after cardiac arrest and hypothermia: a prospective study. Ann Neurol 67:301–307
7. Fugate JE, Wijdicks EF, Mandrekar J et al (2010) Predictors of neurologic outcome in hypothermia after cardiac arrest. Ann Neurol 68:907–914
8. Synek VM (1990) Value of a revised EEG coma scale for prognosis after cerebral anoxia and diffuse head injury. Clin Electroencephalogr 21:25–30
9. Synek VM, Shaw NA (1989) Epileptiform discharges in presence of continuous background activity in anoxic coma. Clin Electroencephalogr 20:141–146
10. Rundgren M, Rosen I, Friberg H (2006) Amplitude-integrated EEG (aEEG) predicts outcome after cardiac arrest and induced hypothermia. Intensive Care Med 32:836–842
11. Rundgren M, Westhall E, Cronberg T, Rosen I, Friberg H (2010) Continuous amplitude-integrated electroencephalogram predicts outcome in hypothermia-treated cardiac arrest patients. Crit Care Med 38:1838–1844
12. Rossetti AO, Urbano LA, Delodder F, Kaplan PW, Oddo M (2010) Prognostic value of continuous EEG monitoring during therapeutic hypothermia after cardiac arrest. Crit Care 14:R173
13. Thenayan EA, Savard M, Sharpe MD, Norton L, Young B (2010) Electroencephalogram for prognosis after cardiac arrest. J Crit Care 25:300–304
14. Legriel S, Bruneel F, Sediri H et al (2009) Early EEG monitoring for detecting postanoxic status epilepticus during therapeutic hypothermia: A pilot study. Neurocrit Care 11:338–344
15. Rittenberger JC, Popescu A, Brenner RP, Guyette FX, Callaway CW (2012) Frequency and timing of nonconvulsive status epilepticus in comatose post-cardiac arrest subjects treated with hypothermia. Neurocrit Care 16:114–122
16. Rossetti AO, Logroscino G, Liaudet L et al (2007) Status epilepticus: an independent outcome predictor after cerebral anoxia. Neurology 69:255–260

17. Rossetti AO, Oddo M, Liaudet L, Kaplan PW (2009) Predictors of awakening from post-anoxic status epilepticus after therapeutic hypothermia. Neurology 72:744–749
18. Leithner C, Ploner CJ, Hasper D, Storm C (2010) Does hypothermia influence the predictive value of bilateral absent N20 after cardiac arrest? Neurology 74:965–969
19. Rothstein TL (2012) Therapeutic hypothermia and reliability of somatosensory evoked potentials in predicting outcome after cardiopulmonary arrest. Neurocrit Care 17:146–149
20. Cronberg T, Rundgren M, Westhall E et al (2011) Neuron-specific enolase correlates with other prognostic markers after cardiac arrest. Neurology 77:623–630
21. Oksanen T, Tiainen M, Skrifvars MB et al (2009) Predictive power of serum NSE and OHCA score regarding 6-month neurologic outcome after out-of-hospital ventricular fibrillation and therapeutic hypothermia. Resuscitation 80:165–170
22. Rossetti AO, Carrera E, Oddo M (2012) Early EEG correlates of neuronal injury after brain anoxia. Neurology 78:796–802
23. Zandbergen EG, Hijdra A, Koelman JH et al (2006) Prediction of poor outcome within the first 3 days of postanoxic coma. Neurology 66:62–68
24. Tiainen M, Roine RO, Pettila V, Takkunen O (2003) Serum neuron-specific enolase and S-100B protein in cardiac arrest patients treated with hypothermia. Stroke 34:2881–2886
25. Shinozaki K, Oda S, Sadahiro T et al (2009) S-100B and neuron-specific enolase as predictors of neurological outcome in patients after cardiac arrest and return of spontaneous circulation: a systematic review. Crit Care 13:R121
26. Steffen IG, Hasper D, Ploner CJ et al (2010) Mild therapeutic hypothermia alters neuron specific enolase as an outcome predictor after resuscitation: 97 prospective hypothermia patients compared to 133 historical non-hypothermia patients. Crit Care 14:R69
27. Mortberg E, Zetterberg H, Nordmark J, Blennow K, Rosengren L, Rubertsson S (2011) S-100B is superior to NSE, BDNF and GFAP in predicting outcome of resuscitation from cardiac arrest with hypothermia treatment. Resuscitation 82:26–31
28. Hayashida H, Kaneko T, Kasaoka S et al (2010) Comparison of the predictability of neurological outcome by serum procalcitonin and glial fibrillary acidic protein in postcardiac-arrest patients. Neurocrit Care 12:252–257
29. Rundgren M, Friberg H, Cronberg T, Romner B, Petzold A (2012) Serial soluble neurofilament heavy chain in plasma as a marker of brain injury after cardiac arrest. Crit Care 16:R45
30. Choi SP, Park KN, Park HK et al (2010) Diffusion-weighted magnetic resonance imaging for predicting the clinical outcome of comatose survivors after cardiac arrest: a cohort study. Crit Care 14:R17
31. Mlynash M, Campbell DM, Leproust EM et al (2010) Temporal and spatial profile of brain diffusion-weighted MRI after cardiac arrest. Stroke 41:1665–1672
32. Wijman CA, Mlynash M, Caulfield AF et al (2009) Prognostic value of brain diffusion-weighted imaging after cardiac arrest. Ann Neurol 65:394–402
33. Wu O, Sorensen AG, Benner T, Singhal AB, Furie KL, Greer DM (2009) Comatose patients with cardiac arrest: predicting clinical outcome with diffusion-weighted MR imaging. Radiology 252:173–181
34. Kim J, Choi BS, Kim K et al (2012) Prognostic performance of diffusion-weighted MRI combined with NSE in comatose cardiac arrest survivors treated with mild hypothermia. Neurocrit Care 17:412–420
35. Naatanen R, Kujala T, Kreegipuu K et al (2011) The mismatch negativity: an index of cognitive decline in neuropsychiatric and neurological diseases and in ageing. Brain 134:3435–3453
36. Fischer C, Luaute J, Nemoz C, Morlet D, Kirkorian G, Mauguiere F (2006) Improved prediction of awakening or nonawakening from severe anoxic coma using tree-based classification analysis. Crit Care Med 34:1520–1524
37. Tzovara A, Rossetti AO, Spierer L et al (2013) Progression of auditory discrimination based on neural decoding predicts awakening from coma. Brain (in press)

Part IX

Monitoring

Patient Monitoring Alarms in the ICU and in the Operating Room

F. Schmid, M. S. Goepfert, and D. A. Reuter

Introduction

Historically, the word 'alarm' originates from the Latin, 'ad arma', or the French, 'à l'arme', which can be translated into 'to your weapons'. Hence, the word indicates a call for immediate action, for attack or for defense. Alarms have existed ever since humans have lived in groups. Some of the first documented alarms are watchmen on towers in the Middle Ages, who warned of fires or enemies by ringing bells. Warning fires provided a visual alert to enemy attacks, visible across long ranges and enabling an early reaction of armed forces. Today, comparable systems are available that send warning-SMSs (Short Message Service) of nearing tsunamis to mobile phones [1].

In complex fields of work like aviation, mining, anesthesiology, and intensive care medicine – and here particularly with regard to monitoring of vital functions – alarms are ubiquitous and have been the subject of medical, technical, and psychological research for decades [2, 3]. Monitoring of vital functions and function of life-support devices is essential for critically ill patients, although real evidence based data are missing. However, modern patient monitors and implemented risk management (including alarms) must be constructed in accordance to approved

F. Schmid (✉)
Department of Anesthesiology, Center of Anesthesiology and Intensive Care Medicine, Hamburg Eppendorf University Hospital, Martinistr. 52, 20246 Hamburg, Germany
E-mail: feschmid@uke.de

M. S. Goepfert
Department of Anesthesiology, Center of Anesthesiology and Intensive Care Medicine, Hamburg Eppendorf University Hospital, Martinistr. 52, 20246 Hamburg, Germany

D. A. Reuter
Department of Anesthesiology, Center of Anesthesiology and Intensive Care Medicine, Hamburg Eppendorf University Hospital, Martinistr. 52, 20246 Hamburg, Germany

J.-L. Vincent (Ed.), *Annual Update in Intensive Care and Emergency Medicine 2013*,
DOI 10.1007/978-3-642-35109-9_30,

and current international standards IEC 60601-1-11 and IEC 80001-1 [4, 5]. Tinker et al. surveyed 1,175 anesthetic-related closed malpractice claims from 17 professional liability insurance companies. It was determined that 31.5 % of the negative outcomes could have been prevented by use of additional monitors. The authors concluded that monitoring with adequate thresholds appeared able to improve patient outcomes [6]. Cooper et al. showed in the 1980s that 70 % of all anesthesia-related critical incidents were caused by human error [7]. Similar data are available from the aviation industry [8]. Inevitable mistakes may be corrected in time if detected by a monitoring system (including alarms) before physiological variables run out of range.

An alarm is an automatic warning that results from a measurement, or any other acquisition of descriptors of a state, and indicates a relevant deviation from a normal state [9]. Loeb surveyed the reaction of anesthesiologists to relevant changes in monitoring parameters, and showed that anesthesiologists needed a mean time of 61 seconds to recognize a change in the parameters; 16 % of the changes were unrecognized for over 5 minutes [10]. In contrast, Morris and Montano studied the reaction of anesthesiologists to optical and acoustic warnings during maintenance of general anesthesia. The anesthesiologists showed a reaction time of 6 seconds to optical warnings and 1 second to acoustic warnings [11]. An ideal alarm should only detect immediate or threatening danger that requires prompt attention. The alarm design should adequately represent the underlying situation. The announcement of the alarm should be instantly perceptible in critical situations. Additionally, the user should be informed of circumstances that impair the reliability of the alarming system.

In addition to these general properties, device alarms have various goals, which follow a certain hierarchy [12]:

- Detection of life-threatening situations: The detection of life-threatening situations was the original purpose of monitor alarms. False negative alarms are not acceptable in such situations because of the danger of severe patient harm or death.
- Detection of imminent danger: The early detection of gradual change that might indicate imminent danger.
- Diagnostic alarms: These alarms indicate a pathophysiological condition (e. g., shock) rather than warning of 'out-of-range' variables.
- Detection of life-threatening device malfunction: This ability is essential for all life-support devices, which must recognize malfunctions, such as disconnection from the patient, occlusion of the connection to the patient, disconnection from power, gas, or water supply, and internal malfunction.
- Detection of imminent device malfunction: The early detection of device-related problems that could result in malfunction is an integral part of many therapeutic devices. These warning mechanisms range from simple aspects (e. g., low-battery warnings) to complex algorithms and sensors that track the wear of respiratory valves.

Alarm Design

Alarms are typically displayed in two ways or as a combination of both:

1. Acoustic
   The alarm is given as a warning sound. Most manufacturers distinguish the priority of an alarm with different signals. Intuitive alarms with different tone sequences (e. g. 'short-long-short' for 'ven-ti-late') have been the object of research but have not found their way into routine clinical practice. Alarms directly mentioning organ systems, device hardware, or parts of it (e. g., ventilation or circulation) or alarms with direct labeling of the physiological problem ('blood-pressure' or 'oxygen') have also not been introduced into practice [13].
2. Visual
   Visual alarms involve mostly flashing or coloring of the related parameter in an eye-catching manner. Some systems provide integrated displays of several parameters. One example is a spider-display, which shows the relationship of different parameters in a stylized spider web. Such applications can be useful to display different parameters in context. Compared to other professions in industry and aviation, adoption of such new displays in healthcare has been slow.

Alarm-Related Problems

Alarms help to prevent patient harm by providing rapid recognition of and reaction to critical situations, but only if they are not 'false alarms'. Medical progress leads to an increasing number of 'monitorable' parameters and thus an increasing number of possible alarms.

False Alarms

In medicine, false alarms are conventionally defined as alarms without clinical or therapeutic consequence. Today's monitoring systems are still designed using a 'better-safe-than-sorry'-logic: A large number of false alarms are accepted rather than risking missing one valid alarm [14]. Alarms can be differentiated into technically correct/technically false and clinically relevant/clinically not relevant. Alarms can be classified as technically correct, if they are based upon a technically correct measurement. Technically false alarms are not based on a technically correct measurement (e. g., interference with pulse oximetry caused by ambient light). Because not all technically correct alarms are clinically relevant, they can be further differentiated into clinically relevant or not relevant (e. g., inadequate thresholds).

False Alarm Rates

There are several studies in the medical literature about monitoring alarms in anesthesiology and intensive care medicine. Lawless suggested that 94 % of all alarms in a pediatric intensive care unit (PICU) were clinically irrelevant [15]. Tsien and Fackler also found that 92 % of alarms were false alarms in their observation in a PICU [16]. In both studies, all alarms were recorded by the nursing staff, who also assessed their relevance and validity. O'Carroll reported that only 8 of 1,455 alarms were caused by potentially life-threatening situations [17]. An observation by Siebig and co-workers showed that these results are not limited to the PICU. These authors digitally recorded all the alarms for 38 patients on a 12-bed medical ICU and retrospectively assessed their relevance and validity: Only 17 % of the alarms were relevant, with 44 % being technically false [18]. Chambrin et al. conducted a multicenter study in 1999, including 131 medical ICU patients. The medical staff recorded all alarms, which were assessed according to their relevance and the reaction of the medical staff. Twenty-six percent of the alarms had marginal consequences, for example leading to re-positioning of sensors. In only 6 % did the alarm lead to a call for a doctor. Seventeen percent were the result of technical problems and 24 % were caused by staff manipulation [14].

In contrast to ICU observations, there are only a few studies about false alarms in perioperative settings. Comparison between the ICU and the operating room (OR) is limited in part because ICU patients are only sedated and not anesthetized, causing higher rates of patient movement artifacts. Furthermore, in the OR, changes in patients' conditions often occur much more rapidly than in the ICU because of changes in the depth of anesthesia and surgical manipulation (e. g., extensive blood loss).

Schmid et al. [19] studied perioperative alarms in a highly complex surgical setting and included 25 patients undergoing elective cardiac surgery with extracorporeal circulation. All patient monitor and anesthesia workstation alarms were digitally recorded. Additionally, the anesthesiology workplace was videotaped from two angles to allow better assessment of external influences, retrospectively. During 124 hours of monitoring, 8,975 alarms were recorded: 7,556 alarms were hemodynamic alarms, 1,419 alarms were ventilation-related. This corresponded to 359 ± 158 alarms per procedure (1.2 alarms/minute). The reaction time to the alarms was on average 4 seconds. Of all the alarms, 96 % were caused by threshold violations. Of the 8,975 alarms, 6,386 were classified as serious and life-threatening and analyzed further: 4,438 (70 %) of these were labeled as valid, 1,948 (30 %) were caused by artifacts; 1,735 (39 %) of the valid alarms were classified as relevant, 2,703 (61 %) were not relevant.

These results supported earlier studies in less complex settings. Seagull and Sanderson surveyed perioperative alarms in different surgical disciplines (arthroscopic, cardiac surgery, abdominal surgery, and neurosurgery) with 6 cases in each discipline. The authors found 72 % of alarms had no clinical consequences [20]. A study by Kestin et al. [21] included 50 pediatric patients (1 month to 10 years old) in the OR of a pediatric hospital (pediatric surgery, eye surgery, dental surgery, orthopedic surgery) and also found that 75 % alarms had no therapeutic consequences (1 alarm per 4.5 minutes on average). Only 3 % of all alarms indicated critical situations [21]. However, the studies by Kestin [21] and Seagull [20] were limited by the fact that 5 and 6 different monitors, respectively, were used in these observational studies.

Artifacts: A Common Source of False Alarm

Many false alarms are caused by artifacts. The main sources of artifact are well known and are of physiological and non-physiological origin. Most of these artifacts directly influence the measured signals [22], leading to incorrect measurements and this, in turn, triggers the alarm. The most common artifacts and their sources are listed in Table 1.

Table 1 Monitoring parameters and related artifacts

Signal	Artifact source	Parameter
Ventilatory alarms		
Pulse oximetry	Movement Injection of contrast dye Interruption of blood-flow by non-invasive blood pressure measurement Ambient light	Oxygen saturation Pulse frequency
Capnography	Occlusion of CO_2-line (by kinking or built up fluid) Ventilator circuit leakage Atmospheric pressure variations Suctioning Dead space in measurement circuit	End-tidal CO_2 Inspired CO_2 Respiratory rate
Hemodynamic Alarms		
EKG	Electrosurgical interference Power-line interference Movement artifacts (patient movement, positioning) Electrode instability or electrode distortion EMG/neuromonitoring interference Incorrect connection or lead contact Pacing/defibrillation Abnormally tall T-waves mistaken as QRS-complex MRI interference	Heart rate, ST-values Arrhythmia detection
Non-invasive blood pressure	Movement Inadequate size or cuff position Compression of cuff by external forces (surgeon or equipment pressing against the cuff Kinked cuff tubing and leaking cuff bladder	Systolic, diastolic blood pressure Mean arterial pressure
Other Alarms		
Temperature	Dislocated sensor	Temperature

EKG: electrocardiogram, EMG: electromyogram, MRI: magnetic resonance imaging, CO_2: carbon dioxide

Consequences of False Alarms

The story of "the shepherd who cried wolf" appears in Aesop's Fables and, with some minor variations, can be found in the folklore of many different cultures. "One day, just to stir up excitement, the shepherd boy rushed down from the pasture, crying 'Wolf! Wolf!' The villagers heard the alarm and came running to help chase the marauder away, only to find the sheep peaceful and no wolf in sight. But there came a day when a wolf really came. The boy screamed and called for help. But all in vain! The neighbors, supposing him to be up to his old tricks, paid no heed to his cries, and the wolf devoured the sheep!" [23].

Based on this Fable, Breznitz formed the phrase "Crying-Wolf-Phenomenon" for the desensitization caused by high false alarm rates, with the possible consequence of ignoring relevant alarms [24]. The high incidence of false alarms in anesthesiology and intensive care medicine is not only a disturbance but a risk factor when relevant alarms in critical situations are ignored. That this phenomenon is not limited to monitoring alarms was impressively demonstrated by the attack of the Japanese air force on the United States Navy at Pearl Harbor, Hawaii on December 7, 1941. Despite a valid advance warning by the new radar technology, no appropriate reaction followed. The simultaneous report of a contact and the destruction of an enemy submarine also did not lead to a reaction because the commanding admiral wanted to wait for confirmation due to frequent false alarms [25].

Various studies have shown that anesthesiologists' reaction times to alarms increases in situations where there is low alarm validity [26, 27]. The annoyance from false alarms may also lead to complete inactivation of alarms or to inappropriately wide threshold settings by the clinical user to limit alarms as much as possible. Thereby, the 'mesh of the alarm-net' gets wider and the risk of missed relevant alarm increases [28].

Medical Staff and Alarms

Alarms in the ICU and in the OR frequently lead to sound levels up to 70 dB(A). This level corresponds to heavy traffic. Sound levels up to 90 dB are not rare [29]. In a study by Hagerman et al., 94 patients with chest pain were retrospectively distributed into a good and poor acoustic group. Acoustics were altered during the study period by changing the ceiling tiles throughout the ICU from sound-reflecting (poor acoustics) to sound-absorbing tiles (good acoustics) of similar appearance. The patients were asked to complete a questionnaire about the quality of care. The patients considered the staff attitude was much better in the good acoustics period [30]. Increased sound levels caused by alarms can impact on the health of the medical personnel. In 1988, Topf and Dillon demonstrated the relationship between increased sound levels in ICUs and burn-out syndromes in ICU nurses [31].

Patients and Alarms

For undisturbed night-sleep, sound levels below 40 dB(A) are recommended. As sound levels on the ICU are frequently above this level, sleep deprivation in ICU patients is well recognized [32]. Sleep deprivation in ICU patients leads to an impairment of the immune response and increased sympathetic nervous system activity: Catecholamine secretion increases heart rate, metabolism, and oxygen consumption [33]. Frequent arousal from sleep may lead to cardiac arrhythmias in patients with pre-existing heart disease but also in healthy patients [34]. Minckley reported significantly increased opioid needs when noise levels were high in her observation of 644 postoperative patients [35]. In the study by Hagerman et al., patients during the good acoustic (sound-absorbing ceiling tiles) period had lower pulse amplitude values than those in the bad acoustic group; patients in the bad acoustics group also had higher rates of re-hospitalization after 1 (18 % vs. 10 %) and 3 months (48 % vs. 21 %) [30]. In a recent study, Van Rompaey et al. found reduced rates and later onset of delirium in patients who slept with earplugs at night [36].

Technical Approaches for False Alarm Reduction

Essentially, there are three technical approaches to help reduce false alarms: (1) Improving signal extraction (prevention or detection of artifacts); (2) improving algorithms for alarm generation; (3) improving alarm validation. An algorithm for alarm generation can be based on a single parameter (e. g., heart-rate or mean arterial pressure) or on several parameters simultaneously (e. g., heart rate detection from elecrocardiogram [EKG], pulse oximetry oxygen saturation [SpO_2] and arterial line). Most devices are equipped with alarms based on a single parameter. In recent years, different approaches for false alarm reduction have been developed.

Phase Specific Settings

Observations, especially in surgical settings, have shown that different phases of the surgical procedure are characterized by different numbers and types of false alarms and also different patterns of alarms and specific reactions by the medical staff (e. g., during induction and emergence of anesthesia, during extracorporeal circulation, or single lung ventilation, or suctioning of patients). Schmid et al. found different characteristic patterns and density of alarms in 4 different intraoperative phases (beginning of surgery, start of extracorporeal circulation [ECC], end of ECC, end of surgery) [19].

Seagull and Sanderson also differentiated three different phases in anesthesia procedures (introduction, maintenance and emergence) and found characteristic patterns of alarms and alarm reactions in each phase [20].

This knowledge could be used for the development of phase specific settings to reduce false alarms (e. g., for specific settings for surgery or on the ICU).

Integrated Validation of Alarms (Cross Checking)

Matching of different parameters can be used for the reduction of false alarms: e. g., a 'ventricular fibrillation' alarm can be assumed to be false in the presence of undisturbed pulse oximetry and arterial blood pressure waveforms. Aboukhalil et al. [37] were able to reduce the incidence of false arrhythmia-related alarms from 42.7 % to 17.2 % in an offline application on a database of 447 patients (5,386 arrhythmia alarms). However, 9.7 % of the true cases of ventricular fibrillation were not detected; this situation is inadmissible for a lethal arrhythmia. Removal of ventricular arrhythmias from the algorithm still resulted in reduction in the incidence of false alarms to 22.7 % [37].

Implementation of Time Delays

Görges et al. [38] showed in an ICU setting and Schmid et al. [19] in an intraoperative setting that a great number of false alarms are caused by only mild threshold violations of short duration. In an offline validation, Görges et al. showed that the implementation of a 14-second delay reduced false alarms by 50 %; a 19-second delay reduced false alarms by 67 %. However, a simple delay carries the risk of unrecognized critical situations of short duration (e. g., short self-limiting tachycardia). The implementation of a graduated delay brings additional safety and flexibility to that approach. First, severe deviations are alarmed faster; this results in improved patient safety. Second, the graduation offers the possibility of a prolonged delay (more than 14 seconds) in cases of only moderate and clinically not-relevant deviations. However, studies using such an approach are still missing.

Statistical Approaches for False Alarm Reduction

Improved signal extraction is an essential approach for reduction of false alarms caused by artifacts. Several approaches have been developed over the last decades.

Autoregressive Models and Self-Adjusting Thresholds

An autoregressive model describes measurement values as a linear transformation and integrates previous values plus a random error. An autoregressive model is appropriate for the observation of values in steady-state and for alarm generation caused by deviation from steady-state. It is also used for generation of self-adjusting thresholds, because of integration of the individual patient's condition. However, self-adjusting thresholds always have to be elaborated and confirmed by the user [9].

Statistical Process Control

Statistical approaches are commonly used in alarm systems to detect 'out-of-control' states in a process. The original applications were in industrial production processes but they are also used for alarm generation. Kennedy used a process control approach to detect the onset of changes in systolic blood pressure [39]. The algorithm was tested on an existing database and detected 94 % of changes correctly, whereas anesthesiologists only detected 85 %.

Median Filters

The median filter is a non-linear, signal processing method used for removal of short-term noise in measurement signals without influencing the baseline signal. For this purpose, the median is calculated for a defined interval. Thus, the signal is 'smoothed' and short noises, such as movement artifacts or interference from electro-surgery, are eliminated. This method is limited in long-lasting interferences that exceed the adjusted duration of the filter. Mäkivirta et al. [40] evaluated the effectiveness of a combination of a "short" (15 seconds) and a "long" (2.5 minutes) filter in a database of 10 cardiac surgery patients. The use of the filter increased the alarms that had therapeutic consequences from 12 to 49 %; the authors declared that no relevant alarms were missed.

Artificial Intelligence

Although statistical approaches are predominantly used for the reduction of artifacts, artificial intelligence offers the possibility of integrating more complex contexts. This approach tries to validate alarms by imitating human thinking. Artificial intelligence can be embedded into decision-making systems. A paper by Imhoff and Kuhls provides an overview of artificial intelligence use in intensive care monitoring [9].

Rule-Based Expert Systems

Rule-based expert systems are based on an integrated expert knowledge database. Some early rule-based expert systems were developed for medical use in the 1970s (MYCIN-System, ONCOCIN-System) [41]. These early systems applied expert knowledge from a database into a new context and simulated expert decisions in oncology and therapy of infectious diseases. In 1993, Sukuvaara et al. [42] developed an alarm system for the detection of hypovolemia, hyperdynamic circulation, left-heart failure, and hypoventilation. Although results showed that rule-based expert systems work well in the context of pathologic conditions, they have not been introduced into the clinical arena. The expansion of rule-based expert systems by so-called machine-learning is possible, whereby the pre-existing database is updated by actual patient data.

Neural Networks

Neural networks were developed to imitate the neuronal process of human thinking. They are able to anticipate the presence of diseases on the basis of advance information (e. g., hemodynamic data from a myocardial infarction study group). Baxt and Skora [43] developed a neural network for early detection of myocardial infarction in patients admitted to a hospital with chest pain. The system was "trained" to detect specific changes in patients with myocardial infarction by implementation of a database (350 patients, 120 of whom had myocardial infarction). The results showed that the neural network was able to detect or to exclude infarction with a sensitivity and specificity of 96 %. The doctors at the respective emergency department achieved an average sensitivity of 73.3 % and specificity of 81.1 %. Neural networks have also been used for alarm generation in anesthesia ventilators [44].

Fuzzy Logic

Fuzzy logic was introduced by Zadeh in the 1960s [45]. A common problem in clinical routine is the aim for objectivity and precision when the information does not allow an explicit conclusion. Fuzzy logic allows diffuse processing of exact data. Fuzzy logic is widely used in industry (e. g., for picture stabilization in cameras). Goldman and Cordova [46] demonstrated a patient monitor that was able to diagnose a simulated cardiac arrest by evaluation of EKG, capnography, and arterial blood pressure using fuzzy logic.

Bayesian Networks

Bayesian networks have been used for estimation of event occurrence. In patient monitoring, they can be used for decision support. Laursen developed software for cardiac event detection [47]. The software continuously compared different physiologic parameters and their changes; thus, it was possible to check values against each other for plausibility and to anticipate cardiac events.

Conclusion

Medical progress has led to obvious improvements in ICU and perioperative monitoring over recent decades. With the increase in 'monitorable' parameters, rates of alarms have also increased. But technical progress has rarely affected the rates of false alarms. In addition to noise-related increase in burn-out rates, false alarms lead to desensitization of medical staff to alarms with the risk of critical situations potentially being ignored despite correct alarming. Patients are also directly affected by alarm-related sleep disorders with subsequent development of delirium and increased sympathetic nervous system activity and catecholamine secretion. In recent years, many promising approaches using statistical methods and artificial intelligence have been developed for the reduction of false alarms without obvious changes in false alarm rates in our clinical reality.

References

1. Tsunami Alarm System. Available at: http://www.tsunami-alarm-system.com/en/index.html. Accessed Oct 2012
2. Billings CE, Raynard WD (1984) Human factors in aircraft incidents: results of a 7-years study. Aviat Space Environ Med 55:960–965
3. Kowalski-Trakofler KM, Vaught C, Mallett LG et al (2004) Safety and health training for an evolving workforce: an overview from the mining industry. Information Circular 9474:1–15
4. International Organization for Standardization (2010) IEC-ISO 60601-1-11. Available at http://www.iso.org/iso/home/store/catalogue_tc/catalogue_detail.htm?csnumber=45605. Accessed August 2012
5. International Organization for Standardization (2010) IEC 80001-1:2010. Available at http://www.iso.org/iso/home/store/catalogue_tc/catalogue_detail.htm?csnumber=44863. Accessed August 2012
6. Tinker JH, Dull DL, Caplan RA, Ward RJ, Cheney FW (1989) Role of monitoring devices in prevention of anesthetic mishaps: A closed claims analysis. Anesthesiology 71:541–546
7. Cooper JB, Newbower RS, Kitz RJ (1984) An analysis of major errors and equipment failures in anesthesia management: considerations for prevention and detection. Anesthesiology 60:34–42

8. Flight Safety Foundation (2003) Flight Safety Digest – The Human Factors Implications for Flight Safety of Recent Developments in the Airline Industry. Available at: http://flightsafety.org/fsd/fsd_mar-apr03.pdf Accessed Oct 2012
9. Imhoff M, Kuhls S (2006) Alarm algorithms in critical care monitoring. Anesth Analg 102:1525–1537
10. Loeb RG (1993) A measure of intraoperative attention to monitor displays. Anesth Analg 76:337–341
11. Morris RW, Montano SR (1996) Response times to visual and auditory alarms during anaesthesia. Anaesth Intensive Care 24:682–684
12. Imhoff M, Kuhl S, Gather U, Fried R (2009) Smart alarms from medical devices in the OR and ICU. Best Pract Res Clin Anaesthesiol 23:39–50
13. Block FE, Rouse JD, Hakala M, Thomson CL (2000) A proposed new set of alarm sounds which satisfy standards and rationale to encode source information. J Clin Monit 16:541–546
14. Chambrin MC, Raveaux P, Calvelo-Aros D, Jaborska A, Chopin C, Boniface B (1999) Multicentric study of monitoring alarms in the adult intensive care unit (ICU): A descriptive analysis. Intensive Care Med 25:1360–1366
15. Lawless ST (1994) Crying Wolf: False alarms in a pediatric intensive care unit. Crit Care Med 22:981–985
16. Tsien CL, Fackler JC (1997) Poor prognosis for existing monitors in the intensive care unit. Crit Care Med 25:614–619
17. O'Carroll TM (1986) Survey of alarms in an intensive care unit. Anaesthesia 41:742–744
18. Siebig S, Kuhls S, Imhoff M et al (2010) Collection of annotated data in a clinical validation study for alarm algorithms in intensive care – A methodologic framework. J Crit Care 25:128–135
19. Schmid F, Goepfert MS, Kuhnt D et al (2011) The wolf is crying in the operating room: patient monitor and anesthesia workstation alarming patterns during cardiac surgery. Anesth Analg 112:78–83
20. Seagull FJ, Sanderson PM (2001) Anesthesia alarms in context: An observational Study. Hum Factors 43:66–78
21. Kestin IG, Miller BR, Lockhart CH (1988) Auditory alarms during anesthesia monitoring. Anesthesiology 69:106–109
22. Takla G, Petre JH, Doyle JD, Horibe M, Gopakumaran B (2006) The problem of artefacts in patient monitor data during surgery: A clinical and methodological review. Anesth Analg 103:1196–1204
23. Aesop (1985) The Shepherd Boy and the Wolf. In: Aesops Fables. Watermill Classic Edition. NJ Watermill Press, Mahwah, pp 116–117
24. Breznitz S (1984) Cry wolf: The Psychology of False Alarms. Psychology Press, New York
25. Barkeley AW, Cooper J, George WF et al (1946) Congressional investigation of the pearl harbor attack. US Government, Washington, pp 141–143
26. Westenskow DR, Orr J, Simon FH, Bender HJ, Frankenberger H (1992) Intelligent alarms reduce anaesthesiologist's response time to critical faults. Anesthesiology 77:1074–1079
27. Bliss JP, Dunn MC (2000) Behavioural implications of alarm mistrust as a function of task workload. Ergonomics 43:1283–1300
28. Block FE, Nuutinen L, Ballast B (1999) Optimization of alarms: A study on alarm limits, alarm sounds and false alarms intended to reduce annoyance. J Clin Monit 15:75–83
29. Kam PCA, Kam AC, Thompson JF (1994) Noise pollution in the anaesthetic and intensive care environment. Anaesthesia 49:982–986
30. Hagerman I, Rasmanis G, Blomkvist V, Ulrich R, Eriksen CA, Theorell T (2005) Influence of intensive coronary care acoustics on the quality of care and physiological state of patients. Int J Cardiol 98:267–270
31. Topf M, Dillon E (1988) Noise induced stress as a predictor of burnout in critical care nurses. Heart Lung 17:567–573

32. Aaron JN, Carlisle CC, Carskadon MA, Meyer TJ, Hill NS, Millman RP (1996) Environmental noise as a cause of sleep disruption in an intermediate respiratory care unit. Sleep 19:707–710
33. Hansell HN (1984) The behavioural effects of the noise on men: The patient with "intensive care psychosis". Heart Lung 13:59–65
34. Smith R, Johnson L, Rothfeld D, Zir L, Tharp B (1972) Sleep and cardiac arrythmias. Arch Intern Med 130:751–753
35. Minckley BB (1968) A study of noise and its relationship to patient discomfort in the recovery room. Nurs Res 17:247–250
36. Van Rompaey B, Elseviers MM, Van Drom W, Fromont V, Jorens PG (2012) The effect of earplugs during the night on the onset of delirium and sleep perception: a randomized controlled trial in intensive care patients. Crit Care 16:R73
37. Aboukhalil A, Nielsen L, Saeed M, Mark RG, Clifford GD (2008) Reducing false alarm rates for critical arrhythmias using the arterial blood pressure waveform. J Biomed Inf 41:442–451
38. Görges M, Markewitz BA, Westenskow DR (2009) Improving alarm performance in the medical intensive care unit using delays and clinical context. Anesth Analg 108:1546–1552
39. Kennedy RR (1995) A modified trigg's tracking variable as an "advisory" alarm during anesthesia. Int J Clin Monit Comput 12:197–204
40. Mäkivirta A, Koski E, Kari A, Sukuvaara T (1991) The median filter as a processor for a patient monitor limit alarm system in intensive care. Comput Methods Programs Biomed 34:139–144
41. Shortliffe EH, Davis R, Axline SG et al (1975) Computer-based consultations in clinical therapeutics: Explanation and rule acquisition capabilities of the MYCIN-System. Comput Biomed Res 8:303–320
42. Sukuvaara T, Koki EM, Mäkivirta A, Kari A (1993) A knowledge-based system for monitoring cardiac operated patients – technical construction and evaluation. Int J Clin Monit Comput 10:117–126
43. Baxt WG, Skora J (1996) Prospective validation of artificial neural network trained to identify acute myocardial infarction. Lancet 347:12–15
44. Orr JA, Westenskow DR (1994) A breathing circuit alarm system based on neural networks. J Clin Monit 10:101–109
45. Zadeh LA (1965) Fuzzy sets. Inform Control 8:338–353
46. Goldman JM, Cordova MJ (1994) Advanced clinical monitoring: Considerations for real-time hemodynamic diagnostics. Proc Annu Symp Comput Appl Med Care:752–756
47. Laursen P (1994) Event detection on patient monitoring data using causal probabilistic networks. Method Inform Med 33:111–115

Bedside Monitoring of Heart-Lung Interactions

F. J. da Silva Ramos, E. L. V. Costa, and M. B. P. Amato

Introduction

Cardiopulmonary interactions are a direct consequence of the anatomy of the heart, lungs, and great vessels. Being intrathoracic structures, the heart, lungs, part of the vena cava, and part of the aorta are affected similarly by changes in pleural pressures. Additionally, the entire cardiac output flows from the right heart through the lungs towards the left heart as in three separate compartments arranged in series. This anatomy leads to: (1) reciprocal effects between the performance of the heart and that of the lung, because right cardiac filling is limited by lung expansion or by increments in pleural pressure; and (2) a delay between acute changes in right ventricular (RV) output and the observed effects in left ventricular (LV) output (Fig. 1).

In patients receiving positive pressure mechanical ventilation, RV output decreases during inspiration because of both a decrease in venous return and an increase in RV afterload [1–5]. The decrease in RV output leads to a delayed fall in the venous return from the lungs to the left heart after a few heartbeats (Fig. 2) [1–5]. This fall in the venous return to the left heart is commonly preceded by an early inspiratory increase in left heart filling, due to squeezing of blood from capillaries to the left heart during thoracic pressurization [6, 7]. Other mechanisms for

F. J. da Silva Ramos
Intensive Care Unit and Research and Education Institute, Hospital Sírio-Libanês,
Cel Nicolau dos Santos 69, 01308-60 São Paulo, Brazil

E. L. V. Costa
Intensive Care Unit and Research and Education Institute, Hospital Sírio-Libanês,
Cel Nicolau dos Santos 69, 01308-60 São Paulo, Brazil
Respiratory Intensive Care Unit, University of Sao Paulo School of Medicine,
Av Dr Arnaldo 455, Room 2206 (2nd floor), 01246-903 São Paulo, Brazil

M. B. P. Amato (✉)
Respiratory Intensive Care Unit, University of Sao Paulo School of Medicine,
Av Dr Arnaldo 455, Room 2206 (2nd floor), 01246-903 São Paulo, Brazil
E-mail: amato@unisys.com.br

J.-L. Vincent (Ed.), *Annual Update in Intensive Care and Emergency Medicine 2013*,
DOI 10.1007/978-3-642-35109-9_31,

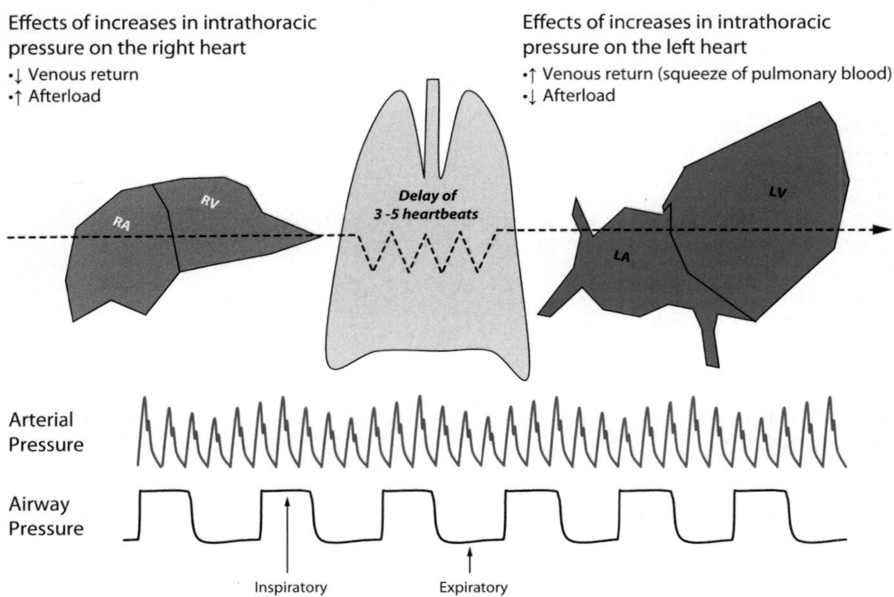

Fig. 1 Schematic representation of the hemodynamic effects of positive pressure ventilation on heart-lung interactions. Thoracic pressurization leads to a decrease in venous return and to an increase in right heart afterload. After a few heartbeats this decrease in right ventricle outflow is transmitted to the left heart. In the left heart, thoracic pressurization leads to increased venous return caused by squeezing of the lungs and to decreased afterload. RA: right atrium, RV: right ventricle, LA: left atrium, LV: left ventricle

the early inspiratory increase in LV stroke volume have been suggested, including a decrease in the afterload of the left ventricle [8] and the longer time the aortic valve stays open during thoracic pressurization [9].

As a consequence of such delays and couplings, breath by breath variation in left stroke volume is commonly found in opposite phase with the systemic venous return: Although representing the effects of the previous lung insufflation, the lowest values for the LV stroke volume will only be observed in the subsequent expiration, despite the maximum surge in venous return to the right chambers at this moment. Conversely, the highest values for LV stroke volume are usually observed at end-inspiration, despite the nadir in venous return to the right chambers at this moment. Such opposite oscillations, however, could be disentangled during an end-expiratory pause [10]; by avoiding the next inspiratory phase, a slow and sustained increase in LV stroke volume would be observed, reflecting the progressive surge in venous return that started a few heartbeats before, at the beginning of exhalation.

The precise duration of the inspiratory or expiratory phase is, therefore, a crucial factor for such cyclic interactions. The nadir of the LV stroke volume does not necessarily coincide with the end-expiration (nor does the peak coincide with end-inspiration) and depends on ventilator settings.

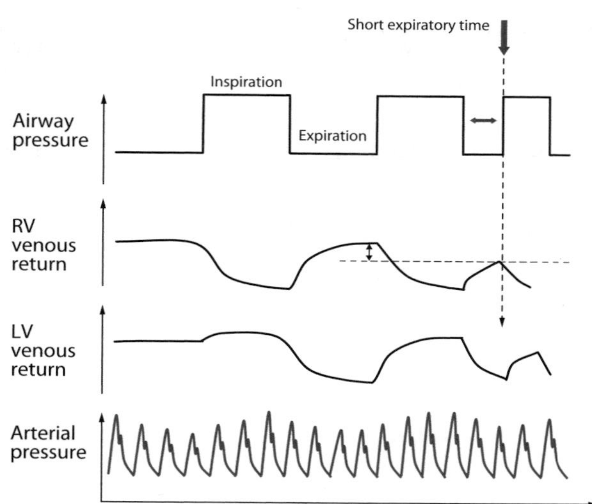

Fig. 2 Schematic representation of the hemodynamic effects of respiratory rate on heart-lung interactions during positive pressure ventilation. The right and left venous return curves are represented devoid of their pulsatile components to facilitate interpretation. Notice that the curve of the venous return to the left heart is delayed in relation to the curve of the right heart. Also notice that a short expiratory time may affect the amplitude of the cyclic change in venous return. RV: right ventricular, LV: left ventricular

Heart-Lung Interactions to Evaluate Fluid Responsiveness in Mechanically Ventilated Patients

Fluid responsiveness is generally defined as an increase in cardiac output or in stroke volume of 15 % or greater after a fluid challenge [11–13]. Positive pressure ventilation induces changes in venous return, which can be used instead of a fluid challenge to assess fluid responsiveness [9]. The logic behind such convenient inference is straightforward: If small increments in pleural pressures caused by cyclic increments in alveolar pressures are enough to cyclically impair venous return, the cardiac output is pre-load dependent; therefore, an increase in pre-load by fluid administration should increase cardiac output.

Cardiac output or stroke volume can be estimated beat-to-beat from analyses of the arterial waveform (PiCCO™ monitor, Pulsion Medical System, Munich, Germany; Vigileo™/FloTrac™, Edwards Lifesciences LLC, Irvine, CA, USA; or LidCO™ plus Ltd, Cambridge, UK). Stroke volume variation (SVV) and its surrogate, pulse pressure variation (PPV), can be calculated as the difference between the maximal and minimal stroke volume (or pulse pressure) during one complete respiratory cycle, divided by the mean stroke volume (or mean pulse pressure). Several studies have demonstrated that SVV and PPV are sensitive indicators of fluid responsiveness in sedated, mechanically ventilated patients without respiratory efforts [14–17]. PPV has the advantage over SVV in that it is easier to measure because it can be calculated in any patient with an arterial line, not requiring special monitors. On the other hand, in order to reliably reflect the changes in stroke volume, PPV requires a fixed compliance of the systemic arteries, a condition that cannot be guaranteed in all circumstances.

Michard et al. [16] used PPV to predict the hemodynamic effects of positive end-expiratory pressure (PEEP) in patients with acute lung injury (ALI) who were sedated and mechanically ventilated with tidal volumes of 8 to 12 ml/kg. PPV on zero end-expiratory pressure (ZEEP) was closely correlated with PEEP-induced decreases in cardiac index. The same group analyzed the value of PPV to predict fluid responsiveness in 40 patients with acute circulatory failure due to sepsis and found a high sensitivity (94 %) and a high specificity (96 %) using a PPV cut-off value of 13 % [17].

Despite initial enthusiasm after the first publications [11, 16, 17], the use of PPV and SVV as tools to evaluate fluid responsiveness of critically ill patients was later shown to have important limitations [18]. Most of these limitations are related to some infringement of at least one of the two basic conditions for PPV or SVV to reflect the pre-load status: (1) The positive pressure ventilation must create a long and strong enough – not excessive – perturbation in pleural pressures to cause a cyclic decrease in venous return to the right heart; and (2) the cyclic changes in LV stroke volume must mainly reflect the cyclic changes in venous return to right heart occurring a few heartbeats before; thus, oscillations in stroke volume from other causes, e. g., oscillations in afterload to the right or left ventricle [19], have to be discarded. Clinical conditions in which at least one of these assumptions is likely to be false, such as during low tidal volume ventilation [20], high respiratory rates [21], high intra-abdominal pressures [22], light sedation, absence of muscle paralysis, RV dysfunction [19, 23], and arrhythmias might preclude correct interpretation of PPV and SVV [18]. In the following sections, we will discuss the recent literature addressing these limitations.

Assumption 1: Enough, But Not Too Much, Perturbation in Pleural Pressure to Cause a Cyclic Decrease in Venous Return to the Right Heart

Tidal Volume

In theory, the higher the tidal volume, the larger are the cyclic changes in pleural pressures, and the larger are the changes in venous return to the right heart. PPV was validated in patients submitted to tidal volumes of 8–12 ml/kg [17]. The influence of tidal volume on PPV was later addressed by De Backer et al. [20]. These authors tested the hypothesis that tidal volume could influence PPV in 60 patients, 10 of whom had acute respiratory distress syndrome (ARDS), and concluded that PPV was a reliable predictor of fluid responsiveness only when tidal volume was at least 8 ml/kg. Oliveira et al. later evaluated the effects of tidal volume, PEEP and inspiratory-to-expiratory time ratio variations on PPV in 10 healthy and hypovolemic pigs [24]. These authors confirmed that increases in tidal volume (from 8 to 16 ml/kg) promoted a substantial increase in PPV. The increase in mean airway pressure caused by PEEP also elevated cardiac filling pressures and PPV, although to a much lesser extent, suggesting that the changes in PEEP were not enough to significantly change chest-wall compliance, and thus to cause substantially different swings in pleural pressure. Finally, the inversion of the inspiratory-to-expiratory time ratio did not induce significant changes in static and functional hemodynamic parameters [24].

More recently, Kim and Pinsky [25] analyzed the influence of tidal volume, cardiac contractility, and the sampling duration of PPV in seven dogs submitted to positive pressure ventilation. The authors found that increasing the sampling duration to include more ventilatory cycles increased the magnitude of PPV up until five breaths, and that increasing tidal volume from 5 to 20 ml/kg promoted a proportional increase in PPV. The first observation likely simply reflects a statistical aspect related to minimum sampling, whereas the second confirms the effect of progressive perturbations in pleural pressures. These authors also showed that impaired contractility decreases PPV (see the explanation provided later), whereas increased contractility does not.

In patients with ARDS, the protective lung ventilation strategy consists of ventilation with low tidal volumes (6 ml/kg), eventually with high PEEP [26]. This strategy likely limits the use of PPV and SVV in this population. da Silva Ramos et al. [27] explored the influence of different ventilatory strategies on hemodynamic parameters in pigs with ALI during normovolemia and hypovolemia. In this study, the tidal volume was the ventilatory parameter that most influenced the functional hemodynamic parameters. In an observational study, Huang et al. [28] evaluated the clinical applicability of PPV and SVV in patients with ARDS ventilated with a protective strategy. In this study, PPV performed better than SVV, and a cut-off value of 12 % was able to predict fluid responsiveness with a sensitivity of 68 % and specificity of 100 %. The authors suggested that, in hypovolemic patients, high PEEPs could extramurally compress the thoracic aorta, decreasing aortic compliance and magnifying the changes in PPV [28].

In an attempt to adjust PPV for different ventilator settings, Vallée et al. [29] compared the accuracies of PPV alone vs. PPV adjusted by driving pressure (plateau pressure – total PEEP), the PPV/dP index, using different tidal volumes. Their hypothesis was that the PPV/dP index would perform better than PPV-alone in patients with tidal volumes less than 8 ml/kg. The results obtained from a group of unselected intensive care unit (ICU) patients failed to show an improved overall prediction of PPV at low tidal volumes, even when adjusted by PPV/dP index. We believe that such results were to be expected, because high driving pressures in these patients are usually a consequence of parenchymal abnormalities, rather than of substantial changes in chest-wall compliance (which means that the swings in pleural pressure do not necessarily follow the driving pressure).

Respiratory Rate

Each inspiration during positive pressure ventilation causes a steep increase in intrathoracic pressure, which is followed by a slower decrease in venous return to the right heart (Fig. 2). When the respiratory rate is too fast, the inspiratory time, the expiratory time, or both may be insufficient to allow for the maximal cyclic decrease in venous return. In these circumstances, this decrease might become respiratory-rate dependent. De Backer et al. [21] investigated the consequence of heart rate (HR), respiratory rate, and the ratio between HR and respiratory rate on indices of fluid responsiveness (PPV and caval index using echocardiography) in a series of hypovolemic patients. Seventeen patients were included in the study. Respiratory variations in LV stroke volume were influenced by respiratory rate, and right and left indices of fluid responsiveness were dissociated in these conditions. An increase in respiratory rate, especially when the HR to respiratory rate ratio was less than 3.6, was accompanied by a significant decrease in PPV, whereas the caval index was unaltered. This dissociation was likely associated with the delay (3–5 heartbeats) in perturbations in the right chambers being transmitted to the left ones. If a new breath disturbs the system (transiently increasing left venous return), before the full propagation of the depressive effects observed in the right heart, the net effect on the left heart is going to be attenuated. The authors concluded that PPV is directly affected by respiratory rate and its use requires caution if high respiratory rates are used.

Monnet et al. [10] assessed whether the hemodynamic effects of a 15-second end-expiratory pause were able to predict fluid responsiveness in ventilated patients with an irregular cardiac rhythm or mild spontaneous respiratory activity. In 34 patients (11 patients with cardiac arrhythmias and 23 with mild spontaneous respiratory activity), the authors evaluated the increase in pulse pressure and in cardiac index during the maneuver and compared it with passive leg raising. They found that the end-expiratory pause promoted an increase in pulse pressure and in cardiac index in responders to a fluid challenge, showing that the expiratory pause allowed for a late increase in venous return to the left heart, increasing left stroke volume in preload responsive patients (note that the cyclic surge in venous return to the right chambers, observed during normal expiration, is not long enough to be propagated to the left heart before the end-expiration, see Fig. 2). An increase in pulse pressure greater than 5 % during the expiratory pause had a sensitivity of 87 % and a specificity of 100 % to predict fluid responsiveness.

Increased Intra-abdominal Pressure

Abdominal distension and visceral edema are common in critically ill patients and lead to increased pleural pressures, potentially limiting diaphragmatic movements [30]. The consequent increase in intrathoracic pressure also reduces venous return and affects heart-lung interactions [30]. Renner et al. [22] investigated the influence of increased intra-abdominal pressure (IAP) on the ability of PPV and SVV to predict the response to a volemic expansion. They evaluated the effect of IAP > 25 mm Hg induced by pneumoperitoneum in 14 pigs during normovolemia and after a fluid challenge. During normovolemia and with normal IAP, the fluid challenge promoted an expected reduction in PPV and SVV. Increasing IAP to

25 mm Hg led SVV, but not PPV, to lose its predictive ability. PPV remained useful only if threshold values were changed (≥ 11.5 % at baseline vs. ≥ 20.5 % during IAP). One possible explanation for these findings is the magnification of swings in pleural pressure promoted by the procedure. Since tidal-volumes were maintained in the context of decreased chest wall compliance, the cyclic swings in pleural pressure were excessive, causing high PPV values even in patients with adequate pre-load. This study illustrates an important principle of functional hemodynamics: With a large enough swing in pleural pressure, it is always possible to get high PPV values, even for patients who are not responsive to fluids [22].

Spontaneous Ventilation

During spontaneous ventilation, there is an inspiratory decrease in pleural pressure, which is transmitted to the heart and increases the gradient for venous return. The perturbation is basically the mirror image of the phenomenon described above for positive pressure ventilation. However, the magnitude of the change in pleural pressure and in venous return is effort-dependent and seldom measured. Perhaps for this reason, the predictive value of PPV as a surrogate for fluid responsiveness in spontaneously breathing patients is much less than in patients under controlled mechanical ventilation [31–33]. Magder et al. [34] suggested that spontaneously breathing patients who decreased their right atrial pressure more than 1 mm Hg during an adequate inspiratory effort were preload responsive. More recently, Heenan et al. [35] failed to confirm these findings. The authors found that neither right atrial pressure variation nor PPV were able to predict fluid responsiveness in 21 patients breathing spontaneously. In this study, it is unclear whether inspiratory efforts were sufficient to cause significant changes in pleural pressure. Measurement of pleural pressure, for example through an esophageal balloon, would have helped to interpret their findings. In view of such difficulties, it has been suggested that PPV should not be routinely used in spontaneously breathing patients. The assessment of pre-load in such patients should be rather guided by maneuvers not dependent on patient effort, like passive leg-raising [36] or prolonged end-expiratory pause [10].

Assumption 2: The Cyclic Changes in Left Ventricular Stroke Volume Must Mainly Reflect the Cyclic Changes in Venous Return to the Right Heart that Occurred a Few Heartbeats Before

RV dysfunction can lead to a decrease in RV ejection during inspiration because of increased RV afterload (increased pulmonary vascular resistance). Thus, cyclic changes in the venous return to the left heart (and in left-heart stroke volume) will also be present, although not related to a decreased pre-load to the right chambers. In this situation, volume expansion will likely fail to increase the venous return to the left heart, in spite of increased venous return to the right heart. Jardin [19] proposed that RV dysfunction can lead to a false positive PPV. Mahjoub et al. [23] subsequently studied 35 mechanically ventilated patients with a PPV greater than 12 %, 12 of whom (34 %) were non-responders (false positive) when a fluid challenge was performed. In these patients, a peak systolic velocity in the tricuspid annulus lower than 0.15 m/s assessed by echocardiography was a good parameter to detect false positive PPV values [23].

Conversely, positive pressure ventilation decreases the LV afterload, because the tidal increases in pleural pressure promote direct compression of the heart facilitating its ejection. This effect is more pronounced in the presence of LV dysfunction and can cause PPV to increase irrespective of the preload responsiveness. In this case, the increased values of PPV are much more a consequence of an increased systolic pressure during inspiration (reflecting an increased left-heart stroke volume caused by the transiently lower afterload) than of a decreased systolic pressure during exhalation. Some maneuvers have been proposed to isolate these two components of the systolic pressure variation, increasing the specificity of the preload assessment [37–39]. After a short period of apnea, the systolic pressure variation can be divided into two components, the delta up (Δup) and the delta down (Δdown) [37]. The Δdown is the difference between the systolic blood pressure during apnea and the lowest value after a mechanical breath. Its magnitude reflects the amount of decrease in the venous return due to the increased intrathoracic pressure [37, 40]. The Δup is the difference between the maximal value of the systolic blood pressure during inspiration and the value during apnea. The Δup represents a transient increase in the LV stroke output due to a combination of increased preload as blood is squeezed out of the lungs, decreased afterload caused by direct pressure of the expanding lungs on the heart, and improved LV compliance due to a transient decrease in the volume of the right heart [40]. Increases in Δup have been related to LV dysfunction [41].

How to Overcome These Limitations

The best way to deal with the current limitations is to evaluate the falsehood of both assumptions. For example, in a patient under mechanical ventilation with low tidal volumes, a false negative PPV or SVV would be avoided by knowing that the low tidal volumes caused little respiratory changes in the stroke volume of the right heart. Echocardiography and electrical impedance tomography (EIT) are non-invasive diagnostic tools that can be useful in these situations.

Echocardiography

Echocardiography enables assessment of the venous return to the right heart (variations in the diameter of the vena cava) [42–45], of RV function and of LV output

[45]. As such, echocardiography might be used as a diagnostic test to identify situations in which PPV and SVV should be used with caution or not at all [23]. Additionally, echocardiography can be used as a monitoring tool to assess fluid responsiveness when PPV and SVV have limited clinical usefulness.

Electrical Impedance Tomography

EIT is a non-invasive monitoring tool that allows real-time imaging of lung ventilation and perfusion [46]. EIT beat-to-beat estimates of pulmonary perfusion are significantly correlated with stroke volume [47]. Until recently, however, dynamic separation of the cardiac-related signal required a breath hold, electrocardiogram (EKG)-gated imaging, or frequency-domain filtering, all of which are unsuitable for real-time analyses during breathing. Filtering using principal components analysis was recently shown to allow for real-time separation of pulmonary from cardiac signals and can potentially be used to assess RV SVV during the respiratory cycle [48]. As illustrated above, there are various clinical situations in which the changes in LV stroke volume are dissociated from the RV output (e. g., LV failure) or in which the RV output is dissociated from venous return to the right chambers (e. g., RV failure). Thus, direct assessment of RV output could be helpful for proper interpretation of PPV or SVV.

Alternatively, EIT could be used to image the impedance changes in the thoracic aorta caused by the LV ejection, provided that the thoracic aorta can be identified in the thoracic images. Recently, Maisch et al. [49], after identifying the aortic region with an unsupervised algorithm [50], showed that SVV estimated with EIT using a frequency-domain analysis was strongly correlated with SVV measured by both aortic blood flow measurement and pulse contour analysis.

Conclusion

The functional parameters, PPV and SVV, are useful predictors of fluid responsiveness. Knowledge of the physiological bases that supports their use, as well as understanding of their pitfalls under specific circumstances, will help clinicians to make better use of them.

References

1. Morgan BC, Martin WE, Hornbein TF, Crawford EW, Guntheroth WG (1966) Hemodynamic effects of intermittent positive pressure respiration. Anesthesiology 27:584–590
2. Jardin F, Farcot JC, Gueret P, Prost JF, Ozier Y, Bourdarias JP (1983) Cyclic changes in arterial pulse during respiratory support. Circulation 68:266–274

3. Pinsky M (1984) Determinants of pulmonary arterial flow variation during respiration. J App Physiol 56:1237–1245
4. Jardin F, Delorme G, Hardy A, Auvert B, Beauchet A, Bourdarias JP (1990) Reevaluation of hemodynamic consequences of positive pressure ventilation: emphasis on cyclic right ventricular afterloading by mechanical lung inflation. Anesthesiology 72:966–970
5. Jardin F, Vieillard-Baron A (2003) Right ventricular function and positive pressure ventilation in clinical practice: from hemodynamic subsets to respirator settings. Intensive Care Med 29:1426–1434
6. Brower R, Wise RA, Hassapoyannes C, Bromberger-Barnea B, Permutt S (1985) Effect of lung inflation on lung blood volume and pulmonary venous flow. J Appl Physiol 58:954–963
7. Vieillard-Baron A, Chergui K, Augarde R et al (2003) Cyclic changes in arterial pulse during respiratory support revisited by doppler echocardiography. Am J Respir Crit Care Med 168:671–676
8. Robotham JL, Cherry D, Mitzner W, Rabson JL, Lixfeld W, Bromberger-Barnea B (1983) A re-evaluation of the hemodynamic consequences of intermittent positive pressure ventilation. Crit Care Med 11:783–793
9. Magder S (2004) Clinical usefulness of respiratory variations in arterial pressure. Am J Respir Crit Care Med 169:151–155
10. Monnet X, Osman D, Ridel C, Lamia B, Richard C, Teboul J (2009) Predicting volume responsiveness by using the end-expiratory occlusion in mechanically ventilated intensive care unit patients. Crit Care Med 37:951–956
11. Michard F, Teboul J (2002) Predicting fluid responsiveness in icu patients: a critical analysis of the evidence. Chest 121:2000–2008
12. Bendjelid K, Romand J (2003) Fluid responsiveness in mechanically ventilated patients: a review of indices used in intensive care. Intensive Care Med 29:352–360
13. Marik PE, Cavallazzi R, Vasu T, Hirani A (2009) Dynamic changes in arterial waveform derived variables and fluid responsiveness in mechanically ventilated patients: a systematic review of the literature. Crit Care Med 37:2642–2647
14. Berkenstadt H, Margalit N, Hadani M et al (2001) Stroke volume variation as a predictor of fluid responsiveness in patients undergoing brain surgery. Anesth Analg 92:984–989
15. Reuter DA, Felbinger TW, Schmidt C et al (2002) Stroke volume variations for assessment of cardiac responsiveness to volume loading in mechanically ventilated patients after cardiac surgery. Intensive Care Med 28:392–398
16. Michard F, Chemla D, Richard C et al (1999) Clinical use of respiratory changes in arterial pulse pressure to monitor the hemodynamic effects of peep. Am J Respir Crit Care Med 159:935–939
17. Michard F, Boussat S, Chemla D et al (2000) Relation between respiratory changes in arterial pulse pressure and fluid responsiveness in septic patients with acute circulatory failure. Am J Respir Crit Care Med 162:134–138
18. Michard F (2005) Volume management using dynamic parameters: the good, the bad, and the ugly. Chest 128:1902–1903
19. Jardin F (2004) Cyclic changes in arterial pressure during mechanical ventilation. Intensive Care Med 30:1047–1050
20. De Backer D, Heenen S, Piagnerelli M, Koch M, Vincent JL (2005) Pulse pressure variations to predict fluid responsiveness: influence of tidal volume. Intensive Care Med 31:517–523
21. De Backer D, Taccone FS, Holsten R, Ibrahimi F, Vincent JL (2009) Influence of respiratory rate on stroke volume variation in mechanically ventilated patients. Anesthesiology 110:1092–1097
22. Renner J, Gruenewald M, Quaden R et al (2009) Influence of increased intra-abdominal pressure on fluid responsiveness predicted by pulse pressure variation and stroke volume variation in a porcine model. Crit Care Med 37:650–658
23. Mahjoub Y, Pila C, Friggeri A et al (2009) Assessing fluid responsiveness in critically ill patients: false-positive pulse pressure variation is detected by doppler echocardiographic evaluation of the right ventricle. Crit Care Med 37:2570–2575

24. Oliveira RH, Azevedo LCP, Park M, Schettino GPP (2009) Influence of ventilatory settings on static and functional haemodynamic parameters during experimental hypovolaemia. Eur J Anaesthesiol 26:66–72
25. Kim HK, Pinsky MR (2008) Effect of tidal volume, sampling duration, and cardiac contractility on pulse pressure and stroke volume variation during positive-pressure ventilation. Crit Care Med 36:2858–2862
26. Amato MB, Barbas CS, Medeiros DM et al (1998) Effect of a protective-ventilation strategy on mortality in the acute respiratory distress syndrome. N Engl J Med 338:347–354
27. da Silva Ramos FJ, de Oliveira EM, Park M, Schettino GPP, Azevedo LCP (2011) Heart-lung interactions with different ventilatory settings during acute lung injury and hypovolaemia: an experimental study. Br J Anaesth 106:394–402
28. Huang C, Fu J, Hu H et al (2008) Prediction of fluid responsiveness in acute respiratory distress syndrome patients ventilated with low tidal volume and high positive end-expiratory pressure. Crit Care Med 36:2810–2816
29. Vallée F, Richard JCM, Mari A et al (2009) Pulse pressure variations adjusted by alveolar driving pressure to assess fluid responsiveness. Intensive Care Med 35:1004–1010
30. Maerz L, Kaplan LJ (2008) Abdominal compartment syndrome. Crit Care Med 36:S212–S215
31. De Backer D, Pinsky MR (2007) Can one predict fluid responsiveness in spontaneously breathing patients? Intensive Care Med 33:1111–1113
32. Teboul J, Monnet X (2008) Prediction of volume responsiveness in critically ill patients with spontaneous breathing activity. Curr Opin Crit Care 14:334–339
33. Magder S (2006) Predicting volume responsiveness in spontaneously breathing patients: still a challenging problem. Crit Care 10:165
34. Magder S, Georgidis G, Cheong T (1992) Respiratory variations in right atrial pressure predict the response to fluid challenge. J Crit Care 7:76–85
35. Heenen S, De Backer D, Vincent JL (2006) How can the response to volume expansion in patients with spontaneous respiratory movements be predicted? Crit Care 10:R102
36. Maizel J, Airapetian N, Lorne E, Tribouilloy C, Massy Z, Slama M (2007) Diagnosis of central hypovolemia by using passive leg raising. Intensive Care Med 33:1133–1138
37. Perel A, Pizov R, Cotev S (1987) Systolic blood pressure variation is a sensitive indicator of hypovolemia in ventilated dogs subjected to graded hemorrhage. Anesthesiology 67:498–502
38. Coriat P, Vrillon M, Perel A et al (1994) A comparison of systolic blood pressure variations and echocardiographic estimates of end-diastolic left ventricular size in patients after aortic surgery. Anesth Analg 78:46–53
39. Beaussier M, Coriat P, Perel A et al (1995) Determinants of systolic pressure variation in patients ventilated after vascular surgery. J Cardiothorac Vasc Anesth 9:547–551
40. Pizov R, Ya'ari Y, Perel A (1989) The arterial pressure waveform during acute ventricular failure and synchronized external chest compression. Anesth Analg 68:150–156
41. Pinsky MR, Matuschak GM, Itzkoff JM (1984) Respiratory augmentation of left ventricular function during spontaneous ventilation in severe left ventricular failure by grunting. An auto-epap effect. Chest 86:267–269
42. Charron C, Caille V, Jardin F, Vieillard-Baron A (2006) Echocardiographic measurement of fluid responsiveness. Curr Opin Crit Care 12:249–254
43. Barbier C, Loubières Y, Schmit C et al (2004) Respiratory changes in inferior vena cava diameter are helpful in predicting fluid responsiveness in ventilated septic patients. Intensive Care Med 30:1740–1746
44. Vieillard-Baron A, Augarde R, Prin S, Page B, Beauchet A, Jardin F (2001) Influence of superior vena caval zone condition on cyclic changes in right ventricular outflow during respiratory support. Anesthesiology 95:1083–1088
45. Beaulieu Y (2007) Bedside echocardiography in the assessment of the critically ill. Crit Care Med 35:S235–249
46. Costa ELV, Lima RG, Amato MBP (2009) Electrical impedance tomography. Curr Opin Crit Care 15:18–24

47. Fagerberg A, Stenqvist O, Aneman A (2009) Monitoring pulmonary perfusion by electrical impedance tomography: an evaluation in a pig model. Acta Anaesthesiol Scand 53:152–158
48. Deibele JM, Luepschen H, Leonhardt S (2008) Dynamic separation of pulmonary and cardiac changes in electrical impedance tomography. Physiol Meas 29:S1–S14
49. Maisch S, Bohm SH, Solà J et al (2011) Heart-lung interactions measured by electrical impedance tomography. Crit Care Med 39:2173–2176
50. Solà J, Adler A, Santos A, Tusman G, Sipmann FS, Bohm SH (2011) Non-invasive monitoring of central blood pressure by electrical impedance tomography: first experimental evidence. Med Biol Eng Comput 49:409–415

Assessment of Volume Responsiveness During Mechanical Ventilation: Recent Advances

X. Monnet and J.-L. Teboul

Introduction

Predicting which patients with acute circulatory failure will respond to fluid by a significant increase in cardiac output is a daily challenge, in particular in the setting of the intensive care unit (ICU). This challenge has become even more crucial because evidence is growing that administering excessive amounts of fluid is a risk factor in critically ill patients, in particular in patients with lung injury. However, some tests and indices allow prediction of fluid responsiveness before intravenous fluids are infused. In patients receiving mechanical ventilation, the arterial pulse pressure variation (PPV) has been used for many years. More recently, other tests, which may overcome some limitations of PPV, have been developed. In addition, recent studies have emphasized how the hemodynamic effects of volume expansion should be assessed once fluid has been administered.

The Concept of Predicting Fluid Responsiveness

Volume expansion is the first-line treatment in the majority of cases of acute circulatory failure. Fluid is administered with the expectation that it will increase cardiac preload and cardiac output to a significant extent. Nevertheless, this can occur only if cardiac output is dependent upon cardiac preload, i. e., if both ventricles operate on the ascending limb of the cardiac function curve [1] (Fig. 1). If this

X. Monnet (✉)
Service de réanimation médicale, Hôpitaux universitaires Paris-Sud, Hôpital de Bicêtre, rue du Général Leclerc 78, F-94270 Le Kremlin-Bicêtre, France
E-mail: xavier.monnet@bct.aphp.fr

J.-L. Teboul
Service de réanimation médicale, Hôpitaux universitaires Paris-Sud, Hôpital de Bicêtre, rue du Général Leclerc 78, F-94270 Le Kremlin-Bicêtre, France

J.-L. Vincent (Ed.), *Annual Update in Intensive Care and Emergency Medicine 2013*, DOI 10.1007/978-3-642-35109-9_32, © Springer-Verlag Berlin Heidelberg and BioMed Central Ltd. 2013

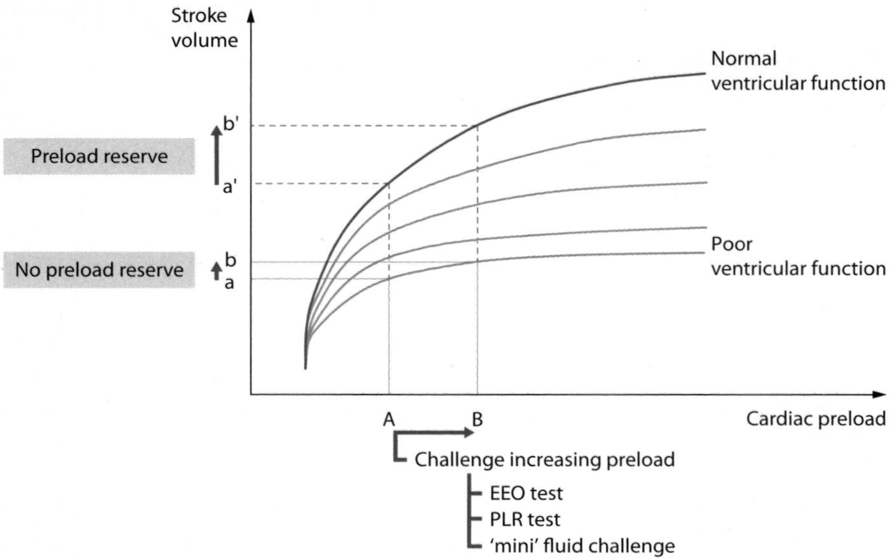

Fig. 1 Functional hemodynamic monitoring for assessing the Frank-Starling relationship in patients with spontaneous breathing activity and/or cardiac arrhythmias and/or low tidal volume and/or low lung compliance. The same increase in cardiac preload (from A to B) induced by volume expansion can result in a significant (from a' to b') or to a negligible (from a to b) increase in stroke volume depending upon the shape of the *curve*. A static value of preload (A) does not predict to which extent stroke volume will respond to increased cardiac preload induced by fluid administration. Functional hemodynamic monitoring consists of observing the resulting effects of a preload variation, as can be induced by an end-expiratory occlusion test (EEO), a passive leg raising test (PLR) or by a 'mini' fluid challenge

is not the case, volume expansion may only exert adverse effects without having any hemodynamic benefit. An important point is that excessive fluid administration has been demonstrated to increase mortality during septic shock [2, 3] and to prolong mechanical ventilation during acute respiratory distress syndrome (ARDS) [4]. In the same context, the amount of extravascular lung water (EVLW), i. e., the volume of lung edema, has been demonstrated to be related to mortality in critically ill patients [5] and, more recently, to be an independent prognostic factor during ARDS [6]. Thus, fluid responsiveness should be detected before deciding to administer volume expansion, especially in patients in whom fluid overload should be particularly avoided, i. e., patients with septic shock and/or ARDS.

For this purpose, 'static' markers of cardiac preload have been used for many years. Nevertheless, a very large number of studies clearly demonstrate that neither pressure nor volume markers of preload can predict fluid responsiveness [7, 8]. This finding is mainly because a given value of preload can correspond to either a large or a negligible response of cardiac output to fluid administration, depending upon the slope of the Frank-Starling curve, which cannot be *a priori* determined in a given patient (Fig. 1). This is the reason why a 'dynamic approach' has been developed for assessing volume responsiveness [9]. The concept is to assess preload-dependency by observing the effects on cardiac output of changes in cardiac preload induced by various tests.

Monitoring Respiratory Variations in Stroke Volume: a Large Base of Evidence

Pulse Pressure Variation

The first application of this 'dynamic' concept consisted of quantifying the variations in stroke volume induced by positive-pressure ventilation [10]. As a result of heart-lung interactions, each mechanical insufflation decreases venous return and, if the right ventricle is preload-dependent, reduces the right ventricular (RV) outflow. Increase in RV afterload induced by increased lung volume contributes to this reduction in RV outflow. In turn, this results in a decrease in left ventricular (LV) preload, which occurs after a delay of a few cardiac cycles, required for the blood to transit through the lungs. In the case of conventional ventilation, this effect should occur at expiration. If the left ventricle is also preload-dependent, the LV stroke volume transiently decreases. As a result, a cyclic variation in stroke volume under mechanical ventilation indicates the existence of preload-dependency of both ventricles [10].

The arterial pulse pressure (systolic minus diastolic arterial pressure) as a surrogate of stroke volume has been proposed to predict fluid responsiveness through its respiratory variation [10]. A number of studies conducted in various clinical settings have repeatedly demonstrated that PPV actually predicts fluid responsiveness [11]. Among the different indicators of fluid responsiveness, PPV is supported by the highest level of evidence. Importantly, PPV is calculated automatically and displayed in real-time by the most recent bedside hemodynamic monitors.

Other Surrogates of Stroke Volume

Almost all indices that provide a beat-to-beat estimation of stroke volume have been investigated for their ability to test fluid responsiveness by their respiratory variation: Aortic blood flow measured by esophageal Doppler [12]; subaortic peak velocity measured by echocardiography [13]; stroke volume estimated from pulse contour analysis [14]. Some recent studies have investigated non-invasive estimations of stroke volume, such as the non-invasive arterial pulse pressure estimated by the volume-clamp method [15, 16] or the amplitude of the plethysmographic waveform [17]. All these non-invasive methods still require confirmatory studies, but they may be of great interest for the perioperative management of low-risk surgical patients, when there is no need for an invasive monitoring device.

Finally, analysis of respiratory variations of the diameter of the inferior vena cava (using transthoracic echocardiography) [18] or of the superior vena cava (using transesophageal echocardiography) [19] can also be used to assess fluid responsiveness in mechanically ventilated patients.

Limitations of the Respiratory Variation in Stroke Volume for Predicting Fluid Responsiveness

The use of respiratory variation of stroke volume or surrogates to predict fluid responsiveness has some limitations that are now clearly identified. The first and most important limitation is the presence of some spontaneous breathing activity [20]. When a patient has some breathing efforts under mechanical ventilation – and even more when the patient is not intubated – the variation in intrathoracic pressure is not regular, neither in rate nor in amplitude, such that the variation in stroke volume cannot relate to preload-dependency [21–23]. Thus, using the respiratory variation of stroke volume to test the preload sensitivity is valid only in cases of coma or deep sedation during mechanical ventilation, a condition that has become less frequent in the ICU.

A second limitation of using the respiratory variation in stroke volume is the presence of cardiac arrhythmias as in these cases, the variation in stroke volume is obviously more related to the irregularity of diastole than to heart-lung interactions.

A third limitation refers to conditions in which the variations in intravascular pressure induced by mechanical ventilation are of small amplitude. In the case of low tidal volume, the small variations in intrathoracic pressure may not be sufficient to trigger significant preload variations, even in cases of preload responsiveness. Some studies have actually shown that PPV loses its predictive value in the case of low tidal volume [24, 25]. The changes in intravascular pressure induced by mechanical ventilation may also be reduced if the transmission of changes in alveolar pressure to the pressure of the intrathoracic structures is attenuated, e. g., in the case of low lung compliance. A recent clinical study demonstrated that if the compliance of the respiratory system is less than 30 ml/cm H_2O, the value of PPV for predicting fluid responsiveness is dramatically reduced, independently of tidal volume [26].

A fourth limitation is the use of high frequency ventilation. If the ratio of heart rate to respiratory rate is low, e. g., if the respiratory rate is elevated, the number of cardiac cycles per respiratory cycle may be too low to allow respiratory stroke volume variation (SVV) to occur [27]; nevertheless, this applies to respiratory rates as high as 40 breaths/min [27].

A fifth limitation is the presence of increased abdominal pressure [28, 29]. In such cases, a higher PPV cut-off value must be considered for the prediction of fluid responsiveness [28]. Finally, open-chest surgery is another situation where the ventilation-induced variation of hemodynamic signals loses its predictive value for fluid responsiveness [30].

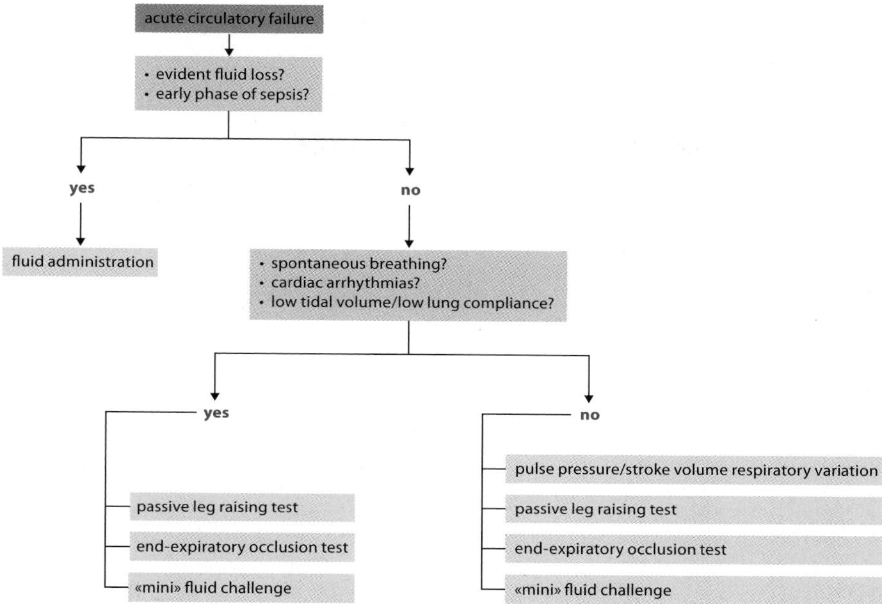

Fig. 2 Decision-making process of fluid administration

Except for open-chest conditions, the limitations of PPV and surrogates as predictors of fluid responsiveness mainly concern the intensive care setting and not the operating room where these heart-lung interaction indices are fully relevant. During recent years, alternative methods have been developed for predicting fluid responsiveness in critically ill patients (Fig. 2).

Alternatives to the Respiratory Variation of Hemodynamic Signals: Recent Advances

The End-Expiratory Occlusion Test

This test is another method that takes advantage of heart-lung interactions to predict fluid responsiveness in ventilated patients. During mechanical ventilation, each insufflation increases the intrathoracic pressure and impedes venous return. Thus, interrupting the respiratory cycle at end-expiration inhibits the cyclic impediment in venous return. The resulting increase in cardiac preload may thus help to test preload responsiveness (Fig. 1). Indeed, it was demonstrated that if a 15-second end-expiratory occlusion test increased the arterial pulse pressure or the pulse contour-derived cardiac output by more than 5 %, the response of cardiac output to a 500 ml saline infusion could be predicted with good sensitivity and specificity

[31]. Noticeably, all patients of the latter study were arrhythmic or had mild spontaneous breathing activity. These initial results were recently confirmed [26].

Beyond its simplicity, the main advantage of the end-expiratory occlusion test is that it exerts its hemodynamic effects over several cardiac cycles and thus remains valuable in case of cardiac arrhythmias [31]. Also, the end-expiratory occlusion test can be used in patients with spontaneous breathing activity, unless marked triggering activity interrupts the test. Another limitation is that the effects of the end-expiratory occlusion test, which must be observed over 15 s, are much easier to observe on a continuous display of cardiac output than on the arterial pulse pressure because the value of the latter is not continuously calculated and displayed by bedside monitors.

The 'Mini' Fluid Challenge

Obviously, the easiest way to test preload responsiveness is to administer fluid and to observe the resulting effect on cardiac output. Nevertheless, the disadvantage of the 'classical' fluid challenge is that it consists of administration of 300–500 ml of fluid [32]. Because it is not reversible, such a fluid challenge may contribute to fluid overload, especially when it is repeated several times a day [33].

In this regard, a new method has been proposed for performing a fluid challenge [34]. It consists of administering 100 ml of colloid over 1 min and observe the effects of this 'mini' fluid challenge on stroke volume, as measured by the subaortic velocity time index using transthoracic echocardiography (Fig. 1). In a clinical study, an increase in the velocity time index of more than 10 % predicted fluid responsiveness with a sensitivity of 95 % and a specificity of 78 % [34].

The first advantage of this test over the classical fluid challenge is obviously that such a small volume of fluid is unlikely to induce fluid overload [33], even if repeated several times a day. Another advantage is that it is easy to perform and that it can be assessed in a non-invasive way [34]. Nevertheless, a strong limitation is that, even in cases of preload-dependency, such a small volume infusion will unavoidably induce only small changes in cardiac output. This test, therefore, requires a very precise technique for measuring cardiac output. Whether non-invasive techniques, such as echocardiography, are precise enough for this purpose is still uncertain. Finally, this method cannot be used in the presence of cardiac arrhythmias. In the study by Muller et al., one fourth of patients were excluded because of this limitation [34].

The Passive Leg-Raising Test

In a lying subject, raising the legs from the horizontal position passively transfers a significant volume of blood from the lower part of the body toward the cardiac chambers: Passive leg-raising (PLR) partially empties the venous reservoir and converts a part of the unstressed blood volume to stressed volume. In this connection, PLR increases right [35–37] and left [22, 35] cardiac preload. Eventually, the increase in left cardiac preload results in an increase in cardiac output depending upon the degree of preload reserve of the left ventricle. The increase in cardiac preload induced by PLR totally reverses once the legs are returned back to the supine position [22, 35, 36]. In summary, PLR acts like a reversible and short-lived 'self' volume challenge [38] (Fig. 1). As a clinical application of this simple physiological concept, several studies reported that the increase in cardiac output induced by the PLR test enables prediction of fluid responsiveness; many of these studies were included in a meta-analysis [39]. These findings have contributed to establish PLR as a reliable and easy way to predict fluid responsiveness at the bedside [40]. Interestingly, since the test exerts its effects over several cardiac and respiratory cycles, it remains a good predictor of fluid responsiveness in patients with spontaneous breathing activity (even non-intubated) or cardiac arrhythmias [22, 31].

The postural change used for performing the PLR test is important [38]. If PLR is started from the 45° semi-recumbent position, the induced increase in central venous pressure is larger than if started from the supine position [36]. In fact, starting PLR from the semi-recumbent position mobilizes blood coming not only from the inferior limbs but also from the large splanchnic compartment. As a consequence, starting PLR from the semi-recumbent posture is more sensitive than starting from the horizontal posture to detect fluid responsiveness [36], so that this method should be considered as a standard.

Another important point concerns the method that can be used for measuring the changes in cardiac output during PLR [38]. A real-time measurement able to track hemodynamic changes in the time frame of PLR effects, i. e., 30–90 s, must be used. Indeed, the increase in cardiac output during PLR is not sustained when the leg elevation is prolonged. This aspect is particularly true in septic patients in whom capillary leak may account for an attenuation of the PLR effects after one minute, as already described [22]. This is why clinical studies that have tested the value of PLR to predict volume responsiveness used real-time hemodynamic measurements, such as aortic blood flow measured by esophageal Doppler [22, 41], pulse contour analysis-derived cardiac output [16, 26, 42], cardiac output measured by bioreactance [43, 44] or endotracheal bioimpedance cardiography [45], subaortic blood velocity measured by echocardiography [46–48], ascending aortic velocity measured by suprasternal Doppler [49] and, more recently, end-tidal carbon dioxide [50, 51].

Beyond its reliability and ease of use, the PLR test has some limitations [38]. First, its effects cannot be assessed by observing the arterial pressure. PLR-induced changes in arterial pulse pressure are less accurate than PLR-induced changes in cardiac output or stroke volume, as found by several studies [39]. This finding is explained by the fact that arterial pulse pressure is only a rough surrogate of stroke volume. This means that correct performance of a PLR test requires a device that allows a more direct estimation of cardiac output. Second, the PLR test cannot be used in instances in which mobilizing the patient is not possible or allowed, e. g., in the operating room or in the case of head injury [52].

How to Assess the Response to Volume Expansion?

Effects of Volume Expansion on Cardiac Output

If the decision is taken to infuse fluid in case of preload reserve, the ensuing question is whether the fluid actually exerts its expected beneficial effects. What is expected from fluid administration is a significant increase in cardiac output. In this regard, it has been recently shown that changes in arterial pressure are relatively imprecise to estimate the effects of fluid infusion on cardiac output [53, 54]. In 228 patients who received a standardized saline infusion, fluid-induced changes in arterial pulse pressure were weakly correlated with the simultaneous changes in cardiac output ($r = 0.56$) [54]. Consequently, the changes in pulse pressure induced by volume expansion detected a positive response to fluid (i. e., an increase in cardiac output $\geq 15\,\%$) with a specificity of 85 % but with a sensitivity of only 65 %; in other words, 22 % of cases were false negatives, meaning that in these patients, fluid administration significantly increased cardiac output whereas the arterial pulse pressure did not change to a large extent. Pierrakos et al. confirmed these results in 51 septic shock patients [54], in whom there was no significant correlation between fluid-induced changes in arterial pulse pressure and fluid-induced changes in cardiac output. These results are explained by the fact that arterial pulse pressure is physiologically related to stroke volume but also inversely correlated with arterial compliance [55], which may differ among patients and may change over time in the same patient. Moreover, the proportionality between pulse pressure and stroke volume is physiologically expected at the aortic level, but not at the peripheral arterial level because of the pulse wave amplification phenomenon.

Another important point emphasized by the above cited studies [53, 54], is that the fluid-induced changes in cardiac output are not reflected at all by the fluid-induced changes in mean arterial pressure (MAP). Physiologically, the changes in MAP are dissociated from the changes in cardiac output because of the sympathetic modulation of the arterial tone, which tends to maintain MAP constant while cardiac output varies. These results suggest that precise assessment of the effects of volume expansion should not rely on simple blood pressure measurements but should rather be based on direct measurements of cardiac output. This may be particularly important in patients at risk of fluid overload during sepsis and/or ARDS.

Effects of Volume Expansion on Tissue Oxygenation

What is really expected from volume expansion in a patient with acute circulatory failure is not only an increase in cardiac output but also an improvement in tissue oxygenation. This can only occur if oxygen consumption depends on oxygen delivery (DO_2). However, this is not always the case. In a recent study, we observed that volume expansion administered in patients with acute circulatory failure increased cardiac output $\geq 15\,\%$ in 49 % of cases ("volume-responders") [56]. Although DO_2 significantly increased in "volume-responders", a significant increase in oxygen consumption occurred in only 56 % of these patients. When looking at variables that could identify patients who would benefit from volume expansion in terms of oxygen consumption, we found that markers of global tissue hypoxia, such as blood lactate, were more relevant than the central venous oxygen saturation ($ScvO_2$). This illustrates the difficulty of using $ScvO_2$ for assessment of fluid therapy [57] because $ScvO_2$ cannot detect preload responsiveness [58] or identify among volume-responders those who will benefit from fluid infusion in terms of tissue oxygenation [56]. Importantly, in our study, DO_2 decreased with volume infusion in the "volume-non-responders" (51 %), owing to development of hemodilution [56]. This latter finding reinforces the message that identifying volume responders before any fluid administration is crucial since volume expansion in patients without preload-dependency can be deleterious not only on lung function but also on peripheral oxygenation.

Conclusion

There is growing evidence suggesting that overzealous fluid administration is deleterious in critically ill patients, particularly in cases of sepsis and/or lung injury. During recent years, several tests have been developed to detect volume responsiveness before administering fluid. These tests can also serve to detect volume unresponsiveness, which could be helpful at any moment of fluid resuscitation to better assess the benefit/risk ratio of continuing such a strategy [59]. The analysis of respiratory variation in stroke volume has received the largest level of evidence, but cannot be used in cases of spontaneous breathing activity, cardiac arrhythmias, low tidal volume or low lung compliance. Some more recently developed tests, such as the end-expiratory occlusion test, the 'mini' fluid challenge and the PLR test can be used as alternative methods, solving the problem of prediction of volume responsiveness in cases of spontaneous breathing activity and/or cardiac arrhythmias. The ideal management of fluid therapy should also include a precise assessment of the effects of volume expansion on cardiac output and tissue oxygen consumption.

References

1. Marik PE, Monnet X, Teboul JL (2011) Hemodynamic parameters to guide fluid therapy. Ann Intensive Care 1:1
2. Vincent JL, Sakr Y, Sprung CL et al (2006) Sepsis in European intensive care units: results of the SOAP study. Crit Care Med 34:344–353
3. Boyd JH, Forbes J, Nakada TA, Walley KR, Russell JA (2011) Fluid resuscitation in septic shock: A positive fluid balance and elevated central venous pressure are associated with increased mortality. Crit Care Med 39:259–265

4. Wiedemann HP, Wheeler AP, Bernard GR et al (2006) Comparison of two fluid-management strategies in acute lung injury. N Engl J Med 354:2564–2575
5. Sakka SG, Klein M, Reinhart K, Meier-Hellmann A (2002) Prognostic value of extravascular lung water in critically ill patients. Chest 122:2080–2086
6. Jozwiak M, Silva S, Persichini R et al (2013) Extra-vascular lung water is an independent prognostic factor in patients with acute respiratory distress syndrome. Crit Care Med (in press)
7. Michard F, Teboul JL (2002) Predicting fluid responsiveness in ICU patients: a critical analysis of the evidence. Chest 121:2000–2008
8. Marik PE, Baram M, Vahid B (2008) Does central venous pressure predict fluid responsiveness? A systematic review of the literature and the tale of seven mares. Chest 134:172–178
9. Michard F, Teboul JL (2000) Using heart-lung interactions to assess fluid responsiveness during mechanical ventilation. Crit Care 4:282–289
10. Michard F, Boussat S, Chemla D et al (2000) Relation between respiratory changes in arterial pulse pressure and fluid responsiveness in septic patients with acute circulatory failure. Am J Respir Crit Care Med 162:134–138
11. Marik PE, Cavallazzi R, Vasu T, Hirani A (2009) Dynamic changes in arterial waveform derived variables and fluid responsiveness in mechanically ventilated patients: a systematic review of the literature. Crit Care Med 37:2642–2647
12. Monnet X, Rienzo M, Osman D et al (2005) Esophageal Doppler monitoring predicts fluid responsiveness in critically ill ventilated patients. Intensive Care Med 31:1195–1201
13. Feissel M, Michard F, Mangin I, Ruyer O, Faller JP, Teboul JL (2001) Respiratory changes in aortic blood velocity as an indicator of fluid responsiveness in ventilated patients with septic shock. Chest 119:867–873
14. Berkenstadt H, Margalit N, Hadani M et al (2001) Stroke volume variation as a predictor of fluid responsiveness in patients undergoing brain surgery. Anesth Analg 92:984–989
15. Biais M, Stecken L, Ottolenghi L et al (2011) The ability of pulse pressure variations obtained with CNAPTM device to predict fluid responsiveness in the operating room. Anesth Analg 113:523–528
16. Monnet X, Dres M, Ferre A et al (2012) Prediction of fluid responsiveness by a continuous non-invasive assessment of arterial pressure in critically ill patients: comparison with four other dynamic indices. Br J Anaesth 109:330–338
17. Sandroni C, Cavallaro F, Marano C, Falcone C, De Santis P, Antonelli M (2012) Accuracy of plethysmographic indices as predictors of fluid responsiveness in mechanically ventilated adults: a systematic review and meta-analysis. Intensive Care Med 38:1429–1437
18. Feissel M, Michard F, Faller JP, Teboul JL (2004) The respiratory variation in inferior vena cava diameter as a guide to fluid therapy. Intensive Care Med 30:1834–1837
19. Vieillard-Baron A, Chergui K, Rabiller A et al (2004) Superior vena caval collapsibility as a gauge of volume status in ventilated septic patients. Intensive Care Med 30:1734–1739
20. Teboul JL, Monnet X (2008) Prediction of volume responsiveness in critically ill patients with spontaneous breathing activity. Curr Opin Crit Care 14:334–339
21. Heenen S, De Backer D, Vincent JL (2006) How can the response to volume expansion in patients with spontaneous respiratory movements be predicted? Crit Care 10:R102
22. Monnet X, Rienzo M, Osman D et al (2006) Passive leg raising predicts fluid responsiveness in the critically ill. Crit Care Med 34:1402–1407
23. Soubrier S, Saulnier F, Hubert H et al (2007) Can dynamic indicators help the prediction of fluid responsiveness in spontaneously breathing critically ill patients? Intensive Care Med 33:1117–1124
24. De Backer D, Heenen S, Piagnerelli M, Koch M, Vincent JL (2005) Pulse pressure variations to predict fluid responsiveness: influence of tidal volume. Intensive Care Med 31:517–523
25. Muller L, Louart G, Bousquet PJ et al (2010) The influence of the airway driving pressure on pulsed pressure variation as a predictor of fluid responsiveness. Intensive Care Med 36:496–503

26. Monnet X, Bleibtreu A, Ferré A et al (2012) Passive leg raising and end-expiratory occlusion tests perform better than pulse pressure variation in patients with low respiratory system compliance. Crit Care Med 40:152–157
27. De Backer D, Taccone FS, Holsten R, Ibrahimi F, Vincent JL (2009) Influence of respiratory rate on stroke volume variation in mechanically ventilated patients. Anesthesiology 110:1092–1097
28. Jacques D, Bendjelid K, Duperret S, Colling J, Piriou V, Viale JP (2011) Pulse pressure variation and stroke volume variation during increased intra-abdominal pressure: an experimental study. Crit Care 15:R33
29. Tavernier B, Robin E (2011) Assessment of fluid responsiveness during increased intra-abdominal pressure: keep the indices, but change the thresholds. Crit Care 15:134
30. de Waal EE, Rex S, Kruitwagen CL, Kalkman CJ, Buhre WF (2009) Dynamic preload indicators fail to predict fluid responsiveness in open-chest conditions. Crit Care Med 37:510–515
31. Monnet X, Osman D, Ridel C, Lamia B, Richard C, Teboul JL (2009) Predicting volume responsiveness by using the end-expiratory occlusion in mechanically ventilated intensive care unit patients. Crit Care Med 37:951–956
32. Vincent JL, Weil MH (2006) Fluid challenge revisited. Crit Care Med 34:1333–1337
33. Vincent JL (2011) "Let's give some fluid and see what happens" versus the "mini-fluid challenge". Anesthesiology 115:455–456
34. Muller L, Toumi M, Bousquet PJ et al (2011) An increase in aortic blood flow after an infusion of 100 ml colloid over 1 minute can predict fluid responsiveness: the mini-fluid challenge study. Anesthesiology 115:541–547
35. Boulain T, Achard JM, Teboul JL, Richard C, Perrotin D, Ginies G (2002) Changes in BP induced by passive leg raising predict response to fluid loading in critically ill patients. Chest 121:1245–1252
36. Jabot J, Teboul JL, Richard C, Monnet X (2009) Passive leg raising for predicting fluid responsiveness: importance of the postural change. Intensive Care Med 35:85–90
37. Monnet X, Jabot J, Maizel J, Richard C, Teboul JL (2011) Norepinephrine increases cardiac preload and reduces preload dependency assessed by passive leg raising in septic shock patients. Crit Care Med 39:689–694
38. Monnet X, Teboul JL (2008) Passive leg raising. Intensive Care Med 34:659–663
39. Cavallaro F, Sandroni C, Marano C et al (2010) Diagnostic accuracy of passive leg raising for prediction of fluid responsiveness in adults: systematic review and meta-analysis of clinical studies. Intensive Care Med 36:1475–1483
40. Antonelli M, Levy M, Andrews PJ et al (2007) Hemodynamic monitoring in shock and implications for management. International Consensus Conference, Paris, France, 27–28 April 2006. Intensive Care Med 33:575–590
41. Lafanechere A, Pene F, Goulenok C et al (2006) Changes in aortic blood flow induced by passive leg raising predict fluid responsiveness in critically ill patients. Crit Care 10:R132
42. Biais M, Vidil L, Sarrabay P, Cottenceau V, Revel P, Sztark F (2009) Changes in stroke volume induced by passive leg raising in spontaneously breathing patients: comparison between echocardiography and Vigileo/FloTrac device. Crit Care 13:R195
43. Benomar B, Ouattara A, Estagnasie P, Brusset A, Squara P (2010) Fluid responsiveness predicted by noninvasive bioreactance-based passive leg raise test. Intensive Care Med 36:1875–1881
44. Marik PE, Levitov A, Young A, Andrews L (2013) The use of NICOM (Bioreactance) and Carotid Doppler to determine volume responsiveness and blood flow redistribution following passive leg raising in hemodynamically unstable patients. Chest (in press)
45. Fellahi JL, Fischer MO, Dalbera A, Massetti M, Gerard JL, Hanouz JL (2012) Can endotracheal bioimpedance cardiography assess hemodynamic response to passive leg raising following cardiac surgery? Ann Intensive Care 2:26

46. Guinot PG, Zogheib E, Detave M et al (2011) Passive leg raising can predict fluid responsiveness in patients placed on venovenous extracorporeal membrane oxygenation. Crit Care 15:R216
47. Lamia B, Ochagavia A, Monnet X, Chemla D, Richard C, Teboul JL (2007) Echocardiographic prediction of volume responsiveness in critically ill patients with spontaneously breathing activity. Intensive Care Med 33:1125–1132
48. Lukito V, Djer MM, Pudjiadi AH, Munasir Z (2012) The role of passive leg raising to predict fluid responsiveness in pediatric intensive care unit patients. Pediatr Crit Care Med 13:e155–e160
49. Thiel SW, Kollef MH, Isakow W (2009) Non-invasive stroke volume measurement and passive leg raising predict volume responsiveness in medical ICU patients: an observational cohort study. Crit Care 13:R111
50. Monge Garcia MI, Gil Cano A, Gracia Romero M, Monterroso Pintado R, Perez Madueno V, Diaz Monrove JC (2012) Non-invasive assessment of fluid responsiveness by changes in partial end-tidal CO2 pressure during a passive leg-raising maneuver. Ann Intensive Care 2:9
51. Monnet X, Bataille A, Magalhaes E et al (2012) End-tidal carbon dioxide is better than arterial pressure for predicting volume responsiveness by the passive leg raising test. Intensive Care Med 39:93–100
52. De Backer D, Pinsky MR (2007) Can one predict fluid responsiveness in spontaneously breathing patients? Intensive Care Med 33:1111–1113
53. Monnet X, Letierce A, Hamzaoui O et al (2011) Arterial pressure allows monitoring the changes in cardiac output induced by volume expansion but not by norepinephrine. Crit Care Med 39:1394–1399
54. Pierrakos C, Velissaris D, Scolletta S, Heenen S, De Backer D, Vincent JL (2012) Can changes in arterial pressure be used to detect changes in cardiac index during fluid challenge in patients with septic shock? Intensive Care Med 38:422–428
55. Chemla D, Hebert JL, Coirault C et al (1998) Total arterial compliance estimated by stroke volume-to-aortic pulse pressure ratio in humans. Am J Physiol 274:H500–H505
56. Monnet X, Julien F, Ait-Hamou N et al (2013) Lactate and veno-arterial carbon dioxide difference/arterial-venous oxygen difference ratio, but not central venous oxygen saturation, predict increase in oxygen consumption in fluid responders. Crit Care Med (in press)
57. Teboul JL, Hamzaoui O, Monnet X (2011) SvO2 to monitor resuscitation of septic patients: let's just understand the basic physiology. Crit Care 15:1005
58. Velissaris D, Pierrakos C, Scolletta S, De Backer D, Vincent JL (2011) High mixed venous oxygen saturation levels do not exclude fluid responsiveness in critically ill septic patients. Crit Care 15:R177
59. Teboul JL, Monnet X (2009) Detecting volume responsiveness and unresponsiveness in intensive care unit patients: two different problems, only one solution. Crit Care 13:175

Point-of-Care Coagulation Management in Intensive Care Medicine

P. Meybohm, K. Zacharowski, and C. F. Weber

Introduction

Coagulopathy in critically ill patients is common and of multifactorial origin [1]. Coagulopathy-associated risk of bleeding and the use of allogeneic blood products are independent risk factors for morbidity and mortality [2, 3]. Therefore, prompt and correct identification of the underlying causes of these coagulation abnormalities is required, since each coagulation abnormality necessitates very different therapeutic management strategies. Standard laboratory tests of blood coagulation yield only partial diagnostic information, and important coagulation defects, e.g., reduced clot stability, platelet dysfunction, or hyperfibrinolysis, remain undetected. Therefore, point-of-care (POC) diagnostics are increasingly being used for rapid specific testing of hemostatic function. Algorithm-based hemotherapy, including POC techniques, reliably corrects coagulopathy, but may also have the potential to reduce blood loss, transfusion requirements and risk of transfusion-related adverse events, prevent thromboembolic events, and save costs.

This article reviews the most frequent coagulation abnormalities in critically ill patients. In particular, we will discuss differential diagnoses, benefits and limitations of POC coagulation management and hemotherapy algorithms.

P. Meybohm
Clinic of Anesthesiology, Intensive Care Medicine and Pain Therapy, Goethe-University Hospital Frankfurt, Theodor-Stern-Kai 7, 60590 Frankfurt am Main, Germany

K. Zacharowski (✉)
Clinic of Anesthesiology, Intensive Care Medicine and Pain Therapy, Goethe-University Hospital Frankfurt, Theodor-Stern-Kai 7, 60590 Frankfurt am Main, Germany
E-mail: kai.zacharowski@kgu.de

C. F. Weber
Clinic of Anesthesiology, Intensive Care Medicine and Pain Therapy, Goethe-University Hospital Frankfurt, Theodor-Stern-Kai 7, 60590 Frankfurt am Main, Germany

J.-L. Vincent (Ed.), *Annual Update in Intensive Care and Emergency Medicine 2013*, DOI 10.1007/978-3-642-35109-9_33, © Springer-Verlag Berlin Heidelberg and BioMed Central Ltd. 2013

Diagnosis of Coagulopathy in Intensive Care Medicine

Coagulopathy in critically ill patients is typically a multifactorial problem involving:

- disturbances in physiological basic conditions for hemostasis (pH, concentration of ionized calcium, temperature and hematocrit)
- disturbances of primary hemostasis, e.g., preexisting or perioperatively acquired disturbances of platelet count and function, due to sepsis, disseminated intravascular coagulation (DIC), heparin-induced thrombocytopenia, massive blood loss, or drug-induced thrombocytopenia;
- abnormalities of blood plasma, e.g., preoperative anticoagulation medication as well as isolated or global clotting-factor deficits (impaired synthesis, massive loss, or increased turnover);
- complex coagulopathies, e.g., DIC or hyperfibrinolysis (Fig. 1) [1].

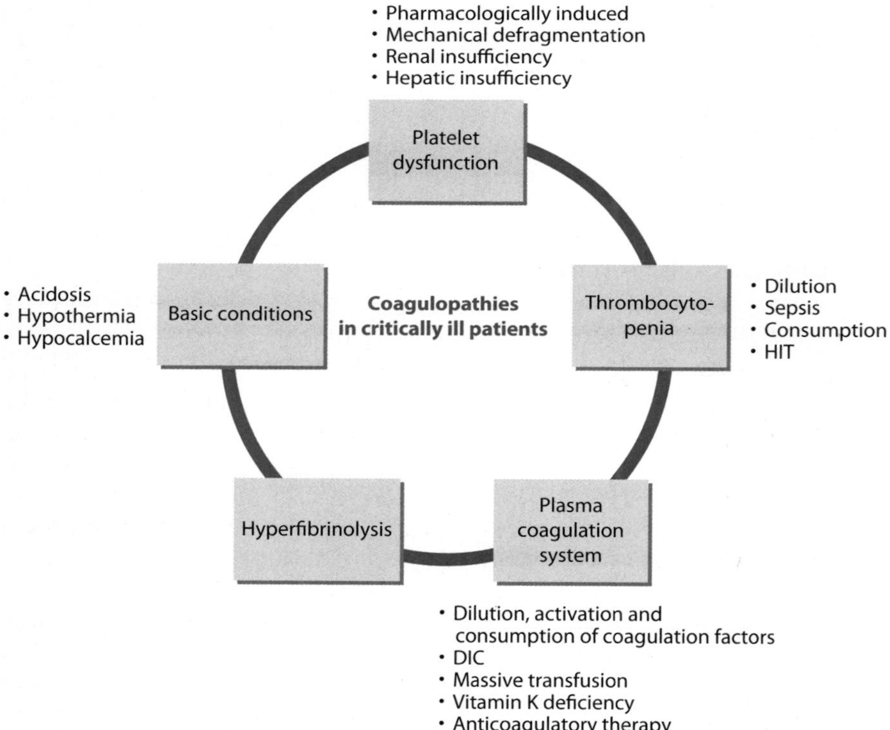

Fig. 1 Overview of coagulopathies typically present in critically ill patients. DIC: disseminated intravascular coagulopathy; HIT: heparin-induced thrombocytopenia

In patients with extracorporeal life support (ventricular-assist devices, extracorporeal membrane oxygenation [4]), the risk of coagulopathy is further increased by:

- therapeutic anticoagulation with the use of heparin to limit clotting;
- dilution, activation and consumption of both coagulation factors and platelets.

Limitations of Conventional Laboratory Coagulation Analyses

The conventional laboratory coagulation analyses (Quick's test, activated partial thromboplastin time (aPTT), platelet count, fibrinogen concentration) may be of limited use for the prediction and detection of coagulopathies and for treatment monitoring, in particular in patients with ongoing bleeding [5]. Analysis at a standardized temperature of 37 °C impedes the detection of coagulopathies induced by hypothermia. The global tests (e.g., aPTT and Quick's test) reflect only the initial formation of thrombin in plasma and are unaffected by any of the corpuscular elements of the blood. The platelet count is purely quantitative and cannot detect preexisting, drug-induced, or perioperatively acquired platelet dysfunction. Moreover, conventional coagulation tests convey no information about clot stability over time, nor do they provide any information regarding (hyper-)fibrinolysis. Thus, it is critically important to recognize that routine coagulation tests cannot detect clinically significant coagulation defects that contribute to bleeding, hypo- or hyperfibrinolysis, hypercoagulability, and platelet aggregation.

Point-of-Care Techniques

In contrast to standard laboratory tests, POC techniques, including whole blood platelet function tests (impedance or turbidimetric aggregometry) and viscoelastic tests (thromboelastometry/-graphy), reflect in detail the hemostatic status of the critically ill patient. The use of POC diagnostics may partly compensate for the methodological limitations of conventional coagulation testing. Test results are also available earlier (analysis time of 20 to 25 minutes [6]) compared to conventional laboratory analyses (turnaround time of 40 to 90 minutes after blood drawing [7]), for which the delayed results may not reflect the current state of the coagulation system and may lead to inappropriate treatment.

However, none of the currently available POC techniques can provide adequate information about all aspects of the complex process of blood clotting. From a pathophysiological point of view, coagulation can be divided into four areas: Primary hemostasis, thrombin generation, clot formation/stabilization, and fibrinolysis.

Aggregometric testing of whole-blood samples is used mainly to study platelet function [8]. In bleeding patients in whom the hematocrit is greater than 30 % and the platelet count exceeds 70–100/nl, aggregometric tests can be used to screen for disorders of primary hemostasis, e.g., von Willebrand syndrome, and to quantify the effect of antiplatelet medications. The available aggregometric POC tests (Multiplate®, PFA-100®, TEG® Platelet Mapping™ Assay, VerifyNow®) differ in the agonists that are used to activate the platelets in the test cells, such as collagen, adenosine phosphate, epinephrine, arachidonic acid, and thrombin, and in the shearing forces that are generated in the test cells.

Viscoelastic POC techniques (ROTEM®, TEG®) are based on thromboelastography, which was described decades ago by Hartert [9]. These tests are used to measure the time until clot formation begins, the dynamics of clot formation, and the solidity and stability of clots over time. They enable parallel measurements to be performed on a single blood sample after clotting has been activated using a variety of agonists. A special advantage of viscoelastic techniques is that they can directly detect hyperfibrinolysis. Aggregometric tests combined with viscoelastic methods yield a far broader diagnostic spectrum than do conventional laboratory testing of coagulation.

Implementation of POC Testing in Intensive Care Medicine

Cardiovascular Surgery

Most of the previous trials related to POC coagulation testing were performed in cardiac surgical patients [10–13]. The majority reported a potential decrease in transfusion requirements following POC diagnostics. In two studies, the authors exclusively focused on coagulopathic patients [13, 14], in whom POC techniques resulted in significantly reduced postoperative blood loss and beneficial effects in terms of clinically relevant endpoints. Nuttall et al. [14] randomized patients to a control group following individual anesthesiologist's transfusion practices or a protocol group using a transfusion algorithm guided by coagulation tests (prothrombin time, aPTT, platelet counts, thromboelastogram maximum amplitude, and fibrinogen concentration). We recently published the results of a prospective study including coagulopathic patients in whom diffuse bleeding was diagnosed after heparin reversal or increased blood loss was observed during the first 24 hours postoperatively; the previous protocol group of Nuttall et al. was now defined as our control group with conventional tests (platelet count, fibrinogen concentration, international normalized ratio [INR], aPTT, and activated clotting time [ACT]), and patients in the POC-guided group received repeated thromboelastometry and whole blood impedance aggregometry [13]. The following endpoints were lower in the POC-guided group: Erythrocyte, frozen plasma and platelet transfusion rates; postoperative mechanical ventilation duration; length of ICU stay; composite adverse events rate; costs of hemostatic therapy; and 6-month mortality (Fig. 2).

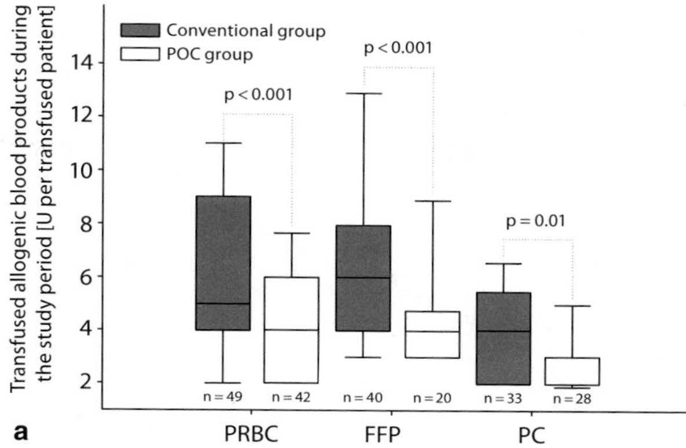

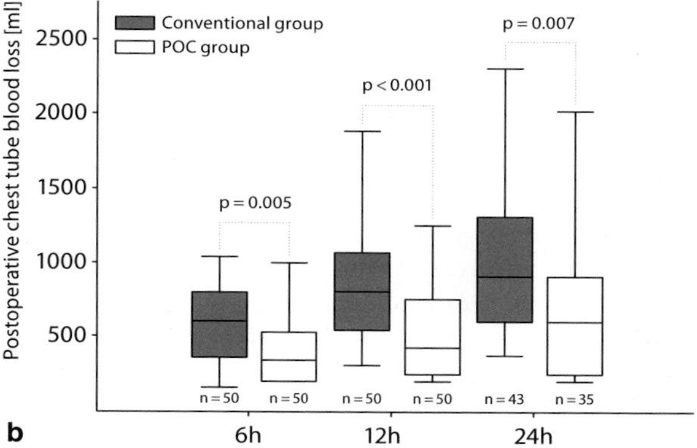

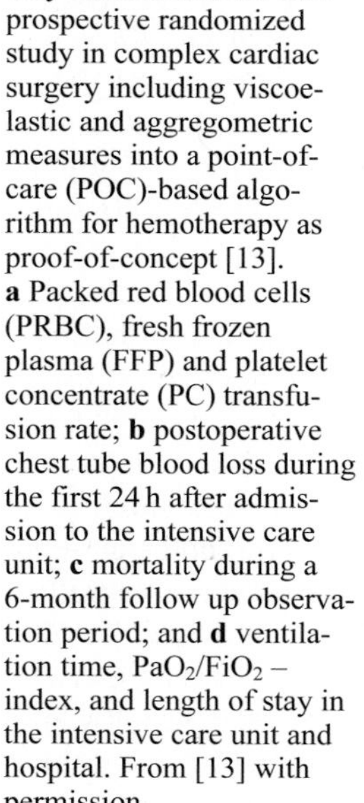
Fig. 2 Primary and secondary outcomes of the first prospective randomized study in complex cardiac surgery including viscoelastic and aggregometric measures into a point-of-care (POC)-based algorithm for hemotherapy as proof-of-concept [13]. **a** Packed red blood cells (PRBC), fresh frozen plasma (FFP) and platelet concentrate (PC) transfusion rate; **b** postoperative chest tube blood loss during the first 24 h after admission to the intensive care unit; **c** mortality during a 6-month follow up observation period; and **d** ventilation time, PaO_2/FiO_2 – index, and length of stay in the intensive care unit and hospital. From [13] with permission

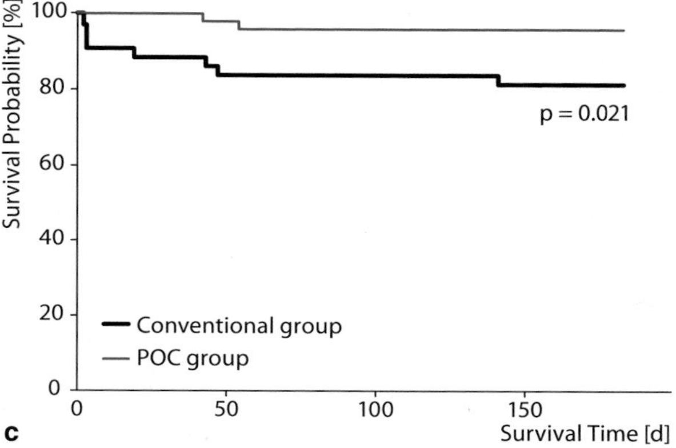

Fig. 2 *Continued*

	Conventional group	POC group	p-value
Postoperative PaO_2/FiO_2–indices			
At ICU admission	323 (201/402) (n=50)	355 (282/460) (n=50)	0.069
2 h after ICU admission	326 (219/393) (n=50)	338 (277/423) (n=50)	0.087
4 h after ICU admission	309 (256/373) (n=50)	358 (300/407) (n=50)	0.015
12 h after ICU admission	299 (222/371) (n=48)	398 (328/467) (n=45)	< 0.001
24 h after ICU admission	228 (137/312) (n=23)	327 (259/468) (n=17)	0.009
Time of mechanical ventilation [min]	827 (440/2835) (n=50)	316 (230/513) (n=50)	< 0.001
ICU period [h]	24 (20/87) (n=50)	21 (18/31) (n=50)	0.019
Hospitalization period [d]	12 (9/23) (n=50)	12 (9/22) (n=50)	0.718

d

Our findings support those of a recently published retrospective study by Gorlinger et al. [15] that included 3,865 cardiac surgery patients in whom POC testing combined with first-line administration of coagulation factor concentrates was associated with decreased incidence of blood transfusion and adverse events. In ICU patients undergoing mechanical circulatory support, monitoring of hemostasis using POC thromboelastometry/-graphy and platelet function analysis is also recommended to reduce the risk of bleeding and thromboembolic complications [4]. Notably, these hemostatic tests should be performed repeatedly during mechanical circulatory support therapy since thrombin generation, clot firmness and platelet response may change significantly over time with marked inter- and intra-individual variability.

Organ Transplantation

In patients with liver transplantation, significant blood loss has been found to be an independent risk factor for postoperative morbidity. To date, there is no consensus as to how to monitor and manage perioperative blood loss. In a prospective randomized study, Wang et al. recently randomized 28 patients undergoing orthotopic liver transplantation either to standard laboratory measures of blood coagulation or thromboelastography analysis. POC-guided transfusion was associated with decreased transfusion of frozen plasma (12.8 ± 7 vs. 21.5 ± 12.7 units), but did not affect 3-year survival [16]. Analyzing more than 18,000 thromboelastography measurements in the context of 642 patients with liver transplantation, the implementation of a POC coagulation management based on early, calculated, goal-directed therapy with fibrinogen concentrate, prothrombin complex concentrate and antifibrinolytic therapy resulted in early detection of hyperfibrinolysis and consequently antifibrinolytic therapy [17], and a reduction in transfusion requirements for erythrocytes, fresh frozen plasma (FFP), and platelets as well as a reduced incidence of massive transfusion [18].

Massive Bleeding and Trauma Patients

When critically ill patients need urgent massive transfusion because of massive blood loss, there may not be enough time to analyze the results of POC testing before the erythrocyte transfusion is given. However, coagulation factor deficiency is the primary cause of coagulopathy in massive transfusion because of dilution of coagulation factors. The level of fibrinogen typically falls below the lower reference range after 150 % blood volume loss, followed by a decrease in other coagulation factors to 25 % activity after 200 % blood loss [19]. FFP alone, if given in sufficient quantity (> 15–20 ml/kg), will most likely correct fibrinogen and most coagulation factor deficiencies, but large volumes may be required, which are further associated with infectious complications [20] and multiple organ failure [21]; therefore goal-directed therapy with coagulation factor concentrates should be preferred [18] in patients outside the clinical setting of 'massive transfusion'.

In major trauma patients, coagulopathy has been shown to be present in approximately 30 % of admitted patients, accounting for up to 40 % of all trauma-related deaths [22]. Although FFP transfusion is often a routine part of transfusion protocols, its efficacy is uncertain. Most notably, FFP administration is also associated with acute lung injury (ALI), volume overload, and nosocomial infection [20, 21]. Additionally, trauma-associated coagulopathy is the consequence of a low admission fibrinogen level, which is independently associated with injury severity score, shock, and mortality at 24 h and 28 days after trauma. In a prospective cohort study of 517 trauma patients, thromboelastography enabled rapid detection of hypofibrinogenemia, and early administration of fibrinogen was related with improved survival [23]. Using rapid thromboelastography, Holcomb et al. recently succeeded in identifying patients with an increased risk of fibrinolysis and erythrocyte, plasma and platelet transfusions out of 1,974 major trauma patients [24]. Schochl et al. [25] retrospectively analyzed the effects of thromboelastometry-guided hemostatic therapy in 131 trauma patients who received ≥ 5 erythrocyte concentrate units within 24 hours after admission. POC-guided hemostatic therapy with fibrinogen concentrate as first-line hemostatic therapy (if maximum clot firmness [MCF] measured by FibTEM [fibrin-based test] was < 10 mm) and additional use of prothrombin complex concentrate (if clotting time measured by extrinsic activation test [EXTEM] > 1.5 times normal) allowed rapid and reliable diagnosis of the underlying coagulopathy, and resulted in a favorable survival rate compared with predicted mortality [25]. Although a recent meta-analysis concluded that use of a thromboelastography- or thromboelastometry-guided transfusion strategy significantly reduced bleeding in massively transfused patients, these POC techniques were not, however, able to improve morbidity or mortality in patients with massive transfusion [26]. Therefore, prospective randomized studies focusing on POC-guided therapy are needed in these patients.

Severe Sepsis

Because hemostatic alterations are a common early event in patients with severe sepsis, and commonly used sepsis biomarkers, such as procalcitonin and interleukin (IL)-6, may also increase in patients with trauma or surgery even without infection, thromboelastometry variables may have potential as early biomarkers of sepsis in critically ill patients. Adamzik and colleagues [27] recently demonstrated, in an observational cohort study of 56 patients with severe sepsis and 52 patients after major surgery, that the thromboelastometry-derived lysis index was a more reliable biomarker of severe sepsis than were procalcitonin, IL-6, and C-reactive protein (CRP). More interestingly, a multivariate analysis of another cohort study of 98 septic patients [28] revealed that the absence or presence of at least one pathological thromboelastometry variable allowed better prediction of 30-day survival in severe sepsis than did the simplified acute physiology system (SAPS) II and sequential organ failure assessment (SOFA) scores, emphasizing the importance of the coagulation system and the future role of POC techniques in sepsis.

Economic Aspects

Results of the currently available trials do not allow any firm conclusions about the putative economic savings resulting from the use of POC coagulation testing. A number of retrospective studies have compared the costs of hemotherapy before and after the implementation of POC-based hemotherapy algorithms, albeit with partially conflicting results. In a study of 1,422 patients undergoing elective cardiac surgery, Spalding et al. found that implementation of POC coagulation testing lowered the cost of allogeneic blood products and other hemotherapeutic agents by about 50 % [29]. The total cost of POC testing (devices, reagents, test tubes, control solutions, maintenance, etc.) exceeds that of conventional coagulation testing, because combined viscoelastic and aggregometric coagulation testing costs about €25 to €35, whereas a conventional test battery (aPTT, fibrinogen, thrombin time, Quick, complete blood count) generally costs less than €10. Taken together, it appears that POC-guided coagulation therapy indeed lowers the rate of transfusion of allogeneic blood products overall (mainly by lowering FFP and platelet transfusion rates), but simultaneously increases the use of clotting-factor concentrates (mainly fibrinogen and prothrombin complex concentrates) [15]. The economic savings from the reduced use of allogeneic blood products, may, however, compensate for or outweigh these increased expenditures in clotting-factor concentrates [13].

Hemotherapy Algorithm Including Point-of-Care Techniques

Coagulation management in intensive care medicine should be based on a hemotherapy algorithm that includes POC techniques, and that is implemented as institutional standard care (Fig. 3). Hemotherapy should involve an assessment of the patient's individual bleeding risk, evaluation and correction of basic physiological conditions required for hemostasis, and repeated evaluation and correction of thrombin and clot formation. If indicated, replacing deficient coagulation factors and improving the hemostatic potential of the primary hemostasis are consecutive steps in therapy escalation. Final options are off label use of factor XIII and recombinant factor VIIa.

Maintain Optimal Physiological Conditions for Hemostasis

The patient's physiological pH and core temperature should be maintained at > 7.3 and > 36 °C, respectively. Calcium is an elementary cofactor in several enzymatic processes during coagulation. It is important to maintain a plasma ionized calcium concentration of > 1.0 mmol/l. With respect to the rheological properties of erythrocytes and the provision of thromboxane A2 and adenosine diphosphate (ADP) for platelet aggregation, hematocrit should be maintained at a concentration of > 25 % [19].

Antagonize Anticoagulant Therapy

In patients with previous heparin therapy (e.g., extracorporeal life support, renal replacement therapy) and ongoing bleeding, it is necessary to exclude any persistent heparin effects. Protamine is routinely used to antagonize heparin. However, if the ACT remains > 130 s or viscoelastic measures indicate persistent heparin effects, it may be necessary to administer additional protamine (30 IU/kg) and to re-evaluate its therapeutic effect.

Newer anticoagulants include both direct and indirect inhibitors of coagulation factors. The indirect (antithrombin-dependent) inhibitors include the low molecular weight heparins (e.g., enoxaparin and dalteparin) and selective factor Xa inhibitors (e.g., fondaparinux and rivaroxaban). The direct thrombin inhibitors (e.g., lepirudin, argatroban, bivalirudin, and dabigatran) directly bind to and inhibit thrombin. Approximately 60 % of the anticoagulant effect of low-molecular-weight heparins can also be neutralized by protamine. In contrast, there are no specific reversal agents for any of the newer anticoagulants; prothrombin complex concentrates might be beneficial for the treatment of anticoagulant-associated coagulation factor deficiencies (dose ranges from 25 to 100 U/kg depending on the product used). In patients with life-threatening bleeding, hemodialysis might be considered to remove selected small-molecule anticoagulants (e.g., lepirudin, dabigatran) [30].

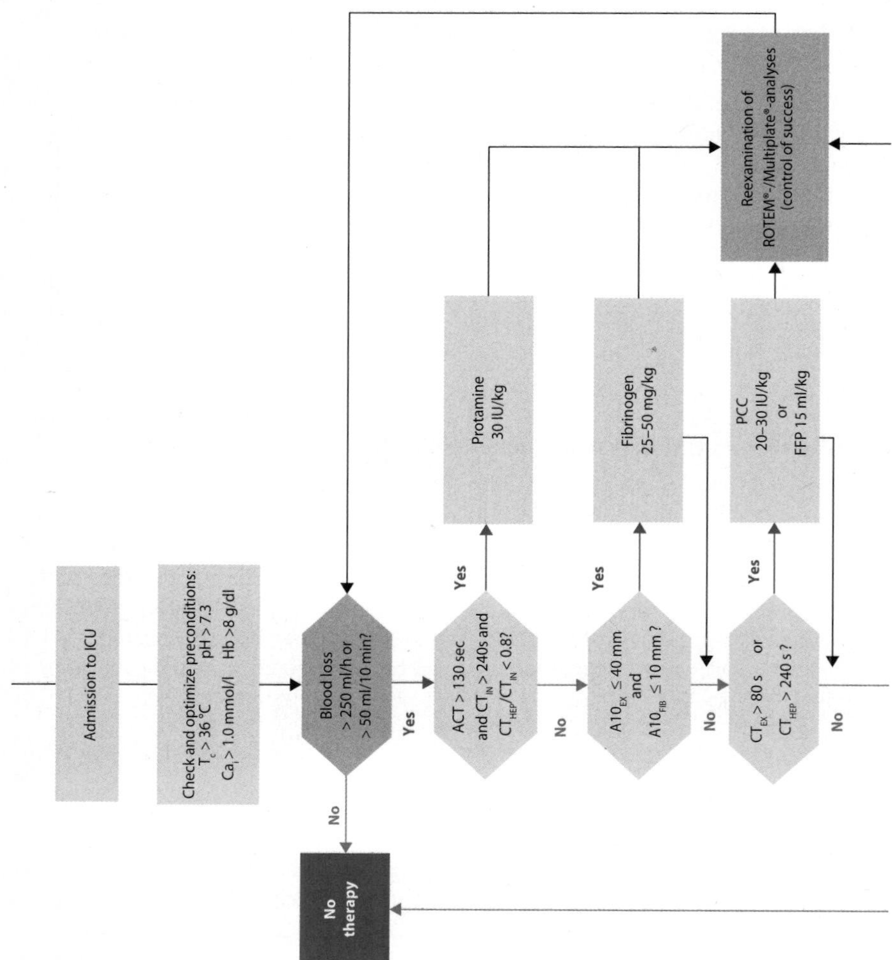

Fig. 3 Hemotherapy algorithm including point-of-care (POC) techniques. ACT: activated clotting time; ADP: ADPtest; ASPI: ASPItest; A10: amplitude of clot firmness 10 min after clotting time; Ca_i: ionized calcium; CT: clotting time; EX: EXTEM; FFP: fresh frozen plasma; FIB: FIBTEM; F XIII: factor XIII concentrate; HEP: HEPTEM; ICU: intensive care unit; IN: INTEM; PC: pooled platelet concentrate; PCC: prothrombin complex concentrate; rFVIIa: activated recombinant factor VII; T_c: core temperature; TRAP: TRAPtest. From [13] with permission

Maintain Adequate Levels of Coagulation Factors

If coagulopathy persists following reversal of the anticoagulant effects, it should be ensured that adequate levels of coagulation factors are maintained. Fibrinogen is

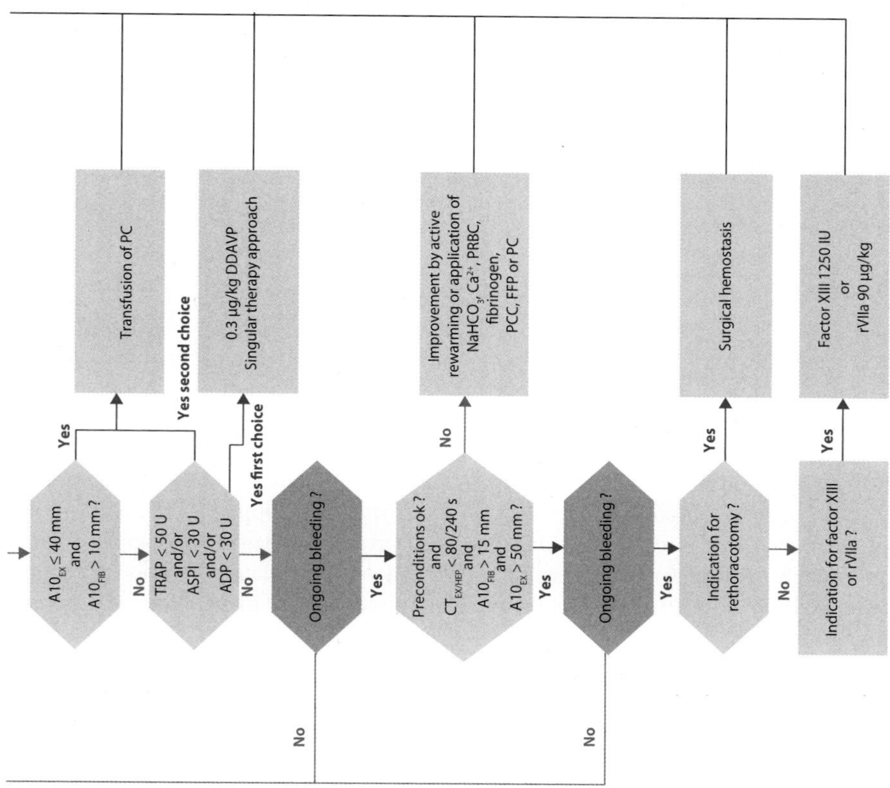

Fig. 3 *Continued*

the first coagulation factor to decrease below lower reference values during bleeding [31]. As the precursor to fibrin, and as a ligand for platelet aggregation, fibrinogen plays a key role in clot formation [32]. Thus, if plasma levels of fibrinogen decrease below 150–200 mg/dl, or if viscoelastic tests indicate a deficiency (if maximum clot firmness measured by FibTEM is < 10 mm), it is necessary to administer fibrinogen substitute. In the past, FFP (15–30 ml/kg) was used as a source of replacement fibrinogen. But again, the transfusion of FFP is, under certain conditions, associated with volume overload, sepsis, multiple organ failure, and increased perioperative mortality [20, 21]. An alternative source of fibrinogen is fibrinogen concentrate, which should be used at a concentration of 25–50 mg/kg. A recent review of trials in which fibrinogen concentrate was used in perioperative settings or in cases of massive hemorrhage suggests that this form of substitution is both effective and well tolerated [33].

If coagulopathy persists even though fibrinogen has been supplemented, and if the INR is >1.4, or if viscoelastic measures reveal a deficiency of prothrombin-complex coagulation factors II, VII, IX, and X, then substitution of these factors is indicated. A dosage of 15–30 ml/kg FFP is necessary to increase the concentration of these factors. However, the use of a prothrombin-complex concentrate, which contains factors II, VII, IX, and X, proteins C and S, heparin, and antithrombin, represents an attractive alternative because of the smaller volumes required to supplement the deficiency (recommended dose 20–30 IU/kg) [34].

Platelets

After the substitution of coagulation factors, the therapy algorithm should lead to a consideration of both platelet count and function. Importantly, temperature has a strong impact on platelet function [35]. Primary hemostasis may further be impaired by preexisting or perioperatively-acquired disturbances of platelet function, or isolated thrombocytopenia from sepsis, DIC, heparin-induced thrombocytopenia, massive blood loss, or drug-induced thrombocytopenia. In addition, use of extracorporeal circulation may also cause irreversible platelet damage mainly as a result of mechanical defragmentation and reduced platelet surface glycoproteins (GPIb and GPIIb/IIIa), which are important for platelet adhesion and aggregation [36].

Routine standard laboratory analyses are of limited informative value as they only provide a quantitative measure of platelet numbers without providing any information regarding platelet functionality. In contrast, aggregometric measures allow assessment of platelet function by measuring the amount of platelet aggregation induced in the presence of common platelet agonists such as thrombin, arachidonic acid, ADP, epinephrine, or collagen. Aggregometric tests help to identify surgical patients at increased risk of bleeding or with resistance to anti-platelet therapy and, therefore, at increased risk of thromboembolism. Moreover, these tests may help to analyze the extent of platelet dysfunction in critically ill patients [37]. However, the clinical outcome benefits of including these tests in hemotherapy algorithms have not yet been investigated.

If platelet function has been shown to be deficient, administration of desamino-D-arginine vasopressin (DDAVP) represents a therapeutic option. DDAVP (0.3 μg/kg) has been shown to induce a three-fold increase in von-Willebrand factor and factor VIII [38]. These factors promote an increase in platelet-endothelial cell adhesion via the GPIb receptor and platelet-platelet aggregation via the GPIIb/IIIa receptor. Hemostatic potential can further be improved by transfusion of platelet concentrates; one unit of platelet concentrate increases the platelet count by approximately 30,000/μl. However, there are inherent risks associated with the transfusion of platelet concentrates, in particular risk of bacterial and/or viral infections. Additionally, the number and functionality of platelets in platelet concentrates decreases with storage time [39].

Ultima Ratio

If coagulopathy persists and surgical causes for bleeding have been ruled out, off-label use of two additional coagulation factor concentrates, factor XIII and activated factor VII, may represent an 'ultima ratio' therapeutic approach. Factor XIII enhances blood clot stability by cross-linking fibrin monomers and integrating alpha 2-antiplasmin into developing clots. There is no routinely available test parameter that can indicate factor XIII deficiency. In addition, there are currently no standardized reference values. However, especially in diffuse bleeding, factor XIII substitution (15–30 IU/kg) may be indicated to achieve a factor XIII activity above 60–70 % [40].

Administration of recombinant factor VIIa (90 µg/kg) induces a so-called 'thrombin burst'. As the final stage of the therapy algorithm, this approach may potentially reverse life-threatening coagulopathy. However, several conditions, such as plasma pH ≥ 7.2, fibrinogen concentration > 150 mg/dl, platelet count > 50,000/µl, hematocrit ≥ 25 %, ionized calcium concentration > 1 mmol/l and body temperature > 36 °C, should be met before factor VIIa is administered. Moreover, as highlighted in a recent systematic review, the effectiveness of recombinant factor VIIa in reducing the transfusion rate of allogeneic blood products or perioperative blood loss remains controversial [41].

Conclusion

In the absence of prospective, randomized trials, adequate data are not yet available regarding the use of POC techniques in critically ill patients in the ICU. Nevertheless, POC coagulation testing is faster and more comprehensive than conventional laboratory tests of blood coagulation, and enables effective and economical hemotherapy. None of the POC techniques covers the whole spectrum of hemostasis, thus the combination of aggregometric and viscoelastic methods is recommended. Hemotherapy should be based on an escalating algorithm including POC diagnostics, which is adapted to the specific bleeding risks of the patient's condition (e.g., cardiovascular surgery, organ transplantation, and trauma surgery). In this respect, POC techniques should be an integral part of a patient blood management program [42]; beyond this, POC analysis may also enable diagnosis of sepsis-induced hemostatic alterations, and may even have the potential to predict mortality in septic patients. Finally, prospective studies are urgently needed to analyze whether hemostatic therapy based on POC testing can provide significant benefits with respect to clinical outcomes for our critical care patients.

References

1. Levi M, Opal SM (2006) Coagulation abnormalities in critically ill patients. Crit Care 10:222
2. Glance LG, Dick AW, Mukamel DB et al (2011) Association between intraoperative blood transfusion and mortality and morbidity in patients undergoing noncardiac surgery. Anesthesiology 114:283–292
3. Murphy GJ, Reeves BC, Rogers CA, Rizvi SI, Culliford L, Angelini GD (2007) Increased mortality, postoperative morbidity, and cost after red blood cell transfusion in patients having cardiac surgery. Circulation 116:2544–2552
4. Gorlinger K, Bergmann L, Dirkmann D (2012) Coagulation management in patients undergoing mechanical circulatory support. Best Pract Res Clin Anaesthesiol 26:179–198
5. Kozek-Langenecker S (2007) Management of massive operative blood loss. Minerva Anestesiol 73:401–415
6. Haas T, Spielmann N, Mauch J et al (2012) Comparison of thromboelastometry (ROTEM(R)) with standard plasmatic coagulation testing in paediatric surgery. Br J Anaesth 108:36–41
7. Toulon P, Ozier Y, Ankri A, Fleron MH, Leroux G, Samama CM (2009) Point-of-care versus central laboratory coagulation testing during haemorrhagic surgery. A multicenter study. Thromb Haemost 101:394–401
8. Jambor C, von Pape KW, Spannagl M, Dietrich W, Giebl A, Weisser H (2011) Multiple electrode whole blood aggregometry, PFA-100, and in vivo bleeding time for the point-of-care assessment of aspirin-induced platelet dysfunction in the preoperative setting. Anesth Analg 113:31–39
9. Hartert H (1951) Thrombelastography, a method for physical analysis of blood coagulation. Z Gesamte Exp Med 117:189–203
10. Avidan MS, Alcock EL, Da Fonseca J et al (2004) Comparison of structured use of routine laboratory tests or near-patient assessment with clinical judgement in the management of bleeding after cardiac surgery. Br J Anaesth 92:178–186
11. Ak K, Isbir CS, Tetik S et al (2009) Thromboelastography-based transfusion algorithm reduces blood product use after elective CABG: a prospective randomized study. J Card Surg 24:404–410
12. Westbrook AJ, Olsen J, Bailey M, Bates J, Scully M, Salamonsen RF (2009) Protocol based on thromboelastograph (TEG) out-performs physician preference using laboratory coagulation tests to guide blood replacement during and after cardiac surgery: a pilot study. Heart Lung Circ 18:277–288
13. Weber CF, Gorlinger K, Meininger D et al (2012) Point-of-care testing: A prospective, randomized clinical trial of efficacy in coagulopathic cardiac surgery patients. Anesthesiology 117:531–547
14. Nuttall GA, Oliver WC, Santrach PJ et al (2001) Efficacy of a simple intraoperative transfusion algorithm for nonerythrocyte component utilization after cardiopulmonary bypass. Anesthesiology 94:773–781
15. Gorlinger K, Dirkmann D, Hanke AA et al (2011) First-line therapy with coagulation factor concentrates combined with point-of-care coagulation testing is associated with decreased allogeneic blood transfusion in cardiovascular surgery: a retrospective, single-center cohort study. Anesthesiology 115:1179–1191
16. Wang SC, Shieh JF, Chang KY et al (2010) Thromboelastography-guided transfusion decreases intraoperative blood transfusion during orthotopic liver transplantation: randomized clinical trial. Transplant Proc 42:2590–2593
17. Gorlinger K (2006) Coagulation management during liver transplantation. Hamostaseologie 26:S64–S76

18. Gorlinger K, Fries D, Dirkmann D, Weber CF, Hanke AA, Schochl H (2012) Reduction of fresh frozen plasma requirements by perioperative point-of-care coagulation management with early calculated goal-directed therapy. Transfus Med Hemother 39:104–113
19. Stainsby D, MacLennan S, Thomas D, Isaac J, Hamilton PJ (2006) Guidelines on the management of massive blood loss. Br J Haematol 135:634–641
20. Sarani B, Dunkman WJ, Dean L, Sonnad S, Rohrbach JI, Gracias VH (2008) Transfusion of fresh frozen plasma in critically ill surgical patients is associated with an increased risk of infection. Crit Care Med 36:1114–1118
21. Watson GA, Sperry JL, Rosengart MR et al (2009) Fresh frozen plasma is independently associated with a higher risk of multiple organ failure and acute respiratory distress syndrome. J Trauma 67:221–227
22. Maegele M, Lefering R, Yucel N et al (2007) Early coagulopathy in multiple injury: an analysis from the German Trauma Registry on 8724 patients. Injury 38:298–304
23. Rourke C, Curry N, Khan S et al (2012) Fibrinogen levels during trauma hemorrhage, response to replacement therapy, and association with patient outcomes. J Thromb Haemost 10:1342–1351
24. Holcomb JB, Minei KM, Scerbo ML et al (2012) Admission rapid thrombelastography can replace conventional coagulation tests in the emergency department: experience with 1974 consecutive trauma patients. Ann Surg 256:476–486
25. Schochl H, Nienaber U, Hofer G et al (2010) Goal-directed coagulation management of major trauma patients using thromboelastometry (ROTEM)-guided administration of fibrinogen concentrate and prothrombin complex concentrate. Crit Care 14:R55
26. Afshari A, Wikkelso A, Brok J, Moller AM, Wetterslev J (2011) Thrombelastography (TEG) or thromboelastometry (ROTEM) to monitor haemotherapy versus usual care in patients with massive transfusion. Cochrane Database Syst Rev CD007871
27. Adamzik M, Eggmann M, Frey UH et al (2010) Comparison of thromboelastometry with procalcitonin, interleukin 6, and C-reactive protein as diagnostic tests for severe sepsis in critically ill adults. Crit Care 14:R178
28. Adamzik M, Langemeier T, Frey UH et al (2011) Comparison of thrombelastometry with simplified acute physiology score II and sequential organ failure assessment scores for the prediction of 30-day survival: a cohort study. Shock 35:339–342
29. Spalding GJ, Hartrumpf M, Sierig T, Oesberg N, Kirschke CG, Albes JM (2007) Cost reduction of perioperative coagulation management in cardiac surgery: value of "bedside" thrombelastography (ROTEM). Eur J Cardiothorac Surg 31:1052–1057
30. Crowther MA, Warkentin TE (2008) Bleeding risk and the management of bleeding complications in patients undergoing anticoagulant therapy: focus on new anticoagulant agents. Blood 111:4871–4879
31. Hiippala ST, Myllyla GJ, Vahtera EM (1995) Hemostatic factors and replacement of major blood loss with plasma-poor red cell concentrates. Anesth Analg 81:360–365
32. Bolliger D, Gorlinger K, Tanaka KA (2010) Pathophysiology and treatment of coagulopathy in massive hemorrhage and hemodilution. Anesthesiology 113:1205–1219
33. Warmuth M, Mad P, Wild C (2012) Systematic review of the efficacy and safety of fibrinogen concentrate substitution in adults. Acta Anaesthesiol Scand 56:539–548
34. Dickneite G, Pragst I (2009) Prothrombin complex concentrate vs fresh frozen plasma for reversal of dilutional coagulopathy in a porcine trauma model. Br J Anaesth 102:345–354
35. Scharbert G, Kalb M, Marschalek C, Kozek-Langenecker SA (2006) The effects of test temperature and storage temperature on platelet aggregation: a whole blood in vitro study. Anesth Analg 102:1280–1284
36. Rinder CS, Mathew JP, Rinder HM, Bonan J, Ault KA, Smith BR (1991) Modulation of platelet surface adhesion receptors during cardiopulmonary bypass. Anesthesiology 75:563–570
37. Picker SM (2011) vitro assessment of platelet function. Transfus Apher Sci 44:305–319
38. Lethagen S (1994) Desmopressin (DDAVP) and hemostasis. Ann Hematol 69:173–180

39. Cauwenberghs S, van Pampus E, Curvers J, Akkerman JW, Heemskerk JW (2007) Hemostatic and signaling functions of transfused platelets. Transfus Med Rev 21:287–294
40. Korte W (2010) F. XIII in perioperative coagulation management. Best Pract Res Clin Anaesthesiol 24:85–93
41. Yank V, Tuohy CV, Logan AC et al (2011) Systematic review: benefits and harms of in-hospital use of recombinant factor VIIa for off-label indications. Ann Intern Med 154:529–540
42. Shander A, Van Aken H, Colomina MJ et al (2012) Patient blood management in Europe. Br J Anaesth 109:55–68

Revisiting Lactate in Critical Illness

M. Nalos, A. S. McLean, and S. Huang

Introduction

The traditional view of lactate as a harmful waste product of anaerobic glycolysis needs to be challenged in the face of new evidence. It is important to differentiate between lactate as a biomarker on one hand and lactate as a metabolic substrate on the other. Here we will review metabolic, protective and potential therapeutic properties of this fascinating molecule.

Elevated plasma lactate levels are common in the critically ill due to increased lactate production and less frequently to reduced lactate clearance [1, 2]. Admission plasma lactate levels and the trend in lactate levels may both be used as a marker of illness severity and prognosis in the critically ill patient [3, 4]. Despite the correlation of lactate with the severity of critical illness, there is no proven causal relationship between elevated lactate *per se* and poor outcome. More accurately, elevated lactate levels serve as a sentinel marker of metabolic stress, which indeed is reflective of illness severity [5, 6]. The associated metabolic acidosis forms the basis of the traditional view of lactic acid as a wasteful byproduct of anaerobic metabolism due to cellular hypoxia. This led to lactate being considered a 'toxic' compound which was both a cause of tissue damage and a direct marker of tissue hypoxia. However, this 'surviving' dogma, based on the correlation between lactate levels and acidosis derived in 1920, has been challenged and largely

M. Nalos (✉)
Department of Intensive Care Medicine, Nepean Hospital & Nepean Medical School, University of Sydney, PO Box 63, Penrith, 2750 NSW, Australia
E-mail: mareknalos@gmail.com

A. S. McLean
Department of Intensive Care Medicine, Nepean Hospital & Nepean Medical School, University of Sydney, PO Box 63, Penrith, 2750 NSW, Australia

S. Huang
Department of Intensive Care Medicine, Nepean Hospital & Nepean Medical School, University of Sydney, PO Box 63, Penrith, 2750 NSW, Australia

J.-L. Vincent (Ed.), *Annual Update in Intensive Care and Emergency Medicine 2013*,
DOI 10.1007/978-3-642-35109-9_34, © Springer-Verlag Berlin Heidelberg 2013

disputed [7–9]. On the contrary, lactate assumes an important role as a metabolic regulator and an easily transferable metabolic substrate between lactate producing and lactate consuming tissues, thus linking tissue energy needs with efficient metabolism [10, 11]. We will first review the role of lactate production and metabolism during exercise, emphasize the importance of lactate for cardiac and cerebral metabolism and comment on lactate significance during ischemia. We will finish by reviewing the therapeutic use of lactate in the critically ill.

Lactate in Exercise

During physical exercise, muscle lactate production increases in proportion to exercise intensity as a result of sympathetic stimulation of muscle glycogenolysis and glycolysis in fast glycolytic muscle fibers [11]. However, lactate production during exercise is not limited to the working muscle, and the concomitant metabolic acidosis in muscle is not caused by lactate production itself. Rather an increased reliance on glycolytic, non-mitochondrial ATP turnover leads to an increased NADH/NAD^+ ratio and a switch from oxidation of pyruvate to reduction of lactate. The main, but not only, cause of non-mitochondrial ATP formation during exercise is reduced oxygen tension in the myocyte. The need for NADH reoxidation in the cytoplasm means that the formation of lactate via lactate dehydrogenase (LDH) is essential for ongoing energy production [9]. Interestingly, the activity of LDH is highest in muscle fibers that have the lowest volume density of mitochondria and the lowest number of capillaries per fiber area [12]. In exercising humans, muscle lactate concentrations may reach 10–30 mmol/l [13, 14]. Because lactic acid is a relatively strong acid with a pKa-value of 3.86, at cellular pH it is almost fully dissociated into a lactate anion and a proton, both of which have marked effects on myocyte function and both have been linked to exercise-induced fatigue. However, lactate *per se* has minimal effects on the muscle contractile apparatus and lactate *in vivo* in fact delays metabolic acidosis while contributing to ATP synthesis via oxidation [9, 11, 15]. To counter proton acidity, myocytes possess transport and buffer systems, the most efficient being bicarbonate, which is an open system allowing proton removal via the circulation and respiration. Formation of lactate also enables the proton to be efficiently removed as a result of: (1) free diffusion of the undissociated acid; (2) exchange of the lactate anion for another anion (e.g., Cl^- or HCO_3^-) on the band 3 protein; and (3) H^+-monocarboxylate symport proteins [9]. The major pathway for the transport of lactate across the sarcolemmal membrane is the monocarboxylate transporter 4 (MCT-4), which transports lactate and proton out of muscle cells [12]. Interestingly, it has been documented that the isoform MCT-1, together with LDH, has also been localized in the mitochondria thus suggesting direct oxidative lactate utilization by myocyte mitochondria [16]. It is, therefore, only when intracellular lactate cannot be removed by oxidation (low PO_2 or mitochondrial dysfunction), cannot be transported across the sarcolemma and cannot be taken up by adjacent muscle fibers for oxidation as well as glycogenesis that lactic acid accumulates in the muscle [11, 17]. Once lactate diffuses into the blood stream, it is distributed between plasma and circulating red blood cells (RBCs), which express MCT-1 and band 3 pathways and function as a lactate sink [18]. Lactate is then transported to heart, brain, liver, kidney, skin and muscle to serve as oxidative or gluconeogenic substrate [11, 19, 20]. The functional interplay of all the above mechanisms leads to improved muscle performance and delay in the occurrence of local metabolic acidosis [9]. Whereas immediate lactate clearance from muscles may be reduced during exhaustive exercise, clearance of exogenous lactate is not compromised during submaximal exercise. On the contrary, lactate is avidly taken up and metabolized via oxidation and gluconeogenesis, leading to preserved blood glucose levels, reduced concentrations of endogenous catecholamines and unchanged perception of fatigue [12, 19, 21]. In humans, approximately half of the produced lactate is oxidized at rest, whereas during exercise 60–80 % of lactate disposal is through oxidative pathways accounting for as much as 25 % of total carbohydrate oxidation [22, 23]. Although the majority of lactate produced is oxidized, it is still a major substrate for gluconeogenesis during exercise. At the same time, fatty acid oxidation is proportionally reduced by direct lactate-mediated (via GPR81 receptor) inhibition of lipolysis in adipocytes as well as reduction of beta oxidation of fatty acids via mass effect and redox control [11].

Exercise training has little effect on the amount of lactate produced during physical activity but it does affect the magnitude of lactate oxidation by changes in mitochondrial biogenesis and by increased expression of lactate transporters on cellular membranes allowing more effective shuttling of lactate [11, 18]. High lactate transport capacity allows trained individuals to achieve better performance and high MCT activities were found in elite athletes [12]. In contrast, humans with MCT deficiency suffer from exercise intolerance [24]. Mitochondrial biogenesis in myocytes is thought to involve lactate-induced production of mitochondrial reactive oxygen species (ROS) leading to induction of MCT-1 and peroxisome proliferator activated receptor γ coactivator-1α (PGC1α) mRNA and protein levels [11, 25]. Interestingly, lactate at high concentrations is able to directly scavenge oxygen atom radicals, thus potentially limiting exercise-induced increases in the production of ROS [26]. Further studies are needed to clarify the role of lactate and its concentrations on ROS production during exercise.

Heart Metabolism and Lactate

The main energy supply for the heart is the oxidation of fatty acids but this organ is a metabolic omnivore, able to metabolize glucose, lactate and amino acids in varying proportions. In a normal heart at rest, approximately 60–90 % of the ATP generated comes from beta-oxidation of fatty acids; 10–40 % comes from pyruvate formed by glycolysis and the conversion of lactate. Although fatty acids have higher yields of ATP per fatty acid molecule, it costs more oxygen in the process –

the ATP per O_2 yield is around 2.85. As a result, in terms of oxygen efficiency, this process is not as efficient as glucose or lactate for which the ATP per O_2 yield is 3.17 and 3.00, respectively. This translates to about 10% higher ATP per O_2 utilized.

Fatty acid metabolism not only results in lower ATP production efficiency, but cardiac mechanical performance is also lower at a given rate of oxygen consumption. For example, increasing the arterial supply of free fatty acids in dogs increased oxygen consumption without improving cardiac mechanical power [27]. This finding is partly explained by uncoupling of oxidative phosphorylation when less ATP is produced. Increased intracellular free fatty acids have been shown to activate uncoupling proteins allowing protons to leak into the mitochondia without generating ATP [28]. Paradoxically, an increase in mechanical efficiency of the left ventricle was observed when the beta-oxidation process was inhibited [29].

The proportion of lactate uptake by the myocardium and its use as a metabolic fuel increases during exercise, beta-adrenergic stimulation, elevated afterload, fast pacing and in experimental hemorrhagic shock [30–32]. Lactate may account for up to 60% of cardiac oxidative substrate utilization and could exceed glucose as a source of pyruvate in the presence of elevated plasma lactate levels [20, 33]. Lactate taken up by the human heart is rapidly oxidized by LDH to pyruvate, decarboxylated by pyruvate dehydrogenase and oxidized to CO_2 by the tricarboxylic acid (TCA) cycle. During exercise and in shock the blood acts as an important source of lactate which the heart utilizes as the predominant source of energy [32, 34]. Whereas the primary oxidative substrates during coronary ischemia are still fatty acids, the uptake of glucose is increased, thereby promoting the oxygen efficient glucose and lactate utilization pathways [35]. However, in rats with ischemia-induced chronic heart failure, maximum lactate influx into isolated cardiomyocytes was increased by 250% and the MCT-1 protein level was increased by 260% without concomitant upregulation of glucose transporters, suggesting increased utilization of lactate in heart failure [36]. Of clinical relevance, sodium lactate infusion has been reported to increase cardiac output in anesthetized pigs after surgery whereas whole body oxygen utilization tended to increase suggesting lactate oxidation [37].

Lactate Metabolism in Brain

The human brain at rest at normal plasma glucose and lactate levels is a net lactate producer [17, 38]. However, during increased demand on brain metabolism lactate is increasingly utilized as an energy substrate [17, 39–41]. Despite earlier concerns about lactate blood brain barrier permeability, lactate can pass through the barrier with an efficiency between 25–50% of that found with glucose, due to the presence of MCTs. When blood lactate levels are around 1 mmol/l, lactate contributes around 10% of the energy supply and at normoglycemia, lactate is preferred to glucose when lactate levels are raised to 4 mmol/l [42]. With progressive increases

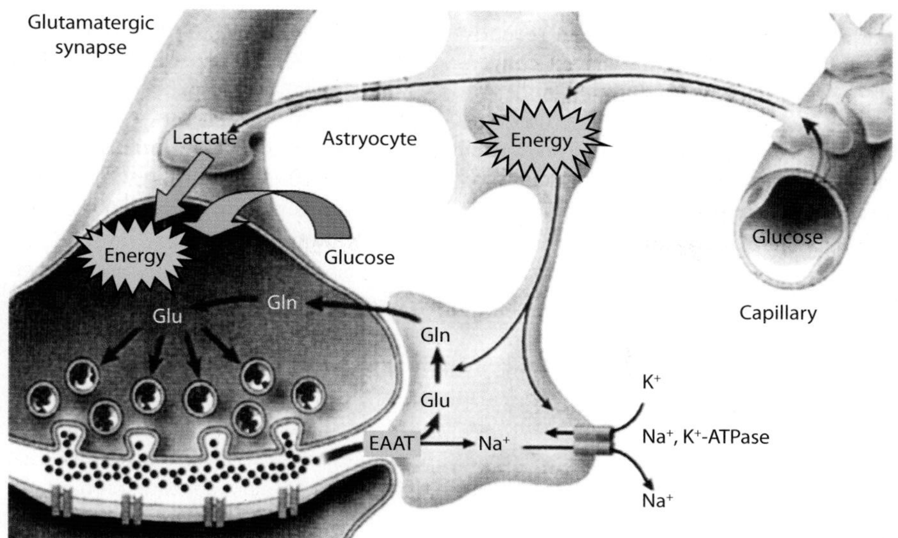

Fig. 1 Astrocyte neuronal lactate shuttle: Lactate derived from glial glycolysis or transported from blood supports neuronal energy needs as well as glutamine resynthesis and cellular sodium extrusion via Na/K-ATPase. From [45] with permission

in blood lactate, net brain lactate uptake and the contribution of lactate to cerebral oxidative substrate utilization (up to 60%) display linear increases [17, 20, 41]. During exercise, brain lactate uptake can reach a maximal rate of 1.3 mmol/min and lactate is almost completely oxidized [41]. Thus, lactate provides a quantitatively important alternative source of energy to the human brain. This is of clinical relevance during starvation, in diabetes and after traumatic brain injury (TBI) or cerebral ischemia [43, 44].

Further support for lactate being a part of normal human brain physiology comes from experimental evidence suggesting the existence of the so-called "astrocyte-neuron lactate shuttle". According to this concept, increased neuronal activity leads to release of the excitatory neurotransmitter glutamate, the uptake of which stimulates astrocyte Na^+-K^+ATPase, glucose uptake and glycolysis. The excess lactate produced in astrocytes is then transported via MCT-4 to adjacent neurons, taken up via MCT-2 present on neuronal cell membrane, converted to pyruvate and oxidized via the TCA cycle (Fig. 1), theoretically leading to production of 18 molecules of ATP [45, 46]. As astrocytes outnumber neurons by a factor of 20, they are able to support neuronal ATP requirements, in particular during hypoglycemia or ischemia [39, 40, 43, 46]. Blood-derived lactate is converted to pyruvate by LDH and may either be directly oxidized in neurons or converted to glycogen in astrocytes, respectively, depending on local intracellular energy needs [17, 45]. At times of increased energy demand from neurons or during neuronal ischemia, glycolysis and glycogenolysis is activated in astrocytes, lactate is formed and transported out of astrocytes.

In animal experiments, administration of exogenous lactate has been shown to reduce structural brain damage in middle cerebral artery stroke and brain trauma [43, 44]. Moreover, lactate ameliorated functional neuronal injury during global ischemia, stroke and TBI, an effect reproduced in severe brain injury patients [45, 47, 48]. The maximum protective effect in animals has been observed when the interstitial lactate concentration was between 4–7 mmol/l [43]. Although the nature of cerebral tissue protection is unclear, several mechanisms are likely to play a role. Exogenously infused lactate, in the form of sodium salt, may correct preexisting metabolic acidosis, increase cerebral blood flow in the ischemic penumbra, lead to reduction in cerebral edema and serve as an ATP-sparing oxidative metabolic substrate [43, 48].

Furthermore, emerging experimental evidence suggests that when lactate supplements pyruvate, potentially more intracellular glucose may be available for diversion out of the glycolytic pathway via a pentose phosphate shunt (PPS). This process may in turn lead to increased substrate availability for the synthesis of protein and lipid molecules, but importantly also to enhanced production of reduced glutathione, the most important cellular oxygen radical scavenger [43, 49]. This indirect antioxidant effect has the potential to reduce oxygen radical induced neuronal injury. Increased flux through the PPS has been demonstrated in experimental brain injury and in patients with severe TBI, especially during the first 48 hours post injury [50, 51].

Lactate and Ischemia

Although elevated lactate levels are associated with anaerobic metabolism, the assumption that elevated lactate represents tissue hypoxia is inaccurate and caution needs to be exercised when treatment decisions are based solely on this paradigm. More accurately, elevated lactate is a marker of 'metabolic crisis', in which, for various reasons, there was a reduction in mitochondrial oxidative metabolism [8, 52]. Although the reduction in mitochondrial metabolism can be due to low oxygen tensions, this is only one cause and not necessarily the most common. Mitochondrial dysfunction, autophagy and a reduction in mitochondrial numbers are common in critical illness [53, 54]. Mitochondrial autophagy is a cellular process whereby dysfunctional mitochondria are removed thus preventing an increase in ROS formed relative to ATP production. Autophagy is increased in critical illness and may serve to preserve cell viability and protect against uncontrolled proliferation (cellular dysplasia) at the expense of cellular function.

Furthermore, rapidly proliferating cells, such as leukocytes and cells participating in wound tissue repair, preferably upregulate glycolysis and glutaminolysis without concomitant increase in mitochondrial activity even in the presence of adequate oxygen tension. The rationale for such apparently wasteful behavior is not energy demands but rather increased flux through the PPS to satisfy needs for

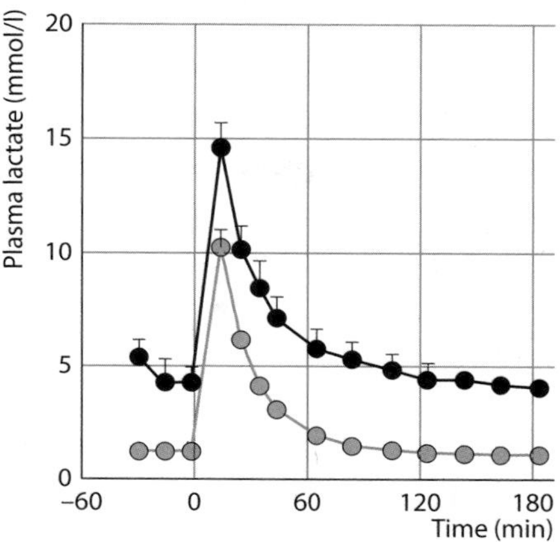

Fig. 2 Evolution of plasma lactate concentration over 3 hours from baseline level (time 0) after 2.5 mmol/kg sodium lactate infused in 15 min in either healthy subjects (*open circles*) or cardiogenic shock patients (*filled circles*). From [2] with permission

synthesis of new macro-molecules, such as nucleic acids, lipid mediators, and biomembranes, with additional benefit from increased production of glutathione. In fact, the high rates of aerobic glycolysis and glutaminolysis are in excess of the actual need for precursor provision in order to maintain high sensitivity to specific regulators of biosynthetic pathways involved in cellular proliferation [55, 56]. Thus, lactate production by rapidly dividing immune cells may not be negligible [57]. In agreement with this concept, preliminary data obtained from whole blood mRNA analysis in septic patients suggest significantly increased gene expression of enzymes and membrane transporters associated with glycolytic and lactate metabolism, namely glucose transporter (GLUT)-1, hexokinase-3, pyruvate kinase (PKM)-2, subunit A of LDH and MCT-4 (unpublished data).

In addition, clinically relevant lactate production in the presence of an ample oxygen supply is clearly documented during beta-2 adrenergic stimulation (salbutamol, epinephrine) and enhanced Na/K-ATPase activity [58]. Critical illness and stress are associated with elevated endogenous catecholamine levels adding yet another source of aerobically produced lactate.

It is commonly perceived that lactate clearance is significantly impaired in shocked patients as was demonstrated in stable septic patients [1]. Many suspect liver ischemia as the culprit although other tissues participate in lactate clearance, such as kidney via gluconeogenesis or heart, brain, muscle and skin via oxidation [10, 32, 59]. Indeed, whole body lactate clearance is not compromised after major hepatectomy [60]. When exogenous sodium lactate is infused in severe cardiogenic shock, lactate clearance is not significantly altered compared to healthy volunteers (Fig. 2). In this elegant study, Chiolero et al. demonstrated that about 60 % of exogenous lactate was metabolized via oxidation whereas most of the remaining lactate increased glucose production via gluconeogenesis [2]. Our preliminary data in critically ill patients with acute heart failure also suggest normal lactate clearance during infusion of sodium lactate (unpublished data).

Exogenous Lactate as Therapy

Evidence as outlined above provides a rationale for administration of lactate with therapeutic intent in several conditions associated with critical illness. Sodium lactate solution has been infused to a variety of healthy volunteers as well as critically ill patients. Half-molar (0.5 M) sodium lactate was well tolerated in patients post major surgery, improved cardiac performance in patients after cardiac bypass surgery and was associated with improved hemodynamics in patients suffering from cardiogenic shock [2, 61, 62]. When infused to treat raised intracranial pressure (ICP) in TBI patients, 0.5 M sodium lactate solution was associated with a sustained reduction of ICP and significantly improved neurological outcome at six months when compared to standard treatment with 20 % mannitol [48]. Although the number of patients in that study was small, results of a larger multicenter trial in TBI patients are keenly awaited. The solution of 0.5 M sodium lactate has also been used as an effective resuscitation fluid in patients suffering from Dengue hemorrhagic shock, a condition characterized by severe endothelial dysfunction (Dadang Hudaya S et al. unpublished data). We have infused 0.5 M sodium lactate solution in critically ill patients with acute non-septic heart failure and preliminary results indicate that it is well tolerated despite a tendency for metabolic alkalosis due to concomitant loop diuretic use while cardiac output increased in some patients.

Conclusion

In summary, the association of serum lactate levels with stress, ischemia and prognosis is well recognized but assuming that raised lactate solely represents tissue hypoxia and by extension is harmful in itself, is misleading. An understanding of the role of lactate in cellular energy production is essential to unraveling the place of this intriguing, potentially therapeutically useful molecule in the management of the critically ill patient.

Acknowledgement We dedicate this chapter to the memory of our friend Professor Xavier M Leverve.

References

1. Levraut J, Ciebiera JP, Chave S et al (1998) Mild hyperlactatemia in stable septic patients is due to impaired lactate clearance rather than overproduction. Am J Respir Crit Care Med 156:1–6
2. Chioléro RL, Revelly JP, Leverve X et al (2000) Effects of cardiogenic shock on lactate and glucose metabolism after heart surgery. Crit Care Med 28:3784–3791
3. Bakker J, Coffernils M, Leon M, Gris P, Vincent JL (1991) Blood lactate levels are superior to oxygen-derived variables in predicting outcome in human septic shock. Chest 99:956–962

4. Nichol AD, Egi M, Pettila V et al (2010) Relative hyperlactatemia and hospital mortality in critically ill patients: a retrospective multi-centre study. Crit Care 14:R25
5. Vespa P, Bergneider M, Hattori N et al (2005) Metabolic crisis without brain ischemia is common after traumatic brain injury: a combined microdialysis and positron emission tomography study. J Cereb Blood Flow Metab 25:763–774
6. Leverve XM (2005) Lactate in the intensive care unit: pyromaniac, sentinel or fireman? Crit Care 9:622–623
7. Hill AV, Long CNH, Lupton H (1924) Muscular exercise, lactic acid, and the supply and utilization of oxygen. Proc R Soc Lond B Biol Sci 16:84–137
8. Philp A, Macdonald AL, Watt PW (2005) Lactate – a signal coordinating cell and systemic function. J Exp Biol 208:4561–4575
9. Robergs RA, Ghiasvand F, Parker D (2004) Biochemistry of exercise-induced metabolic acidosis. Am J Physiol Regul Integr Comp Physiol 287:R502–R516
10. Leverve X, Mustafa I, Péronnet F (1998) Pivotal role of lactate in aerobic metabolism. In: Vincent JL (ed) Yearbook of Intensive Care and Emergency Medicine. Springer-Verlag, Heidelberg, pp 588–596
11. Brooks GA (2009) Cell-cell and intracellular lactate shuttles. J Physiol 587:5591–5600
12. Pösö AR (2002) Monocarboxylate transporters and lactate metabolism in equine athletes: A review. Acta Vet Scand 43:63–74
13. Bangsbo J, Gollnick PD, Graham TE et al (1990) Anaerobic energy production and O2 deficit-debt relationship during exhaustive exercise in humans. J Physiol 422:539–559
14. Brooks GA (1986) Lactate production under fully aerobic conditions: the lactate shuttle during rest and exercise. Fed Proc 45:2924–2929
15. Dutka TA, Lamb GD (2000) Effect of lactate on depolarization-induced Ca^{2+} release in mechanically skinned skeletal muscle fibres. Am J Physiol Cell Physiol 278:C517–C525
16. Brooks GA, Brown MA, Butz CE, Sicurello JP, Dubouchaud H (1999) Cardiac and skeletal muscle mitochondria have a monocarboxylate transporter MCT1. J Appl Physiol 87:1713–1718
17. Van Hall G, Stroemstad M, Rasmussen P et al (2009) Blood lactate is an important energy source for the human brain. J Cereb Blood Flow Metab 29:1121–1129
18. Connes P, Bouix D, Py G et al (2004) Does exercise-induced hypoxemia modify lactate influx into erythrocytes and hemorheological parameters in athletes? J Appl Physiol 97:1053–1058
19. Miller BF, Fattor JA, Jacobs KA et al (2002) Lactate and glucose interactions during rest and exercise in men: effect of exogenous lactate infusion. J Physiol 544:963–975
20. Ide K, Schmalbruch IR, Quistorf B, Horn A, Secher N (2000) Lactate, glucose and O2 uptake in human brain during recovery from maximal exercise. J Physiol 522:159–164
21. Fattor JA, Miller BF, Jacobs KA, Brooks GA (2005) Catecholamine response is attenuated during moderate-intensity exercise in response to the “lactate clamp”. Am J Physiol Endocrinol Metab 288:E143–E147
22. Roef MJ, de Meer K, Kalhan SC, Straver H, Berger R, Reijngoud DJ (2003) Gluconeogenesis in humans with induced hyperlactatemia during low-intensity exercise. Am J Physiol Endocrinol Metab 284:E1162–E1171
23. Miller BF, Fattor JA, Jacobs KA et al (2002) Metabolic and cardiorespiratory responses to “the lactate clamp”. Am J Physiol Endocrinol Metab 283:E889–E898
24. Fishbein WN (1986) Lactate transporter defect: a new disease of muscle. Science 234:1254–1256
25. Hashimoto T, Hussien R, Oommen S, Gohil K, Brooks GA (2007) Lactate sensitive transcription factor network in L6 myocytes: activation of MCT1 expression and mitochondrial biogenesis. FASEB J 21:2602–2612
26. Groussard C, Morel I, Chevanne M, Monnier M, Cillard J, Delamarche A (2000) Free radical scavenging and antioxidant effects of lactate ion: an in vitro study. J Appl Physiol 89:169–175
27. Mjos OD (1971) Effect of free fatty acids on myocardial function and oxygen consumption in intact dogs. J Clin Invest 50:1386–1389

28. Borst P, Loos JA, Christ EJ, Slater EC (1962) Uncoupling activity of long-chain fatty acids. Biochim Biophys Acta 62:509–518
29. Hutter JF, Schweickhardt C, Piper HM, Spieckermann PG (1984) Inhibition of fatty acid oxidation and decrease of oxygen consumption of working rat heart by 4-bromocrotonic acid. J Mol Cell Cardiol 16:105–108
30. Lopaschuk GD, Ussher JR, Folmes CD, Jaswal JS, Stanley WC (2010) Myocardial fatty acid metabolism in health and disease. Physiol Rev 90:207–258
31. Bergman BC, Tsvetkova T, Lowes B, Wolfel EE (2009) Myocardial glucose and lactate metabolism during rest and atrial pacing in humans. J Physiol 587:2087–2099
32. Kline JA, Thornton LR, Lopaschuk GD, Barbee RW, Watts JA (2000) Lactate improves cardiac efficiency after hemorrhagic shock. Shock 14:215–221
33. Stanley WC (1991) Myocardial lactate metabolism during exercise. Med Sci Sports Exerc 23:920–904
34. Gertz EW, Wisneski JA, Stanley WC, Neese RA (1988) Myocardial substrate utilization during exercise in humans. Dual carbon-labelled carbohydrate isotope experiments. J Clin Invest 82:2017–2025
35. Young LH, Renfu Y, Russell R et al (1997) Low-flow ischemia leads to translocation of canine heart GLUT-4 and GLUT-1 glucose transporters to the sarcolemma in vivo. Circulation 95:415–422
36. Johannsson E, Lunde PK, Heddle C et al (2001) Upregulation of the cardiac monocarboxylate transporter MCT1 in a rat model of congestive heart failure. Circulation 104:729–734
37. Barthelmes D, Jakob SM, Laitinen S, Rahikainen A, Ahonen H, Takala J (2010) Effect of site of lactate infusion on regional lactate exchange in pigs. Br J Anaesth 105:627–634
38. Boumezbeur F, Petersen KF, Cline GW et al (2010) The contribution of blood lactate to brain energy metabolism in humans measured by dynamic ^{13}C nuclear magnetic resonance spectroscopy. J Neurosci 30:13983–13991
39. Maran A, Cranston I, Lomas J, Macdonald I, Amiel SA (1994) Protection by lactate of cerebral function during hypoglycaemia. Lancet 343:16–20
40. Schurr A (2002) Lactate, glucose and energy metabolism in the ischemic brain. Int J Mol Med 10:131–136
41. Quistorff B, Secher NH, Van Lieshout JJ (2008) Lactate fuels the human brain during exercise. FASEB J 22:3443–3439
42. Smith D, Pernet A, Hallett WA, Bingham E, Marsden PK, Amiel SA (2003) Lactate: a preferred fuel for human brain metabolism in vivo. J Cereb Blood Flow Metab 23:658–664
43. Berthet C, Lei H, Thevenet J, Gruetter R, Magistretti PJ, Hirt L (2009) Neuroprotective role of lactate after cerebral ischemia. J Cereb Blood Flow Metab 29:1780–1789
44. Holloway R, Zhou Z, Harvey HB et al (2007) Effect of lactate therapy upon cognitive deficits after traumatic brain injury in the rat. Acta Neurochir (Wien) 149:919–927
45. Magistretti PJ (2006) Neuron-glia metabolic coupling and plasticity. J Exp Biol 209:2304–2311
46. Genc S, Kurnaz IA, Ozilgen M (2011) Astrocyte – neuron lactate shuttle may boost more ATP supply to the neuron under hypoxic conditions – in silico study supported by in vitro expression data. BMC Syst Biol 5:162
47. Rice AC, Zsoldos R, Chen T et al (2002) Lactate administration attenuates cognitive deficits following traumatic brain injury. Brain Res 928:156–159
48. Ichai C, Armando G, Orban JC et al (2009) Sodium lactate versus mannitol in the treatment of intracranial hypertensive episodes in severe traumatic brain-injured patients. Intensive Care Med 35:471–479
49. Herrero-Mendez A, Almeida A, Fernandez E, Maestre C, Moncada S, Bolanos JP (2009) The bioenergetic and antioxidant status of neurons is controlled by continuous degradation of key glycolytic enzyme by APC/C-Cdh1. Nat Cell Biol 11:747–752
50. Ben-Yoseph O, Camp DM, Robinson TE, Ross BD (1995) Dynamic measurements of cerebral pentose phosphate pathway activity in vivo using [1,6-$^{13}C_2$,6,6-$^{2}H_2$]glucose and microdialysis. J Neurochem 64:1336–1342

51. Dusick JR, Glenn TC, Paul Lee WN et al (2007) Increased pentose phosphate pathway flux after clinical traumatic brain injury: a [1,2-$^{13}C_2$]glucose labeling study in humans. J Cereb Blood Flow Metab 27:1593–1602
52. Zhou L, Stanley WC, Saidel GM, Yu X, Cabrera ME (2005) Regulation of lactate production at the onset of ischaemia is independent of mitochondrial NADH/NAD^+: insights from in silico studies. J Physiol 569:925–937
53. Watts JA, Kline JA, Thornton LR, Grattan RM, Brar SS (2004) Metabolic dysfunction and depletion of mitochondria in hearts of septic rats. J Mol Cell Cardiol 36:141–150
54. Watanabe E, Muenzer JT, Hawkins WG et al (2009) Sepsis induces extensive autophagic vacuolization in hepatocytes: a clinical and laboratory-based study. Lab Invest 89:549–561
55. Newsholme EA, Crabtree B, Ardawi MS (1985) The role of high rates of glycolysis and glutamine utilization in rapidly dividing cells. Biosci Rep 5:393–400
56. Ahmed N, Williams JF, Weidemann MJ (1993) Glycolytic, glutaminolytic and pentose-phosphate pathways in promyelocytic HL60 and DMSO-differentiated HL60 cells. Biochem Mol Biol Int 29:1055–1067
57. Bauer DE, Harris MH, Plas DR et al (2004) Cytokine stimulation of aerobic glycolysis in hematopoietic cells exceeds proliferative demand. FASEB J 18:1303–1305
58. Levy B, Desebbe O, Montemont C, Gibot S (2008) Increased aerobic glycolysis through beta-2 stimulation is a common mechanism involved in lactate formation during shock states. Shock 4:417–421
59. Joseph SE, Heaton N, Potter D, Pernet A, Umpleby MA, Amiel SA (2000) Renal glucose production compensates for the liver during the anhepatic phase of liver transplantation. Diabetes 49:450–456
60. Chioléro R, Tappy L, Gillet M et al (1999) Effect of major hepatectomy on glucose and lactate metabolism. Ann Surg 229:505–513
61. Mustafa I, Leverve XM (2002) Metabolic and hemodynamic effects of hypertonic solutions: sodium-lactate versus sodium chloride infusion in postoperative patients. Shock 18:306–310
62. Leverve XM, Boon C, Hakim T, Anwar M, Siregar E, Mustafa I (2008) Half-molar sodium-lactate solution has a beneficial effect in patients after coronary artery bypass grafting. Intensive Care Med 34:1796–1803

Part X

Transthoracic Monitoring

Diaphragmatic Ultrasound in Critically Ill Patients

M. Zambon, L. Cabrini, and A. Zangrillo

Introduction

The diaphragm is the most important inspiratory muscle. It is dome-shaped, with the crural portion inserted on the anterior portions of lumbar vertebrae 1 through 3, and the costal portion inserted on the xiphoid process and the upper, inner margins of the lower six ribs. The majority of the muscular portion of the diaphragm lies directly beside the lower rib cage, referred to as the zone of apposition (ZOA) (Fig. 1a).

Diaphragmatic contraction exerts two types of force on the rib cage: First, there is a force related to the shortening of the muscle fibers that are concentrated mainly in the ZOA, which displaces the dome caudally. As the diaphragm moves downwards, intra-abdominal pressure (IAP) increases, and the anterior abdominal wall is displaced ventrally. The net effect is an increase in trans-diaphragmatic pressure (Pdi), with a decrease in pleural pressure and lung expansion. Second, an increase in the tension of the diaphragm dome reduces the curvature, therefore expanding the lungs and the ribcage outwards [1].

Mechanical ventilation is a life-saving supportive therapy that is used essentially to improve gas exchange and support work of breathing. As a consequence, the demand on respiratory muscles is reduced to such an extent that they become inactive. It is now clear that mechanical ventilation itself contributes to atrophy

M. Zambon (✉)
Department of Anesthesia and Intensive Care, Vita-Salute University and San Raffaele Hospital, Via Olgettina 60, Milan, 20132, Italy
E-mail: zambon.massimo@hsr.it

L. Cabrini
Department of Anesthesia and Intensive Care, Vita-Salute University and San Raffaele Hospital, Via Olgettina 60, Milan, 20132, Italy

A. Zangrillo
Department of Anesthesia and Intensive Care, Vita-Salute University and San Raffaele Hospital, Via Olgettina 60, Milan, 20132, Italy

J.-L. Vincent (Ed.), *Annual Update in Intensive Care and Emergency Medicine 2013*,
DOI 10.1007/978-3-642-35109-9_35, © Springer-Verlag Berlin Heidelberg 2013

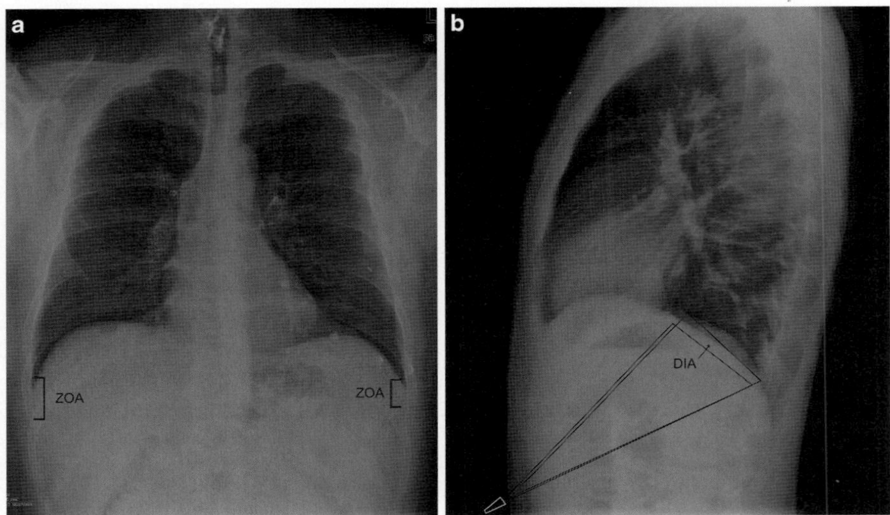

Fig. 1 **a** Anteroposterior chest X-ray showing the zone of apposition (ZOA). **b** Latero-lateral chest X-ray showing the sub-costal view. DIA: Diaphragmatic inspiratory amplitude

and injury of muscle fibers, which further leads to decreased force-generating capacity of the diaphragm, a condition termed ventilator-induced diaphragmatic dysfunction (VIDD) [2, 3]. Several animal models have shown that complete cessation of diaphragmatic activity with controlled mechanical ventilation results in atrophy and injury of diaphragmatic fibers. Muscle function alterations are time-dependent, becoming evident as early as 12 hours after initiation of mechanical ventilation and worsening as mechanical ventilation is prolonged [4–7].

Under mechanical ventilation, the reduced recruitment (and thus metabolic load) of the respiratory muscles promotes atrophy. Current data support a complex underlying pathophysiology involving oxidative stress and the activation of several intracellular proteolytic pathways involved in degradation of the contractile apparatus [8–11]. Furthermore, in critically ill patients, the reduced diaphragm perfusion elicited by mechanical ventilation facilitates effective redistribution of cardiac output to sustain perfusion of vital organs. The net result is a decrease in the ability of the diaphragm to augment blood flow to match oxygen demand in response to contractile activity. The imbalance in oxygen supply-demand will promote muscle fatigue [12].

Interestingly, recent animal studies showed a similar level of atrophy and weakness with assisted (pressure support) ventilation [13]. These data support the existence of mechanisms other than disuse for VIDD. Patients with impaired oxygenation are commonly treated with antibiotics, corticosteroids, sedatives and neuromuscular agents, all of which can weaken respiratory muscles (ICU neuromyopathy) [14, 15]. Furthermore, because the susceptibility to diaphragmatic fatigue *in vivo* is inversely related to maximal strength, diaphragm atrophy will also increase the risk of diaphragmatic fatigue once spontaneous breathing is resumed [16].

Methods to Evaluate Diaphragmatic Function

Measurement of Pdi is generally considered the 'gold standard' for establishing a diagnosis of diaphragmatic dysfunction. Pdi is calculated as the difference between esophageal (Pe) and gastric (Pga) pressures [17, 18]. However, this test is invasive and uncomfortable as it requires placement of esophageal and gastric probes. Moreover, it is insensitive in detecting unilateral diaphragmatic dysfunction; because of contraction of the functioning hemidiaphragm, Pdi may not significantly drop in this condition.

Chest radiography is reasonably sensitive in detecting unilateral diaphragmatic paralysis (sensitivity, 90 %), but its specificity is unacceptably low (44 %), and it is often not sensitive when bilateral diaphragmatic dysfunction is present [19]. Pulmonary function testing is another non-invasive means of assessing patients for diaphragmatic dysfunction. The accuracy and reproducibility of these tests are limited by their dependence on lung volumes, as well as patient effort and ability to cooperate. In addition, there is a wide degree of variability within the normal range and an age-related decrease in normal values [18].

The fluoroscopic evaluation of diaphragm dome motion is perhaps the most commonly used non-invasive diagnostic technique. Descent of the diaphragm is visualized via the sniff test, which consists of a short, sharp inspiratory effort through the nostrils at functional residual capacity (FRC). Reduced or paradoxical motion of the hemidiaphragm is indicative of diaphragmatic dysfunction. In the setting of bilateral diaphragmatic paralysis, apparently normal descent of the diaphragms may be seen during inspiration as a result of compensatory respiratory strategies, leading to a false-negative result. False-positive results are also possible [20, 21]. An additional drawback to fluoroscopy is that it necessitates significant radiation exposure.

Electromyography may also be used to diagnose diaphragmatic dysfunction. Recordings are made during spontaneous breathing or during electrical stimulation of the phrenic nerve. Technical issues include proper electrode placement, the possibility of electromyography 'cross-talk' from adjacent muscles, and variable muscle-to-electrode distances resulting from differences in subcutaneous fat between individuals. However, these tests are particularly helpful in differentiating between neuropathic and myopathic causes of known diaphragmatic dysfunction [22].

In the last few decades, ultrasound devices have been studied in critical care medicine in many settings, such as hemodynamic assessment, trauma, lung/pleural pathology or vascular access. Assessment of diaphragmatic anatomy and function using echography was first described in the 1980s [23–25]. In a seminal study, Wait et al. measured diaphragm thickness with ultrasound at necropsy, verifying the measures of the same segment by ruler. They found a good correlation between anatomic measurements and evaluation with ultrasound. The echographic study was then repeated in ten healthy volunteers, studying diaphragmatic function in terms of variations of diaphragm thickness [25]. Recently other authors have investigated diaphragmatic atrophy or dysfunction in critical care settings using ultrasound.

Ultrasound Technique to Study the Diaphragm

Two acoustic windows have been described for studying the diaphragm with ultrasound:

1. At the Zone of Apposition

To identify the diaphragm, the probe is placed between the 8th and 10th intercostal space in the midaxillary or anteroaxillary line. The ultrasound beam must be directed perpendicular to the rib cage (Fig. 1a). In this area, the inferior border of the costophrenic sinus can be identified as the zone of transition from the artifactual representation of normal lung (lung sliding) to the visualization of the liver (right side) or the spleen (left side). The ZOA is 0.5–2 cm below the costophrenic sinus. After the skin surface and the chest wall, two parallel echogenic layers are identified (Fig. 2): the most superficial line is the parietal pleura, the deeper line is the peritoneum just superficial to the liver or the spleen. These two membranes adhere to the diaphragm and, as a result, the less echogenic structure lying between these two lines is the muscle.

The diaphragm thickness is better measured in time motion mode, as the distance (in millimeters) between the outer edges of the echogenic lines at end-expiration (Fig. 3). In healthy, spontaneously breathing subjects the normal thickness of the diaphragm at the ZOA is 1.7 ± 0.2 mm when relaxing, increasing to

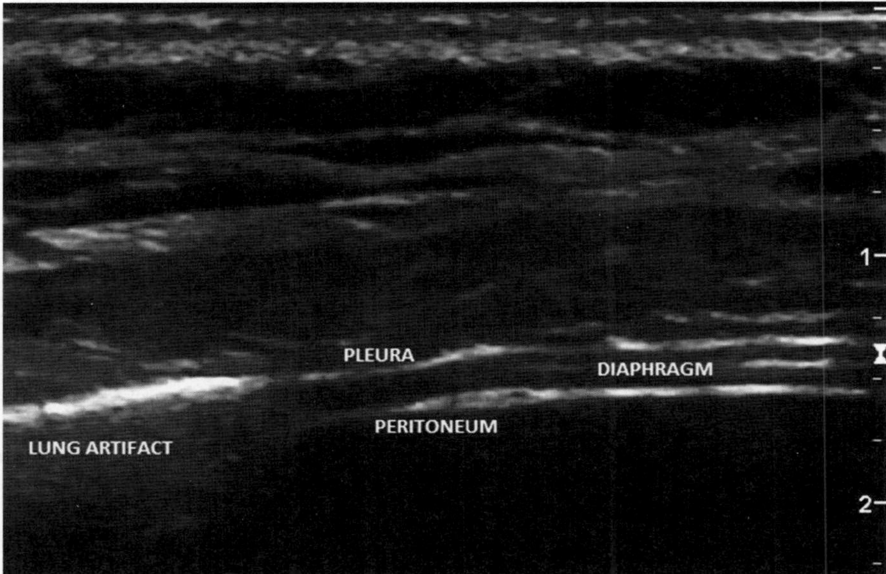

Fig. 2 2D ultrasound imaging of the diaphragm at the zone of apposition (ZOA)

4.5 ± 0.9 mm when breath holding at total lung capacity (TLC) [26]. The change in diaphragm thickness with respiratory movement can be expressed as a percentage called the thickening fraction:

$$\text{Thickening fraction} = \left(T_{EI} - T_{EE}\right) / T_{EE}$$

where T_{EE} is the thickening at end-expiration measured just before the thickening starts and T_{EI} is the thickening at end-inspiration or the maximal thickening [25].

In spontaneously breathing patients, a more precise and reproducible method to estimate thickening fraction is to obtain a deep breath, such as for spirometric tests. Hence, T_{EI} is the thickening at TLC, and T_{EE} is the thickening at FRC. The thickening fraction has a linear correlation with tidal volume in spontaneously breathing subjects [25, 27], whereas in mechanically ventilated patients the relationship is less reliable, being influenced by the level of ventilatory support.

2. Sub-Costal View, Using Liver and Spleen as Acoustic Windows

The probe is placed between the midclavicular and anterior axillary lines, in the subcostal area, and directed medially, cranially, and dorsally, so that the ultrasound

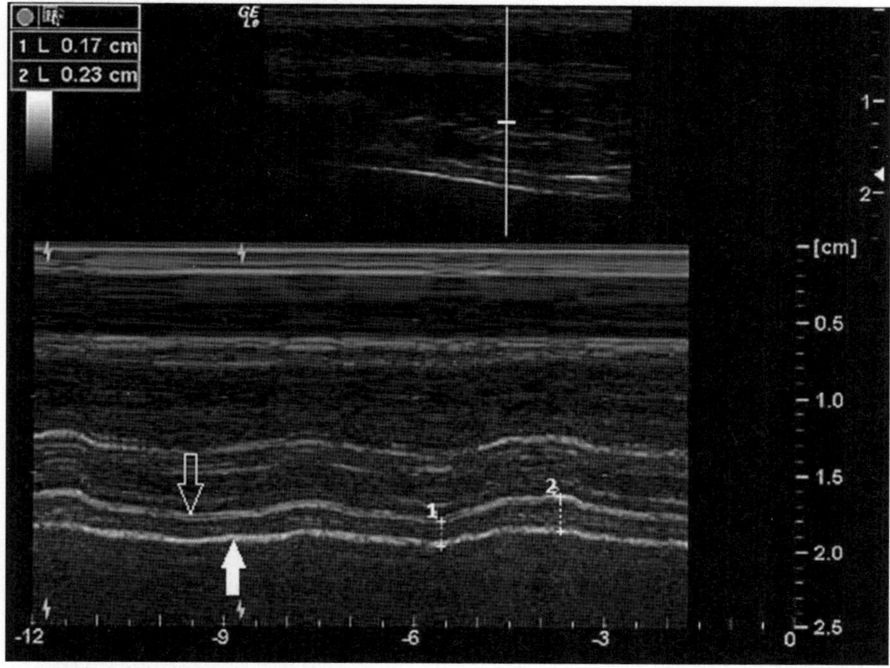

Fig. 3 Measurement of diaphragm thickness in M-mode, at ZOA in a healthy subject. Clear arrow: pleura; solid arrow: peritoneum; 1: thickness at end-expiration (T_{EE}); 2: thickness at end-inspiration (T_{EI})

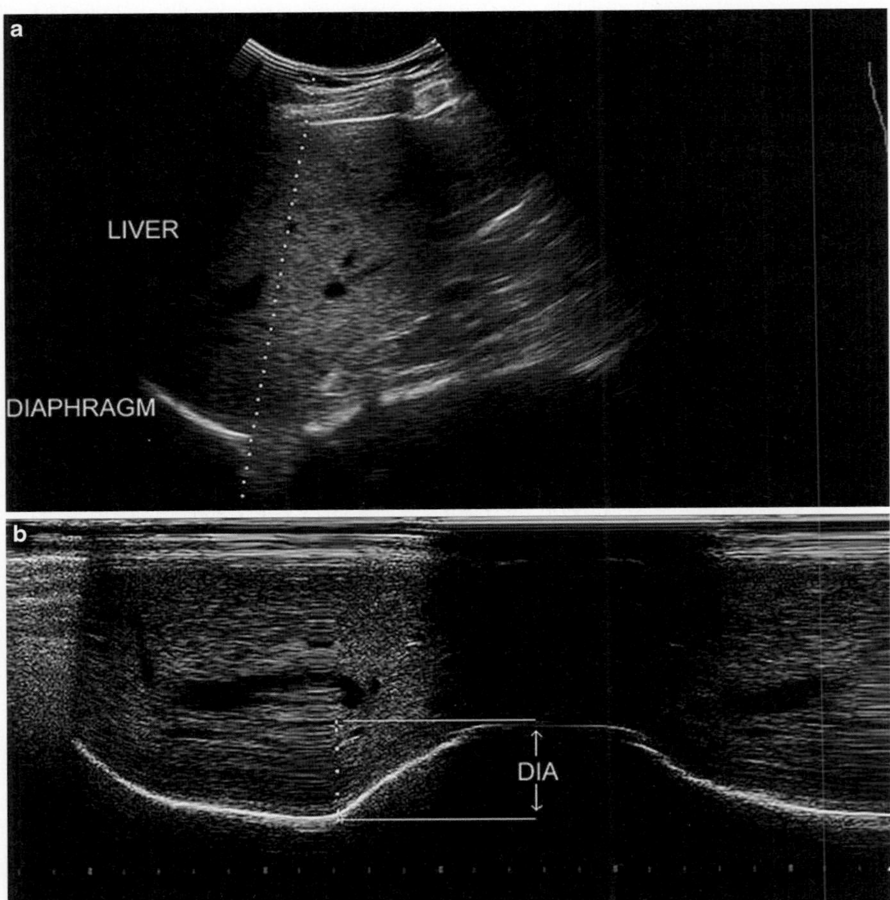

Fig. 4 **a** Sub-costal view of the right hemidiaphragm (see Fig. 1b). **b** M-mode showing diaphragmatic excursion. DIA: Diaphragmatic inspiratory amplitude

beam reaches the posterior third of the diaphragm perpendicularly (Fig. 1b). The inspiratory and expiratory cranio-caudal displacement of the diaphragm respectively shortens and lengthens the probe-diaphragm distance [28] (Fig. 4).

Diaphragmatic movement is usually better appreciated on the right side, because on the left side the descending lung, bowel and gas interposition during inspiration often hides the diaphragm. The diaphragm inspiratory amplitude (DIA) in healthy subjects during quiet spontaneous breathing was found to be 1.34 ± 0.18 cm [28, 29]. DIA was shown to have a linear correlation with inspired volume [30, 31]. A negative inspiratory amplitude (inspiratory peak below the baseline) indicates paradoxic diaphragm movement, a condition associated with severe diaphragmatic dysfunction and use of accessory muscles.

In our experience, the ZOA is the better acoustic window for appreciating diaphragm thickness, because the muscle is closer to the probe, whereas diaphragm excursion (i.e., DIA) is better appreciated with the sub-costal view. In fact, with the latter, M-mode ultrasound can record the cranio-caudal movement of the upper part of the muscle, which is greater than the lateral movement at the ZOA.

Various probes have been used to explore the diaphragm. In our experience a high frequency (7–15 MHz) linear array (such as a vascular probe) is the better choice to explore the ZOA and a 3.5–5 MHz phased array (echocardiographic) probe is better for evaluating diaphragmatic excursion. Higher frequencies provide better resolution and are ideal for imaging a superficial structure, such as the diaphragm, in the area of apposition to the rib cage, whereas lower frequencies travel further but, because of their longer wavelength, have less resolution and are a better choice for the sub-costal view.

We suggest that several breathing cycles be recorded and the widest measurement considered, to avoid possible under-estimation of the DIA or thickening fraction caused by intrinsic respiratory variability.

Clinical Applications of Diaphragmatic Ultrasound

Diaphragm Paralysis

Although uncommon, diaphragm paralysis is an under-diagnosed cause of respiratory failure. Trauma (surgical or nonsurgical) and malignancy involving the phrenic nerve are common causes of diaphragm paralysis [32]. Ultrasonography proved to be a sensitive and specific method for the diagnosis of diaphragm paralysis. A paralyzed diaphragm is atrophic and does not shorten; therefore, when explored with ultrasound at the ZOA, it is thin and shows minimal or absent thickening during inspiration. A thickening fraction of $<20\%$ with inspiration is diagnostic of diaphragm paralysis [33]. Furthermore, ultrasound has proved to be useful during follow up, assessing functional recovery in patients with unilateral or bilateral diaphragm paralysis. Recovery from diaphragm paralysis is defined as the return of normal diaphragmatic thickening during inspiration (thickening fraction $>20\%$) [34].

Post-operative Diaphragmatic Dysfunction: Cardiac Surgery

Post-operative diaphragmatic dysfunction or diaphragm paralysis may be responsible for a number of pulmonary complications, including atelectasis and pneumonia. It is a common alteration in cardiac surgery patients, who have a relatively high incidence of diaphragm paralysis because of some degree of phrenic nerve injury [35].

Early diagnosis (prior to extubation) is mandatory to avoid the risk of extubation failure. A normally positioned diaphragm on chest X-ray does not exclude diaphragmatic dysfunction, nor does an elevated diaphragm always confirm it. A relatively high incidence of motion abnormalities not detected by chest X-rays has been found using diaphragm ultrasound [36]. Ultrasonography has proved to be an effective tool for the early diagnosis of diaphragm paralysis in pediatric [37] and adult patients [38, 39].

Lerolle et al. tried to determine a quantitative ultrasonographic criterion based on diaphragm motion for the diagnosis of severe diaphragmatic dysfunction, using transdiaphragmatic pressure measurements as a reference method. They studied hemidiaphragmatic excursion in patients requiring prolonged mechanical ventilation after cardiac surgery with ultrasonography. Without using M-mode, this study measured diaphragm excursion on 2D echography using pleural effusions, very frequent in these patients, as acoustic windows. They found that a diaphragmatic excursion of <25 mm was associated with severe diaphragmatic dysfunction [40]. Their results obtained an excellent negative likelihood ratio; ultrasonography may thus be considered as an optimal test to exclude severe diaphragmatic dysfunction following cardiac surgery in daily practice.

Post-operative Diaphragmatic Dysfunction: Abdominal Surgery

The reduction in diaphragmatic performance is the main determinant of postoperative pulmonary complications after upper abdominal surgery. This reduction in diaphragm function may be responsible for atelectasis, reduced vital capacity, and hypoxemia in postoperative patients [41, 42]. Mechanisms other than the mechanical muscle wall injury are involved; in fact, diaphragm dysfunction is observed in both laparotomic and laparoscopic surgery [43, 44].

Using M-mode sonography techniques, Ayoub et al. [45] demonstrated that DIA was significantly decreased after laparoscopic or open cholecystectomy. Recently, similar results have been found in patients undergoing open liver lobectomy [46]. Using M-mode sonography, diaphragm excursion was linearly correlated with vital capacity, and appeared a good predictor of pulmonary dysfunction. On postoperative days (POD) 1 and 2, DIA during deep breathing and vital capacity had decreased by 60% from their preoperative values. By POD 7, DIA values during deep breathing had recovered significantly from the values on PODs 1 and 2 but still showed a significant degree of impairment compared with the preoperative values. The authors concluded that the M-mode sonographic technique could be a useful tool to investigate postoperative diaphragmatic dysfunction at the bedside.

Weaning from Mechanical Ventilation

In a recent prospective, observational study, Kim et al. evaluated diaphragmatic dysfunction in 88 patients in a medical intensive care unit (ICU) who were ventilated for more than 48 hours. M-mode ultrasonography was performed during a spontaneous breathing trial. Diaphragmatic dysfunction was diagnosed by a vertical excursion of < 10 mm or paradoxic movements (defined as negative excursions), and a rapid shallow breathing index was simultaneously calculated at the bedside. Diaphragmatic dysfunction was identified in 29 % of patients and there was a correlation with longer duration of mechanical ventilation and with weaning failure. In the diaphragmatic dysfunction group, the median diaphragmatic excursions were 3.0 mm for the right and 2.6 mm for the left diaphragm compared with 17.9 mm and 18.0 mm, respectively, in the non-diaphragmatic dysfunction group. The optimal cut-off values of diaphragmatic excursion for predicting primary weaning failure were 14 mm for the right diaphragm and 12 mm for the left diaphragm. Interestingly, the area under the receiver operating characteristics curve of ultrasonographic criteria to predict weaning failure was similar to that of the rapid shallow breathing index [47].

A considerable amount of research regarding weaning from mechanical ventilation with assisted modes and non-invasive ventilation (NIV) has been focused on the ability of these techniques to reduce the work of breathing. In a recent small observational study, Vivier and colleagues studied patients during NIV after extubation. These authors showed that the assessment of diaphragm thickening in its ZOA was feasible, accurate and reliable [48]. Furthermore, they assessed the usefulness of this approach as an index of respiratory workload. They measured the diaphragmatic pressure-time product per breath (PTPdi), which is the integration of the area under the Pdi curve (obtained by recording gastric and esophageal pressures with a double-balloon catheter) vs. time; this method allows direct measures of respiratory muscle effort in mechanically ventilated patients but its execution is complicated, confining its use to the research setting. Applying increased pressure support levels (spontaneous breathing, then 5, 10, 15 cm H_2O), Vivier et al. showed a parallel decrease in thickening fraction (measured with ultrasound at ZOA) and PTPdi, and reported that the two parameters were significantly correlated. Interestingly, thickening fraction did not correlate with tidal volumes: using different levels of pressure-support ventilation, the tidal volume was determined not only by the respiratory effort, but also by the pressure provided by the ventilator. These results, therefore, show that during NIV, thickening of the diaphragm reflects muscle effort and not the increase in pulmonary volume induced by ventilation.

Conclusion

Exploring diaphragmatic dysfunction with ultrasound is feasible, reliable and accurate at the bedside. Ultrasound provides structural and functional information about the muscle itself and can be repeated if follow-up is required. There is limited, although promising, evidence about the usefulness of diaphragmatic imaging by ultrasound in the critical care setting. Ultrasound is useful in diagnosing and quantifying VIDD as a cause of difficult weaning and may guide adjustments of ventilator settings. Further research is needed to define a possible role of diaphragm ultrasound as a guide in the complex process that leads to weaning from mechanical ventilation. Protocols that take into account diaphragmatic function may lead to improved outcomes, such as reduction of duration of mechanical ventilation.

References

1. Wade OL (1954) Movements of the thoracic cage and diaphragm in respiration. J Physiol 124:193–212
2. Tobin MJ, Laghi F, Jubran A (2010) Narrative review: ventilator-induced respiratory muscle weakness. Ann Intern Med 153:240–245
3. Vassilakopoulos T, Petrof BJ (2004) Ventilator-induced diaphragmatic dysfunction. Am J Respir Crit Care Med 169:336–341
4. Anzueto A, Tobin MJ, Moore G, Peters JI, Seidenfeld JJ, Coalson JJ (1987) Effect of prolonged mechanical ventilation on diaphragmatic function: a preliminary study of a baboon model. Am Rev Respir Dis 135:A201 (abst)
5. Sassoon CS, Caiozzo VJ, Manka A, Sieck GC (2002) Altered diaphragm contractile properties with controlled mechanical ventilation. J Appl Physiol 92:2585–2595
6. Yang L, Luo J, Bourdon J, Lin MC, Gottfried SB, Petrof BJ (2002) Controlled mechanical ventilation leads to remodeling of the rat diaphragm. Am J Respir Crit Care Med 166:1135–1140
7. Powers SK, Shanely RA, Coombes JS et al (2002) Mechanical ventilation results in progressive contractile dysfunction in the diaphragm. J Appl Physiol 92:1851–1858
8. Levine S, Nguyen T, Taylor N et al (2008) Rapid disuse atrophy of diaphragm fibers in mechanically ventilated humans. N Engl J Med 358:1327–1335
9. Hussain H, Mofarrahi M, Sigala I et al (2010) Mechanical Ventilation–induced diaphragm disuse in humans triggers autophagy. Am J Respir Crit Care Med 182:1377–1386
10. Levine S, Biswas C, Dierov J et al (2011) Increased proteolysis, myosin depletion, and atrophic AKT-FOXO signaling in human diaphragm disuse. Am J Respir Crit Care Med 183:483–490
11. Jaber S, Petrof BJ, Jung B et al (2011) Rapidly progressive diaphragmatic weakness and injury during mechanical ventilation in humans. Am J Respir Crit Care Med 183:364–371
12. Uchiyama A, Fujino Y, Hosotsubo K, Miyoshi E, Mashimo T, Nishimura M (2006) Regional blood flow in respiratory muscles during partial ventilatory assistance in rabbits. Anesth Analg 102:1201–1206
13. Hudson MB, Smuder AJ, Nelson WB, Bruells CS, Levine S, Powers SK (2012) Both high level pressure support ventilation and controlled mechanical ventilation induce diaphragm dysfunction and atrophy. Crit Care Med 40:1254–1260
14. McCool FD, Tzelepis GE (2012) Dysfunction of the diaphragm. N Engl J Med 366:932–942
15. Hermans G, Agten A, Testelmans D, Decramer M, Gayan-Ramirez G (2010) Increased duration of mechanical ventilation is associated with decreased diaphragmatic force: a prospective observational study. Crit Care 14:R127
16. Vassilakopoulos T, Zakynthinos S, Roussos C (1998) The tension–time index and the frequency/tidal volume ratio are the major pathophysiologic determinants of weaning failure and success. Am J Respir Crit Care Med 158:378–385
17. Polkey MI, Green M, Moxham J (1995) Measurement of respiratory muscle strength. Thorax 50:1131–1135
18. ATS/ERS (2002) Statement on respiratory muscle testing Am J Respir Crit Care Med 166:518–624

19. Chetta A, Rehman AK, Moxham J, Carr DH, Polkey MI (2005) Chest radiography cannot predict diaphragm function. Respir Med 99:39–44
20. Alexander C (1966) Diaphragm movements and the diagnosis of diaphragmatic paralysis. Clin Radiol 17:79–83
21. Laghi F, Tobin MJ (2003) Disorders of the respiratory muscles. Am J Respir Crit Care Med 168:10–48
22. Saadeh PB, Crisafulli CF, Sosner J, Wolf E (1993) Needle electromyography of the diaphragm: a new technique. Muscle Nerve 16:15–20
23. Harris RS, Giovannetti M, Kim BK (1983) Normal ventilatory movement of the right hemidiaphragm studied by ultrasonography and pneumotachography. Radiology 146:141–144
24. Diament MJ, Boechat M, Kangarloo H (1985) Real-time sector ultrasound in the evaluation of suspected abnormalities of diaphragmatic motion. J Clin Ultrasound 13:539–543
25. Wait JL, Nahormek PA, Yost WT, Rochester DF (1989) Diaphragmatic thickness-lung volume relationship in vivo. J Appl Physiol 67:1560–1568
26. Ueki J, De Bruin PF, Pride NB (1995) In vivo assessment of diaphragm contraction by ultrasound in normal subjects. Thorax 50:1157–1161
27. Cohn D, Benditt JO, Eveloff S, McCool FD (1997) Diaphragm thickening during inspiration. J Appl Physiol 83:291–296
28. Ayoub J, Cohendy R, Dauzat M et al (1997) Non-invasive quantification of diaphragm kinetics using M-mode sonography. Can J Anaesth 44:739–744
29. Boussuges A, Gole Y, Blanc P (2009) Diaphragmatic motion studied by m-mode ultrasonography: methods, reproducibility, and normal values. Chest 135:391–400
30. Houston JG, Angus RM, Cowan MD, McMillan NC, Thomson MC (1994) Ultrasound assessment of normal hemidiaphragmatic movement: relation to inspiratory volume. Thorax 49:500–503
31. Cohen E, Mier A, Heywood P, Murphy K, Boultbee J, Guz A (1994) Excursion-volume relation of the right hemidiaphragm measured by ultrasonography and respiratory airflow measurements. Thorax 49:885–889
32. Qureshi A (2009) Diaphragm paralysis. Semin Respir Crit Care Med 303:315–320
33. Gottesman E, Mc Cool FD (1997) Ultrasound evaluation of the paralyzed diaphragm. Am J Respir Crit Care Med 155:1570–1574
34. Summerhill EM, El-Sameed YA, Glidden TJ, McCool FD (2008) Monitoring recovery from diaphragm paralysis with ultrasound. Chest 133:737–743
35. Efthimiou J, Butler J, Woodham C, Benson MK, Westaby S (1991) Diaphragm paralysis following cardiac surgery: role of phrenic nerve cold injury. Ann Thorac Surg 52:1005–1008
36. DeVita MA, Robinson LR, Rehder J, Hattler B, Cohen C (1993) Incidence and natural history of phrenic neuropathy occurring during open heart surgery. Chest 103:850–856
37. Balaji S, Kunovsky P, Sullivan I (1990) Ultrasound in the diagnosis of diaphragmatic paralysis after operation for congenital heart disease. Br Heart J 64:20–22
38. Manabe T, Ohtsuka M, Usuda Y, Imoto K, Tobe M, Takanashi Y (2003) Ultrasonography and lung mechanics can diagnose diaphragmatic paralysis quickly. Asian Cardiovasc Thorac Ann 11:289–292
39. Fedullo AJ, Lerner RM, Gibson J, Shayne DS (1992) Sonographic measurement of diaphragmatic motion after coronary artery bypass surgery. Chest 102:1683–1686
40. Lerolle N, Guérot E, Dimassi S et al (2009) Ultrasonographic diagnostic criterion for severe diaphragmatic dysfunction after cardiac surgery. Chest 135:401–407
41. Ford GT, Whitelaw WA, Rosenal TW, Cruse PJ, Guenter CA (1983) Diaphragm function after upper abdominal surgery in humans. Am Rev Respir Dis 127:431–436
42. Chuter TAM, Weissman C, Matyews DM, Starker PM (1990) Diaphragmatic breathing maneuvers and movement of the diaphragm after cholecystectomy. Chest 97:1110–1114
43. Erice F, Fox GS, Salib YM, Romano E, Meakins JL, Magder SA (1993) Diaphragmatic function before and after laparoscopic cholecystectomy. Anesthesiology 79:966–975
44. Sharma RR, Axelsson H, Oberg A et al (1999) Diaphragmatic activity after laparoscopic cholecystectomy. Anesthesiology 91:406–413

45. Ayoub J, Cohendy R, Prioux J et al (2001) Diaphragm movement before and after cholecystectomy: a sonographic study. Anesth Analg 92:755–761
46. Kim SH, Na S, Choi JS, Na SH, Shin S, Koh SO (2010) An evaluation of diaphragmatic movement by M-mode sonography as a predictor of pulmonary dysfunction after upper abdominal surgery. Anesth Analg 110:1349–1354
47. Kim WY, Suh HJ, Hong SB, Koh Y, Lim CM (2011) Diaphragm dysfunction assessed by ultrasonography: influence on weaning from mechanical ventilation. Crit Care Med 39:2627–2630
48. Vivier E, Mekontso Dessap A, Dimassi S et al (2012) Diaphragm ultrasonography to estimate the work of breathing during non-invasive ventilation. Intensive Care Med 38:796–803

Two Steps Forward in Bedside Monitoring of Lung Mechanics: Transpulmonary Pressure and Lung Volume

G. A. Cortes and J. J. Marini

Introduction

For many decades, pressure-based respiratory mechanics have served to aid the judgment of clinicians when monitoring mechanical ventilation and making important decisions in respiratory care. However, measurements based on airway pressure (P_{AW}) alone have limited ability to generate individualized insights for a diverse patient population with varied pathologic conditions. While the passive lungs are the primary target of attention, P_{AW}-based interpretations may be influenced by differences in breathing pattern, alterations in chest wall activity (including diaphragmatic function), changes in lung volume, asymmetry of lung disease, abdominal distension, etc. All of these factors may complicate the interpretation of respiratory mechanics and make fixed criteria for safe ventilation difficult to apply.

Functional residual capacity (FRC) and calculated transpulmonary pressure (P_{TP}) are two components of the bedside monitoring array recently introduced into clinical practice. Used separately, and together, they complement and may improve interpretations stemming from parameters of lung mechanics based on P_{AW} alone. As a more physiologic approach, monitoring FRC and P_{TP} represents an opportunity to individualize the interpretation of lung mechanics and guide development of a ventilator strategy tailored to the specifics of a given patient.

In this update, we briefly address the management rationale and technical background for monitoring FRC and calculating P_{TP}, placing major emphasis on the potential clinical applicability of these two missing pieces in bedside monitoring.

G. A. Cortes
Department of Pulmonary and Critical Care, University of Minnesota, Regions Hospital, 640 Jackson Street St. Paul, MN 55101, USA

J. J. Marini (✉)
Department of Pulmonary and Critical Care, University of Minnesota, Regions Hospital, 640 Jackson Street St. Paul, MN 55101, USA (✉)
E-mail: John.J.Marini@HealthPartners.Com

J.-L. Vincent (Ed.), *Annual Update in Intensive Care and Emergency Medicine 2013*, DOI 10.1007/978-3-642-35109-9_36, © Springer-Verlag Berlin Heidelberg and BioMed Central Ltd. 2013

Esophageal Pressure and Calculated Transpulmonary Pressure

P_{TP} (alveolar pressure – esophageal pressure [Pes]) is a conceptual step closer to what is actually needed for monitoring when the object of interest is the lung itself. Pes has been used in the physiology laboratory to estimate pleural pressure for more than five decades [1, 2]. Balloon catheter systems have been shown to be both precise and practical in measuring local Pes [3]. The small quantity of gas within the balloon tends to concentrate where the pressure of the surrounding tissue is most negative. A series of holes in the catheter, arranged in a spiral pattern along a 10 cm length, transmits the most negative pressure surrounding the catheter in a given horizontal plane [4]. Using this system implies that important logistical aspects, such as positioning of the esophageal balloon catheter [5], amount of insufflated gas and compliance of the balloon, have been addressed so as to promote fidelity of the Pes measurements [1].

Baydur's technique for placing the esophageal balloon [5] has been tested and found to be generally valid in spontaneously breathing subjects in sitting, supine, and lateral positions. This maneuver is conducted by occluding the airways at end-expiration and measuring the ratio of changes in esophageal and airway pressure during spontaneous inspiratory efforts made during occlusion. With lung volume unchanging, the fluctuations of both esophageal and airway pressure should be theoretically equivalent [5]. In subjects who are not spontaneously breathing, however, other cues and feedbacks must be used to assure appropriate positioning of the catheter that senses esophageal pressure. The technique used by Talmor, Loring and colleagues in passively ventilated patients [6] involved advancing the catheter into the stomach as a first step. This initial location was verified by transiently increasing balloon pressure with abdominal compression. Subsequently, the catheter was withdrawn into the esophagus, using obvious cardiac oscillations and changes in P_{TP} during tidal ventilation to adjust the esophageal balloon catheter to the correct position [6]. This method may reduce the technical challenges accompanying placement in the clinical setting during passive mechanical ventilation without affecting catheter reliability.

Interpreting Pes Measurements: What Is Pes Really Measuring?

According to observations made by Agostoni et al. [7–9], tidal changes in Pes correlate with those of the pleural pressure applied to the surface of the lung, thereby enabling a valid estimation of P_{TP} based on the difference between estimated alveolar pressure and Pes [7–9]. However, the pressure vector generated by the weight of mediastinal content (mediastinal artifact) may increase Pes in the supine position [10]. Additionally, Pes represents the least positive *local* pressure along its own horizontal (gravitational) plane in the upright position [4]; even with position unchanged, absolute P_{TP} values elsewhere in the chest are theoretically different. For such reasons, the ability of Pes to track *global* average changes in pleural pressure may be limited when supine and in the presence of asymmetrical lung disease [11].

Absolute values of Pes are not only influenced by the 'mediastinal artifact' as a result of re-positioning from sitting to supine, but also by elevation of intra-abdominal pressure (IAP) and position-related lung volume changes. Recently, Owens et al. [12] concluded that Pes measurement artifacts imposed by mediastinal weight and postural effects are within a clinically acceptable range. These authors [12] compared the changes in end-expiratory Pes secondary to position changes in a cohort of overweight/obese spontaneously breathing patients with those occurring in lean subjects. Despite sitting and supine end-expiratory Pes values that were higher in the overweight/obese cohort than in the lean cohort, the observed changes in end-expiratory Pes as a result of re-positioning from sitting to supine were unexpectedly similar in both groups [12]. These results point toward a relatively constant increment in Pes attributable to 'mediastinal artifact' when supine, independent of the body mass index (BMI). Moreover, elevated IAP and reduced chest wall compliance appear to explain components of the higher end-expiratory Pes values encountered in both positions among overweight/obese subjects [12].

After all these considerations, it might be concluded that despite strong studies supporting Pes as a reliable surrogate for pleural pressure [1–3], esophageal balloon estimation of pleural pressure may be influenced by regional characteristics of the sampled horizontal plane when supine, and also by pulmonary and/or extra-pulmonary conditions, such as elevated IAP, obesity, and heterogeneity of lung disease [13, 14]. Whatever the shortcomings of esophageal manometry may be, the reported data support its reliability in sampling a local region surrounding the lung when supine – the potentially critical and clinically relevant dependent zone.

The Role of Transpulmonary Pressure in Acute Lung Injury

Acute lung injury (ALI) and the acute respiratory distress syndrome (ARDS) are challenging respiratory conditions that require careful tuning of mechanical ventilation settings to improve oxygenation without inflicting injury [15]. To achieve adequate physiologic goals and simultaneously prevent ventilator-induced lung injury (VILI), transpulmonary pressure monitoring has been proposed as a promising approach to guide ventilation strategy in ALI/ARDS settings [6]. Airway pressure-based plateau and positive end-expiratory pressure (PEEP) values are simply not enough.

An influential study already mentioned [6] evaluated the value of monitoring Pes and calculating P_{TP} in order to find a level of PEEP that could maintain oxygenation while theoretically preventing lung injury secondary to alveolar collapse or overdistension in patients with ALI/ARDS [6]. Patients in the "esophageal pressure-guided group" underwent mechanical ventilation with PEEP adjusted by

Pes measurements and P_{TP} calculations; the "control group" of patients was mechanically ventilated according to the ARDS Network (ARDSnet) recommendations [15]. PEEP levels were adjusted to achieve an end-expiratory P_{TP} within a positive range of 0–10 cm H_2O and tidal volume was limited to keep end-inspiratory $P_{TP} < 25$ cm H_2O – a threshold never encountered in any of the studied patients. At 72 hours, the patients in the "esophageal pressure-guided group" had a ratio of partial pressure of arterial oxygen to the fraction of inspired oxygen (PaO_2/FiO_2) which averaged 88 mm Hg higher than in the control group. Similarly, improvement in respiratory-system compliance was also observed in the "esophageal pressure-guided group". However, despite trends toward improved survival, this study does not provide uncontestable data supporting reduction in mortality associated with this mechanical ventilation strategy guided by P_{TP} estimations in patients with ALI/ARDS [6].

Other studies suggest Pes measurement as a physiologically defensible and reliable tool for estimating P_{TP} in critically ill patients [13, 14, 16]. As an example of such enthusiastic reports, Grasso et al. [16] evaluated whether keeping end-inspiratory P_{TP} within a theoretically innocuous range might allow safe increases of PEEP in pursuit of improved oxygenation. These authors found that relaxing the excessively prudent P_{AW}-based criteria for safe ventilation (justified by P_{TP} calculations) may avoid unnecessary use of extracorporeal membrane oxygenation (ECMO) in patients with ALI/ARDS from influenza A (H1N1) infection [16]. Although such data are encouraging, we believe that although clinically feasible, measuring P_{ES} and calculating P_{TP} as a strategy for setting the parameters of ventilator support must be embraced with caution, especially in the setting of lung injury, where the tension of the alveolar microenvironment may only be roughly represented by the P_{TP}. Additionally, increasing PEEP using P_{TP} monitoring might be consider 'safe' with regard to the mechanics of pulmonary injury, but may be simultaneously associated with hazardous consequences for hemodynamics [17].

The degree to which Pes is influenced by positioning, abdominal distension, spontaneously breathing efforts, and other conditions associated with reduced chest wall compliance in the setting of ALI/ARDS is still unclear and requires further clinical investigation. For example, estimates of P_{TP} based on Pes measurements are almost certain to imprecisely represent all stresses within an asymmetrically compromised lung [11]. The volume-altering effects of unilateral pleural effusion were radically different for the two lungs of experimental animals, and yet the calculated P_{TP} was little affected by fluid instillation [11]. In other words, we cannot expect a single local pressure to represent stresses everywhere across the topography of a heterogeneous thorax.

Nonetheless, P_{TP} monitoring deserves credit for shifting the attention of clinicians to a more individually-tailored physiologic understanding of the respiratory function changes that occur during ALI and, although not perfect, estimations of P_{TP} are of more help in elucidating the interactions between patient characteristics, disease conditions and ventilator settings than are pulmonary mechanics based on airway pressure alone [17] (Table 1).

Table 1 Potential added values of two newly available tools in bedside monitoring*

Transpulmonary pressure	Functional residual capacity
Non-invasively estimates lung-distending pressure	Non-invasively estimates 'functional' lung size, which refines compliance and resistance calculations
Samples 'local' (but potentially critical) dependent zones of the lungs	Helps monitor disease progression and resolution
Presents a new approach for setting 'effective' PEEP level in ALI/ARDS patients	Allows assessment of the impact of common interventions: PEEP and positioning
Offers the potential for monitoring 'true' driving pressures across the lung (tidal changes in P_{TP}), despite abnormalities of the chest wall and effort	Complements P_{TP} in the setting of non-symmetrical lung and chest wall diseases (e.g., atelectasis, effusion, etc.)
	Optimizes lung-protection strategy by determining the size of the 'baby lung', allowing for calculation of the 'strain ratio'

*see text for limitations. ALI: Acute lung injury; ARDS: Acute respiratory distress syndrome; P_{TP}: Transpulmonary pressure; PEEP: Positive end-expiratory pressure

Monitoring Functional Residual Capacity

Measuring absolute resting gas volume (FRC) is an essential component of the testing battery needed to interpret lung mechanics in the out-patient pulmonary function laboratory. However, the measurement of FRC in the ventilated patient has faced logistical and technical challenges [18]. In a dynamic process of evolution, attempts to monitor FRC that were based on body plethysmography and planimetry (X-ray quantification method) [19] have now migrated to more sophisticated ventilator-integrated systems. These newer methods allow bedside measurement of FRC without interrupting mechanical ventilation, making accurate FRC measurement feasible in the critically ill [20]. Conceptually, FRC provides information to the clinician that cannot be easily inferred from the P_{AW}, tidal flow, and volume data available to this point in time.

Technological Development of Serial FRC Testing

a. **Equilibration method**
   Gas-dilution methods for quantifying FRC were developed as early as 1800 using inspired hydrogen [21]. Closer to the present day, helium gas equilibration methods have been used for research in patients. Such techniques involve manual (bag) ventilation after disconnection of the endotracheal tube from the me-

chanical ventilator, so that a fixed volume and concentration of helium is uniformly distributed between the lungs and bag after approximately 10 breaths taken through a closed circuit. The proportion of helium remaining in the bag after the equilibration period provides a direct dilution estimate of FRC, which has been reported accurate when compared to other methods [22]. This method requires interruption of care to connect the tracer gas, thereby increasing the risk of lung de-recruitment and cannot be conducted in unstable patients. Moreover, accuracy depends on the timing and skill of the operator conducting the measurement.

b. **Wash-out methods**

When tracer gas is added to or washed from the lungs during ventilation with serial fixed tidal volumes, the rate of change to the new concentration relates inversely to FRC. With this rationale, a method for estimating FRC from the wash-in/wash-out rate of a 'tracking' gas was first described by Durig in 1903 [23] and then by Darling et al. in 1940 [24]. Variants of such methods have used changing concentrations of sulfur hexafluoride (SF6), oxygen (O_2) and/or nitrogen (N_2). In 1993, Fretschner et al. [25] measured FRC via integrated nitrogen wash-in/out in a test lung model and in ventilated patients exposed to FiO_2 changes of 0.3 – a method that involved intra-breath signal synchronization of flow and FiO_2. This innovation allowed for the determination of FRC values without ventilator disconnection, but incurred an error of approximately 20 % [25].

Recently, intricate and rapidly responding sensors have used sampling of respired gases from the ventilator circuitry to calculate FRC more safely and with relative accuracy without the need to interrupt ventilation. Gas-automated FRC measurement has been improved by using precise solenoid control and software synchronization of signals (flow and gas concentration) during ventilation. One example (Engstrom Carestation® technology, GE Healthcare Madison, WI) of this approach directly measures the end-expiratory lung volume by slightly altering the delivered FiO_2 level (step changes of only 0.1) for short periods of time using its volumetric O_2 and CO_2 measurement capability [26]. In a previous study we compared this method with ('gold standard') quantitative computer tomographic (CT) imaging and found that this automated method correlated well (across a wide range of end-expiratory lung volumes) [20].

c. **Technical limitations**

Some limitations, however, must be acknowledged regarding the measurement of FRC by gas washout in clinical practice. For example, rapid and/or irregular respiratory rates with large variations in tidal volume may alter FRC values and/or prevent gas-automated methods from performing the measurement [27]. Abnormal metabolic states because of high fever and/or agitation, as well as neurological conditions that alter respiration may also influence FRC measurements by varying CO_2 production and breathing patterns [27, 28].

Rationale for Monitoring FRC in the Critical Care Setting

FRC has been studied in ventilated patients for more than twenty years [29]. The effect of PEEP on FRC has been assessed and quantified by many investigators [30–32], whose work taken together has concluded that PEEP invariably increases FRC determined by gas dilution methods, according to the well known pressure-volume (P-V) relationship of the respiratory system [30–32]. In one study, this incremental effect of PEEP was observed with normal lungs, primary lung disease, and secondary lung disease for PEEP values up to 15 cm H_2O; FRC increased in proportion to the applied PEEP increments [30].

The FRC measured in response to PEEP admixes volumes resulting from recruitment of reopened units and expansion of the already patent ones. Such information, however, if used in conjunction with spirometric P-V information, may theoretically help elucidate actual consequences of PEEP application.

FRC measurements must be evaluated in conjunction with data regarding oxygenation as well as tidal compliance [33–36]. Although the latter relates inversely to the stiffness of the lung and/or chest wall, the tidal compliance traditionally used at the bedside does not necessarily track lung volume, as further increments of PEEP above a specific level may simply cause overdistension – indicated by accompanying increases of elastance [33]. Studies conducted in lung injury models have investigated the relationship between FRC and tidal compliance [33–35]. In a porcine oleic-acid-injury study, Rylander et al. [37] found that FRC was a more sensitive indicator of PEEP-induced aeration than was compliance. Additionally, Lambermont et al. [34] showed that FRC may potentially be useful in identifying an optimal PEEP level when it is associated with the best compliance and lowest dead space to tidal volume ratio [34]. There is still no irrefutable information regarding the range of values of FRC to be expected in the setting of ALI/ARDS. However, much of the available data strongly supports the potential use of FRC in therapeutic decision-making and its utility as a diagnostic tool. Perhaps relating FRC to its expected values is not as important as knowing the response of FRC to interventions or to the course of disease.

Clinical Implications of FRC Measurement

Important information can be extracted from the FRC value, because this measurement correlates with 'functional' (aerated and communicating) lung size [28]. Resting aerated lung volume is tightly correlated with oxygenation [36], estimated risk for VILI [15], work of breathing [38] and gas trapping [39]. As such, FRC could be used as an indicator of disease progression and response to therapy. Finally, FRC can also help monitor the relationship between body position changes and the physiological response of the compromised respiratory system [39]. Clinical experience shows that oxygenation is markedly affected by postural changes in certain patients. These hypoxemic episodes may be the result of position-related

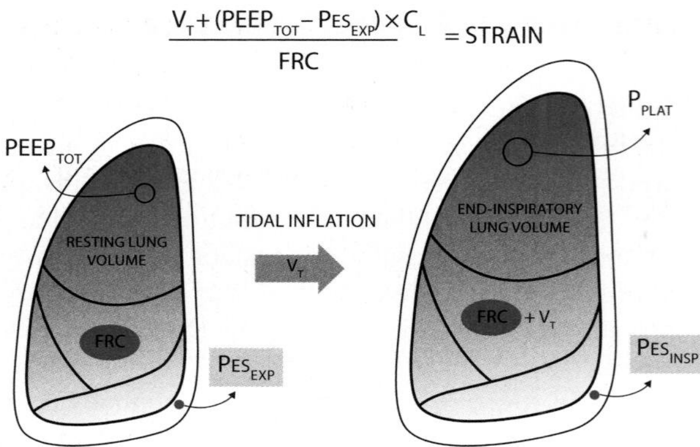

Fig. 1 Potential roles of transpulmonary pressure (P_{TP}) and functional residual capacity (FRC) in bedside monitoring of risk of ventilator-induced lung injury (VILI). Negative values of end-expiratory P_{TP} (total positive end-expiratory pressure [$PEEP_{TOT}$] – end-expiratory esophageal pressure [Pes_{EXP}]) suggest collapse in the region of the balloon. Tidal reversal to positive end-inspiratory P_{TP} values (plateau airway pressure [P_{PLAT}] – end-inspiratory esophageal pressure [Pes_{INSP}]) suggests potentially damaging tidal opening/collapse cycles. Resting lung volume (FRC) may be used in a 'strain' equation (see text and Table 1) in which end-inspiratory and end-expiratory absolute lung volumes are required, in addition to $PEEP_{TOT}$ and Pes_{EXP}. V_T: tidal volume, C_L: lung compliance

ventilation/perfusion changes associated with abrupt reductions in FRC or to regional perfusion changes [40, 41].

Regarding the role of FRC in interpretation of lung mechanics, changes in lung volume could help characterize the nature and severity of lung disease. Resistance and compliance are expressed in absolute terms (cm H_2O/l/s and ml/cm H_2O, respectively) that vary with aerated lung dimensions. Knowing the FRC value facilitates the separation of restrictive from obstructive disease and allows better interpretation of parenchymal gas exchanging efficiency [42]. Additionally, since 'specific compliance' and 'specific elastance' account for the resting size (volume) of the aerated lung, the response of the respiratory system to an imposed stress may be best evaluated when FRC is known [43]. By determining the size of the 'baby lung', FRC has the potential to elucidate the mechanical stress incurred during tidal breathing and the risk for VILI in the setting of ALI/ARDS [43, 44]. We must recognize that FRC values could lead to subject-specific interpretations of lung stress (P_{TP}), and may be integral for assessing lung strain (tidal volume/FRC) – commonly equated with tissue 'stretch' [44]. With current techniques, valid FRC measurements can be obtained to calculate a strain ratio. The latter references the end-tidal volume to its resting level, with strain ratios exceeding 1.5–2.0 signaling concern for lung overstretch [44] (Fig. 1).

Similar principles relate to airway resistance. Whether in obstructive disease, ALI/ARDS, or other volume-reduced states (e.g., surgical reduction of lung tissue, effusion-compressed lung), knowledge of FRC also enables calculation of specific resistance and provides better information regarding airway status [43, 44]. Additionally, non-symmetrical disorders of the chest wall (e.g., unilateral pleural effusion and increased IAP) may cause P_{TP} and FRC to dissociate from each other [11]. Such dissociation may also be characteristic of some other lung disorders (e.g., secretion plugging, unilateral pneumonia, atelectasis, embolism, pneumothorax, etc.). In other words, separations or disconnections among these monitored mechanic variables, especially if trended, graphed and/or indexed, could be valuable in diagnosis and monitoring.

Conclusion

Calculating P_{TP} based on Pes measurements and monitoring FRC are two complementary pieces of the diagnostic/monitoring puzzle to be added to traditional pulmonary mechanics stemming from P_{AW} and tidal air flow. Mechanical ventilation guided by P_{TP} calculations opens possibilities for personalizing and improving the analysis of the mechanics of pulmonary injury. It seems clear that these newly available tools, used separately and/or together, have potential to improve delivery of respiratory care by characterizing the response to interventions or to the course of disease. Moreover, recognizable patterns and trends in correlated indexes of FRC and P_{TP}, in addition to traditional monitoring tools, could help diagnose and/or provide an early warning to the clinician of impending danger in the settings of chest wall abnormalities (e.g., elevated IAP) and the asymmetrically distributed lung diseases often encountered in critical care. Instead of the first response being crisis intervention or expensive testing, earlier evaluation and prevention could be achieved by using and understanding FRC and P_{TP} values. Computer technology already deployed should make such derived information easy to display.

References

1. Milic-Emili J, Mead J, Turner JM, Glauser EM (1964) Improve technique for estimating pleural pressure from esophageal balloons. J Appl Physiol 19:207–211
2. Mead J, Gaensler EA (1959) Esophageal and pleural pressures in man, upright and supine. J Appl Physiol 14:81–83
3. Pelosi P, Goldner M, McKibben A et al (2001) Recruitment and derecruitment during acute respiratory failure: an experimental study. Am J Respir Crit Care Med 164:122–30
4. American Thoracic Society/European Respiratory Society (2002) ATS/ERS Statement on Respiratory Muscle Testing. Am J Respir Crit Care Med 166:518–624
5. Baydur A, Behrakis PK, Zin WA, Jaeger M, Milic-Emili J (1982) A simple method for assessing the validity of the esophageal balloon technique. Am Rev Respir Dis 126:788–791
6. Talmor D, Sarge T, Malhotra A et al (2008) Mechanical ventilation guided by esophageal pressure in acute lung injury. N Engl J Med 359:2095–2104
7. Agostoni E, Miserocchi G (1970) Vertical gradient of transpulmonary pressure with active and artificial lung expansion. J Appl Physiol 29:705–712
8. Agostoni E, D'Angelo E, Bonanni MV (1970) Topography of pleural surface pressure above resting volume in relaxed animals. J Appl Physiol 29:297–306

9. Agostoni E, D'Angelo E, Bonanni MV (1970) The effect of the abdomen on the vertical gradient of pleural surface pressure. Respir Physiol 8:332–346
10. Knowles JH, Hong SK, Rahn H (1959) Possible errors using esophageal balloon in determination of pressure-volume characteristics of the lung and thoracic cage. J Appl Physiol 14:525–530
11. Graf J, Formenti P, Santos A et al (2011) Pleural effusion complicates monitoring of respiratory mechanics. Crit Care Med 39:2294–2299
12. Owens RL, Campana LM, Hess L, Eckert DJ, Loring SH, Malhotra A (2012) Sitting and supine esophageal pressures in overweight and obese subjects. Obesity (Silver Spring) 20:2354–2360
13. Loring SH, O'Donnell CR, Behazin N et al (2010) Esophageal pressures in acute lung injury: do they represent artifact or useful information about transpulmonary pressure, chest wall mechanics, and lung stress? J Appl Physiol 108:515–522
14. Talmor DS, Fessler HE (2010) Are esophageal pressure measurements important in clinical decision-making in mechanically ventilated patients? Respir Care 55:162–172
15. The Acute Respiratory Distress Syndrome Network (2000) Ventilation with lower tidal volumes as compared with traditional tidal volumes for acute lung injury and the acute respiratory distress syndrome. N Engl J Med 342:1301–1308
16. Grasso S, Terragni P, Birocco A et al (2012) ECMO criteria for influenza A (H1N1)-associated ARDS: role of transpulmonary pressure. Intensive Care Med 38:395–403
17. Richard JC, Marini JJ (2012) Transpulmonary pressure as a surrogate of plateau pressure for lung protective strategy: not perfect but more physiologic. Intensive Care Med 38:339–341
18. Rimensberger PC, Bryan AC (1999) Measurement of functional residual capacity in the critically ill. Relevance for the assessment of respiratory mechanics during mechanical ventilation. Intensive Care Med 25:540–542
19. Pierson DJ (1990) Measuring and monitoring lung volumes outside the pulmonary function laboratory. Respir Care 35:660–668
20. Graf J, Santos A, Dries D, Adams AB, Marini JJ (2010) Agreement between functional residual capacity estimated via automated gas dilution versus via computed tomography in a pleural effusion model. Respir Care 55:1464–1468
21. Yernault JC, Pride N, Laszlo G (2000) How the measurement of residual volume developed after Davy (1800). Eur Respir J 16:561–564
22. Suter PM, Schlobohm RM (1974) Determination of functional residual capacity during mechanical ventilation. Anesthesiology 41:605–607
23. Durig A (1903) Über die Größe der Residualluft (About the size of the residual air). Zentralblatt Physiol 17:258–267
24. Darling RC, Cournand A, Richards DW (1940) Studies on the intrapulmonary mixture of gases. An open circuit method for measuring residual air. J Clin Invest 19:609–618
25. Fretschner R, Deusch H, Weitnauer A, Brunner JX (1993) A simple method to estimate functional residual capacity in mechanically ventilated patients. Intensive Care Med 19:372–376
26. Chiumello D, Cressoni M, Chierichetti M et al (2008) Nitrogen washout/washin, helium dilution and computed tomography in the assessment of end expiratory lung volume. Crit Care 12:R150
27. Brewer LM, Orr JA, Sherman MR, Fulcher EH, Markewitz BA (2011) Measurement of functional residual capacity by modified multiple breath nitrogen washout for spontaneously breathing and mechanically ventilated patients. Br J Anaesth 107:796–805
28. Heinze H, Eichler W (2009) Measurements of functional residual capacity during intensive care treatment: the technical aspects and its possible clinical applications. Acta Anaesthesiol Scand 53:1121–1130
29. Hedenstierna G (1993) The recording of FRC – is it of importance and can it be made simple? Intensive Care Med 19:365–366
30. Bikker IG, van Bommel J, Miranda DR, Bakker J, Gommers D (2008) End-expiratory lung volume during mechanical ventilation: a comparison with reference values and the effect of

positive end-expiratory pressure in intensive care unit patients with different lung conditions. Crit Care 12:R145

31. Patroniti N, Saini M, Zanella A et al (2008) Measurement of end-expiratory lung volume by oxygen washin–washout in controlled and assisted mechanically ventilated patients. Intensive Care Med 34:2235–2240
32. Bikker IG, Scohy TV, Bogers A, Bakker J, Gommers D (2009) Measurement of end-expiratory lung volume in intubated children without interruption of mechanical ventilation. Intensive Care Med 35:1749–1753
33. Suter PM, Fairley HB, Isenberg MD (1978) Effect of tidal volume and positive end-expiratory pressure on compliance during mechanical ventilation. Chest 73:158–162
34. Lambermont B, Ghuysen A, Janssen N (2008) Comparison of functional residual capacity and static compliance of the respiratory system during a positive end-expiratory pressure (PEEP) ramp procedure in an experimental model of acute respiratory distress syndrome. Crit Care 12:R91
35. Maisch S, Reissmann H, Fuellekrug B (2008) Compliance and dead space fraction indicate an optimal level of positive end-expiratory pressure after recruitment in anesthetized patients. Anesth Analg 106:175–181
36. Heinze H, Sedemund-Adib B, Heringlake M, Meier T, Eichler W (2010) Relationship between functional residual capacity, respiratory compliance, and oxygenation in patients ventilated after cardiac surgery. Respir Care 55:589–594
37. Rylander C, Hogman M, Perchiazzi G, Magnusson A, Hedenstierna G (2004) Functional residual capacity and respiratory mechanics as indicators of aeration and collapse in experimental lung injury. Anesth Analg 98:782–789
38. Marini JJ, Capps JS, Culver BH (1985) The inspiratory work of breathing during assisted mechanical ventilation. Chest 87:612–618
39. Marini JJ, Tyler ML, Hudson LD, Davis BS, Huseby JS (1984) Influence of head-dependent positions on lung volume and oxygen saturation in chronic air-flow obstruction. Am Rev Respir Dis 129:101–105
40. Rodriguez-Nieto MJ, Peces-Barba G, Gonzalez Mangado N, Paiva M, Verbanck S (2002) Similar ventilation distribution in normal subjects prone and supine during tidal breathing. J Appl Physiol 92:622–666
41. Behrakis PK, Baydur A, Jaeger MJ, Milic-Emili J (1983) Lung mechanics in sitting and horizontal body positions. Chest 83:643–646
42. Agustí A, Barnes PJ (2012) Update in chronic obstructive pulmonary disease 2011. Am J Respir Crit Care Med 185:1171–1176
43. Gattinoni L, Pesenti A (2005) The concept of "baby lung". Intensive Care Med 31:776–784
44. Chiumello D, Carlesso E, Cadringher P et al (2008) Lung stress and strain during mechanical ventilation for acute respiratory distress syndrome. Am J Respir Crit Care Med 178:346–355

Esophageal Pressure Monitoring in ARDS

D. Chiumello, S. Coppola, and S. Froio

Introduction

Acute respiratory distress syndrome (ARDS) remains a disease with high mortality rates despite recent therapeutic advances [1]. Although mechanical ventilation can be lifesaving, inappropriate use of the ventilator can itself promote lung injury. It could be useful to know the mechanics characteristics of the respiratory system in order to be able to set a protective ventilation strategy, because ARDS is a syndrome with marked clinical variability. The assessment of respiratory mechanics is important in mechanically ventilated patients because acute respiratory failure is most often the consequence of severe abnormalities in the mechanical properties of the respiratory system, including its lung and chest wall components [2]. Despite possible technical artifacts, recording of the esophageal pressure (Pes) provides the opportunity of estimating pleural pressure (P_{Pl}), to partition the mechanics and better understand the underlying pulmonary injury.

In this chapter, we will focus on the physiological meaning of Pes monitoring, on the esophageal balloon technique at the bedside, on the role of Pes on the dis-

D. Chiumello (✉)
Dipartimento di Anestesia, Rianimazione (Intensiva e Subintensiva) e Terapia del Dolore, Fondazione IRCCS Ca' Granda – Ospedale Maggiore Policlinico, Via F. Sforza 35, 20122 Milan, Italy
E-mail: chiumello@libero.it

S. Coppola
Dipartimento di Anestesia, Rianimazione (Intensiva e Subintensiva) e Terapia del Dolore, Fondazione IRCCS Ca' Granda – Ospedale Maggiore Policlinico, Via F. Sforza 35, 20122 Milan, Italy

S. Froio
Dipartimento di Anestesia, Rianimazione (Intensiva e Subintensiva) e Terapia del Dolore, Fondazione IRCCS Ca' Granda – Ospedale Maggiore Policlinico, Via F. Sforza 35, 20122 Milan, Italy

J.-L. Vincent (Ed.), *Annual Update in Intensive Care and Emergency Medicine 2013*,
DOI 10.1007/978-3-642-35109-9_37,

tending force of the lung and on the clinical application of Pes monitoring in critically ill patients with acute lung injury (ALI) and ARDS.

Pathophysiology

The respiratory system is composed of the lung and chest wall components, and their individual mechanical properties determine the behavior of the respiratory system as a whole. The applied airway pressure (P_{AW}) is used in part to inflate the lung and in part to inflate the chest wall. The static mechanics characteristics of the respiratory system depend on the ratio between changes in the pressure and the volume applied (elastance of the respiratory system). Because the two components of the respiratory system, the lung and the chest wall, are in series, in mathematical terms it follows that

$$E_{RS} = E_{CW} + E_L$$

where E_{RS} is the total respiratory system elastance, E_{CW} is the chest wall elastance and E_L is the lung elastance.

The distending force of the lung, that is transpulmonary pressure (P_{TP}), is the pressure difference between the alveoli and the pleural pressure, whereas the distending force of the thoracic cage is the P_{Pl} to which all the intrathoracic structures are subjected. In other terms, the airway pressure (P_{AW}) required to inflate the respiratory system is the sum of the pressure required to inflate the lung (P_{TP}) plus the pleural pressure (P_{Pl}), required to inflate the chest wall. In static conditions, when the airway resistance is nil:

$$P_{AW} = P_{TP} + P_{Pl}$$

P_{AW} is easily obtained by measuring the pressure at the airway opening from a side tap in the mouthpiece or tracheal cannula [3]. The distending force of the lung is not the P_{AW}, which is commonly used in clinical practice, but the P_{TP} [4].

P_{Pl} is more difficult to measure, since it would require direct measurement of the pressure in the pleural space with needles. In humans this is not possible. P_{Pl} depends on the pressure applied to the airways (P_{AW}) in static condition, and on the ratio between the chest wall elastance (E_{CW}) and the total elastance of the respiratory system (E_{RS}) as follows:

$$P_{Pl} = P_{AW} \cdot E_{CW} / E_L$$

and

$$P_{TP} = P_{AW} \cdot E_L / E_{RS}$$

Because of the close proximity of the esophagus and the pleural space, Pes is frequently used as a substitute for P_{Pl}. This value can be obtained at the bedside using an esophageal balloon.

Pes is a physiological value that can be influenced by many different forces:[5]

- Elastance of the rib cage (recoil pressure at high lung/thoracic volume)
- Weight of the rib cage, of the mediastinal organs, mainly the heart that may put a constant pressure load on the esophagus
- Weight and elastance of the diaphragm and abdomen (may put a constant load on the esophagus)
- Elastance of the esophageal wall
- Elastance of the esophageal balloon.

In the upright subject, the balloon will be exposed to the pressures caused by the lung, rib cage and diaphragm elastances. In the supine position, the weight of the rib cage, mediastinal organs and abdomen will cause pressure on the balloon, making conclusions regarding E_L and E_{CW} not reliable when you consider the absolute value of Pes.

Pes is relatively more positive in the supine position than in other postures. Talmor et al. [6] and Loring et al. [7] subtracted a mean of 5 cm H_2O to obtain the corresponding P_{Pl} assuming the pressure caused by the weight of the mediastinal organs.

However, it should be remembered that the absolute value of Pes does not provide any information about the mechanical properties of the respiratory system, because this pressure may vary considerably from that existing elsewhere [8]. To study the mechanical characteristics of the lung and the chest wall it is not the absolute value of Pes that is important but its modifications with gas movements in the respiratory system.

Esophageal Balloon Technique

The most widely used method for recording Pes in the study of respiratory mechanics employs an air-containing latex balloon (10 cm long, diameter 3.5 to 4.8 cm, wall thickness 0.1 mm, minimum unstretched volume 0.2 ml and pressure 0 to 0.5 cm H_2O within the balloon when it contains 0.5 ml of air) that transmits the balloon pressures to a manometer [9]. The tip of the balloon should be placed at a constant distance of 45 cm from the nares. The validity of this technique has been questioned by several authors because of the influence of the balloon volume, position and body posture.

The balloon should be inflated with an adequate volume of air so as to transmit the pressure without artifacts: A volume sufficient to prevent the walls of the balloon from occluding all the multiple holes in the end of the catheter, but not so much that there is tension in the balloon walls [10]. The pressure within the balloon placed in the esophagus can be the same as the local P_{Pl} only if the pressure difference across all intervening structures (balloon wall, esophageal wall, and various mediastinal structures) is zero. Over a certain range of balloon volumes there is only a negligible pressure drop across the wall of the balloon itself. Within this range, balloon pressure increases with balloon volume, presumably as a result of distension and displacement of the esophageal wall and surrounding structures. As a result, the pressure in the esophageal balloon tends to be more positive than P_{Pl}. Since the magnitude of this difference is unknown, many authors do not recognize Pes as a measure of absolute P_{Pl} [11]. On the other hand, it has been thought that variations in P_{Pl} would be reliably recorded from these balloons suggesting that even if small errors in absolute pressure were induced, satisfactory measurement of the change in pressure could be obtained [12].

Topography of the Esophageal Pressure

The best place to measure Pes seems to be the middle third of the esophagus because in this position Pes accurately reflects changes in P_{Pl}. Studies have shown that volume-pressure curves for lungs based on Pes vary with the position of the balloon within the esophagus [13]. In approximately the upper third of the esophagus, pressure variations were unrelated to variations in pleural pressure and were probably the result of traction on, or compression of, the esophagus by the trachea. In the lower third of the esophagus, pressures were found to vary markedly from point to point and with body posture [13]. In fact, in the upright subject the classic position of the balloon is in the lower third of the esophagus. This is the location of the heart and in the supine position the heart may exert weight on the balloon. In the supine position, it may be better to locate the balloon in the middle third of the esophagus to avoid or reduce the weight of the heart [5]. It has been concluded that in studies of respiratory mechanics, Pes should be measured in the middle third of the esophagus for subjects in supine position [13].

It is crucial to confirm correct positioning using the occlusion test [10] or by compression of the rib cage. Traditionally, in spontaneously breathing subjects, the balloon position in assessed with an occlusion test. The occlusion test requires that the subject is able to breathe spontaneously: When inspiratory efforts are made against an occluded airway, the deflections in Pes should match P_{AW}. Simultaneous measurement of tracheal and esophageal pressures during occluded inspiratory efforts was used to assess the validity of the esophageal balloon technique in anesthetized subjects in spontaneous breathing. In this setting, the occlusion test was performed by occluding the external airway at end-expiration and recording the esophageal and tracheal pressure changes during the following two or three occluded inspiratory efforts [14].

In paralyzed animals [15], correct positioning can be checked by gently applying pressure to either the abdomen or the rib cage during an expiratory hold: When this is done, the changes in Pes and P_{AW} should be equal, indicating good transmission of pressure from the balloon; if this is not the case, the catheter position must be adjusted.

The measurement of the $\Delta Pes/\Delta P_{AW}$ ratio during an occluded inspiratory effort allows the reliability of the esophageal balloon technique to be tested. During such a maneuver, the changes in P_{Pl} should be identical to the changes in tracheal pressure, apart from a negligible difference resulting from thoracic gas rarefaction. If the $\Delta Pes/\Delta P_{AW}$ is near to unity, then esophageal balloon measurements are a valid measure of the changes in pleural surface pressure. Deviations from the line of identity result from cardiac artifacts. Repositioning of the esophageal balloon may be necessary to obtain a satisfactory $\Delta Pes/\Delta P_{AW}$ ratio during occluded inspiratory efforts [14].

Esophageal Pressure and Transpulmonary Pressure

Pes is frequently used to estimate P_{Pl} to calculate the elastic and resistive forces in the lung in intensive care, anesthesia and in spontaneously breathing subjects. To understand the physiological role of Pes we have to remember the static relationship between pressure and volume systems and its lung and chest wall components. At forced vital capacity – FRC (resting lung volume) – the pressure applied to the whole respiratory system is 0 cm H_2O, no respiratory muscles are active and no external force is applied to the system. At FRC, pressure is needed to keep the lung expanded and the lung would collapse if no pressure is applied to the lung. This pressure comes from the elastic forces in the chest wall that exert a negative pressure at the FRC level. Thus, at FRC, the elastic forces of the lung act to decrease lung volume and the elastic forces in the chest wall act to expand it. With decreasing lung volume the recoil force of the lung decreases. Using a simple analogy with a rubber balloon, the more it is inflated, the stronger is the recoil pressure. On the other hand, the smaller the chest wall circumference, the larger is its expanding force [16, 17].

Lungs inflate and deflate in response to changes in P_{TP}, the distending force of the lung. The potential for damage to the lungs caused by mechanical ventilation, depends on the magnitude of the P_{TP} [18]. Depending on the chest wall's contribution to respiratory mechanics, a given positive end-expiratory and/or end-inspiratory plateau pressure may be appropriate for one patient but inadequate or potentially injurious for another. As explained above, Pes is useful to calculate the P_{TP}. Systematic use of Pes has the potential to improve ventilator management by providing more direct assessment of lung distending pressure.

Clinical Practice

ARDS is known to be characterized by a reduction in FRC and an increase in static elastance of the respiratory system [19]. Given the underlying pulmonary injury that is present in patients with ARDS, the increase in static elastance is thought to reflect mainly alterations of the mechanical properties of the lung rather than those of the chest wall.

Table 1 Clinical studies on esophageal pressure monitoring in patients with acute respiratory distress syndrome (ARDS)

Author, year [ref]	Study design	Type of patient	Number of patients	Clinical use of Pes	Aim	Major Results
Pelosi, 1995 [9]	Case control study	ALI, ARDS, normal	16	To calculate E_{RS} and E_{CW} Δ(Pes plat-Pes exp)/Vt	To partition respiratory mechanics and to verify the effect of PEEP and lung volume changes on lung and chest wall mechanics.	At ZEEP, E_{RS} and E_L were higher in ALI/ARDS patients compared with normal subjects PEEP did not significantly modify E_L in either group
Ranieri, 1997 [22]	Case control study	Early ARDSp and ARDSextrap	27	Δ(Pes plat-Pes rel) to study the static inflation PV curve of the chest wall and lung	Relative contribution of the chest wall and the lung to the impairment of respiratory mechanics	In ARDSp, the inspiratory PV curve of the respiratory system and lung showed a progressive increase in E_{RS} with inflating volume because of alveolar overinflation. ARDSextrap was characterized by increased values of E_{CW}
Gattinoni, 1998 [24]	Prospective observational study	ARDSp and ARDSextrap	21	To calculate E_{CW} (ΔPes/V_T)	To assess mechanics differences between ARDSp and ARDSextrap at different PEEP levels.	At ZEEP, E_{RS} was similar in both groups; E_L was higher in ARDSp; E_{CW} was higher in ARDSextrap. At PEEP 15 cm H_2O, E_{RS} increased in ARDSp and decreased in ARDSextrap
Grasso, 2002 [27]	Prospective multicenter	Early ARDS	22	To study E_{CW} on ZEEP	Effectiveness of RMs on oxygenation could be influenced by the elastic properties of lung and chest wall	E_{CW} and E_L on ZEEP were higher in nonresponders to RMs RMs improved oxygenation in patients without impaired chest wall mechanics
Albaiceta, 2003 [25]	Case series	Early ARDSp and ARDSextrap	10	P_{AW}-V curve Pes-V curve, P_{TP}-V curve during deflation maneuver	To compare deflation PV curve between ARDSp and ARDSextrap	Differences between ARDSp and ARDSextrap are present all along the pressure axis and are related to differences in the Pes-V and in the P_{TP}-V curves

Table 1 *Continued*

Author, year [ref]	Study design	Type of patient	Number of patients	Clinical use of Pes	Aim	Major Results
Talmor, 2006 [6]	Prospective observational study	ARF	70	To estimate end-expiratory and end-inspiratory P_{TP} ($P_{TP} = P_{AW} - Pes + 5$)	To characterize the influence of the chest wall on P_{Pl} and P_{TP}	When Pes values are high, P_{TP} can be underestimated and PEEP applied could be inadequate to maintain end expiratory positive P_{TP}
Talmor, 2008 [28]	Randomized controlled trial	ALI/ARDS	61	End-expiratory P_{TP} to set PEEP; End-inspiratory P_{TP} to keep $P_{TP} < 25$ cm H_2O at end inspiration.	P_{Pl} would be useful to find a PEEP value that could improve oxygenation, by maintaining positive P_{TP}.	Oxygenation and respiratory system compliance improve when mechanical ventilation is directed by absolute values of Pes
Grasso, 2012 [31]	Case series	ARDS (H1N1)	14	ΔPes (Pes plat – Pes exp) to calculate P_{Pl} to obtain P_{TP}	The assessment of P_{TP} could change the ventilatory strategy to reverse refractory hypoxemia and avoid need for ECMO in patients with chest wall impairment	In ARDS patients with a stiff chest wall, targeting PEEP to reach the upper physiological limit of P_{TP} improves oxygenation to an extent that ECMO criteria will no longer be met

ARDSp: pulmonary ARDS; ARDSextrap: extrapulmonary ARDS; ARF: acute respiratory failure; Pes: esophageal pressure; P_{TP}: transpulmonary pressure; P_{Pl}: pleural pressure; PEEP: positive end-expiratory pressure; PV: pressure-volume; P_{AW}: airway pressure; V_T: tidal volume; E_{CW}: chest wall elastance; E_{RS}: respiratory system elastance; E_L: lung elastance; Pes plat: esophageal plateau pressure; Pes exp; end expiratory esophageal pressure; Pes rel: release esophageal pressure; ECMO: extracorporeal membrane oxygenation; ALI: acute lung injury; ZEEP: zero end-expiratory pressure, RM: recruitment maneuver

Clinical studies have been performed using Pes measurements to better understand the respiratory mechanics of underlying disease and eventually influence the management of the mechanical ventilation in ARDS patients. We performed a computerized search of MEDLINE/PubMed using the following search keywords "Esophageal pressure and ARDS". Our search was limited to studies on humans and those published in English. We screened clinical studies concerning esophageal pressure monitoring in ARDS patients for relevance (Table 1).

Katz et al. [20] and Pelosi et al. [21] reported an increase in chest wall elastance in mechanically ventilated patients with different degrees of ALI [22]. The increase in elastance of the chest wall may be attributed to various factors [9]:

- a decrease in FRC, which might produce a decrease in the volume of the thoracic cage, moving it to a less compliant portion of its pressure-volume curve
- abdominal distension
- chest wall edema
- pleural effusion

A direct relationship between FRC and intrathoracic volume does not apply to ALI because a significant portion of the intrathoracic volume is occupied by blood, exudate, edema and pleural fluid [9]. A computed tomography (CT) study demonstrated that, in ALI patients, the thoracic volume was normal despite a significantly lower lung gas volume [21]. Therefore, the hypothesis that the increase in the E_{CW} could be due to a decrease in FRC should be ruled out. This increase may most likely be ascribed to alterations in the intrinsic properties of the chest wall, which seem to appear rapidly after mechanical ventilation is started. During mechanical ventilation, patients are often sedated with opioids, affecting gut pathophysiology and resulting in abdominal distension. It is also important to remember that an individual patient with pulmonary ARDS may have a concomitant increase in intra-abdominal pressure (IAP) [23]. Moreover in ALI patients positive fluid balances and pleural effusions are often present.

The mechanical properties of the chest wall may be influenced by the etiology of ARDS. There are striking differences in chest wall mechanics between patients with pulmonary ARDS (ARDSp), usually due to diffuse pneumonia, and those with extrapulmonary ARDS (ARDSextrap), usually due to abdominal diseases. Although E_{RS} is similar in both groups, the P_{Pl} is normal in ARDSp patients but abnormally high in ARDSextrap patients. The presence of abdominal disease in critically ill patients with ALI/ARDS should be a drive for careful investigation of their respiratory mechanics [23]. The same P_{AW} may generate dramatically different P_{TP} and P_{Pl} with marked consequences on lung distension and on hemodynamics, in patients with pulmonary and extrapulmonary ARDS. The method available to measure P_{Pl} in clinical practice is the measurement of the changes in Pes [5].

Patients with ARDSp and patients with ARDSextrap have different mechanical behavior, different lung morphology and different PEEP response. The chest wall elastance differences explain most of these different behavioral patterns. ARDSextrap patients have diffuse interstitial lung edema due to inflammatory mediators originating in extrapulmonary foci and alveolar collapse. The increase in lung weight causes compression atelectasis of the dependent lung regions. ARDSp patients tend to have less homogeneous lung alteration and predominant consolidation of some lung regions instead of lung collapse. In ARDSextrap patients, the elevated P_{Pl} caused by increased E_{CW} will cause the P_{TP} to be lower than in ARDSp patients with normal elastance. The potential for recruitment is also greater in ARDSextrap patients than in ARDSp patients.

Several groups have used Pes measurement to study these two groups of patients [22, 24, 25]. Gattinoni et al. performed a clinical study to asses mechanical differences between ARDSp and ARDSextrap at different levels of PEEP. They concluded that E_{RS} was similar in both groups without PEEP, whereas at 15 cm H_2O of PEEP, E_{RS} increased in ARDSp and decreased in ARDSextrap [24]. Ranieri et al. investigated the static inflation P-V curve of the chest wall and lung and showed that the flattening of the P-V curve at high pressures observed in some patients with ARDS may be due to an increase in E_{CW} [22]. Albaiceta et al. compared the deflation P-V curves in ARDSp and ARDSextrap in a case series of patients. The differences between the P-V curves of these two groups were present all along the pressure axis and were related to differences not only in the Pes-V curve, but also in the P_{TP}-V curve [25].

Chest wall elastance may be important in the pathogenesis of ventilator-induced lung injury (VILI); for example, we may expect more VILI for a given applied pressure when the E_{CW} is normal. In fact, the primary determinants of VILI are stress, defined as the lung counter force that reacts to an external load, and strain, defined as the deformation of the structure referred to the initial status. Gattinoni at al. reasoned that the clinical equivalent of stress is P_{TP} and the clinical equivalent of strain is the ratio of volume change to FRC [26]. The same tidal volume may result in a completely different P_{TP}, depending on the E_{RS} and on the E_{CW}/E_{RS} ratio, and consequently result in different VILI.

E_{CW} plays an important role when performing recruitment maneuvers because the P_{TP} and not the P_{AW} is determinant for lung opening. The P_{AW} applied to open the lung will be completely different in patients with normal or abnormal E_{CW}. In patients with a stiff or low compliance chest wall, a P_{TP} that is too low will not recruit collapsed lung even if the P_{AW} is high [23]. Therefore, the effectiveness of recruitment maneuvers on oxygenation could be influenced by the elastic properties of lung and chest wall. Grasso et al. showed that recruitment maneuvers improved oxygenation only in patients with early ARDS without impairment of chest wall mechanics and with a large potential for recruitment. In fact non-responders to recruitment maneuvers are characterized by higher values of E_{CW} and E_L [27].

In the same way, titration of PEEP to find the lowest pressure needed to keep the lung open, can be guided by following P_{TP}. The goal of applied PEEP in patients with ARDS is to maintain alveolar recruitment and to prevent cycles of recruitment and derecruitment. PEEP values that are too low allow some lung to be collapsed, values that are too high result in overdistension: An optimal approach to setting applied PEEP has not been established [5].

Talmor et al. [28] reported improved management of ARDS patients if PEEP was applied following P_{TP} rather than P_{AW} alone. These authors titrated applied

PEEP to achieve a P_{TP} of 0 to 10 cm H_2O at end-expiration while maintaining $P_{TP} < 25$ cm H_2O at end-inspiration to avoid alveolar overdistension. End-expiratory and end-inspiratory P_{TP} were calculated using the absolute value of Pes during end-expiratory and during end-inspiratory hold respectively [28]. P_{TP} was negative at end-expiration in some patients. However, when there is some gas in the lung, the distending stress of the lung is equal to the recoil stress. In a non-homogeneous lung, as in ARDS, P_{TP} is the result of all the different local distending stresses, and is either positive or zero in the gas-free lung [3]. If the P_{Pl} is high, it will aid lung emptying. The lung is protected against any negative P_{TP} because its deformation will increase the distending stress, and the bronchioles collapse [29]. However, Vieillard-Baron and Jardin commented that Talmor et al. did not measure Pes, but rather the distending pressure of the esophageal balloon [30].

In a recent case series of patients with influenza A H1N1-associated ARDS, Grasso et al. targeted PEEP to reach the upper physiological limit of P_{TP} (25 cm H_2O) instead of the safe limit of P_{AW} plateau. They calculated P_{Pl} in a different way, considering the pressure applied to the airways and the ratio between E_{CW} and E_{RS}. E_{CW} was estimated using the changes in Pes [31]. Chiumello et al. [4] demonstrated that tidal volume and airway plateau pressure are inadequate surrogates for lung stress and strain, and that Pes variations are the best available surrogates for P_{Pl} variations.

Pes variations enable partitioned respiratory mechanics to be studied in ARDS patients, remembering that the absolute value of Pes gives no reliable information about the severity of disease. In 48 ARDS patients, we compared the esophageal pressure measured after a complete expiration to the elastic equilibrium volume of the respiratory system, with the total lung tissue, volume and gas calculated by the quantitative analysis of CT scans and found no significant correlations (unpublished data). We show the relationship between Pes and total lung tissue in Fig. 1 ($R^2 = 0.01$).

Furthermore the evaluation of hemodynamics calls for special care in cases of increased chest wall elastance. The increased P_{Pl} may lower the cardiac output by reducing the venous return and the cardiac volume. Both the central venous pressure and the wedge pressure may appear 'falsely' elevated in the presence of increased P_{Pl} [32]. Finally E_{CW} may influence the distribution of ventilation and gas-exchange [33]. There is evidence that the characteristics of E_{CW} in the supine position may be useful to predict the oxygenation response in the prone position in patients with ARDS. In the supine position, the higher the E_{CW}, the lower is the oxygenation response. Moreover in the prone position, the improvement in oxygenation is directly related to the associated increase in Ecw. It has been shown that ARDSextrap patients have a greater potential for oxygenation improvement in the prone position than do ARDSp patients [34].

We believe that Pes-guided mechanical ventilation may be helpful in the management of patients with ARDS although at the present time there are few clinical studies that have investigated a safe threshold of P_{TP}. Moreover, nasogastric polyfunctional catheters have recently been evaluated as a good alternative, allowing

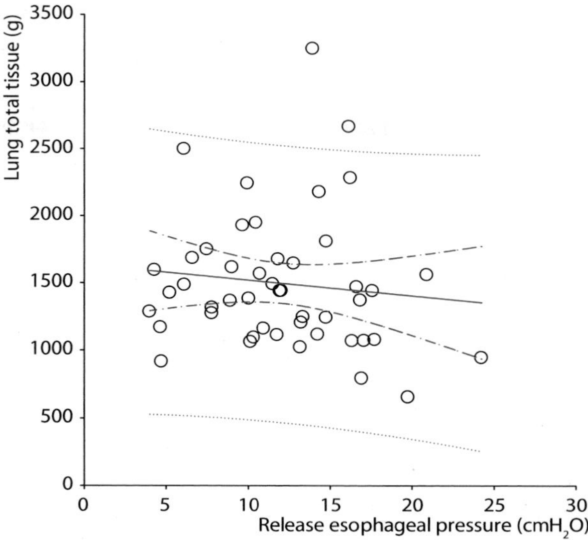

Fig. 1 Linear regression between total lung tissue (g), calculated by quantitative analysis of computed tomography (CT) scan, and esophageal pressure measured at the end of a complete expiration to the elastic equilibrium volume of the respiratory system after the end inspiratory occlusion was released in 48 patients with acute respiratory distress syndrome (ARDS). $R^2 = 0.01$

the possibility of monitoring Pes in patients who require enteral nutrition during mechanical ventilation [35].

Conclusion

A rational approach to the treatment of patients with ALI and ARDS requires knowledge of both E_L and E_{CW}. Pes variations are the best available surrogate of P_{Pl} variations and provide reliable information about the partitioning of respiratory mechanics. It is possible to investigate P_{Pl} and P_{TP} at the bedside using an esophageal balloon. Although it may be difficult and fraught with errors and artifacts, monitoring of Pes permits better characterization of the underlying ARDS pathology and can help to tailor a more physiological mechanical ventilation.

References

1. Ware LB, Matthay MA (2000) The acute respiratory distress syndrome. N Engl J Med 342:1334–1349
2. Polese G, Rossi A, Appendini L et al (1991) Partitioning of respiratory mechanics in mechanically ventilated patients. J Appl Physiol 71:2425–2433
3. Agostoni E, Rahn H (1960) Abdominal and thoracic pressures at different lung volumes. J Appl Physiol 15:1087–1092
4. Chiumello D, Carlesso E, Cadringher P et al (2008) Lung stress and strain during mechanical ventilation for acute respiratory distress syndrome. Am J Respir Crit Care Med 178:346–355

5. Hedenstierna G (2012) Esophageal pressure: benefit and limitations. Minerva Anestesiol 78:959–966
6. Talmor D, Sarge T, O'Donnell CR et al (2006) Esophageal and transpulmonary pressures in acute respiratory failure. Crit Care Med 34:1389–1394
7. Loring SH, O'Donnell CR, Behazin N et al (2010) Esophageal pressures in acute lung injury: do they represent artefact or useful information about transpulmonary pressure, chest wall mechanics, and lung stress? J Appl Physiol 108:515–522
8. Richard JC, Marini JJ (2012) Transpulmonary pressure as a surrogate of plateau pressure for lung protective strategy: not perfect but more physiologic. Intensive Care Med 38:339–341
9. Pelosi P, Cereda M, Foti G et al (1995) Alterations of lung and chest wall mechanics in patients with acute lung injury: effects of positive end-expiratory pressure. Am J Respir Crit Care Med 152:531–537
10. Baydur A, Behrakis PK, Zin WA et al (1982) A simple method for assessing the validity of the esophageal balloon technique. Am Rev Respir Dis 126:788–791
11. Milic-Emili J, Mead J, Turner JM et al (1964) Improved technique for estimating pleural pressure from esophageal balloons. J Appl Physiol 19:207–211
12. Drummond GB, Wright AD (1983) Inaccuracy of oesophageal pressure for pleural pressure estimation in supine anaesthetized subjects. Br J Anaesth 55:585–593
13. Milic-Emili J, Mead J, Turner JM (1964) Topography of esophageal pressure as Topography of esophageal pressure as a function of posture in man. J Appl Physiol 19:212–216
14. Higgs BD, Behrakis PK, Bevan DR et al (1983) Measurement of pleural pressure with esophageal balloon in anesthetized humans. Anesthesiology 59:340–343
15. Lanteri CJ, Kano S, Sly PD (1994) Validation of esophageal pressure occlusion test after paralysis. Pediatr Pulmonol 17:56–62
16. Jonson B, Beydon L, Brauer K et al (1993) Mechanics of respiratory system in healthy anesthetized humans with emphasis on viscoelastic properties. J Appl Physiol 75:132–140
17. Gattinoni L, Pesenti A (2005) The concept of "baby lung". Intensive Care Med 31:776–784
18. Washko GR, O'Donnell CR, Loring SH (2006) Volume-related and volume-independent effects of posture on esophageal and transpulmonary pressures in healthy subjects. J Appl Physiol 100:753–758
19. Marini JJ (1990) Lung mechanics in the adult respiratory distress syndrome. Recent conceptual advances and implications for management. Clin Chest Med 11:673–690
20. Katz JA, Zinn SE, Ozanne GM et al (1981) Pulmonary, chest wall, and lung-thorax elastances in acute respiratory failure. Chest 80:304–311
21. Pelosi P, D'Andrea L, Vitale G et al (1994) Vertical gradient of regional lung inflation in adult respiratory distress syndrome. Am J Respir Crit Care Med 149:8–13
22. Ranieri VM, Brienza N, Santostasi S et al (1997) Impairment of lung and chest wall mechanics in patients with acute respiratory distress syndrome: role of abdominal distension. Am J Respir Crit Care Med 156:1082–1091
23. Gattinoni L, Chiumello D, Carlesso E et al (2004) Bench-to-bedside review: chest wall elastance in acute lung injury/acute respiratory distress syndrome patients. Crit Care 8:350–355
24. Gattinoni L, Pelosi P, Suter PM et al (1998) Acute respiratory distress syndrome caused by pulmonary and extrapulmonary disease. Different syndromes? Am J Respir Crit Care Med 158:3–11
25. Albaiceta GM, Taboada F, Parra D et al (2003) Differences in the deflation limb of the pressure-volume curves in acute respiratory distress syndrome from pulmonary and extrapulmonary origin. Intensive Care Med 29:1943–1949
26. Gattinoni L, Carlesso E, Cadringher P et al (2003) Physical and biological triggers of ventilator-induced lung injury and its prevention. Eur Respir J Suppl 47:15s–25s
27. Grasso S, Mascia L, Del Turco M et al (2002) Effects of recruiting maneuvers in patients with acute respiratory distress syndrome ventilated with protective ventilatory strategy. Anesthesiology 96:795–802
28. Talmor D, Sarge T, Malhotra A et al (2008) Mechanical ventilation guided by esophageal pressure in acute lung injury. N Engl J Med 359:2095–2104

29. Mead J, Takishima T, Leith D (1970) Stress distribution in lungs: a model of pulmonary elasticity. J Appl Physiol 28:596–608
30. Vieillard-Baron A, Jardin F (2009) Esophageal pressure in acute lung injury. N Engl J Med 360:832–833
31. Grasso S, Terragni P, Birocco A et al (2012) ECMO criteria for influenza A (H1N1)-associated ARDS: role of transpulmonary pressure. Intensive Care Med 38:395–403
32. Pinsky MR, Desmet JM, Vincent JL (1992) Effect of positive end-expiratory pressure on right ventricular function in humans. Am Rev Respir Dis 146:681–687
33. Pelosi P, Tubiolo D, Mascheroni D et al (1998) Effects of the prone position on respiratory mechanics and gas exchange during acute lung injury. Am J Respir Crit Care Med 157:387–393
34. Lim CM, Kim EK, Lee JS et al (2001) Comparison of the response to the prone position between pulmonary and extrapulmonary acute respiratory distress syndrome. Intensive Care Med 27:477–485
35. Chiumello D, Gallazzi E, Marino A et al (2011) A validation study of a new nasogastric polyfunctional catheter. Intensive Care Med 37:791–795

Part XI

Lung Cells

Mesenchymal Stem/Stromal Cells: Opportunities and Obstacles in ARDS

G. F. Curley, M. Hayes, and J. G. Laffey

Introduction

The acute respiratory distress syndrome (ARDS) constitutes a major cause of death in critical care worldwide, with mortality rates of 40–60 % even with ongoing advances in care. Despite being the focus of ongoing intensive research efforts for over four decades, there are no pharmacologic therapies for acute lung injury (ALI)/ARDS. The lack of success to date with standard 'pharmacologic' approaches suggests the need to consider more complex therapeutic approaches, aimed at reducing early injury while maintaining host immune competence, and facilitating (or at least not inhibiting) lung regeneration and repair. Mesenchymal stem/stromal cells (MSCs) might fit this new therapeutic paradigm for ARDS and, consequently, are attracting a lot of attention. MSCs are multipotent cells derived from adult tissues that are capable of self-renewal and differentiation into chondrocytes, osteocytes and adipocytes. The origin of MSCs in multiple adult tissues, coupled with their relative ease of isolation and expansion potential in culture make them attractive therapeutic candidates.

G. F. Curley
Department of Anesthesia, Keenan Research Center, Li Ka Shing Knowledge Institute, St. Michael's Hospital, 30 Bond Street, Toronto, ON, M5B 1W8, Canada

M. Hayes
Department of Anesthesia, School of Medicine, Clinical Sciences Institute, National University of Ireland, Newcastle Road, Galway, Ireland

J. G. Laffey (✉)
Department of Anesthesia, Keenan Research Center, Li Ka Shing Knowledge Institute, St. Michael's Hospital, 30 Bond Street, Toronto, ON, M5B 1W8, Canada
Email: laffeyj@smh.ca

J.-L. Vincent (Ed.), *Annual Update in Intensive Care and Emergency Medicine 2013*, DOI 10.1007/978-3-642-35109-9_38, © Springer-Verlag Berlin Heidelberg 2013

Therapeutic Potential of MSCs for ARDS

MSCs offer substantial potential as a novel therapeutic approach to ARDS for several reasons. First, MSCs are immunologically well tolerated, and can be transplanted allogeneically, an important advantage for acute illnesses, such as ARDS. Second, the inflammatory response associated with ARDS is intense but generally short-lived. Whereas previous strategies to simply inhibit this response have been unsuccessful, the more complex, 'immunomodulatory' properties of MSCs may prove more effective. MSCs may be able to 'reprogram' the immune response to reduce the destructive inflammatory elements while preserving the host response to pathogens. Third, MSCs may augment repair processes following ALI [1]. The resolution of ARDS is hindered by damage to the epithelial barrier, which inhibits alveolar fluid clearance and depletes surfactant. MSCs may restore epithelial and endothelial function, in part via secretion of paracrine factors to enhance restoration of these tissues. Fourth, ARDS frequently occurs in association with a generalized process resulting in dysfunction and failure of multiple organs. MSCs have been demonstrated to decrease injury and/or restore function in the kidney [2], liver [3] and heart [4]. Fifth, MSCs may directly attenuate bacterial sepsis, the commonest and most severe cause of ALI/ARDS, via a number of mechanisms, including enhancement of phagocytosis, increased bacterial clearance [5], and anti-microbial peptide secretion [6]. Sixth, recent preclinical evidence suggests that MSCs may strengthen bioenergetics in the injured lung by transferring mitochondria-containing microvesicles [7]. Seventh, it is feasible to access both the distal lung epithelium via the intratracheal route and the pulmonary endothelium via the intravenous route as the entire cardiac output transits the pulmonary vasculature. Finally, stem cells are already being assessed in clinical studies for a wide range of disease processes, with a large body of evidence attesting to their safety and efficacy.

What Are the Active MCS Components?

Role of the MSC Secretome

The MSC "secretome" contains multiple immunomodulatory mediators, including prostaglandin E2 (PGE2) [8], transforming growth factor (TGF)-β [9], indoleamine 2,3-dioxygenase [10], interleukin (IL)-1-receptor antagonist (IL-1ra) [11], tumor necrosis factor (TNF)-α-induced protein (TSG)-6 [12], and IL-10 [13]. Xu et al. performed *ex vivo* co-culture studies of MSCs with endotoxin-injured lung cells and showed that the immunomodulatory effect was paracrine but also enhanced by cell-to-cell contact [14]. Németh et al. found that MSCs attenuated lung injury secondary to cecal ligation and puncture (CLP), at least in part, through secretion of PGE2, which reprograms host macrophages to increase IL-10 production [8]. Endotoxin-induced stimulation of the Toll-like receptor (TLR)4 expressed by the MSCs resulted in increased production of cyclooxygenase-2 and PGE2.

The demonstration by Krasnodembskaya et al. that MSCs secrete the anti-microbial peptide, LL-37, suggests a direct role for MSCs in combating pathogen-mediated sepsis [6].

The beneficial effects of MSCs in lung repair following injury appear to be mediated, at least in part via the secretion of cytoprotective factors [1, 15, 16]. Two of these factors – keratinocyte growth factor (KGF) and angiopoietin – have been shown to restore pulmonary epithelial and endothelial barrier function and enhance repair [1, 15, 16]. Lee et al. showed that restoration of permeability in an explanted endotoxin-injured human lung was mediated mainly by the action of KGF on amiloride-dependent sodium transport in the alveolar epithelium [16]. In primary cultures of human alveolar type II cells, human MSCs grown without cell contact in a Transwell plate restored the increase in epithelial permeability to protein caused by exposure to inflammatory cytokines in part by the secretion of angiopoeitin-1 [17].

Role of MSC-Derived Microvesicles

Microvesicles are small vesicles released by almost all cell types, which carry with them cytoplasmic and membrane constituents derived from the originating cells [18]. A growing body of evidence indicates that microvesicles derived from MSCs may enhance tissue repair in models of acute kidney and liver injury via transfer of gene products (i. e., mRNA and miRNAs) [2] and/or mitochondria [7] to target cells. MSC-derived microvesicles have an *in vitro* anti-apoptotic effect on renal tubular epithelial cells and enhance both structural and functional recovery from glycerol-induced kidney injury in severe combined immunodeficiency (SCID) mice [19]. More recently, Gatti et al. demonstrated that MSC-derived microvesicles administered as a single dose immediately post-induction of ischemia-reperfusion kidney injury improved renal function, promoted renal tubular cell proliferation and inhibited apoptosis [2].

MSC Contact-Dependent Effects

Cell-cell contact, mediated by adhesion molecules, appears to be another important mechanism by which MSCs modulate immune effector cells, such as macrophages [8] and T cells [20]. In a mouse model of endotoxin-induced systemic sepsis, Xu et al. found that the paracrine effect of MSCs in reducing lung inflammation, injury, and edema was enhanced by direct cell-to-cell contact [14]. In a murine model of lipopolysaccharide (LPS)-induced lung injury, Islam et al. [7] demonstrated that MSCs reduced lung injury via mitochondrial transfer to injured cells; human and murine MSCs attached to alveolar epithelial cells following intra-tracheal administration via connexin-43-containing gap junctions and subsequently transferred mitochondria to the injured cells. MSC therapy enhanced cellular ATP levels, restored surfactant secretion in the injured epithelial cells and increased animal survival [7].

How Do MSCs Work? (Table 1)

Immunomodulatory Effects

MSCs interact with a wide range of immune cells and exert multiple effects on the innate and adaptive immune responses. These effects include suppression of T cell proliferation, natural killer (NK) cell function and inhibition of dendritic cell differentiation [21]. MSCs have been shown to prevent neutrophil apoptosis and degranulation in culture without inhibiting their phagocytic or chemotactic capabilities [22]. They also regulate B cell [21] and monocyte function via poorly defined mechanisms. MSCs appear to decrease host damage arising from the inflammatory response, while enhancing host resistance to sepsis. MSCs decrease pro-inflammatory cytokine expression [12, 13], and secrete anti-inflammatory agents, including IL-1ra, IL-10, and PGE2 [8]. MSCs also reduce lung neutrophil recruitment and modulate immune effector cell activity.

Table 1 Postulated mechanisms of action of mesenchymal stem/stromal cells (MSCs) in preclinical models of acute lung injury (ALI)

Study	Lung injury model	MSC delivery route and timing of administration	Postulated mechanism of action
Ortiz, 2007 [11]	Murine bleomycin	i.v.	Secretion of IL-1 receptor antagonist Inhibition of TNF-α production by macrophage and IL-1α dependent T cell line
Xu, 2007 [14]	Murine i.p. LPS	i.v. 1 h/24 h post injury	Production of soluble factors by MSCs that promote an anti-inflammatory cytokine milieu Paracrine effect was enhanced by cell-to-cell contact Production of chemoattractants for MSCs by lung cells
Gupta, 2007 [13]	Murine i.t. LPS	i.t. 4 h/24 h post LPS	Paracrine effect by MSCs in downregulating the inflammatory response Engraftment rate $<5\,\%$
Lee, 2009 [16]	*Ex vivo* perfused human lung	i.t. 1/24 post LPS human MSCs	Secretion of KGF by MSCs resulting in improved endothelial permeability and restoration of alveolar epithelium fluid transport
Nemeth, 2009 [8]	Murine CLP	i.v. 24 h pre-/post-injury	Prostaglandin E2 dependent reprogramming of macrophage to increase production of IL-10

Table 1 *Continued*

Mei, 2010 [5]	Murine CLP	i.v. 6/24 h post-injury	Modification of inflammatory gene transcriptional activity Downregulation of the acute inflammatory response and upregulation of pathways relevant to phagocytosis and bacterial clearance
Krasnodembskaya, 2010 [6]	Murine *E.coli* pneumonia	i.t. 4/24 h post-injury human MSCS	Secretion of the anti-microbial peptide LL-37 resulting in increased bacterial clearance
Danchuk, 2011 [12]	Murine LPS	i.v., OA and IP human MSCs	Secretion of TSG-6 by MSCs resulting in reduced neutrophil recruitment and activation Secretion of KGF
Gupta, 2012 [51]	Murine *E. coli* pneumonia	i.t. 4/24 h post-injury	Reduced mortality and increased bacterial clearance, in part, by upregulation of the antibacterial protein lipocalin 2.
Krasnodembskaya, 2012 [52]	Murine Gram-negative peritoneal sepsis	i.v. 4/24 h post-injury human MSCs	Increased animal survival and bacterial clearance secondary to enhanced monocyte phagocytosis
Islam, 2012 [7]	Murine LPS	i.t. 4/24 h post-injury-human and murine MSCs	Increased alveolar ATP concentrations by transfer of mitochondria-containing microvesicles from MSCs to injured cells

i.v.: intravenous; IL: interleukin; TNF-α: tumor necrosis factor-alpha; i.p.: intra-peritoneal; LPS: lipopolysaccharide; i.t.: intra-tracheal; KGF: keratinocyte growth factor; CLP: cecal ligation and puncture; OA: oropharyngeal aspiration; TSG-6: tumor necrosis factor alpha-induced protein 6; iNOS: inducible nitric oxide synthase; ET-1: endothelin-1; MCP-1: monocyte chemotactic protein-1

Anti-microbial Effects

Several experimental studies have demonstrated beneficial effects of MSCs in the setting of bacteria-induced sepsis [5, 8]. In a murine model of sepsis induced by CLP, MSCs were associated with improved animal survival and organ function, whilst decreasing blood and peritoneal fluid bacterial counts [8]. Another murine CLP study showed reduced organ dysfunction and animal mortality associated with increased bacterial clearance and enhanced host cell phagocytosis by MSCs [5]. These findings are explained in part by the immunomodulatory properties of MSCs, but the mechanism whereby bacterial clearance was enhanced remains unclear. Newer evidence now indicates that MSCs may directly modulate the innate immune response and possess intrinsic anti-microbial properties. MSCs express TLRs and become activated in response to bacterial products [13]. Signaling through TLRs influences MSC-mediated immunomodulation as well as proliferation and migration. Intriguingly, Krasnodembskaya et al. demonstrated that secretion of the anti-microbial peptide, LL-37, by MSCs resulted in inhibition of bacterial growth *in vitro* and *in vivo* [6]. Secretion of LL-37 was upregulated in response to stimulation by bacteria. Intrabronchial administration of human MSCs in a mouse model of *Escherichia coli* pneumonia resulted in improved bacterial clearance from lung homogenates and bronchoalveolar lavage (BAL) fluid [6].

Cytoprotective Effects

ARDS is characterized by extensive damage to the pulmonary epithelium. Repair and recovery of an intact pulmonary epithelium is imperative for restoration of pulmonary homeostasis. Following injury, the lung itself releases many factors that contribute to repair mechanisms including members of the epidermal growth factor and fibroblast growth factor families (TGF, keratinocyte growth factor, hepatocyte growth factor [HGF]), chemokines (monocyte chemoattractant protein [MCP]-1), interleukins (IL-1, IL-2, IL-4, IL-13), and prostaglandins (PGE2). MSCs secrete several growth factors that specifically enhance epithelial repair, including KGF, HGF and angiopoietin-1. In the pulmonary epithelium, human MSCs enhance epithelial wound repair by a mechanism that is dependent, in part, on MSC secretion of KGF [1].

Alveolar Epithelial Fluid Clearance

Resolution of ARDS is impaired by inflammation-mediated destruction of the integrity of the alveolar-capillary barrier. The impairment of alveolar fluid clearance correlates with increased morbidity and mortality in ALI. Several pre-clinical studies on MSCs in ALI models have demonstrated that MSCs reduce pulmonary edema [1, 12, 13, 16]. Lee et al. demonstrated that MSCs improved alveolar barrier function and fluid clearance via a paracrine mechanism in the endotoxin-injured, explanted, perfused human lung [16]. Subsequent studies using small interfering RNA (siRNA) demonstrated that 80 % of the beneficial effects of MSCs were mediated by KGF. *In vivo* studies have suggested that KGF restored permeability, in part by upregulation of amiloride-dependent sodium transport in the alveolar epithelium [16].

Type II pneumocytes play a critical role in alveolar fluid clearance. *In vitro* work by Fang et al. examined the effect of MSCs on alveolar fluid clearance by type II pneumocytes. Primary cultures of human alveolar type II cells were injured by exposure to pro-inflammatory cytokines resulting in increased permeability to protein (^{131}I-labeled albumin). Co-culture of human MSCs resulted in restoration of the epithelial cell permeability to baseline levels. siRNA knockdown of potential paracrine soluble factors in the MSC secretome identified angiopoietin-1 as the active mediator [17]. The beneficial effect of angiopoietin-1 on resolution of pulmonary edema has been replicated in *in vivo* studies by Xu et al. and Mei et al.

who found that MSCs transfected with angiopoietin-1 reduced the severity of lung injury in live bacteria and endotoxin-induced lung injury models [14, 15].

Cellular Transdifferentiation and Engraftment

Cellular differentiation is the process by which a less specialized cell becomes a more specialized cell type. MSCs are capable of differentiation into a variety of 'lineage-specific' (i. e., mesenchymal) tissues, including bone, cartilage, tendon, fat, bone marrow stroma and muscle [23]. Transdifferentiation refers to the potential for adult stem cells to differentiate into cells of other lineages. MSCs were initially considered as a possible therapy for ALI/ARDS because of their potential to replace damaged lung tissue via engraftment and transdifferentiation into epithelial cells. Krause et al. found that a single bone marrow-derived hematopoietic stem cell could give rise to cells of different organs, including the lung, and demonstrated that up to 20 % of lung alveolar cells were derived from this single bone marrow stem cell [24]. Kotton et al. demonstrated that bone marrow-derived cells engrafted into pulmonary epithelium and exhibited characteristics specific to lung epithelial cells [25]. In a bleomycin-induced model of lung injury, Ortiz et al. demonstrated that murine MSCs homed to sites of injury and assumed an epithelium-like phenotype, reducing inflammation and collagen deposition [26]. However, later studies disagreed with this paradigm, demonstrating that functional engraftment of bone marrow-derived stem cells and differentiation into lung epithelial cells is a much rarer event than initially thought and is of unclear therapeutic significance [25].

What Are the Barriers to Clinical Translation for ARDS?

The therapeutic potential of MSCs for patients suffering from ARDS is clear, and MSCs appear close to clinical translation. However, gaps remain in our knowledge, which need to be addressed.

Optimization of Dosage Regimens

The optimal route of delivery for MSCs remains unclear. Most of the experimental studies in ALI have been carried out using intratracheal delivery. However, the pulmonary circulation is an ideal target for intravenous delivery, given it is the first capillary bed encountered by injected cells. Indeed, the pulmonary vascular bed acts as a barrier to MSC delivery to other organs, such as the heart, kidney and brain, such that investigators now utilize local injection techniques to target these organs. MSCs home to injured organs, whether the injury occurs in the liver, kidney, or the lung, and intravenously delivered MSCs may have multiple beneficial effects in ALI with associated multiple organ failure. MSCs have been delivered intravenously in other conditions with a good safety record.

The ideal dose – or doses – of MSCs for critically ill patients with ALI remains a matter of conjecture. Extrapolation from animal studies and from human studies of MSC administration in other disease states may be used as a guide. For example, in a dose-escalation safety trial of MSCs after acute myocardial infarction, Hare et al. administered 0.5–5 million cells/kg [4]. However, such doses will need validation in the critical care setting. It has been suggested that treatment could be given over three consecutive days, as has been used in a trial of autologous endothelial progenitor cells in patients with end-stage pulmonary hypertension [27]. However, the optimal dose of stem cells may differ substantially in different disease states. In addition, the dose may be influenced by other factors, such as the stage of illness, type of MSCs, route of cell delivery, viability and purity of MSCs and condition of the patient.

Timing of MSC delivery is also important. Most pre-clinical studies have demonstrated that MSCs are effective when administered in early phase of injury. However, recent data from our group suggest that MSCs may be effective after the injury has become established [1]. The demonstration that MSCs are effective when administered later in the course of the injury is important in terms of their clinical translation potential.

Incomplete Mechanistic Knowledge

Our understanding of the mechanisms of action of MSCs remains incomplete. This is borne out by the diverse array of paracrine mediators that have been demonstrated to possess therapeutic effects in diverse pre-clinical models. There are marked differences in MSCs from mice and humans in terms of properties, such as cell surface epitopes, ease of expansion, and genomic stability [28]. It is also becoming increasingly apparent that different inflammatory environments can profoundly influence MSC behavior [29]. Furthermore, there is growing evidence that MSCs represent a heterogeneous population of cells and that different MSC subtypes exist [30]. The relative importance of other actions of MSCs, such as mitochondrial and DNA transfer, microvesicle secretion and secretion of antimicrobial peptides remain unclear. Meanwhile the fact that many of the effects of MSCs appear to be mediated via elements of the MSC secretome raises the intriguing possibility of avoiding the need to administer the cells themselves. However, it seems unlikely – though not proven – that all of the beneficial effects of MSC therapy can be realized without administering the cells.

Concerns Regarding *In Vitro* Culture

One of the limitations in translating MSC therapy to the clinical setting is the fact that the numbers of cells that can be directly isolated from tissues is insufficient to achieve a therapeutic effect. This necessitates *ex vivo* MSC passage and expansion to increase MSC numbers. However, repeated passaging can alter the MSC phenotype, and may give rise to more restricted self-renewing progenitors that lose their differentiation potential, thus resulting in loss of efficacy [31]. MSC expression of homing receptors, such as CXCR4, a chemotactic receptor for stromal-derived factor (SDF)-1, which is crucial for their migration capability, might diminish as cells are continually passaged [32]. This may explain why freshly isolated MSCs have greater homing ability compared with their culture-expanded counterparts [33]. Repeated passage in culture may also give rise to chromosomal damage and even malignant transformation [34]. In addition, culture conditions, including culture density, culture surface composition [4], oxygen levels [35] and temperature [36], can profoundly influence phenotype and behavior of MSCs. The demonstration that thawed cryopreserved banked MSCs (used in clinical studies) may be less effective than 'fresh' MSCs (used in pre-clinical studies) may explain inconsistencies in results between clinical and pre-clinical studies [37].

Immunogenicity of MSCs

The possibility of clinical use of allogeneic MSCs as a therapy relies on the concept that MSCs evade or even repress the normal host-mediated immune rejection response. Recent experimental work showing that MSCs can elicit a memory T-cell response resulting in graft rejection in mice has called into question their characterization as "immunoprivileged cells" that can be transferred without immunosuppression of recipients [38]. MSCs are also subject to influence by their microenvironment. There are conflicting results in the literature regarding the effect of host inflammation on allo-MSC immune rejection and MSC-mediated immunomodulation. Some studies indicate that immune rejection of MSCs is more likely in an inflammatory microenvironment. Le Blanc et al. found that interferon (IFN)-γ, a key cytokine in host innate and adaptive immunity, results in upregulation of major histocompatibility complex (MHC) class I and II on MSCs [39]. Cho et al. reported that stimulation of porcine MSCs with IFN-γ augmented host T-cell and antibody responses [40]. However, these data must be weighed against comprehensive evidence that pre-stimulation of MSCs with IFN-γ enhances their immunosuppressive effects in various diseases, including chronic obstructive pulmonary disease (COPD), graft-vs.-host disease and allergic airway disease [41]. Moreover, a large body of preclinical data demonstrates the capacity of MSCs to modulate diverse immune responses and allogeneic cell-based therapies have been safely administered to many thousands of patients [4, 42]. Nevertheless, caution is required in relation to immune-modulating therapy in the aftermath of the anti-

CD28 monoclonal antibody trial [43], particularly given the very limited clinical experience with mesenchymal stem cells in critically ill patients to date.

Safety Concerns Regarding MSCs

Pulmonary Fibrosis

The potential for MSC therapy to contribute to fibroproliferative ARDS remains a potential concern, because bone marrow cells have been implicated in the fibrotic process. In bleomycin-induced pulmonary fibrosis, Hashimoto and colleagues demonstrated that bone marrow progenitor cells were recruited to injured areas and differentiated into fibroblasts [44]. In pulmonary fibrosis induced by irradiation, circulating cells of bone marrow origin contributed to the fibrotic process [45]. However, in animal models of pulmonary fibrosis induced by bleomycin, MSCs ameliorated the fibrotic process, resulting in reduced lung expression of pro-fibrotic cytokines and stimulated production of growth factors involved in endogenous stem cell mobilization from bone marrow, thus helping the repair process [26]. MSCs transfected to overexpress the growth factor KGF also decreased lung fibrogenesis [46].

Malignant Transformation

Potential tumor formation and the long-term effects of 'plasticity' of administered stem cells are legitimate safety concerns. Jeong et al. recently described sarcoma formation in the hind limbs and hearts of mice following MSC transplantation [47]. This study utilized genetically unmodified MSCs that exhibited multiple chromosomal abnormalities at passage 4 [47]. MSCs may increase tumor formation first through potential direct malignant transformation of the MSCs themselves or second through indirect tumor modulatory effects of the MSCs in preventing apoptosis and augmenting tumor growth. Direct malignant transformation of MSCs may occur during *in vivo* expansion [34]. Transduction of MSCs to over-express products of therapeutic value has shown promise in pre-clinical lung-injury models [15]. However, it is possible that genetic manipulation of stem cells will result in further chromosomal instability. Concerns also exist that MSCs may play a role in the development of cancers by contributing to the stromal components of the tumor [48].

Experimental work on the role of MSCs in tumor modulation has produced conflicting results, with some studies reporting an inhibitory effect of MSCs on tumor growth and others indicating a protective effect on tumor progression and metastatic spread through anti-apoptotic effects and other mechanisms [49]. The picture is further complicated by an apparent dual role of MSCs on tumor growth [50]. Tian et al. found that human MSCs caused G1 phase cycle arrest and apoptosis in lung and esophageal cancer cell lines, but when examined *in vivo*, the MSCs augmented tumor growth and formation [50].

Conclusion

The therapeutic potential of MSCs for ARDS is clear from preclinical studies. The mechanisms of action of MSCs are increasingly well understood, and include modulation of the immune response to reduce lung injury, while maintaining host immune-competence and facilitating lung regeneration and repair. The demonstration that human MSCs exert benefit in the injured human lung is particularly persuasive. However, it is important to remember that, despite promising results from preclinical studies in other disease states, clinical trials of cell therapies to date have shown only modest and sometimes inconsistent benefits. In addition, important knowledge gaps exist, and safety concerns have been raised regarding MSC therapy in patients with ARDS; these issues must be addressed prior to embarking on large scale clinical studies of MSCs for ARDS.

Acknowledgement The authors wish to thank Dr. Jeremy A. Scott for his thoughtful critique of the manuscript.

References

1. Curley GF, Hayes M, Ansari B et al (2012) Mesenchymal stem cells enhance recovery and repair following ventilator-induced lung injury in the rat. Thorax 67:496–501
2. Gatti S, Bruno S, Deregibus MC et al (2011) Microvesicles derived from human adult mesenchymal stem cells protect against ischaemia-reperfusion-induced acute and chronic kidney injury. Nephrol Dial Transplant 26:1474–1483
3. Kanazawa H, Fujimoto Y, Teratani T et al (2011) Bone marrow-derived mesenchymal stem cells ameliorate hepatic ischemia reperfusion injury in a rat model. PLoS One 6:e19195
4. Hare JM, Traverse JH, Henry TD et al (2009) A randomized, double-blind, placebo-controlled, dose-escalation study of intravenous adult human mesenchymal stem cells (prochymal) after acute myocardial infarction. J Am Coll Cardiol 54:2277–2286
5. Mei SH, Haitsma JJ, Dos Santos CC et al (2010) Mesenchymal stem cells reduce inflammation while enhancing bacterial clearance and improving survival in sepsis. Am J Respir Crit Care Med 182:1047–1057
6. Krasnodembskaya A, Song Y, Fang X et al (2010) Antibacterial effect of human mesenchymal stem cells is mediated in part from secretion of the antimicrobial peptide LL-37. Stem Cells 28:2229–2238
7. Islam MN, Das SR, Emin MT et al (2012) Mitochondrial transfer from bone-marrow-derived stromal cells to pulmonary alveoli protects against acute lung injury. Nat Med 18:759–765

8. Nemeth K, Leelahavanichkul A, Yuen PS et al (2009) Bone marrow stromal cells attenuate sepsis via prostaglandin E(2)-dependent reprogramming of host macrophages to increase their interleukin-10 production. Nat Med 15:42–49
9. Nemeth K, Keane-Myers A, Brown JM et al (2010) Bone marrow stromal cells use TGF-beta to suppress allergic responses in a mouse model of ragweed-induced asthma. Proc Natl Acad Sci USA 107:5652–5657
10. De Miguel MP, Fuentes-Julian S, Blazquez-Martinez A et al (2012) Immunosuppressive properties of mesenchymal stem cells: advances and applications. Curr Mol Med 12:574–591
11. Ortiz LA, Dutreil M, Fattman C et al (2007) Interleukin 1 receptor antagonist mediates the antiinflammatory and antifibrotic effect of mesenchymal stem cells during lung injury. Proc Natl Acad Sci USA 104:11002–11007
12. Danchuk S, Ylostalo JH, Hossain F et al (2011) Human multipotent stromal cells attenuate lipopolysaccharide-induced acute lung injury in mice via secretion of tumor necrosis factor-alpha-induced protein 6. Stem Cell Res Ther 2:27
13. Gupta N, Su X, Popov B, Lee JW, Serikov V, Matthay MA (2007) Intrapulmonary delivery of bone marrow-derived mesenchymal stem cells improves survival and attenuates endotoxin-induced acute lung injury in mice. J Immunol 179:1855–1863
14. Xu J, Woods CR, Mora AL et al (2007) Prevention of endotoxin-induced systemic response by bone marrow-derived mesenchymal stem cells in mice. Am J Physiol Lung Cell Mol Physiol 293:L131–L141
15. Mei SH, McCarter SD, Deng Y, Parker CH, Liles WC, Stewart DJ (2007) Prevention of LPS-induced acute lung injury in mice by mesenchymal stem cells overexpressing angiopoietin 1. PLoS Med 4:e269
16. Lee JW, Fang X, Gupta N, Serikov V, Matthay MA (2009) Allogeneic human mesenchymal stem cells for treatment of E. coli endotoxin-induced acute lung injury in the ex vivo perfused human lung. Proc Natl Acad Sci USA 106:16357–16362
17. Fang X, Neyrinck AP, Matthay MA, Lee JW (2010) Allogeneic human mesenchymal stem cells restore epithelial protein permeability in cultured human alveolar type II cells by secretion of angiopoietin-1. J Biol Chem 285:26211–26222
18. Tetta C, Bruno S, Fonsato V, Deregibus MC, Camussi G (2011) The role of microvesicles in tissue repair. Organogenesis 7:105–115
19. Collino F, Deregibus MC, Bruno S et al (2010) Microvesicles derived from adult human bone marrow and tissue specific mesenchymal stem cells shuttle selected pattern of miRNAs. PLoS One 5:e11803
20. Augello A, Tasso R, Negrini SM et al (2005) Bone marrow mesenchymal progenitor cells inhibit lymphocyte proliferation by activation of the programmed death 1 pathway. Eur J Immunol 35:1482–1490
21. Corcione A, Benvenuto F, Ferretti E et al (2006) Human mesenchymal stem cells modulate B-cell functions. Blood 107:367–372
22. Raffaghello L, Bianchi G, Bertolotto M et al (2008) Human mesenchymal stem cells inhibit neutrophil apoptosis: a model for neutrophil preservation in the bone marrow niche. Stem Cells 26:151–162
23. Pittenger MF, Mackay AM, Beck SC et al (1999) Multilineage potential of adult human mesenchymal stem cells. Science 284:143–147
24. Krause DS, Theise ND, Collector MI et al (2001) Multi-organ, multi-lineage engraftment by a single bone marrow-derived stem cell. Cell 105:369–377
25. Kotton DN, Fabian AJ, Mulligan RC (2005) Failure of bone marrow to reconstitute lung epithelium. Am J Respir Cell Mol Biol 33:328–334
26. Ortiz LA, Gambelli F, McBride C et al (2003) Mesenchymal stem cell engraftment in lung is enhanced in response to bleomycin exposure and ameliorates its fibrotic effects. Proc Natl Acad Sci USA 100:8407–8411
27. Ghofrani HA, Barst RJ, Benza RL et al (2009) Future perspectives for the treatment of pulmonary arterial hypertension. J Am Coll Cardiol 54:S108–S117

28. Meisel R, Brockers S, Heseler K et al (2011) Human but not murine multipotent mesenchymal stromal cells exhibit broad-spectrum antimicrobial effector function mediated by indoleamine 2,3-dioxygenase. Leukemia 25:648–654
29. Gregory CA, Ylostalo J, Prockop DJ (2005) Adult bone marrow stem/progenitor cells (MSCs) are preconditioned by microenvironmental "niches" in culture: a two-stage hypothesis for regulation of MSC fate. Sci STKE 2005:pe37
30. Lee RH, Hsu SC, Munoz J et al (2006) A subset of human rapidly self-renewing marrow stromal cells preferentially engraft in mice. Blood 107:2153–2161
31. Sarugaser R, Hanoun L, Keating A, Stanford WL, Davies JE (2009) Human mesenchymal stem cells self-renew and differentiate according to a deterministic hierarchy. PLoS One 4:e6498
32. Karp JM, Leng Teo GS (2009) Mesenchymal stem cell homing: the devil is in the details. Cell Stem Cell 4:206–216
33. Rombouts WJ, Ploemacher RE (2003) Primary murine MSC show highly efficient homing to the bone marrow but lose homing ability following culture. Leukemia 17:160–170
34. Rubio D, Garcia S, Paz MF et al (2008) Molecular characterization of spontaneous mesenchymal stem cell transformation. PLoS One 3:e1398
35. Das R, Jahr H, van Osch GJ, Farrell E (2010) The role of hypoxia in bone marrow-derived mesenchymal stem cells: considerations for regenerative medicine approaches. Tissue Eng Part B Rev 16:159–168
36. Stolzing A, Scutt A (2006) Effect of reduced culture temperature on antioxidant defences of mesenchymal stem cells. Free Radic Biol Med 41:326–338
37. Francois M, Copland IB, Yuan S, Romieu-Mourez R, Waller EK, Galipeau J (2012) Cryopreserved mesenchymal stromal cells display impaired immunosuppressive properties as a result of heat-shock response and impaired interferon-gamma licensing. Cytotherapy 14:147–152
38. Nauta AJ, Fibbe WE (2007) Immunomodulatory properties of mesenchymal stromal cells. Blood 110:3499–3506
39. Le Blanc K, Tammik L, Sundberg B, Haynesworth SE, Ringden O (2003) Mesenchymal stem cells inhibit and stimulate mixed lymphocyte cultures and mitogenic responses independently of the major histocompatibility complex. Scand J Immunol 57:11–20
40. Cho PS, Messina DJ, Hirsh EL et al (2008) Immunogenicity of umbilical cord tissue derived cells. Blood 111:430–438
41. Polchert D, Sobinsky J, Douglas G et al (2008) IFN-gamma activation of mesenchymal stem cells for treatment and prevention of graft versus host disease. Eur J Immunol 38:1745–1755
42. Griffin MD, Ritter T, Mahon BP (2010) Immunological aspects of allogeneic mesenchymal stem cell therapies. Hum Gene Ther 21:1641–1655
43. Suntharalingam G, Perry MR, Ward S et al (2006) Cytokine storm in a phase 1 trial of the anti-CD28 monoclonal antibody TGN1412. N Engl J Med 355:1018–1028
44. Hashimoto N, Jin H, Liu T, Chensue SW, Phan SH (2004) Bone marrow-derived progenitor cells in pulmonary fibrosis. J Clin Invest 113:243–252
45. Epperly MW, Guo H, Gretton JE, Greenberger JS (2003) Bone marrow origin of myofibroblasts in irradiation pulmonary fibrosis. Am J Respir Cell Mol Biol 29:213–224
46. Aguilar S, Scotton CJ, McNulty K et al (2009) Bone marrow stem cells expressing keratinocyte growth factor via an inducible lentivirus protects against bleomycin-induced pulmonary fibrosis. PLoS One 4:e8013
47. Jeong JO, Han JW, Kim JM et al (2011) Malignant tumor formation after transplantation of short-term cultured bone marrow mesenchymal stem cells in experimental myocardial infarction and diabetic neuropathy. Circ Res 108:1340–1347
48. Cogle CR, Theise ND, Fu D et al (2007) Bone marrow contributes to epithelial cancers in mice and humans as developmental mimicry. Stem Cells 25:1881–1887

49. Lazennec G, Jorgensen C (2008) Concise review: adult multipotent stromal cells and cancer: risk or benefit? Stem Cells 26:1387–1394
50. Tian LL, Yue W, Zhu F, Li S, Li W (2011) Human mesenchymal stem cells play a dual role on tumor cell growth in vitro and in vivo. J Cell Physiol 226:1860–1867
51. Gupta N, Krasnodembskaya A, Kapetanaki M et al (2012) Mesenchymal stem cells enhance survival and bacterial clearance in murine Escherichia coli pneumonia. Thorax 67:533–539
52. Krasnodembskaya A, Samarani G, Song Y et al (2012) Human mesenchymal stem cells reduce mortality and bacteremia in gram-negative sepsis in mice in part by enhancing the phagocytic activity of blood monocytes. Am J Physiol Lung Cell Mol Physiol 302:L1003–L1013

Stem Cells in Acute and Chronic Lung Injury: Building Evidence for Therapeutic Use

M. A. Antunes, P. R. M. Rocco, and P. Pelosi

Introduction

Beneficial effects of stem cells have been reported in experimental models of acute and chronic lung injury [1]. It has been suggested that both cell-to-cell contact and the release of soluble mediators by stem cells may play a role in promoting immune regulation and cell regeneration. Nevertheless, the mechanisms of stem cell action are not yet fully understood.

Lung diseases are characterized according to epithelial and/or endothelial and/or extracellular matrix damage with reactive fibrogenetic processes as well as structural changes in the airways [2]. Several stem cell sources and lineages have been used to treat lung diseases: Bone marrow-derived cells (whole bone marrow, hematopoietic and mesenchymal stem cells), adipose-derived stem cells, lung-derived stem cells, embryonic stem cells, induced pluripotent stem cells (iPSCs), and endothelial progenitor cells (EPCs) [3] (Table 1). Furthermore, for each type of lung disease, different resident and circulating progenitor cells are activated, producing different effects [2].

In this chapter, we describe and discuss the most recent advances in stem cell biology, focusing on: (1) The role of resident and circulating epithelial, endothelial, and mesenchymal progenitor cells in the lung; (2) the effects of stem cell

M. A. Antunes
Laboratory of Pulmonary Investigation, Carlos Chagas Filho Biophysics Institute, Federal University of Rio de Janeiro, Brazil

P. R. M. Rocco
Laboratory of Pulmonary Investigation, Carlos Chagas Filho Biophysics Institute, Federal University of Rio de Janeiro, Brazil

P. Pelosi (✉)
IRCCS AOU San Martino-IST, Department of Surgical Sciences and Integrated Diagnostics, University of Genoa, L.go R.Benzi, 8-16132, Genoa, Italy
E-mail: ppelosi@hotmail.com

J.-L. Vincent (Ed.), *Annual Update in Intensive Care and Emergency Medicine 2013*,
DOI 10.1007/978-3-642-35109-9_39,

therapy in the context of acute respiratory distress syndrome (ARDS), silicosis, emphysema, and asthma; and (3) advances in clinical trials of cell-based therapy.

Table 1 Summary of experimental studies using stem cell sources and lineages in pulmonary diseases

First Author [ref]	Protocol	Model	Cell Type	Route	Amount
Acute Lung Injury					
Ortiz, 2003 [10]	Bleomycin	C57BL/6	BM-MSC	i.v.	5×10^5
Mei, 2007 [17]	LPS i.t.	C57BL/6	BM-MSC+ ANGPT1	i.v.	2.5×10^5
Xu, 2007 [11]	Bleomycin	C57BL/6	BM-MSC	i.v.	5×10^5
Lam, 2008 [22]	Oleic acid i.v.	New Zealand White rabbits	EPC	i.v.	1×10^5
Aguillar, 2009 [18]	Bleomycin	C57BL/6	HSC/BM-MSC	i.v.	2 doses 5×10^5
Araújo, 2010 [19]	LPS i.t./i.p.	C57BL/6	BMDMC	i.v.	2×10^6
Iyer, 2010 [12]	LPS i.v.	C57BL/6	BM-MSC	i.v.	5×10^5
Lee, 2010 [13]	Bleomycin	Sprague-Dawley rats	BM-MSC	i.v.	1×10^6
Mao, 2010 [6]	LPS i.v.	Sprague-Dawley rats	EPC	i.v.	5×10^6
Mei, 2010 [14]	CLP	C57BL/6	BM-MSC	i.v.	2.5×10^5
Kim, 2011 [15]	LPS i.t.	ICM mice	UCB-MSC	i.t.	1×10^5
Brudecki, 2012 [23]	CLP	BALB/c	HSC	i.v.	5×10^5
Tai, 2012 [16]	LPS i.t.	Kunming mice	BM-MSC	i.v.	5×10^6
Silicosis					
Lassance, 2009 [25]	Silica i.t.	C57BL/6	BMDMC	i.t.	2×10^6
Maron-Gutierrez, 2011 [26]	Silica i.t.	C57BL/6	BMDMC	i.v.	2×10^6
Emphysema					
Zhen, 2010 [34]	Papain	Lewis rats	BM-MSC	i.v.	4×10^6
Schweitzer, 2011 [35]	Cigarette smoking injury	C57BL/6 or DBA/2J	AD-MSC	i.v.	5×10^5
Cruz, 2012 [33]	Elastase	C57BL/6	BMDMC	i.v.	2×10^6
Ingenito, 2012 [1]	Elastase	Sheep	LD-MSC	Intra-bronchial	5×10^7/site

Table 1 *Continued*

First Author [ref]	Protocol	Model	Cell Type	Route	Amount
Asthma					
Abreu, 2010 [43]	Ovalbumin	C57BL/6	BMDMC	i.v.	2×10^6
Bonfield, 2010 [42]	Ovalbumin	BALB/c	BM-MSC	i.v.	1×10^6
Nemeth, 2010 [46]	Ragweed	C57BL/6	BM-MSC	i.v.	7.5×10^5
Brown, 2011 [47]	IgE anti-dinitrophenyl	C57BL/6	BM-MSC	id	0.5×10^6
Goodwin, 2011 [44]	Ovalbumin	BALB/c, C57BL/6	BM-MSC	i.v.	2×10^6
Lee, 2011 [45]	Toluene diisocyanate	BALB/c	BM-MSC	i.v.	1×10^5

ANGPT1: transfection with the vasculoprotective gene angiopoietin 1; BMDMC: bone marrow-derived mononuclear cells; HSC: hematopoietic stem cells; EPC: endothelial progenitor cells; HSC: hematopoietic stem cells; UCB-MSC: umbilical cord blood-derived mesenchymal stem cells; BM-MSC: bone marrow derived mesenchymal stem cells; LD-MSC: lung derived mesenchymal stem cells; AD-MSC: adipose derived mesenchymal stem cells; CLP: cecal ligation puncture; LPS: lipopolysaccharide; i.p.: intraperitoneal; i.v.: intravenous; i.t.: intratracheal. All studies showed beneficial effects.

The Role of Resident and Circulating Progenitor Cells

The lung has defense mechanisms that are critical for survival, including replacement of injured or damaged cells [4]. There are two potential sources of cells for this reparative process: Resident and circulating (epithelial, endothelial and mesenchymal) progenitor cells. Additionally, circulating hematopoietic progenitor cells may play a relevant role (Fig. 1).

Resident lung epithelial progenitor cells encompass: (1) Basal cells from submucosal glands and ducts; (2) the basal epithelial layer of the cartilaginous proximal airway; (3) Clara cells from the bronchoalveolar duct junctions; (4) and type 2 epithelial cells. Resident basal and progenitor epithelial cells, as well as the basal epithelial layer of the cartilaginous proximal airway, are capable of differentiating into all airway epithelial cell types. In addition to a capacity for self-renewal, these cells divide slowly and express markers of early epithelial differentiation. Clara cells act as transit-amplifying cells after injury to ciliated airway epithelial cells. They also present a low proliferative frequency in the steady state, and are broadly distributed throughout the bronchiolar epithelium. Finally, Clara cells contribute to specialized tissue function. In the alveoli, surfactant-producing type 2 alveolar epithelial cells are well recognized as progenitors for type 1 alveolar epithelial cells [4].

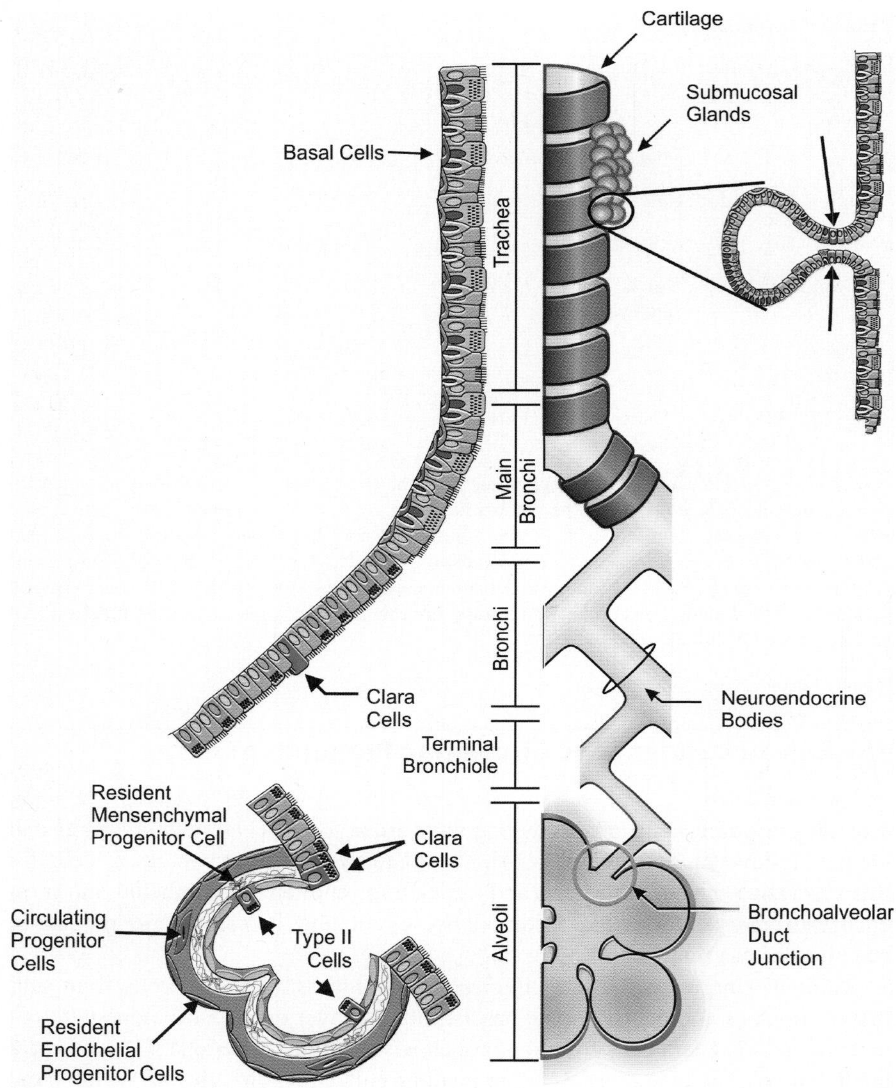

Fig. 1 Lung progenitor cells. Resident (basal cells, Clara cells, epithelial type II cells, mesenchymal progenitor and endothelial progenitor) and circulating progenitor (mesenchymal, epithelial and endothelial progenitors) cells are highlighted in red on the schematic figure. Putative niches of resident progenitor cells are indicated with black arrows (right-side of the figure)

Circulating epithelial progenitor cells migrate to the lungs and contribute to the re-epithelization of the airway and re-establishment of the pseudo-stratified epithelium in the presence of damage. Resident EPCs are located in the lung microvasculature, where it is possible to find at least two different subtypes of cells: (1) Originators of blood vessel endothelial cells; and (2) lymphatic endothelial cells [5]. Circulating EPCs, a specific subtype of hematopoietic stem cells, migrate from the bone marrow or peripheral blood to the damaged lung contributing to the repair of injured endothelium and to the formation of new blood vessels [6, 7].

Resident mesenchymal progenitor cells are preferentially localized in the corners of the alveoli, close to type II alveolar epithelial cells. They have the ability to secrete keratinocyte growth factor (KGF), an important modulator of epithelial cell proliferation and differentiation [8]. However, there is little information regarding the associations of these local mesenchymal progenitors with other resident somatic cells and their potential for therapeutic use.

Circulating mesenchymal progenitor cells (fibrocytes) are involved in the pathogenesis of fibrosis [9]. The role of circulating mesenchymal progenitor cells is controversial, but they might contribute to the regeneration of lung after injury. Circulating hematopoietic progenitor cells derive from the bone marrow. Once homed to the lung, they can differentiate into a variety of inflammatory (eosinophils, basophils, and mast cells) and/or structural cells (fibrocytes and vascular endothelial cells).

Stem Cell Research in Pulmonary Diseases

Acute Respiratory Distress Syndrome

The morbidity and mortality associated with ARDS is still high, despite recent advances in therapeutic strategies. Experimental studies have shown that stem cells may contribute to lung repair and reduce lung edema, alveolar epithelial cell permeability, and local as well as systemic inflammatory response.

Bone marrow-derived mononuclear cells, mesenchymal stem cells (MSCs) from different sources (bone marrow, adipose tissue, umbilical cord), as well as iPSCs have been used in experimental models of lung injury. Pulmonary damage leads to the release of several attractant factors, including granulocyte colony-stimulating factor (G-CSF), granulocyte-macrophage stimulating-factor (GM-CSF) [10], and modulated stromal cell-derived factor (SDF)-1 and its receptor CXCR4 [11], with mobilization of bone marrow cells to the lung. Bone marrow cells act on: (1) Restoration of the systemic redox imbalance by regulating the cysteine and glutathione disulfide redox state [12]; (2) modulation of factors related to angiogenesis, fibrosis, and inflammation (interleukin [IL]-1β, IL-6, IL-8, IL-10, tumor necrosis factor [TNF]-α, macrophage inflammatory protein [MIP]-2, myeloperoxidase [MPO], vascular endothelial growth factor [VEGF], transforming growth factor [TGF]-β, inducible nitric oxide synthase [iNOS], nitrate and nitrite) [13–16]; (3) the reprogramming of macrophages by releasing prostaglandin E(2) and reducing lung inflammation through an increase in IL-10; and (4) reduction of organ dysfunction biomarkers [14] (Fig. 2). These beneficial effects take place despite relatively low levels of engraftment, suggesting a pivotal role of paracrine effects.

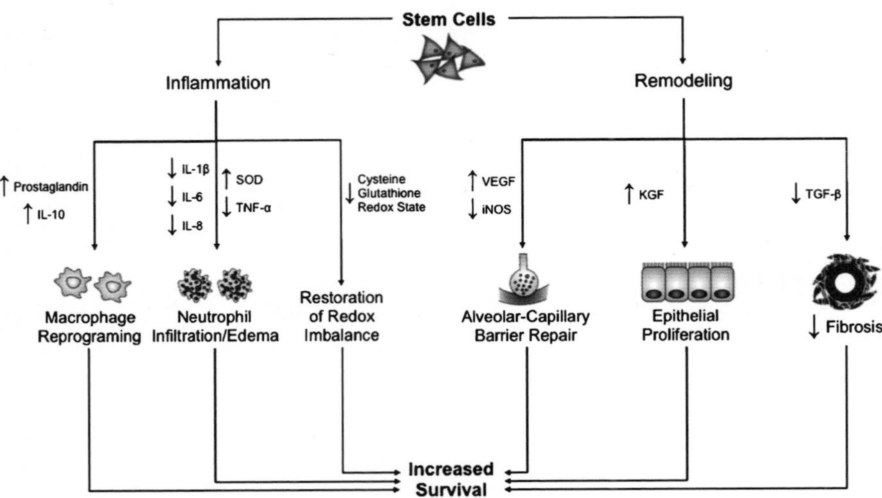

Fig. 2 Stem cells in acute respiratory distress syndrome (ARDS). Summary of described effects of stem cells in experimental studies in ARDS. IL: interleukin; SOD: superoxide dismutase; TNF-α: tumor necrosis factor-α; VEGF: vascular endothelial growth factor; iNOS: inducible nitric oxide synthase; KGF: keratinocyte growth factor; TGF-β: transforming growth factor-β

Bone marrow-derived MSCs also serve as a vehicle for gene therapy. Angiopoietin-1 (Ang1) is a critical factor for endothelial survival and vascular stabilization via the inhibition of endothelial permeability and leukocyte-endothelium interactions. MSC cell-based angiopoietin-1 gene therapy has been reported to reduce alveolar-capillary permeability [17] in lung injury through enhanced expression of KGF and proliferation of endogenous type II pneumocytes [18].

Even though MSCs are widely employed in experimental studies, they present limitations, such as culture conditions that are detrimental for cell transplantation and risk of contamination. Based on these drawbacks, and because ARDS patients require early treatment, bone marrow-derived mononuclear cells, including both hematopoietic and mesenchymal (non-hematopoietic) stem cell types, have been used in some experimental models of lung injury. The potential advantages of bone marrow-derived mononuclear cells are: (1) Easy and safe administration on the day of harvesting; (2) expression of several genes involved in inflammatory response and chemotaxis; (3) lower cost as compared to MSCs [19]; and (4) cellular cross-talk among the multiple cell types [20]. In a lipopolysaccharide (LPS)-induced acute lung injury (ALI) model, therapy with bone marrow-derived mononuclear cells reduced lung inflammation and remodeling, hastened epithelial and endothelial repair [19], and improved lung function. Additionally, the beneficial effects of bone marrow-derived mononuclear cells were more evident in extrapulmonary compared to pulmonary ALI because of the different balance between pro- and anti-inflammatory cytokines and growth factors associated with the etiology of lung disease [19].

In critically ill patients, levels of circulating EPCs are increased and inversely correlated with organ dysfunction and death [21]. Therefore, EPC transplantation has been used in oleic acid-induced lung injury, leading to attenuation of endothelial dysfunction in the pulmonary artery and reduction of iNOS, neutrophil infiltration, water content, hyaline membrane formation, and hemorrhage [22]. In endotoxin-induced lung injury, EPCs reduced pro-inflammatory cytokines, adhesion molecules, iNOS, endothelin-1, and MPO activity, as well as upregulating IL-10, VEGF, and the antioxidant enzyme, superoxide dismutase, decreasing pulmonary edema and neutrophil infiltration, and promoting alveolar-capillary membrane repair [6, 7]. Moreover, EPCs acted in the late phase of lung injury, reconstituting the immunocompetence and phagocytic capacity of peritoneal macrophages [23].

Silicosis

Silicosis is a pneumoconiosis that involves formation of nodules and destruction of large areas of the lung, leading to impaired gas exchange and pulmonary function, which may result in respiratory failure. Despite extensive efforts, no available therapy has been shown to halt or efficiently reverse this disorder [24].

Cell-based therapy has been used in experimental models of silicosis, with beneficial effects on lung morphofunction, inflammation and fibrosis [25, 26]. In a recent study, the early intravenous injection of bone marrow-derived mononuclear cells, immediately after silica administration, minimized lung function impairment and attenuated fibrosis in both nodules (granuloma) and lung parenchyma. These effects were associated with a reduction in IL-β, IL-1α, IL-1 receptor antagonist (IL-1ra), and IL-1 receptor 1, as well as TGF-β [26]. Even though stem cells reduced both lung inflammation and remodeling, they were not able to clear silica particles from the lung, perpetuating the inflammatory and fibrogenic processes. Therefore, we hypothesized that intratracheal instillation of bone marrow-derived mononuclear cells may lead to better effects compared to intravenous administration. In this context, bone marrow-derived mononuclear cells resulted in improved lung mechanics and a significant reduction in the area of granulomatous nodules in a model of silicosis at day 30, but this beneficial effect did not last until day 60 [25]. The absence of therapeutic efficacy at the late phase of silicosis may have been a consequence of the recurring cycle of macrophage phagocytosis and cell death yielding a release of intracellular silica that was engulfed by other macrophages, perpetuating the fibrogenic process [25] (Fig. 3). Together, these data suggest that cell-based therapy may be a promising therapeutic approach for silicosis as a multiple-dose treatment.

Emphysema

Emphysema, defined as irreversible destruction of the alveoli, is one of the leading causes of death in the world. It is characterized by persistent airflow limitation that is usually progressive and associated with an elevated chronic inflammatory re-

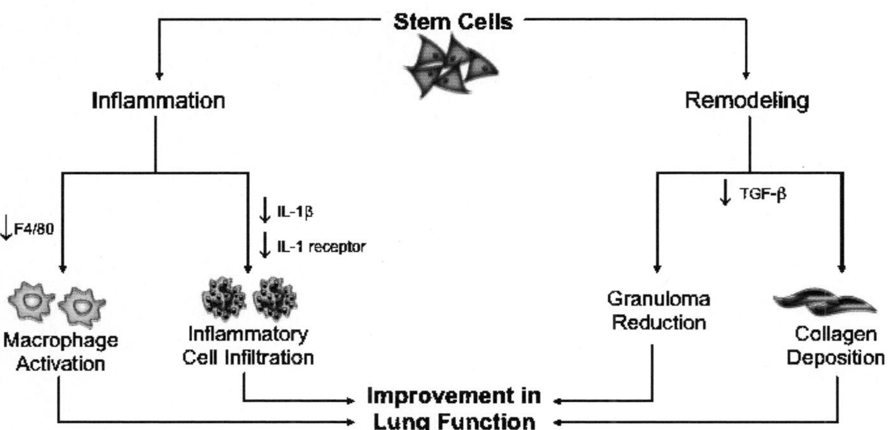

Fig. 3 Stem cells in silicosis. Summary of described effects of stem cells in experimental studies in silicosis. F4/80: extracellular antigen present in mature murine macrophages; IL: interleukin; TGF-β: transforming growth factor-β

sponse, resulting in loss of alveolar septa and enlargement of distal airspace to the terminal bronchiole. In spite of the advances in the prevention and treatment of emphysema symptoms, no effective therapy has been discovered.

Circulating hematopoietic stem cells and EPCs are reduced in emphysema patients as a result of bone marrow impairment, which may explain the low tissue regenerative capacity [27]. Based on the aforementioned, studies have investigated factors that may stimulate the migration of bone marrow progenitor cells to emphysematous lung. In experimental emphysema, hepatocyte growth factor (HGF) has been observed to recruit EPCs to injured lungs, activating endothelial cell migration and proliferation, inducing angiogenesis and re-epithelization [28]. Similarly, adrenomedullin, a potent vasodilator peptide the receptor of which is expressed in the basal cells of airway epithelium and type II pneumocytes, is involved in lung epithelial regeneration, thus improving lung function [29]. Interestingly, factors that mobilize bone marrow cells to injured tissues, including G-CSF and GM-CSF, failed to restore emphysema-like lesions [30]. Together, these data suggest that the factors responsible for the stimulation of homing, proliferation, and differentiation of bone marrow cells may vary according to the pulmonary disease.

Stem cells may have different therapeutic effects on the pathways associated with emphysema pathophysiology (Fig. 4), such as apoptosis, inflammation, and oxidative stress. Intra-bone marrow injection of allogeneic bone marrow cells prevented the progression of emphysema and improved the structure of the lung [31]. Hematopoietic stem cells have been proposed to be a promising candidate for the combination of cell and gene therapies in emphysema, because these cells promote sustained expression of α1-antitrypsin in lung with no activation of cellular or humoral immune response [32]. Bone marrow-derived mononuclear cells reduced lung inflammation and fibrosis, improving lung mechanics and histology, as well as decreasing right ventricle area and thickness in experimental emphysema. These

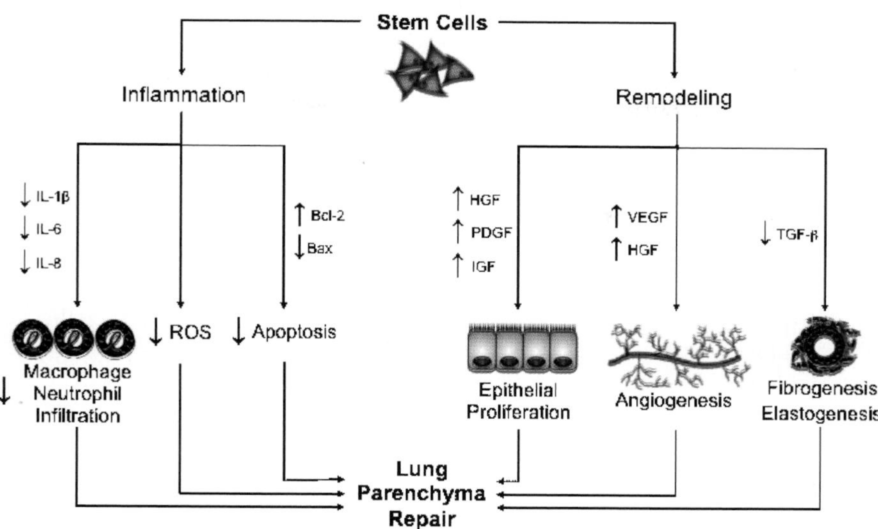

Fig. 4 Stem cells in emphysema. Summary of described effects of stem cells in experimental studies in emphysema. ROS: reactive oxygen species; IL: interleukin; Bcl-2: anti-apoptotic protein; Bax (or Bcl-2-associated X protein): pro-apoptotic protein; HGF: hepatocyte-derived growth factor; PDGF: platelet-derived growth factor; IGF: insulin-like growth factor; VEGF: vascular endothelial growth factor; TGF-β: transforming growth factor-β

effects were associated with the release of several growth factors related to emphysema dysfunction: Platelet-derived growth factor (PDGF), insulin-like growth factor (IGF), TGF-β, and VEGF [33]. The most widely investigated stem cells in emphysema are MSCs [34]. These cells are able to reduce inflammatory mediators, migrate to the lung, engraft, and differentiate into type 2 alveolar epithelial cells; they also inhibit epithelial and endothelial cell apoptosis, stimulate angiogenesis, and reduce oxidative stress [34]. Furthermore, MSCs from other sources may apparently be good candidates for emphysema treatment, including adipose tissue-derived [35] and lung tissue-derived MSCs [1]. Adipose tissue represents an ideal source for obtaining stem cells, because adipose tissue-derived stem cells are abundant, easily harvested with minimal morbidity, and may be transplanted safely and efficaciously. Adipose tissue-derived stem cells are thought to be efficient in emphysema, since this cell type appears to selectively induce HGF expression in injured lung tissue, which favors alveolar and vascular regeneration, enhances epithelial cell proliferation, and promotes angiogenesis in pulmonary vasculature, leading to restoration of lung function. Moreover, adipose tissue-derived stem cells seem to have beneficial effects on pulmonary and systemic injuries induced by cigarette smoke. These cells reduce inflammation, apoptosis, airspace enlargement, restore the cachexia induced by cigarette smoke exposure, and protect lungs by stimulating bone marrow hematopoietic progenitor cell function previously suppressed by cigarette smoke [35]. Adipose tissue-derived stem cells have been detected in the lung parenchyma and large airways after up to 21 days, which may explain their sustained beneficial effects. MSCs derived from lung tissue are highly proliferative, clonogenic mesenchymal cells in adult lung parenchyma, but their benefits may be limited in emphysema, since they increase cell infiltration, as well as collagen and elastin contents, bringing no improvement in lung function [1].

Regardless of the source of stem cells, studies show that the number of cells engrafted and differentiated is minimal, suggesting that the release of paracrine mediators may be responsible for the reduction in lung inflammation and remodeling [33, 36]. Recent evidence shows that the reconstitution of fibroblast capacity to produce extracellular matrix components through stem cells is mediated in part by phosphatidylinositol 3-kinase/Akt pathway [36]. However, the exact mechanisms require clarification.

Asthma

Asthma is a disabling chronic pulmonary inflammatory disease affecting more than 300 million people worldwide. The pathogenesis of asthma is characterized by airway and lung parenchyma inflammation, infiltration of mast cells, basophils, eosinophils, monocytes, and T helper type 2 lymphocytes, stimulating the production of allergen-specific IgE. Following injurious stimuli, rapid repair mechanisms involving proliferation and differentiation of resident progenitor and stem cell pools are necessary in order to maintain lung architecture. However, the ability of the epithelium to properly repair and regenerate [37] is reduced in asthma. Moreover, circulating mesenchymal progenitor cells (fibrocytes) acquire α-smooth muscle actin phenotype, differentiate into myofibroblasts, and have been associated with chronic inflammation and excessive collagen deposition [38], impairing lung function [39]. After allergen challenge, eosinophils stimulate the homing of EPCs, which may lead to angiogenesis [40]. Cell-based therapy would likely be a reasonable strategy to hasten the repair process and attenuate inflammatory and remodeling responses in asthma [41–43]. In this line, both MSCs [44, 45] and bone marrow-derived mononuclear cells [43] are able to reduce eosinophil infiltration, the amount of collagen deposition, and smooth muscle actin content in lung tissue [45], cytokine and growth factor response in bronchoalveolar lavage (BAL) fluid (IL-4, IL-5, IL-13, interferon [IFN]-γ, keratinocyte-derived chemokine and MIP-1α) [42]. Finally, bone marrow-derived mononuclear cells attenuate airway hyperresponsiveness to methacoline [44, 45]. Some mechanisms seem to be mediated by MSCs in asthma (Fig. 5): Modulation of iNOS [42]; systemic isotype-specific IgE production [46]; mast cell suppression caused by up-regulation of cyclooxygenase (COX)2 [47]; increase in the number of regulatory T cells (T-reg) after challenge, because of increased TGF-β-induced T-reg differentiation [46]; and promotion of a Th1 phenotype in antigen-specific CD4T lymphocytes to inhibit Th2-mediated allergic airway inflammation through a process dependent on IFN-γ [44]. Nevertheless, the mechanisms of action of different cell sources in asthma remain con-

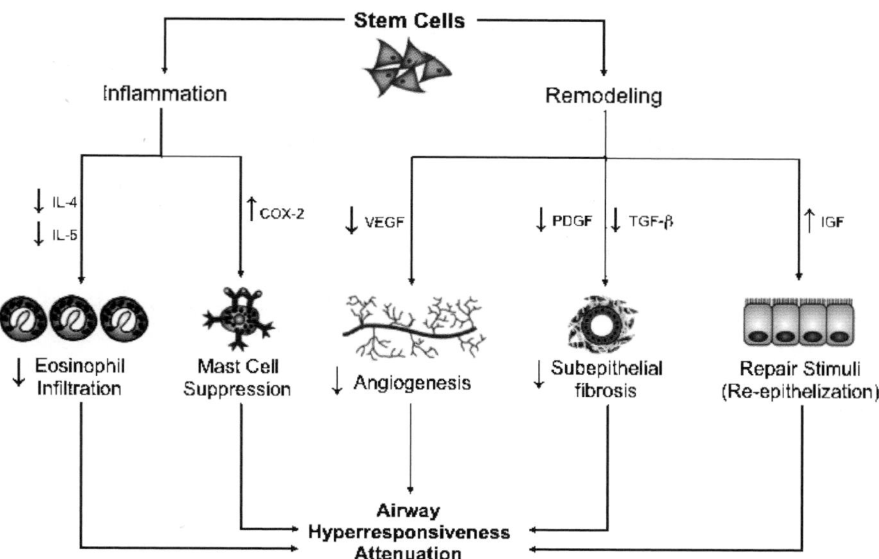

Fig. 5 Stem cells in asthma. Summary of described effects of stem cells in experimental studies in asthma. IL: interleukin; COX-2: cyclooxygenase-2; VEGF: vascular endothelial growth factor; PDGF: platelet-derived growth factor; TGF-β: transforming growth factor-β; IGF: insulin-like growth factor

troversial. For instance, whole bone marrow cell transplantation reduces TGF-β, whereas MSCs increase TGF-β production in allergen-challenged lungs, but both result in reduced inflammation and fibrosis [43, 46].

Clinical Trial Advances in Cell-Based Therapy

Clinical trials have been started to test the safety and the possible effectiveness of stem cells administration to treat lung diseases. In chronic obstructive pulmonary disease (COPD)/emphysema, four clinical trials are currently recruiting or completed. In Brazil, a safety study of bone marrow-derived cell infusion in 4 patients with advanced COPD (stage IV dyspnea) has been published recently [48]. The investigators performed autologous bone marrow-derived cell transplantation and administered G-CSF immediately prior to bone marrow harvest. During a 12-month follow-up, patients reported a significant improvement in quality of life and remained clinically stable with no significant adverse effects. In the USA, a phase II, multicenter, randomized, double-blind, placebo-controlled study was designed to evaluate the safety and efficacy of intravenous infusion of PROCHYMAL™ (*ex vivo* cultured adult human MSCs) in moderate to severe COPD patients (ClinicalTrials.gov ID: NCT01510431). This study has been completed, and has established a 2-year follow-up to test the safety of the transplantation and a 1-year follow-up to evaluate pulmonary function, exercise capability and quality of life. So far, no data have been published. In Mexico, a non-randomized study is currently underway to evaluate the safety and efficacy of autologous adipose-derived stem cell transplantation in GOLD III and IV patients (ClinicalTrials.gov ID: NCT01559051). In a 6-month follow-up, the authors confirmed that the therapy was safe, but lung function and quality of life results remain to be published. In the Netherlands, a phase I study to test the safety and feasibility of administration of MSCs prior to lung volume reduction surgery for severe pulmonary emphysema (GOLD III patients) is currently recruiting patients (ClinicalTrials.gov ID: NCT01306513). This study is estimated to be completed at the end of 2013.

Another Brazilian trial at the Federal University of Rio de Janeiro was performed in patients with chronic and accelerated silicosis. A non-randomized, phase I study was performed to evaluate the safety of intrabronchial instillation of autologous bone marrow derived mononuclear cells. Each patient received 2×10^7 bone marrow-derived cells labeled with 99mTc for posterior tracing. This study analyzed lung function and quality of life data. Some data were presented at the American Thoracic Society meeting in 2010 and 2011 [49, 50], showing the safety of the intrabronchial route for cell administration in patients with silicosis.

Conclusion

The therapeutic use of stem cells for treatment of different lung diseases is open to controversy [2]. Some issues still require clarification: (1) The short and long term beneficial and adverse effects of stem cell therapy in lung diseases, prioritizing patient safety; (2) the efficacy of a single cellular population to regenerate the entire organ remains low, due to surface size and complexity of lung structure. Therefore, studies have to be performed to address the following issues: (1) Identification of resident cell populations that respond to lung damage and of exogenous cells that are able to ameliorate lung disease; (2) the best route of stem cell administration, based on the etiology of lung damage; (3) the dose and timing of cell administration; (4) the identification of specific lineage markers for lung stem and progenitor cells.

More knowledge is required about the therapeutic potential of stem cells and other cell therapies in experimental and clinical trials before we can safely move towards clinical application.

References

1. Ingenito EP, Tsai L, Murthy S, Tyagi S, Mazan M, Hoffman A (2012) Autologous lung-derived mesenchymal stem cell transplantation in experimental emphysema. Cell Transplant 21:175–189
2. Garcia O, Carraro G, Navarro S et al (2012) Cell-based therapies for lung disease. Br Med Bull 101:147–161

3. Abreu SC, Antunes MA, Pelosi P, Morales MM, Rocco PR (2011) Mechanisms of cellular therapy in respiratory diseases. Intensive Care Med 37:1421–1431
4. Weiss DJ, Bertoncello I, Borok Z et al (2011) Stem cells and cell therapies in lung biology and lung diseases. Proc Am Thorac Soc 8:223–272
5. Schniedermann J, Rennecke M, Buttler K et al (2010) Mouse lung contains endothelial progenitors with high capacity to form blood and lymphatic vessels. BMC Cell Biol 11:50
6. Mao M, Wang SN, Lv XJ, Wang Y, Xu JC (2010) Intravenous delivery of bone marrow-derived endothelial progenitor cells improves survival and attenuates lipopolysaccharide-induced lung injury in rats. Shock 34:196–204
7. Gao X, Chen W, Liang Z, Chen L (2011) Autotransplantation of circulating endothelial progenitor cells protects against lipopolysaccharide-induced acute lung injury in rabbit. Int Immunopharmacol 11:1584–1590
8. Badri L, Walker NM, Ohtsuka T et al (2011) Epithelial interactions and local engraftment of lung-resident mesenchymal stem cells. Am J Respir Cell Mol Biol 45:809–816
9. Fujiwara A, Kobayashi H, Masuya M et al (2012) Correlation between circulating fibrocytes, and activity and progression of interstitial lung diseases. Respirology 17:693–698
10. Ortiz LA, Gambelli F, McBride C et al (2003) Mesenchymal stem cell engraftment in lung is enhanced in response to bleomycin exposure and ameliorates its fibrotic effects. Proc Natl Acad Sci USA 100:8407–8411
11. Xu J, Mora A, Shim H, Stecenko A, Brigham KL, Rojas M (2007) Role of the SDF-1/CXCR4 axis in the pathogenesis of lung injury and fibrosis. Am J Respir Cell Mol Biol 37:291–299
12. Iyer SS, Torres-Gonzalez E, Neujahr DC et al (2010) Effect of bone marrow-derived mesenchymal stem cells on endotoxin-induced oxidation of plasma cysteine and glutathione in mice. Stem Cells Int 2010:868076
13. Lee SH, Jang AS, Kim YE et al (2010) Modulation of cytokine and nitric oxide by mesenchymal stem cell transfer in lung injury/fibrosis. Respir Res 11:16
14. Mei SH, Haitsma JJ, Dos Santos CC et al (2010) Mesenchymal stem cells reduce inflammation while enhancing bacterial clearance and improving survival in sepsis. Am J Respir Crit Care Med 182:1047–1057
15. Kim ES, Chang YS, Choi SJ et al (2011) Intratracheal transplantation of human umbilical cord blood-derived mesenchymal stem cells attenuates Escherichia coli-induced acute lung injury in mice. Respir Res 12:108
16. Tai WL, Dong ZX, Zhang DD, Wang DH (2012) Therapeutic effect of intravenous bone marrow-derived mesenchymal stem cell transplantation on early-stage LPS-induced acute lung injury in mice. Nan Fang Yi Ke Da Xue Xue Bao 32:283–290
17. Mei SH, McCarter SD, Deng Y, Parker CH, Liles WC, Stewart DJ (2007) Prevention of LPS-induced acute lung injury in mice by mesenchymal stem cells overexpressing angiopoietin 1. PLoS Med 4:e269
18. Aguilar S, Scotton CJ, McNulty K et al (2009) Bone marrow stem cells expressing keratinocyte growth factor via an inducible lentivirus protects against bleomycin-induced pulmonary fibrosis. PLoS One 4:e8013
19. Araujo IM, Abreu SC, Maron-Gutierrez T et al (2010) Bone marrow-derived mononuclear cell therapy in experimental pulmonary and extrapulmonary acute lung injury. Crit Care Med 38:1733–1741
20. Rafii S, Lyden D (2003) Therapeutic stem and progenitor cell transplantation for organ vascularization and regeneration. Nat Med 9:702–712
21. Cribbs SK, Sutcliffe DJ, Taylor WR et al (2012) Circulating endothelial progenitor cells inversely associate with organ dysfunction in sepsis. Intensive Care Med 38:429–436
22. Lam CF, Liu YC, Hsu JK et al (2008) Autologous transplantation of endothelial progenitor cells attenuates acute lung injury in rabbits. Anesthesiology 108:392–401
23. Brudecki L, Ferguson DA, Yin D, Lesage GD, McCall CE, El Gazzar M (2012) Hematopoietic stem-progenitor cells restore immunoreactivity and improve survival in late sepsis. Infect Immun 80:602–611

24. Leung CC, Yu IT, Chen W (2012) Silicosis. Lancet 379:2008–2018
25. Lassance RM, Prota LF, Maron-Gutierrez T et al (2009) Intratracheal instillation of bone marrow-derived cell in an experimental model of silicosis. Respir Physiol Neurobiol 169:227–233
26. Maron-Gutierrez T, Castiglione RC, Xisto DG et al (2011) Bone marrow-derived mononuclear cell therapy attenuates silica-induced lung fibrosis. Eur Respir J 37:1217–1225
27. Huertas A, Testa U, Riccioni R et al (2010) Bone marrow-derived progenitors are greatly reduced in patients with severe COPD and low-BMI. Respir Physiol Neurobiol 170:23–31
28. Ishizawa K, Kubo H, Yamada M et al (2004) Hepatocyte growth factor induces angiogenesis in injured lungs through mobilizing endothelial progenitor cells. Biochem Biophys Res Commun 324:276–280
29. Murakami S, Nagaya N, Itoh T et al (2005) Adrenomedullin regenerates alveoli and vasculature in elastase-induced pulmonary emphysema in mice. Am J Respir Crit Care Med 172:581–589
30. Ishikawa T, Aoshiba K, Yokohori N, Nagai A (2006) Macrophage colony-stimulating factor aggravates rather than regenerates emphysematous lungs in mice. Respiration 73:538–545
31. Adachi Y, Oyaizu H, Taketani S et al (2006) Treatment and transfer of emphysema by a new bone marrow transplantation method from normal mice to Tsk mice and vice versa. Stem Cells 24:2071–2077
32. Wilson AA, Kwok LW, Hovav AH et al (2008) Sustained expression of alpha1-antitrypsin after transplantation of manipulated hematopoietic stem cells. Am J Respir Cell Mol Biol 39:133–141
33. Cruz FF, Antunes MA, Abreu SC et al (2012) Protective effects of bone marrow mononuclear cell therapy on lung and heart in an elastase-induced emphysema model. Respir Physiol Neurobiol 182:26–36
34. Zhen G, Xue Z, Zhao J et al (2010) Mesenchymal stem cell transplantation increases expression of vascular endothelial growth factor in papain-induced emphysematous lungs and inhibits apoptosis of lung cells. Cytotherapy 12:605–614
35. Schweitzer KS, Johnstone BH, Garrison J et al (2011) Adipose stem cell treatment in mice attenuates lung and systemic injury induced by cigarette smoking. Am J Respir Crit Care Med 183:215–225
36. Kim EK, Lee JH, Jeong HC et al (2012) Impaired colony-forming capacity of circulating endothelial progenitor cells in patients with emphysema. Tohoku J Exp Med 227:321–331
37. Allakhverdi Z, Comeau MR, Smith DE et al (2009) CD34+ hemopoietic progenitor cells are potent effectors of allergic inflammation. J Allergy Clin Immunol 123:472–478
38. Mehrad B, Burdick MD, Zisman DA, Keane MP, Belperio JA, Strieter RM (2007) Circulating peripheral blood fibrocytes in human fibrotic interstitial lung disease. Biochem Biophys Res Commun 353:104–108
39. Schmidt M, Sun G, Stacey MA, Mori L, Mattoli S (2003) Identification of circulating fibrocytes as precursors of bronchial myofibroblasts in asthma. J Immunol 171:380–389
40. Asosingh K, Swaidani S, Aronica M, Erzurum SC (2007) Th1- and Th2-dependent endothelial progenitor cell recruitment and angiogenic switch in asthma. J Immunol 178:6482–6494
41. Doyle TM, Ellis R, Park HJ, Inman MD, Sehmi R (2011) Modulating progenitor accumulation attenuates lung angiogenesis in a mouse model of asthma. Eur Respir J 38:679–687
42. Bonfield TL, Koloze M, Lennon DP, Zuchowski B, Yang SE, Caplan AI (2010) Human mesenchymal stem cells suppress chronic airway inflammation in the murine ovalbumin asthma model. Am J Physiol Lung Cell Mol Physiol 299:L760–L770
43. Abreu SC, Antunes MA, Maron-Gutierrez T et al (2011) Effects of bone marrow-derived mononuclear cells on airway and lung parenchyma remodeling in a murine model of chronic allergic inflammation. Respir Physiol Neurobiol 175:153–163
44. Goodwin M, Sueblinvong V, Eisenhauer P et al (2011) Bone marrow-derived mesenchymal stromal cells inhibit Th2-mediated allergic airways inflammation in mice. Stem Cells 29:1137–1148

45. Lee SH, Jang AS, Kwon JH, Park SK, Won JH, Park CS (2011) Mesenchymal stem cell transfer suppresses airway remodeling in a toluene diisocyanate-induced murine asthma model. Allergy Asthma Immunol Res 3:205–211
46. Nemeth K, Keane-Myers A, Brown JM et al (2010) Bone marrow stromal cells use TGF-beta to suppress allergic responses in a mouse model of ragweed-induced asthma. Proc Natl Acad Sci USA 107:5652–5657
47. Brown JM, Nemeth K, Kushnir-Sukhov NM, Metcalfe DD, Mezey E (2011) Bone marrow stromal cells inhibit mast cell function via a COX2-dependent mechanism. Clin Exp Allergy 41:526–534
48. Ribeiro-Paes JT, Bilaqui A, Greco OT et al (2011) Unicentric study of cell therapy in chronic obstructive pulmonary disease/pulmonary emphysema. Int J Chron Obstruct Pulmon Dis 6:63–71
49. Loivos LP, Lima MA, Szklo A et al (2010) Intrabronchial instillation of bone marrow derived mononuclear cells in silicotic patients. Am J Respir Crit Care Med 181:A1595 (abst)
50. Sergio AL, Souza LPL, Lima MA et al (2011) Lung perfusion scintigraphy in silicotic patients treated with intrabronchial instillation of bone marrow derived mononuclear cells. Am J Respir Crit Care Med 183:A5212 (abst)

Restoration of Alveolar Epithelial Function as a Therapeutic Strategy for Acute Lung Injury

R. Herrero, C. Sanchez, and J. A. Lorente

Introduction

Acute lung injury (ALI), and its severe form, acute respiratory distress syndrome (ARDS), is a common disorder with a high mortality rate (40 %). Only two supportive strategies have shown to improve survival in patients with ALI/ARDS, namely lung protective ventilation that reduces stretch of the lungs and a fluid conservative strategy [1, 2]. Unfortunately, molecular-based therapies aimed at improving the outcome of these patients have so far been unsuccessful.

ALI/ARDS is initiated by direct lung injury or by systemic inflammatory processes, and it is characterized by diffuse alveolar damage with alterations of the alveolar-capillary membrane. These alterations lead to flooding of the alveolar airspaces by protein-rich edema, which is responsible for the radiographic pulmonary infiltrates and the severe arterial hypoxemia that clinically characterize this syndrome [3]. Remarkably, epithelial damage is more prominent than endothelial damage in the pulmonary alveoli of patients who die with ALI/ARDS [4], suggesting that a better understanding of the mechanisms responsible for the alveolar epithelial injury and repair is important in order to develop more effective therapeutic strategies in ALI.

R. Herrero (✉)
Unidad De Cuidados Intensivos, Fundacion Para La Investigacion Biomedica, Hospital Universitario De Getafe, Ciber De Enfermedades Respiratorias, Universidad Europea De Madrid, Getafe, Madrid, Spain
Email: raquelher@hotmail.com

C. Sanchez
Unidad De Cuidados Intensivos, Fundacion Para La Investigacion Biomedica, Hospital Universitario De Getafe, Ciber De Enfermedades Respiratorias, Universidad Europea De Madrid, Getafe, Madrid, Spain

J. A. Lorente
Unidad De Cuidados Intensivos, Fundacion Para La Investigacion Biomedica, Hospital Universitario De Getafe, Ciber De Enfermedades Respiratorias, Universidad Europea De Madrid, Getafe, Madrid, Spain

J.-L. Vincent (Ed.), *Annual Update in Intensive Care and Emergency Medicine 2013*,
DOI 10.1007/978-3-642-35109-9_40, © Springer-Verlag Berlin Heidelberg 2013

Role of the Alveolar Epithelial Injury in ALI

The landmark studies by Bachofen and Weibel identified important alveolar epithelial damage with predominant injury to alveolar epithelial cells in patients who had died with ARDS. Although injury to the lung microvasculature was also detected, the endothelial lesions were not as prominent as the epithelial disruption [4]. The alveolar epithelium preserves the proper water and solute content of the epithelial lining fluid at the alveolar air-liquid interface, which is critical for adequate gas exchange and host defense against viral and bacterial pathogens. If endothelial permeability is the only function altered in the lungs, the extravascular fluid in the interstitial and alveolar spaces is eventually cleared and the lungs heal without fibrosis. In contrast, substantial injury of the alveolar epithelium results in an increase in protein permeability and an impairment of the alveolar fluid clearance and alveolar protein clearance (the ability of alveolar epithelium to remove pulmonary edema fluid and to clear proteins from the airspaces, respectively). These alterations lead to alveolar flooding with high-molecular weight proteins and to a higher likelihood of disordered repair with the consequent worsening of gas exchange [5].

Alveolar epithelial damage has other important consequences, such as the promotion of inflammatory cell accumulation in injured alveoli, the facilitation of septic shock in patients with bacterial pneumonia and the development of pulmonary fibrosis. These events can result in more prolonged mechanical ventilation and the development of multiple organ dysfunction syndrome, which is frequently the cause of death in these patients [5]. Treatments focused on decreasing the initial epithelial injury and accelerating the repair process of the alveolar epithelium may, therefore, become one of the key approaches for improving the outcome of patients with ARDS.

Protein-Rich Edema Formation in ALI

Increased permeability to proteins of the alveolar epithelium and decreased clearance of alveolar fluid and proteins result in the formation of protein-rich edema in the alveolar airspaces.

Increased Epithelial Permeability to Proteins

The lung alveolar epithelium is an extremely tight barrier that restricts the passage of proteins and water from the interstitium into the alveolar spaces. This restricted passage is due to the presence of tight junctions between adjacent alveolar epithelial cells, rendering the epithelial barrier much less permeable than the endothelial barrier [5]. Tight junctions are located at the luminal end of the intercellular space and are the main structure limiting the passive diffusion of proteins, lipids and

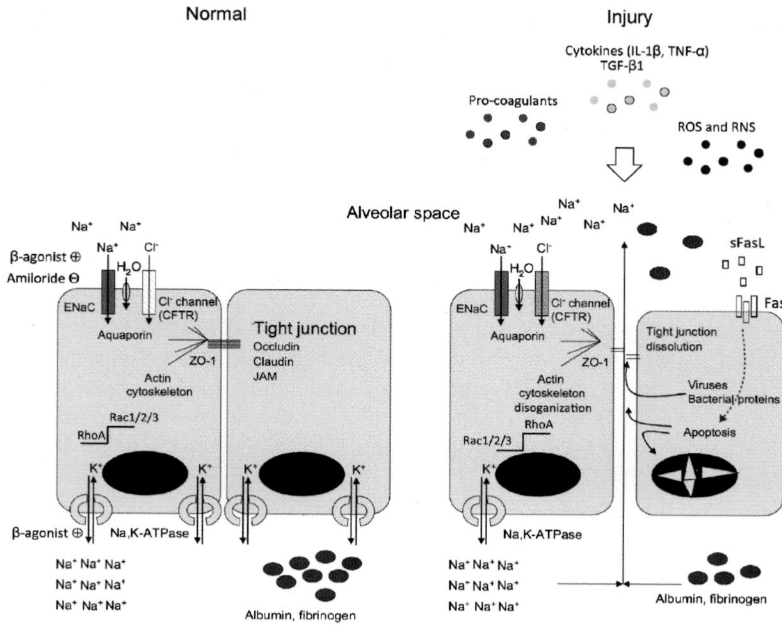

Fig. 1 Scheme of the mechanisms involved in alveolar epithelial injury in ALI (adapted from [48] with permission). IL: interleukin; TNF: tumor necrosis factor; TGF: transforming growth factor; ROS: reactive oxygen species; RNS: reactive nitrogen species

water solutes across the paracellular pathway between two alveolar epithelial cells [6] (Fig. 1). The tight junctions also maintain epithelial polarity and transcellular and paracellular vectorial transport across the epithelium. Therefore, a dysfunction of tight junctions not only leads to an increase in protein permeability, but also worsens the alveolar fluid clearance capacity of the alveolar epithelium, perpetuating protein-rich edema formation. In addition, dysfunction of tight junctions facilitates systemic contamination by microbes and toxins present in the external environment, contributing to the development of multiple organ failure (MOF) [6].

The extracellular component of the tight junctions is comprised of a family of zonula-occludens (ZO) proteins. These proteins interact at the membrane with several scaffolding proteins (occludins, claudins, and junction adhesion molecules) that ultimately link the tight junction to the actin cytoskeleton (Fig. 1). Actin and myosin, the two main components of the anchored cytoskeleton, interact to regulate cell tension and contraction, which also influences epithelial permeability. Disorganization of the tight junctions, as well as disruption of the tight junction-actin interaction and disorganization of actin fibers (formation of peripheral actin stress fibers) result in the dysfunction of tight junctions with a consequent increase in paracellular permeability [6]. Actin remodeling is regulated by members of the Rho family of small GTPases (RhoA and Rac1/2/3), which have opposing effects on epithelial permeability. Whereas activation of Rac1/2/3 preserves epithelial barrier integrity and permeability, activation of RhoA leads to organization of actin stress fibers, formation of large focal adhesions, and interaction of actin and myosin fibers through myosin light chain phosphorylation, resulting in cell contraction and increase in paracellular permeability. A proper balance between the RhoA and Rac1activities is needed to maintain normal epithelial function. In this context, inhibition of RhoA attenuated the development of pulmonary edema and restored alveolar fluid clearance in a murine model of pneumonia by *Pseudomonas aeruginosa* [7] (Fig. 1).

Components of the tight junctions can be direct targets of different insults, such as mechanical stretch, systemic and local inflammation and viral (e.g., adenovirus) and bacterial (e.g., endotoxin) proteins [8, 9]. Other insults can alter tight junctions indirectly by nitric oxide (NO)-dependent mechanisms. NO and peroxynitrite increase epithelial permeability by altering the expression or localization of key tight junction proteins, such as ZO-1 and occludin, and by promoting actin-myosin interaction and cell contraction via Rho kinase activation and myosin light chain phosphorylation [10] (Fig. 1).

Prevention of the extravasation of fluid and proteins across the injured epithelium is important in patients at risk of developing ARDS. Proteins of the tight junction complexes and their interactions with actin fibers of the cytoskeleton are attractive therapeutic targets for maintaining the integrity and function of the alveolar epithelial barrier.

Alteration of Alveolar Fluid Clearance

Alveolar fluid clearance is an integrated function that depends on active ion transport, as well as an intact epithelial physical barrier that prevents back-leak of transported fluid [11]. Fluid clearance occurs following an ionic gradient formed by the alveolar epithelium. Sodium first enters the cell through the amiloride-sensitive (ENaC, epithelial sodium channel) and amiloride-insensitive Na channels, and it is then pumped out of the cell by Na^+-K^+-ATPases located on the basolateral surface of the epithelial cells in both type I and type II alveolar epithelial cells. Cl^- enters the cell mainly via the cystic fibrosis transmembrane conductance regulator (CFTR). Following the ion gradient, liquid passes across the alveolar epithelium through the intercellular spaces and through transcellular water channels named aquaporins [11] (Fig. 1).

The ion and water transport across the alveolar epithelium is regulated by mechanisms that have not been fully defined. The activity of ENaC, CFTR, and Na^+-K^+-ATPase can be upregulated by catecholamine dependent and independent pathways [5, 11]. Catecholamine stimulation of Na^+ channels is mediated via β-adrenoreceptor stimulation of intracellular cAMP and involves protein phosphorylation events by either protein kinase A (PKA) or protein kinase C (PKC). The beta-adrenergic system is also a potent stimulant of Na^+-K^+-ATPase expression in alveolar epithelial cells [12] (Fig. 1). Catecholamine-independent pathways that upregulate alveolar fluid clearance include growth factors, thyroid hormone, and glucocorticoids. The activity of ENaC also depends on channel degradation and stability in the membrane, a process regulated by ubiquitination [13].

The impact of injury stimuli on the Na^+ transport mechanism and alveolar fluid clearance capability of the alveolar epithelium varies depending on the type and severity of epithelial injury and the time after the insult. For example, the alveolar fluid clearance capacity is downregulated in animals with severe septic shock and lung injury associated with important pulmonary endothelial and epithelial damage [5]. Other insults associated with important alveolar epithelial damage, such as severe bacterial pneumonia, mechanical stretch, inflammation, reactive oxygen/nitrogen species, acid or hypoxia/hyperoxia may impair alveolar fluid clearance directly through altered expression and function of Na^+ channels and indirectly through damage of tight junction complexes. Tight junction damage results in a decreased expression of the apical epithelial Na^+ channel and/or basal Na^+-K^+-ATPase [5]. In contrast, the mild interstitial pulmonary edema observed in animal models of endotoxin-induced sepsis associated with endothelial injury but without alveolar epithelial damage was accompanied by augmentation of the alveolar epithelial fluid transport. This enhanced alveolar fluid clearance could be the result of β-agonist stimulation of alveolar epithelial Na^+ transport by endogenous catecholamines released in septic shock [14]. In the recovery stage of lung injury, the epithelial Na^+ transport can also be partly upregulated by the proliferation of alveolar epithelial cells and by the increased activity of ENaC and Na^+-K^+-ATPases in epithelial cells [12].

Alteration of Alveolar Protein Clearance

In addition to alveolar liquid clearance, alveolar protein clearance is an important function of the alveolar epithelium to maintain an adequate air-fluid interface. Inability to clear alveolar protein results in the accumulation of proteins in the alveolar space, which contributes to slow down alveolar fluid clearance because of the increase in protein osmotic pressure [15]. The mechanisms by which the alveolar epithelium clears large molecules, such as serum proteins, from the air space is not totally understood, but it is known that albumin and other macromolecules can be transported actively across the alveolar epithelium through transcellular pathways, probably involving pinocytosis [15].

Mechanisms of Alveolar Epithelial Damage and Potential Therapies

Multiple mechanisms are involved in the alveolar epithelial damage and protein-rich edema formation that are the hallmarks of ALI/ARDS. Clinical studies suggest that the intensity of the alveolar epithelial damage and the decrease in the capacity of the alveolar epithelial barrier to remove alveolar fluid are important determinants of poor outcome in humans [16]. Therefore, strategies aimed at decreasing the initial alveolar epithelial damage and at accelerating the reabsorption of lung edema may be beneficial in patients with ARDS.

β-Adrenergic Stimulation

β-adrenergic agonists accelerate alveolar fluid clearance in normal and injured lungs by modulating the activities of Na^+ channels and Na^+-K^+ATPases and/or by increasing the expression of these proteins [17] (Fig. 1). Vasoactive agents commonly used in critical care, such as dobutamine and dopamine, may also upregulate alveolar fluid clearance. The efficacy of β-adrenergic agonists and vasoactive agents may vary significantly from one patient to another depending on their clinical and pathological conditions, with the intensity of the alveolar epithelial damage being an important factor. The presence of an oxidative environment in the injured alveoli and the endogenous catecholamines released in response to systemic stress are additional factors that affect the response to exogenous catecholamines [14, 17]. It is, therefore, conceivable that pharmacological manipulation of the alveolar epithelium may accelerate the resolution of pulmonary edema in areas where the alveolar epithelium is intact or has been properly repaired.

Several lines of research suggest that β_2-adrenergic agonists not only stimulate alveolar fluid clearance, but also stimulate alveolar epithelial repair and reduce alveolar-capillary permeability in lung injury. Bronchoalveolar lavage (BAL) fluid from patients treated with salbutamol enhanced wound repair responses *in vitro* compared with BAL fluid from placebo treated patients by an IL-1β-dependent mechanism and by autocrine release of epidermal growth factor (EGF) and transforming growth factor (TGF)-α [18]. β_2-agonists stimulate spreading and proliferation of alveolar epithelial cells by mechanisms involving activation of PKA. In addition, β_2-agonists repair endothelial and epithelial permeability by increasing in intracellular cAMP, which relaxes actin-myosin contraction in the cytoskeleton and increases cell-cell contact [18]. Treatment with β_2-adrenergic agonists, has not been associated with increased survival in patients with ALI/ARDS [19], indicating that the use of β_2-adrenergic agonists or vasoactive agents as a single therapy may not be sufficient for rescuing the alveolar epithelium in severe lung injury.

Inflammation

An intense inflammation in the alveoli occurs early in the development of ALI, and it is characterized by marked neutrophil influx, activation of alveolar macrophages, and release of cytokines and chemokines in the airspaces associated with increased airspace epithelial permeability (Fig. 1). Neutrophil influx and their products (proteases and oxidants) are not always associated with alteration of protein permeability in the lungs [20]. The cytokines (tumor necrosis factor [TNF]-α, TNF receptor [TNFR], interleukin [IL]-1, IL-1 receptor antagonist [IL1ra], IL-6, and granulocyte colong-stimualting factor [G-CSF]) and chemokines (IL-8, monocyte chemoattractant protein [MCP]-1, macrophage inflammatory protein [MIP]-1) released into the airspaces are locally produced by endothelial cells, epithelial cells, activated alveolar macrophages and neutrophils. It has been shown that some cytokines modulate alveolar epithelial function in lung injury by increasing protein epithelial permeability and by changing alveolar fluid clearance capacity. IL-1β and TNF-α are the most biologically active cytokines in the pulmonary airspace of patients with ALI [21]. IL-1β increases protein permeability and inhibits fluid transport across the human distal lung epithelium *in vitro* [21]. Inhibition of the TNF pathway resulted in improvement of lung function and restoration of protein permeability in a model of acid-mediated ALI [22]. Not all studies, however, have shown deleterious effects of cytokines on alveolar epithelial function. In this context, TNF-α had a stimulatory effect on alveolar fluid clearance in animal models of pneumonia and ischemia/reperfusion [23]. Therefore, TNF inhibition may not be fully beneficial in injured lungs because it might improve protein permeability but at the same time hinder alveolar fluid clearance.

The mechanisms by which cytokines modify the alveolar fluid clearance capacity and increase epithelial permeability are not completely known. IL-1β and TNF-α alter the alveolar fluid clearance properties of the lung epithelium by affecting the mRNA and protein levels of the major Na^+ and Cl^- transporters [24]. Mechanisms for the increased alveolar epithelial permeability include the formation of actin stress fibers via Rho kinase activation and myosin light chain phosphorylation and the disruption of epithelial tight junctions. In particular, IL-1 receptor-ligand complexes increase epithelial protein permeability through activation of the tyrosine kinase receptor human epidermal growth factor receptor-2 (HER2). This HER2 activation by IL-1β required a disintegrin and metalloproteinase 17 (ADAM17)-dependent shedding of the ligand neuregulin-1 (NRG-1) [25]. Importantly, NRG-1 is detectable and elevated in pulmonary edema samples from patients with ALI, suggesting that this inflammatory signaling pathway in the lung could have diagnostic and therapeutic implications [25].

Growth Factors

Active TGF-β1 is present in the BAL fluid of patients who have ARDS and it has been associated with worsened clinical outcomes. TGF-β induces alveolar epithelial apoptosis and activates fibroblasts leading to the development of lung fibrosis. In addition, it has been shown that TGF-β is required by IL-1β and other cytokines in order to increase alveolar epithelial and endothelial permeability in several models of ALI [26] (Fig. 1). It is believed that the injured epithelium exposes or releases factors that activate TGF-β1. In this regard, latent TGF-β1 in the alveolar

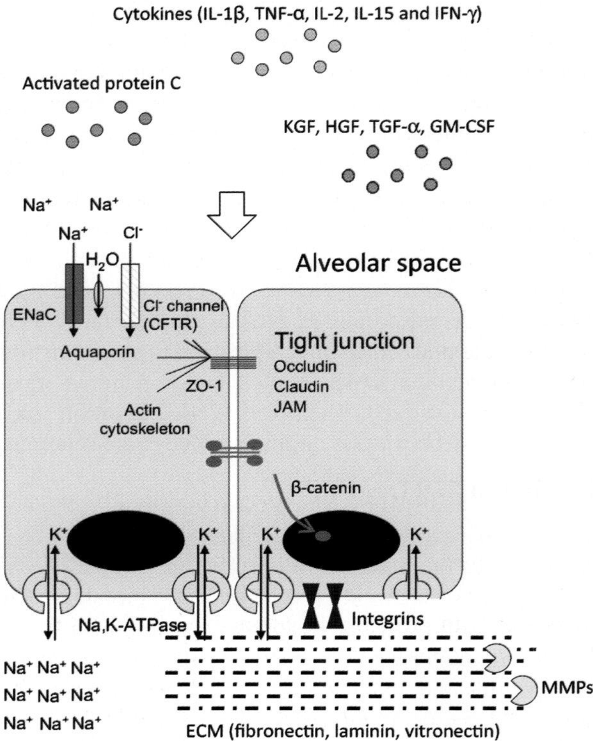

Fig. 2 Scheme of the mechanisms involved in alveolar epithelial repair in ALI (adapted from [48] with permission). IL: interleukin; TNF: tumor necrosis factor; TGF: transforming growth factor; IFN: interferon; KGF: keratinocyte growth factor; HGF: hepatocyte growth factor; GM-CSF: granulocyte-macrophage colony-stimulating factor; MMP: matrix metalloproteinases; ZO: zonula-occludens

interstitium may be activated by exposure to integrin (avb6) on the surface of alveolar epithelial cells [26].

The profibrotic effects of TGF-β require activation of c-abl, a serine/threonine kinase. Inhibition of this kinase by imatinib mesylate prevented bleomycin-induced fibrosis in mice [27], but it did not affect survival or lung function in a randomized clinical trial of patients with idiopathic pulmonary fibrosis [27]. It is unknown whether interventions that antagonize the pro-apoptotic effects of TGF-β1 in epithelial cells or its pro-fibrotic effects in fibroblasts could have beneficial effects on survival in ALI.

Pulmonary edema fluid from ALI/ARDS patients also contains growth factors that have been shown to induce alveolar epithelial repair (Fig. 2). Some of these growth factors such as keratinocyte growth factor (KGF) and hepatocyte growth factor (HGF) are produced by activated fibroblasts, whereas others, such as EGF and TGF-α, are produced by epithelial cells and act in an autocrine-paracrine manner on alveolar epithelial cells. It has been shown that growth factors prevent alveolar epithelial cell apoptosis, promote proliferation of alveolar type II cells, improve alveolar fluid clearance, diminish the increase in protein permeability and prevent the development of fibrosis in *P. aeruginosa*- or ventilator-induced lung injury (VILI, Fig. 2). KGF improved alveolar fluid clearance in part by upregulating Na^+ transport across the alveolar epithelium by enhancing α-ENaC gene expression and by increasing Na^+-K^+-ATPase expression and activity [28]. TGF-α upregulates the production of extracellular matrix protein components and integrin expression on epithelial cells, both being important factors for cell migration and epithelial repair [29]. Other growth factors, such as granulocyte-macrophage-colony stimulating factor (GM-CSF), improve alveolar epithelial function by increasing alveolar fluid clearance and decreasing alveolar epithelial protein levels in the lungs during acute endotoxemia *in vivo*. A clinical trial of GM-CSF therapy has shown promise in reducing ALI in patients with sepsis. Despite all these studies, the potential value of growth factors in patients with ALI/ARDS has not yet been completely defined.

Epithelial Cell Death

Alveolar epithelial cell death could contribute to the disruption of the alveolar barrier in ALI because of epithelial cell shedding and, consequently, flooding of airspaces with protein-rich edematous fluid [30] (Fig. 1). Alveolar epithelial cells can die by apoptosis or necrosis. Both types of cell death have been found in the alveolar wall of lungs from patients who died with ARDS and from animal models of ALI including exposure to hyperoxia, treatment with lipopolysaccharide (LPS) or bleomycin, cecal ligation and puncture (CLP), ischemia-reperfusion injury, and VILI [30, 31]. Necrosis implies disruption of the cell membrane with spilling of intracellular contents, which can cause substantial inflammation. It is thought that necrosis occurs directly by mechanical factors, hyperthermia, local ischemia, or bacterial products in the airspaces. Death by apoptosis is associated with the expression of surface death receptors that allow the clearance of cells with only minimal development of inflammation [30]. Extensive apoptosis and cell detachment of the alveolar epithelium could result in the exposure of the underlying basement membrane to inflammatory products in the alveolar spaces, such as oxidants, proteinases, and inflammatory factors. Moreover, destruction of the alveolar epithelium leads to activation of fibroblast proliferation and collagen production, which can lead to lung fibrosis. In contrast, apoptosis can be beneficial for lung repair by promoting the resolution of type II pneumocyte hyperplasia or the removal of activated inflammatory cells [30]. Despite the fact that apoptosis occurs in alveolar epithelial cells in ALI, its role in the alteration of alveolar epithelial function by affecting protein permeability and alveolar fluid clearance have not been fully elucidated.

Apoptosis can be initiated by activation of a family of death receptors or by direct mitochondrial damage. In the lung, the activation of death receptor-ligand complexes, such as Fas/FasL, TNF-α/TNFR, TGF-β1/TGF-β receptor, and LPS/Toll-like receptor (TLR)4 leads to the activation of a family of cysteinyl aspartate-specific proteases (caspases). Initially, caspase-8 activates the effector caspases (caspase-3 and caspase-7), resulting in cleavage of nuclear DNA and apoptosis. Activation of caspase-8 is often insufficient to induce cell death and requires amplification of the apoptotic signal by the mitochondria. This mitochondrial amplification requires activation of the Bcl-2 family of proteins (Bid, Bax or Bak), which leads to permeabilization of the mitochondrial outer membrane and release of cytochrome c, which enhances the activation of effector caspases. This mitochondrial-dependent apoptotic pathway is important especially in animal models of lung injury induced by hyperoxia/hypoxia, bleomycin, ischemia-reperfusion, VILI and oxidative and nitrosative stress. The role of NO generated from inducible nitric oxide synthase (iNOS) on apoptosis of alveolar epithelial cells is unclear. Some studies suggest that iNOS-derived NO is not detrimental and may even inhibit apoptosis in alveolar and airway epithelial cells in models of sepsis-induced ALI [32]. Many lines of evidence indicate that the Fas/Fas ligand (Fas/FasL) system plays an essential role in the pathogenesis of ALI/ARDS by inducing apoptosis and activation of inflammatory pathways in the early phase, but it also has an important role in lung repair and fibrosis [33] (Fig. 1).

Potential anti-apoptotic therapies could be directed to death-receptor/ligand complexes such as the Fas/FasL system, caspases or the Bcl-2 family of proteins. We need to take into account that the prevention of apoptosis of the alveolar epithelial cells in the early phase of ALI may be beneficial to reduce the progression of this disease and to avoid lung fibrosis, but its inhibition in the proliferative phase when there is epithelial hyperplasia could hinder lung repair. Therefore, the stage of lung injury and the duration of therapies aimed at apoptosis inhibition may be critical factors when designing anti-apoptotic therapies in ALI.

Coagulation

ALI is characterized by the presence of intense procoagulant activity in the alveolar airspaces that can contribute to alveolar epithelial injury [34] (Fig. 1). In the presence of disruption of the alveolar epithelial barrier, plasma proteins, such as fibrinogen and other coagulation factors, enter the alveolar space. In the BAL fluid from patients with ALI, this procoagulant activity is reflected by increased levels of soluble tissue factor, activated factor VII, tissue factor-dependent factor X, thrombin, fibrinopeptide A, D-dimer and fibrinogen. Concomitantly, there is a decrease in fibrinolytic activity, as shown by decreased levels of activated protein C (APC) and urokinase, and increased levels of fibrinolysis inhibitors, such as plasminogen activator inhibitor (PAI) and α2-antiplasmin [34]. Protein C is activated by the thrombin-thrombomodulin complex on the surface of alveolar epithelial cells [35]. Therapies aimed at restoring normal intra-alveolar levels of activated protein C may be of value in patients with clinical ALI/ARDS (Fig. 2).

It has been proposed that increased levels of procoagulant factors in the alveolar space may affect epithelial permeability by changes in the physical forces on cell-cell and cell-matrix interaction due to changes in Rac1/RhoA activity ratio, in cytoskeleton and contraction of the actin-myosin fibers and/or tight junction proteins [36]. In this regard, elevated levels of thrombin cause changes in the contractile machinery of the alveolar epithelial cells with the formation of actin stress fibers, increasing cell contraction and changing intercellular tight junction proteins, such as ZO-1 [36]. In a murine model of *P. aeruginosa* pneumonia, elevation of the APC levels attenuates the increased endothelial and alveolar epithelial protein permeability and improved alveolar fluid clearance via activation of Rac1 and inhibition of RhoA [37]. It is possible, then, that interventions that restitute normal APC levels in the alveolar compartment may have protective effects on the alveolar endothelial/epithelial barrier in ALI (Fig. 2). Some studies in humans suggest that systemic administration of recombinant APC leads to high intra-alveolar levels and has a sustained half-life in the lung. A randomized clinical trial of intravenous infusion of APC for the treatment of ALI in the absence of severe sepsis, however, did not show any beneficial effects in survival or ventilation-free days [38]. In contrast, the nebulized administration of APC attenuated lung injury and reduced pulmonary coagulopathy without systemic anti-coagulant effects in several animal models of ALI [39]. Therefore, the intratracheal administration of APC may represent an alternative treatment for patients with ALI.

Mechanical Stretch

Overdistention of the alveolar epithelium during mechanical ventilation increases the release of inflammatory cytokines [9] and alveolar epithelial cell death. In addition, cyclic stretch of epithelial cells enhances protein permeability associated with reduction of tight junction proteins, disorganization of actin monofilaments, and elevated intracellular calcium concentrations [8]. Therefore, reducing tidal volumes and, thus, the intensity of mechanical stretch on the epithelium, is an important protective strategy of mechanical ventilation for patients with ALI.

Restitution of Alveolar Epithelial Integrity

After injury, restitution of alveolar epithelium integrity is an important step for recovering normal function of the alveolar epithelium and for removing pulmonary edema. Several lines of evidence indicate that there are factors locally produced or released into the alveolar spaces of patients with ALI/ARDS that enhance epithelial repair. These soluble factors derive from fibroblasts, macrophages, endothelial cells, epithelial cells, extracellular matrix and from plasma exudate in the lung of these patients, and comprise cytokines, chemokines, growth factors, prostaglandins, and matrix components. It has been suggested that these factors are present in the alveolar spaces in the early phase of ALI/ARDS [40].

In ALI, there is a predominant injury in type I alveolar epithelial cells as they are more sensitive to injury than type II alveolar epithelial cells [41]. The alveolar epithelial type II cell, which retains stem cell-like properties, is the progenitor for re-epithelialization of the denuded basement membrane [41]. Residual alveolar type II epithelial cells restore the integrity of the alveolar epithelium by spreading and migration, proliferation, and finally by differentiation to alveolar type I cells [41]. However, new evidence has emerged that rat type I cells may also proliferate and show phenotypic plasticity *in vitro* [42].

Part of the epithelial repair activity of the pulmonary edema from ALI/ARDS patients is mediated by IL-1β and by KGF and HGF, which stimulate epithelial cell proliferation and decrease severity of lung injury. Cytokines derived from lymphocytes, such as IL-2, IL-15 and IFN-γ, also promote alveolar epithelial cell growth and migration [43] (Fig. 2).

Re-epithelization on the underlying extracellular matrix involves cell surface receptors, such as integrins. Integrin interaction with extracellular matrix components (fibronectin, laminin, vitronectin) is mediated by specific kinases, such as pp125 FAK (focal adhesion kinase) and I-LK (integrin-linked kinase), and provides traction for the migrating cell to pull forward [44]. Epithelial cell migration is also facilitated by the proteolytical action of matrix metalloproteinases (MMPs), which degrade basement membrane and remodel the extracellular matrix. In human alveolar epithelial cells, MMP-1 decreases cell adhesion and stiffness and increases cell migration on type I collagen in vitro [45].

Lung epithelial repair requires intracellular intermediates that regulate cell migration and proliferation, such as STAT3 (signal transducer and activator of transcription 3) and phosphoinositide-3 kinase (PI3-kinase). PI3-kinase activity is suppressed by PTEN (phosphatase and tensin homolog deleted on chromosome ten), and inhibition of PTEN accelerated wound closure of primary human airway epithelial cells [46]. Another intracellular intermediate is β-catenin, which translocates into the nuclei after epithelial scratch wounding, promoting epithelial cell proliferation *in vitro*. Mitogen-activated protein (MAP) kinases, such as p38, JNK, or the ERK1/2 family, are also involved in this epithelial repair process. Inhibition of MAP kinases decreased lung epithelial cell migration *in vitro* [47].

These extracellular and intracellular signaling intermediates are essential regulators of the repair process of lung epithelium. However, our current knowledge is limited to *in vitro* studies.

Gene Therapy

Gene therapy has demonstrated efficacy in protecting against ALI in animals. In patients, however, there are still technical limitations that prevent the use of gene therapy in human clinical trials. The main reason is the need for the use of viruses to transport the gene of interest into the nucleus. In alveolar epithelial cells, this can be achieved by using adenoviruses as vectors that recognize the adenovirus receptor (CAR) in the tight junction of these cells. Inflammation induced by the viral infection, however, might exacerbate pre-existing lung injury. Whether the use of viruses is sufficiently safe in patients with lung injury remains unclear. One alternative could be the intravenous administration of liposome-encapsulated DNA, which results in relatively high-level expression in the lung. The delivery of a modest electrical voltage creates transient pores in the alveolar epithelial cell membrane that allows entry of plasmid DNA (electroporation). This technique has been successfully used to increase expression of a functional β subunit of the Na^+-K^+-ATPase in the lungs of rats and mice without detectable levels of inflammation [48]. Further studies are required to evaluate the efficacy of these strategies in patients who have ALI.

Cell Therapy

Recent *in vivo* and *in vitro* studies have indicated that mesenchymal stem cells (MSC) may have a therapeutic effect in ALI and on the resolution of pulmonary edema. Despite initial interest in their multipotent properties, engraftment in the lung does not appear to play a major role. The beneficial effects of MSCs derive from their capacity to secrete paracrine soluble factors such as growth factors (KGF) and angiopoietin-1 (Ang-1) that modulate immune responses and protect endothelium or epithelium from injury [49].

The beneficial effects of MSCs on the alveolar epithelial function are due to the improvement in alveolar fluid clearance capacity and the restoration of the alveolar epithelial barrier integrity [49]. MSCs improve alveolar fluid clearance capacity by increasing the apical membrane protein levels of ENaC and the activity of the Na^+-K^+-ATPase leading to an increase in the Na^+ transport across the alveolar epithelium. MSCs may also normalize lung fluid balance and alveolar fluid clearance through therapeutic effects on the lung endothelium [49].

MSCs have the ability to restore protein permeability in injured human alveolar epithelial cells *in vitro*. Secretion of the paracrine-soluble factor, Ang-1, by MSCs seems to be responsible for this beneficial effect. Ang-1 secreted by MSCs protects human alveolar epithelial permeability by preventing the disorganization of tight junction proteins, particularly claudin 18, and blocking actin stress fiber formation upon suppression of nuclear factor-kappa B (NF-κB) activity [50]. Restoration of the receptor-tyrosine kinase, Tie2, is an additional mechanism by which Ang-1 protects epithelial permeability. Therefore, cell-based therapy with MSCs or its soluble factor products are promising tools for the modulation of inflammatory processes and the regeneration of damaged tissues.

Conclusion

Despite considerable research in ALI/ARDS, the mortality of patients with this disease is still high. At the moment, treatment of ARDS remains mainly supportive because none of the pharmacological therapies evaluated so far has reduced morbidity or mortality in controlled clinical trials. One of the main factors that determines the severity and progression of ALI is the extent of the alveolar epithelial damage. Treatments aimed at the alveolar epithelium, either to prevent its initial damage or to improve repair, and resolution of pulmonary edema could be a valuable avenue for improving the outcome of these patients.

Acknowledgements This work was funded by the Centros de Investigación Biomédica en Red de Enfermedades Respiratorias (CIBERES) and the Instituto de Salud Carlos III (Fondo de Investigación Sanitaria, FIS PI0902624, PI0902644, PI1102791).

References

1. Wiedemann HP, Wheeler AP, Bernard GR et al (2006) Comparison of two fluid-management strategies in acute lung injury. N Engl J Med 354:2564–2575
2. The Acute Respiratory Distress Syndrome Network (2000) Ventilation with lower tidal volumes as compared with traditional tidal volumes for acute lung injury and the acute respiratory distress syndrome. N Engl J Med 342:1301–1308
3. Esteban A, Fernandez-Segoviano P, Frutos-Vivar F et al (2004) Comparison of clinical criteria for the acute respiratory distress syndrome with autopsy findings. Ann Intern Med 141:440–445
4. Bachofen M, Weibel ER (1982) Structural alterations of lung parenchyma in the adult respiratory distress syndrome. Clin Chest Med 3:35–56
5. Matthay MA, Robriquet L, Fang X (2005) Alveolar epithelium: role in lung fluid balance and acute lung injury. Proc Am Thorac Soc 2:206–213
6. Schneeberger EE, Lynch RD (2004) The tight junction: a multifunctional complex. Am J Physiol Cell Physiol 286:C1213–C1228
7. Carles M, Lafargue M, Goolaerts A et al (2010) Critical role of the small GTPase RhoA in the development of pulmonary edema induced by Pseudomonas aeruginosa in mice. Anesthesiology 113:1134–1143
8. Cavanaugh KJ, Margulies SS (2002) Measurement of stretch-induced loss of alveolar epithelial barrier integrity with a novel in vitro method. Am J Physiol Cell Physiol 283:C1801–C1808
9. Martinez-Caro L, Lorente JA, Marin-Corral J et al (2009) Role of free radicals in vascular dysfunction induced by high tidal volume ventilation. Intensive Care Med 35:1110–1119
10. Han X, Fink MP, Uchiyama T, Yang R, Delude RL (2004) Increased iNOS activity is essential for pulmonary epithelial tight junction dysfunction in endotoxemic mice. Am J Physiol Lung Cell Mol Physiol 286:L259–L267
11. Mutlu GM, Sznajder JI (2005) Mechanisms of pulmonary edema clearance. Am J Physiol Lung Cell Mol Physiol 289:L685–L695
12. Garty H, Palmer LG (1997) Epithelial sodium channels: function, structure, and regulation. Physiol Rev 77:359–396
13. Staub O, Gautschi I, Ishikawa T et al (1997) Regulation of stability and function of the epithelial Na+ channel (ENaC) by ubiquitination. Embo J 16:6325–6336

14. Pittet JF, Wiener-Kronish JP, McElroy MC, Folkesson HG, Matthay MA (1994) Stimulation of lung epithelial liquid clearance by endogenous release of catecholamines in septic shock in anesthetized rats. J Clin Invest 94:663–671
15. Kim KJ, Malik AB (2003) Protein transport across the lung epithelial barrier. Am J Physiol Lung Cell Mol Physiol 284:L247–L259
16. Ware LB, Matthay MA (2001) Alveolar fluid clearance is impaired in the majority of patients with acute lung injury and the acute respiratory distress syndrome. Am J Respir Crit Care Med 163:1376–1383
17. Matthay MA, Folkesson HG, Clerici C (2002) Lung epithelial fluid transport and the resolution of pulmonary edema. Physiol Rev 82:569–600
18. Perkins GD, Gao F, Thickett DR (2008) In vivo and in vitro effects of salbutamol on alveolar epithelial repair in acute lung injury. Thorax 63:215–220
19. Raghavendran K, Pryhuber GS, Chess PR, Davidson BA, Knight PR, Notter RH (2008) Pharmacotherapy of acute lung injury and acute respiratory distress syndrome. Curr Med Chem 15:1911–1924
20. Martin TR (2002) Neutrophils and lung injury: getting it right. J Clin Invest 110:1603–1605
21. Pugin J, Ricou B, Steinberg KP, Suter PM, Martin TR (1996) Proinflammatory activity in bronchoalveolar lavage fluids from patients with ARDS, a prominent role for interleukin-1. Am J Respir Crit Care Med 153:1850–1856
22. Maniatis NA, Sfika A, Nikitopoulou I et al (2012) Acid-induced acute lung injury in mice associates with p44/42 and c-jun n-terminal kinase activation and requires the function of tumor necrosis factor-alpha receptor I. Shock 38:381–386
23. Rezaiguia S, Garat C, Delclaux C et al (1997) Acute bacterial pneumonia in rats increases alveolar epithelial fluid clearance by a tumor necrosis factor-alpha-dependent mechanism. J Clin Invest 99:325–335
24. Lee JW, Fang X, Dolganov G et al (2007) Acute lung injury edema fluid decreases net fluid transport across human alveolar epithelial type II cells. J Biol Chem 282:24109–24119
25. Finigan JH, Faress JA, Wilkinson E et al (2011) Neuregulin-1-human epidermal receptor-2 signaling is a central regulator of pulmonary epithelial permeability and acute lung injury. J Biol Chem 286:10660–10670
26. Pittet JF, Griffiths MJ, Geiser T et al (2001) TGF-beta is a critical mediator of acute lung injury. J Clin Invest 107:1537–1544
27. Daniels CE, Lasky JA, Limper AH, Mieras K, Gabor E, Schroeder DR (2010) Imatinib treatment for idiopathic pulmonary fibrosis: Randomized placebo-controlled trial results. Am J Respir Crit Care Med 181:604–610
28. Guery BP, Mason CM, Dobard EP, Beaucaire G, Summer WR, Nelson S (1997) Keratinocyte growth factor increases transalveolar sodium reabsorption in normal and injured rat lungs. Am J Respir Crit Care Med 155:1777–1784
29. Berthiaume Y, Lesur O, Dagenais A (1999) Treatment of adult respiratory distress syndrome: plea for rescue therapy of the alveolar epithelium. Thorax 54:150–160
30. Martin TR, Nakamura M, Matute-Bello G (2003) The role of apoptosis in acute lung injury. Crit Care Med 31:S184–S188
31. Lipke AB, Matute-Bello G, Herrero R, Wong VA, Mongovin SM, Martin TR (2011) Death receptors mediate the adverse effects of febrile-range hyperthermia on the outcome of lipopolysaccharide-induced lung injury. Am J Physiol Lung Cell Mol Physiol 301:L60–L70
32. Rudkowski JC, Barreiro E, Harfouche R et al (2004) Roles of iNOS and nNOS in sepsis-induced pulmonary apoptosis. Am J Physiol Lung Cell Mol Physiol 286:L793–L800
33. Herrero R, Kajikawa O, Matute-Bello G et al (2011) The biological activity of FasL in human and mouse lungs is determined by the structure of its stalk region. J Clin Invest 121:1174–1190
34. Welty-Wolf KE, Carraway MS, Ortel TL, Piantadosi CA (2002) Coagulation and inflammation in acute lung injury. Thromb Haemost 88:17–25
35. Ware LB, Fang X, Matthay MA (2003) Protein C and thrombomodulin in human acute lung injury. Am J Physiol Lung Cell Mol Physiol 285:L514–L521

36. Kawkitinarong K, Linz-McGillem L, Birukov KG, Garcia JG (2004) Differential regulation of human lung epithelial and endothelial barrier function by thrombin. Am J Respir Cell Mol Biol 31:517–527
37. Bir N, Lafargue M, Howard M et al (2011) Cytoprotective-selective activated protein C attenuates Pseudomonas aeruginosa-induced lung injury in mice. Am J Respir Cell Mol Biol 45:632–641
38. Liu KD, Levitt J, Zhuo H et al (2008) Randomized clinical trial of activated protein C for the treatment of acute lung injury. Am J Respir Crit Care Med 178:618–623
39. Hofstra JJ, Vlaar AP, Cornet AD et al (2010) Nebulized anticoagulants limit pulmonary coagulopathy, but not inflammation, in a model of experimental lung injury. J Aerosol Med Pulm Drug Deliv 23:105–111
40. Geiser T, Atabai K, Jarreau PH, Ware LB, Pugin J, Matthay MA (2001) Pulmonary edema fluid from patients with acute lung injury augments in vitro alveolar epithelial repair by an IL-1beta-dependent mechanism. Am J Respir Crit Care Med 163:1384–1388
41. Ware LB, Matthay MA (2000) The acute respiratory distress syndrome. N Engl J Med 342:1334–1349
42. Gonzalez RF, Allen L, Dobbs LG (2009) Rat alveolar type I cells proliferate, express OCT-4, and exhibit phenotypic plasticity in vitro. Am J Physiol Lung Cell Mol Physiol 297:L1045–L1055
43. Lesur O, Brisebois M, Thibodeau A, Chagnon F, Lane D, Fullop T (2004) Role of IFN-gamma and IL-2 in rat lung epithelial cell migration and apoptosis after oxidant injury. Am J Physiol Lung Cell Mol Physiol 286:L4–L14
44. Kim HJ, Henke CA, Savik SK, Ingbar DH (1997) Integrin mediation of alveolar epithelial cell migration on fibronectin and type I collagen. Am J Physiol 273:L134–L141
45. Planus E, Galiacy S, Matthay M et al (1999) Role of collagenase in mediating in vitro alveolar epithelial wound repair. J Cell Sci 112:243–252
46. Lai JP, Dalton JT, Knoell DL (2007) Phosphatase and tensin homologue deleted on chromosome ten (PTEN) as a molecular target in lung epithelial wound repair. Br J Pharmacol 152:1172–1184
47. Crosby LM, Waters CM (2010) Epithelial repair mechanisms in the lung. Am J Physiol Lung Cell Mol Physiol 298:L715–L731
48. Budinger GR, Sznajder JI (2006) The alveolar-epithelial barrier: a target for potential therapy. Clin Chest Med 27:655–669
49. Matthay MA, Goolaerts A, Howard JP, Lee JW (2010) Mesenchymal stem cells for acute lung injury: preclinical evidence. Crit Care Med 38:S569–S573
50. Fang X, Neyrinck AP, Matthay MA, Lee JW (2010) Allogeneic human mesenchymal stem cells restore epithelial protein permeability in cultured human alveolar type II cells by secretion of angiopoietin-1. J Biol Chem 285:26211–26222

Part XII

Intravenous Fluids

Colloids for Sepsis: Effectiveness and Cost Issues

A. Farrugia, G. Martin, and M. Bult

Introduction: Sepsis and Fluids

Severe sepsis, defined as acute organ dysfunction secondary to infection, and septic shock, defined as severe sepsis plus hypotension not reversed with fluid resuscitation, originate in the systemic inflammatory response following infection and lead to cardiovascular and organ dysfunction. Sepsis is a major cause of hospital mortality and a considerable economic burden [1]. Resuscitation in sepsis is initially based on goal-directed fluid therapy. This modality remains controversial [2] and a recent randomized trial indicated that bolus fluid therapy in a large population of children with sepsis in a resource-challenged environment [3] increased mortality irrespective of the type of fluid. Nevertheless, this remains an active area of clinical investigation, as evidenced by the large number of registered relevant trials on www.clinicaltrials.gov. The timing, rather than the type, of fluid therapy has been proposed as being crucial [4].

The relative proportion of the different fluids used in sepsis varies between countries [5]. Cost is invariably included as a factor in guidelines on the choice of fluids, with the higher cost of colloids, particularly albumin, being emphasized. Colloids are more expensive than crystalloids, but remain a viable therapeutic option based on their superior hemodynamic properties and plasma volume expanding capacity [6], despite a lack of survival benefit in systematic reviews of heterogeneous patient populations [7], which, notably, did not include septic pa-

A. Farrugia (✉)
School of Surgery, University of Western Australia, 35 Stirling Highway,
Crawley, WA 6009, Australia
E-mail: albert.farrugia@uwa.edu.au

G. Martin
Division of Pulmonary, Allergy and Critical Care, Emory University School of Medicine,
and Grady Memorial Hospital, Atlanta, GA 30303, USA

M. Bult
Plasma Protein Therapeutics Association, 114 Boulevard Brand Whitlock, Brussels, Belgium

J.-L. Vincent (Ed.), *Annual Update in Intensive Care and Emergency Medicine 2013*,
DOI 10.1007/978-3-642-35109-9_41, © Springer-Verlag Berlin Heidelberg 2013

tients. In this chapter, we assess the evidence and cost-effectiveness for colloid therapies in sepsis, focusing particularly on the two most widely used therapies, the natural protein, albumin, and the synthetic product, hydroxyethyl starch (HES).

Human Albumin Solution(s)

Human albumin solutions have been used in acute care for decades. Early observations on service men injured in Pearl Harbor and its apparent safety quickly established albumin as the agent of choice for blood volume expansion after fluid loss. Albumin solutions were adopted by the major regulatory authorities without significant scrutiny or clinical evidence, a situation which changed dramatically with the publication of a meta-analysis from the Cochrane collaboration [8], which claimed to show an increase in mortality when using albumin across a series of randomized controlled trials (RCTs) over a 40-year period. Subsequent meta-analyses of trials using more modern albumin preparations [9] did not confirm the Cochrane meta-analysis findings. In 2005, a large pragmatic RCT of intensive care patients – the Saline vs. Albumin Fluid Evaluation (SAFE) – showed equivalent mortality between resuscitation with albumin and saline [10], and led to all the regulatory reservations regarding albumin's use being withdrawn. Although an observational study suggested that harmful renal effects can ensue from all hyperoncotic colloids [11], a meta-analysis of randomized trials concluded that such renal effects are colloid specific, with albumin displaying renal protection at all formulations [12]. Reviewing the effects of colloid solutions on hemostasis, Van der Linden and Ickx concluded that albumin had no effect [13].

Albumin Solutions in Sepsis

Factors contributing to impaired microcirculatory perfusion in sepsis are shown in Fig. 1 [14] and include features for which albumin is known, on the basis of laboratory and clinical studies, to have a protective effect (reviewed in [15]). Despite the increased microvascular permeability characterizing sepsis, plasma volume is expanded in septic patients given albumin [16] and hypoalbuminemia is corrected [17]. A pre-defined subgroup analysis of patients with sepsis in the SAFE study referred to above indicated a survival benefit for septic patients given albumin [17], a finding supported by a meta-analysis of this and other trials [18]. These findings have contributed to a number of ongoing [19, 20] trials for albumin in sepsis. So far, the data for many of these trials have not been fully published, but data reported in conferences continue to indicate a non-significant survival benefit for albumin vs. crystalloid. Under-powering in these studies may contribute to this consistent finding. A meta-analysis of the three studies conducted so far indicates a significant benefit of albumin on survival (Fig. 2).

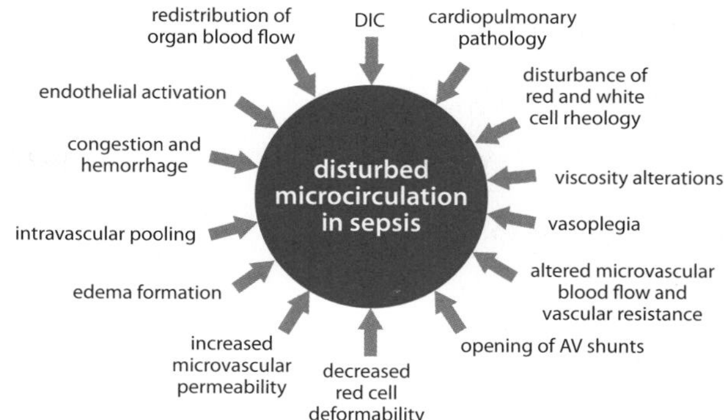

Fig. 1 Factors contributing to microcirculatory impairment in sepsis. From [14]

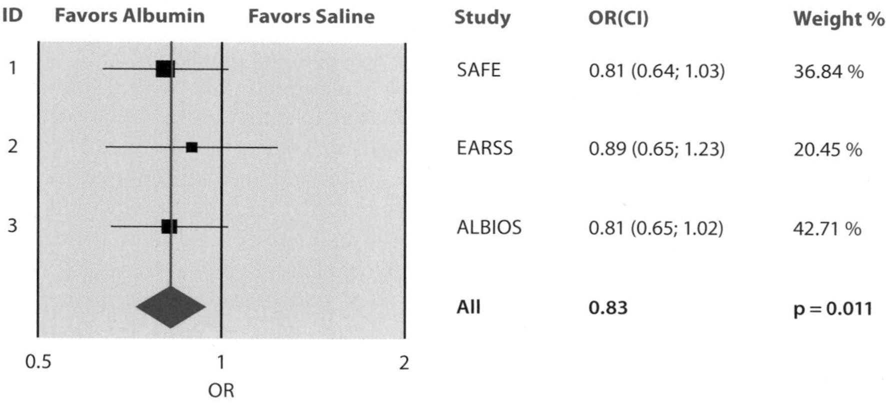

Fig. 2 Meta-analysis of recent clinical trials of albumin vs. crystalloid in sepsis

Hydroxyethyl Starches

HES are a class of colloid solutions that have been used in a range of clinical applications in lieu of albumin. Their pharmacology has been extensively reviewed [21]. Their lower cost per unit compared to albumin has been the main driver for their adoption in clinical practice, and they have assumed a dominant position in the therapeutic colloid market in many countries [5]. HES have been supplied in successive generations of products over the past thirty years, and manufacturers have attempted to develop molecules that do not lead to the adverse events that have been associated with these products since their inception. Over the past decade, a number of HES products with an average molecular weight of 130 kDa and a degree of substitution of 0.4 (low molecular weight HES) have been introduced into therapeutic practice. These properties are claimed by HES manufacturers and clinical advocates to ameliorate or obviate the hemostatic and renal adverse events.

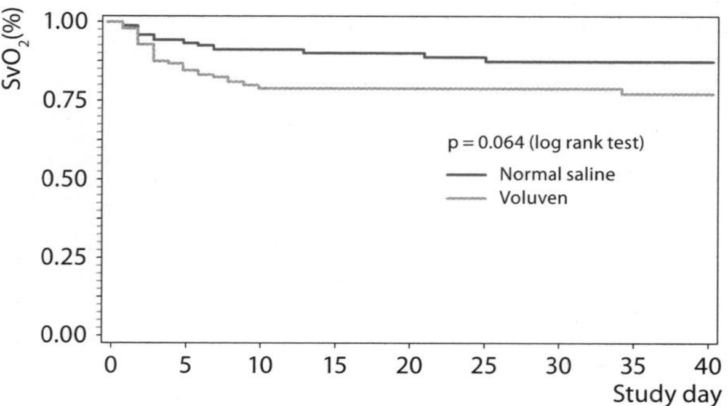

Fig. 3 Renal replacement therapy probability from post-market licensure study for low molecular weight hydroxyethyl starch. From [32]

These claims are now under increasing scrutiny. Two meta-analyses, including a Cochrane review, published in 2009, do not support the claim that septic patients are not at risk of renal dysfunction from low molecular weight HES [22, 23]. Subsequently, the Scandinavian Starch for Severe Sepsis/Septic Shock (6S) trial [24] reported significantly increased mortality and need for renal replacement therapy (RRT) in intensive care unit (ICU) patients with severe sepsis who received low molecular weight HES relative to crystalloid. Increased bleeding reported for the HES arm failed to reach significance. A Task Force of the European Society for Intensive Care Medicine concluded in a Consensus Statement that low molecular weight HES should be used in sepsis only in the context of clinical trials [25]. The evidence base for the safety and efficacy of HES, particularly the low molecular weight HES generation of products, has been dented with the retraction from the peer-reviewed literature of the studies by Joachim Boldt and co-workers [26]. The Boldt issue has stimulated a closer scrutiny of the low molecular weight HES literature by several authors [27–29], who have commented on the paucity of evidence supporting these products. The requirements of regulatory authorities for post-marketing approval for low molecular weight HES have included non-inferiority studies for hemodynamic equivalence or superiority with other fluids rather than safety studies powered to detect differences in, for example, renal dysfunction [30, 31]. Notably, the United States Food and Drug Administration (FDA) included data from one of these studies in the approved product information for the USA, pointing out the trend to an increased risk of RRT with this product [32] (Fig. 3).

Colloid Treatments in Sepsis: Approaching a Decision

Clinical evidence should determine treatment choice, but the global financial pressures on health care inevitably impose cost considerations. As is evident from the present review, certainty regarding many of the key efficacy and safety aspects of

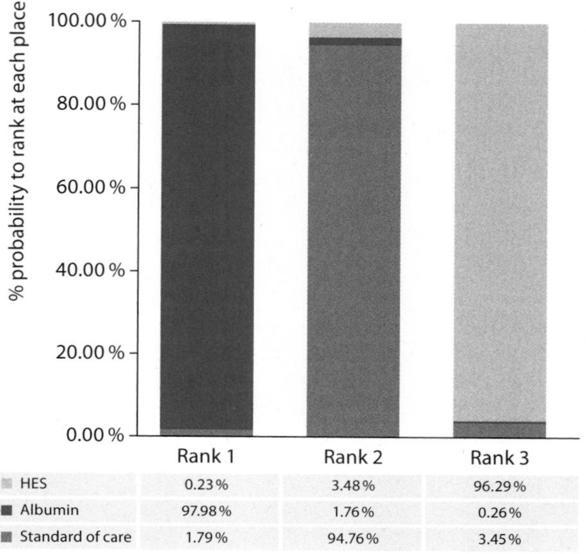

Fig. 4 Multiple treatment meta-analysis for colloid treatments in sepsis extracted from the trials listed in Table 1. Barplots for the ranking probabilities of competing fluid treatments are shown. The horizontal axis is the possible rank of each treatment (from best to worse). A Bayesian framework ranked the treatments and also assigned probability to each rank that a treatment can achieve in terms of lowering the risk of mortality. Ranks are ordered from most effective to least effective. Albumin holds the first rank with hydroxyethyl starch (HES) holding the lowest rank

colloid fluid therapy continues to be elusive. Questions require further clinical investigations, demanding scare funds and time. Given these uncertainties in many of the aspects of fluid therapy and importance of including all healthcare repercussions in providing choices in therapeutics, other tools may be helpful. In the absence of large, high quality, randomized trials comparing different colloids such as albumin and HES, multiple-treatment meta-analysis (or network meta-analysis) allows the indirect comparison of treatments integrating the data from all the available comparisons [33]. The result of combining the data from the studies on fluid treatments in sepsis (Table 1) is shown in Fig. 4, which ranks the treatments and specifies the probability that a treatment can achieve in terms of lowering the risk of mortality: Albumin achieves the highest rank and HES the lowest.

The field of decision analysis is based on assessing situations with uncertainty around multifactorial inputs affect outcomes. Its role in economic analysis in decision making around critical care therapies has been reviewed [47]. Using decision analysis around the use of colloid therapy in sepsis as shown in Fig. 5, a model was populated with the probabilities and costs of the various treatments and outcomes for a hypothetical population of patients using data from the literature [48] to compare the cost-effectiveness of albumin and HES in the specific area of sepsis. Relative to a willingness to pay $10,000 for each incremental life-year gained from using the fluid therapy, in this model albumin is more effective and results in less medical costs than does HES (Table 2).

Table 1 The studies used to perform multiple treatment meta-analysis (mortality estimates) and standard meta-analysis (renal replacement therapy [RRT])

Mortality								Renal Replacement Therapy			
Study	Treatment arms	Crystalloid		Albumin		HES		Crystalloid		HES	
		Deaths	Total	Deaths	Total	Deaths	Total	RRT	Total	RRT	Total
ALBIOS [20]	Crystalloid, Albumin	274	648	244	653						
Bechir [34]	Crystalloid, HES	2	14			7	16				
Brunkhorst [35]	Crystalloid, HES	93	274			107	261	51	272	81	261
Charpentier [19]	Crystalloid, Albumin	103	393	96	399						
Dolecek [36]	Albumin, HES			4	30	6	26				
Finfer [17]	Crystalloid, Albumin	217	615	185	603						
Friedman [37]	Albumin, HES			5	27	10	27				
Guidet [31]	Crystalloid, HES	32	95			40	99	19	95	24	99
Maitland [38]	Crystalloid, Albumin	3	20	4	23						
Maitland [39]	Crystalloid, Albumin	11	61	2	56						
Maitland [3]	Crystalloid, Albumin	126	1,047	128	2,050						
Mcintyre [40]	Crystalloid, HES	6	19			9	21	1	19	3	21
Metildi [41]	Crystalloid, Albumin	11	12	10	12						
Nagy [42]	Crystalloid, HES	2	20			2	21				
Perner 2012 [24]	Crystalloid, HES	172	400			201	398	65	400	87	398

Table 1 *Continued*

Mortality								Renal Replacement Therapy	
Rackow [43]	Crystalloid, Albumin, HES	6	8	6	9	5	9		
Rackow [44]	Albumin, HES			5	10	5	10		
Veneman [45]	Crystalloid, Albumin, HES	5	16	8	15	18	30		
Younes [46]	Crystalloid, HES	3	11			2	12		
OR (albumin vs. HES)	1.8 (95 % CI: 1.295–2.375)							OR (HES vs Control)	1.61 ($p < 0.001$)

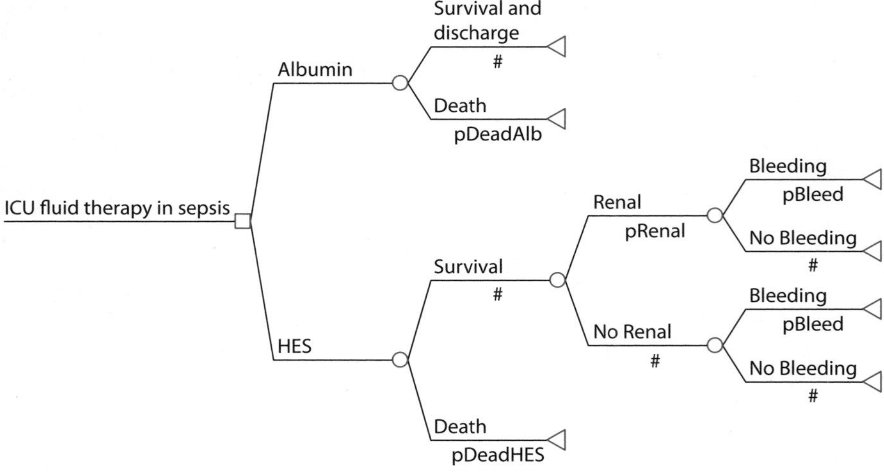

Fig. 5 Structure of a decision analysis model for competing colloid treatments in sepsis

Table 2 Outcomes of the decision analysis model. Albumin is associated with increased survival at lower costs compared to HES

Strategy	Life-years gained	Incremental life-years	Total medical costs	Incremental costs	ICER
HES	–0.69	–1.53	$48,488	$28,085	Dominant
Albumin	0.84		$20,403		

ICER: incremental cost-effectiveness ratio

The mortality rate among sepsis patients post-discharge is high, and the increase in life expectancy predicted by the model represents a 23 % increase relative to standard practice. Crucial to this result is the inclusion of the morbidities associated with HES, particularly the probability of RRT extracted from a standard meta-analysis of trails using HES in sepsis (Fig. 6). These results show the importance of including all the relevant costs associated with a particular therapy, in addition to the specific product cost. This facet is of clear relevance in the current era of cost-containment in health care and hospital costs. With the continuing financial pressures, hospital costs, such as those for fluid therapies, are being apportioned among cost centers, such as pharmacies, with devolved budgets. In terms of drug costs, preference may be given to treatments that are relatively less expensive on an individual basis without assessing their effect on overall treatment outcome [49]. Treatment choice has to take into account the possible adverse effects of the fluids in question. Combining treatment effects, as is done in multiple-treatment meta-analysis and decision analysis, assumes that the drug classes under review, e.g., different albumin and HES solutions, are biopharmaceutically equivalent. Clinical trials do not support the contention that succeeding genera-

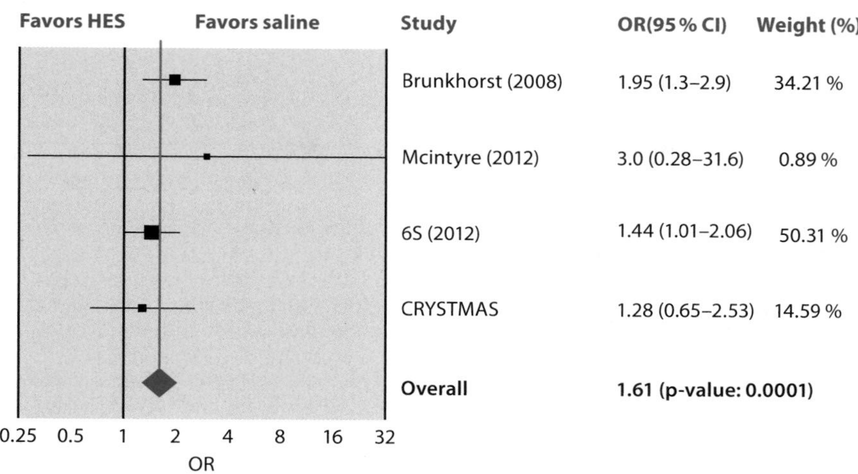

Fig. 6 Standard meta-analysis for trials of hydroxyethyl starch (HES) in sepsis – assessment of renal replacement therapy (RRT) – extracted from Table 1

tions of HES demonstrate safety enhancements in relation to significant adverse events. The FDA has concluded that albumin solutions are biopharmaceutically equivalent [50].

Conclusion

Colloid therapy in sepsis is dominated by the use of either albumin or HES. The safety of albumin appears to be established, and indications of its efficacy in sepsis, assessed as a decrease in mortality, are available mostly from meta-analysis of individual trials which continue to be under-powered. HES are associated with renal and hemostatic problems that affect all the successive generations of these products. The use of multiple-treatment meta-analysis and decision analysis allows the combination of data from all the available studies and indicates that albumin conveys a significant survival benefit over HES in septic patients. The use of albumin in septic patients, when colloid fluid therapy is indicated, shows superior cost-effectiveness to HES when all the medical costs incurred from therapy-associated adverse events are considered. Crude assessments of the basic per unit costs by hospital pharmacies are inadequate and inappropriate tools for decision making. An appreciation of these principles should lead to better and more cost-effective care for patients with sepsis.

Acknowledgment Megha Bansal performed the meta-analyses described in this work. Megha Bansal, Sonia Balboni and Mary Clare Kimber contributed to the decision analysis model.

References

1. Burchardi H, Schneider H (2004) Economic aspects of severe sepsis: a review of intensive care unit costs, cost of illness and cost effectiveness of therapy. Pharmacoeconomics 22:793–813
2. Hilton A, Bellomo R (2012) A critique of fluid bolus resuscitation in severe sepsis. Crit Care 16:302
3. Maitland K, Kiguli S, Opoka RO et al (2011) Mortality after fluid bolus in African children with severe infection. N Engl J Med 364:2483–2495
4. Rivers EP, Katranji M, Jaehne KA et al (2012) Early interventions in severe sepsis and septic shock: a review of the evidence one decade later. Minerva Anestesiol 78:712–724
5. Finfer S, Liu B, Taylor C et al (2010) Resuscitation fluid use in critically ill adults: an international cross-sectional study in 391 intensive care units. Crit Care 14:R185
6. Trof RJ, Sukul SP, Twisk JWR, Girbes ARJ, Groeneveld ABJ (2010) Greater cardiac response of colloid than saline fluid loading in septic and non-septic critically ill patients with clinical hypovolaemia. Intensive Care Med 36:697–701
7. Perel P, Roberts I (2012) Colloids versus crystalloids for fluid resuscitation in critically ill patients. Cochrane Database Syst Rev 6 CD000567
8. Cochrane Injuries Group Albumin Reviewers (1998) Human albumin administration in critically ill patients: systematic review of randomised controlled trials. BMJ 317:235–240
9. Vincent J-L, Wilkes MM, Navickis RJ (2003) Safety of human albumin – serious adverse events reported worldwide in 1998–2000. Br J Anaesth 91:625–630
10. The SAFE Study Investigators (2004) A comparison of albumin and saline for fluid resuscitation in the intensive care unit N Engl J Med 350:2247–2256
11. Schortgen F, Girou E, Deye N, Brochard L (2008) The risk associated with hyperoncotic colloids in patients with shock. Intensive Care Med 34:2157–2168
12. Wiedermann C, Dunzendorfer S, Gaioni L, Zaraca F, Joannidis M (2010) Hyperoncotic colloids and acute kidney injury: a meta-analysis of randomized trials. Crit Care 14:R191
13. Van der Linden P, Ickx B (2006) The effects of colloid solutions on hemostasis. Can J Anesth 53:S30–S39
14. Spronk PE, Zandstra DF, Ince C (2004) Bench-to-bedside review: sepsis is a disease of the microcirculation. Crit Care 8:462–468
15. Quinlan GJ, Martin GS, Evans TW (2005) Albumin: Biochemical properties and therapeutic potential. Hepatology 41:1211–1219
16. Ernest D, Belzberg AS, Dodek PM (1999) Distribution of normal saline and 5 % albumin infusions in septic patients. Crit Care Med 27:46
17. The SAFE Study Investigators (2010) Impact of albumin compared to saline on organ function and mortality of patients with severe sepsis. Intensive Care Med 37:86–96
18. Delaney AP, Dan A, McCaffrey J, Finfer S (2011) The role of albumin as a resuscitation fluid for patients with sepsis: A systematic review and meta-analysis. Crit Care Med 39:386–391
19. Charpentier J, Mira J (2011) Efficacy and tolerance of hyperoncotioc albumin administration in septic patients: The EARSS Study. Intensive Care Med(Suppl 1):S115 (abst)
20. Caironi P (2012) Rimpiazzo dei fluidi nel paziente critico: lo studio Albios. Available at: http://www.smartonweb.org/presentazione/index.php?presentazione_video=si&id=365. Accessed August 2012
21. Jungheinrich C, Neff TA (2004) Pharmacokinetics of hydroxyethyl starch. Clin Pharmacokinet 44:681–99
22. Dart AB, Mutter TC, Ruth CA, Taback SP (2010) Hydroxyethyl starch (HES) versus other fluid therapies: effects on kidney function. Cochrane Database Syst Rev CD007594
23. Zarychanski R, Turgeon AF, Fergusson DA et al (2009) Renal outcomes and mortality following hydroxyethyl starch resuscitation of critically ill patients: systematic review and meta-analysis of randomized trials. Open Med 3:e196

24. Perner A, 6S Trial Group and the Scandinavian Critical Care Trials Group (2012) Hydroxyethyl starch 130/0.4 versus Ringer's acetate in severe sepsis. N Engl J Med 27:1–11
25. Reinhart K, Perner A, Sprung CL et al (2012) Consensus statement of the ESICM task force on colloid volume therapy in critically ill patients. Intensive Care Med 38:368–383
26. Shafer SL (2011) Shadow of doubt. Anesth Analg 112:498–500
27. Hartog CS, Kohl M, Reinhart K (2011) A systematic review of third-generation hydroxyethyl starch (HES 130/0.4) in resuscitation: safety not adequately addressed. Anesth Analg 112:635–645
28. Gattas DJ, Dan A, Myburgh J, Billot L, Lo S, Finfer S (2012) Fluid resuscitation with 6% hydroxyethyl starch (130/0.4) in acutely ill patients: an updated systematic review and meta-analysis. Anesth Analg 114:159–169
29. Hartog CS, Skupin H, Natanson C, Sun J, Reinhart K (2012) Systematic analysis of hydroxyethyl starch (HES) reviews: proliferation of low-quality reviews overwhelms the results of well-performed meta-analyses. Intensive Care Med 38:1258–1271
30. Faraoni D, De Ville A, Hofer A, Heschi M, Gombotz H, van der Linden P (2011) Efficacy and safety of 6% HES 130/0.4 versus 5% HA for volume replacement during pediatric cardiac surgery. Available at: http://www.asaabstracts.com/strands/asaabstracts/abstract.htm;jsessionid=E0BC05F26723C658B921FC24D398E740?year=2011&index=16&absnum=4705. Accessed October 2012
31. Guidet B, Martinet O, Boulain T et al (2012) Assessment of hemodynamic efficacy and safety of 6% hydroxyethylstarch 130/0.4 versus 0.9% NaCl fluid replacement in patients with severe sepsis: The CRYSTMAS study. Crit Care 16:R94
32. Food and Drug Administration (2012) Approved Product Information for Voluven Available at: http://www.fda.gov/downloads/BiologicsBloodVaccines/BloodBloodProducts/ApprovedProducts/NewDrugApplicationsNDAs/UCM083138.pdf. Accessed October 2012
33. Caldwell DM, Ades AE, Higgins JPT (2005) Simultaneous comparison of multiple treatments: combining direct and indirect evidence. BMJ 331:897–900
34. Béchir M, Puhan MA, Neff SB et al (2010) Early fluid resuscitation with hyperoncotic hydroxyethyl starch 200/0.5 (10%) in severe burn injury. Crit Care 14:R123
35. Brunkhorst FM, Engel C, Bloos F et al (2008) Intensive insulin therapy and pentastarch resuscitation in severe sepsis. N Engl J Med 358:125–139
36. Dolecek M, Svoboda P, Kantorová I (2009) Therapeutic influence of 20% albumin versus 6% hydroxyethylstarch on extravascular lung water in septic patients: A randomized controlled trial. Hepatogastroenterology 56:1622–1628
37. Friedman G, Jankowski S, Shahla M (2008) Hemodynamic effects of 6% and 10% hydroxyethyl starch solutions versus 4% albumin solution in septic patients. J Clin Anesth 20:528–533
38. Maitland K, Pamba A, English M et al (2005) Pre-transfusion management of children with severe malarial anaemia: a randomised controlled trial of intravascular volume expansion. Br J Hematol 128:393–400
39. Maitland K, Pamba A, English M et al (2005) Randomized trial of volume expansion with albumin or saline in children with severe malaria: preliminary evidence of albumin benefit. Clin Infect Dis 40:538–545
40. McIntyre LA, Fergusson D, Cook D, Rankin N, Dhingra V, Granton J (2008) Fluid resuscitation in the management of early septic shock (FINESS): a randomized controlled feasibility trial. Can J Anaesth 55:819–826
41. Metildi L, Shackford S, Virgilio R, Peters R (1984) Crystalloid versus colloid in fluid resuscitation of patients with severe pulmonary insufficiency. Surg Gynecol Obstet 158:207–212
42. Nagy K, Davis J, Flides J, Roberts R, Barrett J (1993) A comparison of pentastarch and lactated Ringer's solution in the resuscitation of patients with hemorrhagic shock. Circ Shock 40:289–294
43. Rackow E, Falk J, Fein I (1983) Fluid resuscitation in circulatory shock: A comparison of the cardiorespiratory effects of albumin, hetastarch, and saline solutions in patients with hypovolemic and septic shock. Crit Care Med 11:839–850

44. Rackow E, Mecher C, Astiz M, Griffel M, Falk J, Weil M (1989) Effects of pentastarch and albumin infusion on cardiorespiratory function and coagulation in patients with severe sepsis and systemic hypoperfusion. Crit Care Med 17:394–398
45. Veneman TF, Nijhuis JO, Woittiez AJJ (2004) Human albumin and starch administration in critically ill patients: a prospective randomized clinical trial. Wien Klin Wochenschr 116:305–309
46. Younes R, Yin K, Amino C, Itinoshe M, Rocha e Silva M, Birolini D (1998) Use of pentastarch solution in the treatment of patients with hemorrhagic hypovolemia: randomized phase II study in the emergency room. World J Surg 22:2–5
47. Coughlin MT, Angus DC (2003) Economic evaluation of new therapies in critical illness. Crit Care Med 31:S7
48. Farrugia A, Balboni S, Cassar J, Kimber MC (2003) Colloid treatment in sepsis patients in intensive care – use of albumin vs hydroxyethyl starch (HES) is cost-effective in a decision analysis model. Vox Sang 103(Suppl s1):P547 (abst)
49. Bernard K, Black E, Remtulla S, Schwenger E, Dalen D (2010) Should hospital pharmacy drug budgets be the responsibility of each individual department in an institution, or should such budgets be controlled centrally by the pharmacy department? Can J Hosp Pharm 63:330–332
50. Woodcock J, Griffin J, Behrman R et al (2007) The FDA's assessment of follow-on protein products: a historical perspective. Nat Rev Drug Discov 6:437–442

Risk Factors for Transfusion-Related Lung Injury in ICU Patients

M. C. A. Müller and N. P. Juffermans

Introduction

Multiple observational studies have shown an association between transfusion and lung injury in the critically ill [1–6]. The definition of transfusion-related acute lung injury (TRALI) is the onset of ALI occurring within 6 hours following a blood transfusion. When other risk factors for ALI are present, the term "possible TRALI" is used [7, 8]. Although a temporal relation with a blood transfusion is an obvious requirement for the definition of TRALI, the time frame of 6 hours is arbitrarily chosen. Indeed, it has been recognized that transfusion can result in delayed respiratory complications, termed "delayed TRALI syndrome" [9].

Recent observational studies suggest that the incidence of TRALI is high in several critically ill risk populations. Cohort studies in critically ill patients report a 100-fold higher incidence of TRALI when compared to the general hospital population [10, 11]. Of note, the attributive morbidity and mortality of TRALI is considerable. Up to 70 % of patients who develop TRALI need referral to the intensive care unit (ICU) and invasive mechanical ventilation [12]. When TRALI develops in patients already admitted to the ICU, there is an association with prolonged mechanical ventilation, increased hospital mortality and decreased long-

M.C.A. Müller
Department of Intensive Care and Laboratory of Experimental Intensive Care and Anesthesiology (LEICA), Academic Medical Center, Meibergdreef 9, 1100 AZ, Amsterdam, The Netherlands

N.P. Juffermans (✉)
Department of Intensive Care and Laboratory of Experimental Intensive Care and Anesthesiology (LEICA), Academic Medical Center, Meibergdreef 9, 1100 AZ, Amsterdam, The Netherlands
E-mail: n.p.juffermans@amc.uva.nl

J.-L. Vincent (Ed.), *Annual Update in Intensive Care and Emergency Medicine 2013*,
DOI 10.1007/978-3-642-35109-9_42, © Springer-Verlag Berlin Heidelberg 2013

term survival [10, 11, 13]. Prognosis of the 'delayed TRALI syndrome' is particularly bad, with an estimated mortality of 40 % [9].

Obviously, blood transfusion cannot be avoided altogether. The high incidence and considerable morbidity and mortality of TRALI warrant insight into the risks and benefits of the decision to administer a blood transfusion. This chapter aims to address the susceptibility of critically ill patients to the development of a TRALI reaction. Risk factors for critically ill patients to develop TRALI as well as product-related risk factors will be discussed. Efforts to reduce TRALI have focused to date on modification of blood products, which has resulted in a substantial reduction in TRALI cases, but has not completely mitigated TRALI. In this chapter, we suggest that complete mitigation requires physicians to develop new approaches for patient-specific transfusion practice, aimed at pre-emptively taking action to decrease the risk of TRALI. It may be time to improve our assessment of the critically ill patient in need of a transfusion.

Pathogenesis of TRALI

The high incidence of TRALI reported in critically ill patient populations may be a consequence of its pathogenesis. TRALI is mediated by the interaction of neutrophils with pulmonary endothelial cells and can be caused by any cell-containing or plasma-rich blood product. TRALI is thought to occur as a result of a 'two hit' insult [14, 15]. The first 'hit' is an inflammatory condition of the patient at the time of the transfusion (e.g., sepsis, recent surgery), causing sequestration and priming of neutrophils and the expression of adhesion molecules in the pulmonary compartment. In response to priming, neutrophils undergo changes allowing for close contact with the endothelial surface of the pulmonary vasculature. The second 'hit' is mediated by components within the transfusion product. Donor antibodies against human neutrophil antigens (HNA) or human leukocyte antigens (HLA) present on leukocytes in the lungs of the recipient have been implicated. Bioactive substances that have accumulated during blood storage may also play a role in TRALI. These mediators are thought to stimulate the primed neutrophils to release proteases, resulting in endothelial damage, vascular permeability and the full clinical picture of TRALI [16, 17].

Findings from experimental models support the assumption that in TRALI, neutrophils are primed by inflammation. Priming with a 'first hit' of endotoxin (lipopolysaccharide [LPS]) was found to be a prerequisite for induction of TRALI using plasma from stored blood products [16–19]. In the presence of a priming 'hit', it was demonstrated that lower amounts of antibody were sufficient to elicit the TRALI reaction [20], which supports the notion that the presence of an inflammatory response increases susceptibility to TRALI. Thereby, both transfusion and patient-related factors play a role in TRALI pathogenesis.

Blood Product-Related Risk Factors for TRALI

- Anti-leukocyte Antibodies
  From case series, the presence of donor anti-leukocyte antibodies in the transfused product is thought to be implicated in TRALI. Involved antibodies are mainly directed against HLA class I, HLA class II or HNA. Activation of neutrophils occurs via HLA class I antigens. Mononuclear cells expressing HLA class II are involved by activation through HLA class II antibodies [21]. Recently, a large, prospective, case-controlled multicenter study systematically identified factors associated with an increased risk of TRALI [22]. In this study, blood product-related risk factors were the transfused volume of high titer cognate HLA class II antibody and the volume of high titer HNA antibody. Antibodies not associated with an increased risk of TRALI were non-cognate or weak anti-HLA class II antibody, as well as HLA class I antibodies. The finding that the presence of HLA class II antibodies in plasma of blood donors was of greater importance then class I, underlines results from previous studies [23]. Antibodies against the HNA-3a or 5b antigen appear to be especially important in causing severe cases of TRALI [24].

- Bioactive Response Modifiers
  Bioactive lipids (lysoPCs and neutral lipids) increase during storage of red blood cells (RBCs) and platelet concentrates [25, 26]. These substances were shown to have *in vitro* neutrophil priming capacity and can induce TRALI in animal models [16–18]. A retrospective clinical study of 10 TRALI patients linked the occurrence of TRALI to transfusion of blood products containing lipids with neutrophil-priming activity [27]. However, this finding was not confirmed in a study in cardiac surgery patients developing TRALI [28]. Moreover, in the largest prospective case-control study to date, no association was found between bioactive lipids and TRALI [22]. Other bioactive substances, such as pro-inflammatory cytokines, have not been consistently linked to TRALI [22].

- The Red Cell Storage Lesion
  During storage, RBC products undergo changes that affect their function and *in vivo* survival, which are collectively termed the "storage lesion". *In vitro* experiments have shown increased reactive oxygen species (ROS) formation by endothelial cells upon incubation with aged RBCs but not with fresh cells [29]. Indeed, in a murine 'two hit' transfusion model, aged RBCs were capable of inducing a TRALI reaction [30]. The proposed mechanism is either a decrease in the chemokine scavenging function of the RBC [31] or increased adhesion of the erythrocyte to the endothelium because of deficient anti-adhesive adenosine-5'-triphosphate release from the RBC [32]. Hereby, transfused RBCs may promote or exacerbate microvascular pathophysiology in the lung.

In conclusion, cognate HLA class II antibodies are blood product-related risk factors for TRALI. Bioactive lipids can function as a second 'hit' and are able to induce a TRALI reaction, but clinical data are conflicting. The aged RBC seems to play a role in preclinical models of TRALI. To date, interventions aimed at decreasing TRALI incidence have focused on product-related risk factors.

Mitigating TRALI by Modifying Blood Products

Exclusion of Female Donors

The prevalence of anti-leukocyte antibodies in the donor population depends on donor allo-exposure. Transfusion can lead to sensitization of recipients, albeit with very different reported numbers, ranging from 1 to 12 % [33]. However, pregnancy is the most important cause of sensitization in the donor population. Approximately 10 % of previously pregnant women have HLA antibodies and this number increases to 26–39 % in women who have had three or more pregnancies [33]. In order to prevent antibody-mediated TRALI, a predominantly male donor strategy for preparation of plasma rich products (including fresh frozen plasma and buffy coat-derived pool platelets) was first implemented in the United Kingdom in 2003. Other countries followed. This resulted in a ~ 70 % reduction in reported TRALI cases [33–37]. Hence, it seems that exclusion of female plasma donors prevents the majority of TRALI cases caused by plasma-rich products. However, TRALI cases that occur due to RBC transfusion and pooled platelets are not prevented.

Transfusion of Fresh Red Blood Cells Only

The accumulation of compounds, such as bioactive lipids, during storage suggests that the occurrence of TRALI may be associated with the use of older blood. A meta-analysis of studies on the effect of transfusion of stored blood showed an association between transfusion of stored blood and mortality in various patient populations [38]. In cardiac surgery patients, an association of prolonged storage of blood products and lung injury was found [39]. However, a large prospective study did not find evidence for an association between red cell storage duration and TRALI [22]. In a prospective case-control study in ICU patients, stored RBC products did not have any effect on pulmonary function or gas exchange [40]. Prospective randomized controlled clinical trials investigating the effect of fresh compared to stored RBCs on outcome in the critically ill are currently underway.

Patient-Related Risk Factors for TRALI

Predisposing factors for TRALI presumably lower the recipient's threshold for developing TRALI. Specific host factors have recently been identified (Table 1).

In a mouse model of TRALI, mechanical ventilation synergistically augmented lung injury, which was even further enhanced by the use of injurious ventilator settings [41], supporting the concept that mechanical ventilation aggravates the course of a TRALI reaction. There are also clinical data suggesting that mechanical ventilation may be a risk factor for lung injury following blood transfusion. As many as 33 % of mechanically ventilated critically ill patients developed lung injury within 48 hours after transfusion in an observational study [3]. In accordance, it was found that the presence of mechanical ventilation predisposed to acquiring TRALI in a retrospective study in ICU patients [11]. Furthermore, a recent study confirmed that high peak airway pressures (> 30 cm H_2O) contributed to an increased TRALI risk (OR 5.6 [2.1–14.9]) [22].

In addition to pulmonary hits, systemic inflammatory conditions are often present in critically ill patients. In a retrospective study on risk factors for TRALI in ICU patients, 87 % of the patients that fulfilled the diagnostic criteria for TRALI had a risk factor for ALI prior to onset of (possible) TRALI [11]. Hence, it is not surprising that there is an overlap between risk factors for ALI and TRALI. Of note, comparable to possible TRALI, ALI is a syndrome which occurs as a complication of an inflammatory condition.

Sepsis has been identified as a risk factor for TRALI in several studies in ICU patients [10, 11]. This is in line with animal models showing that endotoxemia reduces the amount of antibodies or bioactive response modifiers needed to induce TRALI [16, 20]. The presence of shock prior to transfusion also increased TRALI risk [22]. Of interest, plasma interleukin (IL)-8 levels in TRALI patients on a general hospital ward were elevated prior to transfusion, underlining the contribution of an inflammatory status to the risk of developing TRALI [22]. In cardiac surgery patients prospectively followed for the onset of TRALI, IL-8 levels prior to transfusion were elevated compared to transfused controls [42]. Because IL-8 has neutrophil-priming capacity, we hypothesize that during an insult, endothelial cells produce IL-8, contributing to attraction of neutrophils to the pulmonary compartment [42]. Whether IL-8 can serve as a biomarker for diagnosing TRALI remains to be determined.

Coronary artery bypass grafting (CABG) was found to be a risk factor for TRALI [11, 43]. In this context, the incidence of TRALI was found to be 2.4 % in a prospective study in cardiac surgery patients [28], which is about 8 to 10-fold higher compared to the general patient population. We speculate that this may be due to a longer time on cardiopulmonary bypass (CPB) [28]. Hematologic malignancy is also a TRALI risk factor in general hospital patient populations as well as in ICU patients [11, 43]. Massive transfusion is a risk factor for acute respiratory distress syndrome (ARDS) [1, 4] as well as for TRALI [11]. In patients admitted to the ICU because of bleeding, the presence of liver failure was a strong risk factor for developing TRALI when compared to transfused patients without liver failure [13]. It is not clear whether these conditions are risk factors solely because these patients commonly receive multiple transfusions, or that fluid overload induces priming. Of note, a prospective case control study in TRALI patients in the general hospital population revealed that an increased TRALI risk was associated with a positive fluid balance [22]. This is in line with findings in ALI patients [44] and indeed suggests that fluid overload may play a role in TRALI pathogenesis.

Table 1 Patient-related risk factors for transfusion-related acute lung injury (TRALI)

	Author, date [ref]	Type of study	Relation between risk factor and TRALI
Sepsis	Rana, 2006 [46]	Retrospective case control	Sepsis in 48 % TRALI patients ($p<0.01$ vs. controls)
	Gajic, 2007 [10]	Prospective case control	Sepsis in 37 % patients developing lung injury after transfusion ($p=0.016$ vs. controls)
	Vlaar, 2010 [11]	Retrospective cohort	Sepsis predisposes to TRALI (OR 2.5 [1.2–5.2])
Shock	Toy, 2012 [22]	Prospective case control	Shock prior to transfusion predisposes to TRALI (OR 4.2 [1.7–10.6])
Mechanical Ventilation	Gajic, 2004 [3]	Retrospective cohort	33 % of ventilated patients develop lung injury within 48 hours after transfusion
	Vlaar, 2010 [11]	Retrospective cohort	Mechanical ventilation predisposes to TRALI (OR 3.0 [1.3–7.1])
	Toy, 2012 [22]	Prospective case control	Peak airway pressure of >30 cm H_2O predisposes to TRALI (OR 5.6 [2.1–14.9])
Cardiac surgery	Vlaar, 2010 [11]	Retrospective cohort	Emergency cardiac surgery predisposes to TRALI (OR 17.6 [1.8–168.5])
	Toy, 2012 [22]	Prospective case control	Cardiac surgery predisposes to TRALI (OR 3.3 [1.21–9.2])
	Vlaar, 2011 [28]	Prospective case control	Time on cardiopulmonary bypass predisposes to TRALI (OR 1.0 [1.0–1.03])
Hematologic malignancy	Rana, 2006 [46]	Retrospective case control	Hematologic malignancy in 25 % TRALI patients ($p<0.01$ vs. controls)
	Vlaar, 2010 [11]	Retrospective cohort	Hematologic malignancy predisposes to TRALI (OR 13.1 [2.7–63.8])
	Silliman, 2003 [43]	Retrospective cohort	Hematologic malignancy in 46 % of TRALI patients ($p=0.0004$ vs. transfused controls)
Massive transfusion	Vlaar, 2010 [11]	Retrospective cohort	Massive transfusion predisposes to TRALI (OR 4.5 [2.1–9.8])
Positive fluid balance	Toy, 2012 [22]	Prospective case control	Fluid balance, increment per liter, predisposes to TRALI (OR 1.17 [1.08–1.28], $p<0.001$)
Liver failure	Benson, 2010 [13]	Retrospective cohort	Liver failure predisposes to TRALI (OR 13.1 [2.7–63.8])
	Toy, 2012 [22]	Prospective case control	Liver transplant surgery predisposes to TRALI (OR 6.7 [1.3–35.7])

Data are percentages or odds ratio (OR) with confidence interval

Taken together, critical illness contributes to increased susceptibility to a TRALI reaction. Of note, in a multivariate analysis of a retrospective study in ICU patients, patient-related risk factors were more important for the onset of TRALI than transfusion-related risk factors, suggesting that development of a TRALI reaction depends more on host factors then on factors in the blood product [11]. This finding suggests that taking an active approach in daily ICU practice may be effective in mitigating the risk of TRALI.

Mitigating TRALI by Individualized Patient Intervention

Appropriate management of critically ill patients has decreased their risk of developing ALI. The same may hold true for TRALI. Given the high number of ICU patients who receive a blood transfusion, the association between blood transfusion and adverse outcome in the critically ill [10, 11, 13], and the recent identification of TRALI risk factors, it is possible and perhaps even mandatory for ICU physicians to take an individualized approach towards their patients in need of a transfusion. Patient-focused strategies that may decrease the risk of TRALI include: Monitoring fluid balance; shock prior to transfusion should be avoided; a restrictive fluid balance should be maintained. Decreasing airway pressures in patients on mechanical ventilation prior to transfusion may also decrease the risk of TRALI. Although not proven in clinical trials, low tidal volume ventilation may further reduce TRALI risk. With the use of electronic medical records, protocols can be developed to further decrease the risk of TRALI. An electronic screening algorithm has been developed which accurately identifies TRALI patients [45]. Improvement in identification may contribute to better patient management of a TRALI case. Electronic health record surveillance may also be a tool for further implementing measures to decrease TRALI.

Conclusion

The presence of an inflammatory condition increases susceptibility to TRALI. Specific patient-related risk factors for TRALI have been identified, empowering the ICU physician to take an individualized approach to the patient in need of a transfusion, which may contribute to mitigating the risk of TRALI.

References

1. Croce MA, Tolley EA, Claridge JA, Fabian TC (2005) Transfusions result in pulmonary morbidity and death after a moderate degree of injury. J Trauma 59:19–23
2. Dara SI, Rana R, Afessa B, Moore SB, Gajic O (2005) Fresh frozen plasma transfusion in critically ill medical patients with coagulopathy. Crit Care Med 33:2667–2671

3. Gajic O, Rana R, Mendez JL et al (2004) Acute lung injury after blood transfusion in mechanically ventilated patients. Transfusion 44:1468–1474
4. Gong MN, Thompson BT, Williams P, Pothier L, Boyce PD, Christiani DC (2005) Clinical predictors of and mortality in acute respiratory distress syndrome: potential role of red cell transfusion. Crit Care Med 33:1191–1198
5. Khan H, Belsher J, Yilmaz M et al (2007) Fresh-frozen plasma and platelet transfusions are associated with development of acute lung injury in critically ill medical patients. Chest 131:1308–1314
6. Kiraly LN, Underwood S, Differding JA, Schreiber MA (2009) Transfusion of aged packed red blood cells results in decreased tissue oxygenation in critically injured trauma patients. J Trauma 67:29–32
7. Goldman M, Webert KE, Arnold DM, Freedman J, Hannon J, Blajchman MA (2005) Proceedings of a consensus conference: towards an understanding of TRALI. Transfus Med Rev 19:2–31
8. Toy P, Popovsky MA, Abraham E et al (2005) Transfusion-related acute lung injury: definition and review. Crit Care Med 33:721–726
9. Marik PE, Corwin HL (2008) Acute lung injury following blood transfusion: expanding the definition. Crit Care Med 36:3080–3084
10. Gajic O, Rana R, Winters JL et al (2007) Transfusion related acute lung injury in the critically ill: prospective nested case-control study. Am J Respir Crit Care Med 176:886–891
11. Vlaar AP, Binnekade JM, Prins D et al (2010) Risk factors and outcome of transfusion-related acute lung injury in the critically ill: A nested case-control study. Crit Care Med 38:771–778
12. Popovsky MA, Moore SB (1985) Diagnostic and pathogenetic considerations in transfusion-related acute lung injury. Transfusion 25:573–577
13. Benson AB, Austin GL, Berg M et al (2010) Transfusion-related acute lung injury in ICU patients admitted with gastrointestinal bleeding. Intensive Care Med 36:1710–1717
14. Bux J, Sachs UJ (2007) The pathogenesis of transfusion-related acute lung injury (TRALI). Br J Haematol 136:788–799
15. Silliman CC (2006) The two-event model of transfusion-related acute lung injury. Crit Care Med 34:S124–S131
16. Kelher MR, Masuno T, Moore EE et al (2009) Plasma from stored packed red blood cells and MHC class I antibodies causes acute lung injury in a 2-event in vivo rat model. Blood 113:2079–2087
17. Silliman CC, Voelkel NF, Allard JD et al (1998) Plasma and lipids from stored packed red blood cells cause acute lung injury in an animal model. J Clin Invest 101:1458–1467
18. Silliman CC, Bjornsen AJ, Wyman TH et al (2003) Plasma and lipids from stored platelets cause acute lung injury in an animal model. Transfusion 43:633–640
19. Tung JP, Fung YL, Nataatmadja M et al (2011) A novel in vivo ovine model of transfusion-related acute lung injury (TRALI). Vox Sang 100:219–230
20. Looney MR, Nguyen JX, Hu Y, Van Ziffle JA, Lowell CA, Matthay MA (2009) Platelet depletion and aspirin treatment protect mice in a two-event model of transfusion-related acute lung injury. J Clin Invest 119:3450–3461
21. Kopko PM, Paglieroni TG, Popovsky MA, Muto KN, MacKenzie MR, Holland PV (2003) TRALI: correlation of antigen-antibody and monocyte activation in donor-recipient pairs. Transfusion 43:177–184
22. Toy P, Gajic O, Bacchetti P et al (2012) Transfusion-related acute lung injury: incidence and risk factors. Blood 119:1757–1767
23. Kopko PM, Popovsky MA, MacKenzie MR, Paglieroni TG, Muto KN, Holland PV (2001) HLA class II antibodies in transfusion-related acute lung injury. Transfusion 41:1244–1248
24. Curtis BR, McFarland JG (2006) Mechanisms of transfusion-related acute lung injury (TRALI): anti-leukocyte antibodies. Crit Care Med 34:S118–S123
25. Silliman CC, Dickey WO, Paterson AJ et al (1996) Analysis of the priming activity of lipids generated during routine storage of platelet concentrates. Transfusion 36:133–139

26. Silliman CC, Moore EE, Kelher MR, Khan SY, Gellar L, Elzi DJ (2011) Identification of lipids that accumulate during the routine storage of prestorage leukoreduced red blood cells and cause acute lung injury. Transfusion 51:2549–2554
27. Silliman CC, Paterson AJ, Dickey WO et al (1997) The association of biologically active lipids with the development of transfusion-related acute lung injury: a retrospective study. Transfusion 37:719–726
28. Vlaar AP, Hofstra JJ, Determann RM et al (2011) The incidence, risk factors, and outcome of transfusion-related acute lung injury in a cohort of cardiac surgery patients: a prospective nested case-control study. Blood 117:4218–4225
29. Mangalmurti NS, Chatterjee S, Cheng G et al (2010) Advanced glycation end products on stored red blood cells increase endothelial reactive oxygen species generation through interaction with receptor for advanced glycation end products. Transfusion 50:2353–2361
30. Vlaar AP, Hofstra JJ, Levi M et al (2010) Supernatant of aged erythrocytes causes lung inflammation and coagulopathy in a "two-hit" in vivo syngeneic transfusion model. Anesthesiology 113:92–103
31. Mangalmurti NS, Xiong Z, Hulver M et al (2009) Loss of red cell chemokine scavenging promotes transfusion-related lung inflammation. Blood 113:1158–1166
32. Zhu H, Zennadi R, Xu BX et al (2011) Impaired adenosine-5'-triphosphate release from red blood cells promotes their adhesion to endothelial cells: A mechanism of hypoxemia after transfusion. Crit Care Med 39:2478–2486
33. Triulzi DJ, Kleinman S, Kakaiya RM et al (2009) The effect of previous pregnancy and transfusion on HLA alloimmunization in blood donors: implications for a transfusion-related acute lung injury risk reduction strategy. Transfusion 49:1825–1835
34. Arinsburg SA, Skerrett DL, Karp JK et al (2012) Conversion to low transfusion-related acute lung injury (TRALI)-risk plasma significantly reduces TRALI. Transfusion 52:946–952
35. Eder AF, Herron R, Strupp A et al (2007) Transfusion-related acute lung injury surveillance (2003–2005) and the potential impact of the selective use of plasma from male donors in the American Red Cross. Transfusion 47:599–607
36. Vlaar AP, Binnekade JM, Schultz MJ, Juffermans NP, Koopman MM (2008) Preventing TRALI: ladies first, what follows? Crit Care Med 36:3283–3284
37. Wright SE, Snowden CP, Athey SC et al (2008) Acute lung injury after ruptured abdominal aortic aneurysm repair: the effect of excluding donations from females from the production of fresh frozen plasma. Crit Care Med 36:1796–1802
38. Wang D, Sun J, Solomon SB, Klein HG, Natanson C (2012) Transfusion of older stored blood and risk of death: a meta-analysis. Transfusion 52:1184–1195
39. Koch CG, Li L, Sessler DI et al (2008) Duration of red-cell storage and complications after cardiac surgery. N Engl J Med 358:1229–1239
40. Kor DJ, Kashyap R, Weiskopf RB et al (2012) Fresh red blood cell transfusion and short-term pulmonary, immunologic, and coagulation status: a randomized clinical trial. Am J Respir Crit Care Med 185:842–850
41. Vlaar AP, Wolthuis EK, Hofstra JJ et al (2010) Mechanical ventilation aggravates transfusion-related acute lung injury induced by MHC-I class antibodies. Intensive Care Med 36:879–886
42. Vlaar AP, Hofstra JJ, Determann RM et al (2012) Transfusion-related acute lung injury in cardiac surgery patients is characterized by pulmonary inflammation and coagulopathy: A prospective nested case-control study. Crit Care Med 40:2813–2820
43. Silliman CC, Boshkov LK, Mehdizadehkashi Z et al (2003) Transfusion-related acute lung injury: epidemiology and a prospective analysis of etiologic factors. Blood 101:454–462
44. Sakr Y, Vincent JL, Reinhart K et al (2005) High tidal volume and positive fluid balance are associated with worse outcome in acute lung injury. Chest 128:3098–3108
45. Clifford L, Singh A, Wilson GA et al (2013) Electronic health record surveillance algorithms facilitate the detection of transfusion-related pulmonary complications. Transfusion (in press)
46. Rana R, Fernandez-Perez ER, Khan SA et al (2006) Transfusion-related acute lung injury and pulmonary edema in critically ill patients: a retrospective study. Transfusion 46:1478–1483

Part XIII

Perioperative Problems

Prevention of Postoperative Pulmonary Problems Starts Intraoperatively

J. Poelaert, L. Szegedi, and S. Blot

Introduction

Pulmonary complications are a burden for the postoperative patient [1]. Atelectasis and pneumonia have been recognized as the most frequent pulmonary problems in critically ill surgical intensive care unit (ICU) patients [2]. However, it is sometimes difficult to differentiate clinically between atelectasis and pulmonary infection. About a century ago, collapse of the lung, related to insufficient inspiratory power was reported [3, 4]. Altered gas exchange was characteristic in these patients [5], and Bendixen et al. used the term "atelectasis" for the very first time in 1963 [6]. Atelectasis occurs with progressive loss of compliance, not least as a consequence of loss of laryngeal muscle tone and disappearance of intrinsic positive end-expiratory pressure (PEEP), after induction of anesthesia, paralysis and bypassing the oropharynx [7]. Atelectasis resolves only with some deep inflations of the lung (recruitment), adequate pain relief, physiotherapy and early mobilization of the patient.

Pulmonary infections are another problem, in particular for high-risk surgical patients [8]. Although preventive measures against ventilator-associated pneumonia (VAP) have a relatively high adherence rate of 72 %, there is consider-

J. Poelaert (✉)
Dept of Anesthesiology and Perioperative Medicine, University Hospital Brussels, Free University of Brussels, Brussels, Belgium
jan.poelaert@uzbrussel.be

L. Szegedi
Dept of Anesthesiology and Perioperative Medicine, University Hospital Brussels, Free University of Brussels, Brussels, Belgium

S. Blot
Dept of Anesthesiology and Perioperative Medicine, University Hospital Brussels, Free University of Brussels, Brussels, Belgium

J.-L. Vincent (Ed.), *Annual Update in Intensive Care and Emergency Medicine 2013*,
DOI 10.1007/978-3-642-35109-9_43,

able variability among countries [9] and disciplines. Moreover, knowledge of these preventive measures is not widespread among non-ICU physicians. Once present, VAP and postoperative pneumonia necessitate antibiotherapy, sometimes in association with prolonged need for mechanical ventilatory support. Both entities, atelectasis and pulmonary infections, increase considerably the length of stay in the hospital and thus costs. Adequate prevention could lead to a significant reduction in cost both at health care and social-economical levels.

In this review, these two clinical entities are critically examined, in particular in the light of preventive measures that could be undertaken in daily practice. We deliberately do not discuss states of acute lung injury (ALI), which can also be present in postoperative patients, often with detrimental consequences. Although some preventive measures can already be initiated intraoperatively, others can be pursued in the ICU setting.

Incidence of Postoperative Pulmonary Complications

The incidence of atelectasis is hard to assess and difficult to calculate. Only imaging can provide a hint of occurrence rates: In patients with normal lungs, 90 % of patients developed atelectatic regions in the most dependent segments, which were still present 1 h after intubation [7, 10]. In 50 % of patients these atelectasis regions remained present until 24 h after intubation. Moreover, they are related to constitutional characteristics [11].

In contrast, postoperative pneumonia and VAP have been studied extensively both in the general ICU and in postoperative cardiac surgical patients. The incidence of VAP after cardiac surgery encompasses 6.3 episodes per 1,000 days of mechanical ventilation [12]. In a meta-analysis, Smetana et al. assessed the risk factors for postoperative pneumonia in non-cardiothoracic surgical patients [13]; congestive heart failure, age, American Society of Anesthesiologists (ASA)-class > 2, and chronic obstructive pulmonary disease (COPD) appeared to be the most important risk factors. Box 1 shows the most important and relevant risk factors for postoperative pulmonary infection. Postoperative pneumonia was associated with a significant 30-day mortality of 21 % in patients undergoing non-cardiac surgery [14], and in a general surgical cohort, 30-day mortality was higher in patients with a postoperative pulmonary complication (19.5 %; 95 % confidence interval (CI), 12.5–26.5 %) than in those without (0.5 %; 95 % CI, 0.2–0.8 %) [2]. Postoperative pneumonia is also associated with larger hospital costs and longer lengths of stay compared with uncomplicated surgery [15]. Patients especially at risk of postoperative pneumonia and VAP are those undergoing high-risk surgery in the presence of extensive co-morbidities, those undergoing cardiac and cardiovascular surgery [16], open thoracic or thoracoplastic surgery [17], and major upper abdominal procedures and prolonged procedures [2].

Box 1
Risk factors for post-operative and ventilator-associated pneumonia

Major and Complicated Surgery	Non-Cardiothoracic Surgery
Cardiac surgery Thoracic surgery Major vascular surgery Major upper abdominal procedure Other high-risk surgeries Extensive co-morbidities	Congestive heart failure Age > 50 years old ASA-class > 2 Chronic obstructive pulmonary disease
ASA: American Society of Anesthesiologists	

Atelectasis

Pathophysiology

Atelectasis is the result of general anesthesia, ventilation and patient-related factors. In large series of postoperative patients (n = 24,000), 0.9 % developed hypoxemia, not resolving with only supplemental oxygen [18]. Intraoperatively, atelectasis is responsible for a large part of hypoxemia. Upon administration of a hypnotic, opioid or neuromuscular blocker, muscular tone is abolished within the first few minutes [1]; during endotracheal suctioning, again, atelectasis may be induced through induction of negative intra-thoracic pressure [19]. Surgical manipulation causing compression and/or traction may be aggravated by type and length of intervention, age and body habitus, bleeding, etc. Cephalic displacement of the diaphragm during general anesthesia in the dorsal recumbent position, sometimes with increased intra-abdominal pressures, as well as the Trendelenburg position, intensifies hypoventilation and compression of the most dorsal lung segments (Box 2). Furthermore, loss of muscle tone and the cardiac weight itself may induce further pulmonary compression or inadequate expansion. Rapidly, the dependent lung segments fill up with fluid, hampering any rapid recruitment [20]. In addition to impaired oxygenation and compliance, microvascular leakage occurs as a witness of damaged endothelial function in anesthetized rats when atelectasis is present [21].

Atelectasis can be classified into three groups: Compression atelectasis occurs during general anesthesia and is caused by chest geometry and diaphragm position and motion [22]; in the case of absorption atelectasis, the greater the inspired oxygen fraction after induction, the faster the collapse of the lung regions [23]; loss-of-surfactant atelectasis collapse occurs within 5 min after a vital capacity maneuver at an inspired oxygen fraction (FiO_2) of 1.0 or immediately after removal of PEEP at FiO_2 of 0.5. Atelectasis in turn impedes surfactant function, making the lung more prone to collapse again after reopening [24].

Box 2
Factors predisposing to atelectasis

- Type and length of surgery
- Age
- Body habitus
- Bleeding
- Loss of muscle tone and cephalic displacement of the diaphragm during general anesthesia
- Increased intra-abdominal pressure
- Cardiac weight
- Increased FiO_2 and low alveolar ventilation
- Intra-tracheal suctioning
- Impaired surfactant

Absorption atelectasis is induced by increased FiO_2 and low alveolar ventilation; in addition, impaired surfactant will also provoke atelectasis (Box 2). In addition to hypoxemia, a fall in functional residual capacity (FRC) and decreased lung compliance, a significant increase in pulmonary resistance may occur, mainly by hypoxic pulmonary vasoconstriction, potentially hampering ejection by the right ventricle.

Diagnosis

Atelectasis is clinically suspected whenever impaired oxygenation and decreased lung compliance occur in a situation that could be related to atelectasis. This clinical diagnosis is particularly important intraoperatively, when active diagnosis is difficult. In situations where imaging is possible, bedside chest radiography appears the first choice.

Typically, signs of volume loss characterize the presence of atelectasis:

- displacement of thoracic structures: Interlobar fissure, hemidiaphragm, shift of mediastinal organs
- compensatory hyperinflation of certain lung segments
- typical triangular shape of collapsed lung segment
- obliteration of a lung segment may opacify adjoining parts of the mediastinum.

A more sensitive and specific diagnosis of atelectasis can be made with computed tomography (CT) scans. Already in 1986, Strandberg et al. described with CT scan the presence of atelectasis after induction of anesthesia [7, 10]. A CT scan depicts areas of increased density [11, 25] with an abrupt decrease in FRC and a lowered inflection point on the pressure-volume relationship. The densities correlate with collapsed lung alveoli [26]. Although CT scans indeed offer a nearly perfect tool for evaluation of the presence of atelectasis [25], this technique is often not very useful because of the need for transportation of an often-hypoxemic patient. All these methods provide regionally specific information, but only as a snapshot in time. Magnetic resonance imaging (MRI) currently has no additional value in the diagnosis of atelectasis. In contrast, ultrasound allows detection of many deviations in lung structure, pleural fluid, etc. In the ICU, this technique has shown value in detecting alveolar collapse [27]. However, intraoperatively ultrasound is often inadequate to visualize properly collapsed lung tissue. Electrical impedance tomography (EIT) is a new technology, which permits continuous visualization of the distribution of ventilation. Data are continuously displayed in the form of images, waveforms and parameters. Measures can be taken to individually tailor ventilator settings. Determining how different lung regions respond to therapeutic interventions over time is challenging without continuous regional information. The use of EIT in ICU settings is well-established; however, intraoperatively its value still has to be demonstrated. Regional ventilation distribution and recruitment has been assessed in experimental models of direct and indirect ALI as well as in normal lungs [28]. Recently, this technology was used to evaluate the effects of PEEP during pneumoperitoneum in laparoscopic surgery. PEEP led to improved aeration of the dorsal lung parts with consequent improved oxygenation and pulmonary compliance [29].

Prevention and Treatment

Experimental and clinical studies suggest recruitment of collapsed alveoli needing peak inspiratory pressures of $>30\,cm\,H_2O$ for >45 s to allow slow alveoli, with a low time constant, to reopen [30]. Table 1 shows the different studies and compares outcomes after recruitment maneuvers. Additional PEEP is obligatory to keep the alveoli open but only after a recruitment maneuver has been applied [19, 25, 30].

Table 1 Recruitment maneuvers and atelectasis in cardiac surgery: Review of the literature

Author	Specimen	Method	Result
Magnusson (1998) [64]	Pigs	ECC	Atelectasis in control Repeat within 6 h
Murphy (2001) [65]	Human	ECC	Earlier extubation
Tschernko (2002) [66]	Human	ECC	Decreased intrapulmonary shunting
Minkovich (2007) [67]	Human	ECC	After ECC and in the ICU
Shim (2009) [68]	Human	Off pump	Earlier extubation; ICU LOS no change

ECC: extracorporeal circulation: LOS: length of stay

In a small group of cardiac surgical patients, a recruitment maneuver induced a rapid decrease in cardiac output, concomitant with a fall in preload conditions [31]. In an animal experimental setting with lung injury, the same findings were described [32]. Furthermore, care should be taken to monitor right ventricular function because of potential overload during the maneuver [32]. Lower peak inspiratory pressures led to less impressive changes in hemodynamics, although equivalent results on oxygenation and compliance recovery [33]. Continuous perioperative monitoring of pressures, volumes and, if available, regional ventilation is necessary during general anesthesia to allow correct adjustment of ventilatory settings.

Postoperative Pneumonia and Ventilator-Associated Pneumonia

Pathophysiology

Postoperative pneumonia and VAP have been described in terms of aspiration of subglottic secretions and gastroesophageal reflux. Bacterial leakage (often 10^{10} bacteria/ml secretion [34]) in conjunction with impaired lung defense, results in tracheobronchial colonization and induction of ventilator-associated tracheobronchitis (VAT) and VAP. This aspiration risk is not a minor issue, as shown by Mahul et al., but can run up to volumes of 150 ml per day [34]; intraoperatively, even in the prone position, drainage from nose and mouth could be as high as 50 ml/h [35]. Risk factors for aspiration include not only the endotracheal tube (ETT), but also mechanical ventilation without PEEP, tracheal suctioning, the presence of a nasogastric tube with gastroesophageal reflux, and various patient-related factors (Box 3).

Box 3
Risk factors for aspiration

- Type of tracheal tube
- Mechanical ventilation without positive end-expiratory pressure
- Intra-tracheal suctioning
- Presence of the nasogastric tube
- Gastroesophageal reflux

Patients suffering from preoperative hypoxemia or a pulmonary infection less than one month before surgery show a significantly increased risk of postoperative pulmonary complications [2].

All types of mechanical ventilation are non-physiological and, in a vicious circle manner, cause further damage to the lungs, with either a biochemical injury (with loss of cytokines, complement, prostanoids, reactive oxygen species, leukotrienes, proteases), and/or a biophysical injury (shear, overdistension, cyclic stretch, increased intrathoracic pressure). Protective tools, such as barrel-shaped polyvinyl chloride (PVC) cuffed ETTs, do not prevent aspiration as demonstrated recently in *in vitro* studies [35, 36]: with an ETT in a rigid cylinder, a dye solution poured above the barrel-shaped PVC cuff of the ETT descended along the channels formed within the PVC.

Diagnosis

VAP is diagnosed on the basis of several criteria. Essential clinical criteria include the presence of fever, purulent sputum and hypoxemia. In addition, a positive Gram-stain, leukocytosis and a positive chest X-ray should be present [37, 38]. The problem occurs after major surgery in patients in whom these criteria are not obvious or overt. Fabregas et al. suggested that the presence of infiltrates on the chest radiograph and two of three clinical criteria (leukocytosis, purulent secretions, fever) had a sensitivity of 69 % and a specificity of 75 % [39], rates that are not worse than those with the clinical pulmonary infection score.

Preventive Measures

Prevention is the cornerstone with respect to abolishing atelectasis and pulmonary infections induced through inadequate sealing and subsequent leakage along the cuff of the endotracheal tube (Fig. 1).

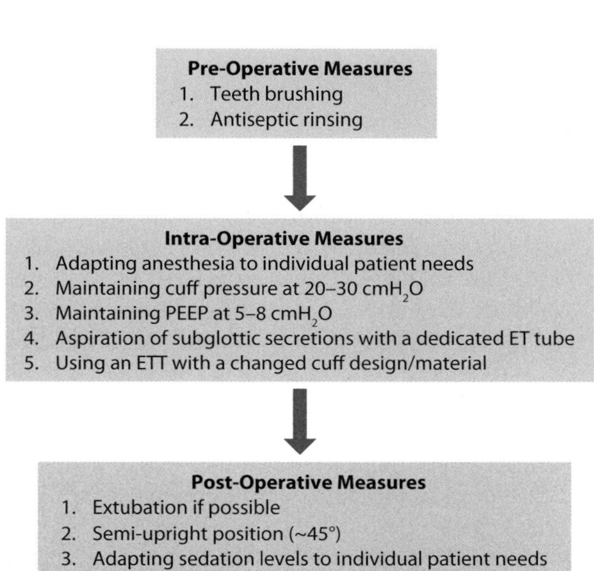

Pre-Operative Measures
1. Teeth brushing
2. Antiseptic rinsing
Intra-Operative Measures
1. Adapting anesthesia to individual patient needs
2. Maintaining cuff pressure at 20–30 cmH2O
3. Maintaining PEEP at 5–8 cmH2O
4. Aspiration of subglottic secretions with a dedicated ET tube
5. Using an ETT with a changed cuff design/material
Post-Operative Measures
1. Extubation if possible
2. Semi-upright position (~45°)
3. Adapting sedation levels to individual patient needs
4. Antiseptic rinsing
5. Teeth brushing if patient is awake

Fig. 1 Measures to prevent post-operative pulmonary complications (see text for details)

Preoperative Measures

In esophageal cancer surgery and in cardiac surgical patients, a clear decline in occurrence rate of postoperative pneumonia was observed with teeth brushing (40, 41). Rinsing of the buccal cavity with a 2% solution of chlorhexidine reduces the frequency of postoperative pneumonia considerably [42]. In a recent meta-analysis, Labeau et al. showed that use of antiseptics resulted in a significant risk reduction of VAP (RR 0.67; 95% CI 0.50–0.88; $p=0.004$) [43]. Chlorhexidine application was shown to be effective (RR 0.72; 95% CI 0.55–0.94; $p=0.02$), in particular in a cardiac surgical subset (RR 0.41, 95% CI 0.17–0.98).

Intraoperative Measures

The rates of VAP and of postoperative pneumonia are time-related: The longer the surgical procedure lasts, the greater the risk of aspiration and thus pulmonary infection. A surgical procedure of more than 2 h increases the risk 4-fold [44]. In this respect, comorbidities play an important role. The sooner the patient can breathe spontaneously and be weaned from the ventilator, the better. This implies that sedation levels in the ICU should be moderate and systematically adapted to the disease state of the patient; the anesthetic level also needs to be adapted in this manner. In addition to these important issues, some preventive measures can be undertaken to reduce intraoperative aspiration.

- Lubrication: In one-lung ventilated thoracic surgery patients, Sanjay et al. demonstrated that lubricated PVC cuffs of a double-lumen tube sealed the trachea nearly twice as long as non-lubricated tubes with a resultant decrease in pulmonary infection rates [45].
- Cuff pressure management: Since the introduction of the high-volume low-pressure tube, cuff pressures have been set considerably lower than with the high-pressure low-volume cuffed ETT. Tracheal damage has decreased considerably, but the risk of underinflation of the cuff has increased [46]. Even with an adequately inflated cuff, the rate of leakage must still be considered. Intervals of a cuff pressure <20 cm H_2O during the first 8 ventilation days significantly increased the risk of postoperative pneumonia (OR 4.23, CI 1.12–15.92).

  Intermittent control of cuff pressure, at least every four hours, to obtain a cuff pressure between 20 and 30 cm H_2O [47, 48], is one approach to this problem. Care should be taken to release the cuff pressure manometer from the valve of the cuff, so that minimal leakage occurs; in this way a slightly increased lower level of, e.g., 24 cm H_2O should be considered. Not controlling the cuff pressure will certainly lead to either underinflation or overinflation and to adequate cuff pressures in less than 20% of cases [49].
- PEEP: Early onset VAP, occurring less than 5 days after intubation, was significantly less frequent in non-hypoxemic patients ventilated with 5–8 cm H_2O PEEP during lung surgery [50]. Prophylactic PEEP was found to be safe and to reduce VAP-rates, including late-onset VAP [51].
- Aspiration of subglottic secretions with a dedicated ETT, with a PVC cuff, may reduce the risk of aspiration [51]. In only 31 patients after cardiac surgery,

Bouza et al. demonstrated a significant difference in VAP-rate, days on ventilator and length of stay in the ICU in those patients needing ventilator support for more than 48 h. Combined use of PEEP and subglottic aspiration reduced the risk of VAP from 48 % in controls to 27 % in patients intubated with this dedicated ET tube [52]. Similarly, Mahul et al. demonstrated, in a mixed medical-surgical ICU population expected to require > 72 h of ventilatory support, that subglottic secretion drainage resulted in a lower frequency of VAP or a later onset [34]. Valles et al. reported a similar reduction in VAP rate without, however, any difference in outcome [53]. Other investigators have described comparable results [12, 54, 55]. Estimating the cost of VAP treatment at €4,300 and a reduction in the VAP-rate of 30 % with a dedicated ETT with subglottic secretion drainage, a cost-benefit equilibrium is present.

The problems and debate associated with the single drainage lumen tube include the correct dorsal position of this lumen and the presence of an open, non-occluded lumen. Indeed, viscous secretions may occlude the sole lumen and suctioning against the tracheal wall may also occlude the lumen of the suction channel [56]. Occlusion was found in 43 % of investigated patients. Introduction of an ET tube with multiple drainage suction holes above the cuff could improve the preventive function of such tubes by less frequent occlusion rates [57], but larger *in vivo* studies are missing.

- Changed cuff design: Several *in vitro* studies have suggested that a modified cuff design could reduce the risk of aspiration and transition of subglottic secretions into the trachea. Indeed, Dullenkopf et al. demonstrated the presence of small channels in the PVC cuff, permitting transit of secretions into the tracheal lumen; the existence of these channels has been shown both with fluoroscopy and with dye solutions [58]. In an *in vitro* investigation, Zanella et al. demonstrated that a tapered-shaped, cuffed ET tube clearly delayed the risk of transit of dye solution up to 12 h on the condition that PEEP (5–8 cm H_2O) was present [36], in contrast to a barrel-shaped cuffed ET-tube, for which the security margin lasted only 2 and maximum 6 h. Finally, Dave et al. demonstrated in three different sized artificial tracheas that the tapered-shaped PVC cuff was more effective in preventing leakage [59]. To the best of our knowledge, published *in vivo* studies are not yet available.

  Theoretically, it is conceivable that a tapered-shaped cuff indeed seals the tracheal lumen much better as this cuff fits perfectly into the lumen at a particular level [60]. The perfect fit is closely related to a particular level of the cuff at which no channels in the PVC are formed. Depending on the tracheal anatomy of a particular patient, this improved sealing can be at an upper or rather lower cuff level.
- Changed cuff material: In the past decade, ETTs with a polyurethane cuff have been developed. Because of the ultra-thin wall, polyurethane cuffs have smaller channels formed by the folds in the cuff. This characteristic has resulted in more favorable research outcomes in comparison with their PVC cuffed counterparts. In an *in vitro* study by Dave et al., it was demonstrated that PVC cuffs always leaked more and faster compared to polyurethane cuffs [59]. In a ran-

domized controlled trial in 134 cardiac surgical patients, it was demonstrated that use of polyurethane cuffed tubes resulted in a reduced prevalence of postoperative pneumonia. The risk of pneumonia was reduced by nearly 50 %, albeit the prevalence of pneumonia in the control group was particularly high [48]. Similarly, Lucangelo et al. showed that a barrel shaped polyurethane cuffed ETT sealed the tracheal lumen better [61]. In children, Dullenkopf et al. demonstrated similar results [62].

Postoperative Measures

Intraoperative measures will certainly diminish considerably the risk of aspiration and, therefore, decrease the potential risk for initial bacterial descent towards the trachea. Preventive measures such as teeth brushing and antiseptic mouth rinsing should be restarted in the postoperative setting. Supine body position is a clear risk factor for pulmonary infections in ventilated patients; in a study comparing supine with semi-recumbent positioning in 86 intubated and mechanically ventilated patients, the rate of microbiologically confirmed pneumonia was significantly lower in the semirecumbent patients ($p=0.018$), and the odds ratio for development of nosocomial pneumonia was 6.8 (1.7–26.7) ($p=0.006$) for supine position [63]. Although the semi-recumbent position is not possible intraoperatively, whenever possible in terms of hemodynamic status, patients should be positioned in a semi-upright position (about 40°) once extubated in the operating room or postoperative care setting.

Conclusion

It is obvious that prevention of (postoperative) pulmonary complications should be a main goal in every perioperative setting. Preventive strategies start already before surgery and should be initiated on the ward with systematic application of oral hygiene. Intraoperatively, anesthesiologists should start more extensive preventive action including optimal cuff pressure and PEEP administration in addition to monitored and individually titrated mechanical ventilator parameters. Using a dedicated ETT is only supported by *in vitro* studies and should be related to the presumed duration of postoperative ventilator support at induction of the anesthetic.

References

1. Hedenstierna G (1989) Mechanisms of postoperative pulmonary dysfunction. Acta Chir Scand Suppl 550:152–158
2. Canet J, Gallart L, Gomar C et al (2010) Prediction of postoperative pulmonary complications in a population-based surgical cohort. Anesthesiology 113:1338–1350
3. Morrow DJ, Stimson PM (1947) Atelectasis in poliomyelitis. Med Clin North Am 31:609–625

4. Sutherland GA (1914) Anterior poliomyelitis; paralysis of abdominal muscles; collapse of lung. Proc R Soc Med 7:31–32
5. Nunn JF (1964) Factors influencing the arterial oxygen tension during halothane anaesthesia with spontaneous respiration. Br J Anaesth 36:327–341
6. Bendixen HH, Hedley-Whyte J, Laver MB (1963) Impaired oxygenation in surgical patients during general anesthesia with controlled ventilation. A concept of atelectasis. N Engl J Med 269:991–996
7. Strandberg A, Tokics L, Brismar B, Lundquist H, Hedenstierna G (1986) Atelectasis during anaesthesia and in the postoperative period. Acta Anaesthesiol Scand 30:154–158
8. Varban OA, McCoy TP, Westcott C (2011) A comparison of pre-operative comorbidities and post-operative outcomes among patients undergoing laparoscopic nissen fundoplication at high- and low-volume centers. J Gastrointest Surg 15:1121–1127
9. Ricard JD, Conti G, Boucherie M et al (2012) A European survey of nosocomial infection control and hospital-acquired pneumonia prevention practices. J Infect 65:285–291
10. Strandberg A, Hedenstierna G, Tokics L, Lundquist H, Brismar B (1986) Densities in dependent lung regions during anaesthesia: atelectasis or fluid accumulation? Acta Anaesthesiol Scand 30:256–259
11. Strandberg A, Tokics L, Brismar B, Lundquist H, Hedenstierna G (1987) Constitutional factors promoting development of atelectasis during anaesthesia. Acta Anaesthesiol Scand 31:21–24
12. Kollef MH, Skubas NJ, Sundt TM (1999) A randomized clinical trial of continuous aspiration of subglottic secretions in cardiac surgery patients. Chest 116:1339–1346
13. Smetana GW, Lawrence VA, Cornell JE (2006) Preoperative pulmonary risk stratification for noncardiothoracic surgery: systematic review for the American College of Physicians. Ann Intern Med 144:581–595
14. Arozullah AM, Khuri SF, Henderson WG, Daley J (2001) Development and validation of a multifactorial risk index for predicting postoperative pneumonia after major noncardiac surgery. Ann Intern Med 135:847–857
15. Dimick JB, Chen SL, Taheri PA, Henderson WG, Khuri SF, Campbell DA Jr (2004) Hospital costs associated with surgical complications: a report from the private-sector National Surgical Quality Improvement Program. J Am Coll Surg 199:531–537
16. Hortal J, Munoz P, Cuerpo G, Litvan H, Rosseel PM, Bouza E (2009) Ventilator-associated pneumonia in patients undergoing major heart surgery: an incidence study in Europe. Crit Care 13:R80
17. Liang J, Qiu G, Shen J et al (2010) Predictive factors of postoperative pulmonary complications in scoliotic patients with moderate or severe pulmonary dysfunction. J Spinal Disord Tech 23:388–392
18. Rose DK, Cohen MM, Wigglesworth DF, DeBoer DP (1994) Critical respiratory events in the postanesthesia care unit. Patient, surgical, and anesthetic factors. Anesthesiology 81:410–418
19. Heinze H, Eichler W, Karsten J, Sedemund-Adib B, Heringlake M, Meier T (2011) Functional residual capacity-guided alveolar recruitment strategy after endotracheal suctioning in cardiac surgery patients. Crit Care Med 39:1042–1049
20. Gattinoni L, Pelosi P, Suter P, Pedoto A, Vercesi P, Lissoni A (1998) Acute respiratory distress syndrome caused by pulmonary and extrapulmonary disease. Different syndromes? Am J Respir Crit Care Med 158:3–11
21. Duggan M, McCaul CL, McNamara PJ, Engelberts D, Ackerley C, Kavanagh BP (2003) Atelectasis causes vascular leak and lethal right ventricular failure in uninjured rat lungs. Am J Respir Crit Care Med 167:1633–1640
22. Warner DO, Warner MA, Barnes RD et al (1996) Perioperative respiratory complications in patients with asthma. Anesthesiology 85:460–467
23. Joyce CJ, Baker AB, Kennedy RR (1993) Gas uptake from an unventilated area of lung: computer model of absorption atelectasis. J Appl Physiol 74:1107–1116

24. Oyarzun MJ, Iturriaga R, Donoso P et al (1991) Factors affecting distribution of alveolar surfactant during resting ventilation. Am J Physiol 261:L210–L217
25. Reinius H, Jonsson L, Gustafsson S et al (2009) Prevention of atelectasis in morbidly obese patients during general anesthesia and paralysis: A computerized tomography study. Anesthesiology 111:979–987
26. Hedenstierna G, Lundquist H, Lundh B et al (1989) Pulmonary densities during anaesthesia. An experimental study on lung morphology and gas exchange. Eur Respir J 2:528–535
27. Karabinis A, Saranteas T, Karakitsos D et al (2008) The "cardiac-lung mass" artifact: an echocardiographic sign of lung atelectasis and/or pleural effusion. Crit Care 12:R122
28. Wrigge H, Zinserling J, Muders T et al (2008) Electrical impedance tomography compared with thoracic computed tomography during a slow inflation maneuver in experimental models of lung injury. Crit Care Med 36:903–909
29. Karsten J, Luepschen H, Grossherr M et al (2011) Effect of PEEP on regional ventilation during laparoscopic surgery monitored by electrical impedance tomography. Acta Anaesthesiol Scand 55:878–886
30. Futier E, Constantin J-M, Pelosi P et al (2010) Intraoperative recruitment maneuver reverses detrimental pneumoperitoneum-induced respiratory effects in healthy weight and obese patients undergoing laparoscopy. Anesthesiology 113:1310–1319
31. Nielsen J, Ostergaard M, Kjaergaard J et al (2005) Lung recruitment maneuver depresses central hemodynamics in patients following cardiac surgery. Intensive Care Med 31:1189–1194
32. Nielsen J, Nilsson M, Freden F et al (2006) Central hemodynamics during lung recruitment maneuvers at hypovolemia, normovolemia and hypervolemia. A study by echocardiography and continuous pulmonary artery flow measurements in lung-injured pigs. Intensive Care Med 32:585–594
33. Odenstedt H, Lindgren S, Olegard C et al (2005) Slow moderate pressure recruitment maneuver minimizes negative circulatory and lung mechanic side effects: evaluation of recruitment maneuvers using electric impedance tomography. Intensive Care Med 31:1706–1714
34. Mahul P, Auboyer C, Jospe R et al (1992) Prevention of nosocomial pneumonia in intubated patients: respective role of mechanical subglottic secretions drainage and stress ulcer prophylaxis. Intensive Care Med 18:20–25
35. Young PJ, Blunt MC (1999) Improving the shape and compliance characteristics of a high-volume, low-pressure cuff improves tracheal seal. Br J Anaesth 83:887–889
36. Zanella A, Scaravilli V, Isgrò S et al (2011) Fluid leakage across tracheal tube cuff, effect of different cuff material, shape, and positive expiratory pressure: a bench-top study. Intensive Care Med 37:343–347
37. Johanson WG Jr, Pierce AK, Sanford JP, Thomas GD (1972) Nosocomial respiratory infections with gram-negative bacilli. The significance of colonization of the respiratory tract. Ann Intern Med 77:701–706
38. Pugin J, Auckenthaler R, Mili N, Janssens JP, Lew PD, Suter PM (1991) Diagnosis of ventilator-associated pneumonia by bacteriologic analysis of bronchoscopic and nonbronchoscopic "blind" bronchoalveolar lavage fluid. Am Rev Respir Dis 143:1121–1129
39. Fabregas N, Ewig S, Torres A et al (1999) Clinical diagnosis of ventilator associated pneumonia revisited: comparative validation using immediate post-mortem lung biopsies. Thorax 54:867–873
40. Akutsu Y, Matsubara H, Shuto K et al (2010) Pre-operative dental brushing can reduce the risk of postoperative pneumonia in esophageal cancer patients. Surgery 147:497–502
41. Stonecypher K (2010) Ventilator-associated pneumonia: the importance of oral care in intubated adults. Crit Care Nurs Q 33:339–347
42. Panchabhai TS, Dangayach NS, Krishnan A, Kothari VM, Karnad DR (2009) Oropharyngeal cleansing with 0.2 % chlorhexidine for prevention of nosocomial pneumonia in critically ill patients: an open-label randomized trial with 0.01 % potassium permanganate as control. Chest 135:1150–1156

43. Labeau SO, Van de Vyver K, Brusselaers N, Vogelaers D, Blot SI (2011) Prevention of ventilator-associated pneumonia with oral antiseptics: a systematic review and meta-analysis. Lancet Infect Dis 11:845–854
44. Delgado-Rodriguez M, Medina-Cuadros M, Martinez-Gallego G, Sillero-Arenas M (1997) Usefulness of intrinsic surgical wound infection risk indices as predictors of postoperative pneumonia risk. J Hosp Infect 35:269–276
45. Sanjay PS, Miller SA, Corry PR, Russell GN, Pennefather SH (2006) The effect of gel lubrication on cuff leakage of double lumen tubes during thoracic surgery. Anaesthesia 61:133–137
46. Rello J, Sonora R, Jubert P, Artigas A, Rue M, Valles J (1996) Pneumonia in intubated patients: role of respiratory airway care. Am J Respir Crit Care Med 154:111–115
47. Valencia M, Ferrer M, Farre R et al (2007) Automatic control of tracheal tube cuff pressure in ventilated patients in semirecumbent position: a randomized trial. Crit Care Med 35:1543–1549
48. Poelaert J, Depuydt P, De Wolf A, Van de Velde S, Herck I, Blot S (2008) Polyurethane cuffed endotracheal tubes to prevent early postoperative pneumonia after cardiac surgery: a pilot study. J Thorac Cardiovasc Surg 135:771–776
49. Nseir S, Brisson H, Marquette CH et al (2009) Variations in endotracheal cuff pressure in intubated critically ill patients: prevalence and risk factors. Eur J Anaesthesiol 26:229–234
50. Ludwig C, Angenendt S, Martins R, Mayer V, Stoelben E (2011) Intermittent positive-pressure breathing after lung surgery. Asian Cardiovasc Thorac Ann 19:10–13
51. Lacherade JC, De Jonghe B, Guezennec P et al (2010) Intermittent subglottic secretion drainage and ventilator-associated pneumonia: A multicenter trial. Am J Respir Crit Care Med 182:910–917
52. Bouza E, Perez MJ, Munoz P, Rincon C, Barrio JM, Hortal J (2008) Continuous aspiration of subglottic secretions in the prevention of ventilator-associated pneumonia in the post-operative period of major heart surgery. Chest 134:938–946
53. Valles J, Artigas A, Rello J et al (1995) Continuous aspiration of subglottic secretions in preventing ventilator-associated pneumonia. Ann Intern Med 122:179–186
54. Lorente L, Lecuona M, Jimenez A, Mora ML, Sierra A (2007) Influence of an endotracheal tube with polyurethane cuff and subglottic secretion drainage on pneumonia. Am J Respir Crit Care Med 176:1079–1083
55. Smulders K, van der Hoeven H, Weers-Pothoff I, Vandenbroucke-Grauls C (2002) A randomized clinical trial of intermittent subglottic secretion drainage in patients receiving mechanical ventilation. Chest 121:858–862
56. Dragoumanis CK, Vretzakis GI, Papaioannou VE, Didilis VN, Vogiatzaki TD, Pneumatikos IA (2007) Investigating the failure to aspirate subglottic secretions with the Evac endotracheal tube. Anesth Analg 105:1083–1085
57. Doyle A, Fletcher A, Carter J, Blunt M, Young P (2011) The incidence of ventilator-associated pneumonia using the PneuX System with or without elective endotracheal tube exchange: A pilot study. BMC Res Notes 4:92
58. Dullenkopf A, Gerber A, Weiss M (2003) Fluid leakage past tracheal tube cuffs: evaluation of the new Microcuff endotracheal tube. Intensive Care Med 29:1849–1853
59. Dave MH, Frotzler A, Spielmann N, Madjdpour C, Weiss M (2010) Effect of tracheal tube cuff shape on fluid leakage across the cuff: an in vitro study. Br J Anaesth 105:538–543
60. Poelaert J (2011) Ventilator-associated pneumonia and cuff shape. Am J Respir Crit Care Med 184:485
61. Lucangelo U, Zin WA, Antonaglia V et al (2008) Effect of positive expiratory pressure and type of tracheal cuff on the incidence of aspiration in mechanically ventilated patients in an intensive care unit. Crit Care Med 36:409–413
62. Dullenkopf A, Gerber AC, Weiss M (2005) Nitrous oxide diffusion into tracheal tube cuffs – efficacy of a new prototype cuff pressure release valve. Acta Anaesthesiol Scand 49:1072–1076

63. Drakulovic MB, Torres A, Bauer TT, Nicolas JM, Nogue S, Ferrer M (1999) Supine body position as a risk factor for nosocomial pneumonia in mechanically ventilated patients: a randomised trial. Lancet 354:1851–1858
64. Magnusson L, Wický S, Tyden H, Hedenstierna G (1998) Repeated vital capacity manoeuvres after cardiopulmonary bypass: effects on lung function in a pig model. Br J Anaesth 80:682–684
65. Murphy GS, Szokol JW, Curran RD, Votapka TV, Vender JS (2001) Influence of a vital capacity maneuver on pulmonary gas exchange after cardiopulmonary bypass. J Cardiothorac Vasc Anesth 15:336–340
66. Tschernko EM, Bambazek A, Wisser W et al (2002) Intrapulmonary shunt after cardiopulmonary bypass: the use of vital capacity maneuvers versus off-pump coronary artery bypass grafting. J Thorac Cardiovasc Surg 124:732–738
67. Minkovich L, Djaiani G, Katznelson R et al (2007) Effects of alveolar recruitment on arterial oxygenation in patients after cardiac surgery: a prospective, randomized, controlled clinical trial. J Cardiothorac Vasc Anesth 21:375–378
68. Shim J, Chun D, Choi Y, Lee J, Hong S, Kwak Y (2009) Effect of early vital capacity manuever on respiratoy variables during multivessel off-pump coronary artery bypass graft surgery. Crit Care Med 37:539–544

Perioperative Hemodynamic Optimization: From Clinical to Economic Benefits

G. Marx and F. Michard

Introduction

Shoemaker et al. [1] were the first to describe the concept of oxygen debt during major surgical procedures and to demonstrate that perioperative hemodynamic optimization has the potential to improve postoperative outcome. Since then, at least 26 other randomized controlled trials (RCTs) [2–27] have shown that perioperative optimization of stroke volume, cardiac output and/or oxygen delivery (DO_2) decreases postoperative morbidity and/or mortality in patients undergoing medium-to-high risk surgery (Table 1).

Several recent meta-analyses have confirmed the ability of perioperative hemodynamic optimization to reduce the rate of postoperative acute kidney injury (AKI) [28], gastrointestinal complications [29], pneumonia, surgical site and urinary tract infections [30], development of at least one postoperative complication [31], and hospital length of stay [32]. The odds ratios reported in these meta-analyses are summarized in Table 2. A large quality improvement evaluation [33] conducted in three UK hospitals confirmed in more than 1,300 patients undergoing abdominal, vascular or orthopedic surgery that implementation of perioperative hemodynamic optimization is not only feasible in real life but also results in a significant decrease in hospital length of stay.

G. Marx (✉)
Klinik für Operative Intensivmedizin und Intermediate Care Universitätsklinikum der RWTH Aachen, Pauwelsstr. 30, 52074 Aachen, Germany
E-mail: gmarx@ukaachen.de

F. Michard
Critical Care, Edwards Lifesciences, 1 Edwards Way, Irvine, CA

J.-L. Vincent (Ed.), *Annual Update in Intensive Care and Emergency Medicine 2013*,
DOI 10.1007/978-3-642-35109-9_44,

Table 1 Randomized controlled trials showing a benefit in perioperative hemodynamic optimization. More than 2,900 patients have been enrolled in these 27 studies

Author, year [reference]	n	Hemodynamic target and treatment	Surgery	Tool	Main clinical benefits
Shoemaker 1988 [1]	310	$DO_2 > 600$ ml/min/m^2 Fluid, dobutamine	General	PAC	Morbidity Mortality (21 vs. 34 %)
Berlauk 1991 [2]	89	CI, PAOP, SVR Not specified	Vascular	PAC	Morbidity
Fleming 1992 [3]	67	$DO_2 > 670$ ml/min/m^2 Fluid, dobutamine	Trauma	PAC	Morbidity
Boyd 1993 [4]	107	$DO_2 > 600$ ml/min/m^2 Fluid, dopexamine	General	PAC	Morbidity Mortality (6 vs. 22 %)
Mythen 1995 [5]	60	SVmax (= plateau value) Fluid	Cardiac	Doppler	Morbidity Hospital LOS
Sinclair 1997 [6]	40	SVmax Fluid	Hip	Doppler	Hospital LOS
Ueno 1998 [7]	34	$DO_2 > 600$ ml/min/m^2 Fluid, dobutamine	Hepatectomy	PAC	Morbidity
Wilson 1999 [8]	138	$DO_2 > 600$ ml/min/m^2 Fluid, dopexamine	General and vascular	PAC	Morbidity Hospital LOS
Polonen 2000 [9]	393	$SvO_2 > 70$ % Fluid, dobutamine	Cardiac	PAC	Morbidity Hospital LOS
Lobo 2000 [10]	37	$DO_2 > 600$ ml/min/m^2 Fluid, dobutamine	General	PAC	Morbidity Mortality (16 vs. 50 %)
Venn 2002 [11]	59	SVmax Fluid	Hip	Doppler	Morbidity
Gan 2002 [12]	100	SVmax Fluid	General	Doppler	Morbidity Hospital LOS
Conway 2002 [13]	57	SVmax Fluid	Bowel	Doppler	Morbidity
McKendry 2004 [14]	174	SVmax Fluid	Cardiac	Doppler	Hospital LOS
Wakeling 2005 [15]	128	SVmax Fluid	Bowel	Doppler	Morbidity Hospital LOS
Pearse 2005 [16]	122	$DO_2 > 600$ ml/min/m^2 Fluid, dopexamine	General	Pulse contour	Morbidity Hospital LOS
Noblett 2006 [17]	108	SVmax Fluid	Bowel	Doppler	Morbidity Hospital LOS

Table 1 *Continued*

Author, year [reference]	n	Hemodynamic target and treatment	Surgery	Tool	Main clinical benefits
Chytra 2007 [18]	162	SVmax Fluid	Trauma	Doppler	Morbidity Hospital LOS
Lopes 2007 [19]	33	PPV < 10 % Fluid	General	A line	Morbidity Hospital LOS
Donati 2007 [20]	135	$ScvO_2 > 73\,\%$ Fluid, dobutamine	General and vascular	CVC	Morbidity Hospital LOS
Mayer 2009 [21]	60	SVV < 12 % Fluid	Abdominal	Pulse contour	Morbidity Hospital LOS
Benes 2010 [22]	120	SVV < 10 % Fluid	Abdominal and vascular	Pulse contour	Morbidity
Jhanji 2010 [23]	135	SVmax or $DO_2 > 600$ ml/min/m^2 Fluid or flu-id + dopexamine	Abdominal	Pulse contour	Morbidity
Cecconi 2011 [24]	40	$DO_2 > 600$ ml/min/m^2 Fluid, dobutamine	Hip	Pulse contour	Morbidity
Pillai 2011 [25]	66	SVmax Fluid	Cystectomy	Doppler	Morbidity
Figus 2011 [26]	104	SVmax Fluid	Flap	Doppler	Morbidity
Ping 2012 [27]	40	11 % < SVV < 13 % Fluid	Abdominal	Pulse contour	Morbidity Hospital LOS

n: number of patients; CI: cardiac index; DO_2: oxygen delivery; SV: stroke volume; SvO_2: mixed venous oxygen saturation, $ScvO_2$: central venous oxygen saturation; PAOP: pulmonary artery occlusion pressure; PPV: arterial pulse pressure variation; SVR: systemic vascular resistance; SVV: stroke volume variation; LOS: length of stay; PAC: pulmonary artery catheter.

Fuelled by this growing body of evidence, recommendations for perioperative hemodynamic optimization have been proposed by the National Health Service (NHS) in the UK and by the French Society of Anesthesiology (SFAR, annual congress, September 2011). Enhanced Recovery after Surgery is a bundle of best evidence-based practices delivered by a multi-professional heathcare team, with the intention of helping patients recover faster after surgery [34]. The Enhanced Recovery Partnership recently recommended: (1) The use of intraoperative fluid management technologies to enhance treatment with the aim of avoiding hypovolemia and fluid excess; and (2) that all anesthetists caring for patients undergoing intermediate or major surgery should have cardiac output measuring technologies immediately available and be trained to use them [34].

Despite this body of scientific evidence, a survey published last year [35] showed that only 16 % of anesthesiologists use perioperative hemodynamic optimi-

Table 2 Odds ratios reported in meta-analyses showing a morbidity reduction with perioperative hemodynamic optimization

Authors [reference]	Benefit	Average odds ratio (confidence interval)
Brienza et al. [28]	Acute kidney injury	0.64 (0.50–0.83)
Giglio et al. [29]	Minor GI complications	0.29 (0.17–0.50)
Giglio et al. [29]	Major GI complications	0.42 (0.27–0.65)
Dalfino et al. [30]	Pneumonia	0.71 (0.55–0.92)
Dalfino et al. [30]	Surgical site infection	0.58 (0.46–0.74)
Dalfino et al. [30]	Urinary tract infection	0.44 (0.22–0.88)
Hamilton et al. [31]	Complication rate*	0.44 (0.35–0.55)

*Proportion of patients developing at least one postoperative complication. GI: gastrointestinal.

zation during major surgical procedures. Reasons for this poor application may include lack of awareness, uncertainty regarding clinical benefits, and difficulties in measuring hemodynamic parameters and/or following treatment protocols in a busy environment where priority is logically given to anesthesia and analgesia [36].

Overcoming Barriers to Adoption

Do We Need More Scientific Evidence?

As mentioned above, clinical evidence is based on multiple single center RCTs, several meta-analyses, and a large quality improvement evaluation performed in the UK. Some of the single center RCTs were conducted more than 10–20 years ago. Because quality of care has likely improved over the last few decades, the validity of their conclusions may now be questioned. Hamilton et al. [31] showed a mortality reduction (odd ratio 0.49) when all published RCTs were taken into account; however, the mortality benefit was no longer visible when selecting only RCTs published after 2000 [31]. A survival benefit is still likely at a global level [37], e.g., when considering emerging countries where mortality rates remain high (Brazil, Russia, India and China represent almost 3 billion people). However, whether a survival benefit still exists for very high-risk procedures in developed countries remains to be confirmed in future clinical studies. Interestingly, Hamilton et al. [31] also showed that the morbidity benefit did not decrease over time, and was as visible in studies published after 2000 (odds ratio 0.38) as in studies published in the nineties (odds ratio 0.62).

Moreover, there is no published large multicenter RCT confirming the clinical value of perioperative hemodynamic optimization. Such a multicenter RCT is ongoing in the UK [38]. The goal of this study, named OPTIMISE, is to enroll more than 730 patients from 11 different hospitals; results should be known in 2013 [38]. One must keep in mind that these large multicenter RCTs, although gold standards for drug trials, are not necessarily the panacea for evaluating new technologies or clinical strategies in anesthesia and critical care [39]. Highly selective enrolment, extra human resources, impossibility to blind the intervention, high compliance rates, and the Hawthorne effect are well known limitations to the extrapolation of RCT results to real life clinical practice [39, 40]. As a result, quality improvement evaluations are increasingly seen as very valuable alternatives to demonstrate that a new therapeutic strategy has an impact on quality of care and patient outcome [40–43].

Using Simple and Less Invasive Hemodynamic Tools

Several positive outcome studies (8 out of the 27 studies listed in Table 1) have been conducted using the pulmonary artery catheter (PAC). Although the PAC is still and by far the most widely used hemodynamic technique (around 2 million PACs are used worldwide every year), it is now often considered too time-consuming and too invasive for the hemodynamic monitoring of patients undergoing non-cardiac surgical procedures (with the notable exception of liver transplantation). Indeed, alternative and less invasive technologies have been developed over recent years. Because these devices are quick to set up and easy to use they fit better with the operating room workflow. Among them, esophageal Doppler and pulse contour methods are leading the way and most recent positive outcome studies have been conducted with these tools (17 of the 27 studies listed in Table 1). The recent development of totally non-invasive solutions may further help to expand the concept of perioperative hemodynamic optimization to a broader patient population.

Simplifying Treatment Protocols

There is now a consensus regarding the fact that no hemodynamic monitoring tool can improve outcome by itself [44]. However, even when clinicians have understood that using a treatment protocol with well defined hemodynamic goals is key, they are often puzzled when they have to select a specific protocol for implementation in their institution. Indeed, many different treatment protocols have been shown to be useful to improve postoperative outcome, from the maximization of DO_2 to the minimization of pulse pressure or stroke volume variation (Table 1), and there is no scientific evidence that one strategy is superior to the other. We believe that it may be wise to select an individual approach (one size does not fit all) and a treatment protocol simple enough to be easily adopted by most (less is

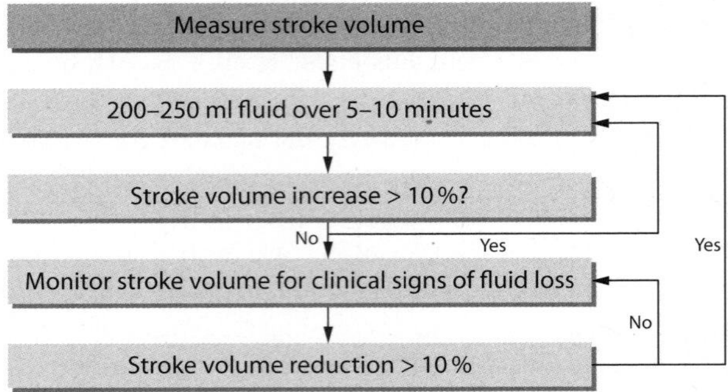

Fig. 1 Intraoperative fluid management protocol using a stroke volume optimization technique. This treatment protocol is recommended by the National Institute for Clinical Excellence in the UK and by the French Society of Anesthesiology (SFAR). It has been used in a large (1,307 patients) quality improvement program, which demonstrated a decrease in hospital length of stay [33]

more). The treatment protocol based on the monitoring and fluid optimization of stroke volume proposed by the NHS and the SFAR has the advantage of meeting these two criteria (Fig. 1) and has been successfully used in a large quality improvement program conducted in the UK [33].

Using Checklists

The use of checklists is another simple but very efficient means of ensuring that therapies are effectively delivered. In 2006, Pronovost et al. [42] demonstrated that a simple checklist could dramatically decrease catheter-related bloodstream infections in critically ill patients. In his best-seller book entitled "The Checklist Manifesto" [45], Dr Gawande nicely described the potential of checklists and justified their need as follows: "the volume and complexity of what we know has exceeded our individual ability to deliver its benefit correctly, safely, or reliably. Knowledge has both saved us and burdened us. That means we need a different strategy for overcoming failure, one that builds on experience and takes advantage of the knowledge people have but somehow also makes up for our inevitable human inadequacies". In 2009, Gawande's team published a study [43] demonstrating the value of a simple perioperative checklist to decrease surgical morbidity and mortality. This Surgical Safety checklist, officially recommended by the World Health Organization (WHO), is now used in many hospitals and countries all over the world. As far as we know, checklists have not yet been developed specifically for perioperative hemodynamic optimization but there is no doubt they could be of value to improve the adoption of and compliance with perioperative hemodynamic optimization strategies and ultimately the outcome of medium-to-high risk surgical patients. Adding a single item to the current "Sign In" section of the Surgical Safety Checklist, such as "The patient's eligibility for perioperative hemodynamic optimization has been considered", may be a very useful first step.

Economic Benefits: Where Are We Today?

The vast majority of perioperative hemodynamic optimization outcome studies showing a significant reduction in postoperative complications were based on the monitoring and optimization of stroke volume and/or cardiac output (Table 1). In other words, perioperative hemodynamic optimization has an inherent cost that may be perceived as a limit to wide adoption. A few studies have investigated the potential economical benefits related to the use of perioperative hemodynamic optimization [1, 46, 47]. All have actually reported cost savings when perioperative hemodynamic optimization is adopted.

Old Cost-Analysis Studies

In their 1988 landmark article, Shoemaker et al. [1] compared the cost of treating high-risk surgical patients with or without a DO_2 optimization treatment protocol (both groups were monitored with a PAC). The average cost was $9,690 lower in the optimization group. In the UK, Guest et al. [46] and Fenwick et al. [47] also reported a cost reduction per patient estimated at £1,259 ($1,889) and £3,467 ($5,201), respectively, when a similar perioperative hemodynamic optimization protocol was used. As far as we know, these are the only prospective studies that have compared the costs of treating high-risk surgical patients with and without perioperative hemodynamic optimization. These studies refer to patients monitored with a PAC and treated one or two decades ago. Anesthesia and surgical practices have changed over the last decades, as have health care costs, making their applicability to current practice somewhat hazardous. Therefore, using the most recent literature we provide a more up to date estimation of potential cost-savings related to the adoption of perioperative hemodynamic optimization.

An Estimation of Potential Cost-Savings Based on Recent Literature

A study published by Boltz et al. in 2012 [48] investigated the effects of postoperative complications on the financial cost of patient care. In 2,250 patients undergoing general and vascular surgery, they showed a synergistic effect, with excess costs of $6,358, $12,802 and $42,790 for patients developing 1, 2, or 3 or more (3+) complications, respectively. For patients developing 1+ postoperative complications, excess costs were $17,949 as compared to patients with no complica-

Table 3 Potential cost-savings related to the use of perioperative hemodynamic optimization. Estimations are shown according to the pre-implementation morbidity rate and based on odds ratios published by Hamilton et al. [31] in 2011 and a cost analysis published by Boltz et al. [48] in 2012

Pre-implementation morbidity rate (%)	10	20	30	40	50	60
Expected morbidity rate after implementation of perioperative hemodynamic optimization (%)	3.5–5.5	7–11	11–17	14–22	18–28	21–33
Expected cost reduction per patient ($)	808–1,167	1,615–2,333	2,423–3,500	3,231–4,667	4,039–5,833	4,846–7,000

tions. The 2011 meta-analysis of 29 RCTS (including a total of 4,805 patients) by Hamilton et al. [31] concluded that perioperative hemodynamic optimization decreased the proportion of patients developing 1+ postoperative complication with an odds ratio ranging between 0.35 and 0.55 (Table 2). From this recent and quite robust clinical and economic information, it becomes possible to provide an estimation of perioperative hemodynamic optimization-induced cost-savings. These savings depend on the pre-implementation morbidity rate and are summarized in Table 3. They range between $808 per patient (for a pre-implementation morbidity rate of 10 % and an odds ratio of 0.55) and $7,000 (for a pre-implementation morbidity rate of 60 % and an odds ratio of 0.35). They are in line with a recent cost simulation [49] suggesting that €1,882 ($2,258) could be saved per patient if perioperative hemodynamic optimization were implemented in elderly hip fracture patients. These amounts are an estimation of what may be considered as the maximum acceptable costs for hemodynamic monitoring technologies in patients undergoing medium-to-high risk surgery. As estimations, they need to be confirmed by prospective studies assessing the real costs of patients treated with and without perioperative hemodynamic optimization.

Cost-Effectiveness Simulation

In many countries, decisions to adopt, reimburse, or issue specific guidance on use of new medical treatments are increasingly based on cost-effectiveness. The term cost-effectiveness has become synonymous with health economic evaluation and has been used to depict the extent to which interventions measure up to what can be considered to represent value for money. Cost-effectiveness analysis has been defined as an economic study design in which consequences of different interventions are measured using a single outcome, usually in 'natural' units (for example, life-years gained, deaths avoided, or complications avoided). Alternative interventions are then compared in terms of cost per unit of effectiveness. A probabilistic

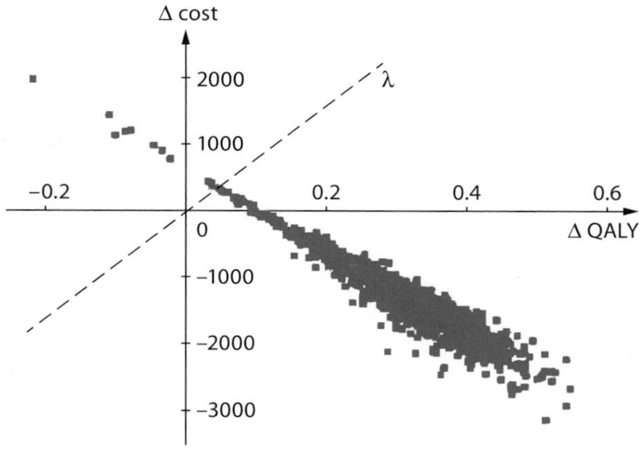

Fig. 2 Simulation of incremental costs and effects (ΔCOST, ΔQALYs) of perioperative hemodynamic optimization (PHO) compared with routine fluid therapy. In 96.5 % of the simulations (each point represents a simulation), PHO was less costly and provided more quality-of-life years (QALYs). From [49] with permission

cost-effectiveness model was recently developed by Bartha et al. [49] for perioperative hemodynamic optimization in elderly hip fracture patients. The model contained a decision tree for the postoperative short-term outcome and a Markov structure for long-term outcome (up to 5 years). Clinical effects estimates, costs, health-related quality-of-life measures, and long-term survival constituted input variables. The data were extracted from previous publications and Swedish databases. Model output consisted of estimated medical care costs related to quality-adjusted life-years (QALYs). In the base case analysis, perioperative hemodynamic optimization reduced costs by €1,882 ($2,258) and gained 0.344 QALYs. In 96.5 % of the simulations, perioperative hemodynamic optimization was less costly and provided more QALYs (Fig. 2). Bartha et al. are currently conducting a prospective clinical and economical evaluation in the same patient population to confirm these simulation data.

Conclusion

Very few strategies have the potential to improve quality of care and to reduce health care costs at the same time. Perioperative hemodynamic optimization is likely one of them; as such, it may become standard of care for patients undergoing medium-to-high risk surgery in the future. The clinical benefits of perioperative hemodynamic optimization are supported by many single center RCTs, several meta-analyses and one large quality improvement evaluation. The economic value makes sense (decreasing complications should logically decrease costs), is supported by a few, dated studies and by simulation models but certainly deserves confirmation in a prospective manner. We expect that OPTIMISE [38], the ongoing multicenter RCT, will confirm both the clinical and economic value of perioperative hemodynamic optimization. Implications for health care systems and societies are potentially huge. There are about 1 million patients in the US who may benefit from perioperative hemodynamic optimization every year (patients undergoing major general and vascular surgery). Assuming a current complication rate of 30 % and a decrease to 19 % with perioperative hemodynamic optimization [31], 110,000 patients could be protected from postoperative complications, leading to around $2 billion savings every year for the US health care system. Estimations are more difficult to make in Europe because of significant discrepancies between health care quality and costs from one country to the other. However, they are likely of the same magnitude and, if confirmed by ongoing studies, should drive the adoption of perioperative hemodynamic optimization in surgical patients at risk of developing postoperative complications.

References

1. Shoemaker WC, Appel PL, Kram HB, Waxman K, Lee TS (1988) Prospective trial of supranormal values of survivors as therapeutic goals in high-risk surgical patients. Chest 94:1176–1186
2. Berlauk JF, Abrams JH, Gilmour IJ et al (1991) Preoperative optimization of cardiovascular hemodynamics improves outcome in peripheral vascular surgery. Ann Surg 214:289–297
3. Fleming A, Bishop M, Shoemaker W et al (1992) Prospective trial of supranormal values as goals of resuscitation in severe trauma. Arch Surg 127:1175–1179
4. Boyd O, Grounds M, Bennett E (1993) A randomized clinical trial of the effect of deliberate perioperative increase of oxygen delivery on mortality in high-risk surgical patients. JAMA 270:2699–2707
5. Mythen MG, Webb AR (1995) Perioperative plasma volume expansion reduces the incidence of gut mucosal hypoperfusion during cardiac surgery. Arch Surg 130:423–429
6. Sinclair S, James S, Singer M (1997) Intraoperative intravascular volume optimisation and length of hospital stay after repair of proximal femoral fracture: a randomised controlled trial. BMJ 315:909–912
7. Ueno S, Tanabe G, Yamada H et al (1998) Response of patients with cirrhosis who have undergone partial hepatectomy to treatment aimed at achieving supranormal oxygen delivery and consumption. Surgery 123:278–286
8. Wilson J, Woods I, Fawcett J et al (1999) Reducing the risk of major elective surgery: randomised controlled trial of preoperative optimisation of oxygen delivery. BMJ 318:1099–1103
9. Polonen P, Ruokonen E, Hippelainen M, Poyhonen M, Takala J (2000) A prospective, randomized study of goal-oriented hemodynamic therapy in cardiac surgical patients. Anesth Analg 90:1052–1059
10. Lobo SMA, Salgado PF, Castillo VG et al (2000) Effects of maximizing oxygen delivery on morbidity and mortality in high-risk surgical patients. Crit Care Med 28:3396–3404
11. Venn R, Steele A, Richardson P, Poloniecki J, Grounds M, Newman P (2002) Randomized controlled trial to investigate influence of the fluid challenge on duration of hospital stay and perioperative morbidity in patients with hip fractures. Br J Anaesth 88:65–71
12. Gan TJ, Soppitt A, Maroof M et al (2002) Goal-directed intraoperative fluid administration reduces length of hospital stay after major surgery. Anesthesiology 97:820–826
13. Conway DH, Mayall R, Abdul-Latif MS, Gilligan S, Tackaberry C (2002) Randomized controlled trial investigating the influence of intravenous fluid titration using oesophageal Doppler monitoring during bowel surgery. Anaesthesia 57:845–849
14. McKendry M, McGloin H, Saberi D, Caudwell L, Brady AR, Singer M (2004) Randomised controlled trial assessing the impact of a nurse delivered, flow monitored protocol for optimisation of circulatory status after cardiac surgery. BMJ 329:258

15. Wakeling HG, McFall MR, Jenkins CS et al (2005) Intraoperative oesophageal Doppler guided fluid management shortens postoperative hospital stay after major bowel surgery. Br J Anaesth 95:634–642
16. Pearse R, Dawson D, Fawcett J, Rhodes A, Grounds RM, Bennett ED (2005) Early goal-directed therapy after major surgery reduces complications and duration of hospital stay. A randomised, controlled trial. Crit Care 9:R687–R693
17. Noblett SE, Snowden CP, Shenton BK, Horgan AF (2006) Randomized clinical trial assessing the effect of Doppler-optimized fluid management on outcome after elective colorectal resection. Br J Surg 93:1069–1076
18. Chytra I, Pradl R, Bosman R, Pelnar P, Kasal E, Zidkova A (2007) Esophageal Doppler-guided fluid management decreases blood lactate levels in multiple-trauma patients: a randomized controlled trial. Crit Care 11:R24
19. Lopes MR, Oliveira MA, Pereira VOS, Lemos IPB, Auler JOC, Michard F (2007) Goal-directed fluid management based on pulse pressure variation monitoring during high-risk surgery: a pilot randomized controlled trial. Crit Care 11:R100
20. Donati A, Loggi S, Preiser JC et al (2007) Goal-directed intraoperative therapy reduces morbidity an length of hospital stay in high-risk surgical patients. Chest 132:1817–1824
21. Mayer J, Boldt J, Mengistu AM, Röhm KD, Suttner S (2010) Goal-directed intraoperative therapy based on autocalibrated arterial pressure waveform analysis reduces hospital stay in high-risk surgical patients: a randomized, controlled trial. Crit Care 14:R18
22. Benes J, Chytra I, Altmann P et al (2010) Intraoperative fluid optimization using stroke volume variation in high-risk surgical patients: results of a prospective randomized study. Crit Care 14:R118
23. Janjhi S, Vivian-Smith A, Lucena-Amaro S, Watson D, Hinds CJ, Pearse RM (2010) Haemodynamic optimisation improves tissue microvascular flow and oxygenation after major surgery: a randomised controlled trial. Crit Care 14:R151
24. Cecconi M, Fasano N, Langiano N et al (2011) Goal-directed haemodynamic therapy during elective total hip arthroplasty under regional anaesthesia. Crit Care 15:R132
25. Pillai P, McEleavy I, Gaughan M et al (2011) A double-blind randomized controlled clinical trial to assess the effect of Doppler optimized intraoperative fluid management on outcome following radical cystectomy. J Urol 186:2201–2206
26. Figus A, Wade RG, Oakey S, Ramakrishmnan VV (2013) Intraoperative esophageal Doppler hemodynamic monitoring in free perforator flap surgery. Ann Plast Surg (in press)
27. Ping W, Hong-Wei W, Tai-Di Z (2013) Effect of stroke volume variability-guided intraoperative fluid restriction on gastrointestinal functional recovery. Hepatogastroenterology (in press)
28. Brienza N, Giglio MT, Marucci M et al (2009) Does perioperative hemodynamic optimization protect renal function in surgical patients? A meta-analytic study. Crit Care Med 37:2079–2090
29. Giglio MT, Marucci M, Testini M et al (2009) Goal-directed haemodynamic therapy and gastrointestinal complications in major surgery: a meta-analysis of randomized controlled trials. Brit J Anaesth 103:637–646
30. Dalfino L, Giglio MT, Puntillo F et al (2011) Haemodynamic goal-directed therapy and postoperative infections: earlier is better. A systematic review and meta-analysis. Crit Care 15:R154
31. Hamilton MA, Cecconi M, Rhodes A (2011) A systematic review and meta-analysis on the use of preemptive hemodynamic intervention to improve postoperative outcomes in moderate and high-risk surgical patients. Anesth Analg 112:1392–1402
32. Corcoran T, Rhodes JEJ, Clarke S et al (2012) Perioperative fluid management strategies in major surgery: a stratified meta-analysis. Anesth Analg 114:640–651
33. Kuper M, Gold SJ, Quraishi T et al (2011) Intraoperative fluid management guided by oesophageal Doppler monitoring. BMJ 342:d3016
34. Mythen MG, Swart M, Acheson N et al (2012) Perioperative fluid management: consensus statement from the enhanced recovery partnership. Perioperative Medicine 1:2

35. Cannesson M, Pestel G, Ricks C, Hoeft A, Perel A (2011) Hemodynamic monitoring and management in patients undergoing high-risk surgery: a survey among North American and European anesthesiologists. Crit Care 15:R197
36. Michard F, Biais M (2012) Rational fluid management: dissecting facts from fiction. Brit J Anaesth 108:369–371
37. Michard F (2011) The burden of high-risk surgery and the potential benefit of goal-directed strategies. Crit Care 15:447
38. UK clinical research network (2012) Study portfolio. Available at http://public.ukcrn.org.uk/search/StudyDetail.aspx?StudyID=6307. Accessed Oct 2012
39. Vincent JL (2010) We should abandon randomized controlled trials in the intensive care unit. Crit Care Med 38:S534–S538
40. Michard F, Cannesson M, Vallet B (2011) Perioperative hemodynamic therapy: quality improvement programs should help to resolve our uncertainty. Crit Care 15:445
41. Cannon CM, Holthaus CV, Zubrow MT et al (2013) The GENESIS project (generalized early sepsis intervention strategies): a multicenter quality improvement collaborative. J Intensive Care Med (in press)
42. Pronovost P, Needham D, Berenholtz S et al (2006) An intervention to decrease catheter-related bloodstream infections in the ICU. N Engl J Med 355:2725–2732
43. Haynes AB, Weiser TG, Berry WR et al (2009) A surgical safety checklist to reduce morbidity and mortality in a global population. N Engl J Med 360:491–499
44. Vincent JL, Rhodes A, Perel A et al (2011) Clinical review: Update on hemodynamic monitoring – a consensus of 16. Crit Care 15:229
45. Gawande A (2010) The checklist manifesto. How to get things right. Profile Books Ltd, London
46. Guest JF, Boyd O, Hart WM et al (1997) A cost analysis of a treatment policy of a deliberate perioperative increase in oxygen delivery in high risk surgical patients. Intensive Care Med 23:85–90
47. Fenwick E, Wilson J, Sculpher M et al (2002) Pre-operative optimisation employing dopexamine or adrenaline for patients undergoing major elective surgery: a cost-effectiveness analysis. Intensive Care Med 28:599–608
48. Boltz MM, Hollenbeak CS, Ortenzi G et al (2012) Synergistic implications of multiple postoperative outcomes. Am J Med Qual 27:383–390
49. Bartha E, Davidson T, Hommel A et al (2012) Cost-effectiveness analysis of goal-directed hemodynamic treatment of elderly hip fracture patients. Anesthesiology 117:519–530

Part XIV

Mechanical Ventilation

Extracerebral Effects of Hyperventilation: What are the Mechanisms?

S. Froio, V. Conte, and N. Stocchetti

Introduction

Hypocapnic hyperventilation is used in neuroanesthesia and in neurointensive care for the treatment of raised intracranial pressure (ICP) in the context of traumatic brain injury (TBI) [1, 2]. The careful and targeted use of hypocapnia for the short-term control of raised ICP remains a useful therapeutic tool [1, 3]. Hypocapnia lowers ICP by the induction of cerebral vasoconstriction with a subsequent decrease in cerebral blood volume. Over the past decade, relatively more attention has been paid to the adverse effects of hyperventilation than to the beneficial and concern seems to exceed enthusiasm because of the potential downside of hyperventilation, i. e., decreasing cerebral blood flow (CBF) to ischemic levels [2]. There is no evidence in the literature unequivocally demonstrating that hyperventilation for the treatment of raised ICP in patients with TBI is related to poorer outcome, and there is also no evidence showing beneficial effects on overall outcome [3, 4].

Potential adverse extracerebral effects have been also suggested to be associated with the harm coming from hyperventilation [1, 2]. Systemic effects affect multiple organs and systems. The risks of systemic adverse effects appear to be greater in patients with preexistent cardiac disease, in patients with absolute or

S. Froio
Neuroscience ICU, Fondazione IRCCS Ca' Granda Ospedale Maggiore Policlinico, Via F. Sforza 35, 20122 Milan, Italy

V. Conte (✉)
Neuroscience ICU, Fondazione IRCCS Ca' Granda Ospedale Maggiore Policlinico, Via F. Sforza 35, 20122 Milan, Italy
E-mail: v.conte@policlinico.mi.it

N. Stocchetti
Neuroscience ICU, Fondazione IRCCS Ca' Granda Ospedale Maggiore Policlinico, Via F. Sforza 35, 20122 Milan, Italy

J.-L. Vincent (Ed.), *Annual Update in Intensive Care and Emergency Medicine 2013*, DOI 10.1007/978-3-642-35109-9_45, relative hypovolemia, and in patients with acute respiratory distress syndrome (ARDS) [1, 2]. When hyperventilation is established by means of artificial ventilation, the effects of hypocapnia are combined with those deriving from positive pressure ventilation and hemodynamics, and often also from sedation, paralysis and increased fluid input. In the clinical setting, in view of the fact that it is impossible to isolate these different components, all of them should be considered when hyperventilation is applied. Conversely, in experimental settings, the independent effects of hypocapnia using different ventilatory modalities have been investigated. In this chapter, we will focus on the mechanisms underlying the effects of hypocapnic hyperventilation on lung, cardiac, renal and splanchnic systems, reviewing the experimental evidence of the last 40 years.

Definition

Hypocapnic hyperventilation may be defined as the induction and/or maintenance of levels of carbon dioxide (CO_2) tension (PCO_2) in the arterial blood below the normal range, which is 40 mm Hg in humans and mammals. The level of CO_2 in the arterial blood depends on the rate of CO_2 production and the rate of CO_2 elimination through the lung and the kidney. At constant CO_2 production, hypocapnia can be achieved by increasing alveolar ventilation. This change in arterial PCO_2 corresponds to an immediate change in arterial pH. Animals *in vivo* and humans in clinical settings are subjected to passive hyperventilation by means of artificial ventilation. Hypocapnia may be achieved by different methods: Increasing the tidal volume and/or the respiratory rate, or decreasing the dead space. Although the most appropriate way for inducing hypocapnia has not been determined, we want to underline the fact that different modalities produce distinctive physiologic changes on organs and systems (Table 1).

Lung and Respiratory System

Positive-pressure ventilation increases lung volume and intrathoracic pressure even when a normal level of arterial PCO_2 is maintained, affecting systemic hemodynamics and lung physiology, reducing venous return, increasing pulmonary resistances and right ventricular afterload because of compression of pulmonary capillaries. This is particularly true when hyperventilation is obtained by increasing tidal volume. In patients with relative or absolute hypovolemia, marked hemodynamic perturbations may be caused [5]. On the other hand, it has been shown that when inducing hypocapnia (24–33 mm Hg) by increasing respiratory rate, pulmonary blood flow does not change [6]. Hypocapnia *per se* exerts effects on muscular tone in the airways, on ventilation/perfusion (V/Q) mismatch, on hypoxic pulmonary vasoconstriction, and on microvascular permeability.

Table 1 Extracerebral effects of hypocapnic hyperventilation

Organs and systems	Reference	Species	$PaCO_2$ (mm Hg)	Effects of increased intrathoracic pressure	Effects of hypocapnic alkalosis
Lung and respiratory system	[7]	rats	*in vitro*	↑ pulmonary vascular resistances ↑ collateral ventilation ↓ V/Q heterogeneity (↑V_T) ↓A-aDO_2 (↑Vt)	↑ bronchoconstriction (phosphatidylinositol) ↑ microvascular permeability ↓ alveolar fluid re-absorption ↑ V/Q heterogeneity and↑A-aDO_2 ↓ hypoxic pulmonary vasoconstriction = pulmonary blood flow = diaphragm contractility
	[10]	rats	10–20		
	[8]	dogs	21		
	[9]	dogs	21		
	[6]	dogs	15–26		
	[11]	rabbits	28		
Cardiovascular system	[17]	ferrets	*in vitro*	↓venous return (↑V_T) ↑ pulmonary vascular resistances (↑V_T) ↑ right ventricular afterload (↑V_T) ↓cardiac output (↑V_T)	↑sensitivity of the myofilaments to Ca^{2+} ↑ intracellular [Ca^{2+}] ↑ inotropism ↓ coronary blood flow = cardiac output
	[18]	dogs	17		
	[8]	dogs	21		
	[13, 16]	dogs	20		
	[14]	monkeys	26		
	[15]	dogs	20		
	[19]	dogs	21		
O_2 transport and utilization	[14]	monkeys	26		↑affinity of Hb for O_2 ↑ glycolysis ↑ O_2 consumption
	[21]	dogs	13		
	[22]	dogs	16		

Table 1 *Continued*

Organs and systems	Reference	Species	$PaCO_2$ (mm Hg)	Effects of increased intrathoracic pressure	Effects of hypocapnic alkalosis
Kidney and electro-lytes	[28, 29, 32]		*in vitro*	↓ renal perfusion ↑ renin production ↑ vasodilator prostaglandins	↑bicarbonate ions excretion ↓ re-absorption of HCO_3^- ions ↓H^+ secretion ↓NH_4 excretion/= NH_4 production ↓Na-K-ATPase activity ↑ K^+ excretion
	[15]	dogs	17		
	[24]	pigs	13		
	[25]	dogs	22		
	[31]	dogs	15		
	[30]	rats	*ex vivo*		
	[33]	rats	23		
	[34]	rats	22		
Gastrointestinal system	[24]	pigs	17	↓ splanchnic perfusion ↓hepatic artery ↓portal vein blood flow ↓hepatic lactic acid utilization	= splanchnic perfusion ↓ mucosal and serosal O_2 delivery =/↓hepatic artery =/↓portal vein blood flow = jejunal electrolyte absorption ↓ ileal/colonic electrolyte absorption
	[36]	dogs	22		
	[37]	dogs	15		
	[40]	rats	22		
	[41]	rabbits	26		
	[42, 43]	rats	23–24		
	[39]	dogs	22		
	[45]	dogs	< 15		

V_T: tidal volume; A-aDO_2: alveolar-arterial difference in oxygen tension; V/Q: ventilation/perfusion; Hb: hemoglobin

Hypocapnia stimulates phosphatidylinositol turnover in the airway smooth muscle *in vitro,* which causes bronchoconstriction of the airways of all sizes [7], and reduces collateral ventilation while inducing dilatation of pulmonary vessels [8]. The resulting effects are altered V/Q, increased V/Q heterogeneity and alveolar-arterial difference in oxygen tension (A-aDO_2). Conversely, when a large tidal volume is used to obtain hypocapnia, hypocapnic bronchoconstriction is completely reversed, V/Q heterogeneity decreases, and A-aDO_2 decreases [8], probably because of the counterbalancing effect of increased intrathoracic pressure. Hypocapnia may alter V/Q also by affecting the adaptive processes that preserve V/Q and oxygenation, i. e., hypoxic pulmonary vasoconstriction [8]. In fact, respiratory alkalosis has been shown to attenuate the hypoxic pulmonary vasoconstriction response in dogs with global alveolar hypoxia and regional hypoxia [9].

Hypocapnia increases microvascular permeability and impairs alveolar fluid reabsorption at the alveolar level because of the reduction in Na^+-K^+ ATPase activity proportionally to the level of hypocapnia (less than 30 mm Hg) [10]. No significant alterations of diaphragm contractility are shown with levels of arterial PCO_2 that are less than normal [11].

The importance of ventilatory management in criticaly ill patients is well-known and the concept that hypocapnia and large volume ventilation might worsen acute lung injury (ALI) and ARDS is also recognized, as a result of the mechanisms described above. The fact that 20 % of patients with severe TBI may develop ALI or ARDS [12] should be taken into account before instituting hyperventilation therapy in patients with TBI.

Cardiovascular System

The effects of hypocapnic alkalosis on cardiovascular function have been investigated in several animal studies; however it might be difficult to appreciate the cardiovascular effects of alterations in PCO_2 *per se* in the presence of increased intrathoracic pressure. During hypocapnic hyperventilation increased intrathoracic pressure is responsible for hemodynamic changes while intracellular pH variations directly affect the contractile machinery.

An increase in intrathoracic pressure leads to a reduction in the venous return to the right side of the heart, an increase in right ventricular afterload, a decrease in the volume and compliance of the left ventricle with a decrease of transmural left ventricle pressure output. In summary, venous return is impaired and the effect of positive pressure ventilation on right ventricular performance depends on the degree of preload and pulmonary vascular resistances [5, 13].

Hypocapnia *per se* did not produce significant changes in cardiac output in monkeys [14] or dogs [15]. Zwillich et al. [16] induced acute hypocapnia (from 38 to 20 mm Hg) in dogs, by increasing respiratory rate, in order to determine the effects on circulatory function. They noted a significant decrease in cardiac output and stroke volume (approximately 10 %). There were no significant changes in heart rate and pulmonary wedge pressure while total systemic resistances increased significantly. However, when animals at the same levels of hypocapnic alkalosis received a fluid load, cardiac output and stroke volume increased significantly. Mechanical hyperventilation is associated with a decreased cardiac output and stroke volume, but both are maintained if left ventricular preload is increased [16].

During acute circulatory failure, venous hypercarbia occurs concomitantly with the decline in cardiac output and tissue perfusion. In a canine model of hemorrhagic shock, mechanical hyperventilation (arterial PCO_2 21 mm Hg) caused a washout of CO_2. Arterial pH, bicarbonate concentration and oxygen saturation remained unchanged in hyperventilated dogs with hemorrhagic shock, whereas cardiac output fell, heart rate increased and stroke index decreased [8].

Myocardial contractility is mainly determined by two factors: The concentration of Ca^{2+} in myocardial cells and the responsiveness of the contractile protein system to Ca^{2+}. Hypocapnic alkalosis rapidly increases left ventricular isovolumetric pressure and the isovolumetric pressure then declines slowly reaching a new steady state within minutes [17, 18]. An increase in intracellular pH increases the sensitivity of the myofilaments to Ca^{2+}. Respiratory alkalosis may produce positive inotropism by: (1) an increase in the intracellular concentration of Ca^{2+}; (2) an increase in the responsiveness of the contractile machinery to Ca^{2+} (3) through the sensitization of contractile protein system to Ca^{2+} [17, 18].

A direct relationship exists between arterial PCO_2 and coronary blood flow [19]. A reduction of blood flow to the left and right ventricles (20 % and 25 % respectively) has been shown using radioactive microspheres and radioisotope activity analysis during hypocapnia [15]. Mild reduction in arterial PCO_2 is associated with a reduction in coronary blood flow and with an increase in oxygen extraction from the coronary blood, leaving adequate oxygenation. In fact neither global nor regional myocardial function changes during hypocapnia [19]. Distal to a critical stenosis, coronary blood flow appears to be unresponsive to hypocapnia, whereas an increase in oxygen extraction and a reduction of the coronary sinus oxygen tension are still detected. Marginal oxygenation is important in determining regional autoregulation [19].

Oxygen Transport and Utilization

Alkalosis increases the affinity of hemoglobin for O_2 and displaces the dissociation curve to the left [20]. As ventilation is increased, the alveolar PO_2 increases, arterial PO_2 increases and, in association with the shift of the oxyhemoglobin dissociation curve to the left, the arterial saturation of hemoglobin rises. 2,3-diphosphoglycerate (DPG) can increase under the influence of alkalosis, but no significant change occurred during 20 minutes of hyperventilation in monkeys [14]. Respiratory alkalosis increases the affinity of hemoglobin for oxygen, and is also associated with increased oxygen uptake. This oxygen uptake is not necessarily associated with changes in cardiac output or evidence of anaerobic metabolism

[14]. Hyperventilation increases oxygen uptake in anesthetized and paralyzed dogs, through extracellular and intracellular pH changes [21, 22]. Intracellular alkalosis increases glycolysis, due to induction of enzymatic activity of phosphofructokinase, increasing the production of lactate and pyruvate, which in the presence of oxygen, is transformed into acetyl-CoA to be utilized in the Krebs cycle [23]. Moreover, pyruvate dehydrogenase (PDH), the first component enzyme of the PDH complex, linking the glycolysis metabolic pathway to the citric acid cycle, might be activated by increased intracellular levels of Ca^{2+} [17, 18].

Kidney and Electrolytes

Particular attention should be paid to the effects of increased intrathoracic pressure on kidney perfusion and to the effects of hypocapnia on the renal compensatory control of pH. A decrease (to 28 % of baseline) of blood flow in the kidney was recorded in pigs under high tidal volume hyperventilation. Changes in kidney perfusion were not observed when hyperventilation was induced by increased respiratory frequency, keeping the tidal volume constant [24]. Boarini et al. observed that kidney blood flow was moderately reduced (8 %) during normotensive hypocapnia (arterial PCO_2 20 mm Hg) [15]. Renal vasodilator prostaglandins increase in response to hypocapnia possibly in order to maintain renal blood flow during vasoconstrictive stimuli. Renin production is also increased during hypocapnic hyperventilation, possibly producing the reduction in renal blood flow observed when normocapnia is restored [25].

The kidney is the main organ involved in the compensatory control of pH during chronic hyperventilation. Respiratory alkalosis is compensated by decreased re-absorption of bicarbonate ions from renal tubules [26]. More bicarbonate ions are excreted in the urine, the plasma concentration of bicarbonate decreases, and the pH returns toward normal levels despite the persistence of low arterial PCO_2 [20, 27].

Studies suggested that the electrolyte excretion patterns observed during hypocapnia may be due to inhibition of H^+ secretion in the kidney in the proximal and distal convoluted tubules [28, 29]. Therefore, acute hyperventilation reduces collecting duct hydrogen secretion and this might be the basis for the reduced net acid excretion observed with more prolonged hypocapnia and the fall in blood bicarbonate associated with chronic hypocapnia [28]. Two renal proton ATPases are responsible for H^+ secretion in the collecting tubule: An electrogenic proton-translocating ATPase and an electroneutral H^+-K^+-ATPase. Significant renal adaptation to hypocapnia occurs within 6 h. The magnitude of bicarbonaturia and the decrease in the activities of both renal proton ATPases are not sufficient to prevent alkalemia after acute hypocapnia. Low PCO_2 slowly induces endocytosis of vesicles containing H^+-ATPases. As the duration of hypocapnia is extended (24 h), renal proton ATPases decrease and bicarbonaturia persists, plasma bicarbonate concentration falls, returning blood pH to a normal level.

A reduction in cellular PCO_2 in tubular cells, therefore, induces an increase in intracellular pH, a reduction in H^+ secretion, and decreased excretion of ammonium (NH_4^+), which is thought to be secondary to inhibition of distal nephron H^+ secretion [20, 28, 29]. Moreover, acute alkalosis inhibits ammonia production by a mechanism that is both slowly activated and reversible. During the first 45 min of hypocapnic perfusion, ammonia production was identical when kidneys subjected to respiratory alkalosis were compared to controls. However, when the perfusate pH was returned to normal, and the observation continued, kidneys that had been previously exposed to respiratory alkalosis produced less ammonia than controls. Since key ammonia-producing enzymes, phosphate-dependent glutaminase and glutamate dehydrogenase, are known to undergo polymerization, this represents one potential explanation for the slow activation [30]. On the other hand, Gougoux et al. demonstrated that in the dog, renal glutamine extraction and ammonia production when expressed per 100 ml of glomerular filtration rate (GFR), remained virtually unchanged following acute respiratory alkalosis (15 mm Hg from 35 mm Hg PCO_2) [31].

Na^+-K^+-ATPase activity decreases within 6 h of hypocapnia, inducing marked natriuresis. The mechanisms are aldosterone and potassium independent, but a direct effect of PCO_2 or pH or change in bicarbonate delivery seems to be involved [32]. In acute respiratory alkalosis, the increase in blood pH is associated with a fall in PCO_2, blood bicarbonate and plasma K^+ [26, 33]. Potassium excretion is known to increase during acute hypocapnia; after 24 hours of persistent hypocapnia, potassium excretion is not different from control [26]. However, during hypocapnic alkalosis, mild hypokalemia is typically observed as a consequence of the shift of H^+ from the cellular to the extracellular compartment together with an opposite movement of K^+.

During respiratory alkalosis, phosphate excretion is also affected in humans, dogs, rats and hamsters. Phosphate concentrations in plasma and whole blood decrease despite a marked increase in re-absorption of phosphate by the kidney. Tissue analysis indicates that phosphate is translocated from the vascular compartment predominantly to muscle and liver. This uptake by muscle may be due to increased glycolysis or glycogenolysis caused by alkalosis. Acute respiratory alkalosis also prevents the phosphaturic effects of parathyroid hormone (PTH) [34, 35].

Gastrointestinal System

During hyperventilation, without increasing intrathoracic pressure, the estimated total splanchnic blood flow does not change significantly over time [24, 36]. Hypocapnia (22 mm Hg), obtained by reducing dead space without changing the tidal volume or the respiratory rate, had no significant effects on the systemic and splanchnic circulations except for a decrease in hepatic artery blood flow [36]. Passive mechanical hyperventilation using intermittent positive pressure ventilation and high tidal volume reduced cardiac output and estimated total splanchnic blood flow. However, the changes in cardiac output and splanchnic blood flow were not observed when hyperventilation (target arterial $PCO_2 \sim 22$ mm Hg) was induced by increased frequency, keeping the tidal volume constant [24].

However, some authors suggest that hypocapnia *per se* alters splanchnic hemodynamics. Gut mucosal and serosal oxygen delivery (DO_2) decrease at the end of a period of hypocapnia of 45 minutes; this mechanism seems to be reversible. After inducing hypocapnia, a net reduction in both mucosal and serosal blood flow occurred. However, a clear redistribution of blood flow in favor of mucosal bed from the serosal layer was observed, probably in an attempt to protect more vulnerable tissues from hypoperfusion [37]. These observations were, however, obtained during vigorous hyperventilation, from 40 mm Hg to 15 mm Hg. Gut intramucosal PCO_2 reflects the balance between tissue CO_2 production and CO_2 removed by the regional circulation. Changes in arterial PCO_2 should result in similar changes in intramucosal PCO_2. An acute decrease in arterial PCO_2 produced comparable changes in tissue PCO_2 under physiological conditions in murine and swine models [38]. The PCO_2 gap between tissues and arterial blood typically increases during shock. This reflects the effect of metabolic acidosis and lactic acidosis during perfusion failure. If hyperventilation is superimposed, there would be an apparent decrease in the PCO_2 gap and potential underestimation of the severity of perfusion failure. Tissue PCO_2 as a marker of the severity of hypoperfusion must be interpreted in relation to concurrent arterial PCO_2 levels. Goldstein et al., using electromagnetic flow transducers in the portal vein and hepatic artery, showed a reduction of both hepatic artery and portal vein blood flow roughly proportional to the degree of respiratory alkalosis [39]. On the other hand, using radioactive spheres Boarini et al. did not find a significant change in splanchnic and hepatic blood flow during hypocapnia [15]. During hypotension combined with hypocapnia there was no statistical change in the blood flows compared to normocapnic hypotension [15].

The primary function of the gastrointestinal tract is to provide the body with a continual supply of water, electrolytes and nutrients. Respiratory alkalosis (PCO_2 22 mm Hg) without altering the respiratory rate, minute volume, or intrathoracic pressure did not affect jejunal net water, sodium, potassium, chloride, bicarbonate movement or the transmural potential difference. Colonic and ileal responses to the respiratory alkalosis were characterized by a decrease in net water, sodium, and chloride absorption and bicarbonate secretion. There was no change in the transmural potential difference [40–43].

The liver has a large capacity for lactate uptake. An increasing blood lactate concentration represents an imbalance between the rates of formation and the rates of disposal of lactic acid in various tissues. Vigorous acute mechanical hyperventilation (less than 10 mm Hg, from 30–40 mm Hg) in dogs, inducing hypotension and splanchnic hypoperfusion, produced marked hyperlactacidemia, with a lactate concentration greater in the hepatic vein than in the aorta. These results suggest that splanchnic lactic acid production is responsible for the rise in blood lactate [44, 45]. Other data support the information that only severe hypotension during hyperventilation produces an increase in blood lactate concentration, resulting from both splanchnic hypoperfusion and decreased hepatic utilization [39].

Overview and Clinical Implications

Hyperventilation has several extracerebral effects. It is extremely difficult to distinguish which are directly caused by hypocapnia and concomitant respiratory alkalosis, from those that are linked to the ventilatory changes superimposed to lower the arterial CO_2 levels. Animal experiments offer a unique opportunity to clarify the different mechanisms, assuming similar physiological mechanisms in different mammalian species.

The evidence reviewed in this paper proves that relevant changes can be detected in the respiratory and cardiovascular systems, together with alterations in the intestinal tract, the kidney and the liver. Some alterations are clearly attributable to artificial ventilation, and highly dependent on the methods used for inducing hypocapnia. Other changes are probably caused by arterial PCO_2 and pH changes, independent from the ventilatory methods.

In animal experiments, CO_2 has usually been decreased to very low levels, but for limited periods. Data from animal studies in which very low levels of hypocapnia ($PCO_2 < 20$ or 10 mm Hg, unlikely to be applied in humans) were used, provide information on the mechanisms involved, rather than quantifying what may happen in patients. Short term changes have been well explored, whereas data on longer term effects are lacking. In general the changes detected, even when obtained with sudden and extreme changes in arterial PCO_2, seem reversible. Hypocapnia in normovolemic animals was in fact always well tolerated.

Conclusion

Knowledge of the extracerebral effects of hyperventilation may help our understanding of clinical management. The simple decision to lower CO_2 may have, in fact, several consequences, such as respiratory alkalosis, electrolyte changes and renal adaptive mechanisms. Moreover, hypocapnia is obtained with ventilatory changes that have hemodynamic consequences. These consequences become more relevant in vulnerable cases, such as hypovolemic patients who may not tolerate increased intrathoracic pressure. Nevertheless, short periods of acute hyperventilation in the context of impending brainstem herniation remain a potentially life-saving therapy [1, 3, 46]. The decision for hypocapnia should be undertaken after careful consideration of the risks and benefits [47].

References

1. Stocchetti N, Maas AI, Chieregato A, van der Plas AA (2005) Hyperventilation in head injury: a review. Chest 127:1812–1827
2. Curley G, Kavanagh BP, Laffey JG (2011) Hypocapnia and the injured brain: more harm than benefit. Crit Care Med 38:1348–1359

3. Bratton SL, Chestnut RM, Ghajar J et al (2007) Guidelines for the management of severe traumatic brain injury. XIV. Hyperventilation. J Neurotrauma 24(suppl 1):S87–S90
4. Muizelaar JP, Marmarou A, Ward JD et al (1991) Adverse effects of prolonged hyperventilation in patients with severe head injury: a randomized clinical trial. J Neurosurg 75:731–739
5. Pinsky MR (1994) Cardiovascular effects of ventilatory support and withdrawal. Anesth Analg 79:567–576
6. Toivonen HJ, Catravas JD (1987) Effects of acid-base imbalance on pulmonary angiotensin-converting enzyme in vivo. J Appl Physiol 63:1629–1637
7. Shibata O, Makita T, Tsujita T et al (1995) Carbachol, norepinephrine, and hypocapnia stimulate phosphatidylinositol turnover in rat tracheal slices. Anesthesiology 82:102–107
8. Domino KB, Swenson ER, Polissar NL, Lu Y, Eisenstein BL, Hlastala MP (1993) Effect of inspired CO2 on ventilation and perfusion heterogeneity in hyperventilated dogs. J Appl Physiol 75:1306–1314
9. Domino KB, Lu Y, Eisenstein BL, Hlastala MP (1993) Hypocapnia worsens arterial blood oxygenation and increases VA/Q heterogeneity in canine pulmonary edema. Anesthesiology 78:91–99
10. Myrianthefs PM, Briva A, Lecuona E et al (2005) Hypocapnic but not metabolic alkalosis impairs alveolar fluid reabsorption. Am J Respir Crit Care Med 171:1267–1271
11. Schnader JY, Juan G, Howell S, Fitzgerald R, Roussos C (1985) Arterial CO2 partial pressure affects diaphragmatic function. J Appl Physiol 58:823–829
12. Mascia L, Zavala E, Bosma K et al (2007) High tidal volume is associated with the development of acute lung injury after severe brain injury: an international observational study. Crit Care Med 35:1815–1820
13. Tsukimoto K, Arcos JP, Schaffartzik W, Wagner PD, West JB (1992) Effects of inspired CO2, hyperventilation, and time on VA/Q inequality in the dog. J Appl Physiol 72:1057–1063
14. Riggs TE, Shafer AW, Guenter CA (1972) Physiologic effects of passive hyperventilation on oxygen delivery and consumption. 1. Proc Soc Exp Biol Med 140:1414–1417
15. Boarini DJ, Kassell NF, Sprowell JA, Olin JJ, Coester HC (1985) Cerebrovascular effects of hypocapnia during adenosine-induced arterial hypotension. J Neurosurg 63:937–943
16. Zwillich CW, Pierson DJ, Creagh EM, Weil JV (1976) Effects of hypocapnia and hypocapnic alkalosis on cardiovascular function. J Appl Physiol 40:333–337
17. Kusuoka H, Backx PH, Camilion de Hurtado M, Azan-Backx M, Marban E, Cingolani HE (1993) Relative roles of intracellular Ca2+ and pH in shaping myocardial contractile response to acute respiratory alkalosis. Am J Physiol 265:H1696–H1703
18. Onishi K, Sekioka K, Ishisu R et al (1996) Decrease in oxygen cost of contractility during hypocapnic alkalosis in canine hearts. Am J Physiol 270:H1905–H1913
19. Coetzee A, Holland D, Foex P, Ryder A, Jones L (1984) The effect of hypocapnia on coronary blood flow and myocardial function in the dog. Anesth Analg 63:991–997
20. Rose BD, Post TW (2001) Clinical Physiology of Acid-Base and Electrolyte Disorders. McGraw Hill, New York
21. Khambatta HJ, Sullivan SF (1973) Effects of respiratory alkalosis on oxygen consumption and oxygenation. Anesthesiology 38:53–58
22. Cain SM (1970) Increased oxygen uptake with passive hyperventilation of dogs. J Appl Physiol 28:4–7
23. Khambatta HJ, Sullivan SF (1974) Carbon dioxide production and washout during passive hyperventilation alkalosis. J Appl Physiol 37:665–669
24. Karlsson T, Stjernstrom EL, Stjernstrom H, Norlen K, Wiklund L (1994) Central and regional blood flow during hyperventilation. An experimental study in the pig. Acta Anaesthesiol Scand 38:180–186
25. Lonigro AJ, Brash DW, Stephenson AH, Heitmann LJ, Sprague RS (1982) Effect of ventilatory rate on renal venous PGE2 and PGF2 alpha efflux in anesthetized dogs. Am J Physiol 242:F38–F45

26. Adrogue HJ, Madias NE (1981) Changes in plasma potassium concentration during acute acid-base disturbances. Am J Med 71:456–467
27. Guyton AC, Hall JE (2000) Textbook of Medical Physiology, 11th edn. Saunders, Philadelphia
28. Giammarco RA, Goldstein MB, Halperin ML, Stinebaugh BJ (1976) The effect of hyperventilation on distal nephron hydrogen ion secretion. J Clin Invest 58:77–82
29. Sehy JT, Roseman MK, Arruda JA, Kurtzman NA (1978) Characterization of distal hydrogen ion secretion in acute respiratory alkalosis. Am J Physiol 235:F203–F208
30. Tannen RL, Goyal M (1984) Response of ammoniagenesis to acute alkalosis. Am J Physiol 247:F827–F836
31. Gougoux A, Vinay P, Cardoso M, Duplain M (1984) Renal metabolism and ammoniagenesis during acute respiratory alkalosis in the dog. Can J Physiol Pharmacol 62:1129–1135
32. Eiam-ong S, Laski ME, Kurtzman NA, Sabatini S (1994) Effect of respiratory acidosis and respiratory alkalosis on renal transport enzymes. Am J Physiol 267:F390–F399
33. Unwin R, Stidwell R, Taylor S, Capasso G (1997) The effects of respiratory alkalosis and acidosis on net bicarbonate flux along the rat loop of Henle in vivo. Am J Physiol 273:F698–F705
34. Hoppe A, Metler M, Berndt TJ, Knox FG, Angielski S (1982) Effect of respiratory alkalosis on renal phosphate excretion. Am J Physiol 243:F471–F475
35. Berndt TJ, Knox FG (1985) Nephron site of resistance to phosphaturic effect of PTH during respiratory alkalosis. Am J Physiol 249:F919–F922
36. Fujita Y, Sakai T, Ohsumi A, Takaori M (1989) Effects of hypocapnia and hypercapnia on splanchnic circulation and hepatic function in the beagle. Anesth Analg 69:152–157
37. Guzman JA, Kruse JA (1999) Splanchnic hemodynamics and gut mucosal-arterial PCO(2) gradient during systemic hypocapnia. J Appl Physiol 87:1102–1106
38. Pernat A, Weil MH, Tang W et al (1999) Effects of hyper- and hypoventilation on gastric and sublingual PCO(2). J Appl Physiol 87:933–937
39. Goldstein PJ, Simmons DH, Tashkin DP (1972) Effect of acid-base alterations on hepatic lactate utilization. J Physiol 223:261–278
40. Feldman GM, Charney AN (1982) Effect of acute respiratory alkalosis and acidosis on intestinal ion transport in vivo. Am J Physiol 242:G486–G492
41. Charney AN, Arnold M, Johnstone N (1983) Acute respiratory alkalosis and acidosis and rabbit intestinal ion transport in vivo. Am J Physiol 244:G145–G150
42. Kurtin P, Charney AN (1984) Intestinal ion transport and intracellular pH during acute respiratory alkalosis and acidosis. Am J Physiol 247:G24–G31
43. Kurtin P, Charney AN (1984) Effect of arterial carbon dioxide tension on amiloride-sensitive sodium absorption in the colon. Am J Physiol 247:G537–G541
44. Berry MN, Scheuer J (1967) Splanchnic lactic acid metabolism in hyperventilation, metabolic alkalosis and shock. Metabolism 16:537–547
45. Zborowska-Sluis DT, Dossetor JB (1967) Hyperlactatemia of hyperventilation. J Appl Physiol 22:746–755
46. Laffey JG, Kavanagh BP (1999) Carbon dioxide and the critically ill – too little of a good thing? Lancet 354:1283–1286
47. Laffey JG, Kavanagh BP (2002) Hypocapnia. N Engl J Med 347:43–53

Endotracheal Tube Biofilm and Ventilator-Associated Pneumonia

A. Coppadoro, J. G. Thomas, and L. Berra

Introduction

Ventilator associated pneumonia (VAP) is one of the most relevant infections in intensive care unit (ICU) patients, and its occurrence increases with duration of mechanical ventilation. It is widely accepted that VAP is associated with increased duration of ventilation, hospital stay and health care costs [1]. However, the impact of VAP on mortality is currently under debate; in a cohort of patients with acute respiratory distress syndrome (ARDS), VAP diagnosis was not associated with increased mortality after adjustment for factors, such as age or severity at admission [2]. Because of the pathogenesis of VAP, in recent years, focus has moved to the endotracheal tube (ETT), to the extent that some authors have suggested changing the name from ventilator-associated to ETT-associated pneumonia [3]. When the ETT is in place, the cough reflex is not effective; cuff inflation reduces secretion clearance by altering ciliary activity, as shown in animal models [4]. One of the main mechanisms to explain the inoculum of pathogens into the lungs is related to the presence of a biofilm on the inner lumen of the ETT; microbes can detach from the biofilm and reach the lower airways, leading to lung colonization and VAP. Key biofilm characteristics and possible VAP preventive measures focusing on biofilm reduction will be presented in this chapter.

A. Coppadoro
Department of Experimental Medicine, University of Milano-Bicocca, Monza, Italy

J. G. Thomas
Department of Pathology, West Virginia University School of Medicine, Morgantown, USA

L. Berra (✉)
Massachusetts General Hospital, Harvard Medical School, Boston, USA
E-mail: lberra@partners.org

J.-L. Vincent (Ed.), *Annual Update in Intensive Care and Emergency Medicine 2013*,
DOI 10.1007/978-3-642-35109-9_46, © Springer-Verlag Berlin Heidelberg 2013

Biofilm General Features

Biofilm forms when bacteria adhere to surfaces and excrete a wide variety of substances, particularly in moist environments. A typical example of biofilm is dental plaque. Biofilm can be formed by a singular bacterial colony, but usually many different bacteria are present at the same time. A glycocalyx matrix, collectively named 'extracellular polymeric substances', facilitates surface adhesion and composes the slime-like medium in which microbes are encased [5]. In general, microbial cells can be found in planktonic and sessile forms. The planktonic form is the floating form of microbes, such as that needed for bacterial identification on Petri plates where single-species colonies grow. However, microbes in biofilms are normally present in the sessile form, where microbes grow in communities firmly attached to a surface into a glycoproteic medium [6]. Biofilms need to be thought of as tri-dimensional structures, where many colonies of microbes are in close relation. With time, biofilm thickness tends to increase and the internal structure changes. In the interior part of the biofilm, the environment is anaerobic and bacterial metabolic activity reduces; however, although nutrients and pH are different, the pathogenetic activity remains preserved. Thanks to the visco-elastic properties of the biofilm, some aggregates of bacteria can detach from the biofilm and migrate over the surface. Four "life stages" have been recognized to describe the process of biofilm extension over a surface (Table 1) [7].

In the sessile form, the same bacteria express a different set of genes than in the planktonic form. Because of the different genetic activation and the thick protective extracellular matrix, bacterial antibiotic resistance is increased in the sessile form [8]. Extracellular biochemical signaling within the microbe community is believed to be responsible for the modulation of gene expression; these phenomena are reduced in the planktonic form, because of the increased distance between colonies.

Table 1 Biofilm life stages

Life stage	Form	Features
I – Lag	Loose surface adhesion	Bacterial first contact with surface
II – Log	Firm adhesion	Inclusion of bacteria in EPS
III – Stationary	Colony growth	3D structure, signaling between colonies
IV – Apoptosis/detachment	Aggregate detachment	Migration of 'communities' over the surface

EPS: extracellular polymeric substances

Biofilm in the ETT

The growth of biofilm on the inner lumen of the ETT occurs soon after intubation; at extubation, almost all ETT are colonized [9]. ETT are commonly made of polyvinylchloride (PVC), a plastic material to which bacteria readily adhere [8]. PVC adherence of bacteria present in the oral cavity and transported by the ETT itself during the intubation maneuver is thought to be the first step in biofilm formation. The inner side of the ETT also provides an ideal surface for bacterial proliferation, because of the reduced immunologic stress on the biofilm, as compared to the tracheal mucosa where host defense systems are active. Multiple host mechanisms exist to reduce airway pathogen colonization, but the effectiveness of these mechanisms is reduced inside the complex matrix of the ETT biofilm, where antibiotic resistance is also enhanced [10]. The biofilm inside the ETT is subject to airflow shear forces, which can promote detachment of bacterial aggregates and bacterial spread along the ETT lumen [11]. In animal models, biofilm flow has been shown to be subject to gravitational forces, with a continuous movement towards the lungs in the semi-recumbent position. With time, the biofilm layer increases in thickness, as a result of the accumulation of saliva leaked from the hypopharynx, mucosal secretions, red blood cells and neutrophils (Fig. 1) [12]. The lumen section available to airflow reduces, increasing resistances and the possibility of pathogen embolization into the lower airways. However, the increase in ETT resistance is highly variable and is not related to the duration of intubation when comparing different patients [13].

Biofilm and VAP

ETT biofilm is believed to be one of the main culprits for VAP development. The same bacteria present in the ETT biofilm can often be found in tracheal aspirates,

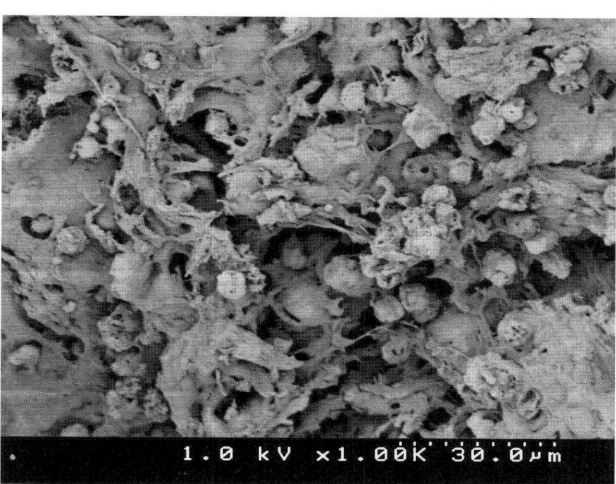

Fig. 1 A large variety of cells, visible on scanning electron microscopy, is dispersed into the glycoproteic material composing the endotrachel tube (ETT) biofilm

suggesting that ETT colonization and tracheal colonization are closely related events [14]. Moreover, Adair et al. showed that in patients diagnosed with VAP, the pathogens cultured in the lower airways are frequently present in the ETT biofilm [15]. These data suggest that initial ETT biofilm colonization may play a fundamental role in VAP pathogenesis, serving as a reservoir of bacteria that detach from the ETT to reach the lower airways. Bacterial detachment is typical of biofilm stage 4, while is not believed to be relevant in other stages (Table 1). This theory is corroborated by the observation that ETT biofilm stage 4, and not duration of intubation, has been associated with increased occurrence of pneumonia [7].

Another interesting feature of ETT biofilm related to VAP development regards microbial interaction within the biofilm. *Candida* species are often present in the ETT, and enhance biofilm formation [16]. *Candida* can interact with many pathogens typically involved in VAP, such as *Pseudomonas aeruginosa*, *Staphylococcus aureus* and *Escherichia coli*, increasing virulence and altering host immune response [17]. In a population of immunocompetent critically ill patients, Azoulay et al. showed an increased risk for *P. aeruginosa* VAP development in the presence of *Candida* airway tract colonization [18]. The mechanisms at the basis of *Candida*-pathogen interaction are not completely elucidated, and future studies on this topic may help to understand the complex VAP pathogenetic processes, which involve several pathogens.

As described above, microbes typically grow in the biofilm in the sessile form. However, standard bacterial isolation in microbiology laboratories occurs through planktonic growth, possibly reducing the number of pathogens identified. Cairns et al. used polymerase chain reaction (PCR) techniques for amplification of 16 rRNA, a phylogenetically preserved bacterial molecule, to analyze microbial communities of ETT biofilms [19]. The authors demonstrated a large number of bacteria within the ETTs, greater than the number obtained with standard microbiological isolation techniques. These data suggest that many pathogens, other than the usual ones, may be involved in VAP development, and that sophisticated techniques should be used for biofilm analysis.

Preventing Biofilm Formation

Many preventive strategies have been proposed to prevent ETT biofilm formation, and to reduce biofilm microbial burden in order to prevent VAP. Some of these strategies have already shown a benefit in clinical trials, whereas others still need to be tested in a real-life environment.

Nanoroughness

The material of which standard ETTs is composed is PVC, which offers an ideal surface for bacterial adhesion. Recent research has focused on the surface properties of PVC, showing that material hydrophobicity and surface roughness can influence bacterial adhesion [20]. Reduced bacterial growth on the ETT lumen was demonstrated in a bench airway model after the PVC surface was treated to create roughness at a nanometric scale (nanoroughness) [21]. The addition of a layer of fructose to the nanorough PVC led *in vitro* to a further reduction of bacterial adhesion, because of a change in the electrical surface properties [22]. Although these novel material modifications appear promising, their clinical usefulness still needs to be assessed.

Coatings

Several agents have been proposed to coat ETT for VAP prevention, typically silver or an association of silver with an antimicrobial agent, such as sulfadiazine, chlorhexidine, gardine [23, 24]. Although many of these coatings have shown promising results *in vitro*, only silver and silver-sulfadiazine showed relevant effects in clinical trials. The action of silver depends on silver ion penetration into the microbial cell; ions interfere with bacterial nucleic acid and prevent replication. Silver-sulfadiazine prevented ETT bacterial colonization and reduced biofilm thickness in a randomized clinical trial on 46 patients [23]. In a large randomized clinical trial (NASCENT), the use of silver-coated ETTs was associated with reduced VAP incidence and delayed VAP occurrence [25]. Coated ETT use appears clinically effective; however, the bactericidal effect may decrease with time, because of the accumulation of secretions on the ETT lumen. When a thick layer of secretions is present on the silver coating, silver ion diffusion is impaired and bacteria can grow on the luminal side of the biofilm. Thus, the clinical effect of coated ETTs tends to reduce with time, resulting in delayed VAP occurrence rather than long-acting VAP prevention, as suggested by the NASCENT trial.

Cleaning Tube Devices

Biofilms can be effectively removed from the ETT with devices designed for this purpose. The Mucus Shaver consists of an inflatable balloon that can be retracted within the ETT. Special rubber rings on the balloon mechanically remove the biofilm [26]. In a small randomized clinical trial, the Mucus Shaver was shown to be safe and effective in reducing ETT bacterial colonization [27]. Biofilm removal with devices similar to the Mucus Shaver is a promising strategy for VAP prevention; if the bacterial reservoir is frequently removed, pathogen inoculation into the lower airways could be reduced. However, no data are currently available about the VAP preventive effects with this or other devices. The use of ETT cleaning devices could also be used in conjunction with coated ETTs, leading to preserved antimicrobial activity of the coating layer even long after intubation [28].

Photodynamic Therapy

A different strategy to reduce bacterial growth within the ETT is based on the use of light. A methylene blue photosensitizer is sprayed into the ETT lumen through a small-bore catheter and absorbed by pathogens. A source of specific-wavelength light is then inserted into the lumen, which activates the photosensitizer agent, generating oxygen radical products. These products lead to DNA interference, membrane lysis and finally cell disruption. In a bench model, use of a single treatment of photodynamic therapy resulted in a reduction in ETT biofilm of up to 99.9% [29]. No data are available about the effectiveness and safety of this technique in a clinical setting.

Preventing Biofilm Dissemination

As described above, the surface of the biofilm is subject to flow shear forces; aggregates of bacteria can detach from the biofilm, particularly in stage 4, to reach the lower airways. Several factors can affect the movement of dislodged biofilm particles to the lower airways; among them, gravity and ventilator settings appear the most relevant.

Ventilator Settings

Biofilm movement follows peak airflow direction: Outward movement is promoted when peak expiratory flow exceeds peak inspiratory flow, and vice-versa [30]. A recent paper by Li Bassi et al. focused on biofilm movement in animal models placed in the semirecumbent position [31]. Outward movement of biofilm was promoted with prolongation of duty cycle, whereas no relevant effects of positive end-expiratory pressure (PEEP) were demonstrated.

Promoting the movement of ETT biofilm outwards may be an effective strategy to reduce VAP rates. However, an increase in duty cycle may not be feasible in all patients, because of occurrence of intrinsic-PEEP caused by air trapping; clinical data regarding the use of specific ventilator settings for VAP prevention are not currently available.

Gravity

The physiological movement of mucus, directed from the lower airways to the glottis by ciliary movement and cough reflex, is impaired after intubation. In animal models, biofilm flow within the ETT was studied with radio opaque particles and shown to be reversed (directed to the lungs) in the semirecumbent position [31]. However, when the animals were placed in the head-down position, biofilm moved towards the glottis again. In a different experiment, the group of animals with the trachea below the glottis developed bacterial colonization of the lung, whereas the group with the trachea above the glottis did not [32]. These findings show that biofilm movements are subject to gravitational forces, and depend on tracheal orientation relative to the horizontal plane. The movement of biofilm towards the lungs, which is associated with lung bacterial colonization in animal models, may also be relevant in the clinical setting.

On the basis of these preclinical data, changing a patient's position to favor gravitational biofilm movement away from the airways has been proposed as a measure to prevent VAP [33]. Current evidence suggests that patients should be placed in the semirecumbent position, based on the observation that elevating the head of the bed prevents gastric aspiration, as compared to the supine position [34]. However, this position promotes leakage of oral content across the ETT cuff, due to incomplete cuff sealing. As an alternative, the lateral horizontal position has been tested and appears to be a safe and feasible approach [35]. Although the risk of gastric reflux in this alternative position is similar to that in the prone position and higher than in the semirecumbent position, the rationale is that maintaining the trachea above the glottis prevents aspiration within the airways, protecting from VAP. A clinical trial investigating the superiority of the lateral Trendelenburg position compared to the semirecumbent position in the prevention of VAP is currently ongoing [36].

Conclusion

ETT biofilm is implicated in the pathogenesis of VAP, one of the most important hospital-acquired infections. Detachment of biofilm bacteria and dislodgment to the lower airways is the proposed pathogenetic mechanism. The biofilm acts as a reservoir of bacteria, which adhere to the inner lumen of the ETT and are protected by a glycoprotein matrix where antibiotic resistance may develop. Gravity and airflow shear forces promote the movement of bacteria to the lungs. ETT modifications, such as internal coatings, prevent biofilm growth and are effective in VAP prevention. Physical removal of biofilm reduces bacterial growth within the ETT, representing a possible VAP preventive measure. Patient position, other than semirecumbent, can promote biofilm movement away from the airways and may be beneficial for reducing VAP rates; a clinical trial is ongoing to prove this hypothesis.

References

1. Chastre J, Fagon JY (2002) Ventilator-associated pneumonia. Am J Respir Crit Care Med 165:867–903
2. Forel JM, Voillet F, Pulina D et al (2012) Ventilator-associated pneumonia and ICU mortality in severe ARDS patients ventilated according to a lung-protective strategy. Crit Care 16:R65
3. Pneumatikos IA, Dragoumanis CK, Bouros DE (2009) Ventilator-associated pneumonia or endotracheal tube-associated pneumonia? An approach to the pathogenesis and preventive strategies emphasizing the importance of endotracheal tube. Anesthesiology 110:673–680
4. Sackner MA, Hirsch J, Epstein S (1975) Effect of cuffed endotracheal tubes on tracheal mucous velocity. Chest 68:774–777
5. Stewart PS, Costerton JW (2001) Antibiotic resistance of bacteria in biofilms. Lancet 358:135–138
6. Donlan RM (2001) Biofilm formation: a clinically relevant microbiological process. Clin Infect Dis 33:1387–1392
7. Wilson A, Gray D, Karakiozis J, Thomas J (2012) Advanced endotracheal tube biofilm stage, not duration of intubation, is related to pneumonia. J Trauma Acute Care Surg 72:916–923
8. Gorman SP, McGovern JG, Woolfson AD, Adair CG, Jones DS (2001) The concomitant development of poly(vinyl chloride)-related biofilm and antimicrobial resistance in relation to ventilator-associated pneumonia. Biomaterials 22:2741–2747
9. Sottile FD, Marrie TJ, Prough DS et al (1986) Nosocomial pulmonary infection: possible etiologic significance of bacterial adhesion to endotracheal tubes. Crit Care Med 14:265–270
10. Bauer TT, Torres A, Ferrer R, Heyer CM, Schultze-Werninghaus G, Rasche K (2002) Biofilm formation in endotracheal tubes. Association between pneumonia and the persistence of pathogens. Monaldi Arch Chest Dis 57:84–87
11. Inglis TJ (1993) Evidence for dynamic phenomena in residual tracheal tube biofilm. Br J Anaesth 70:22–24
12. Inglis TJ, Lim TM, Ng ML, Tang EK, Hui KP (1995) Structural features of tracheal tube biofilm formed during prolonged mechanical ventilation. Chest 108:1049–1052
13. Wilson AM, Gray DM, Thomas JG (2009) Increases in endotracheal tube resistance are unpredictable relative to duration of intubation. Chest 136:1006–1013
14. Gil-Perotin S, Ramirez P, Marti V et al (2012) Implications of endotracheal tube biofilm in ventilator-associated pneumonia response: a state of concept. Crit Care 16:R93
15. Adair CG, Gorman SP, Feron BM et al (1999) Implications of endotracheal tube biofilm for ventilator-associated pneumonia. Intensive Care Med 25:1072–1076
16. Kojic EM, Darouiche RO (2004) Candida infections of medical devices. Clin Microbiol Rev 17:255–267
17. Peleg AY, Hogan DA, Mylonakis E (2010) Medically important bacterial-fungal interactions. Nat Rev Microbiol 8:340–349
18. Azoulay E, Timsit JF, Tafflet M et al (2006) Candida colonization of the respiratory tract and subsequent pseudomonas ventilator-associated pneumonia. Chest 129:110–117
19. Cairns S, Thomas JG, Hooper SJ et al (2011) Molecular analysis of microbial communities in endotracheal tube biofilms. PLoS One 6:e14759
20. Tang H, Cao T, Liang X et al (2009) Influence of silicone surface roughness and hydrophobicity on adhesion and colonization of Staphylococcus epidermidis. J Biomed Mater Res A 88:454–463
21. Machado MC, Tarquinio KM, Webster TJ (2012) Decreased Staphylococcus aureus biofilm formation on nanomodified endotracheal tubes: a dynamic airway model. Int J Nanomedicine 7:3741–3750

22. Durmus NG, Taylor EN, Inci F, Kummer KM, Tarquinio KM, Webster TJ (2012) Fructose-enhanced reduction of bacterial growth on nanorough surfaces. Int J Nanomedicine 7:537–545
23. Berra L, Curto F, Li Bassi G et al (2008) Antimicrobial-coated endotracheal tubes: an experimental study. Intensive Care Med 34:1020–1029
24. Raad II, Reitzel RA, Mohamed JA et al (2011) The prevention of biofilm colonization by multidrug-resistant pathogens that cause ventilator-associated pneumonia with antimicrobial-coated endotracheal tubes. Biomaterials 32:2689–2694
25. Kollef MH, Afessa B, Anzueto A et al (2008) Silver-coated endotracheal tubes and incidence of ventilator-associated pneumonia: the NASCENT randomized trial. JAMA 300:805–813
26. Kolobow T, Berra L, Li Bassi G, Curto F (2005) Novel system for complete removal of secretions within the endotracheal tube: the Mucus Shaver. Anesthesiology 102:1063–1065
27. Berra L, Coppadoro A, Bittner EA et al (2012) A clinical assessment of the Mucus Shaver: a device to keep the endotracheal tube free from secretions. Crit Care Med 40:119–124
28. Berra L, Curto F, Li Bassi G, Laquerriere P, Baccarelli A, Kolobow T (2006) Antibacterial-coated tracheal tubes cleaned with the Mucus Shaver: a novel method to retain long-term bactericidal activity of coated tracheal tubes. Intensive Care Med 32:888–893
29. Biel MA, Sievert C, Usacheva M et al (2011) Reduction of endotracheal tube biofilms using antimicrobial photodynamic therapy. Lasers Surg Med 43:586–590
30. Volpe MS, Adams AB, Amato MB, Marini JJ (2008) Ventilation patterns influence airway secretion movement. Respir Care 53:1287–1294
31. Li Bassi G, Zanella A, Cressoni M, Stylianou M, Kolobow T (2008) Following tracheal intubation, mucus flow is reversed in the semirecumbent position: possible role in the pathogenesis of ventilator-associated pneumonia. Crit Care Med 36:518–525
32. Panigada M, Berra L, Greco G, Stylianou M, Kolobow T (2003) Bacterial colonization of the respiratory tract following tracheal intubation-effect of gravity: an experimental study. Crit Care Med 31:729–737
33. Berra L, Sampson J, Fumagalli J, Panigada M, Kolobow T (2011) Alternative approaches to ventilator-associated pneumonia prevention. Minerva Anestesiol 77:323–333
34. Drakulovic MB, Torres A, Bauer TT, Nicolas JM, Nogue S, Ferrer M (1999) Supine body position as a risk factor for nosocomial pneumonia in mechanically ventilated patients: a randomised trial. Lancet 354:1851–1858
35. Mauri T, Berra L, Kumwilaisak K et al (2010) Lateral-horizontal patient position and horizontal orientation of the endotracheal tube to prevent aspiration in adult surgical intensive care unit patients: a feasibility study. Respir Care 55:294–302
36. Gravity VAP-trial. Available at: http://compartint.net/gravityvaptrial/joomla. Accessed Oct 2012

High-Frequency Percussive Ventilation in ARDS

H. Spapen, J. De Regt, and P. M. Honoré

Introduction

Despite remarkable progress in understanding its complex physiopathology and considerable efforts to improve medical and ventilatory treatment, intensive care unit (ICU) and hospital mortality rates for the acute respiratory distress syndrome (ARDS) remain unacceptably high [1]. Lung protective ventilation, the only intervention with a proven mortality benefit in ARDS [2], is commonly underused [3] and the inherent 'permissive' hypercapnia may be harmful for patients with compromised cardiac function or brain injury. Moreover, the pattern of ARDS has changed over time. Patients with ARDS are now older and more severely ill and the incidence of sepsis-related ARDS is increasing steadily, whereas cases associated with trauma and transfusion have declined [4].

High-frequency ventilation (HFV) has been proposed as an alternative for patients failing conventional ventilation. HFV is defined as any application of mechanical ventilation with a respiratory rate exceeding 100 breaths/minute. Supposed clinical advantages of the physiology behind HFV include improved gas exchange, minimal cardiovascular interference, and less risk for barotrauma as compared with conventional ventilation.

H. Spapen (✉)
Intensive Care Department, University Hospital, Vrije Universiteit, Laarbeeklaan 101, 1090 Brussels, Belgium
E-mail: herbert.spapen@uzbrussel.be

J. De Regt
Intensive Care Department, University Hospital, Vrije Universiteit, Laarbeeklaan 101, 1090 Brussels, Belgium

P. M. Honoré
Intensive Care Department, University Hospital, Vrije Universiteit, Laarbeeklaan 101, 1090 Brussels, Belgium

J.-L. Vincent (Ed.), *Annual Update in Intensive Care and Emergency Medicine 2013*,
DOI 10.1007/978-3-642-35109-9_47, © Springer-Verlag Berlin Heidelberg 2013

Rationale for High-Frequency Percussive Ventilation in ARDS

High-frequency percussive ventilation (HFPV) is a mode of HFV that was developed in the early 1980s. In the ICU, HFPV is delivered by the VDR™ 4 (Volumetric Diffusive Respirator) (Fig. 1). The VDR is a pneumatically powered, time-cycled, pressure-limited ventilator that combines conventional ventilation and HFV. The most unique feature of the VDR is the Phasitron™ which is a piston mechanism providing a dynamic airway interface through which pulsatile flow is delivered into the lungs. Essentially, the lungs are ventilated with continuous percussive subtidal diffusive gas exchange while the convective lung volume changes in a sinusoidal wave format. Percussive frequency, inspiratory and expiratory times, plateau and positive end-expiratory pressure, and the inspiratory/expiratory (I/E) ratio are determinant factors of mean airway pressure and are, either alone or in combination, able to modify gas exchange. An additional benefit is that HFPV generates intrabronchial vibrations, airway turbulence and higher airflow, all of which may enhance mobilization and clearance of airway debris and secretions. HFPV has shown promising results in neonatal and pediatric ARDS and in adult patients with inhalational lung injury [5]. HFPV also significantly improved gas exchange at similar levels of mean airway pressure as in conventional ventilation

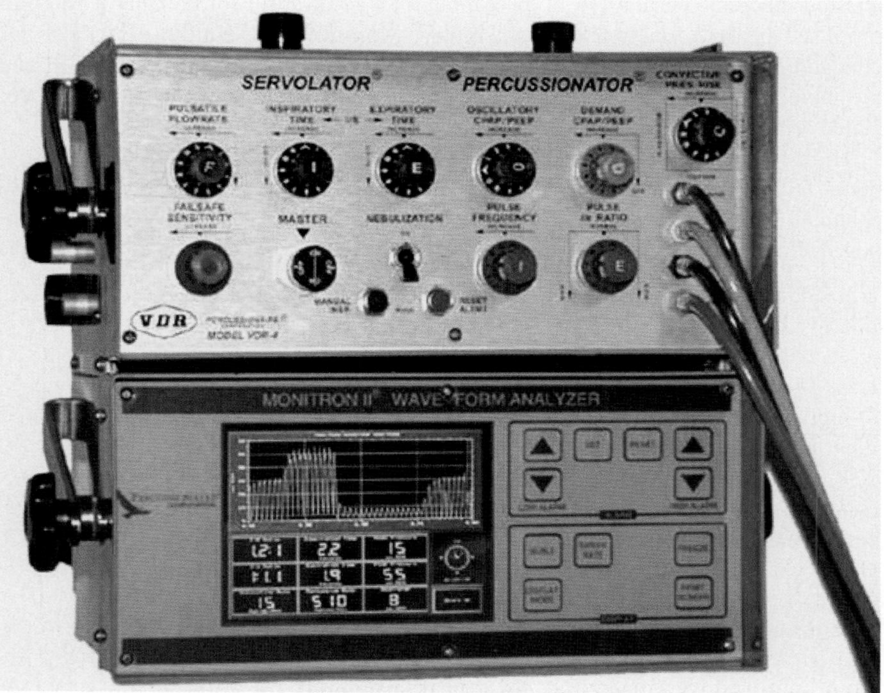

Fig. 1 Volumetric diffusive respirator, VDR™ 4

in adult ARDS patients [6, 7], but is not currently recommended as part of the therapeutic strategy for severe acute lung injury (ALI) [8]

Studies of High-Frequency Percussive Ventilation in ARDS

In an animal model of burn/smoke-induced ARDS, HFPV produced dramatic improvement in oxygenation and ventilation and increased short-term survival as compared to conventional ventilation [9]. To date, two prospective randomized trials have compared conventional ventilation with HFPV in adult burn patients with inhalation injury [10, 11]. In 35 subjects, Reper et al. demonstrated early improvement in oxygenation but no difference in lung infection and mortality [10]. More recently, Chung et al. compared HFPV with low-tidal volume ventilation in 62 burn patients admitted with respiratory failure (nearly half of them diagnosed as ARDS). These authors confirmed early improvement in oxygenation with HFPV. However, the difference in oxygenation was not sustained and similar clinical outcomes (ventilator-free days, pulmonary infection, and mortality) were observed between both ventilation modalities [11].

One prospective randomized trial, conducted 25 years ago, compared conventional ventilation with HFPV in surgical ICU patients with ALI [12]. Both patient groups were ventilated to the same therapeutic endpoints ($pH > 7.35$, $PaCO_2$ 35–45 mm Hg, and $PaO_2/FiO_2 > 225$). In patients with documented ARDS, HFPV improved oxygenation and ventilation at lower peak, mean, and end-expiratory pressures as compared with conventional ventilation. No statistically significant differences in mortality, duration of ICU and hospital stay or incidence of barotrauma were observed between the study groups. Notably, this study does not match current standards of care since it compared the now obsolete intermittent mandatory ventilation mode with HFPV delivered by a non-commercialized VDR device.

Several observational studies have evaluated HFPV in critically ill adult patients with ARDS [13–16]. In general, these studies were retrospective, not protocolized, mainly included surgical and trauma patients, and used HFPV as a rescue therapy in patients failing conventional ventilation. Velmahos et al. [13] reported a series of 32 medical and trauma patients who were switched to HFPV after at least 48 h of conventional ventilation. HFPV significantly improved oxygenation at higher mean airway and lower peak inspiratory pressures; 11 trauma and 8 medical patients died, accounting for an overall mortality rate of 59 %. Paulsen et al. [14] assessed respiratory parameters before and 24 h after initiation of HFPV in 7 trauma and 3 surgical patients. HFPV achieved significant improvement in gas exchange at comparable peak inspiratory pressures; mortality was 30 %. Eastman et al. [15] studied 12 trauma patients and found a nearly 3-fold increase in PaO_2/F_iO_2 ratio after 24 h of HFPV without concomitant increase in mean airway pressure. Finally, Salim et al. [16] described comparable amelioration of the PaO_2/FiO_2 ratio in 10 ARDS patients with severe traumatic brain injury (TBI). Apart from improved oxygenation at lower peak inspiratory pressures, a significant decrease in intracranial pressure (ICP) was observed; only one patient died.

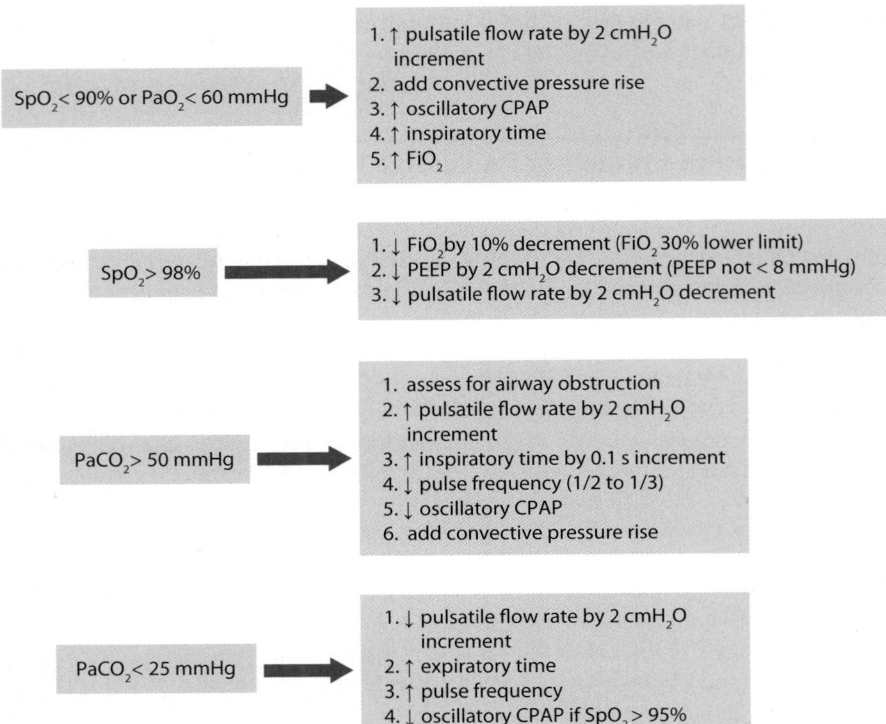

Fig. 2 High-frequency percussive ventilation protocol. CPAP: continuous positive airway pressure; PEEP: positive end-expiratory pressure

We recently conducted the largest observational study of HFPV in a mixed adult trauma, surgical, and medical ARDS population [unpublished results]. Our study design differed considerably from earlier studies. Patients were switched to HFPV within 12 h of developing ARDS (defined as moderate to severe according to the recently published Berlin criteria [17]). Ventilation and oxygenation were adapted according to a predefined protocol (Fig. 2) under supervision of a dedicated team of trained physicians and respiratory therapists. Patients were followed for up to 6 days of HFPV treatment. When stable on HFPV, they could be switched at the physician's discretion to conventional pressure-controlled ventilation and subsequently weaned. Forty-three patients were evaluable, 21 with sepsis-related and 22 with non-sepsis-related ARDS. As expected, HFPV rapidly restored and maintained normal pH and $PaCO_2$ and significantly improved oxygenation in the whole patient cohort. Barotrauma never occurred during HFPV and, except for two septic ARDS patients who developed refractory shock, hemodynamic parameters were not significantly altered. Interestingly, oxygenation improved more in non-septic subjects. Patients with sepsis-related ARDS also spent more days on HFPV than did their non-septic counterparts (6.6 vs. 4.9 days, $p<0.05$). Overall mortality at 30 days and in-hospital mortality were 33 % and 42 %, respectively. A more striking observation was the much higher 30-day (52 % vs. 18 %; p = 0.01) and hospital (62 % vs. 27 %; p = 0.03) mortality rates in sepsis-related as compared with sepsis-unrelated ARDS. Most deaths in the septic subgroup were observed during HFPV (38 % vs. 4.5 %; p = 0.009) and were due to intractable septic shock and multi-organ failure. Although these preliminary findings are difficult to explain, it is conceivable that HFPV adversely propagated reactive pathways that promoted or enhanced local and/or remote organ damage. Sepsis- and non-sepsis-related ARDS may represent different entities with regard to pathophysiology, clinical features and outcome [18]. Septic ARDS patients indeed had more acute inflammation and a higher degree of endothelial cell and coagulation activation than did their non-septic counterparts. Clinically, sepsis-related ARDS was linked to higher mortality, lower successful extubation rates and fewer ventilator-free and ICU-free days [18]. This apparent ARDS heterogeneity may explain why a valuable (ventilatory) treatment may not be suitable and even be detrimental for a distinct patient subgroup (e.g., septic patients with pneumonia) whilst being beneficial for another (e.g., trauma patients).

Conclusion

Globally, the use of HFPV as an alternative ventilation strategy in moderate to severe adult ARDS results in rapid and sustained improvement in oxygenation and ventilation at low risk of hemodynamic complications or barotrauma. However, the lack of randomized studies comparing HFPV with adequately performed conventional lung-protective ventilation does not support the routine use of HFPV. Moreover, the unexpected worse outcome of septic ARDS patients undergoing HFPV needs to be further evaluated.

References

1. Villar J, Blanco J, Añón JM et al (2011) The ALIEN study: incidence and outcome of acute respiratory distress syndrome in the era of lung protective ventilation. Intensive Care Med 37:1932–1941
2. The Acute Respiratory Distress Syndrome Network (2000) Ventilation with lower tidal volumes as compared with traditional tidal volumes for acute lung injury and the acute respiratory distress syndrome. N Engl J Med 342:1301–1308
3. Camporta L, Hart N (2012) Lung protective ventilation. BMJ 344:e2491
4. Pierrakos C, Vincent JL (2012) The changing pattern of ARDS over time: A comparison of two periods. Eur Respir J 40:589–595
5. Salim A, Martin M (2005) High-frequency percussive ventilation. Crit Care Med 33(Suppl):241–245
6. Gallagher TJ, Boysen PG, Davidson DD, Miller JR, Leven SB (1989) High-frequency percussive ventilation compared with conventional mechanical ventilation. Crit Care Med 17:364–366

7. Lucangelo U, Zin WA, Fontanesi L et al (2012) Early short-term application of high-frequency percussive ventilation improves gas exchange in hypoxemic patients. Respiration 84:369–376
8. Diaz JV, Brower R, Calfee CS, Matthay MA (2010) Therapeutic strategies for severe acute lung injury. Crit Care Med 38:1644–1650
9. Wang D, Zwischenberger JB, Savage C et al (2006) High-frequency percussive ventilation with systemic heparin improves short-term survival in a LD100 sheep model of acute respiratory distress syndrome. J Burn Care Res 27:463–471
10. Reper P, Wibaux O, Van Laeke P, Vandeenen D, Duinslaeger L, Vanderkelen A (2002) High frequency percussive ventilation and conventional ventilation after smoke inhalation: a randomised study. Burns 28:503–508
11. Chung KK, Wolf SE, Renz EM et al (2010) High-frequency percussive ventilation and low tidal volume ventilation in burns: a randomized controlled trial. Crit Care Med 38:1970–1977
12. Hurst JM, Branson RD, Davis Jr K, Barrette RR, Adams KS (1990) Comparison of conventional mechanical ventilation and high-frequency ventilation. A prospective, randomized trial in patients with respiratory failure. Ann Surg 211:486–491
13. Velmahos GC, Chan LS, Tatevossian R et al (1999) High-frequency percussive ventilation improves oxygenation in patients with ARDS. Chest 116:440–446
14. Paulsen SM, Killyon GW, Barillo DJ (2002) High-frequency percussive ventilation as a salvage modality in adult respiratory distress syndrome: a preliminary study. Am Surg 68:852–856
15. Eastman A, Holland D, Higgins J et al (2006) High-frequency percussive ventilation improves oxygenation in trauma patients with acute respiratory distress syndrome: a retrospective review. Am J Surg 192:191–195
16. Salim A, Miller K, Dangleben D, Cipolle M, Pasquale M (2004) High-frequency percussive ventilation: an alternative mode of ventilation for head-injured patients with adult respiratory distress syndrome. J Trauma 57:542–554
17. Ranieri VM, Rubenfeld GD, Thompson BT et al (2012) Acute respiratory distress syndrome: the Berlin Definition. JAMA 307:2526–2533
18. Sheu CC, Gong MN, Zhai R et al (2010) Clinical characteristics and outcomes of sepsis-related vs non-sepsis-related ARDS. Chest 138:559–567

NAVA: Applications and Limitations

N. Patroniti, G. Grasselli, and G. Bellani

Introduction

In recent years there has been an increasing interest in the use of partial ventilatory support modes not only as weaning techniques but also in the acute phases of respiratory failure. During assisted spontaneous breathing, a variable proportion of the work of breathing is provided by the ventilator, to unload the patient's respiratory muscles [1]. Multiple ventilator modes are currently available for assisted spontaneous breathing: among these, neurally-adjusted ventilator assist (NAVA) is undergoing extensive clinical evaluation. NAVA is conceptually different from any other mode of ventilation, since the ventilator is not controlled by the 'pneumatic' output of respiratory muscles (i. e., a change in airway pressure or flow) but directly by the neural activity of respiratory centers, expressed by the diaphragm electromyogram (EAdi) [2].

EAdi is recorded through a modified nasogastric tube equipped with multiple-array esophageal electrodes positioned in the lower esophagus, near the crural portion of the diaphragm. Several studies have demonstrated that EAdi provides

N. Patroniti (✉)
Department of Experimental Medicine, University of Milan-Bicocca, Ospedale San Gerardo, via Cadore 48, 20048 Monza, Italy
Department of Perioperative Medicine and Intensive Care, Ospedale San Gerardo, via Cadore 48, 20048 Monza, Italy
E-mail: nicolo.patroniti@unimib.it

G. Grasselli
Department of Perioperative Medicine and Intensive Care, Ospedale San Gerardo, via Cadore 48, 20048 Monza, Italy

G. Bellani
Department of Experimental Medicine, University of Milan-Bicocca, Ospedale San Gerardo, via Cadore 48, 20048 Monza, Italy
Department of Perioperative Medicine and Intensive Care, Ospedale San Gerardo, via Cadore 48, 20048 Monza, Italy

J.-L. Vincent (Ed.), *Annual Update in Intensive Care and Emergency Medicine 2013*,
DOI 10.1007/978-3-642-35109-9_48, © Springer-Verlag Berlin Heidelberg 2013

a reliable estimate of inspiratory timing [3] and drive [4] and that electrical activity of the crural diaphragm is related to global inspiratory efforts in healthy subjects [5, 6] and in patients with acute or chronic respiratory failure [7, 8]. As shown by Sinderby et al. in the first report published in 1998 [2], NAVA uses the EAdi to trigger, cycle off, and adjust the intrabreath assist profile in proportion to the EAdi, according to a proportionality factor called the "NAVA level" (measured in cm $H_2O/\mu V$).

In the first part of this chapter we will summarize the expected potential benefits associated with the use of NAVA in adult patients. We will then review the available published clinical data, focusing on the advantages and the limitations of the technique in different groups of patients.

Expected Benefits of NAVA

Because of its innovative mode of function, NAVA is expected to be associated with several clinical benefits compared to other conventional ventilation modes:

1. Improvement of patient-ventilator interaction: During assisted ventilation modes, interaction between the patient and the ventilator is of paramount importance. Many studies have shown that a high rate of patient-ventilator asynchrony is associated with prolonged duration of mechanical ventilation and ultimately a worse clinical outcome [10, 11]. The use of the neural output from the respiratory centers (EAdi) to fully control the ventilator is expected to: (a) significantly reduce the inspiratory trigger delay, especially in patients with dynamic hyperinflation and intrinsic positive end-expiratory pressure (PEEPi); (b) reduce the incidence and severity of expiratory asynchrony; (c) solve the problem of ineffective triggering and wasted efforts; and (d) eliminate asynchronies due to airleaks (because the neural trigger is independent of pneumatic signals), which should be particularly important in the setting of non-invasive ventilation (NIV). These expectations have been confirmed by studies in animal models [12] and humans, showing a significant decrease in the incidence of asynchronies and improved patient-ventilator interaction with NAVA compared to other conventional modes of ventilation. The findings of the clinical studies will be summarized in a dedicated paragraph later in the chapter.
2. Lung protection and reduction of ventilator-induced lung injury (VILI): Preclinical studies have shown that NAVA is a potentially lung-protective strategy because the delivery of excessive tidal volume (V_T) and transpulmonary pressure is limited by the neural feedback from pulmonary stretch receptors. In a rabbit model of acute lung injury (ALI), Brander et al. [9] showed that, during NAVA, the animals spontaneously chose a protective V_T (around 3–4 ml/kg); in addition, different biological markers of lung injury and inflammation were analyzed and NAVA was at least as protective as low-V_T controlled ventilation. Studies in humans have confirmed that increasing the NAVA level is not associated with an increase in V_T, because when the assist level is increased the

EAdi is downregulated with the net result of reducing the risk of overassistance and hyperinflation [13–17].

3. Prevention of diaphragmatic dysfunction: In theory, NAVA minimizes the risk of ventilator-induced diaphragmatic atrophy because it is based on the continuous coupling between ventilator assistance and the patient's neural output. During pressure support ventilation (PSV), a progressive increase in support ultimately leads to disappearance of a detectable EAdi signal, clearly indicating over-assistance [18]. In contrast, increasing the NAVA level can efficiently unload the respiratory muscles without abolishing the EAdi; in a study on healthy subjects performing maximal inspiratory maneuvers during NAVA at increasing levels of assist, Sinderby et al. showed that despite maximal unloading of the diaphragm at high NAVA levels, EAdi was still present (reduced to about 40 % of baseline values) and able to control the ventilator [19]. Preservation of adequate muscle function should be particularly important to facilitate weaning from mechanical ventilation, and many clinical trials are currently exploring this hypothesis.
4. Maintenance of the 'physiological' variability of breathing pattern: Complex mathematical analyses have demonstrated that the normal breathing pattern in humans is highly variable and exhibits a chaos-like complexity [20]. Unfortunately, almost all the available conventional modes of ventilation tend to impose a monotonous pattern. It has been suggested that restoring a 'physiological' variability of the breathing pattern during mechanical ventilation could be beneficial [21]. Moreover, it has been observed that reduced breathing variability is associated with an increased rate of weaning failure [22, 23]. Studies in humans have clearly demonstrated that NAVA is characterized by a significant increase in breathing pattern variability and complexity compared to PSV, but the clinical relevance of this has to be assessed.

NAVA in Critically Ill Patients

Most physiological and clinical studies available in the literature have been conducted in a general population of critically ill patients recovering from the acute phase of illness or during the weaning phase. Because PSV is the most frequently used mode of partial ventilator assistance, all these studies have compared NAVA with PSV. When applied at equal peak inspiratory pressure levels, NAVA has shown comparable unloading of inspiratory muscles but better patient-ventilator synchrony and less risk of over-assistance [13–17].

Respiratory Pattern and Muscle Unloading

As for all modes of partial ventilatory support, the main ventilator setting variable is the level of assistance. According to a specific clinical target (unloading of

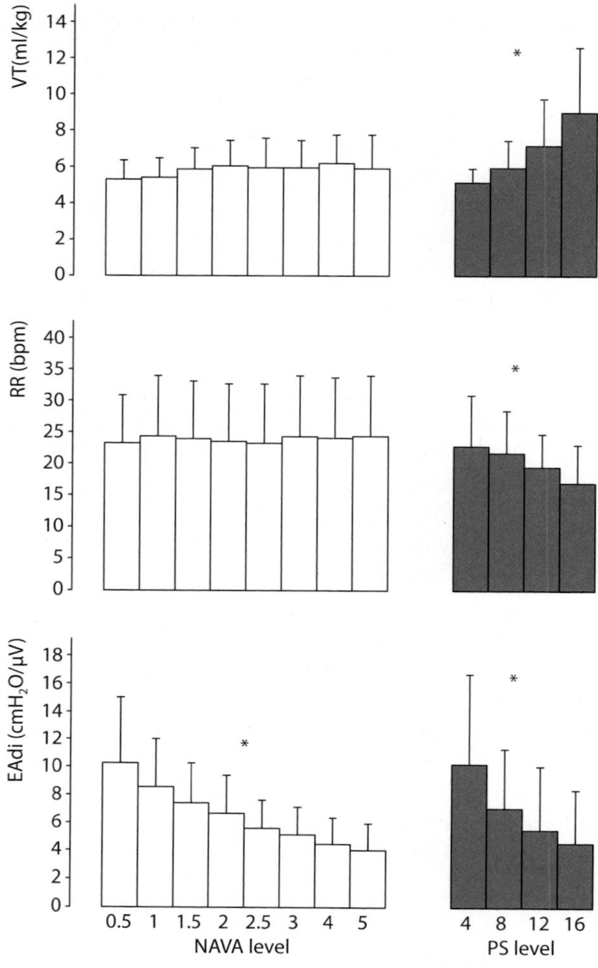

Fig. 1 Effect of the level of assistance during neutrally-adjusted ventilator assist (NAVA, white histograms) and pressure support ventilation (PSV, gray histograms) on tidal volume (V_T), peak of diaphragm electrical activity ($EAdi_{peak}$), and respiratory rate (RR). * $p < 0.05$ effect of NAVA or PS level

inspiratory muscle, support of ventilatory needs, weaning) the level of assistance should be set to preserve the inspiratory muscle activity with a work of breathing that the patient can handle while avoiding over assistance, disuse atrophy of the diaphragm, and minimizing VILI. In the clinical setting, the level of assistance is often based on indirect measurements of muscle unloading, such as occlusion pressure (P0.1), integrated by arterial gas exchange, respiratory pattern variables such as respiratory rate and V_T and clinical signs of patient comfort or distress. During NAVA, the EAdi amplitude is also available to estimate the respiratory drive and work of breathing [7, 8]. Physiological studies comparing NAVA with PSV found that while increasing assistance levels was associated with comparable muscle unloading, the physiologic response in respiratory pattern during NAVA was different than that commonly observed during PSV [5, 7–8]. With PSV, increasing the level of assistance is associated with a reduction in respiratory rate and often an increase in V_T [24, 25]. The decrease in respiratory rate is particularly important in the clinical setting since it is interpreted as a sign of relief from respiratory distress [11, 26]. Several authors have observed that, contrary to PSV, during NAVA increased levels of assistance are associated with scarce or null increase in V_T and no change in respiratory rate [13–17] (Fig. 1). As a consequence, during NAVA, evidence of muscle unloading and patient comfort may not be accompanied by a decrease in respiratory rate, and respiratory rates higher than those commonly accepted in the clinical setting may be observed.

Should the absent response in respiratory rate be interpreted as the inability of NAVA to effectively relieve respiratory distress in some patients, or should the high respiratory rate be accepted as an expression of the patient's best mechanical compromise? Although we lack physiological and clinical data in patients with acute respiratory distress, two considerations support the second possibility: First, when PSV is set to obtain a protective V_T, NAVA set to obtain equivalent peak inspiratory pressure produces respiratory rates similar to PSV (13–17); second, lower respiratory rates during PSV are obtained with a concomitant increase in V_T and possibly with the occurrence of over assistance [11, 13, 17]. Thus acceptance of respiratory rates above 30 bpm may represent the result of the best compromise between patient comfort, protective ventilation and avoidance of over assistance not just during NAVA but also with other modes of partial ventilatory support.

Only a few long-term NAVA studies are available [26–28]. In a study by Barwing et al., application of NAVA for 6 hours was well tolerated by mechanically ventilated patients able to sustain spontaneous breathing [26]. Coisel et al. ventilated 15 postoperative abdominal surgery patients with NAVA and PSV for 24 h each in a randomized order. NAVA was tolerated in all patients [27]. It is worth noting that this is the only study in humans that has reported better oxygenation during NAVA [27].

Patient-Ventilator Interaction

In the commercially available system, inspiration during NAVA may be triggered either from the EAdi signal or from a standard flow trigger on a first-come first-served algorithm. In a recent study by Piquilloud et al., NAVA showed shorter inspiratory and expiratory trigger delays and fewer asynchronies than did PSV [29]; 11 to 42 % of the respiratory cycles in NAVA were triggered by the flow-trigger [29]. Although the 50 to 100 ms shorter delay observed in NAVA is certainly an improvement in patient-ventilator interaction, in our opinion the better synchrony of inspiratory cycle-off is probably the most advantageous aspect of NAVA. Colombo et al. [13] and Patroniti et al. [17] applied different assistance levels during NAVA and PSV. In both studies, the ventilator inspiratory time increased compared to the neural one at increasing pressure support level whereas the difference between neural and ventilator inspiratory time remained constant during NAVA irrespective of the gain level. The ventilator inspiratory time was always longer than the neural one suggesting that delayed inspiratory cycle-off accounts for most of the difference between ventilator and neural time. Considering that a delayed inspiratory cycle-off is strictly related to over-assistance and plays a major role in patient-ventilator interaction during PSV [11], the independency of the cycling-off delay from the assistance level explains the relative protection of NAVA from the risk of over-assistance.

In all physiological studies NAVA was associated with a markedly lower incidence of all type of asynchrony events [13–17, 29]. Piquilloud et al. specifically investigated asynchrony events during NAVA. Compared to PSV, the incidence of ineffective efforts, premature cycling and autotriggering were negligible or absent. The most frequent type of asynchrony was double triggering. The authors also described a type of double triggering specific to NAVA (type 1 double trigger), defined as two pneumatic cycles as a consequence of a biphasic EAdi signal. In this type of asynchrony if, during the expiration, the EAdi increases above the set trigger threshold, even very shortly, the ventilator abruptly closes the expiratory valve and delivers inspiratory flow attempting to pressurize the airway. The incidence of this asynchrony was low [29].

Breathing Variability and Protective Ventilation

Most physiological studies have shown higher variability in EAdi amplitude, V_T and respiratory rate and a better match between variability at the neural level (EAdi) and variability of the output variables (V_T and respiratory rate) [14–17]. Barwing et al. explained the better oxygenation they observed during NAVA compared to PSV as the result of better perfusion-ventilation matching and delivering of periodical sighs [26]. Schmidt et al., who investigated the effect of NAVA levels from 1 to 4 cm H_2O/μV on respiratory pattern variability in patients with acute respiratory failure, found similar variability in EAdi between NAVA and PSV, higher variability of V_T during NAVA, and increased variability of V_T with increasing NAVA levels [14]. Although statistically significant, the increase in EAdi variability was considered negligible and the authors concluded that during NAVA, neural variability is unaffected by the level of assistance [14]. This idea has been partially challenged by a more recent study by Patroniti et al. who found increases in the EAdi coefficient of variation ranging between 0 and 57 % in response to increasing NAVA levels from 0.5 to 5 cm H_2O/μV [17]. In four patients at the highest NAVA levels, these authors observed an unstable pattern associated with periodical delivering of high V_T and peak airway pressure with patient discomfort, eventually requiring discontinuation of the study (Fig. 2). The authors interpreted the observed pattern as a form of over-assistance specific to NAVA, over amplifying the neural variability beyond the expected output variability, with a kind of oscillatory feedback behavior. It is worth nothing that in the presence of

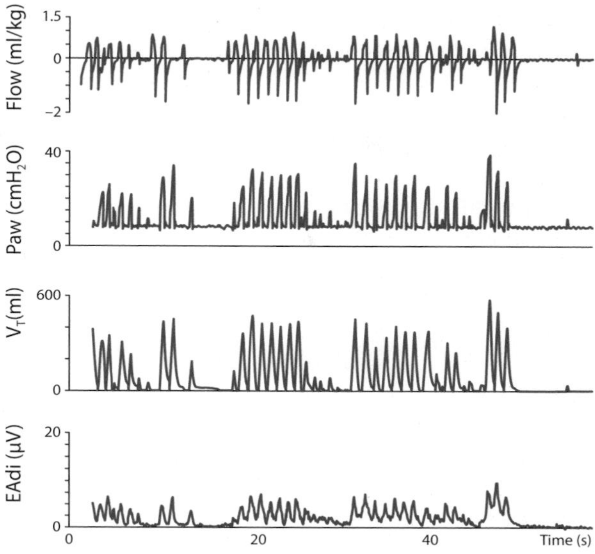

Fig. 2 Example of a patient ventilated with a NAVA level of 5 cm H_2O/μV showing an unstable pattern associated with periodical delivering of high tidal volume (V_T) and peak airway pressure with patient discomfort that required discontinuation of NAVA. Flow: airway flow; Paw: airway pressure; V_T: tidal volume; EAdi: diaphragm electrical activity

excessive V_T variability, there is also an increased risk of delivering a higher proportion of V_T outside a protective range [17].

Role of NAVA During Weaning from Mechanical Ventilation

Weaning is defined as the process of separating the patient from the support of the mechanical ventilator. This process can be challenging in up to 30 % of patients, requiring prolonged ventilation; of note it has been shown that the presence of patient-ventilator asynchronies is associated with prolonged duration of mechanical ventilation and intensive care unit (ICU) stay [10]. Whereas a simple reduction in pressure support can significantly decrease the rate of asynchronies [30], in selected patients (e.g., with unfavorable mechanical properties of the respiratory system or muscle weakness), NAVA could offer further synchrony improvement.

In 15 patients being weaned from mechanical ventilation, Rozé et al. [28] performed a daily spontaneous breathing trial (with PEEP 0 and pressure support 7 cm H_2O), during which the patient's Eadi was measured ($Eadi_{max}$) and NAVA was subsequently applied, with a "NAVA level" yielding an Eadi equal to 60 % of $Eadi_{max}$. This approach could be successfully applied in all patients, none of whom had to be switched back to PSV. The $Eadi_{max}$ increased significantly between day 1 and the day of extubation (possibly indicating improved diaphragmatic function), whereas the NAVA level could be progressively decreased from 2.4 ± 1 to 1 ± 0.7, with a consequent decrease in inspiratory pressure level above PEEP from 20 ± 5 to 10 ± 5 cm H_2O.

Critical illness polyneuropathy is a condition that greatly impairs a patient's weanability. In 13 out of 15 patients with an electrophysiological diagnosis of critical illness polyneuropathy, NAVA was successfully applied for a total of 61 hours (range 37–64 hours) [31].

These studies, albeit preliminary and conducted on a relatively small number of patients, demonstrate the feasibility of ventilating patients with NAVA for days during a difficult weaning process. Hopefully, in the near future, larger studies will demonstrate whether this approach translates into an improved outcome.

Role of NAVA in Non-invasive Ventilation

NIV is beneficial in some patients with acute respiratory failure or exacerbation of chronic obstructive pulmonary disease (COPD), improving gas exchange, decreasing the work of breathing and delaying or preventing the need for endotracheal intubation [32]. In order to effectively support the patients and avoid an increased work of breathing, good synchrony between patient and ventilator is mandatory. In 2012, Schmidt et al. compared the effects of NAVA and pressure support for 'prophylactic' NIV in 17 patients, immediately after extubation [33]. All patients could successfully tolerate both ventilatory modes. The global asynchrony index was lower in NAVA (10.8 %) than in pressure support (26.3 %), but this did not result in improved patient comfort, as assessed by the visual analog scale. NAVA was also characterized by a shorter delay between the initiation of patient effort and the pressurization rate. Asynchrony, however, was not absent in NAVA, which showed 'Type I double triggers' [29]. This study also underlines (both for pressure support and NAVA) the relevant advantages of NIV-specific algorithms in reducing the air leaks and avoiding prolonged airway pressurization after termination of patient effort.

Similar results were reported by Piquilloud et al. [34] in 13 ICU patients (6 with a history of COPD) undergoing NIV for various reasons. The total number of asynchrony events tended to be reduced during NAVA compared to PSV: 4.4 events/min during PSV versus 1.0 events/min during NAVA. The asynchrony index was significantly lower during NAVA with a median value of 4.9 % versus 15.8 % during PSV. The improved synchrony did not, however, affect gas exchange, respiratory rate or respiratory drive (as assessed by peak inspiratory EAdi).

In comparison with a face mask, a head helmet is generally better tolerated by patients and allows longer periods of treatment [35], but it imposes additional synchrony problems, because of its larger internal volume and elevated compliance, which delays the trigger activation and airway pressurization [36]. Using this interface, Moerer et al. [37] compared pressure support based on pneumatic trigger and cycle-off against pressure support based on Eadi-based ('neural') trigger and cycle-off criteria, in seven healthy volunteers instructed to breathe at different respiratory rates and receiving increasing levels of support. The authors showed that the use of a neural trigger led to a shorter (from 5 to 60 times) delay between the volunteer's effort and ventilator assistance and no wasted efforts which were, instead, numerous (up to 50 % of total 'neural breaths') when a pneumatic trigger was used. At the same time, the use of a neural cycle-off improved recognition by the ventilator of the end of the inspiratory effort, leading to shorter expiratory delays. The benefits of neural trigger as compared to a pneumatic one increased at higher respiratory rates and levels of assistance, including a greater 'comfort of breathing' as subjectively reported by the subjects on a visual analog scale. Encouraged by these findings, Cammarota et al. compared NAVA and PSV in 10 patients with acute respiratory failure [38]. NAVA was set to achieve the same peak airway pressure as during PSV. While no differences were observed in terms of gas exchange, NAVA was characterized by a longer inspiratory time and a shorter time required to trigger the ventilator after the initiation of the inspiratory effort. At the same time, NAVA led to disappearance of wasted efforts, and to a decrease in the asynchrony index, which in no patient exceeded 10 % (as opposed to 70 % of patients exceeding the 10 % threshold with PSV). Surprisingly, however, the improved synchrony with the ventilator did not decrease the patient's 'neural' drive, as indicated by the similar peak EAdi values between NAVA and PSV.

NAVA and ECMO: Clinical Studies

Until recently, extracorporeal membrane oxygenation (ECMO) and other forms of extracorporeal respiratory support have been considered as last-resource therapies to be applied in patients with refractory impairment of gas exchange unresponsive to any 'rescue' therapy. In addition, because of the technical complexity and the high incidence of complications, the use of ECMO has been restricted to very few and highly specialized centers [39]. In the last few years, technical improvements, the publication of the results of the CESAR trial [40], and the huge experience accumulated during the H1N1 pandemic [41, 42], have contributed to reawaken interest in this technique, which is now applied with increasing frequency worldwide.

One of the most challenging problems that we have to face when treating a patient on ECMO is how to manage the ventilation of the patient's native lung. Some clinicians believe that an assisted spontaneous breathing mode should be implemented soon, and for this purpose NAVA should (at least in theory) offer some additional benefits compared to other conventional modes. Many researchers are exploring this hypothesis, but only limited data are available from the literature. At the time of writing, only one paper has been published on a small group of 6 patients ventilated with NAVA during ECMO support [43]. Gas exchange and ventilation were studied at different sweep gas flows and during temporary discontinuation of ECMO. During ECMO, V_T was kept between 3 and 5 ml/kg and increased up to 8 ml/kg when ECMO was inactivated; after gas flow reduction, the patients rapidly increased their minute ventilation to restore a physiological pH value but tended to maintain a 'protective' V_T. The authors concluded that "the combination of NAVA and ECMO may permit a closed-loop ventilation with automated protected ventilation".

In addition to the paper by Karagiannidis et al. [43], a few single case reports have been published and two of them deserve, in our opinion, to be cited. Mauri et al. reported the case of a patient on ECMO with severe ARDS and extremely low compliance of the respiratory system (7 ml/cm H_2O): In such situations, PSV is very difficult to implement because, due to lung stiffness, the peak inspiratory flow is reached rapidly and the ventilator starts expiration while the patient is still inspiring [44]. The consequence is a high incidence of asynchronies and, in particular, of double triggering, even after reducing the expiratory trigger criterion of PSV to 1 % of peak inspiratory flow. When NAVA was started, the incidence of asynchronies dropped significantly and it was possible to maintain assisted spontaneous breathing [44]. Another very interesting report of an uncommon but really challenging situation was recently published by Rozé and Ouattara describing the case of a patient with a large air leakage from a broncho-pleural fistula [45]. PSV could not be used, because of the continuous autotriggering caused by the suction pressure of the chest tube: The only way to ventilate the patient was to set an extremely insensitive pressure trigger (lower than the drainage suction pressure), thus imposing an unacceptable workload on the patient. The problem was solved by switching the patient to NAVA, in order to use neural triggering instead of pneumatic triggering; indeed, as explained earlier, neural triggering is not affected by air leakage nor by the suction pressure of the chest drain. With NAVA, assisted spontaneous breathing became possible with good patient-ventilator synchronization [45].

In conclusion, we expect that NAVA, by allowing the maintenance of protective ventilation and significantly improving the interaction between the patient and the mechanical ventilator, may represent a means of increasing the number of spontaneously breathing patients during ECMO support. Moreover, NAVA may be particularly indicated in specific groups of patients, such as those with extremely stiff lungs or with large airleaks. However, specific studies including an adequate number of patients are needed to verify this hypothesis.

Open Issues, Potential Limitations and Future Research

All physiological studies have confirmed the expected benefits of NAVA. However, most studies have been conducted in patients already recovering from respiratory distress or with clinically stable conditions. Thus, we lack long-term clinical studies and, more importantly, we lack studies addressing the effectiveness of NAVA to adequately support patients with impending acute respiratory distress (low respiratory system compliance, high airway resistance, COPD, high ventilatory needs/respiratory drive, severe metabolic acidosis, hemodynamic instability). A crucial issue will be to understand in which of the above listed clinical condi-

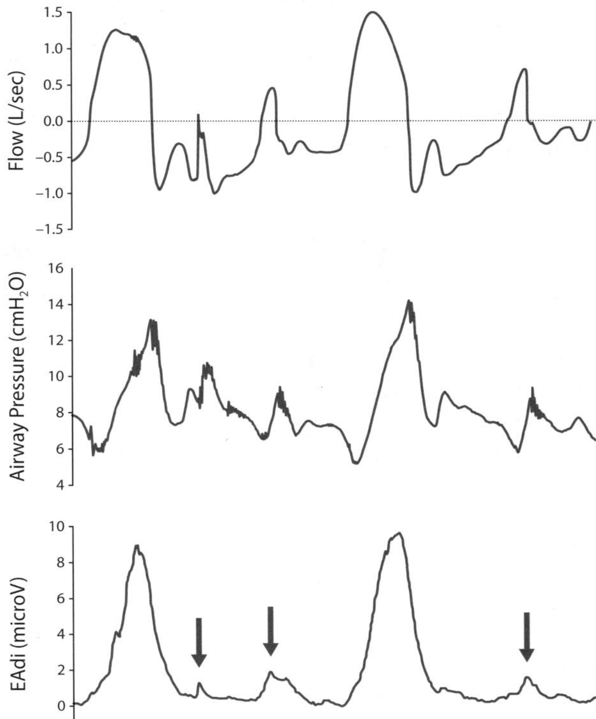

Fig. 3 The figure shows one peculiar asynchrony pattern during NAVA, arising from the presence of unfiltered cardiac electric activity (blue arrows) on the signal of the electrical diaphragmatic activity (Eadi). This can be recognized on Eadi as small spikes, characterized by a much lower amplitude than the regular Eadi peaks and a frequency similar to the patient's heart rate. During the expiratory phase, if these spikes reach the threshold of neural trigger, the ventilator abruptly interrupts the expiratory flow and sometimes a small inspiratory flow is delivered

tions it may be counterproductive and not desirable to follow respiratory center commands.

Another open question is the setting of the NAVA level. Contrary to PSV, given the negligible effect of NAVA on the 'classical' respiratory pattern parameters, changes in respiratory rate and V_T are less informative. Brander et al. observed a two-phase response to increasing NAVA levels, characterized by an initial steep increase in both peak airway pressure and V_T. These authors identified the optimal NAVA level in each patient at the transition between the two phases [46]. A main limitation of this procedure is that the NAVA level is chosen arbitrarily outside any clinical objective. The daily titration procedure proposed by Rozè et al. is certainly more practical and more clinically oriented [28]. A key aspect of the method of Rozè is the use of EAdi as the guiding variable. The possibility of using the EAdi signal not only to drive ventilation but also to quantitate the amount of muscle unloading and respiratory drive is fascinating and will certainly be the subject of future studies.

Another crucial issue remains the quality of the signal and the interpretation of EAdi values. Several factors may affect the signal quality, such as, for example, the catheter position or a poorly filtered electrocardiogram (EKG) signal (Fig. 3). Other possible limitations may arise in patients breathing predominantly through accessory inspiratory muscles. In these patients, the amplitude of the EAdi signal may underestimate the real amount of muscular effort and inspiration may be more easily triggered by the flow than by the EAdi signal. Similar behavior could be observed in patients with high airway respiratory resistance and flow limitation who force expiration. In these patients, the first part of the inspiratory flow may be generated by releasing expiratory muscle, the flow trigger may respond faster than the EAdi trigger and the amplitude of the EAdi trigger may underestimate the generated inspiratory pressure and the effective work of breathing.

Conclusion

NAVA is a promising technique. Physiological studies have proved its superiority in terms of patient-ventilator interaction and preservation of patient respiratory pattern. However, clinical data are scanty. Future research should focus on clinical studies to explore the possibility of extending the potential benefits of NAVA to patients in respiratory distress or in clinical conditions where other partial ventilatory modes frequently fail or provide unsatisfactory ventilatory support. Potential indications for NAVA are numerous, but several issues, including the correct setting of NAVA level according to a patient's characteristics and clinical objectives, need to be explored.

References

1. Putensen C, Muders T, Varelmann D, Wrigge H (2006) The impact of spontaneous breathing during mechanical ventilation. Curr Opin Crit Care 12:160–165
2. Sinderby C, Navalesi P, Beck J et al (1999) Neural control of mechanical ventilation in respiratory failure. Nat Med 5:1433–1436
3. Parthasarathy S, Jubran A, Tobin MJ (2000) Assessment of neural inspiratory time in ventilator-supported patients. Am J Respir Crit Care Med 162:546–552
4. Lourenco RV, Cherniack NS, Malm JR et al (1966) Nervous output from the respiratory centers during obstructed breathing. J Appl Physiol 21:527–533
5. Beck J, Sinderby C, Lindstrom L et al (1998) Effects of lung volume on diaphragm EMG signal strength during voluntary contractions. J Appl Physiol 85:1123–1134
6. Beck J, Sinderby C, Lindstrom L et al (1998) Crural diaphragm activation during dynamic contractions at various inspiratory flow rates. J Appl Physiol 85:451–458
7. Beck J, Gottfried SB, Navalesi P et al (2001) Electrical activity of the diaphragm during pressure support ventilation in acute respiratory failure. Am J Respir Crit Care Med 164:419–424
8. Sinderby C, Beck J, Spahija J et al (1998) Voluntary activation of the human diaphragm in health and disease. J Appl Physiol 85:2146–2158
9. Brander L, Sinderby C, Lecomte F et al (2009) Neurally adjusted ventilatory assist decreases ventilator-induced lung injury and non-pulmonary organ dysfunction in rabbits with acute lung injury. Intensive Care Med 35:1979–1989
10. de Wit M, Miller KB, Green DA et al (2009) Ineffective triggering predicts increased duration of mechanical ventilation. Crit Care Med 37:2740–2745

11. Thille AW, Rodriguez P, Cabello B et al (2006) Patient-ventilator asynchrony during assisted mechanical ventilation. Intensive Care Med 32:1515–1522
12. Beck J, Campoccia F, Allo JC et al (2007) Improved synchrony and respiratory unloading by neurally adjusted ventilatory assist (NAVA) in lung-injured rabbits. Pediatr Res 61:289–294
13. Colombo D, Cammarota G, Bergamaschi V et al (2008) Physiologic response to varying levels of pressure support and neurally adjusted ventilatory assist in patients with acute respiratory failure. Intensive Care Med 34:2010–2018
14. Schmidt M, Demoule A, Cracco C et al (2010) Neurally adjusted ventilatory assist increases respiratory variability and complexity in acute respiratory failure. Anesthesiology 112:670–681
15. Terzi N, Pelieu I, Guittet L et al (2010) Neurally adjusted ventilatory assist in patients recovering spontaneous breathing after acute respiratory distress syndrome: physiological evaluation. Crit Care Med 38:1830–1837
16. Spahija J, de Marchie M, Albert M et al (2010) Patient-ventilator interaction during pressure support ventilation and neurally adjusted ventilatory assist. Crit Care Med 38:518–526
17. Patroniti N, Bellani G, Saccavino E et al (2012) Respiratory pattern during neurally adjusted ventilator assist in acute respiratory failure patients. Intensive Care Med 38:230–239
18. Sinderby C, Beck J (2008) Proportional assist ventilation and Neurally Adjusted Ventilatory Assist: better approaches to patient-ventilator synchrony? Clin Chest Med 29:329–342
19. Sinderby C, Beck J, Spahija J et al (2007) Inspiratory muscle unloading by neurally adjusted ventilatory assist during maximal inspiratory efforts in healthy subjects. Chest 131:711–717
20. Wysocki M, Fiamma MN, Straus C et al (2006) Chaotic dynamics of resting ventilatory flow in humans assessed through noise titration. Respir Physiol Neurobiol 153:54–65
21. Suki B, Alencar AM, Sujeer MK et al (1998) Life-support system benefits from noise. Nature 393:127–128
22. Bien MY, Hseu SS, Yien HW et al (2004) Breathing pattern variability: a weaning predictor in postoperative patients recovering from systemic inflammatory response syndrome. Intensive Care Med 30:241–247
23. Wysocki M, Cracco C, Teixeira A et al (2006) Reduced breathing variability as a predictor of unsuccessful patient separation from mechanical ventilation. Crit Care Med 34:2076–2083
24. Brochard L, Harf A, Lorino H, Lemaire F (1989) Inspiratory pressure support prevents diaphragmatic fatigue during weaning from mechanical ventilation. Am Rev Respir Dis 139:513–521
25. Tokioka H, Saito S, Kosaka F (1989) Effects of pressure support ventilation on breathing pattern and respiratory work. Intensive Care Med 15:491–494
26. Barwing J, Linden N, Ambold M, Quintel M, Moerer O (2011) Neurally adjusted ventilatory assist vs. pressure support ventilation in critically ill patients: an observational study. Acta Anaesthesiol Scand 55:1261–1271
27. Coisel Y, Chanques G, Jung B et al (2010) Neurally adjusted ventilatory assist in critically ill postoperative patients: a crossover randomized study. Anesthesiology 113:925–935
28. Rozé H, Lafrikh A, Perrier V et al (2011) Daily titration of neurally adjusted ventilatory assist using the diaphragm electrical activity. Intensive Care Med 37:1087–1094
29. Piquilloud L, Vignaux L, Bialais E et al (2011) Neurally adjusted ventilatory assist improves patient-ventilator interaction. Intensive Care Med 37:263–271
30. Thille AW, Cabello B, Galia F, Lyazidi A, Brochard L (2008) Reduction of patient-ventilator asynchrony by reducing tidal volume during pressure-support ventilation. Intensive Care Med 34:1477–1486
31. Tuchscherer D, Z'graggen WJ et al (2011) Neurally adjusted ventilatory assist in patients with critical illness-associated polyneuromyopathy. Intensive Care Med 37:1951–1961
32. Nava S, Hill N (2009) Non-invasive ventilation in acute respiratory failure. Lancet 374:250–259

33. Schmidt M, Dres M, Raux M et al (2012) Neurally adjusted ventilatory assist improves patient-ventilator interaction during postextubation prophylactic noninvasive ventilation. Crit Care Med 40:1738–1744
34. Piquilloud L, Tassaux D, Bialais E (2012) Neurally adjusted ventilatory assist (NAVA) improves patient-ventilator interaction during non-invasive ventilation delivered by face mask. Intensive Care Med 38:1624–1631
35. Bellani G, Patroniti N, Greco M, Foti G, Pesenti A (2008) The use of helmets to deliver non-invasive continuous positive airway pressure in hypoxemic acute respiratory failure. Minerva Anestesiol 74:651–656
36. Racca F, Appendini L, Gregoretti C et al (2005) Effectiveness of mask and helmet interfaces to deliver noninvasive ventilation in a human model of resistive breathing. J Appl Physiol 99:1262–1271
37. Moerer O, Beck J, Brander L et al (2008) Subject-ventilator synchrony during neural versus pneumatically triggered non-invasive helmet ventilation. Intensive Care Med 34:1615–1623
38. Cammarota G, Olivieri C, Costa R et al (2011) Noninvasive ventilation through a helmet in postextubation hypoxemic patients: physiologic comparison between neutrally adjusted ventilatory assist and pressure support ventilation. Intensive Care Med 37:1943–1950
39. Pesenti A, Zanella A, Patroniti N (2009) Extracorporeal gas exchange. Curr Opin Crit Care 15:52–58
40. Peek GJ, Mugford M, Tiruvoipati R et al (2009) Efficacy and economic assessment of conventional ventilatory support versus extracorporeal membrane oxygenation for severe adult respiratory failure (CESAR): a multicentre randomised controlled trial. Lancet 374:1351–1363
41. Australia and New Zealand Extracorporeal Membrane Oxygenation (ANZ ECMO) Influenza Investigators (2009) Extracorporeal membrane oxygenation for 2009 influenza A(H1N1) acute respiratory distress syndrome. JAMA 302:1888–1895
42. Patroniti N, Zangrillo A, Pappalardo F et al (2011) The Italian ECMO network experience during the 2009 influenza A(H1N1) pandemic: preparation for severe respiratory emergency outbreaks. Intensive Care Med 37:1447–1457
43. Karagiannidis C, Lubnow M, Philipp A et al (2010) Autoregulation of ventilation with neurally adjusted ventilatory assist on extracorporeal lung support. Intensive Care Med 36:2038–2044
44. Mauri T, Bellani G, Foti G et al (2011) Successful use of neurally adjusted ventilatory assist in a patient with extremely low respiratory system compliance undergoing ECMO. Intensive Care Med 37:166–167
45. Rozé H, Ouattara A (2012) Use of neural trigger during neurally adjusted ventilatory assist in a patient with a large broncho-pleural fistula and air leakage. Intensive Care Med 38:922–923
46. Brander L, Leong-Poi H, Beck J et al (2009) Titration and implementation of neurally adjusted ventilatory assist in critically ill patients. Chest 135:695–703

Extracorporeal Gas Exchange: Present and Future

T. Mauri, A. Zanella, and A. Pesenti

Introduction

Extracorporeal gas exchange allows carbon dioxide removal and oxygenation by circulating blood outside the patient's body through an artificial membrane lung [1]. Extracorporeal gas exchange has been used for many years (it was first developed in the cardiac surgery field in the 1940s [2]) to replace heart and lung functions. In the late 1960s, the idea of using extracorporeal gas exchange to support lung function, rather than to completely substitute it, was raised [3]. In 1971, successful use of extracorporeal membrane oxygenation (ECMO) as lung support in a patient with 'adult' (now 'acute') respiratory distress syndrome (ARDS) was reported for the first time [4]. In this case and in others immediately following, ECMO was instituted as a rescue therapy when maximal ventilation support (i. e., high tidal volume controlled mechanical ventilation) was not sufficient to obtain viable oxygenation. However, after the start of ECMO, ventilatory settings were left unchanged [4] and this may be the main reason why, in subsequent years, two multicenter randomized trials of ECMO in patients with severe ARDS [5, 6] failed to demonstrate any clinical benefit compared to mechanical ventilation alone.

T. Mauri
Department of Perioperative Medicine and Intensive Care, San Gerardo Hospital, Via Pergolesi 33, 20900 Monza, Italy

A. Zanella
Department of Perioperative Medicine and Intensive Care, San Gerardo Hospital, Via Pergolesi 33, 20900 Monza, Italy

A. Pesenti (✉)
Department of Perioperative Medicine and Intensive Care, San Gerardo Hospital, Via Pergolesi 33, 20900 Monza, Italy
E-mail: antonio.pesenti@unimib.it

J.-L. Vincent (Ed.), *Annual Update in Intensive Care and Emergency Medicine 2013*,
DOI 10.1007/978-3-642-35109-9_49,

Meanwhile, evidence was growing on the association between high tidal volume ventilation and ventilator-induced lung injury (VILI) [7]. ECMO then appeared as a powerful tool to support lung function, reduce ventilatory support and prevent VILI even in the most severe cases of ARDS [8–9]. Removing CO_2 and adding O_2 through the artificial lung substantially reduced ventilation volumes, allowing the lung to rest, and minimizing VILI both in experimental animal models and in ARDS patients [9]. Thus, despite the initial negative clinical trials [5, 6], research continued on this 'alternative' use of extracorporeal gas exchange coupled with reduced mechanical ventilation in ARDS patients [10]. Over time, sufficient clinical experience and scientific data were available such that ECMO and ultra-protective ventilation can now be considered as first-line therapy in severely hypoxic ARDS patients not responding to conventional mechanical ventilatory support [11]. In the present chapter, we discuss the evidence supporting ECMO use in severely hypoxic ARDS patients and outline future developments in extracorporeal gas exchange and their application in VILI prevention, in patients waiting for lung transplant and in acute exacerbation of chronic obstructive pulmonary disease (COPD) as an alternative to intubation.

Extracorporeal Gas Exchange: Where Are We?

Technical Aspects

Over the last few years, a large number of technical improvements have enhanced the safety and applicability of ECMO [12]. Roller pumps have been largely abandoned in favor of centrifugal pumps, which greatly decrease the risk of hemolysis [12]. Percutaneous, rather than surgical, vascular cannulation techniques have been adopted and hemorrhagic complications have decreased [13]. Newly designed cannulas permit larger extracorporeal blood flows, while double lumen cannulas allow single vessel cannulation for both blood drainage and reinfusion. Surface coatings with heparin or nitric oxide-releasing materials were introduced on cannulas, connector tubing, pump and oxygenator to improve biocompatibility and to reduce the need for systemic anticoagulation [12]. Original ECMO silicone membrane artificial lungs were made of a large spiral surface membrane permeable to gas [4]. A large blood volume was used for priming and resistance to blood flow was high. With time, consistent plasma leakage was common. New hollow-fiber membrane oxygenators made of polymethylpentene have resolved many of these issues; they have a much lower priming volume and resistance to blood flow, and plasma leakage rarely happens even after prolonged use (i. e., 2–3 weeks) [12]. Thus, new materials have enabled safer, more efficient ECMO treatment with much smaller set-up, allowing interhospital transfer of patients undergoing ECMO by standard ambulance [14].

Evidence Supporting ECMO Use in Severe ARDS: Case Series

Karolinska University Hospital is an active ECMO center and published an important case series in 2000 [15]. Sixteen patients with severe ARDS and a very high lung injury score (average 3.5) were managed with ECMO and assisted pressure support ventilation (PSV), while being only minimally sedated and accepting arterial saturation as low as 70 %. The survival rate in this study was surprisingly high (76 %), suggesting that ECMO could also reduce complications related to heavy sedation and controlled ventilation (e.g., respiratory muscle atrophy).

The Extracorporeal Life Support Organization (ELSO) [16] is a spontaneous worldwide aggregation of more than 130 centers performing ECMO, which has kept a detailed ECMO patient registry since 1986. Data from the ELSO database has over time helped physicians to manage ECMO and suggested strategies to solve problems. In 2009, ELSO data from 1,473 consecutive adult ARDS patients treated with ECMO between 1986 and 2006 were published. At the start of ECMO, patients were young (median ages were 32 years old for survivors and 37 for non-survivors), had severe ARDS (median PaO_2/FiO_2 was 57 mm Hg) and were on high inspiratory pressure mechanical ventilation. After institution of ECMO, inspiratory pressure decreased by more than 20 % and the survival rate was quite high (50 %). Interestingly, survival was associated with a shorter duration of mechanical ventilation prior to ECMO start. This report suggests that ECMO in severe ARDS patients is feasible and associated with an acceptably low mortality; moreover, the advantages of ECMO may be more evident when it is instituted early.

The recent outbreak of H1N1 influenza was a watershed for early use of ECMO in ARDS patients. A considerable percentage of H1N1 patients were young, otherwise healthy and had severe ARDS with a potentially treatable cause; indeed, they were perfect candidates for ECMO. The Australia and New Zealand Intensive Care (ANZIC) Influenza Investigators group published the first series of H1N1 patients admitted to the intensive care unit (ICU), and ECMO was used in 12 % of all mechanically ventilated subjects [17]. The same group then specifically reported outcomes of the 53 H1N1 patients treated with ECMO: Median age was 34, PaO_2/FiO_2 before ECMO was 56 mm Hg, but after a median duration of extracorporeal support of 10 days, the overall mortality was very low (21 %) [18].

Aware of these and other reports, in view of the expected H1N1 influenza pandemic, several countries set up networks of referral ECMO centers. In Italy, for example, health authorities organized a national referral network of selected ICUs to provide advanced respiratory care, including ECMO, for patients with ARDS [19]. Eight of the fourteen ECMO centers were also able to transfer ECMO patients from peripheral to referral hospitals. Between August 2009 and March 2010, 60 patients (48 referred patients, 49 with a confirmed H1N1 diagnosis) received ECMO. All the referred patients were successfully transferred to the ECMO centers without major complications and the authors did not report any specific ECMO-related accident. Survival to hospital discharge in patients receiving ECMO was 68 %. Finally, in keeping with the data from the ELSO registry [16], non-survivors had a longer duration of mechanical ventilation prior to ECMO [19]. These results are now prompting studies on early ECMO institution (i. e., within one week of mechanical ventilation) in ARDS patients, thus switching the concept of ECMO from last-resort rescue therapy to advanced early treatment.

On the other hand, the published literature also includes case series of severe ARDS patients undergoing ECMO with very poor outcomes [20], most likely because of limited experience of the center (as the authors themselves acknowledge). In this respect, we believe that, although highly encouraging, results on ECMO in severe ARDS should not lead to widespread use of this technique but to identification of national advanced respiratory care centers that are able to deliver ECMO to which severe ARDS patients can be referred.

Evidence Supporting ECMO Use in Severe ARDS: Comparative Outcome Studies

Recently, two large studies demonstrated a survival benefit associated with ECMO use in severe ARDS patients. In 2009, results of the Conventional ventilation or ECMO for Severe Adult Respiratory failure (CESAR) trial were published [21]. This study was conducted in the United Kingdom between 2001 and 2006 and was a pragmatic trial: Adult patients with severe respiratory failure (lung injury score ≥ 3, or uncompensated hypercapnia with $pH < 7.20$) were enrolled. Patients were then transferred either to an ECMO center based in Leicester or to a hospital able to provide advanced respiratory care but no ECMO. Patients admitted to the ECMO center were treated with advanced optimal protective ventilation plus ECMO if needed (75 % treated with ECMO), whereas control patients continued conventional treatment according to the best available clinical practice. One hundred and eighty patients were enrolled in the study, 90 in each arm. Sixty-three percent of the ECMO arm patients were alive at 6 months without evidence of severe disability whereas the same was true for only 47 % of the controls. This difference accounted for one life saved for every six patients treated. The study has several limitations, as acknowledged by the authors. However, this was the first controlled trial showing a survival benefit associated with referral of severe ARDS patients to a center able to provide advanced ventilation support including ECMO.

Another recent study conducted in the United Kingdom (a cohort study) compared the outcome of H1N1-related severe ARDS patients referred to an ECMO center versus matched H1N1 severe ARDS patients treated, over the same time period, in other centers that could not perform ECMO. Using three different sophisticated statistical matching techniques (based on demographic, physiological, and comorbidity data), the authors showed that hospital mortality for ECMO-referred patients was almost one half that of non-ECMO-referred patients (≈ 25 % vs. 50 %) [22]. Again, major limitations affect this study: It was not a prospective randomized controlled trial and not all ECMO-referred patients actually received ECMO. However, looking at the whole picture, we believe the amount of pathophysiological knowledge, clinical experience and comparative research outcome data is enough to support the evidence that ECMO and ultra-protective ventilation (performed in selected high-volume referral centers) may be a treatment of choice for severe ARDS patients.

Extracorporeal Gas Exchange: Where Do We Go from Here?

These exciting results have pushed clinical research centers to expand the field of application of extracorporeal gas exchange and to use it in other forms of acute respiratory failure.

Extracorporeal CO_2 Removal

Almost all patients with ARDS are hyperventilated [23] because they do not have only a problem of oxygenation but they also have impaired CO_2 elimination. ARDS, indeed, is also a microvascular disease, as elevated pulmonary pressures are common and many patients develop right heart failure, and increased pulmonary dead space in ARDS is so clinically relevant that it is an extremely strong predictor of mortality [24]. High minute ventilation, necessary to obtain acceptable CO_2 values, also means a greater risk of VILI. In fact, in spite of proven efficacy in terms of patient outcome by reduction of tidal volume from 12 to 6 ml/kg [23], recently Terragni et al. demonstrated that tidal volumes of 6 ml/kg could also induce severe lung hyperdistension [25]. Bellani et al. also showed in ARDS patients undergoing lung protective ventilation that the inflammatory activity measured by positron emission tomography (PET) scan of the normally aerated lung regions was directly correlated with both the plateau pressure and with regional tidal volume normalized by end-expiratory lung gas volume [26]. Hence, ultra-protective mechanical ventilation, with extremely low tidal volumes, would limit VILI but an extracorporeal CO_2 removal strategy is required to contrast the concomitant rise in CO_2 [10]. Since the 1970s, Kolobow and Gattinoni have studied oxygenation and CO_2 removal as separate lung functions. In humans, oxygenation is proportional to pulmonary blood flow whereas CO_2 removal is associated with tidal ventilation. A similar physiology applies to extracorporeal gas exchange [21]. Thus, hypoxia would benefit from high blood flow ECMO whereas hypercapnia may be treated by a CO_2 removal strategy with a much lower blood flow. Lower blood flow also means smaller cannulas and less invasivity. Today, several extracorporeal CO_2 removal systems are already available [27–30]. Terragni et al. applied one of these systems to ARDS patients ventilated with protective tidal volume (6 ml/kg) but with elevated plateau pressure (i. e., 28–30 cmH_2O) and showed that further reduction of the tidal volume to 4.2 ml/kg (plateau pressure $\approx$ 25 cmH_2O) enhanced lung protection while the consequent respiratory acidosis was successfully managed by extracorporeal CO_2 removal [27]. However, the performance of these systems is still suboptimal; either

Table 1 Features of different extracorporeal gas exchange systems

	V-A ECMO	A-V ECMO	V-V ECMO	V-V $ECCO_2R$	V-V low-flow $ECCO_2R$	V-V low flow $ECCO_2R$ + acidification*
Indications	Severe heart failure	Severe ARDS	Severe ARDS	ARDS	Respiratory failure	Respiratory failure
Need for pump	Yes	No	Yes	Yes	Yes	Yes
Blood flow range, l/min	3–5	1–2	3–5	1–2	0.5–1	0.25–0.5
Cardiac support	Yes	No	No	No	No	No
Oxygenation	+++	+	+++	+	–	–
CO_2 removal	+++	++	+++	+++	++	+++
Level of evidence	High	Medium	High	Medium	Low	Experimental

V-A: venoarterial; A-V: arteriovenous; V-V: venovenous; ECMO: extracorporeal membrane oxygenation; $ECCO_2R$: extracorporeal CO_2 removal; * blood acidification before membrane lung increases blood-air CO_2 gradient and enhances CO_2 removal (see text for details)

they remove only a small portion of a patient's CO_2 production or, to achieve complete CO_2 removal, they require blood flows as high as 2 l/min [31] (Table 1). Thus, researchers are aiming to achieve substantial CO_2 removal from very low extracorporeal blood flows (i. e., as low as that commonly employed during hemofiltration). Since the partial CO_2 pressure difference across the membrane guides the CO_2 transfer in the artificial lung, increasing the CO_2 dissolved in blood (and hence its partial pressure) by acidification may enhance the membrane lung performance [32]. We were able, in an animal model, to use a technique of enhanced extracorporeal CO_2 removal based on acidification of blood entering the membrane lung for 48 hours. Acidification increased extracorporeal CO_2 removal by 70 %, extracting about 100 ml/min of CO_2 (near 50 % of total CO_2 production of an adult man) from a blood flow as low as 250 ml/min [33] (Table 1). This strategy was shown to be efficient and no adverse effects were recorded. If these results could be replicated in patients, significant CO_2 removal obtained at blood flows of 250–500 ml/min could achieve natural lung rest, prevent intubation, and avoid VILI and heavy sedation in a broader population of patients with acute respiratory failure.

ECMO as a Bridge to Lung Transplant

Despite the increasing number of lung transplants [34] and the increased number of available lungs, the waiting period on the lung transplant list is still a global problem and waiting list mortality appears to have increased during the past 3 years [34]. The clinical condition of patients with end-stage pulmonary disease may often deteriorate and demand mechanical ventilation; nevertheless, adequate gas exchange may not be achievable [35]. Furthermore, mechanical ventilation may lead to ventilator-associated pneumonia (VAP), VILI, worsening of right heart failure and the criteria for lung transplantation may be lost.

ECMO support has not been considered as a treatment option for patients waiting for lung transplantation until recently, because of significant bleeding complications. In fact, the elevated number of transfusions required could jeopardize the patient's outcome, and ECMO was applied rarely and only as a rescue treatment [36]. Nowadays, the abovementioned technological improvements have significantly decreased bleeding complications; hence, several case reports of patients supported with ECMO as a bridge to lung transplantation have been published [37, 38]. Not only has ECMO been applied in the early phase of mechanical ventilation, but some authors are also employing ECMO as an alternative to endotracheal intubation and mechanical ventilation with encouraging results. In a retrospective analysis, Fuehner et al. [39] compared ECMO in awake and spontaneously breathing patients, with historical non-matched control patients treated with invasive mechanical ventilation. This new strategy was feasible and safe and was associated with improved survival at 6 months after lung transplantation (80 % vs. 50 %).

The benefits of ECMO in awake patients, in addition to gas exchange improvement, could be related to VILI and VAP prevention, and may allow patients to communicate, eat, and receive active rehabilitation and physical therapy up to ambulation. Since the number of donors is still less than the number of patients awaiting lung transplantation, a careful selection of patients is required and criteria for ECMO institution as a bridge to lung transplantation are still under evaluation. Moreover, the number of case reports is still small and some authors have suggested the need for a prospective controlled trial [40] to compare this new strategy versus traditional care. Young patients waiting for lung transplantation who are free from multiple-organ dysfunction and with a good prospective for rehabilitation, could be considered as good candidates for awake ECMO institution.

Extracorporeal Gas Exchange in COPD

COPD, a leading cause of death and morbidity, is characterized by progressive limitation of air flow and recurrent episodes of acute respiratory failure (exacerbation), which may seriously impact quality of life [41]. Lungs of COPD patients, characterized by expiratory flow limitation and increased compliance, are generally hyperinflated and, during exacerbations, the increased ventilatory demand further worsens hyperinflation leading to increased work of breathing and, ultimately, to CO_2 retention [41]. The additional effort of the patient to eliminate CO_2 may even be counterproductive (increased ventilation workload increases CO_2 production), hence mechanical ventilatory support is often required [42]. To this end, extremely good results have been obtained with the use of non-invasive ventilation (NIV), which interrupts this vicious cycle by decreasing the patient's work of breathing [43]. When NIV is not applicable (e.g., intolerance to NIV devices, altered level of consciousness) or insufficient (e.g., deranged pH values), endotracheal intubation and invasive mechanical ventilation are instituted. However, these interventions are not free from complications and may further deteriorate patient outcome [44].

A low extracorporeal CO_2 removal strategy coupled with NIV could fit this scenario perfectly, since it could further unload patients' respiratory muscles and avoid endotracheal intubation. The group of Dr. Zwischenberger, almost ten years ago [45], foresaw a future in which an ambulatory extracorporeal CO_2 removal technique could be applied to severe COPD patients to facilitate ambulation and rehabilitation and thus to enhance suitability for lung transplantation or recovery from an acute exacerbation of the disease. The same group treated a woman with COPD exacerbation using a veno-venous CO_2 removal technique (a low flow pediatric extracorporeal circuit with an adult membrane lung and minimal anticoagulation) [46]. The authors used an 18F pediatric double-lumen cannula in the right jugular vein and a blood flow of 800 ml/min to achieve an extracorporeal CO_2 removal of 60–75 ml/min. The patient's minute ventilation decreased by nearly 30 %, hence hyperinflation decreased and arterial blood gases improved. More recently, Crotti et al. [31] reported the case of a patient with severe COPD exacerbation not responsive to NIV and successfully treated with extracorporeal CO_2 removal technology while conscious and breathing spontaneously.

A pumpless extracorporeal CO_2 removal technique (PECLA: pumpless extracorporeal lung-assist) (Table 1) has been employed in COPD exacerbations not responding to NIV [47]. The device consists of an arterial-venous bypass featured with a membrane lung. Nineteen patients (90 %) treated with PECLA did not require intubation. $PaCO_2$ and pH significantly improved following PECLA institution and, when compared with the historic matched-controls (treated with invasive ventilation), the patients treated with PECLA showed a trend toward a shorter hospital stay but no differences in 28-day or 6-month mortality. The PECLA group had two major and seven minor bleeding complications related to the device.

Extracorporeal gas exchange applied to awake non-intubated patients can avoid endotracheal intubation and mechanical ventilation and prevent the onset of deleterious complications (e.g., VAP, VILI). However, VILI can occur also during spontaneous breathing. Hence, monitoring ventilation in spontaneously breathing patients undergoing extracorporeal gas exchange is crucial. Thus, reliable non-invasive methods to monitor accurately and precisely spontaneous breathing are mandatory [31].

Conclusion

Extracorporeal gas exchange represents a powerful tool to prevent VILI and unload the respiratory muscles of critically ill patients experiencing acute respiratory distress from different etiologies. Evidence is growing related to major clinical benefits associated with ECMO for severe ARDS performed in experienced high-volume centers. Moreover, case series and observational studies have suggested exciting new fields of application for extracorporeal lung support (e.g., CO_2 removal in acute COPD exacerbation patients), but more controlled studies are needed.

References

1. Pesenti A, Zanella A, Patroniti N (2009) Extracorporeal gas exchange. Curr Opin Crit Care 15:52–58
2. Lillehei CW (1957) Surgical treatment of congenital and acquired heart disease by use of total cardiopulmonary bypass; analysis of result in 350 patients. Acta Chir Scand 113:496–501
3. Replogle RL, Arcilla RA, Kolobow T, Haller Jr JA (1968) Prolonged extracorporeal pulmonary support using a new miniature membrane oxygenator. Surg Forum 19:129–130
4. Hill JD, De Leval MR, Fallat RJ et al (1972) Acute respiratory insufficiency. Treatment with prolonged extracorporeal oxygenation. J Thorac Cardiovasc Surg 64:551–562
5. Zapol WM, Snider MT, Hill JD et al (1979) Extracorporeal membrane oxygenation in severe acute respiratory failure. A randomized prospective study. JAMA 242:2193–2196
6. Morris AH, Wallace CJ, Menlove RL et al (1994) Randomized clinical trial of pressure-controlled inverse ratio ventilation and extracorporeal CO2 removal for adult respiratory distress syndrome. Am J Respir Crit Care Med 149:295–305
7. Kolobow T, Moretti MP, Fumagalli R et al (1987) Severe impairment in lung function induced by high peak airway pressure during mechanical ventilation. An experimental study. Am Rev Respir Dis 135:312–315
8. Fumagalli R, Kolobow T, Arosio P, Chen V, Buckhold DK, Pierce JE (1986) Successful treatment of experimental neonatal respiratory failure using extracorporeal membrane lung assist. Int J Artif Organs 9:427–432
9. Gattinoni L, Agostoni A, Pesenti A et al (1980) Treatment of acute respiratory failure with low-frequency positive-pressure ventilation and extracorporeal removal of CO_2. Lancet 2:292–294
10. Gattinoni L, Kolobow T, Damia G, Agostoni A, Pesenti A (1979) Extracorporeal carbon dioxide removal (ECCO2R): a new form of respiratory assistance. Int J Artif Organs 2:183–185
11. Mauri T, Foti G, Zanella A et al (2011) Long-term extracorporeal membrane oxygenation with minimal ventilatory support: a new paradigm for severe ARDS? Minerva Anestesiol 78:385–389
12. Sidebotham D, Allen SJ, McGeorge A, Ibbott N, Willcox T (2012) Venovenous extracorporeal membrane oxygenation in adults: practical aspects of circuits, cannulae, and procedures. J Cardiothorac Vasc Anesth 26:893–909
13. Grasselli G, Pesenti A, Marcolin R et al (2010) Percutaneous vascular cannulation for extracorporeal life support (ECLS): a modified technique. Int J Artif Organs 33:553–557
14. Isgrò S, Patroniti N, Bombino M et al (2011) Extracorporeal membrane oxygenation for interhospital transfer of severe acute respiratory distress syndrome patients: 5-year experience. Int J Artif Organs 34:1052–1060
15. Lindén V, Palmér K, Reinhard J et al (2000) High survival in adult patients with acute respiratory distress syndrome treated by extracorporeal membrane oxygenation, minimal sedation, and pressure supported ventilation. Intensive Care Med 26:1630–1637
16. Brogan TV, Thiagarajan RR, Rycus PT, Bartlett RH, Bratton SL (2009) Extracorporeal membrane oxygenation in adults with severe respiratory failure: a multi-center database. Intensive Care Med 35:2105–2114

17. ANZIC Influenza Investigators, Webb SA, Pettilä V et al (2009) Critical care services and 2009 H1N1 influenza in Australia and New Zealand. N Engl J Med 361:1925–1934
18. Australia and New Zealand Extracorporeal Membrane Oxygenation (ANZ ECMO) Influenza Investigators, Davies A, Jones D et al (2009) Extracorporeal membrane oxygenation for 2009 influenza A(H1N1) acute respiratory distress syndrome. JAMA 302:1888–1895
19. Patroniti N, Zangrillo A, Pappalardo F et al (2011) The Italian ECMO network experience during the 2009 influenza A(H1N1) pandemic: preparation for severe respiratory emergency outbreaks. Intensive Care Med 37:1447–1457
20. Ma DS, Kim JB, Jung S, Choo SJ, Chung CH, Lee JW (2012) Outcomes of venovenous extracorporeal membrane oxygenation support for acute respiratory distress syndrome in adults. Korean J Thorac Cardiovasc Surg 45:91–94
21. Peek GJ, Mugford M, Tiruvoipati R et al (2009) Efficacy and economic assessment of conventional ventilatory support versus extracorporeal membrane oxygenation for severe adult respiratory failure (CESAR): a multicentre randomised controlled trial. Lancet 374:1351–1363
22. Noah MA, Peek GJ, Finney SJ et al (2011) Referral to an extracorporeal membrane oxygenation center and mortality among patients with severe 2009 influenza A(H1N1). JAMA 306:1659–1668
23. The Acute Respiratory Distress Syndrome Network (2000) Ventilation with lower tidal volumes as compared with traditional tidal volumes for acute lung injury and the acute respiratory distress syndrome. N Engl J Med 342:1301–1308
24. Nuckton TJ, Alonso JA, Kallet RH et al (2002) Pulmonary dead-space fraction as a risk factor for death in the acute respiratory distress syndrome. N Engl J Med 346:1281–1286
25. Terragni PP, Rosboch G, Tealdi A et al (2007) Tidal hyperinflation during low tidal volume ventilation in acute respiratory distress syndrome. Am J Respir Crit Care Med 175:160–166
26. Bellani G, Guerra L, Musch G et al (2011) Lung regional metabolic activity and gas volume changes induced by tidal ventilation in patients with acute lung injury. Am J Respir Crit Care Med 183:1193–1199
27. Terragni PP, Del Sorbo L, Mascia L et al (2009) Tidal volume lower than 6 ml/kg enhances lung protection: role of extracorporeal carbon dioxide removal. Anesthesiology 111:826–835
28. Livigni S, Maio M, Ferretti E et al (2006) Efficacy and safety of a low-flow veno-venous carbon dioxide removal device: results of an experimental study in adult sheep. Crit Care 10:R151
29. Wearden PD, Federspiel WJ, Morley SW et al (2012) Respiratory dialysis with an active-mixing extracorporeal carbon dioxide removal system in a chronic sheep study. Intensive Care Med 38:1705–1711
30. Batchinsky AI, Jordan BS, Regn D et al (2011) Respiratory dialysis: reduction in dependence on mechanical ventilation by venovenous extracorporeal CO2 removal. Crit Care Med 39:1382–1387
31. Crotti S, Lissoni A, Tubiolo D et al (2012) Artificial lung as an alternative to mechanical ventilation in COPD exacerbation. Eur Respir J 39:212–215
32. Zanella A, Patroniti N, Isgrò S et al (2009) Blood acidification enhances carbon dioxide removal of membrane lung: an experimental study. Intensive Care Med 35:1484–1487
33. Zanella A, Mangili P, Redaelli S, Ferlicca D, Patroniti N, Pesenti A (2012) Blood acidification enhances extracorporeal carbon dioxide removal: long term animal study. Am J Respir Crit Care Med 185:A6020 (abst)
34. Scientific registry of transplant recipients. Available at: http://www.srtr.org. Accessed Nov 2012
35. Mascia L, Pasero D, Slutsky AS et al (2010) Effect of a lung protective strategy for organ donors on eligibility and availability of lungs for transplantation: a randomized controlled trial. JAMA 304:2620–2627
36. Javidfar J, Brodie D, Iribarne A et al (2012) Extracorporeal membrane oxygenation as a bridge to lung transplantation and recovery. J Thorac Cardiovasc Surg 144:716–721

37. Javidfar J, Bacchetta M (2012) Bridge to lung transplantation with extracorporeal membrane oxygenation support. Curr Opin Organ Transplant 17:496–502
38. Shafii AE, Mason DP, Brown CR et al (2012) Growing experience with extracorporeal membrane oxygenation as a bridge to lung transplantation. ASAIO J 58:526–529
39. Fuehner T, Kuehn C, Hadem J et al (2012) Extracorporeal membrane oxygenation in awake patients as bridge to lung transplantation. Am J Respir Crit Care Med 185:763–768
40. Cypel M, Keshavjee S (2012) Extracorporeal membrane oxygenation as a bridge to lung transplantation. ASAIO J 58:441–442
41. Hogg JC (2004) Pathophysiology of airflow limitation in chronic obstructive pulmonary disease. Lancet 364:709–721
42. Ward NS, Dushay KM (2008) Clinical concise review: mechanical ventilation of patients with chronic obstructive pulmonary disease. Crit Care Med 36:1614–1619
43. Squadrone E, Frigerio P, Fogliati C et al (2004) Noninvasive vs invasive ventilation in COPD patients with severe acute respiratory failure deemed to require ventilatory assistance. Intensive Care Med 30:1303–1310
44. Berkius J, Sundh J, Nilholm L, Fredrikson M, Walther SM (2010) Long-term survival according to ventilation mode in acute respiratory failure secondary to chronic obstructive pulmonary disease: a multicenter, inception cohort study. J Crit Care 25(539):e13–e18
45. Wang D, Lick S, Alpard SK et al (2003) Toward ambulatory arteriovenous CO2 removal: initial studies and prototype development. ASAIO J 49:564–567
46. Cardenas Jr VJ, Lynch JE, Ates R, Miller L, Zwischenberger JB (2009) Venovenous carbon dioxide removal in chronic obstructive pulmonary disease: experience in one patient. ASAIO J 55:420–422
47. Kluge S, Braune SA, Engel M et al (2012) Avoiding invasive mechanical ventilation by extracorporeal carbon dioxide removal in patients failing noninvasive ventilation. Intensive Care Med 38:1632–1639

Recent Advances and Novel Applications of Modern ECMO

R. Roncon-Albuquerque Jr. and J. A. Paiva

Introduction

For more than 30 years, extracorporeal membrane oxygenation (ECMO) has been used in critical care medicine to support patients with severe respiratory and circulatory failure. Until recently, however, its use has been restricted to a small number of patients in highly specialized ECMO centers [1]. Several aspects have contributed to a renewed interest and wider utilization of ECMO in recent years. First, modern ECMO systems have enhanced biocompatibility, are miniaturized and portable, rendering the provision of this technique simpler and safer [2]. Second, high-quality scientific evidence was published related to the role of venovenous (VV)-ECMO for patients with severe acute respiratory distress syndrome (ARDS), in parallel with an increased demand for ECMO during the H1N1 pandemic [3, 4]. Third, technological advances have enabled the emergence of novel applications for ECMO support, e.g., VV-ECMO in spontaneously breathing patients as a bridge to lung transplantation ('awake ECMO') [5], and the use of out-of-hospital veno-arterial (VA)-ECMO for out-of-hospital refractory cardiac arrest [6].

Recent Advances in ECMO Technology

Technological advances have significantly improved the practice of 'modern' ECMO. Polymethylpentene oxygenators and centrifugal pumps have higher bio-

R. Roncon-Albuquerque Jr.
Department of Intensive Care Medicine, Centro Hospitalar S. João, Al. Prof. Hernâni Monteiro, 4200–319, Porto, Portugal
E-mail: rra_jr@yahoo.com

J. A. Paiva
Department of Intensive Care Medicine, Centro Hospitalar S. João, Al. Prof. Hernâni Monteiro, 4200–319, Porto, Portugal

J.-L. Vincent (Ed.), *Annual Update in Intensive Care and Emergency Medicine 2013*, 621
DOI 10.1007/978-3-642-35109-9_50, © Springer-Verlag Berlin Heidelberg 2013

compatibility and durability compared to older silicone membrane oxygenators and roller pumps. This allows less systemic anticoagulation, less blood product consumption, and reduced circuit component exchange, enhancing ECMO safety [7].

Another important step in the improvement of ECMO support was the development of miniaturized and portable ECMO circuits. Hand-held adaptors [8] and ultra-compact mobile systems [9] are now available allowing *in loco* ECMO implantation and safe interhospital transportation of patients who otherwise could not be transferred to a referral ECMO center. Miniature, portable ECMO systems are also useful for intrahospital transportation (e.g., to computerized tomography [CT] scan, operating room). With an experienced team, it was shown that CT imaging of patients on ECMO could be performed safely, providing valuable information for subsequent management [10].

Percutaneous cannulation with the Seldinger technique has been shown to be safe [11] and has become the standard method to establish vascular access for adult ECMO. This allows simple cannulation at the patient's bedside, which is particularly useful for emergent ECMO implantation. The introduction of a bicaval dual-lumen cannula for the internal jugular vein allows provision of adult VV-ECMO with single-site cannulation [12]. The advantages of the single-site approach include avoidance of the femoral access site, improved patient mobility, and considerably reduced recirculation when the cannula is properly positioned [13]. However, for safe and correct placement of the bicaval dual-lumen cannula, image guidance should be performed. Fluoroscopy and transesophageal echocardiography (TEE) are recommended during initial use. As proficiency improves, TEE at the bedside provides an excellent standard of care [14].

Taken together, these improvements led an increasing number of ECMO referral centers to manage patients using the single caregiver model. With this model, the ICU nurse primarily manages the patient, whereas the ECMO specialist team is responsible for managing equipment and supplies, circuit preparation, patient transportation, troubleshooting, daily rounds, education and service administration [15]. This approach shifts the emphasis of care from device management to disease management.

Classical Applications of Modern ECMO

VV-ECMO for Severe ARDS

Use of ECMO for severe acute respiratory failure was hampered for some time by the results of early randomized controlled trials in which the benefit of extracorporeal life support was not apparent [16, 17]. Neither of these studies, however, is relevant to modern ECMO because case selection, ventilation strategies, extracorporeal circuit design and disease management were completely different from modern standards. VV-ECMO is now the standard extracorporeal life support mode for severe respiratory failure. Alternatives to VV-ECMO include VA-ECMO, in which the pump returns blood to the arterial system, thus providing additional hemodynamic support [18]; and extracorporeal CO_2 removal ($ECCO_2R$), using lower extracorporeal blood flows, adequate to remove CO_2 but not suited for oxygenating the patient [19]. Although $ECCO_2R$ removal may be used to facilitate lung-protective ventilation, its use in severe ARDS should still be considered experimental [20, 21].

To clarify the role of modern ECMO for severe acute respiratory failure, the Conventional ventilation or ECMO for Severe Adult Respiratory failure (CESAR) trial was undertaken [3]. In this multicenter randomized clinical trial, 180 patients with severe (Murray score > 3.0 or pH < 7.20) but potentially reversible respiratory failure were randomly allocated to consideration for treatment with ECMO or to receive conventional management. Patients with high pressure (> 30 cmH_2O peak inspiratory pressure) or high inspired oxygen fraction ($FiO_2 > 0.8$) ventilation for more than 7 days, intracranial bleeding or any other contraindication to limited heparinization were excluded. Sixty-three percent of patients allocated to consideration for ECMO survived to 6 months without disability, compared with 47 % of those allocated to conventional management (relative risk 0.69; $p = 0.03$). Referral for consideration for ECMO treatment led to a gain of 0.03 quality-adjusted life-years (QALYs) at 6-month follow-up. Although only 75 % patients referred for ECMO actually received ECMO, the results suggest that patients with severe ARDS should be referred to a center with an ECMO-based management protocol.

The role of modern ECMO for severe acute respiratory failure was further clarified during the H1N1 pandemic and first post-pandemic influenza season. During this period, ECMO was used in a significant number of patients with influenza A (H1N1)-related severe ARDS. Initial experience was gathered in the 2009 southern hemisphere winter [22]. ECMO was also used for respiratory support in H1N1 infection in North American and European ECMO centers during the 2009 and 2010 northern hemisphere winters [23]. A cohort study of patients with H1N1-related severe ARDS in the United Kingdom compared survival to hospital-discharge of patients transferred to ECMO centers with non-ECMO-referred patients [4]. Of 80 ECMO-referred patients, 86 % received ECMO. The hospital mortality rate was 24 % for ECMO-referred patients vs. 52 % for non-ECMO-referred patients (relative risk [RR], 0.45 [95 % CI, 0.26–0.79]; $p = 0.006$) when individual matching was used; 24 % vs. 47 % (RR, 0.51 [95 % CI, 0.31–0.81]; $p = 0.008$) when propensity score matching was used; and 24 % vs. 51 % (RR, 0.47 [95 % CI, 0.31–0.72]; $p = 0.001$) when GenMatch matching was used. These results further support referral and transfer to an ECMO center of adult patients with severe ARDS.

VA-ECMO for Refractory Cardiogenic Shock

VA-ECMO is a valuable option for short-term mechanical circulatory support of patients with refractory cardiogenic shock (e.g., post-acute myocardial infarction

[AMI], postcardiotomy, acute myocarditis) [24]. In a recent report, Sheu et al. evaluated the impact of early VA-ECMO in patients (n=46) with acute ST-segment elevation AMI (STEMI) complicated by profound cardiogenic shock who were undergoing primary percutaneous coronary intervention (PCI), using historical controls [25]. In this study, the use of VA-ECMO was associated with lower 30-day mortality (39% vs. 72%). In another study using historical controls, VA-ECMO (n=33) was associated with improved 1-year survival (24% vs. 64%) in patients with AMI complicated by profound cardiogenic shock [26]. These results are even more relevant given that a recent randomized clinical trial showed no benefit with the use of intraaortic balloon support for AMI with cardiogenic shock, strongly challenging the level I guideline recommendation [27]. Taken together, these results should reestablish equipoise and foster development of randomized clinical trials on the role of modern VA-ECMO for cardiogenic shock.

Several technical aspects favor the short-term use of modern VA-ECMO systems in refractory cardiogenic shock: (i) immediate availability; (ii) bedside implantation; (iii) possibility of patient transportation during ECMO support (e.g., transfer to a center that provides definitive care; transportation to the catheterization laboratory); (iv) biventricular support; (v) respiratory support; and (vi) low cost (compared with ventricular assist devices [VAD]). Therefore, VA-ECMO should be considered for: Short-term bridge-to-decision (e.g., post-AMI cardiogenic shock with cardiac arrest reversed); short-term bridge-to-bridge (e.g., VAD); short-term bridge-to-definitive care (e.g., heart transplant); or short-term bridge-to-recovery (e.g., acute myocarditis). Moreover, pilot studies using VA-ECMO to rescue patients with refractory cardiogenic shock hospitalized in remote hospitals demonstrate the feasibility of providing mechanical circulatory support distant from specialized ECMO centers [28, 29].

Despite the usefulness of VA-ECMO for short-term circulatory support, its use is not recommended for mid-(weeks) or long-(months) term support. First, most patients on VA-ECMO cannot be managed without invasive mechanical ventilation and deep sedation. Second, several complications are frequently associated with prolonged VA-ECMO (e.g., leg ischemia, hemorrhage). Finally, although short-term VA-ECMO could be successfully used as a bridge to high-urgency heart transplantation [30], the use of VADs as a bridge to heart transplant has been shown to be superior to the use of VA-ECMO for mid- and long-term support [31].

VA-ECMO for Refractory Cardiac Arrest

ECMO support can be used for cardiopulmonary resuscitation (CPR) in refractory cardiac arrest. In fact, emergent VA-ECMO for ECMO-assisted CPR (E-CPR) is feasible for both out-of-hospital and in-hospital refractory cardiac arrest. Nevertheless, considerable uncertainty remains regarding patient selection and absolute contraindications for E-CPR. Chen et al. performed a 3-year prospective observational study on the use of E-CPR for witnessed in-hospital cardiac arrest of cardiac origin [32]. Of the 975 patients with in-hospital cardiac arrest events who underwent CPR for longer than 10 min, 113 were enrolled in the conventional CPR group and 59 were enrolled in the E-CPR group. Propensity-score matching was performed to equalize potential prognostic factors. Patients submitted to E-CPR had better short-term (hazard ratio [HR] 0.51, 95 % CI 0.35–0.74, $p<0.0001$) and long-term (HR 0.53, 95 % CI 0.33–0.83, $p=0.006$) survival, when compared to matched conventional CPR. More recently, a multicenter cohort study from Japan reported favorable outcomes for combined E-CPR and intra-arrest PCI in patients with acute coronary syndrome [33]. In this study, rapid-response E-CPR was performed in 86 patients with AMI. Emergency coronary angiography was performed in 81 patients (94 %), and intra-arrest PCI was performed in 61 patients (71 %). The rates of return of spontaneous heartbeat, 30-day survival, and favorable neurological outcomes were 88 %, 29 %, and 24 %, respectively. All of the patients who received intra-arrest PCI achieved return of spontaneous heartbeat. In patients who survived up to day 30, the rate of out-of-hospital cardiac arrest was lower (58 % vs. 28 %; $p=0.01$), the intra-arrest PCI was higher (88 % vs. 70 %; $p=0.04$), and the time interval from collapse to the initiation of ECMO was shorter (40 [25–51] vs. 54 minutes [34–74 minutes]; $p=0.002$).

Clinical outcome seems to be more favorable when E-CPR is used for in-hospital cardiac arrest compared to out-of-hospital cardiac arrest. This seems to be related to the different timings of VA-ECMO implantation. For in-hospital E-CPR, emergent cannulation can be performed almost immediately by a 24/7 in-house ECMO team, whereas in out-of-hospital cardiac arrest, VA-ECMO is normally initiated in the emergency department after prolonged conventional CPR [34, 35]. A report has been published on the feasibility of out-of-hospital emergent VA-ECMO implantation in out-of-hospital refractory cardiac arrest, using modern miniaturized and highly portable ECMO systems to partially circumvent this limitation [36].

A special clinical scenario that merits further consideration for E-CPR is accidental hypothermia, where survival without neurologic damage is still possible after prolonged cardiac arrest if deep hypothermia develops before asphyxia [37]. ECMO was shown to be the preferred method of active internal rewarming because it provides sufficient circulation and oxygenation while the core temperature is effectively increased, reducing the risk of refractory cardiorespiratory failure commonly observed after rewarming [38]. It also allows immediate induction of controlled therapeutic hypothermia after successful resuscitation. In fact, favorable neurologic outcomes with the use of E-CPR and therapeutic hypothermia for cardiac arrest patients with profound hypothermia have been recently described [39]. However, ECMO is not always available and prehospital referral mechanisms for direct transfer of patients with profound hypothermia to hospitals with an established E-CPR program should be implemented [40].

Finally, it should be emphasized that the efficacy of E-CPR should take into account not only patient survival without significant neurological sequelae, but also candidacy for heart transplantation or VAD implantation and, eventually, organ donation. Maj et al. [41] recently published their results on 20 patients submitted to E-CPR at their institution. Only three patients (15 %) survived without any neurological sequelae. Nine patients died on ECMO or the system was withdrawn in anticipation of death. Among these 9 patients, 5 developed brain death and, among these, 4 were suitable for organ donation (20 %). One patient was suitable for VAD implantation. Therefore, the overall survival rate (15 %) should be compounded with 1 patient implanted with a VAD and with 4 patients who were brain dead organ donors owing to the organ perfusion with ECMO. This roughly doubles the E-CPR success rate and the composite outcome (survivors, organ donors, and VAD/transplantation candidates) increases to 40 % of the study population.

Novel Applications of Modern ECMO

Awake ECMO as a Bridge to Lung Transplantation

Many patients on lung transplant lists die from acute exacerbations of their underlying chronic lung disease before they can receive a lung transplant. Although the initial experience and outcomes were unconvincing, modern ECMO technology has allowed significant improvements in patient management, redefining the role of ECMO as bridge-to-lung transplantation [42]. In this context, early mobilization of patients on ECMO is an important goal, because it facilitates participation in physical therapy, encourages oral enteral intake, and improves overall patient conditioning for lung transplantation. The use of the bicaval double-lumen cannula permits early ambulation on VV-ECMO support.

Fuehner et al. recently performed a retrospective, single-center, intention-to-treat analysis of 26 consecutive lung transplantation candidates with terminal respiratory or cardiopulmonary failure receiving 'awake ECMO' support. The outcomes were compared with a historical control group of patients treated with conventional invasive mechanical ventilation as bridge to transplant. The duration of ECMO support or invasive mechanical ventilation, respectively, was comparable in the two groups ('awake ECMO', median 9 [range 1–45] days; mechanical ventilation, median 15 [1–71] days; $p = 0.25$). Six (23 %) of 26 patients in the 'awake ECMO' group and 10 (29 %) of 34 patients in the invasive mechanical ventilation group died before a donor organ was available ($p = 0.20$). Survival at 6 months after lung transplantation was 80 % in the 'awake ECMO' group vs. 50 % in the invasive mechanical ventilation group ($p = 0.02$). Patients in the 'awake ECMO' group required shorter duration postoperative invasive mechanical ventilation ($p = 0.04$) and showed a trend toward a shorter postoperative hospital stay ($p = 0.06$).

ECMO for Refractory Septic Shock

The use of ECMO for refractory septic shock remains controversial. Significant differences in the hemodynamic response to sepsis exist between neonates, children and adults with impact on prognosis, potential benefit and rationale of ECMO support in these different patient populations.

Neonatal septic shock is often complicated by a lack of the physiological transition from fetal to neonatal circulation [43]. The acidosis and hypoxia associated with sepsis increase pulmonary vascular resistance and pulmonary artery pressures leading to patent ductus arteriosus, persistent pulmonary hypertension and persistent fetal circulation in the newborn. Neonatal septic shock with persistent pulmonary hypertension is associated with increased right ventricular afterload, cardiac failure, tricuspid regurgitation and hepatomegaly. This probably explains the favorable outcomes associated with the use of VA-ECMO in refractory septic shock [44].

In contrast, almost 90 % of adult patients present with 'hyperdynamic shock syndrome'. The hemodynamic response includes low systemic vascular resistance, hypotension and normal or increased cardiac output [43]. Despite the hyperdynamic state, these patients have myocardial depression characterized by decreased ejection fraction, ventricular dilatation and flattening of the Frank-Starling curve after fluid resuscitation. Tachycardia and reduction in systemic vascular resistance (SVR) are the main compensatory mechanisms for the declining of cardiac output.

In comparison, the hemodynamic response to sepsis is remarkably different in children and infants. Severe hypovolemia is a hallmark of pediatric septic shock; therefore, children frequently respond well to aggressive volume resuscitation. Almost 50 % of children with septic shock have low cardiac output and elevated SVR often referred to as 'cold shock'. Moreover, children have limited cardiac reserve compared to adults. The adult resting heart rate is 70 bpm; therefore, a two-fold increase in heart rate from 70 to 140 beats per minute can be easily tolerated to maintain cardiac output when stroke volume is decreased. Similar mechanisms are not possible in children and infants. A resting heart rate of 140 beats per minute cannot be doubled to 280 beats per minute because there is not enough time for diastolic filling. Therefore, the predominant response to a decreasing cardiac output is vasoconstriction. This elevated SVR makes hypotension a late sign of shock [45].

In this context, the report by MacLaren et al. with the use of central (atrioaortic) VA-ECMO in refractory pediatric septic shock to achieve higher flow rates and to reverse shock more quickly is noteworthy [46]. Twenty-three patients (median age 6 years) over a 9-year period were included. All patients had microbiological evidence of infection, and meningococcemia was the most common diagnosis. Twenty-two patients had failure of at least three organ systems. Eight (35 %) patients suffered cardiac arrest and required external cardiac massage before ECMO. Eighteen (78 %) patients survived to be weaned from ECMO, and 17 (74 %) children survived to hospital discharge. These results suggest that central ECMO is associated with better survival than conventional ECMO in pediatric septic shock.

However, in a recent report, Huang et al. described the use of conventional VA-ECMO for refractory septic shock at a referral ECMO center in Taiwan [47]. Of the 52 patients included, 75 % had failure of at least 3 organ systems and 40 %

had developed cardiac arrest and received E-CPR. Only 15 % survived to hospital discharge. Non-survivors were older than survivors (59 vs. 44 years; p = 0.009), and none of the patients older than 60 years survived. Therefore, the use of ECMO for adult refractory septic shock remains experimental and should only be considered on an individual basis. According to the favorable pediatric experience and taking into account the current dismal prognosis of adult refractory septic shock, high-flow central VA-ECMO merits evaluation in future studies.

Miniaturized VA-ECMO in the Catheterization Laboratory

Procedures in the cardiac catheterization laboratory have continuously expanded to include high-risk patients with poor left ventricular function, multivessel disease, AMI, multiple comorbidities and advanced age. In this context, circulatory arrest can occur during lifesaving interventions. Mechanical chest compression can severely affect working conditions in this situation or, in extreme cases, lead to break down of the intervention. In contrast, E-CPR may allow procedures in the catheterization laboratory to be completed without mechanical disturbance. Although percutaneous left VADs, such as the Tandem Heart device (Cardiac Assist Inc. Pittsburgh, USA) or the Impella system (Abiomed, Danvers, USA), may be beneficial, they cannot take over the gas exchange function [48]. In order to offer emergent cardiocirculatory and gas exchange function, the use of percutaneous VA-ECMO is necessary. Advances in ECMO technology with the availability of highly miniaturized and portable ECMO systems make VA-ECMO a powerful resuscitation tool in the catheterization laboratory.

In a recent report, Arlt et al. published a case series of 10 PCI and 4 transcatheter aortic valve implantation (TAVI) patients submitted to E-CPR in the catheterization laboratory [49]. With ECMO assistance, return to spontaneous circulation could be rapidly reestablished in all patients. In the PCI group the procedure was successfully completed in all patients, whereas two patients in the TAVI group were bridged on ECMO to surgical aortic valve replacement. In the clinical follow-up, 50 % survived to hospital discharge.

Extracorporeal CO_2 Removal to Avoid Intubation in Type 2 Acute Respiratory Failure

Endotracheal intubation and subsequent mechanical ventilation are often necessary and life-saving treatments for patients with severe respiratory failure. However, the adverse effects of the endotracheal tube, the invasive mechanical ventilation itself and the accompanying analgosedation may trigger a vicious cycle leading to prolonged weaning, and may even contribute to mortality. The main underlying pathophysiological mechanisms are ventilator-associated pneumonia

(VAP) and ventilator-induced lung injury (VILI), and a range of neurological disorders associated with prolonged analgosedation.

In selected populations, especially in patients with acute hypercapnic respiratory failure, non-invasive ventilation (NIV) is a well-established tool to support the failing ventilatory pump and thus to avoid intubation and invasive mechanical ventilation [7, 8]. However, this approach often fails for a variety of reasons and is, therefore, followed by intubation and invasive mechanical ventilation. The prognosis of these patients depends on the severity of the chronic underlying respiratory disease. For example, intubated patients with cystic fibrosis or advanced chronic obstructive pulmonary disease (COPD) have a poor prognosis.

Recently, extracorporeal life support technology has evolved with the development of low blood flow systems for $ECCO_2R$. Two types of $ECCO_2R$ system exist: (i) arteriovenous $ECCO_2R$ (AV-$ECCO_2R$), consisting of a pumpless extracorporeal circuit with an arterial inflow and a venous outflow cannula, with flows (1–2 l/min) driven by the patient's own cardiac output; (ii) venovenous $ECCO_2R$ (VV-$ECCO_2R$), consisting of a low-flow (300–800 ml/min) pump-driven extracorporeal circuit using a double-lumen catheter. A recent paper was published on the use of AV-$ECCO_2R$ to avoid invasive mechanical ventilation in patients with acute respiratory failure failing NIV [50]. In this multicenter, retrospective study, 21 AV-$ECCO_2R$ patients were compared with respect to survival and procedural outcomes to 21 matched controls submitted to conventional invasive mechanical ventilation. Of the 21 patients treated with AV-$ECCO_2R$, 19 did not require intubation. Within 24 h, median $PaCO_2$ levels and pH had significantly improved with the use of AV-$ECCO_2R$. Two major and seven minor bleeding complications related to the device occurred. Further complications were one pseudoaneurysm and one episode of heparin-induced type 2 thrombocytopenia. Compared to the matched control group, there was a trend toward a shorter hospital length of stay in the AV-$ECCO_2R$ group (adjusted $p = 0.056$). There were no group differences in the 28-day (24 % vs. 19 %, adjusted $p = 0.845$) or 6-month (33 % vs. 33 %) mortality. In this study, use of AV-$ECCO_2R$ removal enabled intubation and invasive mechanical ventilation to be avoided in the majority of patients with acute on chronic respiratory failure not responding to NIV. Compared to conventional invasive ventilation, short- and long-term survivals were similar.

Conclusion

Significant technological advances have improved the practice of 'modern' ECMO and expanded its clinical applications (Fig. 1). ECMO support is no longer restricted to a few specialized ECMO centers, being also an important management tool outside the ICU (e.g., E-CPR, ECMO-assisted PCI or TAVI, and interhospital rescue of patients with advanced respiratory and circulatory failure). Moreover, ECMO is no longer an option of last resort and should be considered early in the progression of severe acute respiratory and/or circulatory failure. ECMO referral

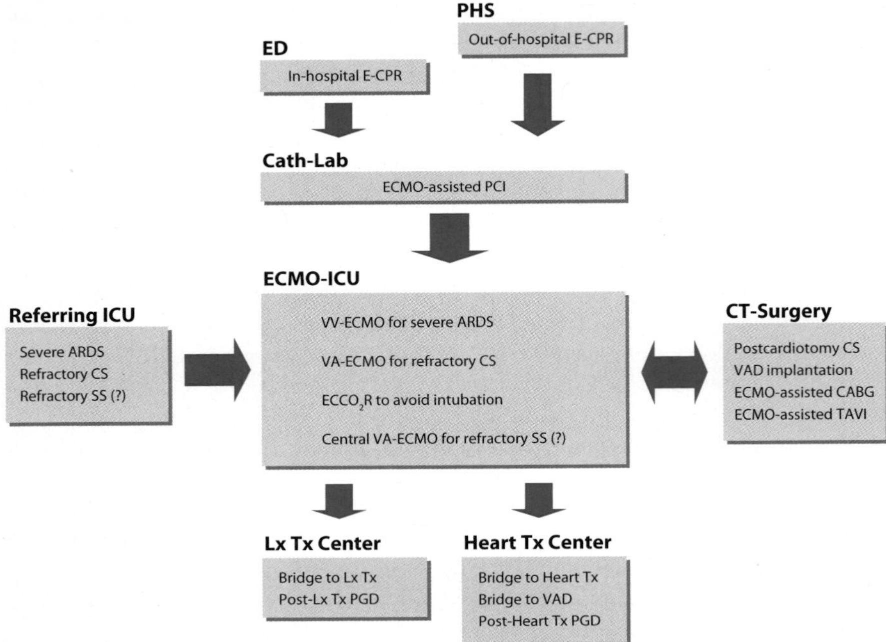

Fig. 1 Extracorporeal membrane oxygenation (ECMO) referral center activity in the future: The ECMO-hub. ARDS: acute respiratory distress syndrome; CABG: coronary artery bypass graft surgery; Cath-Lab: catheterization laboratory; CS: cardiogenic shock; CT-Surgery: cardiothoracic surgery; $ECCO_2R$: extracorporeal CO_2 removal; E-CPR: ECMO-assisted cardiopulmonary resuscitation; ED: emergency department; Lx: lung; PCI: percutaneous coronary intervention; PGD: primary graft dysfunction; PHS: pre-hospital service; SS: septic shock; TAVI: transcatheter aortic-valve implantation; Tx: transplant; VAD: ventricular assist device; VA-ECMO: venoarterial ECMO; VV-ECMO: venovenous ECMO

centers in the future will most probably be converted into ECMO-hubs, and ECMO support will represent an essential part of specialized critical care outreach.

Acknowledgements The authors are grateful to the ECMO specialist team from the Hospital S. João ECMO Center for their dedication to the development of our ECMO program. The authors are also in debt to all medical and nursing staffing from the Department of Critical Care Medicine of Hospital S. João and from the Intensive Care Unit of the Department of Infectious Diseases of Hospital de S. João, for all their commitment in the care of our ECMO patients.

References

1. Fortenberry J (2012) The history and development of extracorporeal support. In: Bartlett R, Lynch W, Wilson J (eds) Extracorporeal cardiopulmonary support in critical care, 4th edn. Extracorporeal Life Support Organization, Ann Arbor, Michigan, pp 1–10

2. Roncon-Albuquerque Jr R, Basilio C, Figueiredo P et al (2012) Portable miniaturized extracorporeal membrane oxygenation systems for H1N1-related severe acute respiratory distress syndrome: A case series. J Crit Care 27:454–463
3. Peek GJ, Mugford M, Tiruvoipati R et al (2009) Efficacy and economic assessment of conventional ventilatory support versus extracorporeal membrane oxygenation for severe adult respiratory failure (CESAR): a multicentre randomised controlled trial. Lancet 374:1351–1363
4. Noah MA, Peek GJ, Finney SJ et al (2011) Referral to an extracorporeal membrane oxygenation center and mortality among patients with severe 2009 influenza A(H1N1). JAMA 306:1659–1668
5. Fuehner T, Kuehn C, Hadem J et al (2012) Extracorporeal membrane oxygenation in awake patients as bridge to lung transplantation. Am J Respir Crit Care Med 185:763–768
6. Peek GJ (2011) Community extracorporeal life support for cardiac arrest – when should it be used? Resuscitation 82:1117
7. Combes A, Bacchetta M, Brodie D, Muller T, Pellegrino V (2012) Extracorporeal membrane oxygenation for respiratory failure in adults. Curr Opin Crit Care 18:99–104
8. Haneya A, Philipp A, Foltan M et al (2009) Extracorporeal circulatory systems in the interhospital transfer of critically ill patients: experience of a single institution. Ann Saudi Med 29:110–114
9. Philipp A, Arlt M, Amann M et al (2011) First experience with the ultra compact mobile extracorporeal membrane oxygenation system Cardiohelp in interhospital transport. Interact Cardiovasc Thorac Surg 12:978–981
10. Jepson SL, Harvey C, Entwisle JJ, Peek GJ (2010) Management benefits and safety of computed tomography in patients undergoing extracorporeal membrane oxygenation therapy: experience of a single centre. Clin Radiol 65:881–886
11. Pranikoff T, Hirschl RB, Remenapp R, Swaniker F, Bartlett RH (1999) Venovenous extracorporeal life support via percutaneous cannulation in 94 patients. Chest 115:818–822
12. Wang D, Zhou X, Liu X, Sidor B, Lynch J, Zwischenberger JB (2008) Wang-Zwische double lumen cannula-toward a percutaneous and ambulatory paracorporeal artificial lung. ASAIO J 54:606–611
13. Brodie D, Bacchetta M (2011) Extracorporeal membrane oxygenation for ARDS in adults. N Engl J Med 365:1905–1914
14. Javidfar J, Wang D, Zwischenberger JB et al (2011) Insertion of bicaval dual lumen extracorporeal membrane oxygenation catheter with image guidance. ASAIO J 57:203–205
15. Bartlett R, MacLaren G, Annich GM (2012) The future of extracorporeal life support. In: Bartlett R, Lynch W, Wilson J (eds) Extracorporeal cardiopulmonary support in critical care, 4th edn. Extracorporeal Life Support Organization, Ann Arbor, Michigan, pp 435– 437
16. Zapol WM, Snider MT, Hill JD et al (1979) Extracorporeal membrane oxygenation in severe acute respiratory failure. A randomized prospective study. JAMA 242:2193–2196
17. Morris AH, Wallace CJ, Menlove RL et al (1994) Randomized clinical trial of pressure-controlled inverse ratio ventilation and extracorporeal CO2 removal for adult respiratory distress syndrome. Am J Respir Crit Care Med 149:295–305
18. Nair P, Davies AR, Beca J et al (2011) Extracorporeal membrane oxygenation for severe ARDS in pregnant and postpartum women during the 2009 H1N1 pandemic. Intensive Care Med 37:648–654
19. Jung C, Lauten A, Pfeifer R, Bahrmann P, Figulla HR, Ferrari M (2011) Pumpless extracorporeal lung assist for the treatment of severe, refractory status asthmaticus. J Asthma 48:111–113
20. Nierhaus A, Frings D, Braune S et al (2011) Interventional lung assist enables lung protective mechanical ventilation in acute respiratory distress syndrome. Minerva Anestesiol 77:797–801
21. Bein T, Scherer MN, Philipp A, Weber F, Woertgen C (2005) Pumpless extracorporeal lung assist (pECLA) in patients with acute respiratory distress syndrome and severe brain injury. J Trauma 58:1294–1297

22. Davies A, Jones D, Bailey M et al (2009) Extracorporeal membrane oxygenation for 2009 Influenza A(H1N1) acute respiratory distress syndrome. JAMA 302:1888–1895
23. Patroniti N, Zangrillo A, Pappalardo F et al (2011) The Italian ECMO network experience during the 2009 influenza A(H1N1) pandemic: preparation for severe respiratory emergency outbreaks. Intensive Care Med 37:1447–1457
24. Sayer GT, Baker JN, Parks KA (2012) Heart rescue: the role of mechanical circulatory support in the management of severe refractory cardiogenic shock. Curr Opin Crit Care 18:409–416
25. Sheu JJ, Tsai TH, Lee FY et al (2010) Early extracorporeal membrane oxygenator-assisted primary percutaneous coronary intervention improved 30-day clinical outcomes in patients with ST-segment elevation myocardial infarction complicated with profound cardiogenic shock. Crit Care Med 38:1810–1817
26. Tsao NW, Shih CM, Yeh JS et al (2012) Extracorporeal membrane oxygenation-assisted primary percutaneous coronary intervention may improve survival of patients with acute myocardial infarction complicated by profound cardiogenic shock. J Crit Care 27:530.e1–530.e11
27. Thiele H, Zeymer U, Neumann FJ et al (2012) Intraaortic balloon support for myocardial infarction with cardiogenic shock. N Engl J Med 367:1287–1297
28. Beurtheret S, Mordant P, Paoletti X et al (2013) Emergency circulatory support in refractory cardiogenic shock patients in remote institutions: a pilot study (the cardiac-RESCUE program). Eur Heart J (in press)
29. Arlt M, Philipp A, Voelkel S et al (2011) Hand-held minimised extracorporeal membrane oxygenation: a new bridge to recovery in patients with out-of-centre cardiogenic shock. Eur J Cardiothorac Surg 40:689–694
30. Barth E, Durand M, Heylbroeck C et al (2012) Extracorporeal life support as a bridge to high-urgency heart transplantation. Clin Transplant 26:484–488
31. Karamlou T, Gelow J, Diggs BS et al (2013) Mechanical circulatory support pathways that maximize post-heart transplant survival. Ann Thorac Surg (in press)
32. Chen YS, Lin JW, Yu HY et al (2008) Cardiopulmonary resuscitation with assisted extracorporeal life-support versus conventional cardiopulmonary resuscitation in adults with in-hospital cardiac arrest: an observational study and propensity analysis. Lancet 372:554–561
33. Kagawa E, Dote K, Kato M et al (2012) Should we emergently revascularize occluded coronaries for cardiac arrest?: rapid-response extracorporeal membrane oxygenation and intra-arrest percutaneous coronary intervention. Circulation 126:1605–1613
34. Haneya A, Philipp A, Diez C et al (2012) A 5-year experience with cardiopulmonary resuscitation using extracorporeal life support in non-postcardiotomy patients with cardiac arrest. Resuscitation 83:1331–1337
35. Kagawa E, Inoue I, Kawagoe T et al (2010) Assessment of outcomes and differences between in- and out-of-hospital cardiac arrest patients treated with cardiopulmonary resuscitation using extracorporeal life support. Resuscitation 81:968–973
36. Arlt M, Philipp A, Voelkel S, Graf BM, Schmid C, Hilker M (2011) Out-of-hospital extracorporeal life support for cardiac arrest-A case report. Resuscitation 82:1243–1245
37. Soar J, Perkins GD, Abbas G et al (2010) European Resuscitation Council Guidelines for Resuscitation 2010 Section 8. Cardiac arrest in special circumstances: Electrolyte abnormalities, poisoning, drowning, accidental hypothermia, hyperthermia, asthma, anaphylaxis, cardiac surgery, trauma, pregnancy, electrocution. Resuscitation 81:1400–1433
38. Ruttmann E, Weissenbacher A, Ulmer H et al (2007) Prolonged extracorporeal membrane oxygenation-assisted support provides improved survival in hypothermic patients with cardiocirculatory arrest. J Thorac Cardiovasc Surg 134:594–600
39. Wanscher M, Agersnap L, Ravn J et al (2012) Outcome of accidental hypothermia with or without circulatory arrest: Experience from the Danish Praesto Fjord boating accident. Resuscitation 83:1078–1084
40. Gordon L, Peek GJ, Ellerton JA (2010) Extracorporeal life support. Is recommended for severe accidental hypothermia. BMJ 341:c7411

41. Maj G, De Bonis M, Pieri M, Melisurgo G, Pappalardo F (2012) Extracorporeal life support for refractory cardiac arrest: what is a good outcome? Intensive Care Med 38:2083–2085
42. Javidfar J, Bacchetta M (2012) Bridge to lung transplantation with extracorporeal membrane oxygenation support. Curr Opin Organ Transplant 17:496–502
43. Aneja R, Carcillo J (2011) Differences between adult and pediatric septic shock. Minerva Anestesiol 77:986–992
44. Schaible T, Hermle D, Loersch F, Demirakca S, Reinshagen K, Varnholt V (2010) A 20-year experience on neonatal extracorporeal membrane oxygenation in a referral center. Intensive Care Med 36:1229–1234
45. Ceneviva G, Paschall JA, Maffei F, Carcillo JA (1998) Hemodynamic support in fluid-refractory pediatric septic shock. Pediatrics 102:e19
46. MacLaren G, Butt W, Best D, Donath S (2011) Central extracorporeal membrane oxygenation for refractory pediatric septic shock. Pediatr Crit Care Med 12:133–136
47. Huang CT, Tsai YJ, Tsai PR, Ko WJ (2013) Extracorporeal membrane oxygenation resuscitation in adult patients with refractory septic shock. J Thorac Cardiovasc Surg (in press)
48. Westaby S, Anastasiadis K, Wieselthaler GM (2012) Cardiogenic shock in ACS. Part 2: Role of mechanical circulatory support. Nat Rev Cardiol 9:195–208
49. Arlt M, Philipp A, Voelkel S et al (2012) Early experiences with miniaturized extracorporeal life-support in the catheterization laboratory. Eur J Cardiothorac Surg 42:858–863
50. Kluge S, Braune SA, Engel M et al (2012) Avoiding invasive mechanical ventilation by extracorporeal carbon dioxide removal in patients failing noninvasive ventilation. Intensive Care Med 38:1632–1639

Part XV

Renal Failure

Measurement of Kidney Perfusion in Critically Ill Patients

A. G. Schneider, M. D. Goodwin and R. Bellomo

Introduction

Acute kidney injury (AKI) is a major complication of critical illness [1] occurring in 30 to 40 % of all critically ill patients and in its severe form requires renal replacement therapy (RRT), in approximately 5 % of patients [2]. AKI has been shown to be an independent predictor for mortality [3] and is associated with invasive therapy and substantial costs [4].

Despite its importance, the pathophysiology of AKI is still poorly understood. AKI is most commonly associated with systemic diseases, such as septic shock, major surgery and cardiogenic shock [1], but a specific mechanism causing AKI to develop in specific patients can rarely be determined. Since the early description of an "acute uremia syndrome" in crush injury victims during World War II [5, 6] and its association with histopathological findings similar to those found in experimental renal artery ligation, ischemia or some form of alteration in renal blood flow has been thought to play a pivotal role in the pathogenesis of AKI. This paradigm that essentially all AKI in critically ill patients is the result of some form or degree of ischemia remains of continuing conceptual dominance to this day [7]. Despite such dominance, there are only very limited data supporting this concept. In a recent systematic review, Prowle et al. [8] highlighted the extraordinary fact

A. G. Schneider
Department of Intensive Care, Austin Health, 145 Studley Road, Heidelberg 3084, Melbourne, Australia

M. D. Goodwin
Department of Radiology, Austin Health, 145 Studley Road, 3084 Heidelberg, Melbourne, Australia

R. Bellomo (✉)
Department of Intensive Care, Austin Health, 145 Studley Road, Heidelberg 3084, Melbourne, Australia
E-mail: rinaldo.bellomo@austin.org.au

J.-L. Vincent (Ed.), *Annual Update in Intensive Care and Emergency Medicine 2013*,
DOI 10.1007/978-3-642-35109-9_51, © Springer-Verlag Berlin Heidelberg and BioMed Central Ltd. 2013

that renal blood flow measurement, irrespective of the technique used, has only been reported in 46 critically ill patients (five studies) within the last sixty years. Thus, our knowledge, understanding, and theoretical constructs regarding global renal perfusion in critically ill patients with RRT-treated AKI (an estimated 5 % of all ICU admissions for a total of approximately a quarter of a million such patients each year in developed countries alone) is, like an inverted pyramid, based on extremely weak evidence.

Furthermore, given the complex and heterogeneous nature of the renal vasculature, evaluating the flow in the main renal arteries (macrocirculation) might not provide sufficient information to adequately understand perfusion alterations in complex diseases, such as septic or cardiogenic shock. Indeed, some pathophysiological processes may be associated with increased global renal blood flow [9, 10] despite loss of function. In such instances, there is experimental evidence that, at least in sepsis, this phenomenon may be caused by intra-renal shunting [11]. Hence, correlation between macroscopic renal blood flow and function is far from linear. Therefore, techniques allowing the study of microcirculatory parameters, such as cortico-medullary perfusion ratio and regional tissue oxygenation measurement, and assessment of their relative change over time may be more valuable in increasing our understanding of the pathophysiology of AKI.

In this state-of-the art review, we discuss the value, challenges, limitations, safety and feasibility of different techniques for the measurement of kidney perfusion in critically ill patients. The advantages of each technique will be weighed against its disadvantages in the context of the critically ill patient with AKI. Particular emphasis will be placed upon techniques enabling some evaluation of the microcirculation, because emerging experimental evidence suggests that these are the techniques that are the most likely to improve our understanding of the disease and help clinicians develop and apply physiologically logical interventions.

Non-Imaging Methods for Renal Blood Flow Quantification

Microsphere Deposition Methods

Microsphere distribution methods [12–14] can provide very detailed information on regional perfusion between and within organs. After intravascular injection of radioactively labeled microspheres, their tissue deposition is proportional to blood supply. Several tracers can be used to evaluate changes after pharmacological intervention. The tissue needs to be harvested and sectioned to allow measurement of radioactivity, which is proportional to the quantity of microspheres deposited and, hence, to the organ perfusion [15]. Results are typically reported in 'flow per gram of whole tissue'. This method is obviously limited to animal research as it involves tissue collection. It is, however, very often used as a comparator in studies validating organ flow measurement.

Paraamino-hippurate Clearance

The classic physiological method to estimate renal plasma flow is by calculation of paraamino-hippurate (PAH) clearance. PAH is an amide derivative of the amino acid glycine and para-aminobenzoic acid. PAH is almost fully removed from the plasma during its first pass though the kidney. Its renal clearance can, therefore, be used as an estimate of the renal plasma flow (ERPF). Typically, this technique involves a bolus followed by a continuous infusion of PAH. PAH concentration is then measured in blood and urine samples. ERPF is then calculated using the classic clearance formula ($RPF \sim Cl_{PAH} = U_{PAH} \times V/P_{PAH}$).

Unfortunately, PAH is not used in clinical practice as the chemical analysis procedure is very cumbersome, not widely available and cannot provide information in 'real-time'. Additionally, as they rely on urine concentration measurement, PAH clearance methods cannot be applied in oligo-anuric patients and its non-invasive use in AKI is, therefore, limited. On the other hand, PAH clearance can be used to measure ERPF for research purposes even in oligo-anuric patients. Such measurement, however, becomes invasive and requires renal vein canulation and sampling.

Renal Vein Thermodilution Methods

Renal thermodilution methods were first described in the 1970s [16, 17], but have gained increased attention in critically ill patients more recently [18, 19]. These methods involve the insertion of an indwelling catheter into one of the renal veins. Renal blood flow calculation is based on measured changes in temperature of the renal vein blood after injection of a bolus of isotonic saline at room temperature [19]. Using such methods, Ricksten et al. have conducted several elegant studies of global renal perfusion in cardiac surgery patients [20–22]. For example, they demonstrated that restoring mean arterial pressure (MAP) from 60 to 75 mm Hg improved the renal oxygen supply/demand relationship after cardiac surgery in patients with vasodilatory shock and AKI [21]. This technique, however, remains highly invasive and, because of the risk of renal vein thrombosis, can only be applied for a limited period of time.

Xenon Washout

Xenon washout techniques were used for research purposes in the seventies [23]. This invasive technique relies on intra-arterial injection of a radioactively marked tracer (Xe^{133}) and external counting with a scintillation probe. Mean renal blood flow is calculated from the initial slope of the disappearance curve. This method was very useful to establish renal vasculature reactivity to different pharmacologic agents [24, 25]. However, it has currently been replaced by less invasive, more precise imaging techniques.

Intravascular Doppler

Blood flow velocity can be evaluated invasively using an intra-arterial Doppler wire. This technique enables calculation of renal blood flow provided that the diameter of the vessel can be estimated [26]. Accurate measurements can be made in small straight tubes (<4.76 mm) and if the flow rate is <200 ml/min [27]. The utility of this technique in humans, in whom renal blood flow is typically in the range of 300 ml/min, is therefore limited. Similarly, this technique cannot account for the presence of collateral vessels and can, therefore, grossly underestimate flow.

Given these technical limitations and its invasiveness, intravascular Doppler is not currently applicable to critically ill patients even in the setting of a research protocol. It can be used as a comparator in animal studies in order to validate newer methods.

Nuclear Medicine Techniques

Scintigraphy

Scintigraphy relies on the injection of radiolabeled isotopes and the capture of the emitted radiation by external gamma cameras generating 2D images. Using isotopes such as iodine-131 (^{131}I) coupled to orthoiodohippurate (OIH), scintigraphy is able to accurately quantify renal blood flow. This technique can be coupled with simultaneous measures of glomerular filtration rate (GFR) with the ability to determine relative function for each kidney.

Several isotopes have been used and although ^{131}I labeled OIH still represents the gold standard for renal blood flow quantification, it is not used clinically because it is associated with high radiation exposure, particularly in patients with renal failure. Therefore, 99mTc-mercapto-acetylglycyl-glycyl-glycine (^{99m}Tc-MAG3) is currently the marker of choice for this purpose [28, 29]. This molecule is mainly excreted via tubular secretion at the distal part of the proximal tubule with a very high first-pass elimination [30]. Semi-quantitative measurement of renal blood flow can be obtained using the first-pass time-activity curve generated from a region of interest over the kidney [31]. Other techniques expressing renal blood flow as a fraction of cardiac output have been proposed [32]. Because of its high and unpredictable (75–90 %) plasma protein binding properties, ^{99m}Tc-MAG3 based techniques are not as accurate as those based on ^{131}I-OIH (75–90 %) to estimate renal blood flow [33]. In addition, ^{99m}Tc-MAG3 is not purely eliminated by the renal route and the percentage eliminated via the hepatobiliary pathway increases in renal dysfunction. Other technetium based molecules (99mTc-Ethylene-l-dicysteine [99mTc-EC] or ^{99m}Tc-tricarbonyl nitrilotriacetic acid [99mTc(CO)3NTA]) [34] with lower hepatobiliary elimination and higher kidney to background ratio have been proposed.

Overall, 99mTc-diethylenetriaminepentaacetic acid (DTPA) is most commonly used for GFR measurement. It delivers slightly lower values as compared with standard inulin clearance but is easier to prepare and more readily available. However, the results generated by the so-called Gates methods [35] have not been shown to be superior to creatinine-based formulas [36].

Renal scintigraphy finds most of its clinical application in renal transplantation medicine. In this context, it can help differentiate acute tubular necrosis from transplant rejection [31]. In AKI, renal scintigraphy is usually of little value for the identification of the mechanism of renal dysfunction, although some patterns can be identified (ureteric obstruction, ischemia) [37]. Renal scintigraphy can be used to determine the symmetry of the disease and provide information on organ size and overall perfusion. Unfortunately, it does not provide information on intrarenal flow distribution.

Positron-Emission Tomography

Positron-emission tomography (PET) scans rely on the injection of a positron-emitting isotope tracer, such as 18-fluorine in the most commonly used PET tracer, 18-F fluorodeoxyglucose (FDG). Many other isotopes also emit positrons, including rubidium-82, 11-carbon and 15-O labeled H_2O. The emitted positron interacts with an electron, emitting a pair of high-energy photons in the annihilation process. These photons are detected by scintillators in the scanner generating 3D images. PET can be coupled with computed tomography (CT) and can then provide significantly better spatial resolution than scintigraphy alone.

Two fundamental approaches have been proposed to measure renal perfusion with PET: Dynamic imaging following bolus injection and static imaging at steady state using an ultra-short-lived tracer. The first technique makes use of a highly extracted blood flow tracer such as rubidium-82 [38]. This method has been used in animal models of renal artery obstruction, occlusion and reperfusion [39]. The second technique makes use of ultra-short-lived tracers, such as oxygen-15-labelled water (half-life of 2 min) [40]. This compound was studied by Juillard et al. [41], who showed an excellent correlation with microsphere techniques in an animal model and by Alpert et al. [42], who used O-15 water to measure renal blood flow in healthy volunteers. Other potential applications include measurements of renal blood flow in renovascular disease, in rejection or in acute tubular necrosis of transplanted organs, in drug-induced nephropathies, ureteral obstruction before and after revascularization and before and after placement of ureteral stents [40].

Despite its theoretical large potential, there has been very little use of PET in functional imaging. More importantly, its use in critically ill patients is likely to be very limited even for research purposes. Indeed, PET protocols are long and require extensive mobilization, which, in unstable patients is often labor intensive and can be associated with safety hazards. This adds to the general limitations associated with the difficulty of producing and handling non-standard tracers, their cost and the requirement for many of them for a nearby cyclotron (because of their extremely short half life). Finally, PET involves radioactivity exposure (although minimal), which might make acceptance by ethics committees, next of kin or ICU staff more difficult in the context of a clinical study.

Magnetic Resonance Imaging

Magnetic resonance imaging has gained immense popularity over the last few decades as it allows generation of very high-resolution images, including 3D reconstructions, without ionizing radiation. Imaging is based on the imaging of protons, using measurement of a radiofrequency signal emitted by protons regaining their thermodynamic equilibrium after their spins have been aligned in a large magnetic field. Protons in different tissues return to their equilibrium state at different relaxation rates.

Among the numerous MRI techniques available, some enable renal blood flow quantification and, importantly, some enable a degree of parametric mapping of intra-organ blood flow distribution or tissue oxygenation. These properties make MRI very appealing to study renal perfusion alterations in critical illness. Unfortunately, these approaches are likely to be limited to research protocols as they involve a lengthy and potentially hazardous transfer, considerable costs and are limited by the availability of MRI machines.

Contrast-Enhanced MRI Modalities

MRI based perfusion studies have classically been based on contrast-enhancement by gadolinium-based solutions. Gadolinium agents produce contrast on MRI scans because gadolinium is a paramagnetic substance, which therefore has a marked local effect on the speed at which adjacent protons return to their thermodynamic equilibrium. Fast acquisition techniques allow sufficient temporal resolution to monitor intra-renal signal changes during first pass of the agent. Approaches have been described [43] enabling quantification of absolute cortical and medullary perfusion. This would make gadolinium-based MRI technology of great interest for the assessment of renal perfusion.

Unfortunately, the discovery of nephrogenic systemic fibrosis and its probable association with gadolinium accumulation in renal failure (acute or chronic) [44] greatly limits its interest in AKI and critically ill patients. The warnings for gadolinium contrast agents have recently been updated and three agents are currently contraindicated in patients with AKI or with chronic renal impairment and a GFR < 30 ml/min. The other agents do not have this contraindication although extensive precautions are still advised [45].

Newer contrast agents based on ultra-small particles of iron oxide (USPIO) molecules have been presented and seem to be safe and potentially useful for renal blood flow measurement [46]. However, their safety profile is not yet fully established and their clinical role is still to be established, in particular since other MRI techniques, which do not need intravenous contrast agents, are now available.

Cine Phase-Contrast MRI

Cine phase-contrast MRI is a magnetic resonance angiographic technique that allows measurement of renal flow in both renal arteries without a contrast agent. Central to the technique is the fact that protons that are moving along the direction of a magnetic field gradient receive a phase shift proportional to their velocity: Static protons are unaffected and receive no phase shift, but moving protons will have their phase changed. The amplitude of this change is dependent on the velocity of the proton. Phase-contrast MRI has been very well validated to measure aortic flow rate but less so for renal arteries because of their small size and issues related to respiratory movements [47–49] (Fig. 1).

Renal blood flow measurements by cine phase-contrast MRI are well correlated with simultaneous PAH clearance measurement [50] and the results are reproducible [51]. King et al. [52] used this method as a tool to predict clinical response after percutaneous angioplasty in renal artery stenosis. This technique has recently been used in critically ill patients to determine renal blood flow in sepsis [53]. To the best of our knowledge, this study was the first to measure global renal blood flow non-invasively in critically ill patients with sepsis associated AKI. Values for renal blood flow varied markedly from 392 to 1,337 ml/min (normal values range according to size and cardiac output from 800 to 1,200 ml/min). This study provided a clear demonstration that, in septic critically ill patients with AKI, renal blood flow can range from low to supranormal and confirmed what animal studies had long suggested: Septic AKI is not a uniform disease and is not reliably associated with decreased renal blood flow (so-called ischemia). Even more importantly, and in keeping with experimental observations, these values correlated well with the patient's cardiac index and renal vascular resistance but not with the patient's GFR. This clear dissociation between global perfusion and global function is important because it implies changes in microvascular perfusion (shunting or changes in intra-glomerular pressure dynamics or both).

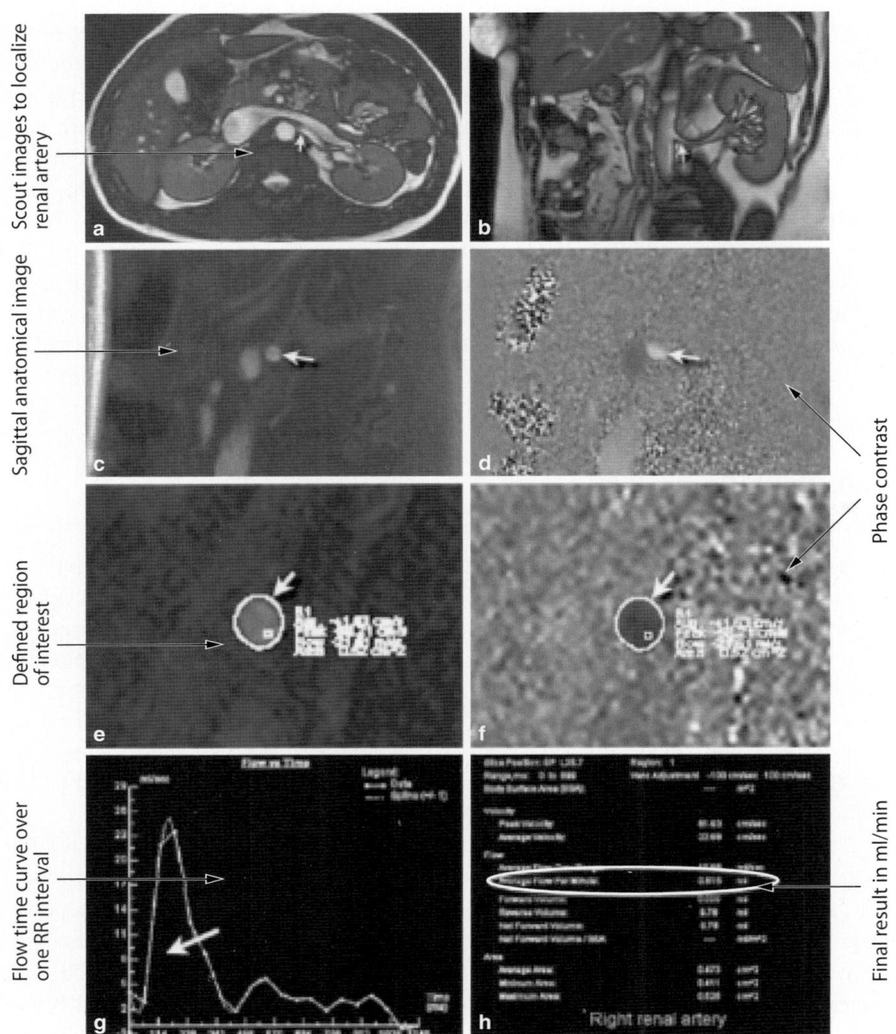

Fig. 1 Cine phase-contrast imaging. **a** and **b** Initial acquisition of scout images enabling localization of renal arteries (*white arrows*); **c** Sagittal image of the renal artery on phase compensated image (*white arrow*); **d** phase contrast image of the renal artery (*white arrow*) at the same level; **e** and **f** magnified views of (c) and (d) where the investigator has placed a region of interest over the renal artery; **g** time intensity curve for one RR interval; h: the area under the curve multiplied by the heart rate approximates the renal blood flow

Arterial Spin Labeling

Arterial spin labeling (ASL) is an MRI modality typically used for cerebral perfusion studies [54]. In an analogy with cine phase-contrast techniques, ASL uses

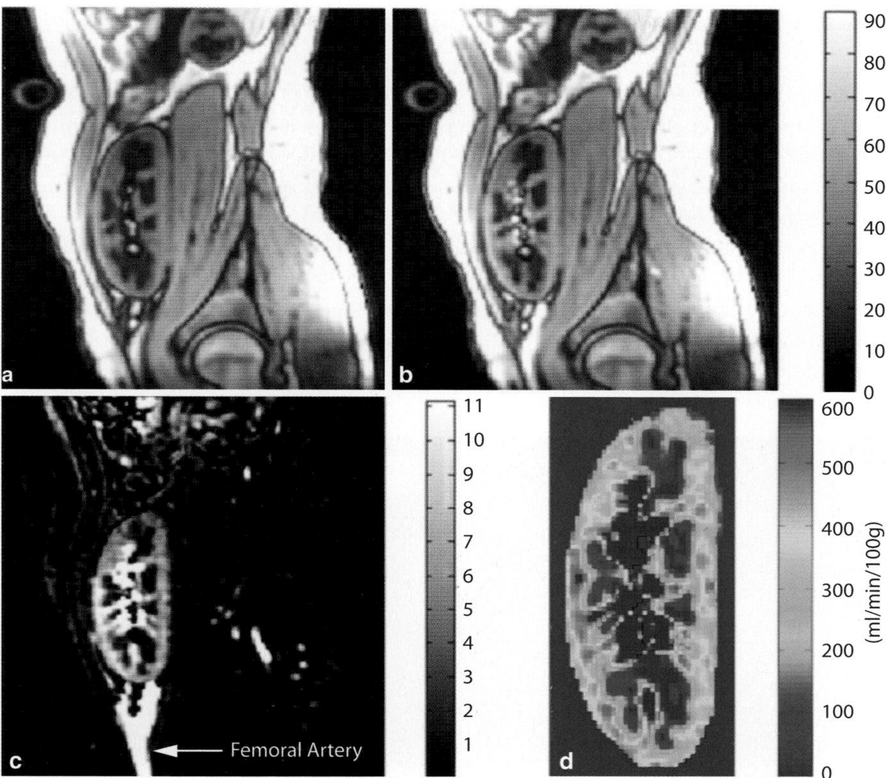

Fig. 2 Arterial spin labeling in a transplant kidney. Tagged image **a** with moving spins labeled; control image **b**; difference between a and b representing the perfusion-weighted image **c**; and resulting perfusion map **d** shown in units of ml/min per 100 g (adapted from [55] with permission)

blood as an endogenous contrast agent. Blood flowing towards a tissue is selectively labeled to have an opposite magnetization compared to this tissue. A perfusion-weighted image can be produced by subtracting an image in which inflowing spins have been labeled from an image in which spin labeling has not been used (Fig. 2). [55]. ASL allows imaging of the renal arteries despite their complex orientation [56]. A fairly good correlation of ASL with PAH clearance has been reported [57] and some applications after renal transplantation or in renal artery stenosis [55, 58] have been proposed. One of the main interests of ASL is its ability to draw parametric maps of relative perfusion (Fig. 2) enabling clinicians to study geographical intra-organ differences in perfusion as opposed to overall organ blood flow. All pixels in a specific tissue can be averaged to provide mean perfusion. Such maps could enable the study of differential perfusion between cortex and medulla in critical illness and to identify ischemic and hyperemic areas within the kidney.

Blood Oxygen Level-Dependent (BOLD) MRI

BOLD MRI takes advantage of the different magnetic properties between oxygenated and deoxygenated hemoglobin. Oxyhemoglobin (the principal form found in arterial blood) has no major magnetic properties, but deoxyhemoglobin is strongly paramagnetic, generating local magnetic field inhomogeneities corresponding to an increase in relaxivity defined as R2*. The amount of deoxyhemoglobin functions as a biological contrast agent and can be related to the strength of R2* weighted pulse sequences. BOLD MRI generates images, the signal intensity of which is a reflection of tissue metabolism representing the balance between oxygen consumption and delivery. Relatively low spatial resolution is a problem inherent to the technique.

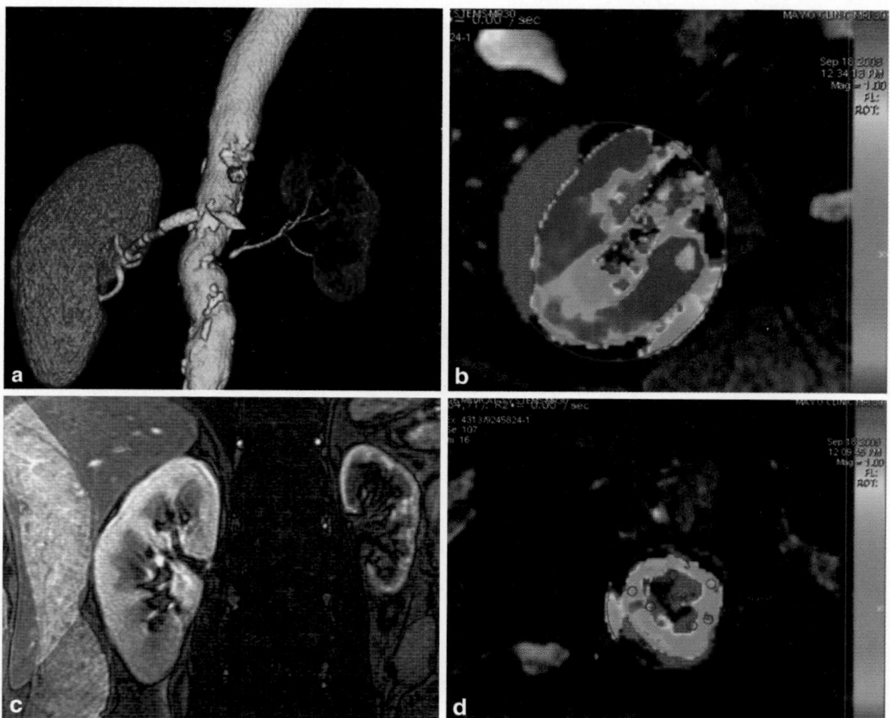

Fig. 3 Blood oxygen level-dependent magnetic resonance imaging (BOLD MRI) in severe occlusive disease of the left kidney. T2 imaging by CT angiogram **a** and T2 MRI **b** demonstrating severe renal-artery stenosis (*left kidney*) and presence of a stent in the contralateral kidney. **c** and **d** Parametric maps of R2* (reflecting the deoxyhemoglobin level) from BOLD MRI in the same patient. In the right kidney ([c] normal, well-perfused), most of the cortex shows low R2* signal (*blue*) and there are some small areas with a high R2* signal in the medulla (*red*). Conversely, in the *left kidney* ([d] vascular compromise), there are higher levels of cortical R2* indicating the presence of more deoxygenated blood and a large, deep area with a high R2* signal (deoxygenated hemoglobin) in the medulla (from [75] with permission)

BOLD enables the generation of parametric maps (Fig. 3) of oxygenation in the kidney as illustrated by Textor et al. [59] in kidneys with renal artery stenosis. This technique has been used to demonstrate an increase in tissue oxygenation after administration of diuretics, particularly in the medullary areas and confirmed by implanted oxygen probes [60]. Similarly, Pruijm et al. [61], showed an increase in medullary oxygenation in healthy volunteers after a decrease in their salt intake. Although not a direct measure of renal blood flow, BOLD MRI might deliver valuable information as it delivers data integrating oxygen delivery and consumption.

Although the various MRI-based techniques discussed above offer promise in our ability to investigate changes in renal perfusion in critically ill patients, it is difficult to imagine how they could be widely applied at this stage. The MRI environment is hostile to the critically ill and carries some significant safety concerns during transport and during a prolonged period in the magnet. In addition, obtaining high quality MRI scans in the critically ill is also often very challenging. The high cost adds a further degree of difficulty, which makes repeated assessment logistically very difficult.

Ultrasonography

Ultrasonography is the most commonly used imaging modality in the initial evaluation of patients with acute or chronic kidney diseases. It is widely available, easy to use, free of complication and can be performed at the bedside.

Standard ultrasound provides information on kidney size (a small kidney suggests possible atrophy in the context of chronic kidney disease, a large kidney might suggest the presence of infiltrative disease), cortical thickness and echogenicity and enables imaging of the excretory tract to diagnose outflow obstruction. In AKI, however, standard ultrasound examination is normal most of the time. Assessment of renal perfusion by ultrasound can be approached by Doppler techniques or with microbubble-based contrast agents (contrast-enhanced ultrasound).

Doppler Ultrasound

Conventional ultrasound can be enhanced by using the Doppler effect. The Doppler effect occurs because the frequency of a reflected sound wave changes according to whether it is moving towards the ultrasound probe or away from it. The speed and direction of flow in a specific scanned volume can be calculated. Doppler ultrasound enables the generation of time-velocity curves from which peak systolic and end-diastolic velocities can be obtained. Based on these values different indices can be calculated and associated with a measurement of the renal artery diameter, renal blood flow can be estimated. The most commonly reported index is called the resistive index (RI). RI is calculated according to the formula:

$$\text{RI} = (\text{peak systolic velocity} - \text{lowest diastolic velocity})/\text{peak systolic velocity}.$$

These measurements, however, have several limitations: Measurements are sensitive to numerous parameters, such as vessel stiffness, heart rate (increased rate over-estimates end diastolic velocity), heart rhythm (difficult to obtain reliable values during atrial fibrillation), external compression by transducer (in particular in a transplanted kidney) or Valsalva maneuvers that can decrease flow velocity [62]. These indices were poorly correlated with invasive measurement of renal blood flow in a sheep model [63]. However, Lerolle et al. demonstrated that Doppler indices on admission could predict AKI in critically ill patients [64]. Unfortunately, because of the way it is calculated, an increased RI may indicate the presence of increased renal vascular resistance with decreased flow or the presence of normal renal resistance with increased flow or even the presence of decreased resistance with markedly increased flow. Ureteric obstruction also significantly affects measurement of RI. The RI alone is, therefore, easily confounding.

Ultrasound-Doppler studies are routinely performed during the follow-up of renal transplant patients where the absence of a decrease of RI could be a sign of early rejection [65].

Altogether, ultrasound-Doppler has many advantages, is non-invasive, can be performed at the bedside, and can be repeated to evaluate changes after an intervention. However, ultrasound-Doppler is inherently patient- and operator-dependent. Its overall reliability and the relationship between derived indices and renal perfusion require further investigation.

Contrast-Enhanced Ultrasound

Gases are ideal contrast agents for ultrasonography as they are highly compressible and their density is 1,000-fold less than blood. Embedded within a shell they can be made to form microbubbles [66], which are extremely potent ultrasound reflectors. Microbubbles change shape when they interact with ultrasound waves resulting in the generation of non-linear signals. Microbubbles can be obtained rapidly by agitating saline. Such microbubbles are used to diagnose right-to-left shunt during cardiac echocardiography. However, these bubbles are very heterogeneous in size and shape, their half-life is very short and they can be associated with cerebral ischemic events [67].

In the last decade, commercial preparations of contrast agents for ultrasound have become available. These agents demonstrate increased stability and have uniform sizes. Microbubbles found in commercial preparations of ultrasound contrast agents (UCA) have very uniform sizes about that of a red blood cell. This property enables the bubbles to circulate through the pulmonary capillaries, hence to be visualized in arterial beds. Although some initial concerns were raised, UCA can now be considered safe after post-marketing experience from over 1 million patients has been reported [68, 69].

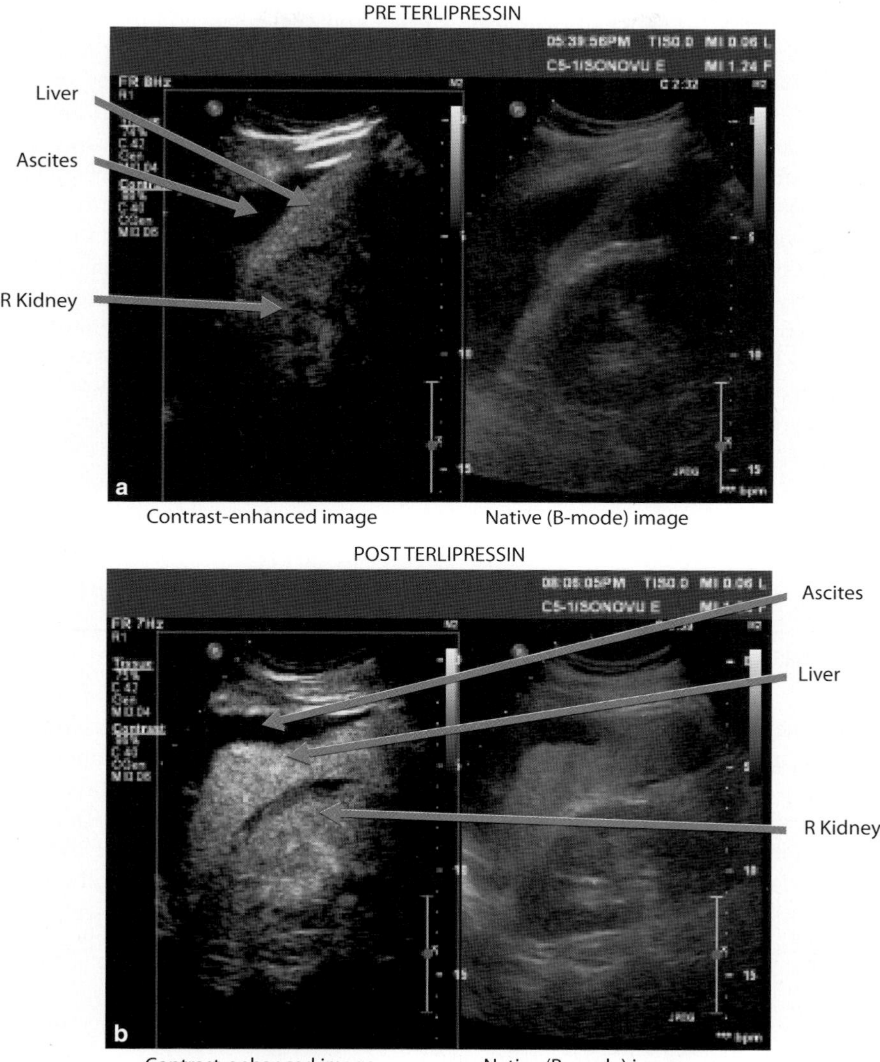

Fig. 4 Example of microcirculatory changes as seen with contrast-enhanced ultrasound images taken during a contrast-enhanced ultrasound study performed on a patient with chronic liver disease and hepatorenal syndrome. The image is centered on the patient's right kidney. Two images are shown: the first **a** was taken just before the intravenous administration of 1 mg of terlipressin and the second **b** 2 hours after. This study demonstrates increased renal perfusion in response to terlipressin administration, as indicated by a brighter signal within the renal cortex on the right image.

Blood flow quantification using contrast-enhanced ultrasound was first described by Wei et al. [70] in a canine model. The same technique was used by Kishimoto et al. to measure renal blood flow, demonstrating a good correlation with changes in renal blood flow as estimated by PAH clearance [71]. Schwenger [72] and Benozzi [73] et al. demonstrated that contrast-enhanced ultrasound was able to distinguish acute rejection from acute tubular necrosis. Another study, in healthy volunteers demonstrated that contrast-enhanced ultrasound was able to detect a 20 % decrease in renal blood flow as induced by an angiotensin II infusion [74]. Above all, contrast-enhanced ultrasound can provide real time visualization of the renal microcirculation. Because it is very well tolerated and can be applied at the bedside, it could in theory be used to determine changes in microcirculation after therapeutic interventions. This would enable us to better understand the intra-renal microcirculatory changes following our common interventions and potentially drive our practice in patients at risk of AKI. As an example, as illustrated in Fig. 4, contrast-enhanced ultrasound was able to confirm a strong microcirculatory response to terlipressin in a patient with hepatorenal syndrome.

Although in its early stages of validation, contrast-enhanced ultrasound seems to be a promising technique to evaluate renal perfusion in critical illness. Indeed, it can be performed at the bedside, is minimally invasive and safe. Contrast-enhanced ultrasound provides information on the microcirculation and, potentially, could improve our understanding of flow alterations in critical illness associated AKI.

Conclusion

Assessment of renal blood flow is important but difficult in AKI. Most techniques are not applicable at the bedside and require extensive patient manipulation, which, in the critically ill patient greatly reduces the practical applicability of any given technique. Furthermore, most techniques only enable global organ flow estimation, whereas information on the microcirculation is perhaps more likely to be useful in understanding the pathogenesis of AKI. Contrast-enhanced ultrasound is the first technique to overcome most of these limitations. Contrast-enhanced ultrasound may soon play a significant role in our ability to investigate microcirculatory changes in AKI.

References

1. Uchino S, Kellum JA, Bellomo R et al (2005) Acute renal failure in critically ill patients: a multinational, multicenter study. JAMA 294:813–818
2. Bagshaw SM, George C, Dinu I, Bellomo R (2008) A multi-centre evaluation of the RIFLE criteria for early acute kidney injury in critically ill patients. Nephrol Dial Transplant 23:1203–1210

3. Chertow GM, Levy EM, Hammermeister KE, Grover F, Daley J (1998) Independent association between acute renal failure and mortality following cardiac surgery. Am J Med 104:343–348
4. Parikh A, Shaw A (2012) The economics of renal failure and kidney disease in critically ill patients. Crit Care Clin 28:99–111
5. Bywaters EG, Beall D (1941) Crush injuries with impairment of renal function. BMJ 1:427–432
6. Darmady EM (1947) Renal anoxia and the traumatic uraemia syndrome. Br J Surg 34:262–271
7. Schrier RW, Wang W (2004) Acute renal failure and sepsis. N Engl J Med 2004 351:159–169
8. Prowle JR, Ishikawa K, May CN, Bellomo R (2009) Renal blood flow during acute renal failure in man. Blood Purif 28:216–225
9. Ishikawa K, Calzavacca P, Bellomo R, Bailey M, May CN (2012) Effect of selective inhibition of renal inducible nitric oxide synthase on renal blood flow and function in experimental hyperdynamic sepsis. Crit Care Med 40:2368–2375
10. Morimatsu H, Ishikawa K, May CN, Bailey M, Bellomo R (2012) The systemic and regional hemodynamic effects of phenylephrine in sheep under normal conditions and during early hyperdynamic sepsis. Anesth Analg 115:330–342
11. O'Connor PM, Evans RG (2010) Structural antioxidant defense mechanisms in the mammalian and nonmammalian kidney: different solutions to the same problem? Am J Physiol Reg Integ Comp Physiol 299:R723–727
12. Rudolph AM, Heymann MA (1967) Validation of the antipyrine method for measuring fetal umbilical blood flow. Circ Res 21:185–190
13. McDevitt DG, Nies AS (1976) Simultaneous measurement of cardiac output and its distribution with microspheres in the rat. Cardiovasc Res 10:494–498
14. Mendell PL, Hollenberg NK (1971) Cardiac output distribution in the rat: comparison of rubidium and microsphere methods. Am J Physiol 221:1617–1620
15. Prinzen FW, Bassingthwaighte JB (2000) Blood flow distributions by microsphere deposition methods. Cardiovasc Res 45:13–21
16. Leivestad T, Brodwall EK, Simonsen S (1978) Determination of renal blood flow by thermodilution method. Scand J Clin Lab Invest 38:495–499
17. Hornych A, Brod J, Slechta V (1971) The measurement of the renal venous outflow in man by the local thermodilution method. Nephron 8:17–32
18. Brenner M, Schaer GL, Mallory DL, Suffredini AF, Parrillo JE (1990) Detection of renal blood flow abnormalities in septic and critically ill patients using a newly designed indwelling thermodilution renal vein catheter. Chest 98:170–179
19. Sward K, Valsson F, Sellgren J, Ricksten SE (2004) Bedside estimation of absolute renal blood flow and glomerular filtration rate in the intensive care unit. A validation of two independent methods. Intensive Care Med 30:1776–1782
20. Sward K, Valsson F, Sellgren J, Ricksten SE (2005) Differential effects of human atrial natriuretic peptide and furosemide on glomerular filtration rate and renal oxygen consumption in humans. Intensive Care Med 31:79–85
21. Redfors B, Bragadottir G, Sellgren J, Sward K, Ricksten SE (2011) Effects of norepinephrine on renal perfusion, filtration and oxygenation in vasodilatory shock and acute kidney injury. Intensive Care Med 37:60–67
22. Redfors B, Bragadottir G, Sellgren J, Sward K, Ricksten SE (2010) Dopamine increases renal oxygenation: a clinical study in post-cardiac surgery patients. Acta Anaesthesiol Scand 54:183–190
23. Hollenberg NK, Adams DF, Solomon H et al (1975) Renal vascular tone in essential and secondary hypertension: hemodynamic and angiographic responses to vasodilators. Medicine 54:29–44
24. Hollenberg NK, Sandor T (1984) Vasomotion of renal blood flow in essential hypertension. Oscillations in xenon transit. Hypertension 6:579–585

25. Hollenberg NK, Sandor T, Holtzman E, Meyerovitz MF, Harrington DP (1989) Renal vasomotion in essential hypertension: influence of vasodilators. Hypertension 14:9–13
26. Elkayam U, Mehra A, Cohen G et al (1998) Renal circulatory effects of adenosine in patients with chronic heart failure. J Am Coll Cardiol 32:211–215
27. Doucette JW, Corl PD, Payne HM et al (1992) Validation of a Doppler guide wire for intravascular measurement of coronary artery flow velocity. Circulation 85:1899–1911
28. Fritzberg AR, Kasina S, Eshima D, Johnson DL (1986) Synthesis and biological evaluation of technetium-99 m MAG3 as a hippuran replacement. J Nucl Med 27:111–116
29. Itoh K (2001) 99mTc-MAG3: review of pharmacokinetics, clinical application to renal diseases and quantification of renal function. Ann Nucl Med 15:179–190
30. Trejtnar F, Laznicek M (2002) Analysis of renal handling of radiopharmaceuticals. Q J Nucl Med 46:181–194
31. Hilson AJ, Maisey MN, Brown CB, Ogg CS, Bewick MS (1978) Dynamic renal transplant imaging with Tc-99 m DTPA (Sn) supplemented by a transplant perfusion index in the management of renal transplants. J Nucl Med 19:994–1000
32. Peters AM, Gunasekera RD, Lavender JP et al (1987) Noninvasive measurement of renal blood flow using DTPA. Contrib Nephrol 56:26–30
33. Jafri RA, Britton KE, Nimmon CC et al (1988) Technetium-99 m MAG3, a comparison with iodine-123 and iodine-131 orthoiodohippurate, in patients with renal disorders. J Nucl Med 29:147–158
34. Verbruggen AM, Nosco DL, Van Nerom CG, Bormans GM, Adriaens PJ, De Roo MJ (1992) Technetium-99 m-L,L-ethylenedicysteine: a renal imaging agent. I. Labeling and evaluation in animals. J Nucl Med 33:551–557
35. Gates GF (1982) Glomerular filtration rate: estimation from fractional renal accumulation of 99mTc-DTPA (stannous). AJR Am J Roentgenol 138:565–570
36. Fawdry RM, Gruenewald SM, Collins LT, Roberts AJ (1985) Comparative assessment of techniques for estimation of glomerular filtration rate with 99mTc-DTPA. Eur J Nucl Med 11:7–12
37. Haufe SE, Riedmuller K, Haberkorn U (2006) Nuclear medicine procedures for the diagnosis of acute and chronic renal failure. Nephron Clin Pract 103:c77–c84
38. Mullani NA, Ekas RD, Marani S, Kim EE, Gould KL (1990) Feasibility of measuring first pass extraction and flow with rubidium-82 in the kidneys. Am J Physiol Imaging 5:133–140
39. Tamaki N, Rabito CA, Alpert NM et al (1986) Serial analysis of renal blood flow by positron tomography with rubidium-82. Am J Physiol 251:H1024–H1030
40. Szabo Z, Xia J, Mathews WB, Brown PR (2006) Future direction of renal positron emission tomography. Semin Nucl Med 36:36–50
41. Juillard L, Janier MF, Fouque D et al (2000) Renal blood flow measurement by positron emission tomography using 15O-labeled water. Kidney Int 57:2511–2518
42. Alpert NM, Rabito CA, Correia DJ et al (2002) Mapping of local renal blood flow with PET and H(2)(15)O. J Nucl Med 43:470–475
43. Vallee JP, Lazeyras F, Khan HG, Terrier F (2000) Absolute renal blood flow quantification by dynamic MRI and Gd-DTPA. Eur Radiol 10:1245–1252
44. Marckmann P, Skov L, Rossen K et al (2006) Nephrogenic systemic fibrosis: suspected causative role of gadodiamide used for contrast-enhanced magnetic resonance imaging. J Am Soc Nephrol 17:2359–2362
45. Perazella MA (2009) Current status of gadolinium toxicity in patients with kidney disease. Clin J Am Soc Nephrol 4:461–469
46. Neuwelt EA, Hamilton BE, Varallyay CG et al (2009) Ultrasmall superparamagnetic iron oxides (USPIOs): a future alternative magnetic resonance (MR) contrast agent for patients at risk for nephrogenic systemic fibrosis (NSF)? Kidney Int 75:465–474
47. Debatin JF, Ting RH, Wegmuller H et al (1994) Renal artery blood flow: quantitation with phase-contrast MR imaging with and without breath holding. Radiology 190:371–378
48. Sommer G, Corrigan G, Fredrickson J et al (1998) Renal blood flow: measurement in vivo with rapid spiral MR imaging. Radiology 208:729–734

49. Prowle JR, Molan MP, Hornsey E, Bellomo R (2010) Cine phase-contrast magnetic resonance imaging for the measurement of renal blood flow. Contrib Nephrol 165:329–336
50. Wolf RL, King BF, Torres VE, Wilson DM, Ehman RL (1993) Measurement of normal renal artery blood flow: cine phase-contrast MR imaging vs clearance of p-aminohippurate. AJR Am J Roentgenol 161:995–1002
51. de Haan MW, Kouwenhoven M, Kessels AG, van Engelshoven JM (2000) Renal artery blood flow: quantification with breath-hold or respiratory triggered phase-contrast MR imaging. Eur Radiol 10:1133–1137
52. King BF, Torres VE, Brummer ME et al (2003) Magnetic resonance measurements of renal blood flow as a marker of disease severity in autosomal-dominant polycystic kidney disease. Kidney Int 64:2214–2221
53. Prowle JR, Molan MP, Hornsey E, Bellomo R (2012) Measurement of renal blood flow by phase-contrast magnetic resonance imaging during septic acute kidney injury: a pilot investigation. Crit Care Med 40:1768–1776
54. Golay X, Hendrikse J, Lim TC (2004) Perfusion imaging using arterial spin labeling. Top Magn Reson Imaging 15:10–27
55. Artz NS, Sadowski EA, Wentland AL et al (2011) Arterial spin labeling MRI for assessment of perfusion in native and transplanted kidneys. Magn Reson Imaging 29:74–82
56. Spuentrup E, Manning WJ, Bornert P, Kissinger KV, Botnar RM, Stuber M (2002) Renal arteries: navigator-gated balanced fast field-echo projection MR angiography with aortic spin labeling: initial experience. Radiology 225:589–596
57. Ritt M, Janka R, Schneider MP et al (2010) Measurement of kidney perfusion by magnetic resonance imaging: comparison of MRI with arterial spin labeling to para-aminohippuric acid plasma clearance in male subjects with metabolic syndrome. Nephrol Dial Transplant 25:1126–1133
58. Fenchel M, Martirosian P, Langanke J et al (2006) Perfusion MR imaging with FAIR true FISP spin labeling in patients with and without renal artery stenosis: initial experience. Radiology 238:1013–1021
59. Textor SC, Glockner JF, Lerman LO et al (2008) The use of magnetic resonance to evaluate tissue oxygenation in renal artery stenosis. J Am Soc Nephrol 19:780–788
60. Warner L, Glockner JF, Woollard J, Textor SC, Romero JC, Lerman LO (2011) Determinations of renal cortical and medullary oxygenation using blood oxygen level-dependent magnetic resonance imaging and selective diuretics. Invest Radiol 46:41–47
61. Pruijm M, Hofmann L, Maillard M et al (2010) Effect of sodium loading/depletion on renal oxygenation in young normotensive and hypertensive men. Hypertension 55:1116–1122
62. Heine GH, Gerhart MK, Ulrich C, Kohler H, Girndt M (2005) Renal Doppler resistance indices are associated with systemic atherosclerosis in kidney transplant recipients. Kidney Int 68:878–885
63. Wan L, Yang N, Hiew CY et al (2008) An assessment of the accuracy of renal blood flow estimation by Doppler ultrasound. Intensive Care Med 34:1503–1510
64. Lerolle N, Guerot E, Faisy C, Bornstain C, Diehl JL, Fagon JY (2006) Renal failure in septic shock: predictive value of Doppler-based renal arterial resistive index. Intensive Care Med 32:1553–1559
65. Rodrigo E, Lopez-Rasines G, Ruiz JC et al (2010) Determinants of resistive index shortly after transplantation: independent relationship with delayed graft function. Nephron Clin Pract 114:c178–186
66. Schneider A, Johnson L, Goodwin M, Schelleman A, Bellomo R (2011) Bench-to-bedside review: Contrast enhanced ultrasonography – a promising technique to assess renal perfusion in the ICU. Crit Care 15:157
67. Romero JR, Frey JL, Schwamm LH et al (2009) Cerebral ischemic events associated with "bubble study" for identification of right to left shunts. Stroke 40:2343–2348
68. Main ML, Ryan AC, Davis TE, Albano MP, Kusnetzky LL, Hibberd M (2008) Acute mortality in hospitalized patients undergoing echocardiography with and without an ultrasound contrast agent (multicenter registry results in 4,300,966 consecutive patients). Am J Cardiol 102:1742–1746

69. Dolan MS, Gala SS, Dodla S et al (2009) Safety and efficacy of commercially available ultrasound contrast agents for rest and stress echocardiography a multicenter experience. J Am Coll Cardiol 53:32–38
70. Wei K, Jayaweera AR, Firoozan S, Linka A, Skyba DM, Kaul S (1998) Quantification of myocardial blood flow with ultrasound-induced destruction of microbubbles administered as a constant venous infusion. Circulation 97:473–483
71. Kishimoto N, Mori Y, Nishiue T et al (2003) Renal blood flow measurement with contrast-enhanced harmonic ultrasonography: evaluation of dopamine-induced changes in renal cortical perfusion in humans. Clin Nephrol 59:423–428
72. Schwenger V, Korosoglou G, Hinkel UP et al (2006) Real-time contrast-enhanced sonography of renal transplant recipients predicts chronic allograft nephropathy. Am J Transplant 6:609–615
73. Benozzi L, Cappelli G, Granito M et al (2009) Contrast-enhanced sonography in early kidney graft dysfunction. Transplant Proc 41:1214–1215
74. Schneider AG, Hofmann L, Wuerzner G et al (2012) Renal perfusion evaluation with contrast-enhanced ultrasonography. Nephrol Dial Transplant 27:674–681
75. Textor SC, Lerman L (2010) Renovascular hypertension and ischemic nephropathy: state of the art. Am J Hypertens 23:1159–1169

Perioperative Acute Kidney Injury After Fluid Resuscitation

Z. Ricci, S. Romagnoli, and C. Ronco

Introduction

Indications for major surgery have increased significantly in the last decade due to marked improvements in surgical techniques, advances in percutaneous and radiological procedures, and enhanced minimally invasive surgery, e.g., laparoscopy, thoracoscopy, etc. This evolution has certainly been associated with a significant improvement in the surgical standard of care and in surgical outcomes. However, as a consequence, older and more severely ill patients are scheduled for surgical procedures. Finally, perioperative care and patient optimization has also evolved and has currently become a specific field of intensive care, aimed at reducing postoperative complications, length of stay and mortality [1].

In this context, it is now clear that preoperative comorbidity is no longer a contraindication to most surgical procedures and acute postoperative organ failures have become common for higher risk patients. Acute kidney injury (AKI) is certainly the most common perioperative acute organ failure, in all surgical fields, including catheterization procedures, minimally invasive surgery and major abdominal and thoracic surgery [2, 3]. In this chapter we will address several aspects of perioperative AKI, focusing on the recently evidenced association between fluid replacement and renal dysfunction.

Z. Ricci (✉)
Department of Cardiology and Cardiac Surgery, Pediatric Cardiac Intensive Care Unit, Bambino Gesù Children's Hospital, IRCCS, Piazza S. Onofrio 4, 00165 Rome, Italy
E-mail: z.ricci@libero.it

S. Romagnoli
Department of Cardiac and Vascular Anesthesia and Post-Surgical Intensive Care Unit, Careggi Hospital, Florence, Italy

C. Ronco
Department of Nephrology, Dialysis and Transplantation, St. Bortolo Hospital, Vicenza, Italy
International Renal Research Institute, Vicenza, Italy

J.-L. Vincent (Ed.), *Annual Update in Intensive Care and Emergency Medicine 2013*,
DOI 10.1007/978-3-642-35109-9_52, © Springer-Verlag Berlin Heidelberg 2013

Etiology of Perioperative Acute Kidney Injury

The risk factors for postoperative AKI include preoperative comorbidities (diabetes, heart failure and chronic kidney disease), emergent surgery, exposure to nephrotoxic drugs (antibiotics and contrast media), hemodynamic instability, hypothermia, inflammatory response to surgery, and hospital-acquired infections [3, 4]. The abdominal compartment syndrome, which develops after persistent intraabdominal hypertension, may result in development of AKI [5]. Postoperative AKI, hence, has a multifactorial etiology and the impact provided by the single variables is impossible to assess. However, one event is surely common to all surgical procedures: The need for fluid replacement, secondary to fluid losses (blood, urine and preoperative fasting) and to hemodynamic management (mostly perioperative hypotension). The European Society of Intensive Care Medicine (ESICM) has recently highlighted that fluid choice may severely affect critically ill patient outcomes [6]. In particular, as fluid replacement during major surgery is commonly provided by crystalloids, colloids and hemoderivatives (albumin, packed red blood cells [RBCs] and fresh frozen plasma [FFP]), the impact of each of these fluid types on postoperative AKI will be detailed.

The Role of Colloids on Perioperative Acute Kidney Injury

The rationale for intraoperative colloid administration (with or instead of crystalloid fluid replacement) would be to achieve the highest volume expansion with a limited amount of fluids. The saline versus albumin fluid evaluation (SAFE) trial clearly showed that the same degree of intravascular fluid replacement was achieved with a significantly lower volume in the albumin group [7]. However, the SAFE authors did not find significant differences relative to all other investigated outcomes (mortality, proportion of patients with new single-organ and multiple-organ failure, length of mechanical ventilation, length of renal replacement therapy, length of hospital stay). The use of different types of colloid solutions (gelatins, dextrans, hydroxyethyl starches [HES]) for volume replacement, in both operating rooms and intensive care units (ICUs), has dramatically increased in recent years, despite the frequently described adverse effects and lack of clear evidence of efficacy [8]. A Cochrane meta-analysis of 86 trials, with a total of 5,484 participants, concluded that there is no evidence that one colloid solution is more effective or safe than any other, although the confidence intervals were wide and did not exclude clinically significant differences between colloids [9]. Recent data on AKI occurrence associated with colloid use has emerged and the most recent trial on about 800 critically ill patients randomized to receive either HES 130/0.4 or Ringer's acetate (33 ml/kg in both cases) for fluid resuscitation, concluded that the colloid group had a significantly greater risk of dying (relative risk [RR] 1.17), of receiving renalreplacement therapy (RR 1.35) and of bleeding

(RR 1.52) [10]. It must be acknowledged that, in contrast, a similar study showed that HES was safe compared to 0.9 % saline, and that there was no difference in Acute Kidney Injury Network (AKIN) and RIFLE (Risk-Injury-Failure-Loss-Endstage renal disease) criteria among groups of septic critically ill patients, and no differences in mortality, coagulation, or pruritus up to 90 days after treatment initiation [11]. The ongoing debate has not definitely elucidated to date whether colloids or crystalloids should be preferentially infused and whether colloids can be safely used in critically ill patients, especially in the light of their potential nephrotoxic role [12]. The exact mechanism of renal damage is not fully understood: It may include reabsorption of the macromolecule into renal tubular cells leading to osmotic nephrotic lesions or renal plugging due to hyperviscous urine [13]. An *in vitro* investigation on cell viability of human proximal tubular (HK-2) cells elegantly showed that HES 130/0.4 significantly decreased cell viability in a concentration-dependent manner. Human albumin, as well as gelatin, also showed deleterious effects on HK-2 cells but, in lower concentrations, human albumin and the crystalloid solution, Sterofundin ISO, were cytoprotective compared with the NaCl control [14]. However, since colloid use has not been shown to clearly improve clinical outcomes, the question remains whether they should be used in patients at risk of AKI [15, 16].

The Role of Fluid Balance in Perioperative Acute Kidney Injury

Dehydration is a very well-known cause of AKI, but fluid overload may also be an important predisposing factor for kidney damage [17]. A systematic review of all randomized controlled studies on goal-directed therapy (GDT)-based fluid resuscitation, focused on renal outcomes and fluids administered during perioperative care, was recently published [18]. The authors identified 24 perioperative studies where GDT was associated with a decreased risk of postoperative AKI (odds ratio [OR] = 0.59) but additional fluid given was limited (median: 555 ml). Surprisingly, the decrease in AKI was greatest (OR = 0.47) in the 10 studies where fluid resuscitation was the same between the GDT and control groups. In line with these findings, inotropic drug use in GDT patients was associated with decreased AKI (OR = 0.52), whereas studies not involving inotropic drugs found no effect of GDT on AKI (OR = 0.75). The greatest protection from AKI occurred in patients with no differences in total fluid delivery and use of inotropes (OR = 0.46). Based on these results, the authors concluded that GDT-based fluid resuscitation may decrease AKI in surgical patients; however, this effect appears most effective when little overall fluid resuscitation is required and most support is from inotropic drugs [18]. Modern perioperative fluid administration, different from past practice, hence suggests that intraoperative fluid therapy should be tailored to two broad clinical contexts: Low-risk patients undergoing low-risk surgery should receive liberal crystalloid infusions in the range of 10–30 ml/kg in order to improve outcomes such as pain, nausea, dizziness, and to accelerate hospital discharge. On the other hand, high-risk patients undergoing major surgery seem to benefit from a more 'restrictive' fluid regimen. This remains to be clearly defined, but from a practical point of view, in a patient with normal renal function, fluid administration should be kept low as long as urine output is maintained between 0.5 and 1.0 ml/kg/h. Studies on dynamic indices of fluid responsiveness (stroke volume variation [SVV] and pulse pressure variation [PPV]) in perioperative settings, aimed at optimizing fluid therapy, have shown that GDT using hemodynamic monitoring to optimize stroke volume by volume loading during high-risk surgery decreases the incidence of postoperative complications [1, 19]. Therefore, rather than roughly categorizing patients into a risk-box and applying a corresponding fluid administration regimen, it may be recommended to give fluids according to specific patients' needs either in the operating room or in the ICU.

Red Blood Cells and Acute Kidney Injury: Not To Transfuse

The ultimate goal of RBC transfusion, a common practice in critically ill patients and patients undergoing surgery, is to increase the oxygen delivery (DO_2 = cardiac output × arterial oxygen content) to improve tissue oxygenation in anemic patients. Although the risks of erythrocyte transfusion have substantially decreased as a result of improvements in testing and storage, it is unclear whether transfusions improve cell oxygen supply and clinical status or not, since several studies have reported increased mortality, lung failure, infections, prolonged hospital length of stay, and renal insufficiency [20]. In fact, observational studies on blood transfusion practices in critically ill patients reported that RBC transfusions were associated with an increased risk of death and organ dysfunction [21, 22] in different clinical settings, including trauma patients [23], burns [24] and, in most cases, in cardiac surgery [25] where a large proportion of the patients receive transfusions and where AKI is a frequent complication occurring during and after surgery [26]. Three specific factors seem to be most likely involved in the development of postoperative AKI: Anemia, hemoglobin concentration and hematocrit. In 2005, Habib et al. [27], in a population of 1,760 patients undergoing coronary artery bypass grafting (CABG), observed that a reduction in hematocrit below 24 % during cardiopulmonary bypass (CPB), increased the likelihood of postoperative renal dysfunction. As a consequence, erythrocyte transfusions, by limiting dilutional anemia during CPB, were found to worsen renal outcome, rather than reducing the incidence of AKI. This paradoxical effect was attributed to the so-called 'storage lesions', alterations already suspected, in other studies, to be responsible for many of several harmful effects of transfusions, including AKI [28]. As an explanation, stored RBCs may impair renal function and contribute to AKI development because of a series of structural and functional modifications; the most important are summarized in Box 1. In addition to chemical and metabolic alterations, stored cells are less deformable, because of a loss of structural protein chains that makes them less able to proceed into the microcirculation thus reducing the ability to transport and deliver oxygen to cells [29]. In addition, old erythrocytes have an increased tendency to adhere to endothelium promoting vasoconstriction and microvascular jamming with further reduction in RBC flow into the capillary circuits.

Box 1
Characteristics of storage lesions

- Depletion of adenosine triphosphate and 2,3-diphosphoglycerate
- Loss of ability to generate nitric oxide (increased adhesiveness to vascular endothelium)
- Release of procoagulant phospholipids
- Decrease in membrane sialic acid
- Accumulation of pro-inflammatory molecules
- RBC lipid peroxidation
- Loss of cellular antioxidant capability
- Changes in the storage medium with decreased pH
- Increased potassium
- Release of pro-inflammatory cytokines
- Increase in free hemoglobin due to hemolysis
- Decrease in S-nitrosohemoglobin concentration

A significant contribution to this issue was brought by a large prospective, randomized, controlled clinical trial (Transfusion Requirements After Cardiac Surgery; TRACS) [30]. The study was conducted to define whether a restrictive perioperative RBC transfusion strategy (hematocrit ≥24 %) was as safe as a liberal strategy (hematocrit ≥30 %). A total of 502 patients were enrolled in the study (253 liberal and 249 restricted, respectively). The mean hemoglobin was 10.5 g/dl (hematocrit 31.8 %) in the liberal group and 9.1 g/dl (hematocrit 28.4 %) in the restricted one. Seventy-eight percent of patients in the liberal group received transfusions (total 613; median 2 U; IQR 1–3) compared to 47 % in the restricted group (total 258; median 0; IQR 0–2). Importantly, there was no difference in the median storage age of RBC units between the groups (median three days). At the end of the study there were no differences in 30-day mortality or organ failure (ARDS, cardiogenic shock and renal failure requiring dialysis or hemofiltration: 5 % vs 4 %). Therefore, the restricted strategy was shown to be as safe as the liberal one according to the primary outcomes. Nonetheless, multiple logistic regression analysis demonstrated that the number of transfused RBC units was an independent risk factor for the occurrence of several clinical complications, including mortality and renal complications (OR = 1.26).

Shashaty et al. [31] explored risk factors for AKI in a cohort of 400 prospectively enrolled critically ill trauma patients followed for five days after ICU admission. During the first five days after ICU admission, 36.8 % of patients developed AKI. The population of patients with AKI was characterized as follows: 14.8 % by creatinine only, 13.3 % by urine output only, and 8.8 % by both criteria and only five of them required dialysis. In the multivariate statistical analysis, the authors found that together with African American race, body mass index, diabetes mellitus, and Abbreviated Injury Scale score for abdomen of 4 or greater, transfusion of unmatched RBC units was independently associated with AKI (OR = 1.13 per unit). The authors considered the possibility of kidney injury after transfusion as potentially derived from two well identified mechanisms: (1) Number of RBCs should be considered as a marker of hypovolemia and, therefore, inadequate DO_2 to the kidney; (2) transfusions may have increased the systemic inflammation and injured the kidney by means of the cytokine-mediated nephrotoxicity. Unmatched RBCs had a much stronger association with AKI than did cross-matched RBCs probably because the administration of unmatched blood products was performed in the most critically ill patients.

Another important issue related to RBC transfusions is the increased circulating free iron due to the shortened RBCs lifespan. This undesired epiphenomenon had already been observed in previous studies [32] that demonstrated a primary role of free iron in oxidative stress and oxidative organ injury. Iron catalyzes several oxidative reactions (Haber-Weiss and Fenton reactions), generating hydroxyl radicals and oxidative stress, which have been demonstrated to be associated with organ injury [33]. In a cardiac surgery population, sources of iron responsible for AKI can be identified in stored old RBCs and in erythrocytes damaged by CPB. Hod et al. [32], in a prospective interventional study on healthy volunteers, evaluated this crucial aspect of RBC transfusion. The aim of Hod's study was to evaluate whether the transfusion of older RBCs produced acute delivery of iron from the monocyte-macrophage system phagocytosis. The basic assumption of the study was that about 25 % of each transfused RBC is rapidly cleared within the first hour and, consequently, a total of 60 mg of iron per RBC unit is delivered to the monocyte-macrophage system and that iron load produces the potent hydroxyl radical ($OH^•$), which can attack proteins, nucleic acids, carbohydrates, and lipids (Fenton reaction) with a specific role in tubular cell damage. The main finding was a significant increase in serum iron and transferrin saturation 4 hours after transfusion with older RBCs (40–42 days) in 13/14 volunteers but not after fresh RBCs (3–7 days). Therefore, transfusion of fresh bank blood produced no detected laboratory evidence of hemolysis and did not significantly alter serum iron, transferrin saturation, or circulating non-transferrin-bound iron. In contrast, when older blood was transfused, an increase in unconjugated bilirubin and serum iron and transferrin saturation was observed. Hod's study confirmed the potential risk of organ failure related to transfusions observed in the cardiac surgery population. In a retrospective study, moderately injured trauma patients (Injury Severity Score < 25), received, in a 7.5-year period, "old" (14 days or more) or "young" (fewer than 14 days) erythrocyte units. Interestingly, all RBC units had undergone pre-storage leukoreduction within 24 hours of collection using high-efficiency filters. A mean of 5.2 units were transfused (median 3.0 units; range, 1–104). As expected, acute respiratory distress syndrome (ARDS), acute renal dysfunction, pneumonia, and in-hospital mortality were all significantly higher in the transfused patients versus those who were not transfused. The OR (95 % CI) for renal dysfunction was 2.08 (0.94–4.60) but when divided into "young" and "old" blood, ORs were 0.97 (0.88–1.07) and 1.18 (1.07–1.29), respectively, demonstrating an association between mortality, pneumonia and renal dysfunction with older blood [34].

Red Blood Cells and Acute Kidney Injury: To Transfuse

Even if RBC transfusions have been shown to be deleterious for renal function, the roles of anemia and/or low DO_2 on postoperative AKI are not clear. Karkouti et al. [35] performed a large cohort study on patients who underwent cardiac surgery with CPB. The effects of preoperative anemia and/or intraoperative transfusions on the day of surgery on AKI (defined as a decrease by more than 50 % of the estimated glomerular filtration rate [GFR] from preoperative to postoperative day 3–4) was evaluated in 12,388 patients who received three units or less of erythrocytes. Patients who received more than three units were excluded to reduce the confounding effect of excessive blood loss (hypovolemia as direct renal injury). The main finding of Karkouti's study was that AKI occurred in 4.1 % of anemic patients and 1.6 % of non-anemic patients suggesting that the risk of AKI was nearly twofold higher in anemic than in non-anemic patients. In addition, as a confirmation of previous studies, the risk of AKI increased in direct proportion to the number of erythrocyte units transfused. Three main reasons were postulated by the authors to explain this higher sensitivity of anemic patents to transfusion-related AKI: (1) Anemic patients develop more severe anemia during the intervention reducing their DO_2 (cellular hypoxia); (2) in spite of normal creatinine values, many anemic patients have subclinical kidney disease (acute on chronic renal failure); (3) anemic patients have abnormal iron metabolism that make them more sensitive to iron load (storage lesions) [35]. Sakr et al. performed a retrospective study in 5,925 surgical ICU patients [36] and showed that lower hemoglobin concentrations were associated with higher morbidity and mortality, whereas higher hemoglobin concentrations and blood transfusions were independently associated with a lower risk of in-hospital death, especially in patients aged from 66 to 80 years and other subgroups of patients. Specifically, transfused patients had higher ICU and in-hospital mortality rates but, after adjustment for confounders and severity of illness, blood transfusions were associated with a lower risk of in-hospital death. The authors considered the discrepancy between these observations and those from other studies to be the result of implementation of leukoreduction and the different case-mix (only surgical ICU patients). Romano and coworkers [37] specifically investigated the effects of leukoreduction on the incidence of cardiac surgery-associated AKI in 1,034 cardiac surgery patients (on-pump CABG). The study demonstrated that after introduction of leukoreduction, mortality rates decreased from 11.4 % to 5.4 % and AKI class R (or greater of the RIFLE criteria [38]) decreased from 51.7 % to 41.5 %. Non-leukodepleted transfusion emerged as an independent predictor (together with intra-aortic balloon pump) of AKI [37].

Conclusion

In conclusion, renal injury risk is minimized by optimal surgery, by reduced bleeding and fluid losses, by accurate systemic perfusion delivery and hemoglobin control and by lower requirements for blood transfusion. As far as is currently evident, in the perioperative phase colloid use should be limited overall and especially avoided in patients at high risk of renal injury. When blood transfusion is required, hemoglobin targets and quality of RBC units should be tailored to the patient's clinical condition: The higher the surgical risk, the narrower will be the 'safe' hemoglobin level and the younger the transfused units should be. Finally, future efforts should be spent in assessing new blood storage methods.

References

1. Hamilton MA, Cecconi M, Rhodes A (2011) A systematic review and meta-analysis on the use of preemptive hemodynamic intervention to improve postoperative outcomes in moderate and high-risk surgical patients. Anesth Analg 112:1392–1402
2. Uchino S, Kellum JA, Bellomo R et al (2005) Acute renal failure in critically ill patients: a multinational, multicenter study. JAMA 17 294:813–818
3. Shiao CC, Wu VC, Li WY et al (2009) Late initiation of renal replacement therapy is associated with worse outcomes in acute kidney injury after major abdominal surgery. Crit Care 13:R171
4. Kheterpal S, Tremper KK, Englesbe MJ et al (2007) Predictors of postoperative acute renal failure after noncardiac surgery in patients with previously normal renal function. Anesthesiology 107:892–902
5. McNelis J, Soffer S, Marini CP et al (2002) Abdominal compartment syndrome in the surgical intensive care unit. Am Surg 68:18–23
6. Reinhart K, Perner A, Sprung CL et al (2012) Consensus statement of the ESICM task force on colloid volume therapy in critically ill patients. Intensive Care Med 38:368–383
7. Finfer S, Bellomo R, Boyce N et al (2004) A comparison of albumin and saline for fluid resuscitation in the intensive care unit. N Engl J Med 350:2247–2256
8. Hartog CS, Skupin H, Natanson C et al (2012) Systematic analysis of hydroxyethyl starch (HES) reviews: proliferation of low-quality reviews overwhelms the results of well-performed meta-analyses. Intensive Care Med 38:1258–1271
9. Bunn F, Trivedi D (2012) Colloid solutions for fluid resuscitation. Cochrane Database Syst Rev 7 CD001319
10. Perner A, Haase N, Guttormsen AB et al (2012) Hydroxyethyl starch 130/0.42 versus Ringer's acetate in severe sepsis. N Engl J Med 367:124–134
11. Guidet B, Martinet O, Boulain T et al (2012) Assessment of hemodynamic efficacy and safety of 6 % hydroxyethylstarch 130/0.4 vs. 0.9 % NaCl fluid replacement in patients with severe sepsis: The CRYSTMAS study. Crit Care 16:R94
12. Hartog CS, Brunkhorst FM, Engel C et al (2011) Are renal adverse effects of hydroxyethyl starches merely a consequence of their incorrect use? Wien Klin Wochenschr 123:145–155
13. Hartog CS, Bauer M, Reinhart K (2011) The efficacy and safety of colloid resuscitation in the critically ill. Anesth Analg 112:156–164
14. Neuhaus W, Schick MA, Bruno RR et al (2012) The effects of colloid solutions on renal proximal tubular cells in vitro. Anesth Analg 114:371–374
15. Dart AB, Mutter TC, Ruth CA, Taback SP (2010) Hydroxyethyl starch (HES) versus other fluid therapies: effects on kidney function. Cochrane Database Syst Rev 20 CD007594

16. Perel P, Roberts I (2012) Colloids versus crystalloids for fluid resuscitation in critically ill patients. Cochrane Database Syst Rev 6 CD000567
17. Doherty M, Buggy DJ (2012) Intraoperative fluids: how much is too much? Br J Anaesth 109:69–79
18. Prowle JR, Chua HR, Bagshaw SM, Bellomo R (2012) Clinical review: volume of fluid resuscitation and the incidence of acute kidney injury – a systematic review. Crit Care 16:230
19. Gurgel ST, do Nascimento Jr P (2011) Maintaining tissue perfusion in high-risk surgical patients: a systematic review of randomized clinical trials. Anesth Analg 112:1384–1391
20. Lelubre C, Vincent JL (2011) Red blood cell transfusion in the critically ill patient. Ann Intensive Care 1:43
21. Vincent JL, Baron JF, Reinhart K et al (2002) ABC (Anemia and Blood Transfusion in Critical Care) Investigators. Anemia and blood transfusion in critically ill patients. JAMA 288:1499–1507
22. Corwin HL, Gettinger A, Pearl RG et al (2004) The CRIT Study: Anemia and blood transfusion in the critically ill – current clinical practice in the United States. Crit Care Med 32:39–52
23. Malone DL, Dunne J, Tracy JK et al (2003) Blood transfusion, independent of shock severity, is associated with worse outcome in trauma. J Trauma 54:898–905
24. Palmieri TL, Caruso DM, Foster KN et al (2006) American Burn Association Burn Multicenter Trials Group: Effect of blood transfusion on outcome after major burn injury: a multicenter study. Crit Care Med 34:1602–1607
25. Koch CG, Li L, Duncan AI et al (2006) Morbidity and mortality risk associated with red blood cell and blood-component transfusion in isolated coronary artery bypass grafting. Crit Care Med 34:1608–1616
26. Reeves BC, Murphy GJ (2008) Increased mortality, morbidity, and cost associated with red blood cell transfusion after cardiac surgery. Curr Opin Cardiol 23:607–612
27. Habib RH, Zacharias A, Schwann TA et al (2005) Role of hemodilutional anemia and transfusion during cardiopulmonary bypass in renal injury after coronary revascularization: implications on operative outcome. Crit Care Med 33:1749–1756
28. Van de Watering L (2011) Red cell storage and prognosis. Vox Sang 100:36–45
29. Marik PE, Sibbald WJ (1993) Effect of stored-blood transfusion on oxygen delivery in patients with sepsis. JAMA 269:3024–3029
30. Hajjar LA, Vincent JL, Galas FR et al (2010) requirements after cardiac surgery: the TRACS randomized controlled trial. Transfusion JAMA 304:1559–1567
31. Shashaty MG, Meyer NJ, Localio AR et al (2012) African American race, obesity, and blood product transfusion are risk factors for acute kidney injury in critically ill trauma patients. J Crit Care 27:496–504
32. Hod EA, Zhang N, Sokol SA et al (2010) Transfusion of red blood cells after prolonged storage produces harmful effects that are mediated by iron and inflammation. Blood 115:4284–4292
33. Haase M, Bellomo R, Haase-Fielitz A (2010) Novel biomarkers, oxidative stress, and the role of labile iron toxicity in cardiopulmonary bypass-associated acute kidney injury. J Am Coll Cardiol 55:2024–5033
34. Weinberg JA, McGwin Jr G, Marques MB et al (2008) Transfusions in the less severely injured: Does age of transfused blood affect outcomes? J Trauma 65:794–798
35. Karkouti K, Wijeysundera DN, Yau TM et al (2012) Advance targeted transfusion in anemic cardiac surgical patients for kidney protection. Anesthesiology 116:613–621
36. Sakr Y, Lobo S, Knuepfer S et al (2010) Anemia and blood transfusion in a surgical intensive care unit. Crit Care 14:R92
37. Romano G, Mastroianni C, Bancone C et al (2010) Leukoreduction program for red blood cell transfusions in coronary surgery: Association with reduced acute kidney injury and in-hospital mortality. J Thorac Cardiovasc Surg 140:188–195
38. Bellomo R, Ronco C, Kellum JA et al (2004) Acute Dialysis Quality Initiative workgroup. Acute renal failure – definition, outcome measures, animal models, fluid therapy and information technology needs: the Second International Consensus Conference of the Acute Dialysis Quality Initiative (ADQI) Group. Crit Care 8:R204–R212

Acute Kidney Injury in Intensive Care: A Role for Backpressure?

J. Bardon, M. Legrand, and A. Mebazaa

Introduction

Acute kidney injury (AKI) occurs in approximately two-thirds of intensive care unit (ICU) patients [1] and is associated with increased mortality, length of stay and cost [2]. It is, therefore, essential to better understand its pathogenesis, and to prevent its occurrence. Renal hypoperfusion is thought to worsen the kidney function in situations in which the kidney is already being injured. Many experimental and clinical studies have focused on forward pressure determinants to improve mean arterial pressure (MAP) and cardiac output [3, 4]. There is, however, increasing evidence that backpressure (venous pressure) plays an important role when the kidney is under aggression. Indeed, high levels of central venous pressure (CVP) are associated with AKI suggesting that CVP can detect renal congestion. We will further discuss the potential role of renal venous congestion in the relationship between fluid overload and prognosis in critically ill patients.

J. Bardon
Department of Anesthesiology and Critical Care and SAMU, AP-HP, Lariboisière Hospital, 75475 Paris, France

M. Legrand (✉)
Department of Anesthesiology and Critical Care and SAMU, AP-HP, Lariboisière Hospital, 75475 Paris, France
E-mail: matthieu.m.legrand@gmail.com

A. Mebazaa
Department of Anesthesiology and Critical Care and SAMU, AP-HP, Lariboisière Hospital, 75475 Paris, France

J.-L. Vincent (Ed.), *Annual Update in Intensive Care and Emergency Medicine 2013*, DOI 10.1007/978-3-642-35109-9_53, © Springer-Verlag Berlin Heidelberg 2013

Recent Advances in the Understanding of AKI with Respect to Renal Hemodynamics

Several factors, including microcirculatory dysfunction, renal hypoxia, renal infiltration by inflammatory cells, oxidative stress, inadequate renal perfusion, and direct toxicity of drugs, contrast products or endogenous proteins (e.g., myoglobin, hemoglobin, immunoglobulin), have been identified as contributors of renal injury [5]. Among these, one of the main concerns of intensivists is to insure adequate renal perfusion and hence adequate renal tissue oxygenation; this is, however, a difficult task to achieve as there are no reliable tools to monitor the adequacy between the demand and the actual oxygen delivery to the kidneys in the clinical setting [6].

The Role of Renal Blood Flow in the Development of AKI

Renal blood flow and glomerular filtration rate (GFR) are autoregulated, which means that despite variations in arterial blood pressure, renal blood flow and GFR are maintained. This autoregulation is possible due to different mechanisms, one of which is tubuloglomerular feedback, which acts by modulating the tonicity of the afferent arteriole, keeping the renal blood flow relatively stable. However, this system has its limits: When the arterial blood pressure decreases below a threshold or when autoregulation is impaired, renal blood flow and glomerular filtration will diminish proportionally to the decrease in renal perfusion pressure. Renal autoregulation can be altered under certain circumstances, such as hypertension, diabetes, atherosclerosis, AKI or during cardiopulmonary bypass (CPB). In this context, a good correlation has been observed between renal blood flow and cardiac output in patients with AKI, contrasting with the inconstant correlation between renal blood flow and GFR. This point illustrates the complex regulation of GFR involving various mechanisms mainly at the arteriolar level [7]. Therefore, a preserved cardiac output does not rule out tissue damage nor does a preserved GFR rule out on-going occurrence of renal tissue damage. Hence, measurement of markers of glomerular function with markers of tissue injury has gained interest. Recently, Nejat et al. [8] reported that patients with pre-renal injury, defined as AKI recovering within 48 h and fractional sodium excretion $< 1\,\%$, had evidence of structural injury (i. e., increased renal biomarkers: Kidney injury molecule [KIM]-1, cystatin C and interleukin [IL]-18), suggesting that 'pre-renal' AKI and 'established' AKI represent a continuum of injury. The classification of AKI as pre-renal and intrarenal, still taught in many textbooks, does not seem to represent the reality.

Reaching normal values of mixed venous oxygen saturation (SvO_2) or supranormal cardiac index (CI) values did not reduce the incidence of acute renal failure in the recent meta-analysis by Corcoran et al. [9], illustrating the complex relationship between systemic hemodynamics, renal hemodynamics and renal function.

Gattinoni et al. [10] did not observe any difference in terms of kidney function when increasing CI or SvO_2 to supranormal values in 762 critically ill patients. Increasing renal blood flow at all costs by giving fluids may, therefore, not be the correct means of preventing or correcting AKI. Crystalloid-based fluid resuscitation induces hemodilution, which increases renal oxygen consumption and decreases oxygen delivery to the kidney, thus inducing renal hypoxia [11, 12]. Fluid resuscitation using normal saline (NaCl 0.9 %) can further compromise the renal hemodynamics by decreasing renal blood flow throughout activation of the tubuloglomerular feedback and afferent arteriole vasoconstriction [13].

Cardio-renal Syndromes

There is a strong interaction between the heart and the kidneys, due to neurohormonal stimulation, mainly of the renin-angiotensin-aldosterone system, and inflammatory signaling. The cardio-renal syndromes (CRS) are entities characterized by Ronco et al. [14] and Ismail et al. [15], stating the relationship between kidney injury and heart failure. These groups have established different subgroups depending on the acute or chronic nature and whether the primary failing organ is either the heart or the kidney; type 1 CRS being defined as acute heart failure that leads to AKI. The central role of venous congestion in its development has regained interest over recent years.

Increasing Evidence for a Role of Backpressure in the Development of AKI

The pathophysiology of renal congestion (or increased backpressure) relies on three major elements: Function of the right heart, blood volume and venous capacitance, in which the neurohormonal system plays an important role.

Under normal conditions, an increase in atrial pressure diminishes the secretion of arginine vasopressin (AVP) and sympathetic activity enhancing diuresis and augmenting atrial natriuretic secretion; however patients with heart failure have an overactivated neurohormonal system inducing water and salt reabsorption, which increases the blood volume, CVP transmitted to the renal veins, thus worsening the congestion.

Experimental Studies

Although the exact underlying pathophysiology of renal congestion is not fully understood, some experimental studies have highlighted potential contributing mechanisms:

Increased Interstitial Pressure and Inflammation

As early as 1931, Winton [16] showed in a dog's isolated kidney model that increase in renal venous pressure diminishes urine output and renal blood flow; part of the explanation being that the transmission of vein pressure to the distal portion of the tubules diminishes urine excretion by venous compression of the tubules. However, this study was performed *ex vivo* on dog kidneys connected to a blood pump, raising the venous pressure over 24 mm Hg and excluding the influence of abdominal pressure, renal capsule pressure on the parenchyma and hemodynamic autoregulation mechanisms. It was further shown that backward pressure increases renal interstitial pressure [17] inducing hypoxia, which may impair glomerular filtration. Herrler et al. [18] studied a murine ischemia-reperfusion kidney model, monitoring subcapsular pressure and evaluating kidney function using 99mTc-MAG3 scintigraphy and laser Doppler perfusion. These authors found that after ischemia, a 0.3 mm incision in the lower pole of the kidney capsule prevented loss of tubular excretion rate and maintained renal blood flow. This suggests that interstitial edema and increased interstitial pressure play an important role in the development of post-ischemic AKI. Tanaka et al. [19] studied histological kidney tissue from patients with heart failure and AKI, some of whom had a dilated inferior vena cava; they found dilated peritubular capillaries as well as an increase in local oxidative stress, infiltration of macrophages in the interstitium and interstitial fibrosis but no proteinuria or histopathological glomerular damage. One of the possible mechanisms for increased inflammation in the congestive kidney is the hypoxia induced by the backpressure, as shown in liver congestion [20].

In a pig model of septic shock, Benes et al. [21] and Chvojka et al. [22] showed that despite an MAP maintained above 70 mm Hg with norepinephrine, the renal perfusion pressure was diminished in the sepsis group, partly due to an increase in renal venous pressure. Interestingly, the renal vascular resistance increased only in the group who developed AKI. Finally, in a rat model of arterial or venous renal occlusion [23], the venous obstruction group showed higher serum creatinine levels as well as a stronger inflammatory response with macrophage activation and infiltration by neutrophils.

Neurohormonal Stimulation

In a denervated rat model with sympathetic stimulation (myocardial infarction) developed by Kon et al. [24] to study the influence of the neurovegetative system on renal perfusion, sympathetic stimulation decreases the GFR by changing the glomerular capillary ultrafiltration coefficient. Heart failure, a frequent cause of rise in CVP, increases angiotensin II concentrations thus decreasing the GFR directly or via sympathetic activation. On the other hand, Kastner et al. [25] showed in a dog's kidney that the renin-angiotensin-aldosterone system played an important role in maintaining the GFR when renal venous pressure increased. However, this study was performed on healthy dogs with no previous renal injury and the effect was significant only for high levels of venous pressure (>30 mm Hg). Finally, Morsing et al. [26] showed a diminution in the sensitivity of the tubuloglomerular feedback after injection in rats of atrial natriuretic peptide (ANP), frequently increased in heart failure, inducing water and salt excretion. However, this mechanism is blunted by the activation of the renin-angiotensin-aldosterone and sympathetic nervous systems, increasing fluid retention, which participates in the renal congestion.

Clinical Studies

There is increasing evidence that fluid overload or a high CVP are independent factors associated with increased mortality [27, 28] and AKI in ICU patients (Table 1). Eight observational studies have reported CVP or measurements related to CVP (inferior vena cava diameter, signs of congestion) as independent factors related to altered renal function. Damman et al. [29] reported that among 51 potential recipients for lung transplant because of pulmonary hypertension, multivariate analysis showed that low renal blood flow and high CVP were independently associated with alteration in the GFR (Fig. 1). The same group confirmed this result [30] in a larger population of 2,557 patients who underwent right heart catheterization. Once again, CVP was associated with kidney dysfunction and independently related to mortality. Finally, the study by Damman et al. [31] focusing on clinical signs of congestion (presence of elevated jugular venous pressure, orthopnea, ascites, or edema) reported that these symptoms were independent factors related to altered GFR in a multivariate analysis. The symptoms had a better association with diminished GFR than did LVEF < 30 %; GFR worsened from patients with no signs of congestion to patients with three or more signs of congestion, showing a strong association between clinical signs of congestion and altered renal function. However, due to the retrospective nature of the study, direct causality could not be established despite the potential confounding factors taken into account in the multivariate analysis.

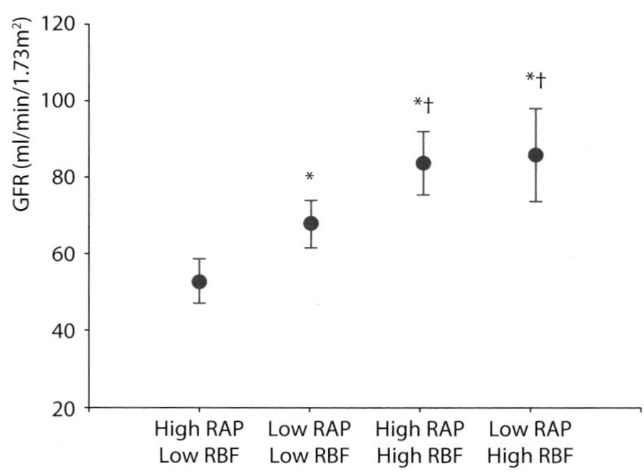

Fig. 1 Relative contributions of right atrial pressure (RAP) and renal blood flow (RBF) to glomerular filtration rate (GFR). Error bars represent 95 % confidence interval. *$p < 0.001$ for difference with High RAP, Low RBF. †$p < 0.01$ for difference with Low RAP, Low RBF. From [29] with permission

Table 1 Clinical studies investigating the association between venous congestion of fluid overload and acute kidney injury

Authors [ref]	Year	Parameter investigated	Study design	No of patients	Population	Main results
Van Biesen [45]	2005	CVP	Prospective monocenter observational study	257	ICU patient with sepsis and AKI	Patients developing AKI had higher CVP on day 1 and day 2
Damman [29]	2007	RAP	Prospective monocenter observational study, multivariate regression analysis	51	Patients with pulmonary hypertension candidates for lung transplantation	RBF and RAP are predictors of AKI
Nohria [46]	2008	RAP	Prospective randomized controlled base	433	Patients hospitalized with HF randomized in PAC group or standard care	Only RAP was correlated to renal function in patients with advanced decompensated HF
Mullens [47]	2009	CVP	Prospective observational study	145	ADHF patient admitted to ICU with pulmonary arterial catheter	CVP was the most important hemodynamic parameter associated with worsening in renal function in ADHF
Damman [30]	2009	CVP	Retrospective observational study	2,557	Patients who underwent right heart cauterization	CVP was independently associated with GFR and mortality
Damman [31]	2010	Clinical signs of congestion	Retrospective analysis of Cardiac Insufficiency Bisoprolol Study II	2,647	NYHA 3/4 chronic HF	Clinical signs of congestion were independently associated with alteration of GFR ($p = 0.012$)
Tanaka [19]	2011	Inferior vena cava diameter	Retrospective monocenter observational study	20	Patients with dilated or hypertrophic HF and renal dysfunction	The rate of decrease of GFR was correlated to IVC diameter ($r = 0.5$, $p = 0.02$)

Table 1 *Continued*

Authors [ref]	Year	Parameter investigated	Study design	No of patients	Population	Main results
Guglin [48]	2011	CVP	Retrospective mono-center observational study	178	Patients scheduled for right heart catheterization	GFR was correlated to CVP
Payen [33]	2008	Fluid balance	Prospective cohort multicenter observational study	1,120	ICU adult patient in the SOAP data base	Patients developing AKI had significantly more fluid balance than those not developing AKI
Bouchard [34]	2009	Fluid accumulation (> 10 % increase body weight)	Prospective multicenter observational study	618	ICU adult patient	Patients with fluid overload had increased mortality, patients with fluid overload were less likely to recover
Grams [49]	2011	Fluid balance	Retrospective database analysis	306	Patients with ALI	Positive fluid balance (adjusted to mean CVP, severity illness, shock, fluid strategy) was associated with increased mortality at 60 days in patients with AKI
Bellomo [32]	2012	Fluid balance	Prospective multicenter observational study from RCT	1,453	ICU patients undergoing renal replacement therapy	Negative mean daily fluid balance was independently associated with a decreased risk of death at 90 days and increased renal replacement-free days

RAP: right atrial pressure; CVP: central venous pressure; NYHA: New York Heart Association; HF: heart failure; ALI: acute lung injury; GFR: glomerular filtration rate; ADHF: acute decompensated heart failure; RCT: randomized controlled trial; PAC: pulmonary artery catheter; IVC: inferior vena cava

Bellomo et al. [32] recently reported that critically ill patients with a negative fluid balance had a significantly reduced risk of death at 90 days and more days free of renal replacement therapy (RRT), adjusted for severity scores, and Payen et al. [33] showed in the large SOAP database that among patients with acute renal failure, those who died had significantly greater daily fluid balance than the survivors (0.98 vs 0.15 l). Bouchard et al. reported a similar observation [34]. We have to acknowledge, however, that such an association between fluid overload and outcome may only reflect that the most severely ill patients received more fluid rather than confirming a causal relationship. However, the results from randomized controlled trials of goal-directed therapy (GDT) in the perioperative setting shed some light on this controversy. Using GDT based on MAP, urine output and CVP (objective < 12 mm Hg) applied to patients in septic shock, the GDT group had decreased in-hospital mortality and risk of renal dysfunction compared to the "standard care" group [35]. Furthermore, the recent meta-analysis by Prowle et al. [36] reported that fluid resuscitation based on GDT resulted in fewer cases of postoperative AKI and was only associated with slightly larger fluid volume administration compared with standard management (the median of the extra fluid volume was 555 ml in the GDT group). Interestingly, AKI protection was reported in the studies where there was an equivalent amount of fluid administration; and the difference was mainly due to the early use of inotropes. In this meta-analysis, four studies reported that fluid overload was an independent factor for mortality or acute renal failure.

In summary, fluid loading associated with fluid monitoring, including regular CVP measures, is associated with a good outcome. However, any excessive fluid load will markedly increase venous pressure and alter kidney function.

Role of Venous Congestion on Extra-renal Organs

Venous congestion may not only affect the kidneys but other organs, such as the liver. Nikolaou et al. [37] studied the prognostic value of liver function tests during acutely decompensated heart failure among the cohort of the SURVIVAL study. They found that abnormal liver function tests were present in approximately half of the patients presenting with acutely decompensated heart failure treated with inotropes and that increased alkaline phosphatase was associated with marked signs of systemic congestion and higher 180-day mortality. Its role on endothelial inflammation was highlighted by Ganda et al. [38], inducing neurohormonal activation, which in turn affects other organs including the heart and the kidneys (Fig. 2).

Fig. 2 Schematic integrative view of the role of venous congestion on the development of organ failure. In response to heart failure and increase venous pressure, (1) the renin-angiotensin-aldosterone system (RAAS) and the sympathetic systems are activated, one system activating the other, enhancing sodium and water absorption, inducing high vascular resistance, high blood volume, thus contributing to the increase in venous pressure. Venous congestion promotes (2) liver congestion and the development of (3) acute kidney injury (AKI). Liver failure induces

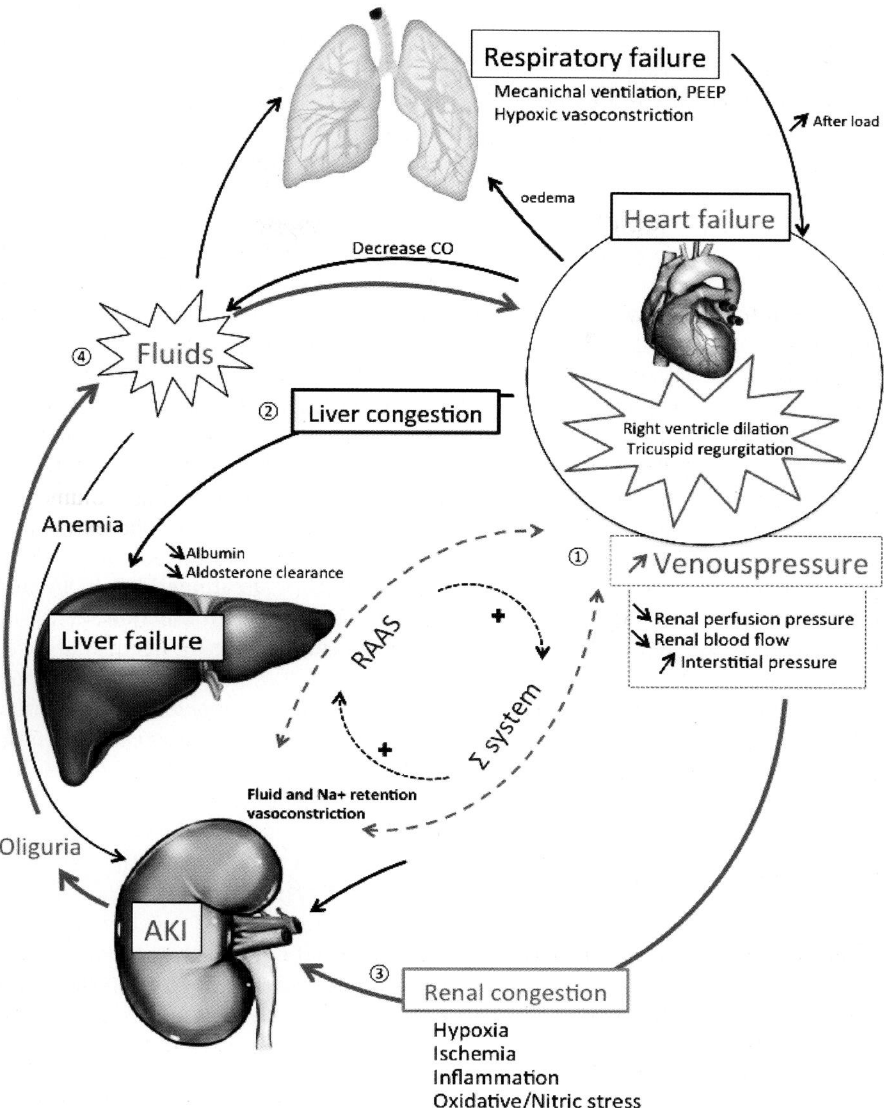

decreased aldosterone clearance, which participates in the hyperactivation of the RAAS while reduced albumin secretion promotes interstitial edema. A vicious circle develops, with AKI having systemic consequences inducing inflammation, apoptosis and capillary leak on remote organs [44]. (4) Fluid therapy in response to hypotension, low cardiac output or oliguria may worsen venous congestion. In addition, metabolic consequences of AKI have an impact on cardiac function: Acidemia has a negative inotropic effect and induces pulmonary vasoconstriction altering the right side heart failure, hyperkalemia contributes to arrhythmia, hyperuremia has a negative effect on myocardial contraction [14]. Σ system: sympathetic system; CO: cardiac output; PAP: pulmonary artery pressure; PvO_2: venous partial pressure of oxygen; PEEP: positive end-expiratory pressure

Prevention and Management of Renal Congestion

Echocardiography provides unique information in showing right ventricular dilation, tricuspid regurgitation and dilatation of the inferior vena cava. Cardiac output, together with CVP monitoring, guides fluid resuscitation indicating when the limit of cardiac compliance has been reached and that fluid administration should be stopped because of the risk of venous congestion and further organ damage (i. e., sustained increase in CVP after fluid loading). Prevention of hypervolemia and fluid overload, define the place for GDT, not so much for reducing fluid volume, but to tailor fluid volume according to the cardiovascular response and detect the need to start vasopressors or inotropes. A conservative fluid administration strategy in surgical patients with acute lung injury (ALI) or acute respiratory distress syndrome (ARDS), targeting a CVP ≤ 4 mm Hg in the absence of shock, has been shown to be safe, associated with no more episodes of severe AKI and to result in more ventilator-free and ICU-free days compared to a liberal strategy [39]. On the other hand, an elevated CVP above 8–12 mm Hg has been associated with AKI and poor outcome. However, as far as we know, there are no studies specifically investigating the diagnostic and therapeutic strategies of renal congestion. In case of suspected or identified venous congestion, treatment should aim to: (1) reduce volemia; (2) improve right ventricular or global heart function.

Fluid overload can be treated by volume depletion either by using diuretics, slow continuous ultrafiltration [40] or regular ultrafiltration [41]. However, one should take particular care concerning the amount of volume depletion, since high loop diuretic doses independently predicted a higher risk for decrease in renal function [42] and were associated with higher mortality [43], and the intensity of ultrafiltration can turn a non-oliguric into an oliguric patient.

Preventing and treating the cause of inflammation should also be a goal, as well as optimizing renal oxygen delivery (prevent hypoxia and anemia) and avoiding nephrotoxins. The treatment of global or right heart dysfunction is not the topic of this review but should be a main concern in the treatment of renal congestion. Strategies aimed at reducing right ventricular afterload (e.g., decreased pulmonary vascular resistances) and improving right ventricular perfusion pressure appears central in this setting. Finally, renal vascular Doppler could explore renal hemodynamics at the bedside but has not been specifically evaluated in the context of venous congestion in critically ill patients.

Conclusion

Although optimization of cardiac output and MAP have long been considered central to the prevention and treatment of AKI in critically ill patients, experimental and clinical studies strongly suggest that elevated venous pressure also compromises renal function. Although hypovolemia should be corrected, hypervolemia and fluid overload have been associated with poor outcome in critically ill patients and patients with acutely decompensated heart failure. A liberal attitude toward fluid resuscitation should be avoided and fluid loading should be guided by relevant hemodynamic parameters. In this way, CVP monitoring appears of tremendous value to detect venous congestion.

References

1. Hoste EA, Kellum JA (2006) Acute kidney injury: epidemiology and diagnostic criteria. Curr Opin Crit Care 12:531–537
2. Chertow GM, Burdick E, Honour M, Bonventre JV, Bates DW (2005) Acute kidney injury, mortality, length of stay, and costs in hospitalized patients. J Am Soc Nephrol 16:3365–3370
3. Langenberg C, Wan L, Egi M, May CN, Bellomo R (2007) Renal blood flow and function during recovery from experimental septic acute kidney injury. Intensive Care Med 33:1614–1618
4. Prowle JR, Molan MP, Hornsey E, Bellomo R (2012) Measurement of renal blood flow by phase-contrast magnetic resonance imaging during septic acute kidney injury: a pilot investigation. Crit Care Med 40:1768–1776
5. Legrand M, Bezemer R, Kandil A, Demirci C, Payen D, Ince C (2011) The role of renal hypoperfusion in development of renal microcirculatory dysfunction in endotoxemic rats. Intensive Care Med 37:1534–1542
6. Legrand M, Almac E, Mik EG et al (2009) L-NIL prevents renal microvascular hypoxia and increase of renal oxygen consumption after ischemia-reperfusion in rats. Am J Physiol Renal Physiol 296:1109–1117
7. Hall JE, Guyton AC, Cowley Jr AW (1977) Dissociation of renal blood flow and filtration rate autoregulation by renin depletion. Am J Physiol 232:215–221
8. Nejat M, Pickering JW, Devarajan P et al (2012) Some biomarkers of acute kidney injury are increased in pre-renal acute injury. Kidney Inter 81:1254–1262
9. Corcoran T, Rhodes JE, Clarke S, Myles PS, Ho KM (2012) Perioperative fluid management strategies in major surgery: a stratified meta-analysis. Anesth Analg 114:640–651
10. Gattinoni L, Brazzi L, Pelosi P et al (1995) A trial of goal-oriented hemodynamic therapy in critically ill patients. N Engl J Med 16:1025–1032
11. Legrand M, Mik EG, Balestra GM et al (2010) Fluid resuscitation does not improve renal oxygenation during hemorrhagic shock in rats. Anesthesiology 112:119–127
12. Legrand M, Mik EG, Johannes T, Payen D, Ince C (2008) Renal hypoxia and dysoxia after reperfusion of the ischemic kidney. Mol Med 14:502–516
13. Chowdhury AH, Cox EF, Francis ST, Lobo DN (2012) A randomized, controlled, double-blind crossover study on the effects of 2-L infusions of 0.9 % saline and plasma-lyte® 148 on renal blood flow velocity and renal cortical tissue perfusion in healthy volunteers. Ann Surg 256:18–24
14. Ronco C, Haapio M, House AA, Anavekar N, Bellomo R (2008) Cardiorenal Syndrome. J Am Coll Cardiol 52:1527–1539
15. Ismail Y, Kasmikha Z, Green HL, McCullough PA (2012) Cardio-Renal Syndrome Type 1: Epidemiology, Pathophysiology and Treatment. Semin Nephrol 32:49–56
16. Winton FR (1931) The influence of venous pressure on the isolated mammalian kidney. J Physiol 72:49–61
17. Fiksen-Olsen MJ, Strick DM, Hawley H, Romero JC (1992) Renal effects of angiotensin II inhibition during increases in renal venous pressure. Hypertension 19:137–141
18. Herrler T, Tischer A, Meyer A et al (2010) The intrinsic renal compartment syndrome: new perspectives in kidney transplantation. Transplantation 89:40–46

19. Tanaka M, Yoshida H, Furuhashi M et al (2011) Deterioration of renal function by chronic heart failure is associated with congestion and oxidative stress in the tubulointerstitium. Intern Med 50:2877–2887
20. Seeto RK, Fenn B, Rockey DC (2000) Ischemic hepatitis: clinical presentation and pathogenesis. Am J Med 109:109–113
21. Benes J, Chvojka J, Sykora R et al (2011) Searching for mechanisms that matter in early septic acute kidney injury: an experimental study. Crit Care 15:R256
22. Chvojka J, Sykora R, Krouzecky A et al (2008) Renal haemodynamic, microcirculatory, metabolic and histopathological responses to peritonitis-induced septic shock in pigs. Crit Care 12:R164
23. Park Y, Hirose R, Dang K et al (2008) Increased severity of renal ischemia reperfusion injury with venous clamping compared to arterial clamping in a rat model. Surgery 143:243–251
24. Kon V, Yared A, Ichikawa I (1985) Role of renal sympathetic nerves in mediating hypoperfusion of renal cortical microcirculation in experimental congestive heart failure and acute extracellular fluid volume depletion. J Clin Invest 76:1912–1920
25. Kastner PR, Hall JE, Guyton AC (1982) Renal hemodynamic responses to increased renal venous pressure: role of angiotensin II. Am J Physiol 243:260–264
26. Morsing P, Stenberg A, Casellas D et al (1992) Renal interstitial pressure and tubuloglomerular feedback control in rats during infusion of atrial natriuretic peptide (ANP). Acta Physiol Scand 146:393–398
27. Schrier RW (2010) Fluid administration in critically ill with acute kidney injury. Clin J Am Soc Nephrol 5:733–739
28. Boyd JH, Forbes J, Nakada TA, Walley KR, Russell JA (2011) Fluid resuscitation in septic shock: A positive fluid balance and elevated central venous pressure are associated with increased mortality. Crit Care Med 39:259–265
29. Damman K, Navis G, Smilde TDJ et al (2007) Decreased cardiac output, venous congestion and the association with renal impairment in patients with cardiac dysfunction. Eur J Heart Fail 9:872–878
30. Damman K, van Deursen VM, Navis G, Voors AA, van Veldhuisen DJ, Hillege HL (2009) Increased central venous pressure is associated with impaired renal function and mortality in a broad spectrum of patients with cardiovascular disease. J Am Coll Cardiol 53:582–588
31. Damman K, Voors AA, Hillege HL et al (2010) Congestion in chronic systolic heart failure is related to renal dysfunction and increased mortality. Eur J Heart Fail 12:974–982
32. Bellomo R, Cass A, Cole L et al (2012) An observational study fluid balance and patient outcomes in the Randomized Evaluation of Normal vs. Augmented Level of Replacement Therapy trial. Crit Care Med 40:1753–1760
33. Payen D, de Pont AC, Sakr Y, Spies C, Reinhart K, Vincent JL (2008) Sepsis Occurrence in Acutely Ill Patients (SOAP) Investigators: A positive fluid balance is associated with a worse outcome in patients with acute renal failure. Crit Care 12:R74
34. Bouchard J, Soroko SB, Chertow GM et al (2009) Program to Improve Care in Acute Renal Disease (PICARD) Study Group: Fluid accumulation, survival and recovery of kidney function in critically ill patients with acute kidney injury. Kidney Int 76:422–427
35. Lin SM, Huang CD, Lin HC, Liu CY, Wang CH, Kuo HP (2006) A modified goal-directed protocol improves clinical outcomes in intensive care unit patients with septic shock: a randomized controlled trial. Shock 26:551–557
36. Prowle JR, Chua HR, Bagshaw SM, Bellomo R (2012) Clinical review: volume of fluid resuscitation and the incidence of acute kidney injury – a systematic review. Crit Care 16:230
37. Nikolaou M, Parissis J, Yilmaz B et al (2013) Liver function abnormalities, clinical profile and outcome in acute decompensated heart failure. Eur Heart J (in press)
38. Ganda A, Onat D, Demmer RT et al (2010) Venous congestion and endothelial cell activation in acute decompensated heart failure. Curr Heart Fail Rep 2010 7:66–74
39. Wiedemann HP, Wheeler AP, Bernard GR et al (2006) Comparison of two fluid-management strategies in acute lung injury. N Engl J Med 354:2564–2575

40. Canaud B, Leblanc M, Leray-Moragues H, Delmas S, Klouche K, Beraud JJ (1998) Slow continuous ultrafiltration for refractory congestive heart failure. Nephrol Dial Transplant 13(Suppl 4):51–55
41. Felker GM, Mentz RJ (2012) Diuretics and ultrafiltration in acute decompensated heart failure. J Am Coll Cardiol 59:2145–2153
42. Butler J, Forman DE, Abraham WT et al (2004) Relationship between heart failure treatment and development of worsening renal function among hospitalized patients. Am Heart J 147:331–338
43. Hasselblad V, Gattis Stough W, Shah MR et al (2007) Relation between dose of loop diuretics and outcomes in a heart failure population: results of the ESCAPE trial. Eur J Heart Fail 9:1064–1069
44. Payen D, Lukaszewicz AC, Legrand M et al (2012) A multicentre study of acute kidney injury in severe sepsis and septic shock: association with inflammatory phenotype and HLA genotype. PLoS One 7:e35838
45. Van Biesen W, Yegenaga I, Vanholder R et al (2005) Relationship between fluid status and its management on acute renal failure. J Nephrol 18:54–60
46. Nohria A, Hasselblad V, Stebbins A et al (2008) Cardiorenal interactions insights from the ESCAPE trial. J Am Coll Cardiol 51:1268–1274
47. Mullens W, Abrahams Z, Francis GS et al (2009) Importance of venous congestion for worsening of renal function in advanced decompensated heart failure. J Am Coll Cardiol 53:589–596
48. Guglin M, Rivero A, Matar F, Garcia M (2011) Renal dysfunction in heart failure is due to congestion but not low output. Clin Cardiol 34:113–116
49. Grams ME, Estrella MM, Coresh J (2011) Fluid balance, diuretic use, and mortality in acute kidney injury. Clin J Am Soc Nephrol 6:966–973

Renal Oxygenation in Clinical Acute Kidney Injury

S.-E. Ricksten, G. Bragadottir, and B. Redfors

Introduction

Renal oxygenation is defined as the relationship between renal oxygen delivery (DO_2) and renal oxygen consumption (VO_2) and it can easily be shown that the inverse of this relationship is equivalent to renal extraction of O_2 (O_2Ex). An increase in renal O_2Ex means that renal DO_2 has decreased in relation to renal VO_2, i. e., renal oxygenation is impaired, and *vice versa*. When compared to other major organs, renal VO_2 is relatively high, second only to the heart. In sedated, mechanically ventilated patients, renal VO_2 is two-thirds (10 ml/min) that of myocardial oxygen consumption (15 ml/min) (Table 1) [1, 2]. Renal blood flow, which accounts for approximately 20 % of cardiac output, is three times higher than myocardial blood flow in this group of patients. Renal O_2Ex in the non-failing kidney is therefore low, 10 %, compared with, e.g., the heart, in which O_2E_X is 55 % (Table 1).

S.-E. Ricksten (✉)
Department of Anesthesiology and Intensive Care Medicine, Sahlgrenska Academy, University of Gothenburg, Sahlgrenska University Hospital, 413 45 Gothenburg, Sweden
E-mail: sven-erik.ricksten@aniv.gu.se

G. Bragadottir
Department of Anesthesiology and Intensive Care Medicine, Sahlgrenska Academy, University of Gothenburg, Sahlgrenska University Hospital, 413 45 Gothenburg, Sweden

B. Redfors
Department of Anesthesiology and Intensive Care Medicine, Sahlgrenska Academy, University of Gothenburg, Sahlgrenska University Hospital, 413 45 Gothenburg, Sweden

J.-L. Vincent (Ed.), *Annual Update in Intensive Care and Emergency Medicine 2013*, DOI 10.1007/978-3-642-35109-9_54, © Springer-Verlag Berlin Heidelberg and BioMed Central Ltd. 2013

Table 1 Renal and myocardial oxygen/demand supply relationship in postoperative mechanically ventilated patients

	Kidney	Heart
Oxygen consumption (ml/min)	10	15
Blood flow (ml/min)	750	250
Oxygen extraction (%)	10	55

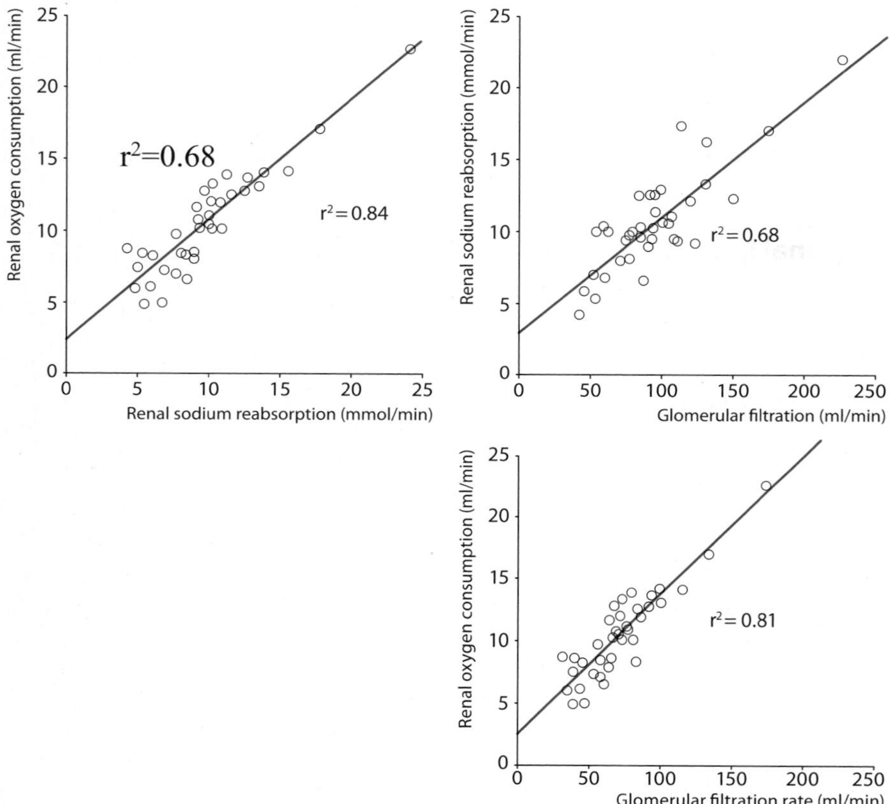

Fig. 1 Demonstrates the close relationships between renal sodium reabsorption, renal oxygen consumption and glomerular filtration rate in postoperative patients (n = 37) undergoing uncomplicated cardiac surgery. Data from [2]

Determinants of Renal Oxygenation

It is well known from experimental studies that tubular sodium reabsorption is the major determinant of renal VO_2 [3] and that under normal physiological conditions, approximately 80 % is used to drive active tubular transport of particularly sodium, but also glucose, amino acids and other solutes. Tubular transport processes are highly load-dependent and it has been shown in experimental studies [4] and in patients [2, 5–7] that there is a close linear correlation between glomerular filtration rate (GFR), renal sodium reabsorption and renal VO_2 (Fig. 1). The filtered load of sodium is, thus, an important determinant of renal VO_2 and maneuvers that decrease GFR and the tubular sodium load act to decrease tubular sodium reabsorption and renal VO_2, and *vice versa* [8]. It has been shown that renal O_2Ex remains stable over a wide range of renal blood flows, which means that changes in renal DO_2, caused by changes in renal blood flow, are directly offset by changes in renal VO_2 [9], i. e., renal VO_2 is flow-dependent. Thus, unlike other organs where increases in blood flow will improve oxygenation, increased renal blood flow augments GFR and the filtered load of sodium, which will increase renal VO_2. Due to this flow-dependency of renal VO_2, renal oxygenation will remain constant, as long as renal blood flow and GFR change in parallel.

Regional Intrarenal Oxygenation and Medullary Hypoxia

The relatively high renal blood flow is directed preferentially to the cortex to optimize the filtration process and solute reabsorption. In contrast, blood flow in the outer medulla is less than 50 % of the cortical blood flow to preserve osmotic gradients and to enhance urinary concentration [10]. The combination of low medullary perfusion, high oxygen consumption of the medullary thick ascending limbs (mTAL) and the countercurrent exchange of oxygen within the vasa recta, results in a poorly oxygenated outer medulla [11]. Oxygen availability is, therefore, low in the outer medulla, which has an oxygen tissue partial pressure (PO_2) of 10–20 mm Hg compared to 50 mm Hg in the cortex. Thus, as the outer medulla is on the border of hypoxia already under normal conditions, it is particularly sensitive to prolonged or intermittent episodes of low renal DO_2, caused by hypoperfusion or hemodilution. This condition may occur, in particular, after major surgery (especially cardiac or vascular surgery) or severe heart failure, which are common causes of ischemic acute kidney injury (AKI) in the intensive care unit (ICU).

Cardiovascular surgery is a 'clinical model' of human AKI. Because it is known when postoperative AKI may occur, in this group of patients, timely, therapeutic interventions for prevention and treatment of early AKI could be instituted. In this situation, it would be logical to improve the renal oxygen supply/demand relationship by augmenting renal DO_2 and/or reducing renal VO_2, i. e., to improve renal oxygenation.

Effects of Diuretics on Renal Oxygenation in the Postoperative Patient

It has repeatedly been shown in experimental studies that furosemide and other loop-diuretics (ethacrynic acid, bumetanide) inhibit renal sodium reabsorption and

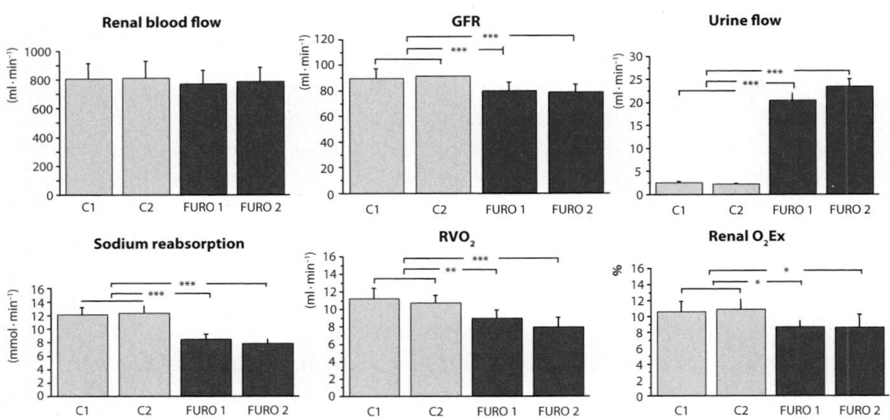

Fig. 2 Renal effects of furosemide 0.5 mg/kg bolus + 0.5 mg/kg/h infusion on renal blood flow, glomerular filtration rate (GFR), urine flow, sodium reabsorption, renal oxygen consumption (RVO_2) and renal oxygen extraction (renal O_2Ex). Furosemide improves renal oxygenation by a decrease in renal sodium reabsorption and RVO_2. Data from [5]

VO_2 in the mTAL (e.g., [12]). This decrease in reabsorptive work will increase oxygen availability and consequently increase the tissue PO_2 of the medulla [11]. Because of this decrease in renal oxygen demand, furosemide could potentially exert preventive renoprotective effects. Indeed, several reports have demonstrated that furosemide causes renoprotection in experimental ischemic AKI (e.g., [13, 14]). Most likely this is mediated by a decrease in medullary VO_2 which will increase the tolerance to renal ischemia, but it has also been suggested that the greater urine flow may 'flush out' tubular casts and thereby reduce intratubular obstruction and the back-leak of filtered urine [15].

Prasad et al. demonstrated in conscious volunteers that 20 mg of furosemide increased medullary oxygenation, using the blood oxygen level-dependent magnetic resonance imaging technique (BOLD MRI) [16]. In contrast, acetazolamide, which inhibits tubular reabsorption of the proximal tubules in the cortex and which does not affect medullary PO_2 in experimental studies, did not affect medullary oxygenation.

Swärd et al. evaluated the renal effects of a bolus dose of furosemide (0.5 mg/kg) followed by an infusion (0.5 mg/kg/h) in the early period after cardiac surgery with cardiopulmonary bypass (CPB), using the retrograde renal vein thermodilution technique and renal extraction of ^{51}chromium-ethylene-diaminetetraacetic acid (^{51}Cr-EDTA) for rapid bedside estimation of RBF and GFR without the need for urine collection [5] (Fig. 2). Furosemide increased fractional excretion of sodium (excreted sodium/filtered sodium) from 2 % to 25 % and caused a 10-fold increase in urine flow because of a 28 % decrease in tubular sodium reabsorption. These changes were in turn associated with a 23 % decrease in renal VO_2. Thus, furosemide decreased renal O_2Ex and improved renal oxygenation as renal blood flow was not significantly affected by the diuretic. Interestingly, GFR decreased by 12 % with furosemide, which could be explained by an increased delivery of sodium to the distal tubules activating the tubuloglomerular feedback mechanism, eventually inducing a constriction of the afferent arterioles and a decrease in GFR [17]. This mechanism could explain the findings of Lassnigg et al., who demonstrated in low-risk cardiac surgery patients with normal renal function that furosemide lowered creatinine clearance postoperatively [18]. The authors, therefore, suggested that loop-diuretics could be detrimental to the patients in terms of renal function and outcome. Another hypothesis would be that furosemide improves the renal oxygen demand/supply relationship and, thus, could increase the tolerance to perioperative renal ischemia, and that the mild to moderate fall in GFR with furosemide is a direct pharmacological consequence (tubuloglomerular feedback activation) of the agent which, if anything, would further decrease renal VO_2. In future studies, the potential preventive renoprotective effects of furosemide should be evaluated in high-risk surgical patients. Furthermore, GFR or creatinine clearance should not be used as the early primary end-point in such studies, because of the furosemide-induced pharmacological activation of the tubuloglomerular feedback mechanism, which will *per se* decrease GFR. Instead markers of tubular injury should be measured, to evaluate whether or not the improved renal oxygenation with furosemide could prevent tubular ischemic cell injury in high-risk surgical patients.

Effects of Dopaminergic Agents on Renal Oxygenation in the Postoperative Patient

Dopamine has been used to prevent acute renal dysfunction in cardiac surgery in the belief that dopamine increases renal blood flow. The preventive effect has, however, been questioned [19–21]. A prospective, randomized controlled trial showed that low-dose dopamine did not affect renal outcome in septic patients with early AKI [22]. It has also been speculated that a dopamine-induced inhibition of proximal tubular Na^+ reabsorption may increase delivery of Na^+ to potentially ischemic distal tubular cells in the medulla, which would increase their oxygen demands [19]. Thus, a dopamine-induced increase in renal VO_2 may have the potential to impair renal oxygenation, which could be detrimental in the treatment of early ischemic acute renal failure [19].

Redfors et al. recently studied the effects of low-dose (2–4 μg/kg/min) dopamine on renal blood flow, GFR, tubular sodium reabsorption, renal VO_2 and the renal oxygen demand/supply relationship in post-cardiac surgery patients [23]. Renal blood flow was estimated by two independent techniques, the retrograde renal vein thermodilution technique and the paraaminohippuric acid (PAH) infusion clearance technique, with correction for renal extraction of PAH. Interestingly, low-dose dopamine induced pronounced renal vasodilation with a 45–55 % increase in renal blood flow. One would expect that such a marked increase in renal blood flow would be accompanied by a proportional increase in GFR (Fig. 3).

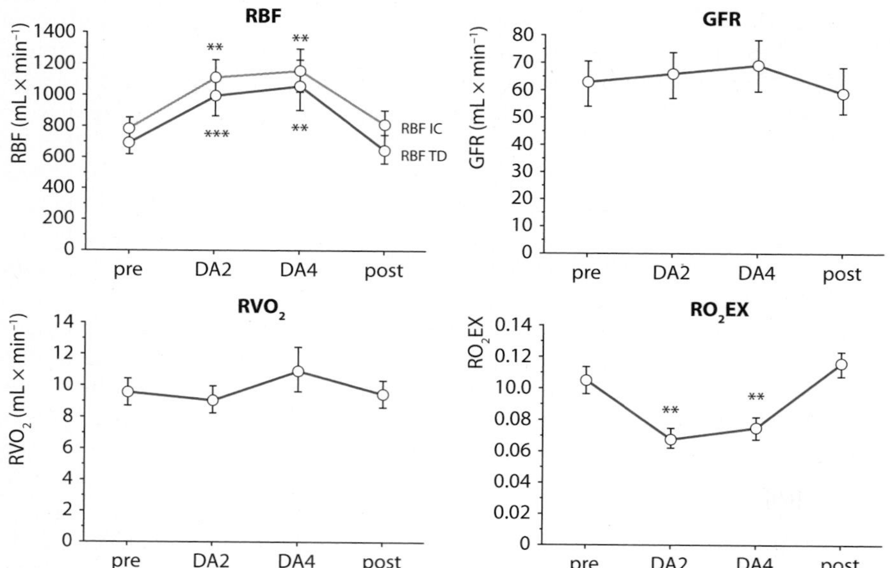

Fig. 3 Effects of 2 and 4 μg/kg/min of dopamine (DA2, DA4) on renal blood flow (RBF), glomerular filtration rate (GFR), renal oxygen consumption (RVO_2) and renal oxygen extraction (RO_2Ex) in postoperative patients. RBF was measured by two independent techniques, retrograde renal vein thermodilution (RBF-TD) and infusion clearance for paraaminohippuric acid (PAH), with correction for renal extraction of PAH (RBF-IC). Note that low-dose dopamine improved renal oxygenation by a profound renal vasodilation with no changes in GFR or RVO_2. From [23] with permission

However, GFR was not significantly affected by dopamine. Thus, because of the lack of effect of dopamine on GFR, renal VO_2 was not affected and, consequently, renal oxygenation was improved (Fig. 3). Thus, the hypothesis put forward by Jones and Bellomo [19], that dopamine may impair renal oxygenation is not supported by the data from Redfors et al. [23].

The lack of effect of dopamine on GFR in postoperative patients highlights the common misunderstanding that an increase in renal blood flow by a renal vasodilator is always accompanied by an increase in GFR. The effect of a renal vasodilator on GFR is dependent on its effect on the longitudinal distribution of renal vascular resistance. The dopamine-induced increase in renal blood flow with no significant effect on GFR is explained by a renal vasodilatory action on pre- and postglomerular resistance vessels. Experimental studies have revealed that dopamine-mediated renal vasodilation predominantly is effected at the post-synaptic dopamine-1 (DA-1) receptors and that dopamine and other DA-1-receptor agonists dilate afferent and efferent arterioles to the same degree [24]. Studies on the effects of low-dose dopamine in volunteers or patients on renal plasma flow and GFR, as measured by clearance techniques are listed in Table 2. Note that in all studies, renal plasma flow increased, whereas in half the studies, GFR was not

Table 2 Effects of low-dose dopamine on renal plasma flow (RPF) and glomerular filtration rate (GFR) in healthy volunteers and patients, as assessed by clearance techniques

Author [ref]	Year	Patients	RPF	GFR
Ter Wee [51]	1986	Volunteers	Increase	Increase
Schoors [52]	1990	Volunteers	Increase	No effect
Olsen [53]	1993	Volunteers	Increase	No effect
Olsen [54]	1993	Volunteers	Increase	Increase
Olsen [55]	1994	Volunteers	Increase	No effect
Richer [56]	1996	Volunteers	Increase	No effect
McDonald [57]	1964	Heart failure	Increase	Increase
Rosenblum [58]	1972	Heart failure	Increase	Increase
Schwartz [59]	1988	Vascular surgery	Increase	Increase
Graves [60]	1993	Burn injury	Increase	No effect
Ungar [61]	2004	Heart failure	Increase	Increase
Redfors [23]	2010	Cardiac surgery	Increase	No effect

affected; in the remaining half, the increase in GFR was considerably lower than the increase in renal plasma flow.

The capacity of dopamine to improve renal oxygenation in postoperative patients would make it suitable for prevention of AKI, as it would increase the tolerance to renal ischemia in major surgery. However, the potential preventive effect of dopamine has not been evaluated in high-risk cardiovascular surgery. Although interest in the use of dopamine for renoprotection has decreased, interest in the use of another dopaminergic agent, fenoldopam, which exerts the same renal effects as dopamine [24], is, strangely enough, increasing. Fenoldopam is a selective dopamine-1 receptor agonist with no ß-1 or α-adrenergic receptor agonistic effects and similar to dopamine, it increases renal plasma flow with no effects on GFR, as demonstrated in healthy volunteers [25]. In three preventive, randomized controlled trials in abdominal aortic surgery [26] and high-risk cardiac surgery [27], fenoldopam improved creatinine clearance compared to placebo. These beneficial effects on renal outcome with fenoldopam and the lack of similar beneficial effects with dopamine (see above), despite similar pharmacological actions, could be explained by the fact that the potential preventive renal effects with dopamine and fenoldopam were evaluated in low-risk and high-risk patients, respectively. Bove et al. compared the preventive effects of fenoldopam and dopamine (2.5 μg/kg/min) on renal excretory function in high-risk cardiac surgery and found, not surprisingly, no difference between the two dopaminergic agents on percentage postoperative increase in serum creatinine [28].

Renal Oxygenation in Clinical Ischemic Acute Kidney Injury

Patients undergoing cardiac surgery with CPB are at high risk of developing postoperative AKI, with a reported incidence of 15–30 %, causing significant morbidity and mortality [29, 30]. In patients undergoing major cardiovascular surgery, even minor changes in serum creatinine are associated with increased in-patient mortality [31]. Postoperative AKI in this group of patients is considered a consequence of impaired renal DO_2, in turn caused by intra-operative hypotension and hemodilution-induced anemia [32], as well as perioperative low cardiac output [29].

It has provocatively been stated that "acute renal failure is acute renal success" [33, 34], as a reduction in GFR in AKI should lead to a reduction in the renal reabsorptive workload, thus preserving medullary oxygenation with a reduced risk of further aggravation of ischemia. In patients with AKI, there are few data on renal VO_2, renal blood flow, GFR and renal oxygenation and current views on renal oxygenation are presumptive and largely based on experimental studies.

Redfors et al. recently studied renal perfusion, filtration and oxygenation in patients with preoperative normal renal function developing early AKI (50–200 % increase in serum creatinine) after complicated cardiac surgery [2]. Renal blood flow was measured by renal vein retrograde thermodilution and by infusion clearance of PAH corrected for renal extraction of PAH. In spite of a normalization of cardiac index (CI) with inotropic treatment with or without intra-aortic balloon pump (IABP), renal oxygenation was severely impaired in patients with early AKI, as demonstrated by a 70 % relative increase in renal O_2Ex, compared to uncomplicated post-cardiac surgery patients with normal renal function This was, in turn, caused by a pronounced renal vasoconstriction and a 40 % lower renal blood flow, in combination with a renal VO_2 that was not significantly different from the control group, despite the 60 % decrease in GFR and renal tubular sodium reabsorption (Table 3). Thus, the renal VO_2 of the AKI patients was 1.9 ml/mmol reabsorbed sodium, a value that was 2.4 times higher than in the uncomplicated control group (0.82 ml/mmol reabsorbed sodium). Figure 4 shows the close correlation between GFR and renal VO_2 in patients with early AKI after cardiac surgery versus those undergoing uncomplicated surgery with no renal impairment. According to the "acute renal success"-hypothesis [42–44], as put forward by several researchers, AKI patients should operate on the lower part of the regression line of the control patients. However, the regression line of the AKI patients is clearly shifted to the left, i. e., at a certain GFR, renal VO_2 is higher, speaking against this hypothesis. On the contrary, the 40 % decrease in renal DO_2 in combination with a tubular sodium reabsorption at a high oxygen demand, suggests that renal hypoxia is present after the initiation phase of ischemic AKI.

One can only speculate on the mechanisms underlying the leftward shift of the GFR/renal VO_2 relationship in AKI patients. A potential explanation could be loss of epithelial cell-polarization and tight junction integrity in AKI, as has been shown in experimental studies and after human renal transplantation [35], making tubular sodium reabsorption less efficient [36]. Another explanation may be diminished renal nitric oxide (NO) generation because of endothelial damage and

Table 3 Renal perfusion, filtration and oxygenation in postoperative acute kidney injury (AKI) [2]

	Control group (n = 37)	AKI group (n = 12)	p-value
Mean arterial pressure (mm Hg)	73.9 ± 1.1	73.5 ± 0.7	ns
Cardiac index (l/min/m^2)	2.63 ± 0.08	2.77 ± 0.16	ns
RBF (ml/min)	758 ± 40	477 ± 54	<0.001
RVR (mm Hg/ml/min)	0.097 ± 0.005	0.146 ± 0.015	<0.01
GFR (ml/min)	74.7 ± 4.7	32.3 ± 3.6	<0.001
Sodium reabsorption (mmol/min)	9.7 ± 0.7	4.0 ± 0.4	<0.001
Renal oxygen consumption (ml/min)	10.4 ± 0.6	11.0 ± 1.1	ns
Renal oxygen extraction	0.097 ± 0.004	0.163 ± 0.009	<0.001

RBF: renal blood flow assessed by the thermodilution technique; RVR: renal vascular resistance; GFR: glomerular filtration rate. Values are means ± SEM.

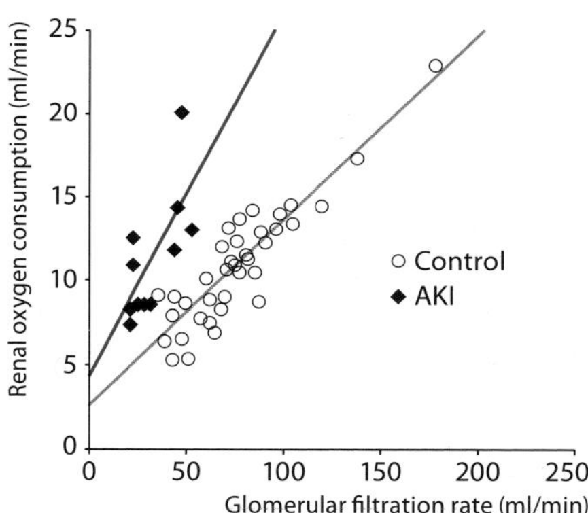

Fig. 4 Close correlation between glomerular filtration rate and renal oxygen consumption in uncomplicated post-cardiac surgery patients (controls, n = 37) and in patients with postoperative acute kidney injury (AKI). Note that the slope of the regression line is steeper in the AKI group. Thus filtration and reabsorbtion of sodium consumes approximately 2.5 times more oxygen in the AKI group. From [2] with permission

downregulation of endothelial NO synthase (eNOS/NOS-3). NO is a major regulator of microvascular oxygen supply and renal VO_2 [37]. Through vasodilation, NO increases renal blood flow and hence DO_2. Furthermore, contemporary work suggests that NO acts as a 'brake' on oxidative metabolism at various sites, including direct competition of NO with oxygen for mitochondrial respiration and inhibition of cytochrome c oxidase [38].

Treatment of Clinical Ischemic AKI

The major goal in the management of early AKI is to increase GFR. However, because of the close association between GFR, tubular sodium reabsorption and renal VO_2 in humans [5–7], a pharmacologically-induced increase in GFR will

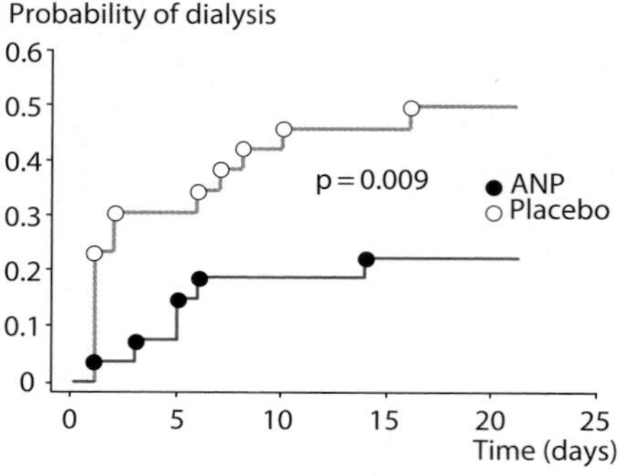

Fig. 5 Effects of atrial natriuretic peptide (ANP) vs placebo on probability of dialysis in post-cardiac surgery patients with early acute kidney injury. Modified from [40] with permission

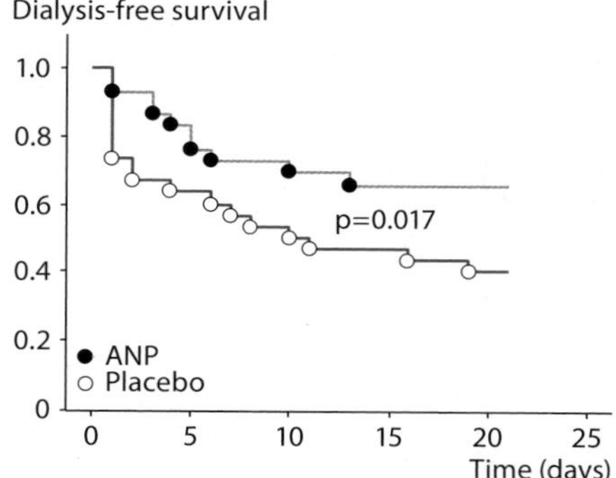

Fig. 6 Effects of atrial natriuretic peptide (ANP) vs placebo on dialysis-free survival in post-cardiac surgery patients with early acute kidney injury. Modified from [40] with permission

increase renal VO_2 and potentially further impair renal oxygenation in patients with AKI. Thus, an ideal agent to treat ischemic AKI would be one that increases both renal blood flow and GFR, i. e., an agent that preferentially induces vasodilation of the preglomerular resistance vessels. Such an agent will not only increase GFR but also meet the increased renal metabolic demand of the medulla by an increase in renal DO_2. It is not likely that the potent renal vasodilator, dopamine, will improve GFR in early clinical ischemic AKI as it exerts a non-specific renal vasodilation of pre- and postglomerular resistance vessels with a pronounced effect on total renal vascular resistance and renal blood flow but with no or minor effects on glomerular hydraulic pressure and GFR (see above). This could explain why low-dose dopamine (2 µg/kg/min) does not improve renal outcome, measured as peak serum creatinine, in ICU patients with systemic inflammatory response syndrome and early AKI [22].

Atrial natriuretic peptide (ANP) is a renal vasodilator, which causes a balanced 30–40 % increase in both renal blood flow and GFR in patients with early ischemic AKI after complicated cardiac surgery [39]. Although, the effects of ANP on renal oxygenation have not been studied, it is less likely that ANP would impair renal oxygenation because of its preferential action on the preglomerular resistance vessels. This is further supported by the findings from a prospective, randomized, blinded trial by Swärd et al., who showed that infusion of ANP en-

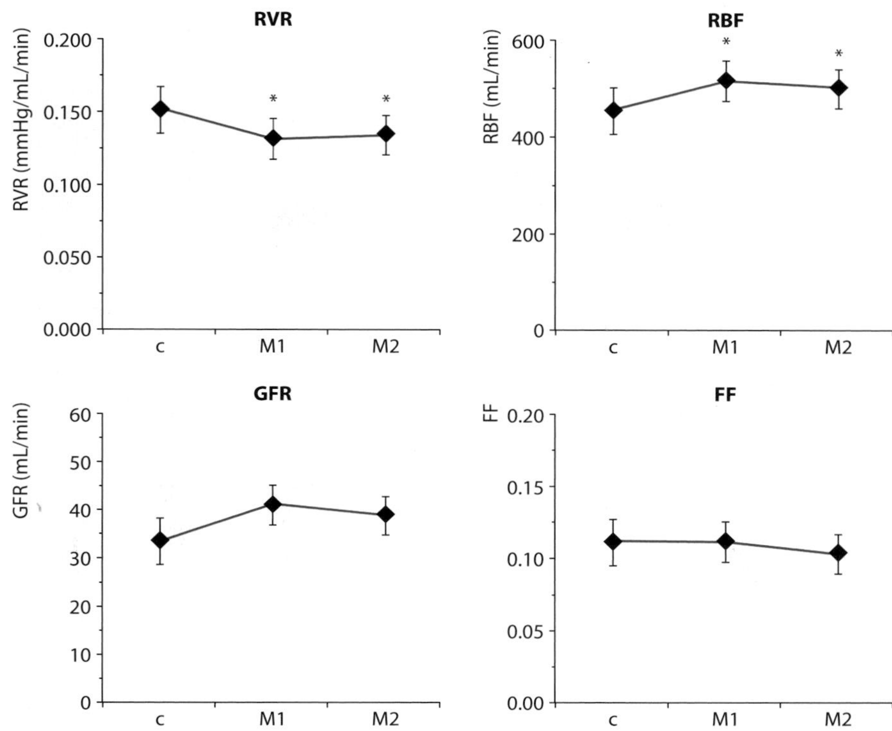

Fig. 7 Effects of mannitol (M1, M2) on renal vascular resistance (RVR), renal blood flow (RBF), glomerular filtration rate (GFR) and renal filtration fraction (FF) in patients with early acute kidney injury after cardiac surgery. * $p < 0.05$ Modified from [44]

hanced renal excretory function, decreased the probability of dialysis and improved dialysis-free survival in early, ischemic AKI after complicated cardiac surgery [40] (Figs. 5 and 6).

Another approach for the treatment of clinical ischemic AKI would be to target the vascular endothelium and tubular epithelium. Experimental studies have shown that mannitol may decrease ischemia-induced swelling of tubular cells, which might obstruct the tubular lumen [41]. Mannitol treatment has been shown to increase GFR in patients after severe trauma or surgery [42]. In addition, our group has shown that mannitol increases GFR in postoperative cardiac surgery patients possibly by a de-swelling effect on tubular cells [6]. Furthermore, it has been suggested that outer medullary hypoxia may cause endothelial ischemic injury and endothelial cell swelling contributing to congestion and impaired perfusion of this region [43], which could, at least to some extent, explain the high renal vascular resistance seen in clinical early AKI [2]. The effects of mannitol treatment on renal perfusion, filtration and oxygenation were recently studied in patients with normal preoperative creatinine, who developed early AKI after complicated cardiac surgery, requiring inotropic support with or without IABP [44].

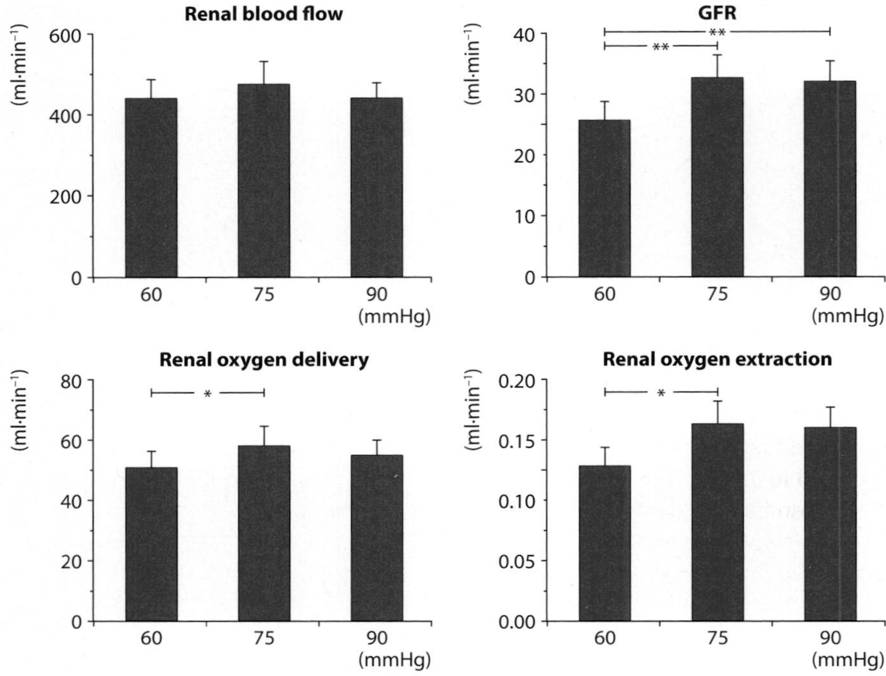

Fig. 8 Renal effects of norepinephrine (NE)-induced variations in target mean arterial pressures (MAP) in post-cardiac surgery patients with NE-dependent vasodilatory shock and acute kidney injury. Restoration of MAP from 60 to 75 mm Hg improves renal oxygen delivery, GFR and the renal oxygen supply/demand relationship. This pressure-dependent renal perfusion, filtration and oxygenation at levels of MAP below 75 mm Hg reflect a more or less exhausted renal autoregulatory reserve. Data from [47]

Mannitol induced a 60 % increase in diuresis, which was accompanied by decrease in renal vascular resistance and a 12–15 % increase in renal blood flow, while no effects were seen on cardiac index or cardiac filling pressures. Mannitol did not affect filtration fraction or renal oxygenation, suggestive of balanced increases in perfusion/filtration and renal oxygen demand/supply (Fig. 7).

Vasodilatory Shock and AKI: Role of Norepinephrine

Vasodilatory shock is not uncommon after complicated cardiac surgery with CPB and occurs often in conjunction with postoperative heart failure [45]. The recommended agent for treatment of volume-resuscitated vasodilatory shock is norepinephrine [46]. Patients with vasodilatory shock after cardiac surgery with CPB may suffer from concomitant AKI. The use of norepinephrine for treatment of vasodilatory shock in patients with ischemic AKI with impaired renal oxygenation is a "two-edged sword" as it may further aggravate renal ischemia. On the other hand, too low a dose of norepinephrine may result in an arterial blood pressure that may be below the limit of renal autoregulation, i. e., when renal blood flow becomes pressure-dependent.

In a recent study in post-cardiac surgery patients with norpinephrine-dependent vasoplegia and concomitant AKI, the effects of norepinephrine on renal perfusion, filtration and oxygenation were evaluated [47]. Norepinephrine infusion rate was randomly and sequentially titrated to target a mean arterial pressures (MAP) of 60, 75 and 90 mm Hg. At each target MAP, data on renal blood flow, GFR and renal O_2Ex were obtained by the renal vein thermodilution technique and by renal extraction of ^{51}Cr-EDTA. At a target MAP of 75 mm Hg, renal DO_2 (13 %), GFR (27 %) and urine flow were higher and renal O_2Ex was lower (–7.4 %) compared with a target MAP of 60 mm Hg. However, the renal variables did not differ when compared at target MAPs of 75 and 90 mm Hg (Fig. 8). Thus, restoration of MAP from 60 to 75 mm Hg improves renal DO_2, GFR and renal oxygenation in patients with vasodilatory shock and AKI. The pressure-dependent renal perfusion, filtration and oxygenation at levels of MAP below 75 mm Hg reflect a more or less exhausted renal autoregulatory reserve.

Low-Dose Vasopressin and Renal Oxygenation

Resistance to norepinephrine and other catecholamines may develop in vasodilatory shock because of adrenergic receptor downregulation and endogenous vasodilators. Furthermore, plasma levels of vasopressin are low in post-cardiotomy vasodilatory shock and in septic shock in contrast to hypovolemic and cardiogenic shock [48]. Vasopressin has, therefore, been suggested as an additional or an alternative therapy in catecholamine-dependent vasodilatory shock [49]. It has also been reported that vasopressin increases creatinine clearance, a surrogate variable of GFR, in these patients [50]. A more detailed analysis on the effects of low-dose vasopressin on renal oxygenation is lacking.

Bragadottir et al. evaluated the renal effects of low-doses (1.2, 2.4, 4.8 U/h) of vasopressin in post-cardiac surgery patients, doses that did not affect systemic blood pressure [7]. Vasopressin exerted a dose-dependent increase in GFR, sodium reabsorption, renal VO_2, renal O_2Ex and renal vascular resistance, whereas renal blood flow decreased. Thus, vasopressin considerably impaired renal oxygenation by postglomerular vasoconstriction, which induced a decrease in renal blood flow and an increase in both GFR and renal VO_2 (Fig. 9). From a renal point of view, vasopressin should be used with caution in the treatment of vasodilatory shock, because it has the potential to cause considerable renal oxygen supply/demand mismatch.

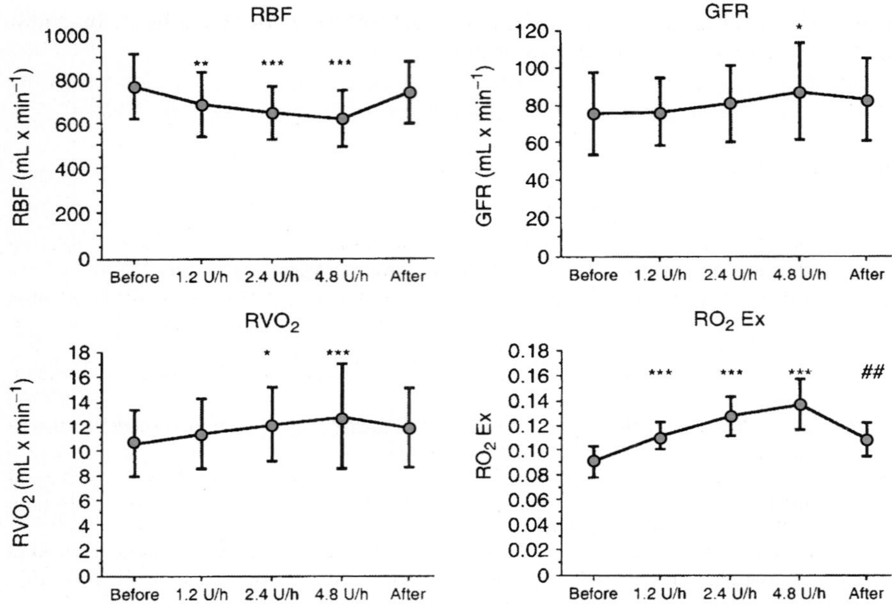

Fig. 9 Effects of incremental infusion rates of vasopressin (1.2, 2.4 and 4.8 units/hour) on renal blood flow (RBF), glomerular filtration rate (GFR), renal oxygen consumption (RVO_2) and renal oxygen extraction (RO_2Ex) in post-cardiac surgery patients. Vasopressin causes a constriction of renal efferent arterioles with a decrease in RBF and an increase in GFR and RVO_2.Vasopressin impairs the renal oxygen demand/supply relationship as reflected by the increase in RO_2Ex. From [7] with permission

Conclusion

In spite of the apparent luxury oxygenation of the kidneys, with a high renal DO_2 in relation to renal VO_2, the outer medulla is on the border of hypoxia in the normal situation. Outer medullary hypoxia, caused by low medullary perfusion, high VO_2 of the medullary thick ascending limbs and the countercurrent exchange of oxygen, is the price the kidneys have to pay for the urine concentration mechanism. The outer medulla is, therefore, particularly sensitive to prolonged or intermittent episodes of low renal DO_2. Dopaminergic agents (dopamine/fenoldopam) and loop-diuretics improve renal oxygenation, and potentially prevent ischemic AKI, whereas vasopressin impairs renal oxygenation in postoperative patients.

Renal oxygenation is impaired in early clinical ischemic AKI because of a low renal blood flow, caused by vasoconstriction and endothelial swelling, in combination with a tubular reabsorption at a high oxygen demand. ANP is ideally suited for treatment of ischemic AKI, as it preferentially dilates the preglomerular resistance vessels; this will increase GFR but also renal blood flow, meeting the increased oxygen demand of the medulla by an increase in renal DO_2. Mannitol increases renal blood flow and GFR in clinical ischemic AKI most likely by endothelial and epithelial de-swelling effects.

References

1. Zäll S, Milocco I, Ricksten SE (1991) Effects of adenosine on myocardial blood flow and metabolism after coronary artery bypass surgery. Anesth Analg 73:689–695
2. Redfors B, Bragadottir G, Sellgren J, Swärd K, Ricksten SE (2010) Acute renal failure is NOT an "acute renal success" – a clinical study on the renal oxygen supply/demand relationship in acute kidney injury. Crit Care Med 38:1695–1701
3. Kiil F, Aukland K, Refsum HE (1961) Renal sodium transport and oxygen consumption. Am J Physiol 201:511–516
4. Torelli G, Milla E, Faelli A, Costantini S (1966) Energy requirement for sodium reabsorption in the in vivo rabbit kidney. Am J Physiol 211:576–580
5. Swärd K, Valsson F, Sellgren J, Ricksten SE (2004) Differential effects of human atrial natriuretic peptide and furosemide on glomerular filtration rate and renal oxygen consumption in humans. Intensive Care Med 31:79–85
6. Redfors B, Swärd K, Sellgren J, Ricksten SE (2009) Effects of mannitol alone and mannitol plus furosemide on renal oxygen consumption, blood flow and glomerular filtration after cardiac surgery. Intensive Care Med 35:115–122
7. Bragadottir G, Redfors B, Nygren A, Sellgren J, Ricksten SE (2009) Low-dose vasopressin increases glomerular filtration rate, but impairs renal oxygenation in post-cardiac surgery patients. Acta Anaesthesiol Scand 53:1052–1059
8. O'Connor PM (2006) Renal oxygen delivery: matching delivery to metabolic demand. Clin Exp Pharmacol Physiol 33:961–967
9. Levy MN (1960) Effect of variations of blood flow on renal oxygen extraction. Am J Physiol 199:13–18
10. Chou SY, Porush JG, Faubert PF (1990) Renal medullary circulation: hormonal control. Kidney Int 37:1–13
11. Brezis M, Rosen S (1995) Hypoxia of the renal medulla – its implications for disease. N Engl J Med 332:647–655
12. Aukland K, Johannesen J, Kiil F (1969) In vivo measurements of local metabolic rate in the dog kidney. Effect of mersalyl, chlorothiazide, ethacrynic acid and furosemide. Scand J Clin Lab Invest 23:317–330
13. Kramer HJ, Schuurmann J, Wassermann C, Dusing R (1980) Prostaglandin-independent protection by furosemide from oliguric ischaemic renal failure in conscious rats. Kidney Int 17:455–464
14. Bayati A, Nygren K, Kallskog O, Wolgast M (1990) The effect of loop diuretics on the long-term outcome of post-ischaemic acute renal failure in the rat. Acta Physiol Scand 139:271–279
15. Shilliday I, Allison ME (1994) Diuretics in acute renal failure. Ren Fail 16:3–17
16. Prasad PV, Edelman RR, Epstein FH (1996) Noninvasive evaluation of intrarenal oxygenation with BOLD MRI. Circulation 94:3271–3275
17. Cupples WA, Braam B (2007) Assessment of renal autoregulation. Am J Physiol Renal Physiol 292:F1105–F11223
18. Lassnigg A, Donner E, Grubhofer G, Presterl E, Druml W, Hiesmayr M (2000) Lack of renoprotective effects of dopamine and furosemide during cardiac surgery. J Am Soc Nephrol 11:97–104
19. Jones D, Bellomo R (2005) Renal-dose dopamine: from hypothesis to paradigm to dogma to myth and, finally, superstition? J Intensive Care Med 20:199–211

20. Marik PE (2002) Low-dose dopamine: a systematic review. Intensive Care Med 28:877–883
21. Woo EB, Tang AT, el-Gamel A et al (2002) Dopamine therapy for patients at risk of renal dysfunction following cardiac surgery: science or fiction? Eur J Cardiothorac Surg 22:106–111
22. Bellomo R, Chapman M, Finfer S, Hickling K, Myburgh J (2000) Low-dose dopamine in patients with early renal dysfunction: a placebo-controlled randomised trial. Australian and New Zealand Intensive Care Society (ANZICS) Clinical Trials Group. Lancet 356:2139–2143
23. Redfors B, Bragadottir G, Sellgren J, Swärd K, Ricksten SE (2010) Dopamine increases renal oxygenation: a clinical study in post-cardiac surgery patients. Acta Anaesthesiol Scand 54:183–190
24. Edwards RM (1986) Comparison of the effects of fenoldopam, SK & F R-87516 and dopamine on renal arterioles in vitro. Eur J Pharmacol 126:167–170
25. Mathur VS, Swan SK, Anjum S, Lambrecht LJ et al (1999) The effects of fenoldopam, a selective dopamine receptor agonist, on systemic and renal hemodynamics in normotensive subjects. Crit Care Med 27:1832–1837
26. Halpenny M, Rushe C, Breen P, Cunningham AJ, Boucher-Hayes D, Shorten GD (2002) The effects of fenoldopam on renal function in patients undergoing elective aortic surgery. Eur J Anaesthesiol 19:32–39
27. Cogliati AA, Vellutini R, Nardini A et al (2007) Fenoldopam infusion for renal protection in high-risk cardiac surgery patients: a randomized clinical study. J Cardiothorac Vasc Anesth 21:847–850
28. Bove T, Landoni G, Calabrò MG et al (2005) Renoprotective action of fenoldopam in high-risk patients undergoing cardiac surgery: a prospective, double-blind, randomized clinical trial. Circulation 111:3230–3235
29. Mangano CM, Diamondstone LS, Ramsay JG, Aggarwal A, Herskowitz A, Mangano DT (1998) Renal dysfunction after myocardial revascularization: risk factors, adverse outcomes, and hospital resource utilization. The Multicenter Study of Perioperative Ischemia Research Group. Ann Intern Med 128:194–203
30. Englberger L, Suri RM, Li Z et al (2011) Clinical accuracy of RIFLE and Acute Kidney Injury Network (AKIN) criteria for acute kidney injury in patients undergoing cardiac surgery. Crit Care 15:R16
31. Lassnigg A, Schmidlin D, Mouhieddine M et al (2004) Minimal changes of serum creatinine predict prognosis in patients after cardiothoracic surgery: a prospective cohort study. J Am Soc Nephrol 15:1597–1605
32. Kanji HD, Schulze CJ, Hervas-Malo M et al (2010) Difference between pre-operative and cardiopulmonary bypass mean arterial pressure is independently associated with early cardiac surgery-associated acute kidney injury. J Cardiothorac Surg 5:71
33. Thurau K, Boylan JW (1976) Acute renal success. The unexpected logic of oliguria in acute renal failure. Am J Med 61:308–315
34. Rosenberger C, Rosen S, Heyman SN (2006) Renal parenchymal oxygenation and hypoxia adaptation in acute kidney injury. Clin Exp Pharmacol Physiol 33:980–988
35. Molitoris BA, Falk SA, Dahl RH (1989) Ischemia-induced loss of epithelial polarity. Role of the tight junction. J Clin Invest 84:1334–1339
36. Molitoris BA (1993) Na(+)-K(+)-ATPase that redistributes to apical membrane during ATP depletion remains functional. Am J Physiol 265:F693–697
37. Laycock SK, Vogel T, Forfia PR et al (1998) Role of nitric oxide in the control of renal oxygen consumption and the regulation of chemical work in the kidney. Circ Res 82:1263–1271
38. Cleeter MW, Cooper JM, Darley-Usmar VM, Moncada S, Schapira AH (1994) Reversible inhibition of cytochrome c oxidase, the terminal enzyme of the mitochondrial respiratory chain, by nitric oxide. Implications for neurodegenerative diseases. FEBS Lett 345:50–54
39. Valsson F, Ricksten SE, Hedner T, Lundin S (1996) Effects of atrial natriuretic peptide on acute renal impairment in patients with heart failure after cardiac surgery. Intensive Care Med 22:230–236

40. Sward K, Valsson F, Odencrants P, Samuelsson O, Ricksten SE (2004) Recombinant human atrial natriuretic peptide in ischemic acute renal failure: a randomized placebo-controlled trial. Crit Care Med 32:1310–1315
41. Burke TJ, Cronin RE, Duchin KL, Peterson LN, Schrier RW (1980) Ischemia and tubule obstruction during acute renal failure in dogs: mannitol in protection. Am J Physiol 238:F305–F314
42. Valdes ME, Landau SE, Shah DM et al (1979) Increased glomerular filtration rate following mannitol administration in man. J Surg Res 26:473–477
43. Molitoris BA, Sandoval R, Sutton TA (2002) Endothelial injury and dysfunction in ischemic acute renal failure. Crit Care Med 30:S235–S240
44. Bragadottir G, Redfors B, Ricksten SE (2012) Mannitol increases renal blood flow and maintains filtration fraction and oxygenation in postoperative acute kidney injury – a prospective interventional study. Crit Care 16:R159
45. Kristof AS, Magder S (1999) Low systemic vascular resistance in patients undergoing cardiopulmonary bypass. Crit Care Med 27:1121–1127
46. Dellinger RP, Levy MM, Carlet JM et al (2008) Surviving sepsis campaign: international guidelines for management of severe sepsis and septic shock. Intensive Care Med 34:17–60
47. Redfors B, Bragadottir G, Sellgren J, Sward K, Ricksten SE (2011) Effects of norepinephrine on renal perfusion, filtration and oxygenation in vasodilatory shock and acute kidney injury. Intensive Care Med 37:60–67
48. Landry DW, Oliver JA (2001) The pathogenesis of vasodilatory shock. N Engl J Med 345:588–595
49. Landry DW, Levin HR, Gallant EM et al (1997) Vasopressin pressor hypersensitivity in vasodilatory septic shock. Crit Care Med 25:1279–1282
50. Patel BM, Chittock DR, Russell JA, Walley KR (2002) Beneficial effects of short-term vasopressin infusion during severe septic shock. Anesthesiology 96:576–582
51. ter Wee PM, Smit AJ, Rosman JB, Sluiter WJ, Donker AJ (1986) Effect of intravenous infusion of low-dose dopamine on renal function in normal individuals and in patients with renal disease. Am J Nephrol 6:42–46
52. Schoors DF, Dupont AG (1990) Further studies on the mechanism of the natriuretic response to low-dose dopamine in man: effect on lithium clearance and nephrogenic cAMP formation. Eur J Clin Invest 20:385–391
53. Olsen NV, Lund J, Jensen PF et al (1993) Dopamine, dobutamine, and dopexamine. A comparison of renal effects in unanesthetized human volunteers. Anesthesiology 79:685-594
54. Olsen NV, Hansen JM, Kanstrup IL, Richalet JP, Leyssac PP (1993) Renal hemodynamics, tubular function, and response to low-dose dopamine during acute hypoxia in humans. J Appl Physiol 74:2166–2173
55. Olsen NV, Lang-Jensen T, Hansen JM et al (1994) Effects of acute beta-adrenoceptor blockade with metoprolol on the renal response to dopamine in normal humans. Br J Clin Pharmacol 37:347–353
56. Richer M, Robert S, Lebel M (1996) Renal hemodynamics during norepinephrine and low-dose dopamine infusions in man. Crit Care Med 24:1150–1156
57. Mc Donald RH, Goldberg LI, McNay JL, Tuttle EP (1964) Effect of dopamine in man: Augmentation of sodium excretion, glomerular filtration rate and renal plasma flow. J Clin Invest 43:1116–1124
58. Rosenblum R, Tai AR, Lawson D (1972) Dopamine in man: cardiorenal hemodynamics in normotensive patients with heart disease. J Pharmacol Exp Ther 183:256–263
59. Schwartz LB, Bissell MG, Murphy M, Gewertz BL (1988) Renal effects of dopamine in vascular surgical patients. J Vasc Surg 8:367–374
60. Graves TA, Cioffi WG, Vaughan GM et al (1993) The renal effects of low-dose dopamine in thermally injured patients. J Trauma 35:97–102
61. Ungar A, Fumagalli S, Marini M et al (2004) Renal, but not systemic, hemodynamic effects of dopamine are influenced by the severity of congestive heart failure. Crit Care Med 32:1125–1129

NGAL in Acute Kidney Injury

O. Rewa and S. M. Bagshaw

Introduction

Acute kidney injury (AKI) represents an abrupt deterioration in kidney function and is a frequently encountered phenomenon in hospitalized patients [1, 2]. The impact of AKI is most profound among patients admitted to intensive care units (ICU). The incidence of AKI among hospitalized and critically ill patients appears to be increasing. This is likely attributable to demographic transition (i. e., older patients; more comorbid illness; greater prevalence of chronic kidney disease) coupled with admissions associated with increasingly complex medical and/or surgical diseases and the need for multi-faceted diagnostic and therapeutic interventions. The development of AKI now complicates the course in an estimated two-thirds of critically ill patients [3–5]. For those with more severe forms of AKI, an estimated 50–70 % will require support with acute renal replacement therapy (RRT), which represents a small, but important subgroup of all critically ill patients (4–8 %) [6]. The initiation of RRT can contribute to a considerable escalation in both the complexity of illness and associated costs of care. Indeed, these critically ill patients experience substantial morbidity, including non-recovery of kidney function and long-term chronic kidney disease or dialysis dependence [7–9] as well as excess mortality, with hospital mortality rates commonly exceeding 60 % [6, 8].

O. Rewa
Department of Critical Care Medicine, Faculty of Medicine, University of Toronto, Canada

S. M. Bagshaw (✉)
Division of Critical Care Medicine, Faculty of Medicine and Dentistry, University of Alberta, 3C1.12 Walter C. Mackenzie Center, 8440-112 ST NW, Edmonton, T6G287, Canada
E-mail: bagshaw@ualberta.ca

J.-L. Vincent (Ed.), *Annual Update in Intensive Care and Emergency Medicine 2013*,
DOI 10.1007/978-3-642-35109-9_55,

Classification of AKI

The diagnostic classification of AKI has evolved considerably in the last several years. In 2004, a consensus definition, the RIFLE classification scheme (Acronym: Risk, Injury, Failure, Loss and End-stage renal disease), was published by the Acute Dialysis Quality Initiative (ADQI) group [10]. This classification defined three grades of severity of AKI (Risk, Injury, Failure), based on relative changes to serum creatinine (sCr) and changes in urine output, and two outcome categories (Loss and End-Stage Kidney Disease) based on the duration of RRT. This novel classification scheme has been validated and widely integrated into the medical literature. The RIFLE classification was later refined by the Acute Kidney Injury Network (AKIN), a consortium uniting representatives from all major nephrology and critical care societies. This adaption specified a 48-hour timeline during which the acute changes in kidney function had to occur to fulfill the definition of AKI. The AKIN modification also simplified the stages of severity of AKI, with the first two representing worsening renal dysfunction and the third stage characterized by kidney failure and encompassing any patients initiated on RRT. The RIFLE/AKIN classification schemes have now been consolidated into the KDIGO Clinical Practice Guidelines for Acute Kidney Injury definition for AKI [11] (Table 1).

Although the development of this consensus classification scheme has been an important landmark for clinical care and research in AKI, it has recognized limitations. The integration of urine output criteria may be confounded by numerous factors unrelated to the severity of underlying kidney injury (e.g., inability to measure outside of intensive monitoring settings; diuretic therapy). In addition, the stages associated with severity of urine output and sCr criteria may not be aligned in terms of prognosis (e.g., Stage 2 by sCr criteria associated with higher mortality

Table 1 Acute kidney injury (AKI) definition (KDIGO Clinical Practice Guidelines for Acute Kidney Injury) [11]

Stage	Serum creatinine criteria	Urine output criteria
1	Increase in sCr $\geq$ 26.4 µmol/l or Increase in sCr to 1.5–1.9 times baseline	$<$0.5 ml/kg/h for 6–12 hours
2	Increase in sCr to 2.0–2.9 times baseline	$<$0.5 ml/kg/h for $\geq$ 12 hours
3	Increase in sCr $\geq$ 3 times baseline or Increase in sCr $\geq$ 354 µmol/l or Initiation of RRT or For patients $<$ 18 years, decrease in eGFR to $<$35 ml/min per 1.73 m^2	$<$0.3 ml/kg/h for $\geq$ 24 hours or anuria $\geq$ 12 hours

sCr: serum creatinine; RRT: renal replacement therapy; eGFR:

than Stage 2 by urine output criteria). Likewise, the use of sCr has limitations. Because sCr is a surrogate marker of kidney function and not a biomarker of kidney damage, changes to sCr may occur long after the injury stimulus has occurred (i. e., changes in sCr after injury may not rise significantly until there is a 50 % decline in glomerular filtration rate [GFR]) [12]. Serum creatinine is known to be influenced by a number of non-renal factors including patient age, sex, muscle mass, nutritional status and metabolism, medications, and extravascular fluid balance. Finally, baseline sCr values are often unknown (in ~30 % of ICU patients). This presents challenges for interpretation and attributing an elevated sCr solely to AKI rather than representing pre-existing chronic kidney disease or a combination of both.

Accordingly, the integration of novel biomarkers that may be sensitive and specific to the detection of early and acute kidney damage would be welcome and are likely essential to appropriately identify, triage and intervene in patients with AKI at increased risk for less favorable outcomes. Similar to conventional markers, such as sCr, these novel biomarkers need to be minimally invasive, easily detectable, reliable and inexpensive, but also need to be a direct biomarker of kidney damage (not a surrogate for function) and show correlation with clinically meaningful and potentially actionable outcomes, such as worsening AKI, need for initiation of RRT, non-recovery of function or a composite of these [13].

Biomarkers in AKI

The concept of novel biomarkers for the accurate and timely diagnosis of AKI brings much promise. However, as with any new information available to the clinician, we must ensure that it will positively inform our decision making process, and not simply provide more 'noise' for the clinician to sift through when trying to reach a diagnostic conclusion. For example, when deciding on whether to initiate RRT, the decision is rarely made based solely on biochemical grounds and rather is more likely to be the integration of a number of variables in the setting of a deteriorating clinical picture. It is with all likelihood that biomarkers will eventually play an increasing role in the diagnosis and management of AKI, but integrated into existing decision-making tools and clinical judgment (Table 2). In August 2011, the Acute Dialysis Quality Initiative (ADQI) held a multi-disciplinary consensus conference specifically focused on the evaluation of biomarkers in acute kidney injury (http://www.adqi.net/).

Neutrophil Gelatinase-Associated Lipocalin

Neutrophil gelatinase-associated lipocalin (NGAL) is a 25 kDa protein bound to gelatinase and is typically expressed in several human tissues including the kidney, trachea, lungs, stomach and colon [13, 14]. NGAL is one of the first and most

Table 2 A summary of potential actions that clinicians could take in response to elevated kidney-damage biomarkers, such as NGAL

Action/Decision	Description
Triage	Longer observation in the ED; transition to higher acuity monitoring unit (i. e., HDU or ICU)
Consultation/Referral	Nephrology; intensive care
Diagnostic evaluation	Further evaluation for diagnosis, etiology, reversible contributing factors (e.g., renal ultrasound; urine microscopy; nephrotoxin exposure)
Initiate renal protective strategies	Restore arterial filling; hemodynamic optimization; discontinue or dose-adjust nephrotoxic medications
Monitoring	Surveillance for development of AKI; worsening AKI; complications of AKI and overt renal failure; RRT planning
Context-specific interventions	Dependent on the key contributing factor for AKI
Follow-up	Surveillance for longer-term decline in kidney function and development of CKD

ED: emergency department; HDU: high dependency unit; ICU: intensive care unit; AKI: acute kidney injury; CKD: chronic kidney disease; RRT: renal replacement therapy

rapidly upregulated transcripts in renal tubular epithelial cells following acute injury [14–16]. The protein by-product of this gene upregulation, NGAL, is easily measured in the urine and plasma, where its concentration increases in a dose-dependent relationship with the severity and duration of acute tubular injury. Numerous observational studies have evaluated urine and serum NGAL for the diagnosis and prognosis of AKI in adult critically ill patients and will be the primary focus of this review (Table 3).

Diagnosis of AKI

In pediatric populations, NGAL has been shown to be an early marker of kidney damage, rising significantly as early as two hours after cardiac surgery with cardiopulmonary bypass (CPB) and predictive of development of conventionally defined AKI [17, 18]. However, translation of these findings to adult populations has been variable [12]. This is likely attributable to the added confounding influences in adult patients, such as burden of comorbid illness (e.g., cardiovascular disease, chronic kidney disease) and the multiple heterogeneous contributing factors for AKI [14]. Several studies have examined the validity of NGAL for the diagnosis of AKI in adult critically ill patients [19–23]. Cruz et al. evaluated serum NGAL in 301 consecutive patients admitted to a general medical/surgical ICU. AKI, defined by the RIFLE criteria, occurred in 133 patients (44 %). NGAL was higher in those developing AKI (185 ng/ml vs. 82 ng/ml, $p < 0.001$) and had good

Table 3 Selected prospective cohort studies examining NGAL in adult patients (studies inclusive of > 100 patients).

Author	Year	Design	Patient Population	N	NGAL	Outcome	AUC ROC
Doi et al [30]	2011	Single center	Mixed	339	Urine	AKI Death	0.70 0.83
de Geus et al [20]	2011	Single center	Mixed	632	Urine and Serum	AKI RRT	0.77 0.88
Endre et al [21]	2011	Multicenter	Mixed	529	Urine	AKI RRT Death	0.66 0.79 0.66
Cruz et al [19]	2010	Single center	Mixed	307	Serum	AKI RRT	0.78 0.82
Kumpers et al [31]	2010	Single center	Mixed + RRT	109	Serum	Death	0.74
Parikh et al [35]	2011	Multicenter	Post-CPB	1,219	Urine and Serum	AKI LOS Death	0.67 and 0.70
Koyner et al [36]	2010	Single center	Post-CPB	123	Urine and Serum	AKI	0.69 and 0.69
Haase-Fieltz [12]	2009	Single center	Post-CPB	100	Serum	AKI RRT	0.79 0.83
Liangos et al [37]	2009	Multicenter	Post-CPB	103	Urine	–	–
Wagener et al [38]	2008	Single center	Post-CPB	426	Urine	AKI	0.60
Torregrosa et al [39]	2012	Single center	Cardiac ICU	135	Urine	AKI	0.98
Shapiro et al [22]	2011	Multicenter	ED + Sepsis	661	Serum	AKI	0.96; 0.51‡
Nickolas et al [29]	2008	Single center	ED	635	Urine	AKI Composite†	0.90; 0.99‡

ICU: intensive care unit; mixed: medical/surgical ICU; ED: emergency department; CPB: cardiopulmonary bypass; AUROC: area under the receiving operator characteristic curve; AKI: acute kidney injury; †Nephrology consultation, RRT initiation, ICU admission; ‡ Sensitivity and specificity.

discrimination for predicting AKI in the subsequent 48 hours (area under receiver operative characteristic curve [AUROC] 0.78), implying a lead-time benefit for the diagnosis of those at elevated risk for AKI [19]. In another large single-center prospective observational study, de Geus et al. [20] measured urine and serum NGAL at ICU admission in 632 consecutive critically ill patients to evaluate its utility to predict development of AKI, defined by the RIFLE criteria, within 1 week. In this study, the discrimination of urine and serum NGAL were higher for more severe AKI (AUROC for RIFLE – Failure 0.88 and 0.86, respectively). Whereas crude prediction was similar to that of admission estimated GFR (eGFR, AUROC 0.84), the integration of urine and serum NGAL in the best clinical prediction model improved discrimination. In addition, urine NGAL was superior to serum NGAL for discriminating between the development of transient and sustained AKI (AUROC 0.80) and added net discrimination improvement to the best clinical prediction model [24]. In another prospective observational study of several novel biomarkers including urine NGAL, in which 529 critically ill patients admitted to two ICUs were enrolled, the diagnostic performance of urine NGAL was improved when stratified by baseline kidney function and time from onset of injury [21].

Subclinical AKI

In a recent pooled analysis of 10 prospective observational studies, detectable elevations in urine and/or plasma NGAL, in the absence of detectable changes in sCr fulfilling the conventional diagnosis of AKI, identified a unique cohort of patients with 'subclinical AKI' [25]. These patients were at greater risk of adverse events, a more complicated clinical course and less favorable clinical outcome, including RRT initiation, higher mortality, longer durations of stay in the ICU and hospital when compared to those without evidence of detectable elevations in NGAL. These findings were consistent regardless of whether NGAL was measured in the urine or serum. It has also recently been suggested that NGAL be used as a marker of kidney damage without evident dysfunction and concomitant elevations in sCr in patients undergoing radiographical procedures involving contrast dyes to better define and treat contrast-induced nephropathy [26]. These observations imply the existence of a clinically important state of subclinical kidney 'damage' detectable only by injury-specific biomarkers, such as NGAL, that occurs without significant loss to GFR and that may be completely missed by our current diagnostic paradigm for AKI [27].

Prognosis in AKI

NGAL has been investigated in numerous studies across a range of clinical settings (e.g., ICU, emergency department [ED], postoperative) as a prognostic biomarker to discriminate and predict clinically important outcomes. A large systematic review and meta-analysis showed that NGAL had value for predicting not only the development of AKI, but also RRT initiation and mortality [28]. Two studies have recently shown that urine NGAL has high predictive value for the diagnosis of AKI within 72 hours for patients presenting to the ED [22, 29]. Indeed, a single elevated urine NGAL > 130 ng/mg was associated with a 24-fold increased risk of treatment escalation, including nephrology consultation, RRT initiation or ICU admission [29]. In the critically ill, several studies have shown that an elevated NGAL at the time of ICU admission predicts RRT initiation (AUROC 0.82–0.88); prolonged stay in ICU and hospital; and/or increased risk of death; however, prediction of mortality was only fair (AUROC 0.68) [19, 20, 30]. Plasma NGAL has also been shown to correlate with the severity and duration of AKI, as well as overall illness severity (e.g., Acute Physiology and Chronic Health Evaluation II [APACHE II] score), implying it may have value as a valuable global biomarker of prognosis [19]. In addition, when measured in critically ill patients with severe AKI started on RRT, serum NGAL concentrations at the time of RRT initiation were higher in non-survivors compared to survivors, and independently predicted 28-day survival [31]. Elevated NGAL after cardiac surgery not only predicts the development of AKI, but is also associated with improved discrimination for hospital stay, RRT initiation or death (AUROC 0.75). Serum NGAL has also been shown to have value for prediction of worsening or progressing of AKI in the postoperative period [32]. Recently, two studies have shown that NGAL may have value for predicting kidney recovery after an episode of severe AKI [33, 34]. Recovery may depend on a number of independent factors, including baseline kidney function, the severity of the initial insult and whether there are ongoing insults. In a small substudy of critically ill patients from the ATN trial, serial measures of a composite of biomarkers, including NGAL, cystatin C, and hepatocyte growth factor (HGF), when integrated with the best clinical prediction model, showed excellent discrimination for recovery to dialysis independence (AUROC 0.90), implying incremental value for integrating a panel of biomarkers for predicting renal recovery [34].

Conclusion

AKI remains a common and challenging clinical problem for clinicians. Indeed, AKI may be largely iatrogenic and may be partly attributable to the advent of modern ICU support. Importantly, its incidence continues to rise, its associated outcomes are poor, and there are currently few, if any, preventative and/or therapeutic interventions that can modify this prognosis once established. Currently, the standard tools we have to diagnose and monitor AKI (i. e., sCr and urine output) have remained unchanged for several decades and are clearly suboptimal. There are now numerous conventional and novel kidney-injury specific biomarkers that have been characterized and are undergoing clinical validation for the diagnosis and clinical outcome prediction across a spectrum of at-risk patients. This list also includes a reappraisal of conventional measures of kidney function, such as urine output, sCr, and urine microscopy; but also importantly highlights a growing list of novel biomarkers, such as interleukin-18, kidney injury molecule-1, L-type fatty acid binding protein, HGF, *N*-acetyl-β-D-glucosaminidase, α-glutathione S-transferase,

π-glutathione S-transferase and matrix metalloproteinase-9. NGAL remains one of the most well-described biomarkers of kidney damage. While numerous ongoing clinical studies are pursuing further clinical validation, available data imply that this biomarker holds promise to better inform on the early diagnosis and provide important prognostic information (e.g., worsening AKI, need for RRT, renal recovery), in particular when integrated with clinical prediction models.

References

1. Chertow GM, Burdick E, Honour M, Bonventre JV, Bates DW (2005) Acute kidney injury, mortality, length of stay, and costs in hospitalized patients. J Am Soc Nephrol 16:3365–3370
2. Liangos O, Wald R, O'Bell JW, Price L, Pereira BJ, Jaber BL (2006) Epidemiology and outcomes of acute renal failure in hospitalized patients: a national survey. Clin J Am Soc Nephrol 1:43–51
3. Bagshaw SM, George C, Bellomo R (2007) Changes in the incidence and outcome for early acute kidney injury in a cohort of Australian intensive care units. Crit Care 11:R68
4. Bagshaw SM, George C, Dinu I, Bellomo R (2008) A multi-centre evaluation of the RIFLE criteria for early acute kidney injury in critically ill patients. Nephrol Dial Transplant 23:1203–1210
5. Hoste EA, Clermont G, Kersten A et al (2006) RIFLE criteria for acute kidney injury are associated with hospital mortality in critically ill patients: a cohort analysis. Crit Care 10:R73
6. Uchino S, Kellum JA, Bellomo R et al (2005) Acute renal failure in critically ill patients: a multinational, multicenter study. JAMA 294:813–818
7. Ahlstrom A, Tallgren M, Peltonen S, Rasanen P, Pettila V (2005) Survival and quality of life of patients requiring acute renal replacement therapy. Intensive Care Med 31:1222–1228
8. Bagshaw SM, Laupland KB, Doig CJ et al (2005) Prognosis for long-term survival and renal recovery in critically ill patients with severe acute renal failure: a population-based study. Crit Care 9:R700–R709
9. Wald R, Quinn RR, Luo J et al (2009) Chronic dialysis and death among survivors of acute kidney injury requiring dialysis. JAMA 302:1179–1185
10. Bellomo R, Ronco C, Kellum JA, Mehta RL, Palevsky P (2004) Acute renal failure – definition, outcome measures, animal models, fluid therapy and information technology needs: the Second International Consensus Conference of the Acute Dialysis Quality Initiative (ADQI) Group. Crit Care 8:R204–R212
11. Kidney Disease: Improving Global Outcomes (2012) KDIGO Clinical Practice Guidelines for Acute Kidney Injury. Kidney Int(Suppl 2):1–138
12. Haase-Fielitz A, Bellomo R, Devarajan P et al (2009) Novel and conventional serum biomarkers predicting acute kidney injury in adult cardiac surgery – a prospective cohort study. Crit Care Med 37:553–560
13. Cowland JB, Borregaard N (1997) Molecular characterization and pattern of tissue expression of the gene for neutrophil gelatinase-associated lipocalin from humans. Genomics 45:17–23
14. Devarajan P (2008) NGAL in acute kidney injury: from serendipity to utility. Am J Kidney Dis 52:395–399
15. Bolignano D, Coppolino G, Campo S et al (2008) Urinary neutrophil gelatinase-associated lipocalin (NGAL) is associated with severity of renal disease in proteinuric patients. Nephrol Dial Transplant 23:414–416

16. Bolignano D, Donato V, Coppolino G et al (2008) Neutrophil gelatinase-associated lipocalin (NGAL) as a marker of kidney damage. Am J Kidney Dis 52:595–605
17. Dent CL, Ma Q, Dastrala S et al (2007) Plasma neutrophil gelatinase-associated lipocalin predicts acute kidney injury, morbidity and mortality after pediatric cardiac surgery: a prospective uncontrolled cohort study. Crit Care 11:R127
18. Mishra J, Dent C, Tarabishi R et al (2005) Neutrophil gelatinase-associated lipocalin (NGAL) as a biomarker for acute renal injury after cardiac surgery. Lancet 365:1231–1238
19. Cruz DN, de Cal M, Garzotto F et al (2010) Plasma neutrophil gelatinase-associated lipocalin is an early biomarker for acute kidney injury in an adult ICU population. Intensive Care Med 36:444–451
20. de Geus HR, Bakker J, Lesaffre EM, le Noble JL (2011) Neutrophil gelatinase-associated lipocalin at ICU admission predicts for acute kidney injury in adult patients. Am J Respir Crit Care Med 183:907–914
21. Endre ZH, Pickering JW, Walker RJ et al (2011) Improved performance of urinary biomarkers of acute kidney injury in the critically ill by stratification for injury duration and baseline renal function. Kidney Int 79:1119–1130
22. Shapiro NI, Trzeciak S, Hollander JE et al (2010) The diagnostic accuracy of plasma neutrophil gelatinase-associated lipocalin in the prediction of acute kidney injury in emergency department patients with suspected sepsis. Ann Emerg Med 56:52–59
23. Soni SS, Ronco C, Katz N, Cruz DN (2009) Early diagnosis of acute kidney injury: the promise of novel biomarkers. Blood Purif 28:165–174
24. de Geus HR, Woo JG, Wang Y et al (2011) Urinary neutrophil gelatinase-associated lipocalin measured on admission to the intensive care unit accurately discriminates between sustained and transient acute kidney injury in adult critically ill patients. Nephron Extra 1:9–23
25. Haase M, Devarajan P, Haase-Fielitz A et al (2011) The outcome of neutrophil gelatinase-associated lipocalin-positive subclinical acute kidney injury: a multicenter pooled analysis of prospective studies. J Am Coll Cardiol 57:1752–1761
26. Ronco C, Stacul F, McCullough PA (2013) Subclinical acute kidney injury (AKI) due to iodine-based contrast media. Eur Radiol 23:319–323
27. Ronco C, Kellum JA, Haase M (2012) Subclinical AKI is still AKI. Crit Care 16:313
28. Haase M, Bellomo R, Devarajan P, Schlattmann P, Haase-Fielitz A (2009) Accuracy of neutrophil gelatinase-associated lipocalin (NGAL) in diagnosis and prognosis in acute kidney injury: a systematic review and meta-analysis. Am J Kidney Dis 54:1012–1024
29. Nickolas TL, O'Rourke MJ, Yang J et al (2008) Sensitivity and specificity of a single emergency department measurement of urinary neutrophil gelatinase-associated lipocalin for diagnosing acute kidney injury. Ann Intern Med 148:810–819
30. Doi K, Negishi K, Ishizu T et al (2011) Evaluation of new acute kidney injury biomarkers in a mixed intensive care unit. Crit Care Med 39:2464–2469
31. Kumpers P, Hafer C, Lukasz A et al (2010) Serum neutrophil gelatinase-associated lipocalin at inception of renal replacement therapy predicts survival in critically ill patients with acute kidney injury. Crit Care 14:R9
32. Koyner JL, Garg AX, Coca SG et al (2012) Biomarkers predict progression of acute kidney injury after cardiac surgery. J Am Soc Nephrol 23:905–914
33. Srisawat N, Murugan R, Lee M et al (2011) Plasma neutrophil gelatinase-associated lipocalin predicts recovery from acute kidney injury following community-acquired pneumonia. Kidney Int 80:545–552
34. Srisawat N, Wen X, Lee M et al (2011) Urinary biomarkers and renal recovery in critically ill patients with renal support. Clin J Am Soc Nephrol 6:1815–1823
35. Parikh CR, Coca SG, Thiessen-Philbrook H et al (2011) Postoperative biomarkers predict acute kidney injury and poor outcomes after adult cardiac surgery. J Am Soc Nephrol 22:1748–1757
36. Koyner JL, Vaidya VS, Bennett MR et al (2010) Urinary biomarkers in the clinical prognosis and early detection of acute kidney injury. Clin J Am Soc Nephrol 5:2154–2165

37. Liangos O, Perianayagam MC, Vaidya VS et al (2007) Urinary N-acetyl-beta-(D)-glucosaminidase activity and kidney injury molecule-1 level are associated with adverse outcomes in acute renal failure. J Am Soc Nephrol 18:904–912
38. Wagener G, Gubitosa G, Wang S, Borregaard N, Kim M, Lee HT (2008) Urinary neutrophil gelatinase-associated lipocalin and acute kidney injury after cardiac surgery. Am J Kidney Dis 52:425–433
39. Torregrosa I, Montoliu C, Urios A et al (2012) Early biomarkers of acute kidney failure after heart angiography or heart surgery in patients with acute coronary syndrome or acute heart failure. Nefrologia 32:44–52

Understanding Acute Kidney Injury in Adult Patients with Thrombotic Thrombocytopenic Purpura

L. Zafrani and É. Azoulay

Introduction

Thrombotic microangiopathies (TMA) are defined by the association of thrombocytopenia, microangiopathic hemolytic anemia, absence of diffuse intravascular coagulation and microvascular thrombosis that can cause visceral ischemic manifestations [1]. Thrombotic thrombocytopenic purpura (TTP) and hemolytic uremic syndrome (HUS) are the classical diseases associated with TMA (Fig. 1). TTP is a life-threatening disorder with a mortality rate of up to 90 % if left untreated. The advent of life-saving plasma therapy and the identification of an inhibitor to ADAMTS13 in TTP and its absence in diarrheal HUS have had a major impact on our current classification of TMA.

TTP and HUS, the two basic clinical forms of TMA, encompass a wide range of primary and secondary forms. Basically, HUS is defined as a TMA syndrome associated with renal impairment. Typical HUS occurs in up to 30 % of infected children about a week after an episode of bloody diarrhea caused by enterohemorrhagic *Escherichia coli* O157:H7 or other *E. coli* serotypes, *Shigella dysenteriae*, or even other microbes. Atypical HUS (the majority of cases of HUS in adults) defines non Shiga-toxin-HUS, which designates a primary disease due to a disorder in complement alternative pathway regulation. At presentation, the clinical distinction between idiopathic adult TTP, various forms of secondary TMA, and atypical HUS can be problematic because the symptoms and laboratory findings often overlap.

L. Zafrani
Dept of Medicine, AP-HP, Hôpital Saint-Louis, Medical ICU; Université Paris-Diderot, 1 avenue Claude Vellefaux, 75010 Paris, France

É. Azoulay (✉)
Dept of Medicine, AP-HP, Hôpital Saint-Louis, Medical ICU; Université Paris-Diderot, 1 avenue Claude Vellefaux, 75010 Paris, France
E-mail: elie.azoulay@sls.aphp.fr

J.-L. Vincent (Ed.), *Annual Update in Intensive Care and Emergency Medicine 2013*,
DOI 10.1007/978-3-642-35109-9_56, © Springer-Verlag Berlin Heidelberg 2013

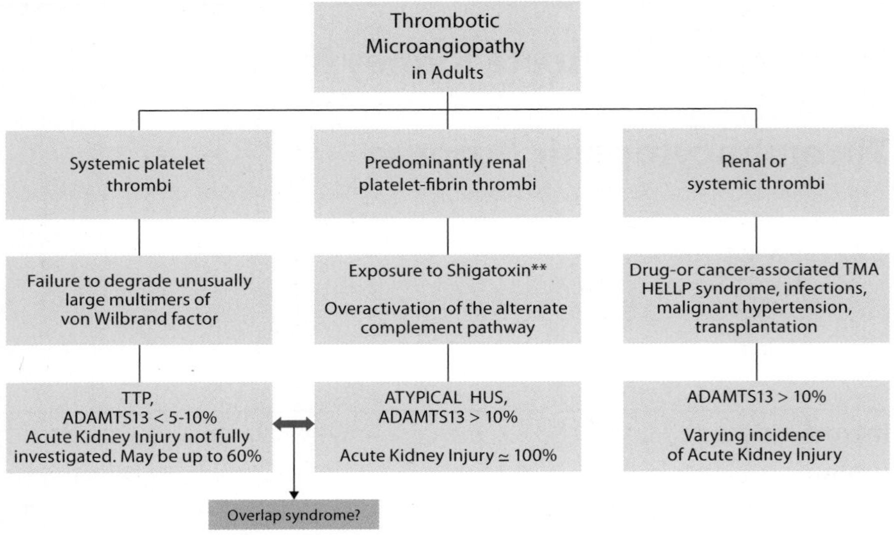

TTP: thrombotic thrombocytopenic purpura; HUS: Hemolytic and uremic syndrome.
** bloody diarrhea in children and thrombotic microangiopathy define typical HUS

Fig. 1 Overview of thrombotic microangiopathies (TMA). Adapted from [1]

Hence, whereas kidney injury is a hallmark feature of HUS, its incidence in TTP remains to be evaluated. In contrast with renal abnormalities which have been thoroughly described in HUS, clinical, biological and pathophysiological aspects of kidney injury in TTP have been scarcely characterized. In this chapter, we will focus on renal involvement in TTP.

TTP and HUS: Pathophysiology

TTP is a life-threatening disorder, typically characterized by neurological, cardiac and renal dysfunction which often requires intensive care unit (ICU) management [2]. Microvascular thrombi occur in most organs in patients with TTP and consist of platelet aggregates with little or no fibrin. The platelet thrombi contain abundant von Willebrand factor (vWf) antigen but no fibrinogen (or fibrin), whereas the platelet thrombi in disseminated intravascular coagulation (DIC) contain fibrin but not vWf [1]. vWF is important for primary hemostasis, inducing platelet aggregation and thrombus formation at sites of endothelial injury. Initially secreted by endothelial cells and megakaryocytes as large multimers, vWF is degraded into progressively smaller circulating forms by a plasma metalloprotease, named ADAMTS13 (a disintegrin and metalloprotease with thrombospondin type 1 domains, member 13) under the influence of shear stress. Failure to cleave these multimers leads to the accumulation of ultralarge vWf in plasma, which induces,

Table 1 Genetic abnormalities in atypical hemolytic uremic syndrome (HUS)

Gene	Protein and function	Effect
CFH	Factor H Cofactor for cleavage of C3b	Inability of factor H to bind to the endothelial surface and to C3b → reduced C3b inactivation
MCP	Membrane cofactor protein Cofactor for cleavage of C3b	No expression of MCP → reduced C3b inactivation
CFI	Factor I Serine protease: cleavage of C3b	Low activity or low level of Factor I
CFB	Factor B C3 convertase stabilization	Gain of function: C3 convertase stabilization
C3	Complement C3	Resistance to C3b inactivation
CFHR1/3	Factor HR1, R3	Anti-factor H antibodies
THBD	Thrombomodulin Membrane-bound anticoagulant glycoprotein: facilitates complement inactivation by CFI	Reduced C3b inactivation

in turn, platelet aggregation and formation of microthrombi in the circulation [1]. Patients with TTP are deficient in ADAMTS13. In most cases, severe ADAMTS13 deficiency is acquired via auto-antibodies to ADAMTS13 [3]; more rarely, severe ADAMTS13 deficiency is related to compound heterozygous or homozygous mutations of the ADAMTS13 gene (Upshaw-Schulman syndrome) [4]. Assessment of ADAMTS13 deficiency (e.g., ADAMTS13 activity < 5–10 %) is now an essential tool for the diagnosis of TTP.

HUS manifests as severe kidney disease with acute renal failure, thrombocytopenia and hemolytic anemia. Typical HUS, which more commonly affects children, is caused by infection, primarily Shigatoxin-producing *E. coli* [5]. In contrast, atypical HUS predominantly affects adults and its pathogenesis involves a defective regulation of complement in renal endothelial cells. Defects in complement regulation can lead to cellular damage, which in turn can activate the blood coagulation cascade and cause thrombosis. An overactivation of the complement alternate pathway secondary to a heterozygote deficiency of regulatory proteins (factor H, factor I or MCP [membrane cofactor protein] or to an activating mutation of factor B or C3) can result in HUS (Table 1) [6, 7].

Definitions and Incidence of Acute Kidney Injury During TTP

Before the widespread availability of ADAMTS13 assessment, the distinction between TTP and HUS relied mainly on whether renal or neurologic dysfunction predominated. Thus, profound renal failure was deemed sufficient to definitely rule out the diagnosis of TTP. As a result, studies focusing on TTP invariably included patients with normal or barely altered kidney function. This may have misled physicians into underestimating the true incidence of AKI in TTP. Also, TTP patients with impaired renal function may have been considered as HUS, with possible dramatic consequences related to delayed plasma therapy.

In critically ill patients with TMA, the incidence of AKI-associated TTP is difficult to establish as most studies in this setting were published before routine ADAMTS13 measurement considered TTP and HUS as a whole. Pene et al. described clinical features of a cohort of patients with severe thrombotic microangiopathies in ICU. Thirty patients (48 %) had a serum creatinine level above 250 μmol/l at admission [2]. Darmon et al. studied 36 adults admitted to our medical ICU with TMA between 2000 and 2003: Renal function ranged from normal to acute failure with anuria; median creatinine clearance was 55.2 ml/min (IQR 28.8–75.4), and the creatinine clearance was 60 ml/min in 55.4 % of patients [8].

In an attempt to better characterize TTP patients, Coppo et al. compared two groups of patients on the basis of ADAMTS13 activity (undetectable or detectable): Patients with TTP, as defined by severe ADAMTS13 deficiency, were characterized by mild renal involvement compared to patients with detectable ADAMTS13 activity. Hemodialysis was more frequently required in non-TTP patients with detectable ADAMTS13 activity (46.7 %) compared to TTP patients with severe ADAMTS13 deficiency (9.7 %) ($p = 0.008$) [9]. Similarly, in a prospective cohort of 142 patients, Vesely et al. showed a relatively low frequency of acute renal failure in patients with severe ADAMTS13 deficiency compared with the other patients with a clinical diagnosis of TMA [10]. However, definitions of acute renal failure were restrictive (creatinine > 350 μmol/l or an increasing serum creatinine > 45 μmol per day for 2 consecutive days), thus AKI of a lesser degree may have been missed.

In recognition of the potential clinical importance of even the smallest changes in kidney function, standardized definitions of AKI are now widely used [11–13]. Based on these new recommendations, we reported that 64 % of patients fulfilled AKI criteria in a cohort of 83 patients admitted to the ICU with TTP defined by TMA and ADAMTS13 activity < 10 %. Using the RIFLE criteria [12], 43 % of patients with AKI were in the Risk category, 17 % in the Injury category, 34 % in the Failure category, 3 % in the Loss category and 1 % in the End-stage category. Seventeen percent of patients with TTP received renal replacement therapy (RRT) during their ICU stay (unpublished data). This high incidence of AKI in our cohort may be explained in part by the use of the more recent definitions of AKI, but may also be the result of selection bias, as patients admitted to the ICU are sicker and more likely to present with multiple organ failure.

Strikingly, there is a lot to learn from hereditary TTP. Indeed, these patients are more prone to develop acute and chronic renal failure than are patients with acquired TTP, regardless of their ADAMTS13 genotype [14, 15]. One possible explanation for this discrepancy between hereditary and acquired TTP has been provided by Manea et al. who first investigated the presence of ADAMTS13 (which is synthesized by the liver) in the kidneys from normal and hereditary TTP patients

[16]. Real-time polymerase chain reaction (PCR) demonstrated the presence of ADAMTS13 mRNA in the normal kidneys. ADAMTS13 was detected in the glomeruli and tubules of normal and TTP kidneys. In the glomeruli, expression was localized to podocytes and endothelium. Electron microscopy detected ADAMTS13 in podocytes, endothelium and glomerular basement membrane. Podocyte-derived ADAMTS13 may offer local protection in the high-shear microcirculation of the glomerulus. The mutations in the two TTP patients studied, enabled protein expression in the podocytes but affected protease secretion. In contrast to patients with hereditary TTP, patients with acquired TTP retain a significant local production of ADAMTS13 in the kidney that may in part protect these patients from glomerular microangiopathy [14].

Characteristics of TTP-associated AKI

Urinalysis

Although a great number of case-reports suggest that abnormalities of urinalysis (hematuria and proteinuria) are common in TTP [14], their actual prevalence is unclear. In our cohort, we found microscopic hematuria in 28 % of patients and proteinuria (defined as proteinuria/creatininuria > 50 mg/mmol) in 66 % of patients at ICU admission. Although in many cases proteinuria/creatininuria exceeded 300 mg/mmol during the first week of hospitalization, it generally decreased after one week and in most cases disappeared at 3 months.

Histology

Because of marked thrombocytopenia and reluctance to platelet transfusions, there is a paucity of histopathological data in TTP. Most data stem from autopsy studies. These studies show that, despite clinical similarities, there are different renal histological patterns in TTP and HUS. Hosler et al. performed a review of autopsied patients with TTP or HUS: In 25 patients classified as having TTP, platelet-rich thrombi were present in the kidney and other organs, such as heart, pancreas or brain. In 31 patients with HUS, fibrin/red cell-rich thrombi were present, but were largely confined to the kidney. Furthermore, the extent of renal lesions was far more severe than in patients with TTP with many cases of bilateral cortical necrosis [17]. However, it is important to note that distinction between TTP and HUS was based on clinical data (mainly on renal and neurologic dysfunction) and not on ADAMTS13 activity assessment which means that some of the TTP patients may have been misclassified as HUS because of the presence of severe renal failure. Now that ADAMTS13 is widely available, new clinical and histological studies are needed in order to understand the pathophysiology of kidney injury in TTP.

Outcome of TTP-associated AKI

Current evidence indicates that, unlike HUS, renal dysfunction is transient in most cases of acquired TTP [14]. In our cohort, among 53 patients with AKI only 4 patients had chronic renal failure with creatinine clearance < 60 ml/min at 6 months with only 1 requiring dialysis. All of them had an underlying autoimmune disease (3 systemic lupus erythematosus, 1 Gougerot-Sjogren syndrome). Moreover, patients with TTP who developed AKI during the first episode of TTP were prone to develop AKI during relapse, suggesting susceptibility for AKI in these patients.

Severe AKI requiring dialysis and leading to chronic renal failure occurs more frequently in hereditary TTP. In 2007, Tsai reported that 9/75 cases published in the literature developed chronic renal failure, including 5 who required dialysis [14]. However, it is noteworthy that all of these patients did not receive adequate therapy (e.g., plasma exchange). Veyradier et al. reported signs of permanent renal lesions in approximately half the pediatric patients with hereditary TTP who did not receive preventive plasma therapy, including chronic proteinuria, chronic renal failure or end-stage renal disease occurring at adolescence or adult age, usually after multiple relapses [18].

Relapses are common during TTP and mortality remains high despite advances in therapy [19, 20]. In a prospective study carried out between 2000 and 2010, Benhamou et al. identified prognostic factors associated with 30-day mortality in TTP patients with severe acquired ADAMTS13 deficiency: Outcome was correlated with age, cerebral manifestations, lactate dehydrogenase level. Interestingly, serum creatinine levels were higher in non-survivors [20]. Renal involvement has also been reported as an adverse prognostic factor in previous studies [21, 22]. Thus, physicians should consider thorough renal assessment, and close monitoring during follow-up of patients affected by TTP-associated AKI.

However, although AKI has been shown to be associated with an increased likelihood of death, it is usually not the direct cause of death in itself. The leading causes of death in the ICU in patients with TMA remain acquired infections, myocardial infarction, stroke, and pulmonary embolism [22].

Causes of TTP-associated AKI

It is important to determine the causes of AKI during TTP (Tables 2 and 3) as they require specific treatments. Distinct causes and pathophysiologic mechanisms, which are not mutually exclusive, can be involved, namely, TMA, acute tubular necrosis secondary to hemodynamic instability, hemolysis-induced tubular damage, drug-induced nephrotoxicity, and glomerulopathy as a manifestation of an underlying autoimmune disease in an acquired TTP with IgG anti-ADAMTS13. Figure 2 summarizes the pathophysiology of TTP-associated AKI and Table 4 summarizes the main differences between TTP-associated AKI and HUS-associated AKI.

Table 2 Laboratory investigations in thrombotic thrombocytopenic purpura (TTP)-associated acute kidney injury (AKI)

Evaluation of hemodynamic and cardiac status	Clinical examination, blood pressure, electrocardiogram, troponin, echocardiography
Investigations related to an infectious disease	Blood cultures, urine culture, thoracic radiography. More investigations in immunocompromised patients
Urinalysis	Hematuria, proteinuria, hemoglobinuria
In case of persistent proteinuria or renal failure	Kidney biopsy (after TTP remission and after aspirin withdrawal)
In case of severe renal failure	Investigation of the complement system: C3, C4, factor H and factor I plasma concentration, MCP expression on leukocytes and anti-factor H antibodies
Investigations related to atypical HUS or overlap syndrome	Genetic screening (factor H ++) to identify risk factors

HUS: hemolytic uremic syndrome; MCP: membrane cofactor protein

Table 3 Renal lesions in thrombotic thrombocytopenic purpura (TTP)-associated acute kidney injury (AKI)

	Histopathological lesions
Thrombotic microangiopathy	Hyaline thrombi in terminal arterioles and capillaries. Endothelial proliferation and detachment.
Acute tubular necrosis	Epithelial cell damage and necrosis: loss of proximal tubule brush border, tubular dilatation, distal tubule casts.
Renal sideropathy	Diffuse intratubular deposition of hemosiderin Tubular damage: distention of tubules, cell debris in the lumen, tubular atrophy

- TMA is a process of microvascular thrombosis affecting various organs, including the kidney: As described above, characteristic pathological features for TTP include hyaline thrombi in terminal arterioles and capillaries. Thrombotic lesions are associated with endothelial proliferation and detachment. Platelet thrombi are rich in vWf, but contain little fibrinogen or fibrin deposition in the lesions [23].
- Acute tubular necrosis: Altered renal hemodynamics leads to prerenal acute renal failure and, if hypoperfusion is severe and prolonged, ischemic acute tubular necrosis. Hemodynamic instability can occur during TTP in a context of cardiogenic shock secondary to cardiac microangiopathy [24]. Septic shock should also be considered in these patients who are frequently placed on immunosuppressive regimen. Moreover, notwithstanding the patient's immune status, bacterial infections may act as a trigger for TTP and screening for infection is required in patients with TTP, mostly in immunocompromised ones [25].

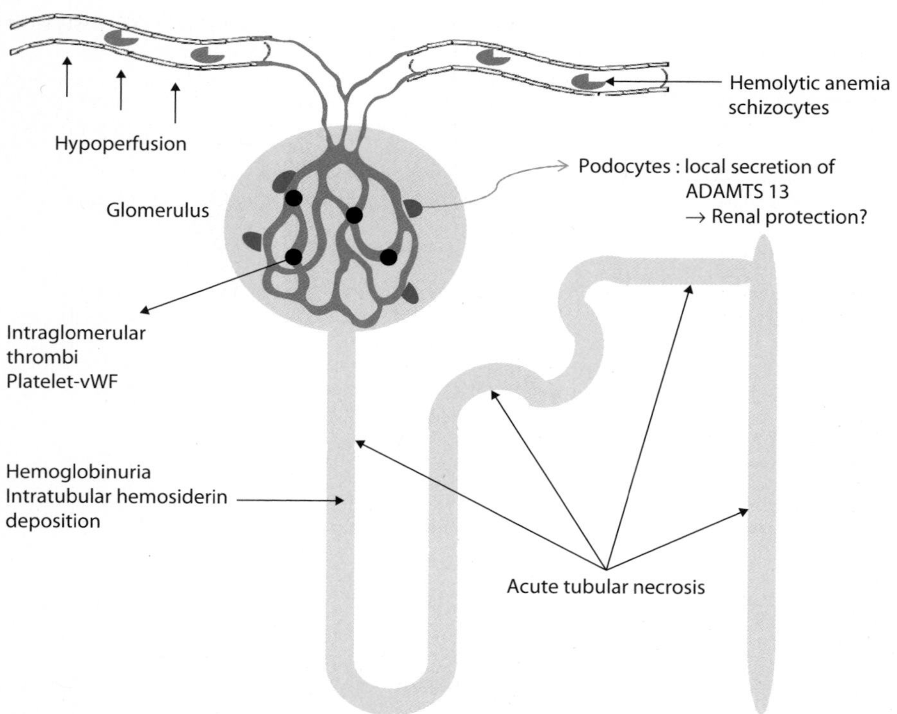

Fig. 2 Pathophysiology of thrombotic thrombocytopenic purpura (TTP)-associated acute kidney injury

- Hemolysis-induced tubulopathy: Considering the high incidence of hemoglobinemia and hemoglobinuria due to acute intravascular hemolysis in TTP, hemolysis-induced tubular damage may be responsible for AKI in this setting. Indeed, investigations conducted in the setting of cardiac surgery (cardiopulmonary bypass [CPB]) have disclosed meaningful insights into the involvement of hemolysis as a major determinant of AKI [26]. Free hemoglobin combines with haptoglobin to form a complex, which is carried to the liver, bypassing the kidney, and is then metabolized. In the presence of oxidants, such as hydrogen peroxide and superoxide, free iron is released from heme molecules into the circulation. Free labile iron is capable of inducing multiple changes in renal tubular epithelial function, including impaired proliferation and the induction of free radical injuries [27, 28]. The association between hemoglobinuria and the development of AKI has been acknowledged in other hemolytic diseases, such as paroxysmal nocturnal hemoglobinuria [29]. In the specific setting of TTP, there is a paucity of data regarding the potential implications of these mechanisms in AKI. However, we believe that TTP-induced AKI may be, at least in part, a renal sideropathy with free iron as the central toxic element.

Table 4 Main differences between thrombotic thrombocytopenic purpura (TTP)-associated acute kidney injury (AKI) and hemolytic uremia syndrome (HUS)-associated AKI

	TTP	Atypical HUS
ADAMTS13	<5–10 %	>10 %
Complement	Usually normal	Overactivation of complement alternative pathway
Incidence of AKI	+++	+++++
Severity of AKI during acute episode	+	+++
Proteinuria	+	+
Hematuria	+	+
Histopathological renal lesions	Platelet thrombi rich in vWF	Fibrin/red cell-rich thrombi
Main causes of AKI	Thrombotic microangiopathy acute tubular necrosis renal sideropathy autoimmune glomerulonephritis	Thrombotic microangiopathy
Renal outcome towards end stage renal failure	<5 %	25 % [42]
Mortality in 2012	10–20 %	2–10 % [42]
Main therapy	Plasma exchange, steroids, blood pressure control Rituximab	Plasma exchange, steroids Eculizumab

- Acquired TTP can be a manifestation of an autoimmune disease, mostly as systemic lupus erythematosus or Gougerot-Sjogren syndrome [9, 30–31]. Hence, TTP patients may display glomerulopathies or interstitial nephropathies related to these autoimmune diseases. An association between TTP and anti-glomerular basement membrane disease has also been reported [32].
- Genetic predisposition to TTP-related AKI: Noris et al. reported two sisters with hereditary TTP; one presented with exclusive neurologic symptoms, whereas her sister presented with severe renal failure that required chronic dialysis [33]. Laboratory investigations unraveled ADAMTS13 deficiency as a result of two heterozygous mutations in both sisters; however, the authors found an additional heterozygous mutation in the factor H of a complement gene in the patient who developed chronic renal failure [33]. In other words, the genetic background that predisposes patients to TTP may also favor the occurrence of AKI. This case, in which one sibling had an additional underlying susceptibility factor for HUS, namely a heterozygous mutation of a regulatory protein of the complement alternative pathway, remains didactical.

Management of TTP

TTP is a medical emergency. Plasma therapy should be provided using plasma exchange as it provides higher plasma volumes. According to hospital practice, ICU admission may be the place where plasma exchanges are easiest to organize 24/7. However, patients may also require mandatory ICU admission for cardiac TMA, neurological involvement, RRT, or severe hypertension. Patients should be admitted early to the ICU, as soon as an organ failure occurs. TTP and HUS are difficult to distinguish and results of ADAMTS13 assessment are not available 24/7. However, because of the risk of sudden clinical deterioration, plasma therapy should be started as soon as possible when patients display biological features of TMA, with or without renal failure, neurologic abnormalities or cardiac dysfunction. Importantly, when a TMA is diagnosed in an adult, after excluding infections (immunocompromised), drug-related TMA, malignant hypertension, preeclampsia, or metastatic cancer-related TMA, urgent life-saving plasma therapy is in order. This is true both in case of obvious TTP, or atypical HUS.

Plasma Exchange

Before plasma therapy, survival of patients with TTP was poor. Therapeutic plasma exchange is now considered to be the standard of care in TTP. In 1991, the Canadian Apheresis Group Analysis showed a significant improvement in response and mortality among patients treated with exchange rather than infusion [34]. Darmon et al. observed that patients treated with plasma infusion had a higher mortality or an increased likelihood of relapse after achieving a response to initial therapy compared to patients treated with plasma exchange. Patients treated with plasma exchange had a faster recovery from organ failure and fewer problems due to inadequate fluid balance [8]. However, as plasma exchange requires apheresis equipment, one can administer plasma infusion to provide temporary benefit pending plasma exchange [35].

Platelet Transfusions

Dramatic case reports indicate that platelet transfusions can be followed by rapid clinical deterioration that may lead to sudden death [36, 37]. The mechanism by which platelet transfusions worsen the disease is unclear. Post-mortem analysis of patients who have died after platelet transfusions showed extensive platelet aggregates in central nervous system [37]. Thus, infused platelets may add to the extent and the severity of the microvascular thrombi formation. For these reasons and even though the contribution of platelet transfusions in the worsened outcome in TTP patients is still controversial [35], we strongly recommend that platelet transfusions be avoided in TTP.

Immunosuppressive Therapy

Corticosteroids

The decision to give corticosteroid during the acute stage of TTP depends on clinical criteria. The aim of corticosteroid administration is the suppression of autoantibodies inhibiting ADAMTS13 activity. George suggests that patients who are unlikely to have severe ADAMTS13 deficiency, such as patients with a history and clinical features suggesting drug-associated TTP or a Shigatoxin-producing *E. coli* infection, should not be treated with corticosteroids. Conversely, patients in whom the etiology is unclear should be treated with corticosteroids [35]. We believe that in adult patients, steroids should be given routinely in TMA patients at a dose of 1 mg/kg for at least 21 days. Pulse steroids may help improve outcomes in severe TTP.

Other Immunosuppressive Therapies

Rituximab is emerging as a major adjunctive drug in patients with severe TTP. In a prospective study conducted between 2005 and 2008, Froissart et al. showed that rituximab was effective and safe in adults with severe TTP who responded poorly to therapeutic plasma exchange [38]. In patients with relapsing TTP, rituximab is now the standard of care. Trials are ongoing on potential benefits from early rituximab in TMA patients.

Other agents, such as vincristine or cyclophosphamide, may also be used as second line therapies after failure to attain sustained remission with plasma exchange [39–40].

Splenectomy

In patients who do not improve with plasma exchange, steroids, rituximab, vincristine or cyclophosphamide, or if organ failures are too severe to wait for immunosuppressive treatment to take effect, physicians should consider splenectomy [40].

Antiplatelet Agents

Antiplatelet agents are usually not recommended for patients with TTP when bleeding is observed or when they also have severe thrombocytopenia. However, it may be advisable for these patients to start treatment with aspirin once platelet counts rise again in response to plasma exchange. The Society for Hemostasis and Thrombosis recommends aspirin after the platelet count has risen to greater than 50,000/μl [41].

Management of TTP-associated AKI

There is no specific guideline for managing AKI in patients with TTP. However, when taking into account the specificities of TTP-associated AKI described above and the usual recommendations for management of AKI in the ICU [13], the following suggestions can be proposed:

- The underlying cause of AKI should first be determined (Table 2) in order to adjust therapy.
- Hemodynamic and fluid status should be assessed. Diuretics should not be used except in the management of volume overload. Fluid administration with either isotonic sodium chloride or sodium bicarbonate solutions is crucial in patients with hemoglobinuria.
- If possible, avoid nephrotoxic drugs, such as aminoglycosides or iodinated contrast media.
- Hypertension can cause endothelial injury and worsen kidney damage in TTP and, thus, may be treated aggressively to achieve systolic blood pressure under 125 mm Hg.
- In cases of severe AKI, consider exploring the alternative complement pathway in order to identify an additional susceptibility factor. This may prompt physicians to consider in the near future complement-directed therapy, such as eculizumab (humanized monoclonal antibody inhibiting C5 activation) for patients with a clinical syndrome overlapping with HUS. In these cases of atypical HUS in adults with no deficient ADAMTS13 activity, eculizumab may become an alternative that needs to be evaluated thoroughly in the near future.
- In patients requiring RRT, given the increased risk of bleeding due to thrombocytopenia, regional citrate anticoagulation rather than heparin may be a preferred option.
- Urinalysis and renal function should be monitored during remission: If severe renal failure or proteinuria persists despite improvement in other markers of TTP (e.g., platelet count), one should consider performing a renal biopsy in order to identify an underlying autoimmune disease that may require specific therapy.

Conclusion

The occurrence of AKI in the setting of TTP is likely to be more frequent than commonly believed and remains largely underestimated owing to the confusion that has prevailed for a long time between TTP and HUS. Routine ADAMTS13 activity assessment has allowed for a more precise distinction between TTP and HUS. In TTP, AKI-related outcomes are fairly good. However, it is not only a factor of ominous prognosis *per se*, but its occurrence should alert physicians to alternative diagnoses and the likelihood of an underlying auto-immune disease. TTP associated with kidney injury represents a daunting challenge, which warrants collaborative and multidisciplinary management, including intensivists, nephrologists and pathologists.

References

1. Moake JL (2002) Thrombotic microangiopathies. N Engl J Med 347:589–600
2. Pene F, Vigneau C, Auburtin M et al (2005) Outcome of severe adult thrombotic microangiopathies in the intensive care unit. Intensive Care Med 31:71–78
3. Tsai HM, Lian EC (1998) Antibodies to von Willebrand factor-cleaving protease in acute thrombotic thrombocytopenic purpura. N Engl J Med 339:1585–1594
4. Levy GG, Nichols WC, Lian EC et al (2001) Mutations in a member of the ADAMTS gene family cause thrombotic thrombocytopenic purpura. Nature 413:488–494
5. Noris M, Remuzzi G (2005) Hemolytic uremic syndrome. J Am Soc Nephrol 16:1035–1050
6. Ruggenenti P, Noris M, Remuzzi G (2001) Thrombotic microangiopathy, hemolytic uremic syndrome, and thrombotic thrombocytopenic purpura. Kidney Int 60:831–846
7. Martinez-Barricarte R, Pianetti G, Gautard R et al (2008) The complement factor H R1210 C mutation is associated with atypical hemolytic uremic syndrome. J Am Soc Nephrol 19:639–646
8. Darmon M, Azoulay E, Thiery G et al (2006) Time course of organ dysfunction in thrombotic microangiopathy patients receiving either plasma perfusion or plasma exchange. Crit Care Med 34:2127–2133
9. Coppo P, Bengoufa D, Veyradier A et al (2004) Severe ADAMTS13 deficiency in adult idiopathic thrombotic microangiopathies defines a subset of patients characterized by various autoimmune manifestations, lower platelet count, and mild renal involvement. Medicine (Baltimore) 83:233–244
10. Vesely SK, George JN, Lammle B et al (2003) ADAMTS13 activity in thrombotic thrombocytopenic purpura-hemolytic uremic syndrome: relation to presenting features and clinical outcomes in a prospective cohort of 142 patients. Blood 102:60–68
11. Chertow GM, Burdick E, Honour M, Bonventre JV, Bates DW (2005) Acute kidney injury, mortality, length of stay, and costs in hospitalized patients. J Am Soc Nephrol 16:3365–3370
12. Bellomo R, Ronco C, Kellum JA, Mehta RL, Palevsky P (2004) Acute renal failure – definition, outcome measures, animal models, fluid therapy and information technology needs: the Second International Consensus Conference of the Acute Dialysis Quality Initiative (ADQI) Group. Crit Care 8:R204–R212
13. Singbartl K, Kellum JA (2012) AKI in the ICU: definition, epidemiology, risk stratification, and outcomes. Kidney Int 81:819–825
14. Tsai HM (2007) The kidney in thrombotic thrombocytopenic purpura. Minerva Med 98:731–747
15. Loirat C, Girma JP, Desconclois C, Coppo P, Veyradier A (2009) Thrombotic thrombocytopenic purpura related to severe ADAMTS13 deficiency in children. Pediatr Nephrol 24:19–29
16. Manea M, Kristoffersson A, Schneppenheim R et al (2007) Podocytes express ADAMTS13 in normal renal cortex and in patients with thrombotic thrombocytopenic purpura. Br J Haematol 138:651–662
17. Hosler GA, Cusumano AM, Hutchins GM (2003) Thrombotic thrombocytopenic purpura and hemolytic uremic syndrome are distinct pathologic entities. A review of 56 autopsy cases. Arch Pathol Lab Med 127:834–839
18. Veyradier A, Obert B, Haddad E et al (2003) Severe deficiency of the specific von Willebrand factor-cleaving protease (ADAMTS 13) activity in a subgroup of children with atypical hemolytic uremic syndrome. J Pediatr 142:310–317

19. Frawley N, Ng AP, Nicholls K, Cohney S, Hogan C, Grigg A (2009) Thrombotic thrombocytopenic purpura is associated with a high relapse rate after plasma exchange: a single-centre experience. Intern Med J 39:19–24
20. Benhamou Y, Assie C, Boelle PY et al (2012) Development and validation of a predictive model for death in acquired severe ADAMTS13 deficiency-associated idiopathic thrombotic thrombocytopenic purpura: the French TMA Reference Center experience. Haematologica 97:1181–1186
21. Dervenoulas J, Tsirigotis P, Bollas G et al (2000) Thrombotic thrombocytopenic purpura/hemolytic uremic syndrome (TTP/HUS): treatment outcome, relapses, prognostic factors. A single-center experience of 48 cases. Ann Hematol 79:66–72
22. Peigne V, Perez P, Resche Rigon M et al (2012) Causes and risk factors of death in patients with thrombotic microangiopathies. Intensive Care Med 38:1810–1817
23. Asada Y, Sumiyoshi A, Hayashi T, Suzumiya J, Kaketani K (1985) Immunohistochemistry of vascular lesion in thrombotic thrombocytopenic purpura, with special reference to factor VIII related antigen. Thromb Res 38:469–479
24. Hawkins BM, Abu-Fadel M, Vesely SK, George JN (2008) Clinical cardiac involvement in thrombotic thrombocytopenic purpura: a systematic review. Transfusion 48:382–392
25. Coppo P, Adrie C, Azoulay E et al (2003) Infectious diseases as a trigger in thrombotic microangiopathies in intensive care unit (ICU) patients? Intensive Care Med 29:564–569
26. Vermeulen Windsant IC, Snoeijs MG et al (2010) Hemolysis is associated with acute kidney injury during major aortic surgery. Kidney Int 77:913–920
27. Sponsel HT, Alfrey AC, Hammond WS, Durr JA, Ray C, Anderson RJ (1996) Effect of iron on renal tubular epithelial cells. Kidney Int 50:436–444
28. Haase M, Bellomo R, Haase-Fielitz A (2010) Novel biomarkers, oxidative stress, and the role of labile iron toxicity in cardiopulmonary bypass-associated acute kidney injury. J Am Coll Cardiol 55:2024–2033
29. Ballarin J, Arce Y, Torra Balcells R et al (2011) Acute renal failure associated to paroxysmal nocturnal haemoglobinuria leads to intratubular haemosiderin accumulation and CD163 expression. Nephrol Dial Transplant 26:3408–3411
30. Yamada R, Nozawa K, Yoshimine T et al (2011) A case of thrombotic thrombocytopenia purpura associated with systemic lupus erythematosus: diagnostic utility of ADAMTS-13 activity. Autoimmune Dis 2011:483642
31. Yamashita H, Takahashi Y, Kaneko H, Kano T, Mimori A (2013) Thrombotic thrombocytopenic purpura with an autoantibody to ADAMTS13 complicating Sjogren's syndrome: two cases and a literature review. Mod Rheumatol (in press)
32. Torok N, Niazi M, Al Ahwel Y, Taleb M, Taji J, Assaly R (2010) Thrombotic thrombocytopenic purpura associated with anti-glomerular basement membrane disease. Nephrol Dial Transplant 25:3446–3449
33. Noris M, Bucchioni S, Galbusera M et al (2005) Complement factor H mutation in familial thrombotic thrombocytopenic purpura with ADAMTS13 deficiency and renal involvement. J Am Soc Nephrol 16:1177–1183
34. Rock GA, Shumak KH, Buskard NA et al (1991) Comparison of plasma exchange with plasma infusion in the treatment of thrombotic thrombocytopenic purpura. Canadian Apheresis Study Group. N Engl J Med 325:393–397
35. George JN (2010) How I treat patients with thrombotic thrombocytopenic purpura: 2010. Blood 116:4060–4069
36. Harkness DR, Byrnes JJ, Lian EC, Williams WD, Hensley GT (1981) Hazard of platelet transfusion in thrombotic thrombocytopenic purpura. JAMA 246:1931–1933
37. Gordon LI, Kwaan HC, Rossi EC (1987) Deleterious effects of platelet transfusions and recovery thrombocytosis in patients with thrombotic microangiopathy. Semin Hematol 24:194–201
38. Froissart A, Buffet M, Veyradier A et al (2012) Efficacy and safety of first-line rituximab in severe, acquired thrombotic thrombocytopenic purpura with a suboptimal response to plasma exchange. Experience of the French Thrombotic Microangiopathies Reference Center. Crit Care Med 40:104–111

39. Ziman A, Mitri M, Klapper E, Pepkowitz SH, Goldfinger D (2005) Combination vincristine and plasma exchange as initial therapy in patients with thrombotic thrombocytopenic purpura: one institution's experience and review of the literature. Transfusion:4541–4549
40. Beloncle F, Buffet M, Coindre JP et al (2012) Splenectomy and/or cyclophosphamide as salvage therapies in thrombotic thrombocytopenic purpura: the French TMA Reference Center experience. Transfusion 52:2436–2444
41. Allford SL, Hunt BJ, Rose P, Machin SJ (2003) Guidelines on the diagnosis and management of the thrombotic microangiopathic haemolytic anaemias. Br J Haematol 120:556–573
42. Loirat C, Fremeaux-Bacchi V (2011) Atypical hemolytic uremic syndrome. Orphanet J Rare Dis 6:60

Acute Kidney Injury Is a Chronic Disease that Requires Long-Term Follow-up

C. J. Kirwan and J. R. Prowle

Introduction

Chronic kidney disease (CKD) is a complex clinical syndrome of diverse etiology. Even mild CKD has been associated with increased long term morbidity and mortality [1] and a wealth of data exists about its prevention, recognition, treatment and outcome. In contrast, acute kidney injury (AKI) has more recently been classified by consensus [2] and information concerning its true epidemiology and long-term outcomes is evolving.

In the critically ill patient, AKI is common, complicating >50 % of all ICU admissions [3], impacts on many other organ systems [4], and is associated with a high mortality (>50 % in those requiring renal replacement therapy [RRT]). As a result, there has been a drive to optimize the prevention, recognition and treatment of AKI.

For patients who survive AKI complicating critical illness, it has traditionally been assumed that renal function will recover in almost all cases [5]. However, even in the 1950s investigators were aware that, when accurate determinations of renal function were made, glomerular filtration rate (GFR) could remain low long after an acute episode of AKI [6, 7]. Following greater clinical interest in the epidemiology of AKI over the last decade, longer-term outcomes of patients who survive AKI have become a focus of investigation and are increasingly being recognized as of key clinical importance [8].

C. J. Kirwan
Adult Critical Care Unit, Royal London Hospital, Barts Health NHS Trust, Whitechapel Road, London E1 1BB, UK

J. R. Prowle (✉)
Adult Critical Care Unit, Royal London Hospital, Barts Health NHS Trust, Whitechapel Road, London E1 1BB, UK
E-mail: John.Prowle@bartshealth.nhs.uk

J.-L. Vincent (Ed.), *Annual Update in Intensive Care and Emergency Medicine 2013*,
DOI 10.1007/978-3-642-35109-9_57,

In this chapter, we briefly review the evidence for the association between AKI and risk of CKD, and the mechanisms underlying this relationship. We discuss difficulties in assessing renal function in critically ill patients after discharge from the ICU and suggest a structure for follow-up of this population. Finally, we highlight the logistic difficulties in identifying and monitoring a diverse spectrum of patients who have experienced AKI and discuss how a networked approach to the management of AKI could allow better pathways for follow-up of these patients.

Evidence that AKI is a Risk Factor for CKD

Over the last 10 years an extensive literature base has developed to support the notion that AKI is a risk factor for CKD [9–12]. A number of publications [10–12] have examined diagnostic coding in large patient databases; however, while these studies are powerful by virtue of their size, the limited nature of the patient information available makes the underlying epidemiology of CKD after AKI difficult to interpret. An analysis of US Medicare records [10] has suggested an eightfold increase in risk of developing end-stage renal disease following an episode of AKI, however, it is not clear what proportion of these patients had pre-existing CKD. Amdur and colleagues [11] reviewed a large database of patients admitted to US Veterans Health Administration Hospitals focusing on a diagnostic coding for "Acute Tubular Necrosis", and again found a significant increase in risk of CKD stage 4 and 5 in these patients. Similarly, a retrospective analysis of a US healthcare insurance database by Lo et al. [12], suggested a 28-fold increase in the risk of developing advanced CKD after episodes of AKI requiring RRT. The severity of AKI has been linked with the risk of subsequent CKD in another analysis of a Veterans Health database [13], with greatest risk of CKD associated with the most severe AKI requiring RRT; in this study additional risk factors for CKD were serum albumin, duration of AKI, age and baseline renal function. Finally, recurrent episodes of AKI may also be a particular risk for progression to CKD; a study conducted in a cohort of patients with diabetes demonstrated a 3.56 hazard ratio for developing CKD stage 4 during follow-up after AKI, with a doubling of risk with each subsequent additional episode of AKI independent of other risk factors [14].

Collectively these studies highlight a group of patients who develop CKD following AKI; however, by definition these patients have had blood tests to measure their renal function during follow-up, which may have been because they had recognized CKD (or other chronic illness) at discharge. Fewer data exist on patients who have appeared to recover back to 'normal' renal function after an episode of AKI. This is a particularly significant group as they are unlikely to receive specific renal follow up, but may still be likely to have an increased risk of developing late CKD [15]. Some information on this group of patients is available from a study by Bucaloiu and co-workers, who followed a cohort of 30,207 patients who were alive at least 90 days after hospital discharge [16]. These authors identified 1,610 patients who had an episode of AKI and recovered to apparently normal renal function and compared them to 3,652 matched controls, finding a 1.9 fold hazard of developing *de novo* CKD in patients who experienced AKI during their hospital admission over a median follow up of 3.3 years, which was associated with an over 50 % prevalence of CKD in the post-AKI population by 36 months after AKI. In addition, AKI during hospitalization was associated with a 1.5 fold hazard ratio for death over this period. This study suggests that decision on renal follow-up for patients surviving AKI cannot be easily based on serum creatinine at hospital discharge.

Pathophysiology of the Relationship Between AKI and Progressive CKD

CKD can be of very varied etiology; however, whatever the cause, substantial nephron loss leads to a common pathological process characterized by proteinuria, systemic hypertension, and a progressive decline in GFR [17]. Tubulo-interstitial fibrosis is the predominant pathology that reflects progression of CKD. This occurs as a consequence of nephron loss through any insult, with chronic inflammation thought to play an important role in this pathophysiology. In AKI, neutrophil cell exudation occurs in the acute phase and a monocytic-lymphocytic infiltrate predominates in later stages as tubules regenerate. Depending on its severity, the early neutrophilic response may contribute to chronic nephron loss; however, the delayed mononuclear cell infiltrate correlates better with pathology during the maintenance and recovery stages of AKI. Depending on the nature of the local inflammatory environment, monocytes may direct repair, regeneration, and tissue remodeling or promote fibroblastic differentiation, proliferation and fibrosis. Once fibrosis is established, a vicious cycle of auto- and paracrine interactions between inflammatory cells, endothelial cells, fibroblasts, and epithelial cells is set up, which, together with peri-tubular capillary rarefaction and hypoxia, causes progressive renal injury. In addition, after nephron loss has occurred, myogenic autoregulation of blood flow becomes impaired, causing unrestricted transmission of systemic pressure to small arterioles. This, together with compensatory neuroendocrine responses, leads to intraglomerular hypertension and hyperfiltration, causing further arteriosclerosis, glomerulosclerosis and tubular atrophy. Thus, irrespective of its etiology, the progression of CKD is largely due to common secondary factors, unrelated to the initiating disease, including race, gender, recurrent AKI, severity of proteinuria, hypertension, sodium intake, obesity, smoking, inflammation and hyperlipidemia [18]. Importantly, removal of risk factors and specific interventions may attenuate these pathophysiological processes and slow the progression of CKD.

Justification for Considering AKI as a Chronic Disease

Incomplete recovery after AKI, leading to progressive CKD is an increasingly recognized phenomenon in adult and pediatric populations [8]. Like all forms of CKD, CKD following AKI is important, as it is associated with long-term morbidity and mortality, including increased cardiovascular morbidity and progression toward end-stage renal disease. Furthermore, as CKD is the foremost risk factor for AKI in acute illness, a vicious cycle of recurrent AKI leading to progressive loss of renal function is often observed [14].

In the treatment of AKI, avoidance of recurrent renal injury is crucial to achieving maximal renal recovery; thus, the treatment of AKI merges into the prevention of CKD. Use of intermittent hemodialysis for RRT in AKI has been associated with poorer renal recovery than continuous modalities of RRT (CRRT), possibly related to intra-dialytic hypotension-induced renal hypoperfusion and recurrent ischemic injury [19]. This factor has been suggested as a justification for the preferred use of CRRT in the treatment of hemodynamically unstable patients with AKI [20]. In addition, it has been suggested recently that in early AKI, rather than the conventional approach of manipulating hemodynamic therapies to preserve urine output, strategies to optimize the renal oxygen supply/demand relationship by reducing glomerular filtration and increasing renal vascular conductance (for example by use of angiotensin-converting enzyme [ACE]-inhibitors) could be beneficial by minimizing renal parenchymal damage, even if this were at the expense of acute need for renal support [21]. In essence, such an approach would represent application of a CKD treatment to the early management of AKI. However, even with these and other potential reno-protective approaches it seems likely that the majority of AKI survivors will be left with some degree of underlying chronic renal damage requiring long-term attention, even if initially there is apparent biochemical recovery.

Detecting CKD as an Outcome After Recovery from AKI

There is thus a strong clinical rationale for identifying, monitoring and treating patients for CKD after AKI; however, practical application of such a policy in ICU survivors is complex. From the earliest studies of recovery from human AKI [6, 7] it has been clear that while many patients make an apparently excellent functional recovery, measured GFR can be persistently below normal, even years later. In a recent pediatric study of 126 patients with recovery from AKI [22], 10 % had developed CKD 1–3 years after AKI; significantly, a further 47 % of patients were identified as having increased risk of developing CKD, as evidenced by mildly decreased GFR, hypertension, and/or hyperfiltration at follow-up. Furthermore, the most common renal sequalae in these patients was microalbuminuria, a finding that is strongly associated with progression in adult CKD and which may precede overt loss of GFR. These finding are supported by animal models of AKI; in a rat model, 4 weeks after ischemia-reperfusion renal injury creatinine levels had returned to normal associated with general restoration of renal morphology and minimal fibrosis; however, when measured there was an underlying reduction in GFR of around 50 % in ischemia-reperfusion exposed rats [23]. When these rats were given a high salt diet, hypertension and proteinuria occurred in ischemia-reperfusion rats, but not in controls [23]. In a similar experiment, system salt loading was associated with reduction in creatinine clearance and a dramatic expansion of interstitial inflammation only in kidneys subjected to ischemia-reperfusion [24]. Pathogenic mechanisms implicated in this model of post-AKI CKD include persistent oxidative stress, altered gene expression and loss of peritubular capillaries [25], while progression of CKD may be mediated by the hemodynamic and fibrotic effects of angiotensin 2 [26]. Thus, after AKI chronic damage may be subtle, present late and may not be associated with obviously abnormal renal biochemistry, but still be of great prognostic significance.

Thus, the first challenge in the management of post-AKI CKD is one of diagnosis. A diverse variety of factors can confound efforts to recognize and stage CKD as an outcome of AKI, particularly in survivors of critical illness (Box 1). In both acute and chronic renal dysfunction the reciprocal relationship between creatinine and GFR means that, at higher GFR, relatively large declines in renal function are accompanied by only small rises in steady state serum creatinine, so that GFR can decrease by almost half before creatinine becomes definitively abnormal. While acutely a GFR of half normal would be adequate to fulfill the physiological roles of the kidney, *persistent* falls in GFR of any degree after AKI are indicative of irreversible nephron loss that can trigger slow, progressive decline in renal function. Thus, the imprecision of creatinine in distinguishing smaller decrements in renal function is of particular significance when assessing recovery after AKI. Even more importantly, acute falls in creatinine generation rate have been demonstrated both in critically ill humans [27] and animal models [28] decreasing both the rate of rise and plateau creatinine in AKI and this, together with the acute effects of hemodilution, makes creatinine an imprecise, delayed and poorly calibrated diagnostic test for AKI in critical illness [29]. Significantly, the greatest decrease in creatinine generation may occur in the sickest patients [27]. The decreased sensitivity of serum creatinine to detect falls in GFR in critical illness suggests that a category of patients with sub-clinical AKI may exist. Analysis of novel biomarkers of renal tubular injury suggests that biomarkers, such as neutrophil gelatinase-associated lipocalin (NGAL), remain associated with an increased risk of death and adverse outcomes even in the absence of diagnostic rises in serum creatinine [30], suggesting that sub-clinical AKI is a genuine and clinically relevant entity. To what extent sub-clinical AKI is a risk factor for CKD is uncertain. The incidence and severity of CKD has been shown to correlate with severity of AKI [13]. However, given that even subtle chronic kidney damage may predispose to adverse long-term outcomes and progressive renal dysfunction, it is likely that a large number of patients may be at risk of developing CKD without ever achieving a biochemical diagnosis of AKI during their critical illness.

Box 1
Impediments to recognition and staging of chronic kidney disease (CKD) after acute kidney injury (AKI).

- Sub-clinical AKI may go unrecognized during acute critical illness.
- Milder interstitial injury after AKI may not be associated with reduction in glomerular filtration rate (GFR) initially, but still be a risk factor for progressive CKD.
- Hyperfiltration and loss of renal reserve may mask reduction in resting GFR, despite being a potential risk factor for CKD progression.
- Significant reduction in GFR from a previously normal baseline may not cause creatinine to rise above the normal range, despite underlying nephron loss.
- Loss of muscle mass after critical illness and in chronic disease may confound ability of serum creatinine to accurately reflect the severity of reduction in GFR.

Even when the AKI is overt, assessing the degree of renal recovery suffers from the same difficulties that confound accurate diagnosis of AKI. Steady-state serum creatinine reflects the equilibrium between creatinine production and creatinine excretion in the kidney, so that a lower serum creatinine can reflect either a higher GFR or a lower creatinine generation. Many patients admitted to the intensive care unit (ICU) have chronically reduced creatinine generation due to reduction in muscle mass associated with chronic illness, or reduction in hepatic creatine production associated with chronic liver disease [31]; in these patients estimation of CKD status will be difficult even at baseline. Creatinine generation rate then falls rapidly in acute critical illness [27, 32] and, importantly, subsequent recovery of creatinine generation is likely to be slow and incomplete. Critical illness is associated with profound loss of skeletal muscle protein [33, 34] and muscle thickness [35, 36]. This is likely to be a progressive ongoing process throughout critical illness and into the recovery phase, as muscle thickness has a strong inverse correlation with time from ICU admission [35, 36]. Thus, estimates of renal function and extent of renal recovery based on ICU or hospital discharge creatinine can fail to detect significant loss of GFR, and will not be directly comparable to premorbid serum creatinine. Recovery of muscle mass after discharge is likely to be slow and incomplete, when weight gain occurs after recovery from critical illness it may be more associated with increase in fat rather than muscle [37], so this effect may persist for many months or even indefinitely.

While serum creatinine may be a poor index for the presence and severity of CKD after critical illness, one might expect formal measures of GFR to more precisely identify patients at risk of CKD progression. However, many patients who have experienced chronic renal scarring after CKD can have relatively normal GFRs for some months or years until overt CKD occurs. It is well established that renal blood flow and GFR increase with physiological stimuli, such as a high protein meal or infusion of amino acids [38]. It has been speculated that loss of this renal functional reserve occurs in early CKD as the kidney lacks capacity to further augment GFR by increasing renal blood flow and intraglomerular pressure [39]. Another way of looking at this phenomenon is that some CKD patients may achieve a normal GFR in the context of systemic and intraglomerular hypertension causing glomerular hyperfiltration [40]; such patients will have no capacity to further increase GFR as their renal reserve is maximally recruited at baseline. Hyperfiltration (increased single nephron GFR) may be triggered by neuroendocrine responses to renal scarring, including local and systemic generation of angiotensin 2, and is a process associated with progressive glomerulosclerosis and progression of CKD. Thus, the very pathophysiological mechanisms that mediate the progression of CKD may, in the short to medium term, mask the severity of CKD as assessed by serum creatinine, or by measurement of resting GFR. Proteinuria is associated with intraglomerular hypertension and hyperfiltration, and persistent proteinuria for >3 months implies a diagnosis of CKD. Even microalbuminuria (urinary albumin:creatinine ratio >3.5 mg/mmol) is associated with increased all cause mortality, cardiovascular mortality, progressive CKD, end-stage renal disease and risk of new episodes of AKI at all levels of GFR, with increasing risk at higher levels of proteinuria [41, 42]. Thus the presence of even mild proteinuria is a key prognostic indicator after recovery from AKI irrespective of serum creatinine and GFR.

Future Directions in Diagnosis

There is considerable interest in the use of renal biomarkers to accelerate and refine the diagnosis of AKI. Plasma NGAL concentrations on the day of diagnosis of AKI have been shown to correlate with degree of renal recovery [43]. This suggests that use of biomarkers as an alternate measure of severity of AKI and systemic inflammation may allow us to prognosticate about renal recovery early in the course of critical illness. Combinations of markers and clinical risk prediction models appear to refine the ability to predict recovery [44]; however, these studies have thus far looked only at prediction of freedom from RRT. Further research is needed to refine the use of biomarkers to discriminate severity of CKD in the majority of patients who come off, or never need, dialysis. Biomarkers of renal recovery might enable the targeting of specific treatments aimed at promoting tubular regeneration and minimizing fibrosis to patients at risk of CKD. Specific markers of renal recovery or fibrosis may refine such decision making; in this regard, urinary hepatocyte growth factor (uHGF), a marker linked to renal tubular epithelial cell regeneration, has been identified as a prognostic marker for recovery after AKI [44]. Additionally, AKI biomarkers could be used to screen for recurrent renal injury in the maintenance and recovery phases of AKI enabling intervention to minimize the impact on recovery.

Managing CKD After AKI

Having discussed the frequency, importance and difficulty of assessing CKD after AKI how then should we follow-up and treat these patients to improve outcomes? Few prospective clinical data exist to guide us in the AKI population. Luckily CKD in general has well-developed clinical guidelines for monitoring and treatment [45] and we should apply these principles to the management of AKI survivors. Given the diagnostic difficulties (Box 1) it seems reasonable to consider all survivors of critical illness at risk of CKD; in particular, those patients who experience significant AKI during critical illness should be specifically screened for development of CKD, irrespective of the apparent degree of renal recovery. Such an assessment should involve measurement of serum creatinine, blood pressure, urinalysis and cardiovascular risk factors. In some patients formal measurement of GFR may be helpful. Even if these investigations are normal, AKI survivors should be regarded as having a risk factor for CKD and should be offered continued screening, whereas in patients with a diagnosis of CKD, its severity and rate of progression should be assessed. The bulk of such work can be performed in primary care following CKD guidelines, such as those provided by the National Institute for Health and Clinical Excellence (NICE) in the UK; however, it is recommended that patients with more severe renal dysfunction or other specific risk factors should have specialist follow-up with a nephrologist [45]. Management will revolve around treatment of hypertension and modification of cardiovascular risk factors. In particular, patients with proteinuria and diabetes or hypertension should be offered ACE inhibitors or angiotensin-2 receptor blocking agents, which may reduce proteinuria and the progression of CKD [46]. In the post-AKI population, a particular concern is patients who experience recurrent episodes of AKI and step-wise loss of renal function; such patients will require closer monitoring and attention to patient-specific risk factors.

Proposed Follow-up Pathway for Patients Surviving AKI Complicating Critical Illness

Given the above concerns, we would like to propose a framework for the ideal follow-up of adult patients surviving critical illness that has been complicated by significant AKI (Fig. 1). Patients with pre-existing CKD before ICU admission should have their CKD stage re-assessed at discharge and CKD follow-up initiated or continued as indicated by their CKD stage; however, as these patients have experienced a new episode of AKI they should at least have CKD criteria re-assessed in 90 days to check for CKD progression if earlier follow-up is not indicated. Significant AKI is that most likely to result in irreversible nephron loss and progressive CKD; in the absence of other evidence we propose that this be defined as occurrence of KDIGO (Kidney Disease: Improving Global Outcomes) AKI-2 or greater, as severity of AKI is often underestimated during critical illness. Clinicians should also be aware, however, that many other survivors of critical illness will be at increased risk of future AKI and CKD, and that patients with other specific risk factors for CKD (diabetes, hypertension, cardiovascular disease) may also warrant monitoring for CKD within the follow-up of their chronic illnesses. Thus, all patients with AKI 2 or greater would be screened for CKD stage at discharge. In addition, any patients with less severe AKI who fail to recover function to an estimated GFR (eGFR) [47] of >60 ml/min/1.73 m^2, who have documented abnormal urinalysis, or who have anatomical renal abnormalities (including renal length <9 cm, single kidney, renal trauma or treatment for obstruction) will meet CKD criteria and should also be followed-up by this pathway. CKD patients meeting criteria for CKD 3b or greater at discharge (eGFR <45 ml/min/1.73 m^2), or with specific indications (Fig. 1), should receive specialist renal follow-up. The choice of a CKD 3b (eGFR <45), rather than a conventional CKD 4 (eGFR <30) cut-off for nephrology referral can be justified in this population as hospital discharge eGFR is likely to significantly underestimate true GFR in survivors of critical illness. In addition a CKD 3b eGFR cut-off has been associated with greater risk of reaching end-stage renal disease in younger patients [48], further justifying contact with a specialist nephrology service at an early stage. Other patients should have their CKD criteria re-assessed after 90 days with measurement of serum creatinine, calculation of eGFR using the Modification of Diet in Renal Disease (MDRD) Study equation [47], measurement of urinary albumin-creatinine ratio, urinalysis for microhematuria, blood pressure measurement and renal ultrasound (if not recently performed). At this stage, patients may require specialist referral, or be deemed appropriate for primary care follow-up at a frequency commensurate with their level of renal dysfunction [45]. Patients with evidence of progressive CKD or recurrent episodes of AKI will require closer monitoring or nephrology referral. Even in the absence of evidence of CKD at 90 days, survivors of significant AKI should have at least one further check for CKD criteria at one year to check for late progression, or indefinite follow-up, depending on the presence of other CKD risk factors.

Identifying Patients for Follow-up

We are some way away from being able to implement such a comprehensive system of AKI follow-up. Systems are required to identify and flag AKI survivors for follow-up. This can be problematic as hospital discharge may be many weeks or months down the line from the episode of AKI or critical illness and the discharging service may not be the one that actively managed the patient during their episode of AKI. Local experience in our institution is that only a fraction of patients who required RRT in the ICU and recovered renal function receive nephrology follow-up. In addition, AKI is frequently omitted from hospital discharge summaries and clinical coding, usually when AKI occurred as a complication of critical

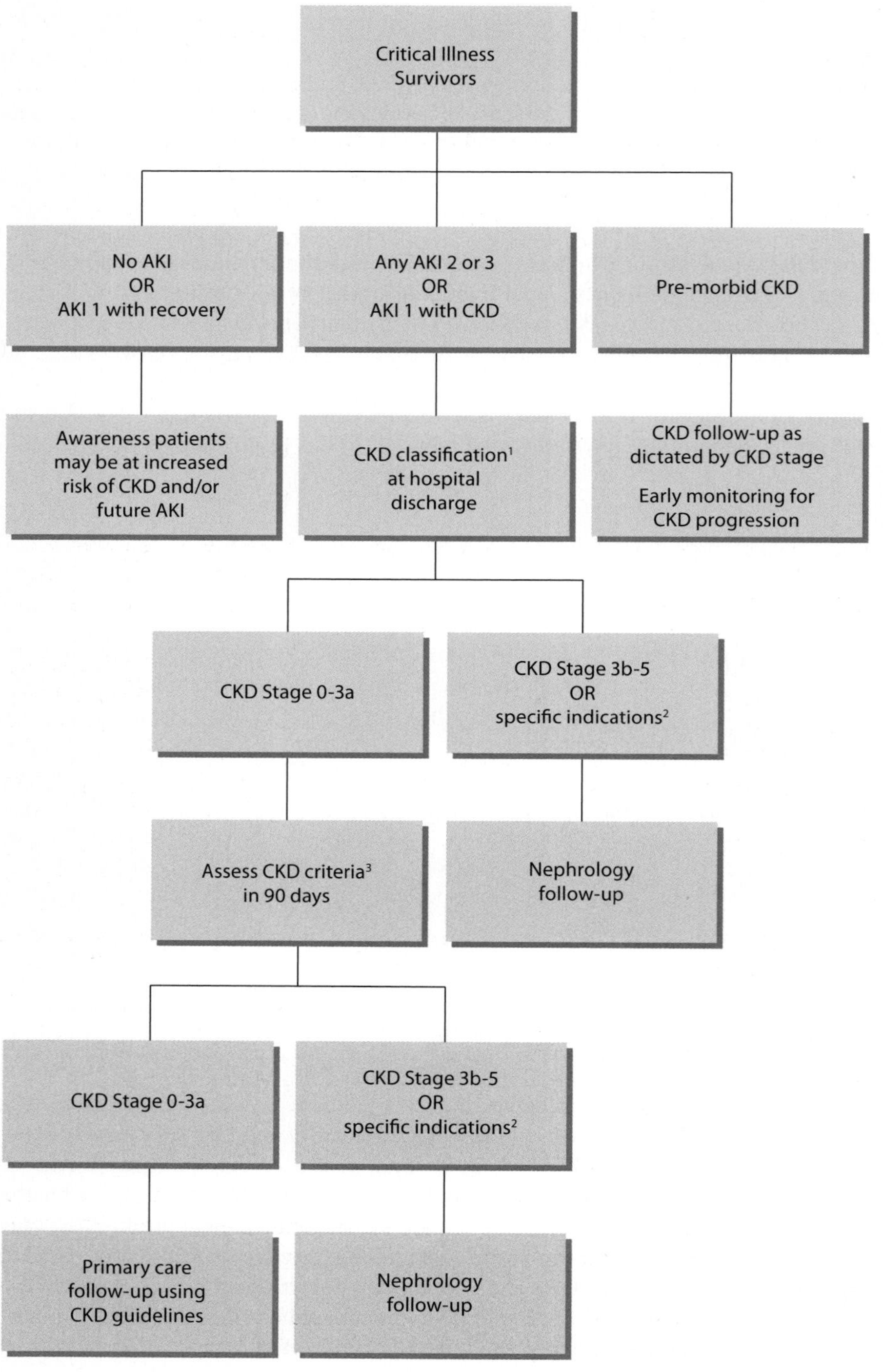
Critical Illness Survivors
No AKI OR AKI 1 with recovery
Any AKI 2 or 3 OR AKI 1 with CKD
Pre-morbid CKD
Awareness patients may be at increased risk of CKD and/or future AKI
CKD classification[1] at hospital discharge
CKD follow-up as dictated by CKD stage
Early monitoring for CKD progression
CKD Stage 0-3a
CKD Stage 3b-5 OR specific indications[2]
Assess CKD criteria[3] in 90 days
Nephrology follow-up
CKD Stage 0-3a
CKD Stage 3b-5 OR specific indications[2]
Primary care follow-up using CKD guidelines
Nephrology follow-up

◀ **Fig. 1** A proposed scheme for follow-up of patients for chronic kidney disease (CKD) after critical illness in adults. [1]CKD staging [50]: Stage 0: No evidence of CKD; Stage 1: kidney damage (proteinuria, hematuria or anatomical abnormality) with estimated glomerular filtration rate (eGFR) > 90 ml/min/1.73 m^2; Stage 2: kidney damage with eGFR 60–90; Stage 3a: eGFR 45–59; Stage 3b: eGFR 30–44; Stage 4: eGFR 15–29; Stage 5: eGFR < 15 or chronic renal replacement therapy (RRT). (Formal diagnosis should be based on 2 measurements > 2 months apart). [2]Specific indications for renal referral may include: Heavy proteinuria, proteinuria and hematuria, rapidly declining eGFR (> 5 ml/min/1.73 m^2 in one year), poorly controlled hypertension, suspected rare or genetic cause of CKD and suspected renal artery stenosis [45]. [3]Basic assessment of CKD includes measurement of serum creatinine, calculation of eGFR using the abbreviated Modification of Diet in Renal Disease (MDRD) formula, measurement of urinary albumin-creatinine ratio, urinalysis for microhematuria, blood pressure measurement and renal ultrasound. Patients with new CKD diagnosis in primary care should have a repeat serum creatinine within 2 weeks and 3 measurements within 90 days to confirm diagnosis and check for CKD progression. In addition, all patients with CKD diagnosis should have a cardiovascular risk assessment.

illness rather than as a presenting complaint. Thus, when patients are seen after discharge in other medical or surgical clinics, renal function is often not assessed. These experiences are not isolated: In an analysis of 3,929 survivors of AKI with CKD at discharge carried out in the USA, one year mortality in this population was 22 %; however, the cumulative incidence of nephrology referral before dying, initiating dialysis, or experiencing an improvement in kidney function was only 8.5 % [15]. Considering the resources that will have been devoted to treatment of the acute critical illness, neglect of simple follow-up and treatment of CKD seems perverse. Unless we adequately identify patients who have had AKI and arrange appropriate monitoring we will be unable to improve outcomes for these patients. As we have described, in many cases appropriate follow-up can be accomplished in primary care, but this will only be possible if primary care providers are made aware of the patient's background and provided with appropriate clinical guidelines. There is, thus, a clear impetus for establishing mechanisms to adequately identify and follow-up patients with AKI across a variety of care environments. In the first instance this should at least involve proper follow-up for patients who received RRT in the ICU, aiming to then build up to a more comprehensive system of follow-up, such as that as suggested above.

Applying a Network Approach to Diagnosis, Management and Follow-up of AKI

In the UK in 2009, the National Patient Safety Agency funded a report by the National Confidential Enquiry into Patient Outcome and Death (NCEPOD) "Adding Insult to Injury – a review of the care of patients who died in hospital with a primary diagnosis of acute kidney injury" [49]. Concerns raised in this report have lead to an upsurge of interest in AKI and many steps have been taken to promote the recognition and prevention of AKI across a range of settings.

Taking forward the successful network approach that has been applied to the management of trauma, cardiac and stroke care, groups of enthusiastic intensivists, nephrologists, acute internal physicians, biochemists and specialist nurses are forming AKI treatment networks. In London we have formed the London Acute Kidney Injury Network (LAKIN). The goal of LAKIN is equitable, high-quality AKI prevention and care in London and aims to achieve this through the collaborative delivery of AKI management and referral pathways, supported by education, audit, innovation and research. There is a comprehensive web site (www.londonaki.net) with open access to guidelines, care bundles and teaching materials to aid the education of primary and secondary care doctors in the importance of AKI, its prevention and treatment. This information is supplemented by a comprehensive, free, handheld mobile device application (App) available through the website.

Collaboration between multidisciplinary teams is essential to education, data collection and conducting clinical trials, and the formation of networks is key to these aspirations. Data from the LAKIN have already shown that AKI is prevalent in many specialties and, as mentioned, poorly followed up. Our hope is that application of a networked approach to AKI will enhance its management in primary, secondary and tertiary care across our region. While the initial focus of the network has been the recognition and treatment of AKI, we believe it also has the potential to naturally facilitate follow-up, by reliably identifying AKI patients and providing a framework within which outcome can be assessed and follow-up achieved, even as patients transition between ward, ICU, rehabilitation facilities and home.

Conclusion

Not only is AKI associated with increased morbidity and mortality in the ICU, it is a significant risk factor for the development of CKD, which is then associated with adverse long-term outcomes. However, the acute and chronic effects of critical illness can complicate the recognition and staging of CKD after AKI. Thus, this important condition is often neglected, despite the fact that appropriate medical follow-up and management can modify risk factors, slow CKD progression, and enable a planned transition to chronic dialysis if required. Current mechanisms of follow-up often fail to identify patients who have experienced AKI during critical illness as at risk of CKD. Robust and effective pathways for monitoring and treating these patients are required and such mechanisms may be most effectively implemented within a networked approach to AKI management.

Acknowledgements: We are grateful to Dr Chris Laing, Consultant Nephrologist, Royal Free Hospital, London, UK and Director, London Acute Kidney Injury Network (LAKIN, www.londonaki.net) for advice and permission to describe LAKIN and its objectives.

References

1. Go AS, Chertow GM, Fan D, McCulloch CE, Hsu CY (2004) Chronic kidney disease and the risks of death, cardiovascular events, and hospitalization. N Engl J Med 351:1296–1305
2. Kidney Disease: Improving Global Outcomes (2012) KDIGO Clinical Practice Guideline for acute kidney injury. Kidney Int Suppl 2:1–138
3. Ostermann M, Chang RW (2007) Acute kidney injury in the intensive care unit according to RIFLE. Crit Care Med 35:1837–1843
4. Hoste EA, De Waele JJ (2005) Physiologic consequences of acute renal failure on the critically ill. Crit Care Clin 21:251–260
5. Kjellstrand CM, Ebben J, Davin T (1981) Time of death, recovery of renal function, development of chronic renal failure and need for chronic hemodialysis in patients with acute tubular necrosis. Trans Am Soc Artif Intern Organs 27:45–50
6. Lowe KG (1952) The late prognosis in acute tubular necrosis; an interim follow-up report on 14 patients. Lancet 1:1086–1088
7. Finkenstaedt JT, Merrill JP (1956) Renal function after recovery from acute renal failure. N Engl J Med 254:1023–1026
8. Chawla LS, Kimmel PL (2012) Acute kidney injury and chronic kidney disease: An integrated clinical syndrome. Kidney Int 82:516–524
9. Mehta RL, Pascual MT, Soroko S, Chertow GM (2002) Diuretics, mortality, and nonrecovery of renal function in acute renal failure. JAMA 288:2547–2553
10. Ishani A, Xue JL, Himmelfarb J et al (2009) Acute kidney injury increases risk of ESRD among elderly. J Am Soc Nephrol 20:223–228
11. Amdur RL, Chawla LS, Amodeo S, Kimmel PL, Palant CE (2009) Outcomes following diagnosis of acute renal failure in U.S. veterans: Focus on acute tubular necrosis. Kidney Int 76:1089–1097
12. Lo LJ, Go AS, Chertow GM et al (2009) Dialysis-requiring acute renal failure increases the risk of progressive chronic kidney disease. Kidney Int 76:893–899
13. Chawla LS, Amdur RL, Amodeo S, Kimmel PL, Palant CE (2011) The severity of acute kidney injury predicts progression to chronic kidney disease. Kidney Int 79:1361–1369
14. Thakar CV, Christianson A, Himmelfarb J, Leonard AC (2011) Acute kidney injury episodes and chronic kidney disease risk in diabetes mellitus. Clin. J Am Soc Nephrol 6:2567–2572
15. Siew ED, Peterson JF, Eden SK et al (2012) Outpatient nephrology referral rates after acute kidney injury. J Am Soc Nephrol 23:305–312
16. Bucaloiu ID, Kirchner HL, Norfolk ER, Hartle 2nd JE, Perkins RM (2012) Increased risk of death and de novo chronic kidney disease following reversible acute kidney injury. Kidney Int 81:477–485
17. Venkatachalam MA, Griffin KA, Lan R, Geng H, Saikumar P, Bidani AK (2010) Acute kidney injury: a springboard for progression in chronic kidney disease. Am J Physiol Renal Physiol 298:F1078–F1094
18. Metcalfe W (2007) How does early chronic kidney disease progress? A background paper prepared for the UK Consensus Conference on early chronic kidney disease. Nephrol Dial Transplant 22(Suppl 9):ix26–ix30
19. Manns M, Sigler MH, Teehan BP (1997) Intradialytic renal haemodynamics – potential consequences for the management of the patient with acute renal failure. Nephrol Dial Transplant 12:870–872
20. Glassford NJ, Bellomo R (2011) Acute kidney injury: how can we facilitate recovery? Curr Opin Crit Care 17:562–568
21. Chawla LS, Kellum JA, Ronco C (2012) Permissive hypofiltration. Crit Care 16:317
22. Mammen C, Abbas AA, Skippen P et al (2012) Long-term risk of CKD in children surviving episodes of acute kidney injury in the intensive care unit: a prospective cohort study. Am J Kidney Dis 59:523–530

23. Pechman KR, De Miguel C, Lund H, Leonard EC, Basile DP, Mattson DL (2009) Recovery from renal ischemia-reperfusion injury is associated with altered renal hemodynamics, blunted pressure natriuresis, and sodium-sensitive hypertension. Am J Physiol Regul Integr Comp Physiol 297:R1358–R1363
24. Basile DP, Leonard EC, Tonade D, Friedrich JL, Goenka S (2012) Distinct effects on long-term function of injured and contralateral kidneys following unilateral renal ischemia-reperfusion. Am J Physiol Renal Physiol 302:F625–F635
25. Basile DP, Donohoe D, Roethe K, Osborn JL (2001) Renal ischemic injury results in permanent damage to peritubular capillaries and influences long-term function. Am J Physiol Renal Physiol 281:F887–F899
26. Basile DP, Leonard EC, Beal AG, Schleuter D, Friedrich J (2012) Persistent oxidative stress following renal ischemia-reperfusion injury increases ANG II hemodynamic and fibrotic activity. Am J Physiol Renal Physiol 302:F1494–F1502
27. Wilson FP, Sheehan JM, Mariani LH, Berns JS (2012) Creatinine generation is reduced in patients requiring continuous venovenous hemodialysis and independently predicts mortality. Nephrol Dial Transplant 27:4088–4094
28. Doi K, Yuen PS, Eisner C et al (2009) Reduced production of creatinine limits its use as marker of kidney injury in sepsis. J Am Soc Nephrol 20:1217–1221
29. Endre ZH, Pickering JW, Walker RJ (2011) Clearance and beyond: the complementary roles of GFR measurement and injury biomarkers in acute kidney injury (AKI). Am J Physiol Renal Physiol 301:F697–F707
30. Haase M, Devarajan P, Haase-Fielitz A et al (2011) The outcome of neutrophil gelatinase-associated lipocalin-positive subclinical acute kidney injury: a multicenter pooled analysis of prospective studies. J Am Coll Cardiol 57:1752–1761
31. Sherman DS, Fish DN, Teitelbaum I (2003) Assessing renal function in cirrhotic patients: problems and pitfalls. Am J Kidney Dis 41:269–278
32. Clark WR, Mueller BA, Kraus MA, Macias WL (1998) Quantification of creatinine kinetic parameters in patients with acute renal failure. Kidney Int 54:554–560
33. Hill AA, Plank LD, Finn PJ et al (1997) Massive nitrogen loss in critical surgical illness: effect on cardiac mass and function. Ann Surg 226:191–197
34. Monk DN, Plank LD, Franch-Arcas G, Finn PJ, Streat SJ, Hill GL (1996) Sequential changes in the metabolic response in critically injured patients during the first 25 days after blunt trauma. Ann Surg 223:395–405
35. Gruther W, Benesch T, Zorn C et al (2008) Muscle wasting in intensive care patients: ultrasound observation of the M. quadriceps femoris muscle layer. J Rehabil Med 40:185–189
36. Reid CL, Campbell IT, Little RA (2004) Muscle wasting and energy balance in critical illness. Clin Nutr 23:273–280
37. Reid CL, Murgatroyd PR, Wright A, Menon DK (2008) Quantification of lean and fat tissue repletion following critical illness: a case report. Crit Care 12:R79
38. Bosch JP, Saccaggi A, Lauer A, Ronco C, Belledonne M, Glabman S (1983) Renal functional reserve in humans. Effect of protein intake on glomerular filtration rate. Am J Med 75:943–950
39. Ronco C, Rosner MH (2012) Acute kidney injury and residual renal function. Crit Care 16:144
40. Brenner BM, Lawler EV, Mackenzie HS (1996) The hyperfiltration theory: a paradigm shift in nephrology. Kidney Int 49:1774–1777
41. Chronic Kidney Disease Prognosis Consortium, Matsushita K, van der Velde M et al (2010) Association of estimated glomerular filtration rate and albuminuria with all-cause and cardiovascular mortality in general population cohorts: a collaborative meta-analysis. Lancet 375:2073–2081
42. Levey AS, de Jong PE, Coresh J et al (2011) The definition, classification, and prognosis of chronic kidney disease: a KDIGO Controversies Conference report. Kidney Int 80:17–28

43. Srisawat N, Murugan R, Lee M et al (2011) Plasma neutrophil gelatinase-associated lipocalin predicts recovery from acute kidney injury following community-acquired pneumonia. Kidney Int 80:545–552
44. Srisawat N, Wen X, Lee M et al (2011) Urinary biomarkers and renal recovery in critically ill patients with renal support. Clin J Am Soc Nephrol 6:1815–1823
45. Royal College of Physicians (2008) The National Collaborating Centre for Chronic Conditions (UK) Chronic Kidney Disease: National Clinical Guideline for Early Identification and Management in Adults in Primary and Secondary Care. Available at: http://www.nice.org.uk/nicemedia/live/12069/42119/42119.pdf. Accessed October 2012
46. Jafar TH, Stark PC, Schmid CH et al (2001) Proteinuria as a modifiable risk factor for the progression of non-diabetic renal disease. Kidney Int 60:1131–1140
47. Levey AS, Coresh J, Greene T et al (2006) Using standardized serum creatinine values in the modification of diet in renal disease study equation for estimating glomerular filtration rate. Ann Intern Med 145:247–254
48. O'Hare AM, Choi AI, Bertenthal D et al (2007) Age affects outcomes in chronic kidney disease. J Am Soc Nephrol 18:2758–2765
49. National Confidential Enquiry into Patient Outcome and Death. Adding Insult to Injury – a review of the care of patients who died in hospital with a primary diagnosis of acute kidney injury. Available at: http://www.ncepod.org.uk/2009aki.htm. Accessed October 2012
50. Levey AS, Coresh J, Balk E et al (2003) National Kidney Foundation practice guidelines for chronic kidney disease: evaluation, classification, and stratification. Ann Intern Med 139:137–147

Part XVI

Renal Replacement Therapy

Regional Citrate Anticoagulation for Renal Replacement Therapy

M. Balik, M. Zakharchenko, and M. Matejovic

Introduction

Compared to heparin, anticoagulation with citrate is associated with almost no bleeding and superior circuit life enabling the delivery of high quality continuous renal replacement therapy (CRRT) [1–5]. The cumulative evidence indicating both the efficacy and safety of regional citrate anticoagulation has also been reflected in recent KDIGO (Kidney Disease: Improving Global Outcomes) guidelines suggesting the use of citrate for prevention of filter clotting in preference to standard heparin, even in patients without an increased bleeding risk [6]. Moreover, with the advent of semiautomated devices for citrate delivery, easy-to-learn operative protocols and the development of commercially available calcium-free CRRT solutions, regional citrate anticoagulation has become the favored modality in many centers. Nevertheless, despite emerging data to support the safety and potential superiority of regional citrate anticoagulation, several important issues remain unclear. These include, for example, the effects of citrate on bivalent cations, energy metabolism, inflammation and interaction of blood elements with the extracorporeal circuit. Another source of concern is the use of citrate in patients with liver failure and cytopathic shock states, when cellular capacity to metabolize citrate is markedly limited. In this chapter, we discuss the homeostatic consequences of var-

M. Balik
Dept. of Anesthesiology and Intensive Care, First Faculty of Medicine, Charles University and General University Hospital, U nemocnice 2, Prague 2, 120 00, Czech Republic

M. Zakharchenko
Dept. of Anesthesiology and Intensive Care, First Faculty of Medicine, Charles University and General University Hospital, U nemocnice 2, Prague 2, 120 00, Czech Republic

M. Matejovic (✉)
Charles University in Prague, Faculty of Medicine in Pilsen, Teaching Hospital Plzen, Czech Republic 1st Medical Department, alej Svobody 80, 304 60 Plzen, Czech Republic
E-mail: matejovic@fnplzen.cz

J.-L. Vincent (Ed.), *Annual Update in Intensive Care and Emergency Medicine 2013*,
DOI 10.1007/978-3-642-35109-9_58,

ious citrate modalities, bioenergetic gains of various forms of citrate-based CRRT, offer emerging insights into the effects of citrate on the blood-hemofilter interactome and address economical aspects of citrate anticoagulation.

Balance Between Blood Flow and Effluent Flow

A very important parameter with every citrate modality is the balance between blood flow and effluent flow, which is the principle of most semi-automated modules. Higher blood flow (Qb) needs higher citrate flow (Qc) to reach the desired 3–4 mmol/l of citrate within the circuit (Fig. 1) [5, 7, 8]. This load of citrate is counterbalanced by the amount of dialysis/filtration. Higher CRRT dosage and effluent flows (Fig. 1) eliminate more of the citrate load [5, 8–11]. To avoid unwanted ion and acid-base derangements under calcium substitution (metabolic alkalosis, hypernatremia, hypomagnesemia) one needs to either reduce blood flow or to increase dialysis/substitution flow.

Recent papers tackling the issue of adequate dosage of dialysis and filtration on morbidity and mortality have found a dose of 20–25 ml/kg/h adequate in critically ill patients [12, 13]. For trisodium citrate (TSC), this dose represents 'flow limited dialysis' [14] and requires slowing blood flow to 80–110 ml/min to limit the dose of citrate, and avoid alkalosis and hypernatremia, which are blood flow related [8, 10]. This approach makes patients stable in terms of homeostasis and the amount of citrate eliminated on the filter in this setting is about 30–36 % [15]. Regardless of citrate anticoagulation, a Qb of 100 ml/min is enough to saturate the dialysate at a flow rate of 2 l/h [14]. However, this low blood flow may limit ultrafiltration in certain situations (pulmonary edema, postdilutional continuous venovenous hemofiltration [CVVH]), because the amount of ultrafiltrated plasma fluid should not exceed 20 % of blood flow for rheological and coagulation reasons.

A blood flow around 150 ml/min requires a higher citrate flow but enables higher ultrafiltration rates to be used. However, increasing dialysis/filtration flows of current commercially available bicarbonate-containing substitution fluids [8, 11, 10] to 2,000–3,000 ml/h may not be sufficient to avoid metabolic alkalosis and hypernatremia when using 4 % TSC [5, 8]. Nevertheless, it may avoid typical metabolic side effects with acid-citrate-dextrose (ACD) and even ordinary calcium-containing lactate-based fluids [16, 17] because part of the ACD (30 %) is given as citric acid. Thus, if higher dose CRRT is prescribed, for example 35 ml/kg, then higher amounts of citrate would be eliminated [9]. The amount lost in the effluent is similar for continuous venovenous hemodiafiltration (CVVHDF) as for CVVH because the sieving coefficient for citrate is about 1 [7, 9, 16] and elimination may be facilitated by the large filter area [18]. The easiest way to calculate the proportion of citrate escaping to the effluent and associated citrate systemic gain is with postdilutional CVVH, where citrate loss can be obtained as prefilter citrate dosage times the filtration fraction [5]. Due to unavailability of direct measures of citrate levels in clinical practice, another means of estimating

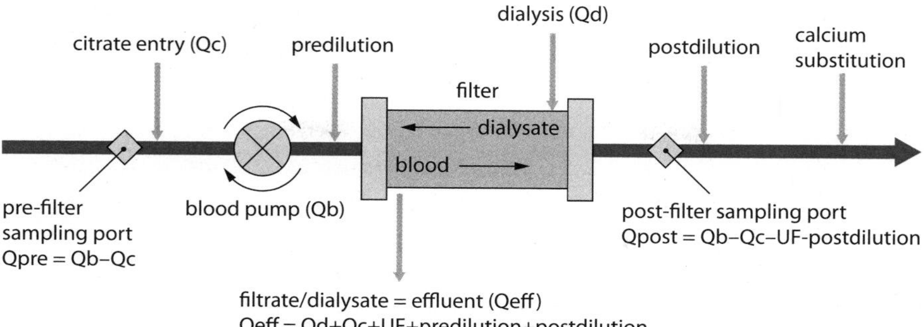

Fig. 1 Configuration of a CRRT circuit under citrate anticoagulation. UF: ultrafiltration, i. e., net fluid removal (l/h); Qb: blood pump speed (l/h); Qc: acid-citrate-dextrose (ACD) pump speed (l/h); Qpre: blood flow at prefilter sampling port (l/h): Qb − Qc; Qpost: blood flow at postfilter sampling port (l/h) = Qb − Qc − UF − postdilution; Qd: dialysis dose (l/h); Qeff: filtrate/dialysate (effluent) production (l/h) = d + UF + Qc + predilution + postdilution

systemic citrate load is to measure the difference in unmeasured anions in the prefilter and postfilter blood [16].

Current Citrate Solutions and Associated Dialysis/Substitution Fluids

There is currently no standard citrate protocol and different solutions and modalities are used. The most frequently used citrate solutions are 4 % TSC [8, 10], 2.2 % ACD [9, 17, 19–21] and an isotonic calcium-free predilution replacement fluid containing citrate in a concentration corresponding to the desired bicarbonate equivalent [22, 23]. There are also other customized, locally prepared solutions, for example, highly concentrated citrate (15 %, 500 mmol/l) for postdilutional CVVH [1].

ACD contains 113 mmol citrate/l and 138.9 mmol glucose/l (2.5 % glucose) which brings a significant load of glucose during CRRT. Thirty percent of the citrate load is provided as citric acid reducing the buffer strength and potential for metabolic alkalosis. Four percent TSC contains 136 mmol/l of TSC salt, which represents a significant load of sodium for a patient. The usual isotonic citrate solution contains 12 mmol/l (0.2 %), which is given in predilution as sodium salt plus citric acid [22]. There are various protocols with citrate concentrations between 12–20 mmol/l, which require infusion of a significant volume of this citrate fluid pre-filter and associated usage of special dialysis/substitution fluid [22, 23]. As with other citrate protocols, the fluids are designed for a similar balance between dialysis/substitution flow and blood flow (i. e., about 3,000–4,000 ml/h for Qb 150 ml/min). Filter survival with these low concentration isotonic citrate solutions is significantly shorter than for the modalities with high concentration citrate

Table 1 Comparison of estimated costs between the three modalities of continuous venovenous hemodiafiltration (CVVHDF): Acid-citrate-dextrose (ACD)/lactate – ACD with calcium-containing and lactate-buffered solution; trisodium citrate (TSC)/bicarbonate – TSC with calcium-free and bicarbonate-buffered solution; Heparin (Hep)/lactate – heparin with lactate-buffered solution. From [15] with permission

	ACD/lactate (Group 1)	TSC/bicarbonate (Group 2)	Hep/lactate (Group 3)	MW-U test p values 1 vs 2	1 vs 3	2 vs 3
Estimated costs (EUR/24 h)						
Citrate solution	53.82 (48.3–55.89)	32.22 (28.43–37.9)	N/A	<0.01	N/A	N/A
Replacement fluids	63 (63–84)	135.3 (135.3–135.3)	79.8 (63–84)	<0.01	0.11	<0.01
Calcium chloride	11.13 (6.36–14.31)	11.13 (9.54–15.9)	N/A	0.38	N/A	N/A
Heparin	N/A	N/A	7.47 (5.81–8.72)	N/A	N/A	N/A
Postfilter Ca^{2+} (6 per 24 h)	13.74	13.74	N/A	N/A	N/A	N/A
Extra aPTT (4 per 24 h)	N/A	N/A	12.56	N/A	N/A	N/A
Total costs/24 h excluding circuits	**142 (128–161)**	**195 (191–224)**	**100 (82–104)**	**< 0.01**	**< 0.01**	**< 0.01**
Daily circuit cost [a]	58 (44–83)	48 (30–75)	85 (64–106)	<0.01	<0.01	<0.01
Total costs/24 h including circuits	**200 (186–219)**	**243 (239–273)**	**185 (167–189)**	**< 0.01**	**< 0.01**	**< 0.01**

[a] estimated from circuit life. The costs of the arterial Ca2+ measurement were not calculated because they were provided with the standard blood gas determination. All values are medians (interquartile range). Daily circuit costs were calculated as 24/circuit lifetime (h) in individual patients and then converted into expenses without correction for circuit down-time. aPTT: activated partial thromboplastin time; MW-U: Mann-Whitney U; N/A: not applicable

[10, 15, 22, 23]. The rationale for minimizing eventual systemic dosage of citrate with these low concentration citrate fluids cannot be supported by the current literature because citrate is readily metabolized in intermediate metabolism [5, 15, 16] and no harm has been shown from a systemic dose of citrate unless alterations of acid-base and ion homeostasis appear.

The available fluids can be bicarbonate or lactate-based. The bicarbonate solution is calcium-free, contains reduced levels of sodium and bicarbonate and is used as a dialysis and/or replacement fluid (for example: Na 133 mmol/l, HCO_3^- 20 mmol/l). Although current recommendations [6] suggest bicarbonate, rather

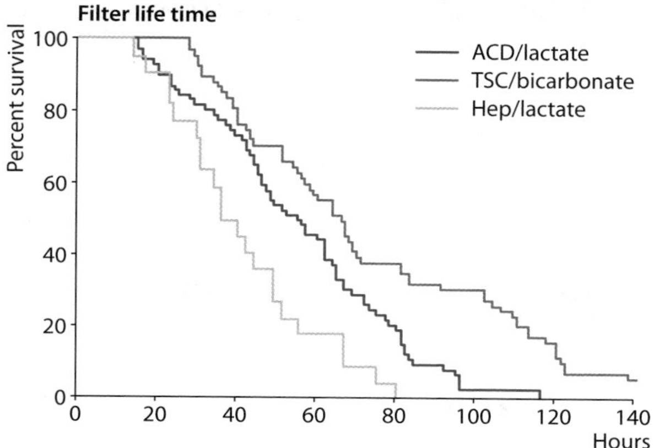

Fig. 2 Kaplan-Meier curves of median circuit survival time in the group with heparin plus calcium-containing lactate buffer (Hep/lactate: 38 h, IQR 30–51); the group with acid-citrate dextrose (ACD) plus calcium-containing fluid (ACD/lactate: 55.5 h, IQR 38.5–74) and in the group with trisodium citrate (TSC) plus calcium-free fluid (TSC/bicarbonate: 64 h, IQR 42.5–107.5). Data from [15]. All $p < 0.01$

than lactate, as a buffer in dialysis and substitution fluids, recent papers have demonstrated good tolerance to lactate-buffered fluids [24, 25]. Patients with primarily elevated lactate levels should be given bicarbonate-buffered fluids; however, the ordinary calcium containing lactate-buffered solutions were apparently well-tolerated in combination with citrate CRRT [16, 17]. Lactate buffers are still widely used because of lack of strong evidence in favor of bicarbonate-buffered solutions, and also because of growing interest in providing lactate as an outstanding metabolic substrate under stress conditions [24–26]. Finally, solution stability and lower cost compared to bicarbonate solutions may also assume importance in this context. If the TSC could be combined with a calcium-free low-lactate buffered solution, patients may tolerate a lactate buffer and still have an acceptable bioenergetic gain. In addition, the cost of the citrate modality (Table 1) may be less than for the heparin one [15]. A customized calcium-free lactate-based fluid has been tested with citrate [11]. The newly commercially available solution needs further clinical testing despite of the first promising results in terms of patient's homeostatic stability [27].

Another important issue is the presence of calcium in dialysis/substitution fluid. Calcium containing solutions are used in postdilution CVVH to replenish the loss of calcium on the filter [1]. In other settings, the presence of calcium in dialysis/substitution fluids neutralizes citrate already in the filter, thereby increasing requirements for prefilter citrate and causing a higher systemic load of citrate, which, in turn, may double the load under calcium-free solutions [9, 15, 16]. Increasing the dosage of citrate has consequences for ion and acid-base changes causing a higher load of sodium and risk of metabolic alkalosis, in particular with TSC [8,10]. This phenomenon is less apparent with ACD, because of the presence of citric acid as part of ACD, which partially compensates the base equivalent of citrate metabolism and reduces sodium cation in ACD compared to the higher load of sodium in TSC [16, 17].

The neutralization of citrate already during passage through the filter with calcium-containing dialysis/substitution fluids not only increases the dosage of prefilter citrate, but also potentiates circuit clotting, particularly at the venous end of an extracorporeal circuit. Application of calcium-free fluids extended the median filter life to 64 h compared to 55.5 h for a calcium containing modality (target postfilter Ca^{2+} concentrations were similar) and to 38 h for the control group on heparin anticoagulation (Fig. 2) [15].

In summary, a slower blood flow and a calcium-free dialysis/substitution fluid requires less citrate infused prefilter compared to higher flows and calcium-containing fluids. Higher citrate flows produce higher citrate levels, which may not be accompanied by apparent acid-base and ion adverse effects if counteracted by appropriate flow of effluent [1, 21, 28].

Homeostatic Implications and Monitoring of Citrate Accummulation

A molecule of citrate gives rise to three molecules of bicarbonate. Metabolic alkalosis may be a result of excessive prefilter infusion of buffer-bases in the form of citrate [8]. Although 20–40 % of the infused amount is eliminated with standard flows of dialysis/hemofiltration on the commonly used polysulfone filters [5, 7, 15], the remaining 60–80 % represents systemic dose of citrate, which may influence the acid-base status. Therefore, the fluids designed for administration with citrate have a reduced concentration of buffer (18–20 mmol/l) and the anionic side of the solution is replaced by chloride (114–116 mmol/l). Metabolic alkalosis may be counteracted by increasing dialysis/substitution fluid at constant blood and citrate flows. Clearance of citrate is similar with diffusive transport (dialysis) and with convective (filtration) mode [15, 20] if a similar dose (effluent flow) is applied, because the sieving coefficient of the molecule is about one in both modalities [16]. Current citrate modalities show low rates of metabolic alkalosis of about 3–4 % [5, 8, 10, 15]. In contrast to metabolic alkalosis, a positive anion gap metabolic acidosis may develop in case of inadequate citrate metabolism. Unfortunately, neither anion gap nor unmeasured anions were sensitive enough to detect changes in citrate levels when assessed in patients' bloodstreams. In contrast, monitoring of unmeasured anions or strong ion difference may be helpful within the extracorporeal circuit as an indirect measure of citrate concentration [16]. In general, metabolic acidosis may be treated by increasing blood flow, associated citrate flow and keeping dialysis/substitution flows constant. Importantly, this should always be done after exclusion of citrate accumulation resulting from impaired citrate metabolism. The most frequent causes of impaired citrate metabolism are liver failure and tissue hypoxia during profound shock. In addition, extreme caution is required in all pathologic states associated with mitochondrial dysfunction and ineffective oxygen utilization (e.g., metformin-associated lactic acidosis).

Calcium is removed from the patient in the form of calcium-citrate complexes through the hemofilter. The calcium loss is proportional to the effluent flow (Fig. 1) and must be balanced by postfilter calcium substitution. If calcium-free fluids are used, the amount of calcium lost on the filter (about 1.7 mmol/l of effluent) approximately doubles the amount lost if calcium-containing fluids are used (0.75 mmol/l of effluent) [10, 16, 17, 30]. Calcium should be substituted by calcium chloride because replacement with calcium gluconate may increase the pool of bicarbonate precursors, thus adding to the risk of unwanted metabolic alkalosis. The usual dose of calcium chloride is about 5–15 ml/h of a 10 % solution. Various citrate protocols have shown either mild accumulation, deficit or even balance of total calcium mostly depending on the intensity of calcium substitution [11, 21, 23, 31]. In addition to the acid-base parameters mentioned above, the calcium index (Ca^{tot}/Ca^{2+}) seems to be the most sensitive parameter of citrate accumulation [5, 7, 29, 32]. Citrate binds to Ca^{2+}, which lowers its detectable level and thus increases the calcium index above 2.25–2.5 in case of failure of citrate metabolism [8, 10, 15–17]. The calcium index seems to be more useful than direct citrate measurement, because no cut-off values for citrate in blood exist. In other words, there are patients with reported high levels and no associated signs of toxicity.

Citrate is at least partially supplied as a sodium salt in all available forms. Therefore, there is always a risk of hypernatremia. This risk is less with ACD and isotonic citrate solutions because part of these solutions is in the form of citric acid. All dialysis/substitution fluids designed for citrate anticoagulation possess low sodium concentrations, between 130–133 mmol/l, allowing for diffusion of sodium to the dialysate to avoid hypernatremia from prefilter citrate infusion [8, 10, 11]. Current citrate modalities show an almost zero incidence of dysnatremia [8, 10, 15–17, 20].

Citrate influences magnesium levels similarly to calcium, although the affinity for ionized magnesium seems to be slightly less than for ionized calcium [11, 30]. The levels of magnesium in available dialysis/substitution fluids (about 0.7–1.0 mmol/l) are insufficient and may lead to depletion of the relatively low body pool of magnesium within a couple of days [34, 35]. The presence of magnesium in dialysis/substitution fluids in citrate-anticoagulated CRRT is a matter of debate [11,23], because magnesium is also chelated by citrate, thus neutralizing a portion of the citrate and increasing the demand for its infusion to lower postfilter Ca^{2+} into a desired range. The importance of removing magnesium for reduction of filter clotting is questionable [36]. In addition, lowering of citrate dosage does not outweigh the risk of hypomagnesemia [34, 35] if magnesium is not replenished properly [11]. Citrate CRRT increases daily requirements for magnesium by an extra 2 to 3 g of magnesium sulfate [30]. This requirement may increase with higher CRRT dosage when more magnesium is eliminated bound to citrate in the effluent.

Standard RRT fluids do not contain phosphorus. However, CRRT in critically ill patients is often indicated earlier when levels are not as high as in chronic dialysis.

Omitting substitution of phosphorous may contribute to development of multiorgan dysfunction [37]. Furthermore, data are lacking on the eventual impact of citrate on phosphorus metabolism through changes in parathormone and ionized calcium.

Bioenergetic Gain During Citrate Anticoagulation

CRRT with citrate anticoagulation has metabolic consequences, including its bioenergetic impact. The bioenergetic equivalents of the substrates are 2.48 kJ/mmol of citrate, 3.06 kJ/mmol of glucose that is part of the ACD solution (2.5 % dextrose) and 1.37 kJ/mmol of lactate if a lactate-based fluid is involved [5, 15, 16, 38].

Recently, several groups have studied bioenergetic gains under various citrate protocols [5, 15, 16]. Similar data for daily citrate systemic gain were reported for predilution CVVH and CVVHDF [15, 16] and for postdilution CVVH [5]. Glucose accounted for the main bioenergetic gain of the ACD modality, up to 6.6 g/h (159 g/24 h) of glucose may enter the patient's circulation [16].

The bioenergetic gain observed with blood flows of about 150 ml/min applied with a combination of ACD as the citrate source and calcium-containing lactate-buffered solutions amounted to about 262.8 kJ/h (59.8 kcal/h), i. e., about 6,000 kJ/day (1,434 kcal/day) not corrected for filter-down time [16]. This CRRT-derived energy load represents an unacceptably high proportion of a patient's daily energy needs. The bioenergetic gain of the combination of ACD anticoagulation and lactate-buffered calcium-containing solutions cannot be applied without reducing the patient's nutritional intake, or at least the carbohydrate load. Ignoring this 'hidden source' of calories may lead to overfeeding with consequent hepatic steatosis and possible deterioration of liver function.

The caloric load of citrate CRRT can be reduced by using TSC as a citrate source (avoiding glucose delivery), by increasing dialysate flow and associated citrate removal, by using bicarbonate-buffered solutions (avoiding lactate delivery), calcium-free solutions (reducing citrate dose), using an isotonic calcium-free citrate-buffered predilution replacement fluid [22], or lowering blood flow (reducing citrate delivery).

If the blood flow is reduced to 100 ml/min, the energy delivery from ACD (glucose and citrate) and lactate buffer would be reduced to about 188 kJ/h, a reduction of 29 %. When ACD is used with bicarbonate-buffered fluids and a blood flow of 100 ml/min, but still containing calcium, the bioenergetic delivery may be further reduced to about 116 kJ/h, i. e., 2,794 kJ/24 h, a reduction of 56 %. If ACD is used with a calcium-free bicarbonate buffered fluid and a blood flow of 100 ml/min, median estimated daily bioenergetic delivery is about 1,910 kJ/24 h (1,120 kJ/24 h from glucose and 816 kJ/24 h from citrate), i. e., a reduction of 68 % (Table 2), although the extrapolated delivery would still require adjustment of daily nutritional intake. In contrast, the total bioenergetic gain from the TSC citrate modality using calcium-free bicarbonate-buffered solutions is about 20 kJ/h (4.8 kcal/h), i. e., about 500 kJ/day, and is solely derived from citrate (Table 2) [15].

Table 2 Comparison of estimated daily citrate anticoagulated continuous venovenous hemodiafiltration (CVVHDF) substrate delivery and bioenergetic gain not corrected for filter down-time and adjusted for the unified blood flow of 100 ml/min. From [15] with permission

	ACD/Ca^{plus}/ lactate (Group 1)	TSC/Ca^{min}/ bicarb (Group 2)	ACD/Ca^{min}/ bicarb (Group 3)	MW-U test p values 1 vs 2	1 vs 3	2 vs 3
Substrate delivery (+) or loss (−), corrected for a Qb of 100 ml/min						
Citrate (mmol/24 h)	455 (416–498)	354 (298–458)	329 (295–360)	<0.01	<0.01	0.33
Glucose (mmol/24 h)	567 (501–613)	-146 (-172– -62)	366 (328–401)	<0.01	<0.01	<0.01
Lactate (mmol/24 h)	1,260 (1,181–1,418)	−67 (-105– -41)	-70 (-110– -43)	<0.01	<0.01	0.35
Bioenergetic gain (+) or loss (−)						
Citrate (kJ/24 h) [a]	1,128 (1,031–1,235)	878 (738–1,136)	816 (732–893)	<0.01	<0.01	0.28
Glucose (kJ/24 h) [a]	1,735 (1,532–1,877)	-447 (-525– -189)	1,120 (1,004–1,227)	<0.01	<0.01	<0.01
Lactate (kJ/24 h) [a]	1,727 (1,618–1,943)	-92 (-144– -57)	-96 (-148– -59))	<0.01	<0.01	0.31
Total (kJ/24 h)a	**4,510 (4,115–4,913)**	**480 (192–602)**	**1,910 (1,568–2,085)**	**< 0.01**	**< 0.01**	**< 0.01**

[a] For conversion to Kcal, divide by 4.184. All values are medians and interquartile ranges. ACD/Ca^{plus}/lactate: acid-citrate-dextrose with calcium-containing and lactate-buffered solution; TSC/Ca^{min}/bicarb: trisodium citrate with calcium-free and bicarbonate-buffered solution; ACD/Ca^{min}/bicarb: ACD with calcium-free and bicarbonate-buffered solution. MW-U: Mann-Whitney U

Continuous is not always continuous, however [39]. Hence, the above estimates of bioenergetic gains should be corrected for filter-down time, which differs between centers and modalities. Estimates of total energy delivery may, therefore, be 10–20 % lower. However, this applies less for the citrate groups, because circuit life with citrate is longer and citrate delivery continues when bags are changed, while the blood pump does not stop.

In summary, the bioenergetic gain of citrate CRRT comes from glucose (in ACD), lactate and citrate. The total amount differs substantially between modalities and is unacceptably high when using ACD as a citrate source in combination with calcium-containing lactate-buffered fluids and an ordinary blood flow of 150 ml/min. With TSC, calcium-free bicarbonate-buffered fluids and blood flow reduced to 100 ml/min, the bioenergetic gain is limited. When calculating the patient's nutritional needs, the energy delivered by CRRT needs to be taken into account.

Impact on the Interaction Between Blood Elements and Extracorporeal Circuit

Interactions of blood with dialysis membranes lead to activation of several pathways, including the complement and contact pathways, and platelet, monocyte and neutrophil activation. However, whether citrate can modulate these complex blood-membrane interactions is largely unknown. We have recently shown that proteomic techniques represent a powerful tool to explore molecular mechanisms of membrane biocompatibility [40, 41]. Using the same approach, we analyzed the composition of blood-membrane interactome under citrate anticoagulation and compared it to heparin. The key difference between citrate and heparin lies in the large content of fibrin alpha chain fragments detected in citrate-associated biofilm (J Mares, personal communication). At the same time, significantly lower amounts of protein (particularly hemoglobin) were found adhering to dialysis membranes after the citrate procedure, despite an equal degree of coagulation activation as documented by D-dimer and thrombin-antithrombin complex production. These findings imply generation of imperfect fibrin clots during citrate anticoagulation. In addition, citrate anticoagulation may have effects reaching far beyond thrombogenicity. In fact, the second most striking feature of the citrate-associated biofilm was adsorption of complement factor H-related protein 3 (FHR3) (J Mares, personal communication). Proteins belonging to the complement factor H family inhibit the membrane attack complex thus protecting self-cells from damage by complement. Several pathogens express surface molecules mimicking these proteins to evade host immunity and an association was noticed between FHR3 and susceptibility to meningococcal disease [42]. Moreover, imbalances in complement regulation related to FHR3 are also linked to the pathogenesis of other diseases such as hemolytic uremic syndrome (HUS) or systemic lupus erythematosus. As all these disorders commonly require RRT, even preferably with regional anticoagulation, it is reasonable to speculate that the choice of anticoagulation may influence the underlying pathology in an unpredictable way. On the other hand, hypocalcemia within the extracorporeal circuit may reduce the inflammatory load by suppressing the release of inflammatory mediators from cells adhered to the membrane [43–45]. Citrate has also been shown to abolish the release of myeloperoxidase (MPO), platelet factor 4 and serotonin from platelets in a calcium-dependent manner [45]. Reduction of platelet activation, however, was not associated with improved intradialytic hemodynamic stability [46]. In summary, the net effect of citrate on molecular mechanisms underlying blood-membrane interactions is highly complex and merits further intensive research.

Cost Efficiency

In addition to metabolic complexity, the costs of the citrate modality are another reason for reluctance of ICU staff to use citrate. A review article [5] and a study published only in abstract form [47] have already suggested that when including treatment of the adverse effects of the heparin modality, the costs of citrate would not be much different. A recent study [15] calculated expenses for anticoagulation, associated monitoring and dialysis/substitution fluids. It showed that the costs of ACD plus lactate-buffered CVVHDF were only slightly higher than the heparin anticoagulated modality, especially when used at the lower blood flow. The use of TSC as the citrate source and calcium-free bicarbonate buffered solutions is a more expensive modality. Thus, reducing bioenergetic gain requires the use of more expensive fluids. It does, however, extend circuit lifetime, which saves costs (Table 1). The median costs of citrate, calcium chloride infusion, dialysis/replacement fluid and 4-hourly postfilter Ca^{2+} measurements for each citrate modality in EUR/ 24 h of CVVHDF are displayed in Table 1. Table 1 also presents overall expenses for the three modalities, including the median circuit cost per 24 hour of CVVHDF; these were estimated from the median circuit lifetime. The expenses for citrate anticoagulation are driven particularly by special calcium-free dialysis/substitution fluids. Based on these data, a single chamber calcium-free lactate buffered bag [27] may make the citrate modality cheaper than the heparin modality with regard to filter longevity.

Conclusion

Because of its efficacy, potential superiority to heparins and availability at affordable costs, citrate has emerged as a useful regional anticoagulant for CRRT. Although its safety has markedly improved with the introduction of well-designed protocols, semiautomated devices and commercially available fluids for citrate-based anticoagulation, there are still many issues to consider and many questions to answer. The use of citrate has important and unrecognized bioenergetic implications that should be included in calculations of patients' nutritional needs and that should take into account the type of citrate and dialysis/substitution solutions. The impact of citrate on calcium and magnesium metabolism, including endocrine changes, needs further clarification, particularly if citrate-based CRRT is provided for a longer time. Furthermore, the safety aspects of citrate under conditions of compromised cellular energy metabolism need to be better defined. Finally, the effect of citrate on the host response, in particular the molecular mechanisms of blood-dialyzer interactions, represents another exciting field both for basic and clinical research.

Acknowledgement: Supported by the Charles University Research Fund (project number P36) and the project CZ.1.05/2.1.00/03.0076 from the European Regional Development Fund.

References

1. Oudemans-van Straaten HM, Bosman RJ, Koopmans M et al (2009) Citrate anticoagulation for continuous venovenous hemofiltration. Crit Care Med 37:545–552
2. Wu MY, Hsu YH, Bai CH, Lin YF, Wu CH, Tam KW (2012) Regional citrate versus heparin anticoagulation for continuous renal replacement therapy: a meta-analysis of randomized controlled trials. Am J Kidney Dis 59:810–818
3. Zhang Z, Hongying N (2012) Efficacy and safety of regional citrate anticoagulation in critically ill patients undergoing continuous renal replacement therapy. Intensive Care Med 38:20–28
4. Hetzel GR, Schmitz M, Wissing H et al (2011) Regional citrate versus systemic heparin for anticoagulation in critically ill patients on continuous venovenous haemofiltration: a prospective randomized multicentre trial. Nephrol Dial Transplant 26:232–239
5. Oudemans-van Straaten HM, Kellum JA, Bellomo R (2011) Clinical review: anticoagulation for continuous renal replacement therapy – heparin or citrate? Crit Care 15:202
6. Global KDI, Group OKAKIW (2012) KDIGO Clinical Practice Guideline for Acute Kidney Injury. Kidney Int 2(Suppl):1–138
7. Oudemans-van Straaten HM (2010) Citrate anticoagulation for continuous renal replacement therapy in the critically ill. Blood Purif 29:191–196
8. Morgera S, Scholle C, Voss G et al (2004) Metabolic complications during regional citrate anticoagulation in continuous venovenous hemodialysis: single-center experience. Nephron Clin Pract 97:c131–c136
9. Mariano F, Morselli M, Bergamo D et al (2011) Blood and ultrafiltrate dosage of citrate as a useful and routine tool during continuous venovenous haemodiafiltration in septic shock patients. Nephrol Dial Transplant 26:3882–3888
10. Morgera S, Schneider M, Slowinski T et al (2009) A safe citrate anticoagulation protocol with variable treatment efficacy and excellent control of the acid-base status. Crit Care Med 37:2018–2024
11. Morgera S, Haase M, Ruckert M et al (2005) Regional citrate anticoagulation in continuous hemodialysis – acid-base and electrolyte balance at an increased dose of dialysis. Nephron Clin Pract 101:c211–c219
12. Bellomo R, Cass A, Cole L et al (2009) Intensity of continuous renal-replacement therapy in critically ill patients. N Engl J Med 361:1627–1638
13. Palevsky PM, Zhang JH, O'Connor TZ et al (2008) Intensity of renal support in critically ill patients with acute kidney injury. N Engl J Med 359:7–20
14. Relton S, Greenberg A, Palevsky PM (1992) Dialysate and blood flow dependence of diffusive solute clearance during CVVHD. ASAIO J 38:M691–M696
15. Balik M, Zakharchenko M, Leden P et al (2013) Bioenergetic gain of citrate anticoagulated continuous hemodiafiltration – a comparison between 2 citrate modalities and unfractionated heparin. J Crit Care 28:87–95
16. Balik M, Zakharchenko M, Otahal M et al (2012) Quantification of systemic delivery of substrates for intermediate metabolism during citrate anticoagulation of continuous renal replacement therapy. Blood Purif 33:80–87
17. Gupta M, Wadhwa NK, Bukovsky R (2004) Regional citrate anticoagulation for continuous venovenous hemodiafiltration using calcium-containing dialysate. Am J Kidney Dis 43:67–73
18. Brunet S, Leblanc M, Geadah D, Parent D, Courteau S, Cardinal J (1999) Diffusive and convective solute clearances during continuous renal replacement therapy at various dialysate and ultrafiltration flow rates. Am J Kidney Dis 34:486–492
19. Mariano F, Tedeschi L, Morselli M, Stella M, Triolo G (2010) Normal citratemia and metabolic tolerance of citrate anticoagulation for hemodiafiltration in severe septic shock burn patients. Intensive Care Med 36:1735–1743
20. Chadha V, Garg U, Warady BA, Alon US (2002) Citrate clearance in children receiving continuous venovenous renal replacement therapy. Pediatr Nephrol 17:819–824

21. Swartz R, Pasko D, O'Toole J, Starmann B (2004) Improving the delivery of continuous renal replacement therapy using regional citrate anticoagulation. Clin Nephrol 61:134–143
22. Palsson R, Niles JL (1999) Regional citrate anticoagulation in continuous venovenous hemofiltration in critically ill patients with a high risk of bleeding. Kidney Int 55:1991–1997
23. Dorval M, Madore F, Courteau S, Leblanc M (2003) A novel citrate anticoagulation regimen for continuous venovenous hemodiafiltration. Intensive Care Med 29:1186–1189
24. Bollmann MD, Revelly JP, Tappy L et al (2004) Effect of bicarbonate and lactate buffer on glucose and lactate metabolism during hemodiafiltration in patients with multiple organ failure. Intensive Care Med 30:1103–1110
25. Leverve X, Mustafa I, Novak I et al (2005) Lactate metabolism in acute uremia. J Ren Nutr 15:58–62
26. Matejovic M, Radermacher P, Fontaine E (2007) Lactate in shock: a high-octane fuel for the heart? Intensive Care Med 33:406–408
27. Balik M, Zakharchenko M, Leden P et al (2013) Novel lactate buffered dialysis and substitution fluid for citrate anticoagulated continuous renal replacement therapy. Intensive Care Med (in press)
28. Monchi M, Berghmans D, Ledoux D, Canivet JL, Dubois B, Damas P (2004) Citrate vs. heparin for anticoagulation in continuous venovenous hemofiltration: a prospective randomized study. Intensive Care Med 30:260–265
29. Hetzel GR, Taskaya G, Sucker C, Hennersdorf M, Grabensee B, Schmitz M (2006) Citrate plasma levels in patients under regional anticoagulation in continuous venovenous hemofiltration. Am J Kidney Dis 48:806–811
30. Zakharchenko MBM, Leden P (2011) Citrate anticoagulated continuous haemodiafiltration: Focus on ionised magnesium. Intensive Care Med 37(Suppl 2):493 (abst)
31. Brain M, Parkes S, Fowler P, Robertson I, Brown A (2011) Calcium flux in continuous venovenous haemodiafiltration with heparin and citrate anticoagulation. Crit Care Resusc 13:72–81
32. Meier-Kriesche HU, Gitomer J, Finkel K, DuBose T (2001) Increased total to ionized calcium ratio during continuous venovenous hemodialysis with regional citrate anticoagulation. Crit Care Med 29:748–752
33. Bakker AJ, Boerma EC, Keidel H, Kingma P, van der Voort PH (2006) Detection of citrate overdose in critically ill patients on citrate-anticoagulated venovenous haemofiltration: use of ionised and total/ionised calcium. Clin Chem Lab Med 44:962–966
34. Soliman HM, Mercan D, Lobo SS, Melot C, Vincent JL (2003) Development of ionized hypomagnesemia is associated with higher mortality rates. Crit Care Med 31:1082–1087
35. Escuela MP, Guerra M, Anon JM et al (2005) Total and ionized serum magnesium in critically ill patients. Intensive Care Med 31:151–156
36. Ames WA, McDonnell N, Potter D (1999) The effect of ionised magnesium on coagulation using thromboelastography. Anaesthesia 54:999–1001
37. Demirjian S, Teo BW, Guzman JA et al (2011) Hypophosphatemia during continuous hemodialysis is associated with prolonged respiratory failure in patients with acute kidney injury. Nephrol Dial Transplant 26:3508–3514
38. Marino PL, Sutin KM (2007) The ICU Book, 3rd edn. Lippincott Williams & Wilkins, Philadelphia, pp 194–208
39. Uchino S, Fealy N, Baldwin I, Morimatsu H, Bellomo R (2003) Continuous is not continuous: the incidence and impact of circuit "down-time" on uraemic control during continuous veno-venous haemofiltration. Intensive Care Med 29:575–578
40. Mares J, Thongboonkerd V, Tuma Z, Moravec J, Matejovic M (2009) Specific adsorption of some complement activation proteins to polysulfone dialysis membranes during hemodialysis. Kidney Int 76:404–413
41. Mares J, Richtrova P, Hricinova A et al (2010) Proteomic profiling of blood-dialyzer interactome reveals involvement of lectin complement pathway in hemodialysis-induced inflammatory response. Proteomics Clin Appl 4:829–838

42. Davila S, Wright VJ, Khor CC et al (2010) Genome-wide association study identifies variants in the CFH region associated with host susceptibility to meningococcal disease. Nat Genet 42:772–776
43. Bos JC, Grooteman MP, van Houte AJ, Schoorl M, van Limbeek J, Nube MJ (1997) Low polymorphonuclear cell degranulation during citrate anticoagulation: a comparison between citrate and heparin dialysis. Nephrol Dial Transplant 12:1387–1393
44. Bohler J, Schollmeyer P, Dressel B, Dobos G, Horl WH (1996) Reduction of granulocyte activation during hemodialysis with regional citrate anticoagulation: dissociation of complement activation and neutropenia from neutrophil degranulation. J Am Soc Nephrol 7:234–241
45. Gritters M, Grooteman MP, Schoorl M et al (2006) Citrate anticoagulation abolishes degranulation of polymorphonuclear cells and platelets and reduces oxidative stress during haemodialysis. Nephrol Dial Transplant 21:153–159
46. Gritters M, Borgdorff P, Grooteman MP et al (2007) Reduction in platelet activation by citrate anticoagulation does not prevent intradialytic hemodynamic instability. Nephron Clin Pract 106:c9–c16
47. Patterson J, Laba D, Blunt M (2011) Economic argument for citrate haemofiltration. Crit Care 15(Suppl 1):P126 (abst)

Does the Choice of Renal Replacement Therapy Affect Renal Recovery?

N. Saxena, A. J. Tolwani, and K. M. Wille

Introduction

Acute kidney injury (AKI) is common in critically ill patients with multiple organ failure (MOF) and is an under-recognized independent predictor of mortality [1]. AKI severe enough to necessitate renal replacement therapy (RRT) in the critically ill patient is associated with a mortality rate over 60 % [2]. Although randomized controlled trials (RCTs) have shown no difference in survival between RRT modalities, renal recovery is another important outcome for patients with AKI and may be affected differently by RRT modality. Roughly 10–20 % of patients who survive an episode of AKI remain dialysis dependent [3]. Failure to recover renal function after AKI has both short-term and long-term implications with respect to morbidity and health care costs. We review the data regarding RRT modality and renal recovery in patients with AKI.

Renal Replacement Therapy Modalities for AKI

AKI can be treated with intermittent hemodialysis (IHD), continuous renal replacement therapy (CRRT), prolonged intermittent renal replacement therapy (PIRRT),

N. Saxena
Division of Nephrology, University of Alabama at Birmingham, 401 19th Street South, Birmingham, AL 35233, USA

A. J. Tolwani (✉)
Division of Nephrology, University of Alabama at Birmingham, 401 19th Street South, Birmingham, AL 35233, USA
E-mail: atolwani@uab.edu

K. M. Wille
Division of Pulmonary, Allergy, and Critical Care Medicine, University of Alabama at Birmingham, 1720 2nd Ave. S, Birmingham, AL 35294–0007, USA

J.-L. Vincent (Ed.), *Annual Update in Intensive Care and Emergency Medicine 2013*,
DOI 10.1007/978-3-642-35109-9_59,

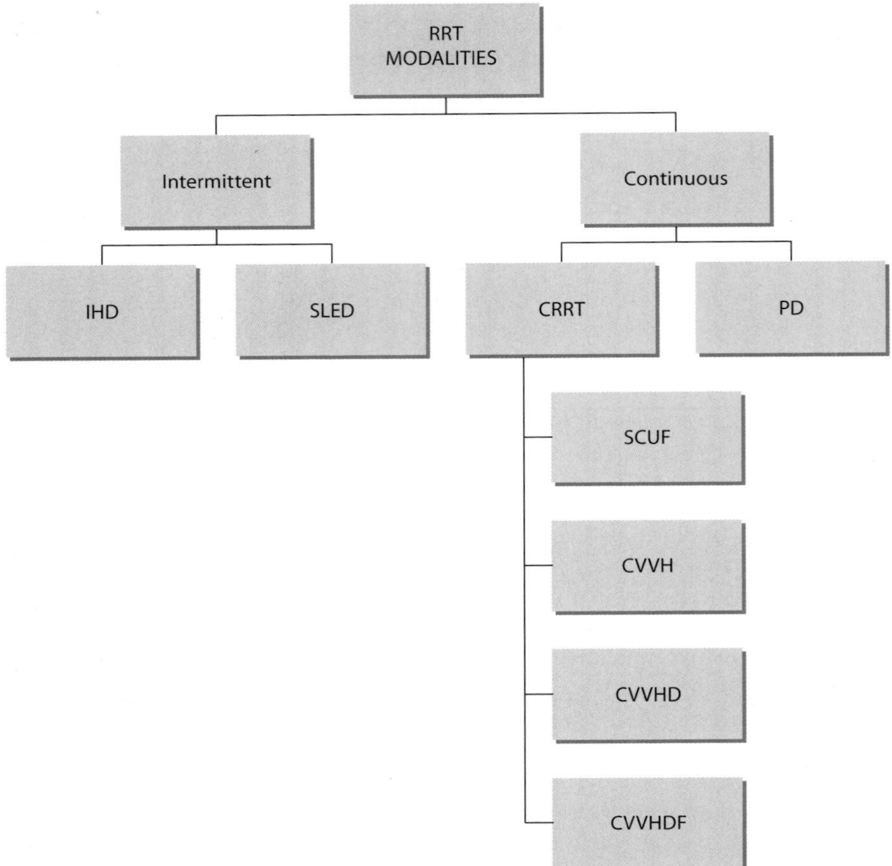

Fig. 1 Approaches to renal replacement therapy (RRT) used in acute kidney injury. This flow chart displays the different modalities of dialysis used to potentially treat acute kidney injury. IHD: intermittent hemodialysis; SLED: sustained low-efficiency dialysis; CRRT: continuous renal replacement therapy; PD: peritoneal dialysis; SCUF: slow continuous ultrafiltration; CVVH: continuous venovenous hemofiltration; CVVHD: continuous venovenous hemodialysis; CVVHDF: continuous venovenous hemodiafiltration

or peritoneal dialysis (PD) (Fig. 1). AKI has been traditionally managed with IHD, delivered 3 to 6 times a week and 3 to 4 hours per session. In IHD, solute clearance occurs mainly by diffusion, whereas volume is removed by ultrafiltration. The main disadvantage of IHD is the risk of hemodynamic instability caused by rapid electrolyte and fluid removal. Intravascular volume depletion, decreased cardiac output, and intercompartmental fluid shifts also contribute to hypotension with IHD [4]. Despite strategies to lessen the chance of hypotension during intermittent therapy, such as dialysate cooling, or decreasing the ultrafiltration rate by increasing the dialysis time or frequency, approximately 10 % of AKI patients cannot be treated with IHD because of hemodynamic instability [5, 6]. Hemodynamic instability can potentially worsen residual renal function and recovery.

CRRT is an 'umbrella' term to describe a variety of continuous modes of RRT used in the intensive care unit (ICU). The different CRRT modalities use diffusion, convection, or a combination of both for solute clearance. Unlike IHD, CRRT is performed continuously (24 h/d) with lower blood, dialysate and ultrafiltration rates. The modalities of CRRT used for AKI are continuous venovenous hemofiltration (CVVH), continuous venovenous hemodialysis (CVVHD), and continuous venovenous hemodiafiltration (CVVHDF). In CVVH, solute clearance occurs by convection. In CVVHD, solute removal occurs by diffusion. CVVHDF combines the convective solute removal of CVVH and the diffusive solute removal of CVVHD. The advantages of CRRT include hemodynamic tolerance caused by slower ultrafiltration and slower solute removal per unit of time. Studies suggest that CRRT is better tolerated in unstable patients with low blood pressure, such as in septic shock or cardiogenic shock [7]. Disadvantages of CRRT include expense, access and filter clotting, need for anticoagulation, and demands on ICU nurse time [8].

PIRRT, also known as sustained low-efficiency dialysis (SLED) and extended daily dialysis (EDD), is a slower dialytic modality run for prolonged periods using conventional hemodialysis machines with modification of blood and dialysate flows. Typically, PIRRT uses low blood-pump speeds of 200 ml/min and low dialysate flow rates of 300 ml/min for 6 to 12 hours daily [8]. PIRRT allows gradual removal of both solute and volume, provides high solute clearance, and obviates the cost of CRRT and its machines, solutions, and the need for trained staff [2]. PIRRT combines the advantages of CRRT and IHD. Studies have demonstrated that PIRRT provides hemodynamic control comparable to CRRT [9].

In PD, the peritoneum is used as a semi-permeable membrane for diffusive removal of solutes. A dialysate solution is administered into the peritoneal cavity through a catheter where it stays for a prescribed period of time and then is drained. The use of PD for AKI is limited by practical considerations. Acute PD requires the surgical insertion of a PD catheter and often is complicated by catheter leakage and malfunction [10]. The use of PD is limited by low solute clearance in critically ill patients and potential pulmonary restriction due to the expansion of the peritoneal cavity [11]. It is contraindicated in postoperative patients who need abdominal surgery or surgical drains. In addition, because PD is less predictive in fluid and solute removal in the ICU, it is used less widely than other therapies. However, there are emerging data that, when used with careful planning, selected ICU patients can be treated with PD [12]. PD is a modality that is inexpensive and often used in places where the technology and resources for IHD and CRRT do not exist.

PD regimens include intermittent, continuous, or tidal PD. The type of PD regimen employed may influence the renal recovery rate. Theoretically, the continuous modality of PD causes less hemodynamic instability by virtue of a low flow continuous system, and, thus, may have important implications for renal recovery. In an observational study, Van Biesen et al. [13] found that PD, when used prior to renal transplant, more favorably influenced post-transplant renal graft recovery compared to IHD. These authors hypothesized that one of the key factors responsible for this effect was differences in volume status at the moment of transplantation, as PD patients have a more stable fluid status and tend to be slightly overhydrated, whereas IHD patients tend to be hypovolemic prior to transplant [13].

Comparison of Renal Recovery in AKI by RRT Modality

Renal recovery is an important outcome measure, as chronic dialysis is associated with significant morbidity, cost, and impairment of quality of life [14]. Complete renal recovery can be defined as the return to baseline kidney function. Partial recovery can be defined when creatinine improves but does not return to its baseline value. Per RIFLE (Risk, Injury, Failure, Loss and End-stage Renal Disease) criteria, as defined by the ADQI (Acute Dialysis Quality Initiative), patients requiring RRT for more than 4 weeks are classified as having AKI and those requiring RRT for more than 3 months as having end-stage renal disease [4]. Most studies evaluating the effect of RRT modality on renal recovery, however, have been observational and have defined renal recovery as no longer requiring RRT.

In a multicenter RCT of 166 patients comparing IHD and CVVHDF for treatment of ICU-related AKI, Mehta et al. [15] found that renal recovery was more frequent with CRRT. The principal outcomes of the study were ICU and hospital mortality and recovery of renal function. Of patients who had IHD as their initial therapy, 17 % developed chronic kidney disease, versus 4 % of patients whose initial therapy was CRRT. Also, a higher number of patients who crossed over from IHD to CRRT recovered renal function than patients who switched from CRRT to IHD (45 % vs. 7 %, $p < 0.01$). CRRT was associated with a significantly higher rate of complete renal recovery in surviving patients who received an adequate trial of therapy with no crossover (92.3 % vs. 59.4 %; $p < 0.01$). Timing and dose of dialysis were not controlled for, nor were other supportive strategies like nutrition and hemodynamic support.

Augustine et al. [16] studied 80 ICU patients with AKI requiring RRT and randomized them to either CVVHD or IHD. These authors reported a significant reduction in mean arterial pressure (MAP) during IHD over the first 3 days of therapy, which was not observed during CVVHD. On day 1 (first IHD treatment), there was a significant decline in MAP in the IHD patients but no change in the CVVHD patients. In addition, more IHD patients (40 %) required an increase in vasopressor support than did CVVHD patients (13 %). On day 3 (second IHD treatment), MAP declined even further in the IHD group, with no change in the CVVHD group. Consequently, after the first 3 days of therapy, MAP was significantly higher in the CVVHD group. The same study found significant differences in fluid balance between the two modalities, even with just a 3-day treatment duration. In the CVVHD group, a net *loss* of 4,005 ml (approximately 4 kg) occurred, while the IHD group sustained a net *gain* of 1,539 ml (approximately 1.5 kg) on an average basis [16]. Thus, not only was net fluid removal greater in the CRRT arm, but it was also achieved with greater hemodynamic stability. Although these findings suggest that IHD may be associated with a higher risk of hypotension-induced renal ischemia, as compared to CRRT, and may delay renal recovery, the authors found no difference in renal recovery between the modalities. This study was limited, however, by the small number of patients included and thus was underpowered for detecting differences in renal recovery between groups.

In 2002, Tonelli et al. [17] published a meta-analysis on the impact of dialysis modality on mortality and renal recovery. The authors evaluated six RCTs comparing IHD to CRRT in critically ill patients with AKI. Of the 6 RCTs, renal recovery data were only available for four, for a total of 401 patients. Neither the incidence of renal death nor the likelihood of dialysis dependence among survivors was significantly different between modalities. The authors stated that the available data were insufficient to draw firm conclusions and that further studies are needed.

In a small Canadian observational study of ICU patients with AKI, Jacka et al. [18] demonstrated greater recovery of renal function after AKI with CRRT as compared with IHD. The study was performed at a single institution where both CRRT and IHD were used for AKI patients. Patients treated with CRRT were significantly more dependent on vasopressors than patients treated with IHD. In this study, of the patients treated with CRRT, 87 % recovered renal function, and only 13 % required chronic dialysis at hospital discharge; conversely, of patients treated with IHD, only 36 % recovered renal function, and 63 % required chronic dialysis at hospital discharge ($p = 0.003$). Another observational study from Canada by Manns et al. [14] evaluated renal recovery at several hospitals in the Alberta region. Similar to Jacka et al. [18], renal recovery was higher in those patients treated with CRRT who survived to hospital discharge; 80 % of the surviving CRRT patients recovered renal function, whereas only 62 % of the surviving IHD patients did ($p = 0.06$). Length of hospital stay was significantly longer, and in-hospital costs higher, for patients who did not recover renal function.

Two large epidemiological studies have also reported increased rates of renal recovery in patients on CRRT. In the Beginning and Ending Supportive Therapy (BEST) kidney trial [19], a multinational, prospective, epidemiological study of AKI in the ICU including over 30,000 patients in 23 countries, 1,218 patients received RRT. Although no mortality difference was detected between patients treated with CRRT as compared to IHD, dialysis independence at hospital discharge was higher after CRRT (85.5 % vs. 66.2 %; $p < 0.0001$).

Bell et al. [1], in a Swedish retrospective cohort study from 1995–2004, evaluated the impact of CRRT and IHD on renal recovery and mortality. A total of 2,202 patients from 32 ICUs were included, and patients with end-stage renal disease were excluded. The primary outcome was the need for chronic dialysis 90 days after dialysis initiation in the ICU for AKI and a secondary outcome was 90-day mortality. In this study, CRRT was more extensively used than IHD, with 86 % (1,911) of patients receiving CRRT and only 14 % (291) receiving IHD as initial therapy. Moreover, as opposed to many other studies, there was very little 'crossover' between the two modalities, with less than 5 % of the patients initially treated with CRRT transitioning to IHD, and no patients initially treated with IHD transitioning to CRRT. Of the patients who survived, AKI patients treated with IHD had a 2-fold higher rate of chronic dialysis dependence at 90 days compared to AKI patients treated with CRRT. Specifically, 16.5 % of the IHD-treated patients did not recover renal function at 90 days compared to 8.3 % for the CRRT group. Multivariate analysis showed that the adjusted odds ratio (OR) of dialysis dependence with IHD compared with CRRT was 2.60 (95 % CI 1.5–4.3). Moreover, in patients who did develop chronic dialysis dependence, the subsequent survival rate was significantly lower for patients treated with IHD.

The VA/NIH Acute Renal Failure Trial Network (ATN) study by Palevsky et al. [20] aimed to determine the optimal intensity of RRT in critically ill patients with AKI and at least one other failing organ or sepsis. The study compared two strategies for the management of RRT in critically ill patients with AKI. Each treatment strategy employed both conventional IHD in patients whose blood pressure was stable and either SLED or CRRT in patients who were hemodynamically unstable. Hypotension was a more serious complication among patients treated with IHD. Approximately 1.7 % of all IHD treatments required discontinuation of therapy due to hypotension as compared to only 0.7 % of CRRT/SLED treatments. These differences were observed despite the fact that the IHD patients were considered hemodynamically stable. Over 70 % of patients in both treatment arms (intensive and less-intensive) had no recovery of kidney function by 28 days and were dialysis dependent. This is quite high compared to other trials, given that patients with chronic kidney disease were excluded. A possible explanation is that the high rate of severe hypotension in the IHD patients may have contributed to the relatively low rate of renal recovery.

The Randomized Evaluation of Normal vs. Augmented Level (RENAL) replacement therapy trial was a multicenter RCT of intensity of CRRT in 1,508 critically ill patients with AKI [2]. In the RENAL trial, patients were randomized to CVVHDF at 25 ml/kg/h versus CVVHDF at 40 ml/kg/h. In contrast to the ATN trial, the RENAL investigators reported that 14 % of patients were dialysis dependent in both treatment arms by 28 days. Unlike the ATN trial, the two intensity arms included only patients on CRRT, and not on other modalities. Moreover, unlike the ATN trial, the RENAL trial included patients with chronic kidney disease. This finding supports the notion that CRRT leads to higher rates of renal recovery.

Most recently, Schneider et al. [21] published a meta-analysis of 50 studies comparing recovery to RRT independence in AKI survivors according to initial RRT modality. The authors reported that among survivors with AKI, dialysis dependency was greater with intermittent RRT (IRRT) than CRRT at hospital discharge, days 28, 60, 90 and after 6 months. After 28 days, RRT dependence among survivors was 19.4 % for CRRT vs. 26.9 % for IRRT ($p < 0.004$); at hospital discharge, it was 10.9 % (CRRT) vs. 20.8 % (IRRT) ($p < 0.0001$); and, at day 90, it was 7.8 % (CRRT) vs. 36.9 % (IRRT) ($p < 0.0001$). The authors concluded that IRRT was associated with higher rates of dialysis dependency.

PD is often the only option available for treatment of AKI in developing countries. Its potential benefits include technical simplicity, lack of need for anticoagulation, cardiovascular stability, and the absence of an extracorporeal circuit. Studies have also compared PD to IHD and CRRT [12]. Gabriel et al. [12] conducted a prospective RCT that compared daily IHD with high-volume PD. High-volume PD was performed continuously, and 120 patients with acute tubular necrosis were randomly assigned to PD or hemodialysis. The primary endpoints were hospital survival and renal recovery. The authors found that mortality and renal function recovery were similar between groups, but patients receiving high volume PD had a shorter time to renal recovery (7.2 ± 2.6 days) compared with those having daily IHD (10.6 ± 4.7 days; $p = 0.04$).

In another study, Phu et al. [22] conducted a RCT of CVVH and intermittent PD in 70 patients with AKI related to infection. Although the primary outcome was correction of metabolic abnormalities, secondary outcomes included renal recovery. PD was conducted by using an intermittent regimen with a rigid catheter. The authors found that the need for further dialysis was higher in survivors who received PD compared to those who received CVVH. Limitations of this study, however, included use of a rigid catheter and an intermittent (rather than continuous high volume) PD regimen, both of which may adversely affect renal recovery.

Data comparing PIRRT to other RRT modalities in terms of renal recovery are lacking.

Conclusion

Optimizing renal recovery is crucial, because end-stage renal disease results in excess morbidity, mortality, and costs. Failure to recover renal function after AKI has both short-term and long-term consequences. Most of the available data suggest that IHD may contribute to worsening renal ischemia and delay of renal recovery due to intradialytic hypotension. Theoretically, CRRT and PD are more physiologic dialysis modalities compared to IHD, and may cause less renal ischemia due to greater hemodynamic stability. PD, however, cannot be used in all instances, and there are many exclusion criteria. Although observational studies have shown CRRT to be associated with higher rates of renal recovery, the evidence is insufficient to support firm recommendations, and most studies evaluated renal recovery only in patients who survived. Studies analyzing combined endpoints of mortality and non-recovery of renal function between RRT modalities have shown no differences in renal recovery. Well-designed RCTs are needed to better define the true effect of each RRT modality on renal recovery following AKI.

References

1. Bell M, SWING, Granath F, Schön S, Ekbom A, Martling CR (2007) Continuous renal replacement therapy is associated with less chronic renal failure than intermittent haemodialysis after acute renal failure. Intensive Care Med 33:773–780
2. Bellomo R, Cass A, Cole L et al (2009) Intensity of continuous renal replacement therapy in critically ill patients. N Engl J Med 361:1627–1638

3. Cartin-Ceba R, Haugen EN, Iscimen R, Trillo-Alvarez C, Juncos L, Gajic O (2009) Evaluation of "Loss" and "End stage renal disease" after acute kidney injury defined by the Risk, Injury, Failure, Loss and ESRD classification in critically ill patients. Intensive Care Med 35:2087–2095
4. Schiffl H (2008) Renal recovery after severe acute renal injury. Eur J Med Res 13:552–556
5. Emili S, Black NA, Paul RV, Rexing CJ, Ullian ME (1999) A protocol-based treatment for intradialytic hypotension in hospitalized hemodialysis patients. Am J Kidney Dis 33:1107–1114
6. Paganini EP, Sandy D, Moreno L, Kozlowski L, Sakai K (1996) The effect of sodium and ultrafiltration modeling on plasma volume changes and hemodynamic stability in intensive care patients receiving hemodialysis for acute renal failure: a prospective, stratified, randomized, crossover study. Nephrol Dial Transplant 11(Suppl 8):32–37
7. Rauf AA, Long KH, Gajic O, Anderson SS, Swaminathan L, Albright RC (2008) Intermittent hemodialysis versus continuous renal replacement therapy for acute renal failure in the intensive care unit: An observational outcomes analysis. J Intensive Care Med 23:195–203
8. O'Reilly P, Tolwani A (2005) Renal replacement therapy III: IHD, CRRT, SLED. Crit Care Clin 21:367–378
9. Kumar VCM, Depner T, Yeun J (2000) Extended daily dialysis: a new approach to renal replacement for acute renal failure in the intensive care unit. Am J Kidney Dis 36:294–300
10. Ansari N (2011) Peritoneal dialysis in renal replacement therapy for patients with acute kidney injury. Int J Nephrol 2011: (article ID: 739794)
11. Goel S, Saran R, Nolph KD (1998) Indications, contraindications and complications of peritoneal dialysis in the critically ill. In: Ronco C, Bellomo R (eds) Critical Care Nephrology. Kluwer Academic Publishers, Dordrecht, pp 1373–1381
12. Gabriel DP, Caramori JT, Martim LC, Barretti P, Balbli AL (2008) High volume peritoneal dialysis vs. daily hemodialysis: A randomized controlled trial in patients with acute kidney injury. Kidney Int (Suppl):S87–S93
13. Van Biesen W, Vanholder R, Van Loo A, Van der Vennet M, Lameire N (2000) Peritoneal dialysis favorably influences early graft function after renal transplantation compared to hemodialysis. Transplantation 69:508–514
14. Manns B, Doig CJ, Lee H et al (2003) Cost of acute renal failure requiring dialysis in the intensive care unit: clinical and resource implications of renal recovery. Crit Care Med 31:449–455
15. Mehta RL, McDonald B, Gabbai FB et al (2001) A randomized clinical trial of continuous versus intermittent dialysis for acute renal failure. Kidney Int 60:1154–1163
16. Augustine JJ, Sandy D, Seifert TH, Paganini EP (2004) A randomized controlled trial comparing intermittent with continuous dialysis in patients with ARF. Am J Kidney Dis 44:1000–1007
17. Tonelli M, Manns B, Feller-Kopman D (2002) Acute renal failure in the intensive care unit: a systematic review of the impact of dialytic modality on mortality and renal recovery. Am J Kidney Dis 40:875–885
18. Jacka MJ, Ivancinova X, Gibney RT (2005) Continuous renal replacement therapy improves renal recovery from acute renal failure. Can J Anaesth 52:327–332
19. Uchino S, Bellomo R, Morimatsu H et al (2007) Continuous renal replacement therapy: a worldwide practice survey. The beginning and ending supportive therapy for the kidney (B.E.S.T. kidney) investigators. Intensive Care Med 33:1563–1570
20. Palevsky PM, Zhang JH, O'Connor TZ et al (2008) VA/NIH Acute Renal Failure Trial Network. Intensity of renal support in critically ill patients with acute kidney injury. N Engl J Med 359:7–20
21. Schneider AG, Bagshaw SM, Glassford N, Bellomo R (2012) Exposure to intermittent hemodialysis and renal recovery after acute kidney injury: a systematic review. Crit Care 16(Suppl 1):P368 (abst)
22. Phu NH, Hien TT, Mai NT et al (2002) Hemofiltration and peritoneal dialysis in infection-associated acute renal failure in Vietnam. N Engl J Med 347:895–902

Part XVII

Neurological Issues

Subarachnoid Hemorrhage: Critical Care Management

M.G. Abate and G. Citerio

Introduction

More than 2,400 years ago, Hippocrates in "*Aphorisms*" (VI, 51) recognized the natural history of spontaneous subarachnoid hemorrhage (SAH) followed by subsequent delayed neurological deterioration *"When persons in good health are suddenly seized with pains in the head, and straightway are laid down speechless, and breathe with stertor, they die in seven days, unless fever come on"*. SAH, nowadays, remains a severe emergency because of the sudden extravasation of blood into the subarachnoid space, still causing, even with modern aggressive medical and surgical therapies, significant morbidity and mortality [1, 2].

The leading cause of non-traumatic SAH is rupture of an intracranial aneurysm, accounting for more than 80 % of SAH cases and for 6 % of total strokes. The general estimated incidence is 8–10 cases per 100,000 inhabitants per year, with important regional differences. Risk factors include hypertension, smoking, alcohol abuse, the use of sympathomimetic drugs (e.g., cocaine) and genetic syndromes, such as autosomal dominant polycystic kidney. The mechanisms of aneurysm formation, growth and subsequent rupture have not yet been fully elucidated. Recent theories recognize an angiogenesis factor, endoglin, as one of the factors involved, but the entire process is probably a multifactorial disease [3–5].

M.G. Abate
Neuroanesthesia and Neurointensive Care Unit, Anesthesia and Intensive Care II, San Gerardo Hospital, via Pergolesi 33, Monza 20900, Milan, Italy

G. Citerio (✉)
Neuroanesthesia and Neurointensive Care Unit, Anesthesia and Intensive Care II, San Gerardo Hospital, via Pergolesi 33, Monza 20900, Milan, Italy
E-mail: g.citerio@hsgerardo.org

J.-L. Vincent (Ed.), *Annual Update in Intensive Care and Emergency Medicine 2013*,
DOI 10.1007/978-3-642-35109-9_60, © Springer-Verlag Berlin Heidelberg 2013

Clinical Features and Outcome of SAH

Aneurysmal SAH is a heterogeneous disease with different clinical exordia and outcomes. The early mortality rate after aneurysmal SAH remains high at 40 %; 10–20 % of these patients never reach medical attention or die during transportation and around half of the survivors retain some neurological deficit. The time course of the disease can be divided into different phases each contributing to the overall outcome:

1. The severity of the initial hemorrhage: Clinical characteristics, e.g., sudden coma and seizures, observed close to the time of presentation with SAH have negative prognostic implications.
2. The intervention to treat the ruptured aneurysm: Surgical or endovascular aneurysm repair must be performed as soon as possible to prevent the rebleeding.
3. Medical management occurs mainly in neurocritical care and is based on the detection and treatment of cerebral and extracerebral complications. The former leads to delayed cerebral vasospasm with or without delayed ischemic neurological deficits. Other medical complications that negatively affect overall morbidity and mortality include cardiac ischemia and neurogenic pulmonary edema.

Clinical Manifestations

The severity of the clinical presentation with compromised neurological status, from seizures, loss of consciousness or focal neurological deficits, is the strongest prognostic factor in aneurysmal SAH, with the more severe cases (defined as poor-grade or high-grade) more likely to develop cerebral and systemic complications, and need longer stays in the intensive care unit (ICU). Validated scales can describe the severity of the clinical presentation [6]: The Hunt and Hess and the World Federation of Neurological Surgeons (WFNS) scales are currently used to categorize the severity of the clinical presentation at the time of bleeding. A retrospective analysis of more than 2,000 cases shows that severity of initial hemorrhage, clinically graded by the WFNS score, was the major determinant of case fatality at 60 days [7].

The Fisher scale [8], modified by Claassen et al. [9], quantifies the additive risk from SAH thickness and accompanying intraventricular hemorrhage (IVH): 0 – none; 1 – minimal SAH without IVH; 2 – minimal SAH with IVH; 3 – thick SAH without IVH; 4 – thick SAH with IVH. The amount of blood is associated with the risk of vasospasm development: SAH completely filling any cistern or fissure and IVH in the lateral ventricles are both risk factors for delayed cerebral ischemia, and their risk is additive.

Prognostic Indicators

Along with the severity of the clinical presentation and the amount of blood seen at the first computed tomography (CT) scan, aneurysm rebleeding is another major predictor of poor outcome. Rebleeding is a complex and multifactorial event involving hemostasis, pathophysiological and anatomical factors [10–12]. Studies investigating the ultra-early phase, within the first 24 h following aneurysmal SAH, have reported rebleeding in as many as 9–17 % of patients, with most cases occurring within 6 h of initial hemorrhage [13]. Several factors are associated with the risk of rebleeding, among these worse neurological status on admission, larger aneurysm size and high systolic blood pressure. There is general consensus on the need for early blood pressure control in these patients until the aneurysm has been secured although no optimal levels of blood pressure have been recommended. Therefore, treat extreme hypertension in patients with an unsecured, recently ruptured aneurysm. Modest elevations in blood pressure (i. e., mean blood pressure < 110 mm Hg) do not require therapy [14]. Pre-morbid baseline blood pressures should be used to refine targets. Hypotension should be avoided.

Other elements are also predictive of poor prognosis. Some are related to patient characteristic, such as older age and pre-existing severe medical illness, and others to systemic complications, such as hyperglycemia, fever, anemia, pneumonia and sepsis [15]. Early global cerebral edema on CT scan [16], intraventricular [17] and intracerebral hemorrhage and, above all, the incidence of cerebral vasospasm with delayed ischemic neurological deficits and cerebral infarction are also related to a negative prognosis. Aneurysm size, location, and complex configuration, may increase the risk of periprocedural complications and affect overall prognosis [18, 19].

Treatment in high-volume centers with availability of neurosurgical and endovascular services is reasonable [20]: Outcome is influenced by patient volume, with better outcomes occurring in high-volume centers treating more than 60 cases per year [21]. Patients treated at low-volume hospitals are less likely to experience definitive treatment and transfer to high-volume centers may be inadequately arranged.

Imaging

Non-contrast head CT scan is a cornerstone in the diagnosis of aneurysmal SAH (Fig. 1). The CT in patients with aneurysmal SAH will show blood in the subarachnoid space, typically in the basal cisterns around the circle of Willis, major fissures, and occasionally intraventricular.

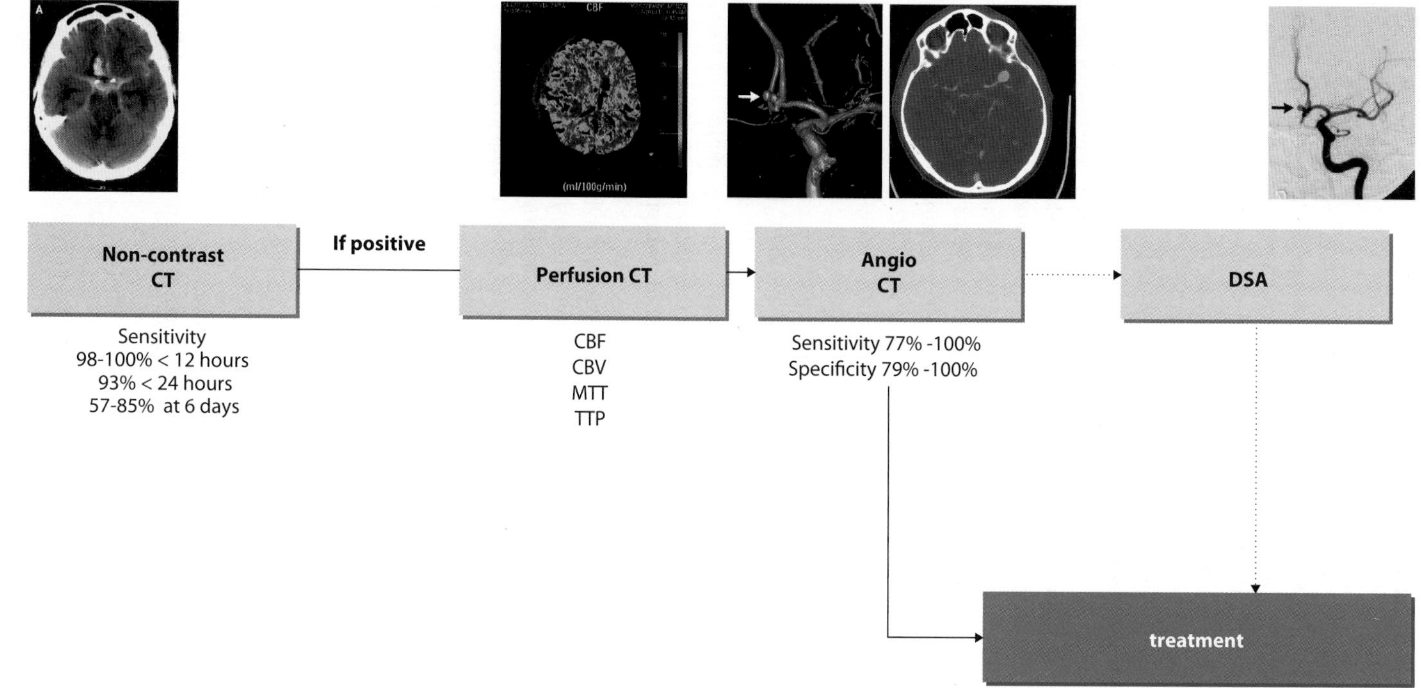
A
CBF
(ml/100g/min)
Non-contrast CT
Sensitivity
98-100% < 12 hours
93% < 24 hours
57-85% at 6 days
If positive
Perfusion CT
CBF
CBV
MTT
TTP
Angio CT
Sensitivity 77% -100%
Specificity 79% -100%
DSA
treatment

◀ **Fig. 1** Diagnostic pathway for aneurysmal subarachnoid hemorrhage (SAH). Non-contrast head computed tomography (CT) scan is a cornerstone in the diagnosis of aneurysmal SAH. If positive, in the same session a perfusion CT and an angio CT may be considered. If an aneurysm is detected by angio CT, this investigation may help guide the decision regarding type of aneurysm repair. If angio CT is inconclusive, digital subtraction angiography (DSA) is recommended. DSA could also be useful for determining whether an aneurysm is amenable to coiling or to expedite microsurgery. CBF: cerebral blood flow; CBV: cerebral blood volume; MTT: mean transit time; TTP: time-to-peak

The latest American Heart Association (AHA)/American Stroke Association (ASA) Guidelines for the Management of Aneurysmal Subarachnoid Hemorrhage [22] suggest, as an updated recommendation, that CT angiography may be considered in defining aneurysmal SAH. If an aneurysm is detected by CT angiography, this investigation may help guide the decision regarding the type of aneurysm repair. If CT angiography is inconclusive, digital subtraction angiography (DSA) is recommended. Moreover, DSA could be useful for determining whether an aneurysm is amenable to coiling or to expedite microsurgery.

Surgical and Endovascular Management

After initial stabilization, aimed at restoring respiratory and cardiovascular function, early aneurysm repair should be undertaken, when possible and reasonable, to prevent rebleeding [22]. If a delay in aneurysm treatment occurs, an early, short course of antifibrinolytic therapy prior to aneurysm repair should be considered to reduce the incidence of rebleeding. Prolonged (> 3 days) antifibrinolytic therapy exposes patients to increased adverse effects when the risk of rebleeding is reduced, and should be avoided [14].

Aneurysm obliteration can be achieved by surgical or endovascular methods. The decision regarding aneurysm treatment should be a multidisciplinary decision based on characteristics of the patient and of the aneurysm. The only multicenter randomized trial comparing microsurgical and endovascular repair, the International Subarachnoid Aneurysm Trial (ISAT) [23], randomized more than 2,000 patients with aneurysmal SAH from 42 neurosurgical centers. In this cohort, the risk of death at 5 years was significantly lower in the coiled group, but the proportion of survivors who were independent was not statistically different between the groups, and rebleeding was higher in the coiled group [24]. ISAT has been a strong driver of change in the management of ruptured aneurysms. Nevertheless, the evidence for the advantage of coiling in the long-term should not be assumed from ISAT data.

Neurosurgical clipping should be considered in patients with large (> 50 ml) intraparenchymal hematomas and middle cerebral artery aneurysms. Endovascular coiling should be considered in the elderly (> 70 years), in those presenting with poor-grade (WFNS classification IV/V) aneurysmal SAH, and in those with aneurysms of the basilar apex.

Neurocritical Care Management

Patients with aneurysmal SAH should be treated in multidisciplinary high-volume centers with experienced cerebrovascular surgeons, neuroradiologists and dedicated neurointensive care. Varelas et al. [25] demonstrated that hospital treatment volumes and availability of both endovascular and neurological intensive care services were strong determinants of improved outcomes in aneurysmal SAH.

Vasospasm and Delayed Cerebral Ischemia

Vasospasm refers to narrowing of cerebral arteries subsequent to aneurysmal SAH and has been widely recognized as an unfavorable complication that can be responsible for delayed cerebral ischemia. Vasospasm frequently occurs between days 4 and 21 after bleeding. The initial trigger for arterial narrowing is the contact between the oxyhemoglobin that accumulates after the bleeding at the abluminal side of the vessels.

Dhar and Diringer [26] showed that systemic inflammatory activation is common after SAH even in the absence of infection. Therefore, aneurysmal SAH triggers immune activation sufficient to induce a systemic inflammatory response syndrome (SIRS). A higher burden of SIRS in the initial four days independently predicted symptomatic vasospasm and was associated with worse outcome. Recently, the focus of research into delayed cerebral ischemia has moved from pure cerebral artery constriction towards a more complex, multifactorial etiology [27, 28]. Novel pathological mechanisms have been advocated, including damage to cerebral tissue in the first 72 h after aneurysm rupture, the so called "early brain injury" [29, 30], cortical spreading depression [31], and microthrombosis [32]. A better evaluation of the impact of these pathophysiological mechanisms is essential, if new methodologies for the prophylaxis, diagnosis and treatment of delayed cerebral ischemia are to be developed.

No effective preventive therapy is currently available. Oral nimodipine administration has been confirmed as being associated with an improved neurological outcome, counteracting processes other than vessel narrowing [33]. Euvolemia is recommended until vasospasm is diagnosed.

Several trials investigated the use of drugs to prevent or treat vasospasm, including clazosentan, an endothelin-1 receptor antagonist, and magnesium. Clazosentan has been associated with a dose-dependent reduction in the incidence of angiographic vasospasm but subsequent trials failed to demonstrate any benefit [34, 35]. A phase 3 trial (Intravenous Magnesium sulfate for Aneurysmal Subarachnoid Hemorrhage [IMASH]) did not support any clinical benefit from magnesium infusion over placebo in aneurysmal SAH [36].

Once vasospasm involves the large arteries and is angiographically visible, approximately 50 % of patients develop delayed cerebral ischemia [37]. Data on prophylactic angioplasty of the basal cerebral arteries and antiplatelet prophylaxis are inconclusive. Neurointensivists must always watch for the occurrence of vasospasm in patients with aneurysmal SAH. We suggest the following sequence to identify vasospasm and delayed ischemic neurological deficits (Fig. 2):

- Frequent clinical examination, looking for a new focal deficit or reduced consciousness. Symptomatic vasospasm is defined as the development of new focal neurological signs, deterioration in level of consciousness, or both, when other possible causes of worsening (for example, hydrocephalus, seizures, metabolic derangement, infection, or over- sedation) have been excluded. Delayed cerebral ischemia is defined as symptomatic vasospasm or the appearance of new infarction on CT or magnetic resonance imaging (MRI) when the cause is felt to be attributable to vasospasm.
- Daily transcranial Doppler (TCD), widely described in the literature as a safe and useful tool to measure increase in cerebral blood flow velocities as a sign of cerebral vessel narrowing. TCD is a simple and non-invasive bedside screening tool to detect vasospasm; its sensitivity and specificity in identifying vasospasm is good for middle cerebral arteries [38]. TCD vasospasm is commonly defined as a mean flow velocity in any vessel > 120 cm/s.
- In selected patients, we use continuously invasive probes (thermal diffusion flowmetry, Hemedex) to quantify regional cerebral blood flow (rCBF) and continuous electroencephalography (cEEG) to trend CBF changes. In fact, CBF more closely reflects fuel delivery than does cerebral perfusion pressure (CPP).

Whenever clinical deterioration is identified, TCD reveals significant increased velocity or thermal diffusion flowmetry shows a flow reduction, we move to the next step, requiring the transport of the patient outside the ICU.

- Perfusion imaging (perfusion CT) may be more accurate for identifying delayed cerebral ischemia than anatomic imaging. Perfusion CT is a promising technology: CBF and MTT (mean transit time) have the highest overall diagnostic accuracy [39, 40]. Threshold values of 35 ml/100 g/min for CBF and 5.5-second MTT are suggestive of delayed cerebral ischemia on the basis of the patient population utility method.
- DSA is still the gold-standard technique but it is invasive and time-consuming. Angiographic vasospasm is defined as moderate-to-severe arterial narrowing on digital subtraction angiography. We move to this next step, after perfusion CT, only when an endovascular treatment is planned.

Once vasospasm occurs, induction of hypertension with high mean arterial pressure (MAP) to counteract vessel narrowing is recommended for patients with delayed cerebral ischemia unless cardiac status excludes it. Cerebral angioplasty and/ or selective intra-arterial vasodilator therapy is reasonable in patients with symptomatic cerebral vasospasm, particularly those who do not respond rapidly to hypertensive therapy. Once delayed cerebral ischemia is likely, other neuroprotective strategies must be employed, including sedation, hypothermia and CPP optimization. Derangements in cerebrovascular autoregulation, the intrinsic capacity of the cerebral arteries to maintain constant CBF despite changes in CPP, are involved in the development of delayed cerebral ischemia following aneurysmal SAH.

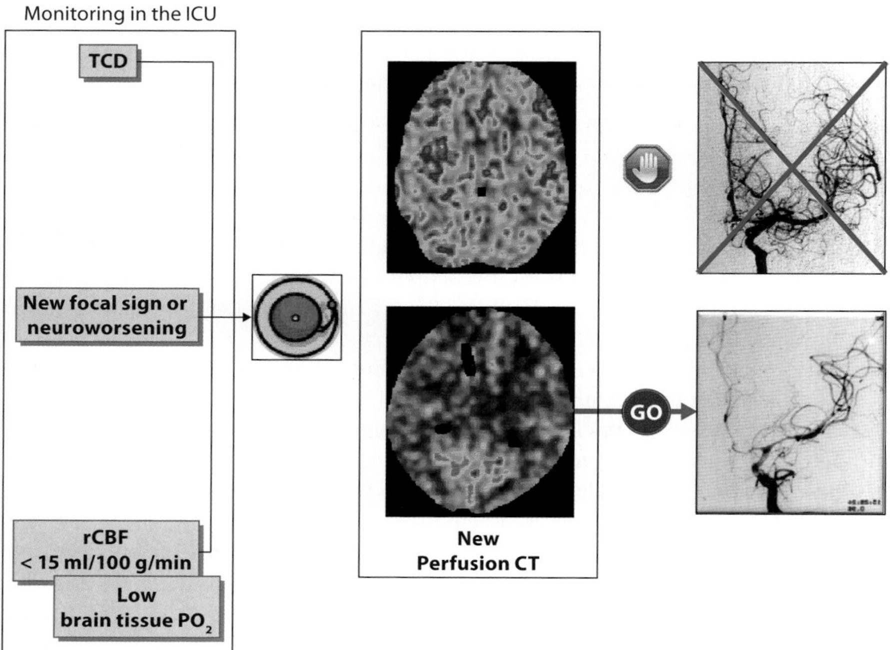

Fig. 2 Sequence to identify vasospasm and delayed ischemic neurological deficit. Each time a clinical deterioration is identified, transcranial Doppler (TCD) reveals significant increased velocity, or thermal diffusion flowmetry shows a flow reduction, we perform perfusion imaging (perfusion computed tomography [CT]) for a better evaluation of cerebral blood flow (CBF) and mean transit time (MTT) (see text). We move to digital subtraction angiography (DSA) after perfusion CT only when a perfusion disturbance is identified or/and an endovascular treatment is planned

High intracranial pressure (ICP) and persistent autoregulatory failure after SAH are independently associated with the occurrence of delayed cerebral infarction and may be an important cofactor in addition to vasospasm itself. Assessment of the status of cerebrovascular autoregulation, measuring the ability of vessels to autoregulate with the pressure reactivity index (PRx), would identify patients with an increased risk of delayed ischemic neurological deficits.

Multimodal brain monitoring is extensively used in various neurocritical care units. Different tools (e.g., brain tissue oxygen tension [PbO_2] and cerebral microdialysis) can help clinicians in detecting metabolic and CBF derangements, mainly in those patients suffering from high-grade aneurysmal SAH. Interestingly, in a recent paper, Chen et al. [41] analyzed a population of patients with low-grade aneurysmal SAH. Patients underwent brain monitoring with PbO_2 and microdialysis. The lactate/pyruvate ratio (LPR) and the frequency of brain hypoxia and energy dysfunction at different ICP and CPP values were analyzed. Interestingly, markers of reduced CBF and metabolic derangements were present in some patients, even in the absence of ICP/CPP disturbance, stressing the importance of these additional tools in managing low grade aneurysmal SAH.

Hydrocephalus and High Intracranial Pressure

Intracranial hypertension (high ICP) can occur in patients with aneurysmal SAH. The pathophysiology can be multifactorial, including acute hydrocephalus, reactive hyperemia and global ischemic insult with brain edema. The latter generally occurs at the onset of the bleeding. Once the aneurysm ruptures, a sudden discharge of blood into the basal cisterns with an acute increase in ICP and reduction in CBF can be immediately fatal. In surviving patients, acute hydrocephalus is likely to occur because the blood clot obstructs CSF flow, or CSF reabsorption is reduced. Acute hydrocephalus has been reported in 15–87 % of patients in different studies [11, 14] and is usually managed by cerebrospinal fluid (CSF) diversion with external ventricular drainage (EVD) or lumbar drainage depending on the clinical scenario.

In patients with high ICP and acute hydrocephalus, ICP monitoring is reasonable and continuous ICP values are desirable as increasing MAP is necessary to sustain CPP and maintain adequate cerebral perfusion.

Seizures

No randomized, controlled trials exist to guide decisions on prophylaxis or treatment of seizures. The majority of SAH patients with seizures had seizure onset before medical evaluation and delayed seizures occurred in 3 % to 7 % of patients. Benefits from prophylactic anticonvulsive therapy are still unclear. Therefore, routine use of anticonvulsant prophylaxis with phenytoin is not recommended after SAH [14].

In the neurocritical care setting, it seems reasonable to monitor the occurrence of seizures with clinical examination and EEG. cEEG is becoming a crucial component of neurocritical care and should be considered in patients with low-grade SAH who fail to improve or who have neurological deterioration of undetermined etiology. Lindgren and co-workers analyzed the frequency of non-convulsive status epilepticus (NCSE) in sedated and ventilated aneurysmal SAH patients. The main finding of this study supported the use of cEEG and showed how continuous sedation in aneurysmal SAH patients in need of controlled ventilation was associated with a low frequency of clinical and subclinical seizures [42].

Claassen et al. described some relationships between constant epileptiform discharges after SAH and mortality [43]. The absence of sleep potentials and the presence of repetitive epileptiform activity in the form of periodic lateralized epileptiform activity are prognostic indicators of a poor neurological outcome as repetitive epileptiform activity is a marker of ischemic damage that cannot be seen on brain imaging. Thus, once seizures and epileptic activity are suspected and diagnosed, treatment is compulsory given the detrimental consequences.

Management of Medical Complications

Sodium Abnormalities

Hyponatremia is frequently seen following aneurysmal SAH. Hyponatremia is a severity marker of SAH, being more frequent in low-grade patients. Hyponatremia is sustained from different mechanisms. A key point to interpret the origin of these abnormalities is the accurate investigation of the volemic state of patients by some combination of central venous pressure (CVP), intrathoracic volume measurements, and fluid balance. The cerebral salt wasting syndrome (CSWS) is the result of excessive secretion of natriuretic peptides and causes sodium reduction from excessive natriuresis. Therefore CSWS, defined as the renal loss of sodium during intracranial disease, is a hypovolemic hyponatremic condition linked with natriuresis and decrease fluid volume. CSWS is more common in patients with low clinical grade, ruptured anterior communicating artery aneurysms, and hydrocephalus, and it may be an independent risk factor for poor outcome [27]. Mineralocorticoid administration has been investigated in different studies and seems to be associated with a better control of hyponatremia and reduced administration of crystalloids.

The syndrome of inappropriate antidiuretic hormone secretion (SIADH) is caused by elevated serum vasopressin activity, and represents a euvolemic hyponatremic state. Fluid restriction in SIADH is indicated but with caution because as it has been associated with an incidence of cerebral infarction. Sodium balance should be calculated on a daily basis and hydrocortisone could be used to overcome the excessive natriuresis [28].

Stunned Myocardium

Cardiac dysfunction after SAH is referred to as 'neurogenic stunned myocardium' and can represent a critical care challenge [2, 44]. Cardiopulmonary complications can develop immediately after the bleeding and clinical findings vary from no symptoms with mildly raised troponin enzymes through to cardiogenic shock, reduced left ventricular function, congestive heart failure and pulmonary edema in approximately 10% of patients. Clinical features of neurogenic stunned myocardium include electrocardiogram (EKG) abnormalities, increase in serum markers that decays within days, chest x-ray suggestive of pulmonary edema, echocardiogram regional wall motions abnormalities (RWMA) and a coronary angiogram with normal coronary arteries. Baseline cardiac assessment with serial enzymes, EKG, echocardiography and cardiac output monitoring is recommended, especially in patients with evidence of myocardial dysfunction [14]. The most widely accepted theory on the pathogenesis of aneurysmal SAH-induced myocardial dysfunction relies on massive catecholamine release [45]. At the time of bleeding, a sudden increase in ICP may cause sympathetic activation via hypothalamic damage. Histological studies have shown myocardial changes, known as myocardial contraction band necrosis, which refers to a specific form of myocyte injury with hypercontracted sarcomeres and interstitial mononuclear inflammatory response. Myocardial stunning can be challenging and carries great implications in terms of therapy [46]. In fact, patients who develop vasospasm are at high risk of delayed cerebral ischemia. Sustaining CBF and adequate oxygen delivery via implementation of CPP is mandatory. Consequently, MAP needs to be sustained by fluid and vasopressors (usually with phenylephrine) given that CPP = MAP – ICP.

However, if catecholamines themselves cause neurogenic stunned myocardium, then phenylephrine, along with other available sympathomimetic drugs, may be harmful [47]. In selected cases, other strategies can be adopted to sustain CPP or cardiac output after aneurysmal SAH (e.g., milrinone, dobutamine and intra-aortic balloon pump counterpulsation).

Fever

Fever is the most common medical complication in patients suffering from aneurysmal SAH and has been widely associated with neurological deterioration in neurocritical care patients [48]. Non-infectious (central) fever has been associated with the amount of blood (the severity of injury) and the development of vasospasm. Fever affects cerebral metabolism and small increases in temperature can exacerbate ischemic brain damage via an imbalance between substrate delivery and metabolic needs. Temperature elevations have also been associated with cerebral hyperemia, edema worsening and elevated ICP. Therefore, temperature monitoring and aggressive fever control is reasonable in the acute phase of aneurysmal SAH in order to reduce the burden of the secondary insult [14]. Core body temperature reduction (hypothermia) as a neuroprotective strategy is still under investigation.

Glucose Control

Hyperglycemia is commonly identified during initial evaluation of patients with aneurysmal SAH. Accurate glycemic control must be part of the general critical care management of patients with aneurysmal SAH. In fact, prolonged hyperglycemia is associated with an increased ICU length of stay, increased risk of death or severe disability and is an independent predictor of death or severe disability. An independent association between hyperglycemia and symptomatic vasospasm has also been described and elevated blood glucose levels at the time of admission were prognostic of unfavorable outcome, defined as death, vegetative state, or severe disability at 12 months.

Hypoglycemia (serum glucose < 80 mg/dl) should be avoided. Serum glucose should be maintained around 140 mg/dl. There are reports of cerebral microdialysis findings of cerebral metabolic crisis and low cerebral glucose in SAH patients being treated with insulin infusions, even in the absence of systemic hypoglycemia

[49]. If microdialysis is being used, serum glucose may be adjusted to avoid low cerebral glucose [14].

Deep Venous Thrombosis

Deep venous thrombosis occurs relatively frequently after aneurysmal SAH, especially in patients immobilized because of poor neurological status. Heparin-induced thrombocytopenia has been described in several studies [22]. Early identification and targeted treatment are recommended and prophylaxis (with subcutaneous heparinoids and external pneumatic compression sleeves) is reasonable for patients who are comatose and admitted to the neurocritical care unit.

Conclusion

Aneurysmal SAH is a complex disease with different degrees of clinical severity. Patients' characteristics and neurological impairment at the time of bleeding can be summarized using international scales. The optimal management of SAH has not been fully established yet. Several topics are still under debate. However, management of patients with aneurysmal SAH requires a multidisciplinary approach in a high volume hospital. Early aneurysm repair is compulsory as rerupture is frequent and associated with poor prognosis.

Recently, the AHA/ASA updated the guidelines for the evaluation and treatment of patients with SAH and the Neurocritical Care Society released guidelines summarizing the current state of art and areas of uncertainty in treatment of aneurysmal SAH [14, 22].

Efforts to improve outcome after aneurysmal SAH should focus on the medical complications that contribute to poor outcome together with delayed cerebral ischemia. Given the multifactorial etiology underling delayed cerebral ischemia and the cascade of events that happen at the onset of bleeding (mainly CBF reduction), new monitoring tools, such as perfusion CT, cEEG, microdialysis and PbO_2 should be routinely promoted to optimize cerebral physiology.

References

1. Suarez JI, Tarr RW, Selman WR (2006) Aneurysmal subarachnoid hemorrhage. N Engl J Med 354:387–396
2. Coppadoro A, Citerio G (2011) Subarachnoid hemorrhage: an update for the intensivist. Minerva Anestesiol 77:74–84
3. Leblanc GG, Golanov E, Awad IA, Young WL (2009) Biology of Vascular Malformations of the Brain. Stroke 40:e694–e702

4. Penn DL, Komotar RJ, Connolly ES (2011) Hemodynamic mechanisms underlying cerebral aneurysm pathogenesis. J Clin Neurosci 18:1435–1438
5. Frösen J, Tulamo R, Paetau A et al (2012) Saccular intracranial aneurysm: pathology and mechanisms. Acta Neuropathol 123:773–786
6. Rosen DS, Macdonald RL (2005) Subarachnoid hemorrhage grading scales: a systematic review. Neurocrit Care 2:110–118
7. Risselada R, Lingsma HF, Bauer-Mehren A et al (2010) Prediction of 60 day case-fatality after aneurysmal subarachnoid haemorrhage: results from the International Subarachnoid Aneurysm Trial (ISAT). Eur J Epidemiol 25:261–266
8. Fisher CM, Kistler JP, Davis JM (1980) Relation of cerebral vasospasm to subarachnoid hemorrhage visualized by computerized tomographic scanning. Neurosurgery 6:1–9
9. Claassen J, Bernardini GL, Kreiter K et al (2001) Effect of cisternal and ventricular blood on risk of delayed cerebral ischemia after subarachnoid hemorrhage: the Fisher scale revisited. Stroke 32:2012–2020
10. Larsen CC, Astrup J (2012) Rebleeding after aneurysmal subarachnoid hemorrhage: a literature review. World Neurosurg (in press)
11. Fountas KN, Kapsalaki EZ, Machinis T, Karampelas I, Smisson HF, Robinson JS (2006) Review of the literature regarding the relationship of rebleeding and external ventricular drainage in patients with subarachnoid hemorrhage of aneurysmal origin. Neurosurg Rev 29:14–18
12. Lord AS, Fernandez L, Schmidt JM et al (2011) Effect of rebleeding on the course and incidence of vasospasm after subarachnoid hemorrhage. Neurology 78:31–37
13. Starke RM, Connolly ES (2011) Rebleeding after aneurysmal subarachnoid hemorrhage. Neurocrit Care 15:241–246
14. Diringer MN, Bleck TP, Claude Hemphill J et al (2011) Critical Care Management of Patients Following Aneurysmal Subarachnoid Hemorrhage: Recommendations from the Neurocritical Care Society's Multidisciplinary Consensus Conference. Neurocrit Care 15:211–240
15. Wartenberg KE, Wartenberg KE, Schmidt JM et al (2006) Impact of medical complications on outcome after subarachnoid hemorrhage. Crit Care Med 34:617–623
16. Claassen J, Carhuapoma JR, Kreiter KT, Du EY, Connolly ES, Mayer SA (2002) Global cerebral edema after subarachnoid hemorrhage: frequency, predictors, and impact on outcome. Stroke 33:1225–1232
17. Kramer AH, Mikolaenko I, Deis N et al (2010) Intraventricular hemorrhage volume predicts poor outcomes but not delayed ischemic neurological deficits among patients with ruptured cerebral aneurysms. Neurosurgery 67:1044–1052
18. Pierot L, Cognard C, Anxionnat R, Ricolfi F, CLARITY Investigators (2010) Ruptured intracranial aneurysms: factors affecting the rate and outcome of endovascular treatment complications in a series of 782 patients (CLARITY study). Radiology 256:916–923
19. Berman MF, Solomon RA, Mayer SA, Johnston SC, Yung PP (2003) Impact of hospital-related factors on outcome after treatment of cerebral aneurysms. Stroke 34:2200–2207
20. Johnston SC (2000) Effect of endovascular services and hospital volume on cerebral aneurysm treatment outcomes. Stroke 31:111–117
21. Vespa P, Diringer MN, The Participants in the International Multi-disciplinary Consensus Conference on the Critical Care Management of Subarachnoid Hemorrhage (2011) High-Volume Centers. Neurocrit Care 15:369–372
22. Connolly ES, Rabinstein AA, Carhuapoma JR et al (2012) Guidelines for the Management of Aneurysmal Subarachnoid Hemorrhage: A Guideline for Healthcare Professionals From the American Heart Association/American Stroke Association. Stroke 43:1711–1737
23. Molyneux AJ, Kerr RSC, Yu L-M et al (2005) International subarachnoid aneurysm trial (ISAT) of neurosurgical clipping versus endovascular coiling in 2143 patients with ruptured intracranial aneurysms: a randomised comparison of effects on survival, dependency, seizures, rebleeding, subgroups, and aneurysm occlusion. Lancet 366:809–817

24. Molyneux AJ, Kerr RSC, Birks J et al (2009) Risk of recurrent subarachnoid haemorrhage, death, or dependence and standardised mortality ratios after clipping or coiling of an intracranial aneurysm in the International Subarachnoid Aneurysm Trial (ISAT): long-term follow-up. Lancet Neurol 8:427–433
25. Varelas PN, Schultz L, Conti M, Spanaki M, Genarrelli T, Hacein-Bey L (2008) The impact of a neuro-intensivist on patients with stroke admitted to a neurosciences intensive care unit. Neurocrit Care 9:293–299
26. Dhar R, Diringer MN (2008) The burden of the systemic inflammatory response predicts vasospasm and outcome after subarachnoid hemorrhage. Neurocrit Care 8:404–412
27. Pluta RM, Hansen-Schwartz J, Dreier J et al (2009) Cerebral vasospasm following subarachnoid hemorrhage: time for a new world of thought. Neurol Res 31:151–158
28. Rowland MJ, Hadjipavlou G, Kelly M, Westbrook J, Pattinson KTS (2012) Delayed cerebral ischaemia after subarachnoid haemorrhage: looking beyond vasospasm. Br J Anaesth 109:315–329
29. Cahill J, Cahill WJ, Calvert JW, Calvert JH, Zhang JH (2006) Mechanisms of early brain injury after subarachnoid hemorrhage. J Cereb Blood Flow Metab 26:1341–1353
30. Cahill J, Zhang JH (2009) Subarachnoid hemorrhage: is it time for a new direction? Stroke 40(3 Suppl):S86–S87
31. Al-Tamimi YZ, Orsi NM, Quinn AC, Homer-Vanniasinkam S, Ross SA (2010) A review of delayed ischemic neurologic deficit following aneurysmal subarachnoid hemorrhage: historical overview, current treatment, and pathophysiology. World Neurol 73:654–667
32. Sabri M, Ai J, Lakovic K, D'Abbondanza J, Ilodigwe D, Macdonald RL (2012) Mechanisms of microthrombi formation after experimental subarachnoid hemorrhage. Neurosci 224:26–37
33. Dorhout Mees SM, Rinkel GJE, Feigin VL et al (2007) Calcium antagonists for aneurysmal subarachnoid haemorrhage. Cochrane Database Syst Rev CD000277
34. Macdonald RL, Higashida RT, Keller E et al (2011) Clazosentan, an endothelin receptor antagonist, in patients with aneurysmal subarachnoid haemorrhage undergoing surgical clipping: a randomised, double-blind, placebo-controlled phase 3 trial (CONSCIOUS-2). Lancet Neurol 10:618–625
35. Wong GKC, Poon WS (2011) Clazosentan for patients with subarachnoid haemorrhage: lessons learned. Lancet Neurol 10:871
36. Wong GKC, Chan MTV, Poon WS, Boet R, Gin T (2006) Magnesium therapy within 48 hours of an aneurysmal subarachnoid hemorrhage: neuro-panacea. Neurol Res 28:431–435
37. Vergouwen MDI, Vermeulen M, van Gijn J et al (2010) Definition of delayed cerebral ischemia after aneurysmal subarachnoid hemorrhage as an outcome event in clinical trials and observational studies: proposal of a multidisciplinary research group. Stroke 41:2391–2395
38. Sloan MA, Alexandrov AV, Tegeler CH et al (2004) Assessment: transcranial Doppler ultrasonography: report of the Therapeutics and Technology Assessment Subcommittee of the American Academy of Neurology. Neurology 62:1468–1481
39. Sanelli PC, Anumula N, Johnson CE et al (2013) Evaluating CT perfusion using outcome measures of delayed cerebral ischemia in aneurysmal subarachnoid hemorrhage. AJNR Am J Neuroradiol (in press)
40. Sanelli PC, Ugorec I, Johnson CE et al (2011) Using quantitative CT perfusion for evaluation of delayed cerebral ischemia following aneurysmal subarachnoid hemorrhage. AJNR Am J Neuroradiol 32:2047–2053
41. Chen HI, Stiefel MF, Oddo M et al (2011) Detection of cerebral compromise with multimodality monitoring in patients with subarachnoid hemorrhage. Neurosurgery 69:53–63
42. Lindgren C, Nordh E, Naredi S, Olivecrona M (2012) Frequency of non-convulsive seizures and non-convulsive status epilepticus in subarachnoid hemorrhage patients in need of controlled ventilation and sedation. Neurocrit Care 17:367–373

43. Claassen J, Mayer SA, Kowalski RG, Emerson RG, Hirsch LJ (2004) Detection of electrographic seizures with continuous EEG monitoring in critically ill patients. Neurology 62:1743–1748
44. Kopelnik A, Zaroff J (2006) Neurocardiogenic injury in neurovascular disorders. Crit Care Clin 22:733–752
45. Lee VH, Oh JK, Mulvagh SL, Wijdicks EFM (2006) Mechanisms in neurogenic stress cardiomyopathy after aneurysmal subarachnoid hemorrhage. Neurocrit Care 5:243–249
46. Temes RE, Tessitore E, Schmidt JM et al (2010) Left ventricular dysfunction and cerebral infarction from vasospasm after subarachnoid hemorrhage. Neurocrit Care 13:359–365
47. Macmillan CSA, Grant IS, Andrews PJD (2002) Pulmonary and cardiac sequelae of subarachnoid haemorrhage: time for active management? Intensive Care Med 28:1012–1023
48. Scaravilli V, Tinchero G, Citerio G, The Participants in the International Multi-disciplinary Consensus Conference on the Critical Care Management of Subarachnoid Hemorrhage (2011) Fever management in SAH. Neurocrit Care 15:287–294
49. Sandsmark DK, Kumar MA, Park S, Levine JM (2012) Multimodal monitoring in subarachnoid hemorrhage. Stroke 43:1440–1445

Recanalization: A Critical Step in Acute Ischemic Stroke

M. Mazighi

Introduction

To date, intravenous tissue-type plasminogen activator (tPA) is still the only pharmacological treatment approved for acute ischemic stroke. Arterial recanalization is a powerful predictor of stroke outcome in patients treated with either intravenous or endovascular therapy [1]. However, complete recanalization (opening of the primary arterial occlusive lesion) may not be associated with favorable clinical outcome if reperfusion (global re-opening of the distal vascular bed) is not obtained (i. e., due to distal clot embolization) or not tolerated (e.g., in case of hemorrhagic transformation). In fact, tissue downstream to the arterial occlusion must be salvageable to obtain any clinical benefit [2].

Time-to-Recanalization: A Critical Goal

Spontaneous recanalization is common in the setting of acute ischemic stroke. Among patients presenting with carotid artery occlusions, 40 % will experience spontaneous recanalization within 24 hours and more than 90 % after three weeks [3]. These data suggest that recanalization is not the end of the road and that time-to-recanalization is a critical issue [4]. Studies monitoring arterial recanalization have shown that complete recanalization is correlated with good outcome if achieved within 300 min of stroke onset [5, 6]. Furthermore, tPA administration is associated with a favorable outcome when the median time-to-recanalization is achieved within 215 min [1]. In other words, shortening the time-to-recanalization should be the main goal [6]. The sooner the recanalization is obtained, the greater

M. Mazighi (✉)
Department of Neurology and Stroke Centre, Bichat University Hospital, 46, rue Henri Huchard, 75018 Paris, France
E-mail: mikael.mazighi@bch.aphp.fr

J.-L. Vincent (Ed.), *Annual Update in Intensive Care and Emergency Medicine 2013*,
DOI 10.1007/978-3-642-35109-9_61, © Springer-Verlag Berlin Heidelberg 2013

the number of cured patients at 3 months [1]. Evidence has shown that recanalization obtained within 3 hours and 30 minutes, is associated with more than 90 % favorable outcome at 3 months (OR: 2.20; 95 % CI 1.24–3.88; $p=0.007$) [1]. Each 30 minute delay to recanalization is followed by a reduction by 20 % in favorable outcome at 3 months. Favorable clinical outcome following successful recanalization is time-dependent [7].

Recanalization Strategies

Intravenous tPA, the only recommended therapy for acute ischemic stroke, cures 40 % of treated patients. Its efficacy is highly dependent on clot location. Recanalization rates will decrease with the site of arterial occlusion (66 % recanalization rate for distal middle cerebral artery [MCA], 35 % for proximal MCA and 8 % for carotid occlusions) [3]. Considering recanalization rates, endovascular therapy is superior to intravenous thrombolysis. In fact, endovascular therapy including mechanical thrombectomy may achieve recanalization rates up to 87 % [1, 8]. One of the first randomized controlled trials evaluating endovascular therapy, was conducted in patients with MCA occlusions (Prolyse in Acute Cerebral Thromboembolism [PROACT] II) [9]. PROACT II showed a 66 % recanalization rate, which translated to a 40 % favorable outcome rate at 3 months. Non-randomized studies comparing intravenous and intra-arterial routes for thrombolysis in patients with MCA occlusions also suggested that patients treated with intra-arterial thrombolysis may have higher rates of favorable outcome [10]. In this context, combined intravenous-intra-arterial approaches may optimize and overcome the disadvantage of the intra-arterial route (i. e., delay in time-to-treatment). A systematic intravenous tPA-endovascular therapy approach compared to an intravenous tPA only approach is associated with greater recanalization rates and may be associated with early neurological improvement as well as improved 90-day favorable outcome [1].

Endovascular thrombus capture (thrombectomy) is now frequently used in acute reperfusion therapies. Several devices are now available and among them the "Mechanical Embolus Removal in Cerebral Ischemia" (MERCI, Concentric Medical, Mountain View, CA) device has probably been evaluated most. MERCI and Multi-MERCI [11, 12] studies reported the use of this device in acute ischemic stroke patients admitted within 8 hours of symptom onset. The recanalization rate was 53.5 % and favorable outcome at 90 days was achieved in 25 % of the patients [11]. In MERCI and Multi-MERCI, patient selection was based only on the status of the primary artery (occluded or not). This point is debatable, because of the existing evidence for therapeutic window enlargement (outside the recommended 4.5 hours of symptom onset), after patient selection based on multimodal brain imaging (e.g., diffusion and perfusion magnetic resonance imaging [MRI]) [13–15]. We cannot exclude that for patients treated close to the 8 hours after symptom onset, the likelihood of being able to reperfuse salvageable brain was low. The same therapeutic window has been used for the evaluation of other devices, such as the Penumbra (device allowing clot fragmentation with aspiration) and the Solitaire (stent retriever). With the Penumbra System (Alameda, CA), 82 % of treated patients may be recanalized but only 25 % of them will achieve a modified Rankin scale (mRS) ≤ 2 [16]. These clinical outcomes are surprisingly low considering the high rate of recanalization. With the new generation of thrombectomy devices, the stent retrievers, up to 90 % of patients will achieve recanalization with a favorable outcome in 45 % at 3 months [17]. The main interest in these new devices using retriever stents is that a temporary bypass is performed (the thrombus is pushed against the arterial wall while a lumen patency within the stent can be observed) when the stent retriever is deployed.

Which Reperfusion Approach, for Which Patient?

Endovascular therapy is still considered an investigational technique and the optimal strategy for reperfusion needs to be defined. Different conditions may be identified. Endovascular therapy may be used as a direct approach (e.g., if tPA is contraindicated) or as rescue approach after failure of intravenous tPA (Fig. 1). Intravenous tPA alone may be a choice, when its efficacy is likely to be high (e.g., in distal cortical occlusions of MCA) [18]. Combined approaches with intravenous tPA and endovascular therapy may be an option for more proximal occlusions. Recent data from the MERCI and Multi-MERCI trials, showed reduced mortality and time-to-recanalization with endovascular therapy in patients treated with intravenous tPA [19]. These findings suggest that intravenous tPA may increase the efficacy of endovascular therapy. However, this positive relationship was found for MCA occlusions and not for carotid occlusions. Thrombus location seems to modify response to therapy, suggesting that reperfusion approaches may vary from anterior to posterior circulations. The vast majority of the data on reperfusion were obtained in the anterior circulation with limited evidence in the posterior circulation. The Basilar Artery International Cooperation Study (BASICS) prospective registry [20] included 592 patients with symptomatic occlusion of the basilar artery. Patients were divided into three therapeutic groups (anti-thrombotic therapy; intravenous thrombolysis; or endovascular therapy including intra-arterial thrombolysis, thrombectomy, stenting or the combination of these different techniques). No therapeutic approach was superior to another, but subgroup analyses showed some differences. Patients with mild neurological deficit (as opposed to those who had severe neurologic deficit including coma, locked-in or tetraplegia) in the endovascular therapy arm had a worse prognosis compared to those in the intravenous thrombolysis group (RR 1.49; 95 % CI 1.00–2.23). For clinically 'severe' (coma, locked-in or tetraplegia) patients, the risk of a bad prognosis was superior in the antithrombotic group compared to the intravenous thrombolysis or endovascular therapy groups. No difference was observed between the intravenous thrombolysis and endovascular therapy groups (RR 1.06; 95 % CI 0.91–1.22). It is

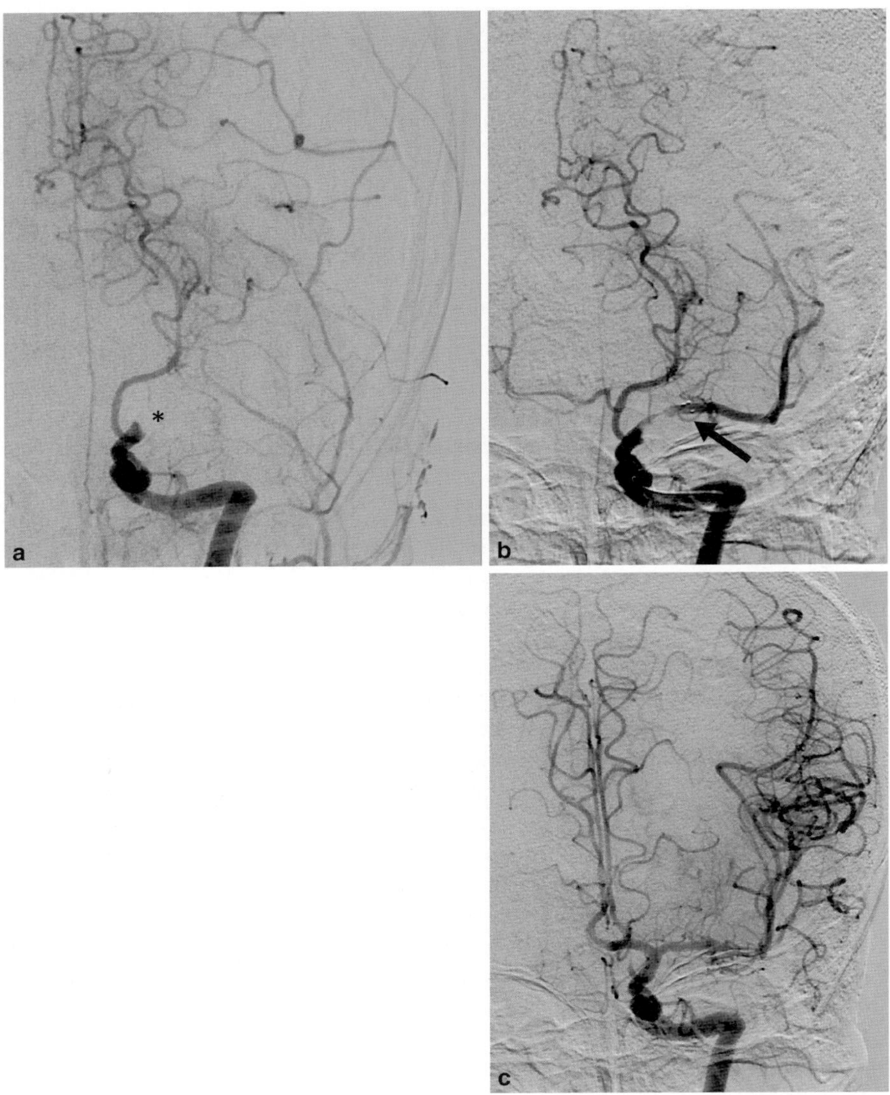

Fig. 1 Anterior view of a left carotid angiogram in a 67-year old female with failed intravenous thrombolysis. **a** Arterial occlusion of the carotid termination (*); **b** deployment of a stent retriever (thrombectomy device, arrow) with partial flow restoration; **c** after clot extraction, restoration of normal flow

important to note that patients in the endovascular therapy group were more often 'severe' and treated later, whereas those of the intravenous thrombolysis group were predominantly treated within 3 hours. Last but not least, symptomatic intracranial bleeding was more frequent in the endovascular therapy group (14 %

[10–18 %]) compared to the intravenous thrombolysis group (6 % [3–11 %]), whereas hemorrhage occurred in less than 1 % of the antithrombotic group. Considering all the limits of a registry, the findings of BASICS suggest that endovascular therapy is not a systematic first line therapy in basilar artery symptomatic occlusions. Another relevant finding from BASICS was the prognosis considering the time-to-treatment. All patients treated 9 hours after symptom onset had a bad prognosis, suggesting that there is no room for reperfusion after 9 hours of symptom onset, unless cerebral imaging shows significant residual salvageable tissue.

Recanalization and Its Consequences

In the setting of acute ischemic stroke, complete recanalization is mandatory but recanalization can cause neurovascular injury, including cerebral edema and brain hemorrhage. Brain hemorrhage has been described as a marker of reperfusion [21], not always associated with clinical deterioration. The low risk of brain hemorrhage in patients with early reperfusion suggests the importance of hypoperfusion in the pathogenesis of brain hemorrhage [22, 23]. In patients with a large area of severe perfusion delay, the risk of brain hemorrhage should be considered, even if brain imaging shows no extensive tissue damage. The Diffusion and Perfusion Imaging for Understanding Stroke Evolution (DEFUSE) trial indicated that a large volume of severe perfusion delay (T max ≥ 8 seconds) was an independent predictor of brain hemorrhage. This has been described as the "malignant profile" (i. e., patients at risk for brain hemorrhage after recanalization therapy) [24]. The perfusion status (severe perfusion delay) rather than tissue status (DWI lesion volume) may be a concern in brain hemorrhage. Blood-brain barrier (BBB) alteration is also common after cerebral ischemia and reperfusion, but its pathogenesis still needs to be clarified. We know that early detection of BBB disruption (detected on post-contrast enhanced T1-weighted MRI) for acute ischemic stroke predicts brain hemorrhage after thrombolysis [25]. Therefore, the assessment of BBB status may be a relevant parameter in the decision-making process for reperfusion therapy.

Conclusion

Early recanalization is a critical target to achieve. In this perspective, endovascular therapy will undoubtedly play a major role in the near future. Evidence from ongoing randomized controlled trials comparing endovascular therapy with the gold standard (intravenous tPA) is needed to change the current guidelines and support endovascular therapy as a first-line therapy. The target population for endovascular therapy will probably be those patients with proximal arterial occlusions, whereas intravenous tPA will probably be indicated for small strokes with distal arterial occlusions. In the future, patient selection will be increasingly based on multimodal imaging to select the best strategy (i. e., the best profile for efficacy and safety). Future challenges will include achieving higher rates of recanalization with limited bleeding and reperfusion injury risk.

References

1. Mazighi M, Serfaty JM, Labreuche J et al (2009) Comparison of intravenous alteplase with a combined intravenous-endovascular approach in patients with stroke and confirmed arterial occlusion (RECANALISE study): a prospective cohort study. Lancet Neurol 8:802–809
2. Khatri P, Neff J, Broderick JP, Khoury JC, Carrozzella J, Tomsick T (2005) Revascularization end points in stroke interventional trials: recanalization versus reperfusion in IMS-I. Stroke 36:2400–2403
3. del Zoppo GJ, Poeck K, Pessin MS et al (1992) Recombinant tissue plasminogen activator in acute thrombotic and embolic stroke. Ann Neurol 32:78–86
4. Lees KR, Bluhmki E, von Kummer R et al (2010) Time to treatment with intravenous alteplase and outcome in stroke: an updated pooled analysis of ECASS, ATLANTIS, NINDS, and EPITHET trials. Lancet 375:1695–1703
5. Saposnik G, Di Legge S, Webster F, Hachinski V (2005) Predictors of major neurologic improvement after thrombolysis in acute stroke. Neurology 65:1169–1174
6. Molina CA, Alexandrov AV, Demchuk AM, Saqqur M, Uchino K, Alvarez-Sabin J (2004) Improving the predictive accuracy of recanalization on stroke outcome in patients treated with tissue plasminogen activator. Stroke 35:151–156
7. Khatri P, Abruzzo T, Yeatts SD, Nichols C, Broderick JP, Tomsick TA (2009) Good clinical outcome after ischemic stroke with successful revascularization is time-dependent. Neurology 73:1066–1072
8. Rha JH, Saver JL (2007) The impact of recanalization on ischemic stroke outcome: a meta-analysis. Stroke 38:967–973
9. Furlan A, Higashida R, Wechsler L et al (1999) Intra-arterial prourokinase for acute ischemic stroke. The PROACT II study: a randomized controlled trial. Prolyse in Acute Cerebral Thromboembolism. JAMA 282:2003–2011
10. Mattle HP, Arnold M, Georgiadis D et al (2008) Comparison of intraarterial and intravenous thrombolysis for ischemic stroke with hyperdense middle cerebral artery sign. Stroke 39:379–383
11. Smith WS, Sung G, Starkman S et al (2005) Safety and efficacy of mechanical embolectomy in acute ischemic stroke: results of the MERCI trial. Stroke 36:1432–1438
12. Smith WS, Sung G, Saver J et al (2008) Mechanical thrombectomy for acute ischemic stroke: final results of the Multi MERCI trial. Stroke 39:1205–1212
13. Chalela JA, Kidwell CS, Nentwich LM et al (2007) Magnetic resonance imaging and computed tomography in emergency assessment of patients with suspected acute stroke: a prospective comparison. Lancet 369:293–298
14. Kane I, Sandercock P, Wardlaw J (2007) Magnetic resonance perfusion diffusion mismatch and thrombolysis in acute ischaemic stroke: a systematic review of the evidence to date. J Neurol Neurosurg Psychiatry 78:485–491
15. Schellinger PD, Thomalla G, Fiehler J et al (2007) MRI-based and CT-based thrombolytic therapy in acute stroke within and beyond established time windows: an analysis of 1210 patients. Stroke 38:2640–2645
16. Penumbra Pivotal Stroke Trial Investigators (2009) The penumbra pivotal stroke trial: safety and effectiveness of a new generation of mechanical devices for clot removal in intracranial large vessel occlusive disease. Stroke 40:2761–2768

17. Castano C, Dorado L, Guerrero C et al (2010) Mechanical thrombectomy with the Solitaire AB device in large artery occlusions of the anterior circulation: a pilot study. Stroke 41:1836–1840
18. del Zoppo GJ, Poeck K, Pessin MS et al (1992) Recombinant tissue plasminogen activator in acute thrombotic and embolic stroke. Ann Neurol 32:78–86
19. Shi ZS, Loh Y, Walker G, Duckwiler GR (2010) Endovascular thrombectomy for acute ischemic stroke in failed intravenous tissue plasminogen activator versus non-intravenous tissue plasminogen activator patients: revascularization and outcomes stratified by the site of arterial occlusions. Stroke 41:1185–1192
20. Schonewille WJ, Wijman CA, Michel P et al (2009) Treatment and outcomes of acute basilar artery occlusion in the Basilar Artery International Cooperation Study (BASICS): a prospective registry study. Lancet Neurol 8:724–730
21. Molina CA, Alvarez-Sabin J, Montaner J et al (2002) Thrombolysis-related hemorrhagic infarction: a marker of early reperfusion, reduced infarct size, and improved outcome in patients with proximal middle cerebral artery occlusion. Stroke 33:1551–1556
22. Kim JH, Bang OY, Liebeskind DS et al (2010) Impact of baseline tissue status (diffusion-weighted imaging lesion) versus perfusion status (severity of hypoperfusion) on hemorrhagic transformation. Stroke 41:e135–e142
23. Saqqur M, Tsivgoulis G, Molina CA et al (2008) Symptomatic intracerebral hemorrhage and recanalization after IV rt-PA: a multicenter study. Neurology 71:1304–1312
24. Albers GW, Thijs VN, Wechsler L et al (2006) Magnetic resonance imaging profiles predict clinical response to early reperfusion: the diffusion and perfusion imaging evaluation for understanding stroke evolution (DEFUSE) study. Ann Neurol 60:508–517
25. Kastrup A, Groschel K, Ringer TM et al (2008) Early disruption of the blood-brain barrier after thrombolytic therapy predicts hemorrhage in patients with acute stroke. Stroke 39:2385–2387

Brain Monitoring in the Intensive Care Unit

M. Srairi, T. Geeraerts, and O. Fourcade

Introduction

Clinical examination of the critically ill patient is essential to assess neurological status, but is limited by the frequent use of sedative agents that affect neurological function [1]. Several life-threatening conditions, such as liver failure or bacterial meningitis, can be associated with brain edema and significant risk of brain ischemia [2–4]. Early diagnosis of brain injury in patients at risk of brain damage is essential to adapt treatments and prevent secondary insults to the brain. Moreover, avoiding excessive sedation has become an important issue in the intensive care unit (ICU) [5]. Several tools are now available at the bedside to diagnose brain ischemia, predict neurological outcome and assess the effect of sedation on neurological function by studying brain electrogenesis, hemodynamics and oxygenation. In this chapter, we will focus on the methods available for brain monitoring at the bedside in the ICU setting. As brain microdialysis is still largely a research tool, it will not be discussed in this article.

M. Srairi
Department of Anesthesia and Intensive Care Medicine, University Hospital of Toulouse, 1 Place Baylac TSA 40031, 31059 Toulouse cedex 9, France

T. Geeraerts (✉)
Department of Anesthesia and Intensive Care Medicine, University Hospital of Toulouse, 1 Place Baylac TSA 40031, 31059 Toulouse cedex 9, France
E-mail: geeraerts.t@chu-toulouse.fr

O. Fourcade
Department of Anesthesia and Intensive Care Medicine, University Hospital of Toulouse, 1 Place Baylac TSA 40031, 31059 Toulouse cedex 9, France

J.-L. Vincent (Ed.), *Annual Update in Intensive Care and Emergency Medicine 2013*, DOI 10.1007/978-3-642-35109-9_62, © Springer-Verlag Berlin Heidelberg 2013

Electrophysiological Monitoring

Electroencephalography

Electroencephalography (EEG) is based on the measurement of a difference in electric potential between two points reflecting neuronal activity. The international ten/twenty-system uses 36 electrodes on the scalp and reflects electrogenesis of only one third of the brain. So-called 'high density EEG' (e.g., using 128 to 264 electrodes) significantly improves spatial resolution of the monitoring. The signal is analyzed with respect to its frequency, amplitude, presence of paroxysmal activity and response to stimuli. The wave frequency allows classification into four bands: The delta band (frequency between 0.5 and 3 Hz) and the theta band (4–7 Hz) are associated with sleep, the alpha band (8–12 Hz) is associated with relaxed wakefulness, and the beta band (13–30 Hz) is seen in awake individuals. Frequency analysis is a method for processing the EEG, which uses fast Fourier transformation (FFT) to decompose the signal into sine waves characterized by a specific frequency, amplitude and power (obtained by squaring the amplitude). This processing produces a spectrum of power where each band of frequency is associated to a specific power of the signal (hence this method is also called 'power spectral analysis' or quantitative EEG [qEEG]). Continuous EEG monitoring (cEEG) coupled with frequency analysis gives interpretable indices and ratios for non-specialists in the ICU, for example, the alpha-delta ratio (ADR, the ratio of the alpha band power to the delta band power) or the composite alpha index (CAI) which is the product of the alpha power in the frontal territory by the alpha power variability.

Indications for EEG use in the intensive care unit

The rationale supporting EEG use in the ICU, apart from looking for paroxysmal activity in epilepsy, is the flow-metabolism coupling leading to variations in electrogenesis with cerebral blood flow (CBF). The commonly accepted indications for EEG in the ICU are:

- during the first 12–24 hours of generalized status epilepticus in order to guide sedation, with a goal of three to five burst-suppression per minute
- diagnosis of non-convulsive status epilepticus responsible for delirium or delayed arousal after sedation withdrawal or in case of severe traumatic brain injury (TBI)
- confirmation of brain death in some countries, e.g., France
- prognosis of post-anoxic encephalopathy
- differential diagnosis between epilepsy and symptoms of psychiatric origin and manifestations of post-anoxic encephalopathy [6]

The American Academy of Neurology (AAN) [7] has listed the electrical patterns predicting poor prognosis in post-anoxic comatose state: Isoelectric EEG or burst-suppression patterns containing generalized epileptiform discharges, generalized periodic complexes on a flat background. A burst-suppression recording is presented in Fig. 1. The majority of EEG studies on post-anoxic encephalopathy report a record during the first 72 hours. These signs are strongly but inconsistently associated with a vegetative state. Therefore, they are considered to have "insufficient prognostic accuracy" to allow an ethical decision to be made [7]. Moreover, the majority of studies were performed before the use of therapeutic hypothermia. Although hypothermia affects the EEG signal, the prognostic value of the electrical pattern does not seem to be affected, as demonstrated by Rossetti et al. [8].

EEG has been proposed for monitoring the sedation level during anesthesia and, by extension, in the ICU. However, the accuracy of EEG seems limited; Roustan et al. [9] found a lack of correlation between qEEG parameters and the level of sedation assessed with a clinical scale in 40 critically ill patients (brain injured patients excluded) sedated with morphine and midazolam. The variability of qEEG parameters between individuals appears to be high [9, 10].

EEG has also been used for the diagnosis of brain ischemia which may be reflected by the following patterns: Reduction in the total power spectrum of EEG, decreased variability of the alpha waves, decreased ADR reflecting a slowdown in the electrogenesis (e.g., slow frequencies prevailing over fast frequencies) [11, 12]. Studies evaluating the sensitivity of EEG for early detection of ischemia linked to vasospasm after aneurysmal subarachnoid hemorrhage (SAH) have the following limits: Limited size, limited to low grade aneurysmal SAH and to non-comatose patients. A recent prospective study of 12 patients at high risk of cerebral vasospasm (Fisher score 3 or higher) revealed a 67 % sensitivity of CAI for the prediction of delayed ischemic neurological deficit [13]. Claassen et al. [14] reported that the ADR was the most sensitive EEG-derived parameter for early diagnosis of vasospasm in 34 patients with high grade aneurysmal SAH, because a more than 10 % decrease in the ADR after stimulation in six successive recordings compared to baseline predicted vasospasm with sensitivity and specificity of 100 % and 76 %, respectively. However, the same electrophysiological patterns can be found in cases of hypothermia or thiopental infusion. Moreover, there is a lack of randomized controlled trials demonstrating the ability of strategies based on EEG monitoring to prevent brain ischemia and improve neurological outcome after aneurysmal SAH. Finally, recent studies have highlighted a potential value of EEG data in the analysis of functional cortico-cortical and cortico-thalamic connections. According to theoretical models, these connections could be part of the substrate of consciousness [15]. The use of measures of 'effective connectivity' obtained by combining high density EEG and transcranial magnetic stimulation methods at the bedside allows identification of electrophysiological patterns that are specific to the patient's neurological state (e.g., persistent vegetative state, minimally conscious state) [16]. These promising data should be confirmed by further studies.

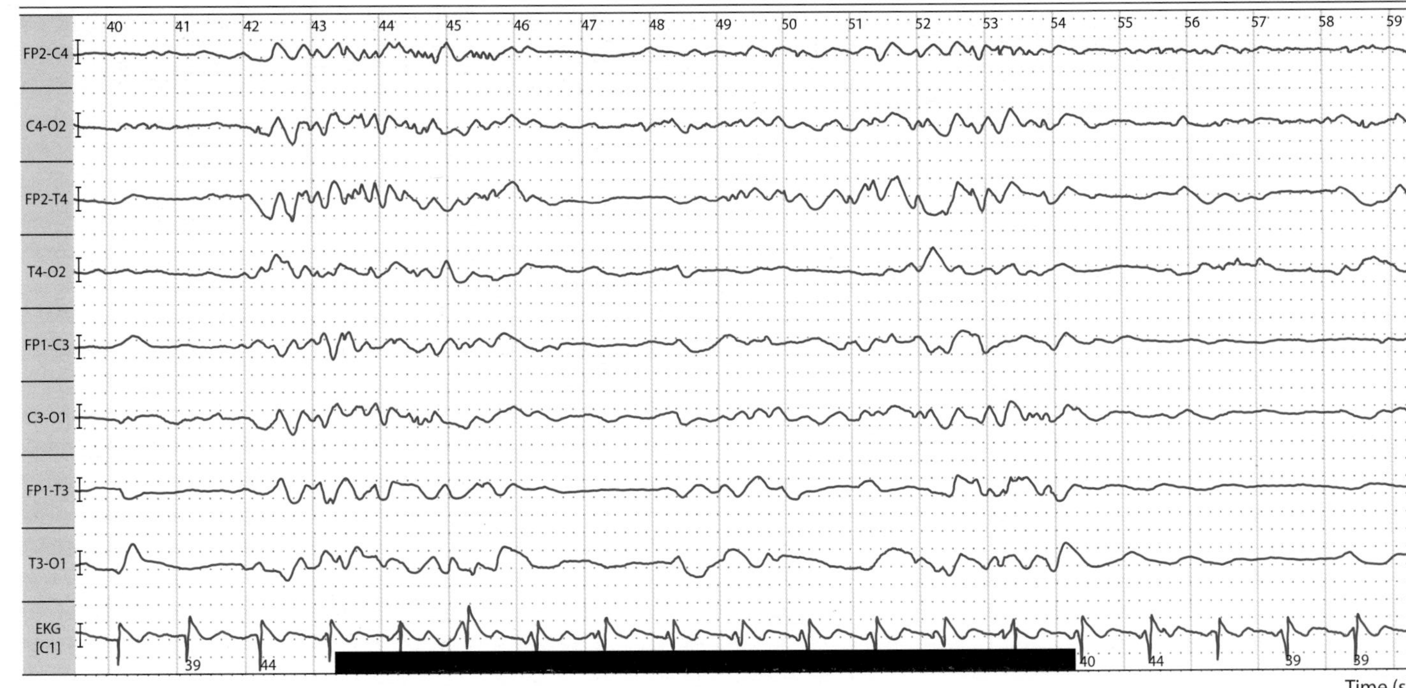

Fig. 1 Electroencephalographic pattern of burst-suppression during deep sedation for convulsive status epilepticus. Burst-suppression is a pattern of high amplitude electrical activity interrupted by low amplitude activity. The recording includes both electrocardiographic (EKG) pattern and electrogenesis. FP: frontoparietal; C: central; T: temporal; O: occipital

Bispectral Index Monitoring

The bispectral index (BIS) is based on the bispectral analysis (derived from the FFT) of the EEG. The relationship between the waves at different frequencies are analyzed to identify harmonic waves (i. e., waves that are correlated) and the degree of 'disorder' of the signal (i. e., represented by the waves that are not correlated), expressed by a variable called synchfastlow. The assumption for use of BIS to monitor sedation is that the higher the level of sedation is, the higher the synchronicity of the waves will be. The BIS algorithm takes into account three parameters: The beta ratio (logarithm of the ratio of the band 30–47 Hz power to the band 11–20 Hz power), the suppression ratio (SR, percentage of time over a period of 4 seconds when the amplitude of the signal is equal to zero or less than a very low cut-off value) and the synchfastlow. BIS values range from 0 (absence of electrical activity) to 100. For a BIS value less than 30, there is a linear relationship between the BIS and the suppression ratio (SR) following this formula: $BIS = 50 - RS/2$.

In patients without brain injury, the use of BIS monitoring during anesthesia enables the consumption of hypnotic to be reduced, and the period of arousal and duration of stay in the recovery room to be shortened [17]. However, perioperative BIS monitoring failed to have any effect in terms of mortality reduction, hospital length of stay and awareness when compared to end-tidal alveolar concentration-guided anesthesia [18]. This result could be explained by the limited amount of information obtained through three surface electrodes and the fact that the BIS monitor is unable to record changes in functional thalamo-cortical and cortico-thalamic connections.

In ICU patient, BIS and clinical sedation scales have been compared, with heterogeneous results. De Deyne et al. [19] reported great variability in the BIS value for the same Ramsay score of 6 in 18 sedated and non-paralyzed patients. In a multicenter prospective study in patients also free from paralyzing drugs, Nasraway et al. [20] found that the BIS value and the Sedation Agitation Scale (SAS) score were not correlated. This result could be related in part to the muscular activity but also to the fact that some patients were not sedated and/or suffered from encephalopathy. In the ICU, the BIS monitoring cannot replace clinical scales for the purpose of sedation level assessment and is not recommended for sedation monitoring in the ICU. BIS monitoring could, however, be of interest when such clinical scales are not appropriate, e.g., during the use of paralyzing agents or in cases of deep sedation. Hence, in a study addressing 12 patients suffering from refractory intracranial hypertension, Riker et al. [21] reported that a range of 3 to 5 burst-suppressions per minute during EEG-guided sedation was associated with a mean BIS value of 15 and an SR of 71. These results are in accordance with the findings of Cottenceau et al. [22], who reported that 2–5 burst-suppressions per minute on the EEG (the usual target for pentobarbital coma) corresponded to BIS values ranging between 6 and 15. The BIS may, therefore, be a surrogate for EEG to assess the level of pentobarbital coma.

Finally, BIS monitoring is not recognized as a valuable test for brain death confirmation [23].

Spectral Entropy

Spectral entropy is a simplified analysis of cortical EEG. It differs from the BIS by a different mathematical processing of the signal. The processing results in two indices:

- State entropy is largely dependent on EEG activity but is also dependent for a small part on the frontal electromyographic (EMG) activity. The state entropy index ranges from 0 to 90.
- Response entropy is an index ranging from 0 to 100 with an algorithm depending to a larger extent on EMG activity than state entropy.

Two prospective studies in the ICU [24, 25] failed to find a correlation of these indices and clinical sedation scales. Therefore, their use for sedation monitoring in the ICU is not supported by a sufficient level of evidence.

Evoked Potentials

Evoked potentials are defined as the recording of an EEG response to a standardized stimulation. Somatosensory evoked potentials (SSEPs) are obtained by electrical stimulation of three nerves (ulnar, median and sural nerves). The analysis takes into account the amplitude and the latency of the response. The short and middle latency evoked potentials (respectively SLEP and MLEP) can be distinguished by the various latencies. The N20 response is a type of SSEP obtained after median nerve stimulation and occurring at 20 ms. The N20 latency is not increased by propofol and thiopental, unlike the other SLEPs. Bilateral absence of the N20 response in case of post-anoxic encephalopathy is predictive of non-awakening with a predictive value of more than 99 % [7]. Hence, N20 use is recommended for the early assessment of neurological outcome in this situation [26]. In contrast, the presence of N20 is not reliably able to predict awareness. Transient bilateral absence of an N20 response in TBI is possible without pejorative meaning. The persistence of SLEPs has a positive predictive value of more than 80 % for good prognosis [26]. Other evoked potentials are available, such as auditory evoked potentials (AEPs). Of note, responses with latencies of more than 300 ms have been demonstrated to have predictive value in brain injured patients [27]. A test of consciousness in non-communicating patients using an auditory paradigm available at the bedside showed encouraging results [28, 29].

Brain Hemodynamic Monitoring

Intracranial Pressure

The association between raised intracranial pressure (ICP) and poor neurological outcome has been clearly established in TBI patients [30–32]. In case of impaired autoregulation of CBF, intracranial hypertension can compromise CBF, contributing to the development of secondary ischemic brain damage. The ICP threshold associated with a poor prognosis is probably 20–25 mm Hg. While the ICP value is important by itself, the time spent above the threshold of 20 mm Hg has a major prognostic value in TBI patients [33, 34].

ICP monitoring is indicated for severe TBI defined by a Glasgow Coma Scale (GCS) score of 8 or less or in case of a GCS above 8 associated with two of the following criteria: Neurological deficit, age over 40 years, episodes of hypotension (defined as systolic arterial blood pressure below 90 mm Hg). Although there is no robust evidence that ICP monitoring improves prognosis in TBI, the Brain Trauma Foundation recommends targeting an ICP level of less than 20 mm Hg (level II evidence) associated with a cerebral perfusion pressure (CPP) between 50 and 70 mm Hg (level III evidence) [35]. However, cerebral ischemia can occur even with 'normal' ICP and CPP since the microcirculation and oxygen diffusion can be impaired in brain injury.

Cerebral Autoregulation Assessment

Mathematical analysis of the ICP waveform has been proposed to explore cerebral autoregulation and brain compliance. Assessment of brain compliance through ICP waveform processing is possible using three indices: ICP amplitude, ICP slope and the correlation of ICP amplitude and mean ICP over a short period of time (also called the RAP index) [36]. High values of RAP index, ICP amplitude and ICP pulse slope are associated with impaired compliance.

Analysis of the variation in ICP in relation to variation in arterial blood pressure, expressed as the regression coefficient between the two parameters, called the pressure reactivity index (PRx), is an approach to monitor autoregulation. When cerebral autoregulation is preserved, ICP and arterial blood pressure are negatively correlated and PRx is therefore negative. On the contrary, a positive PRx is associated with altered autoregulation and poor prognosis. Sorrentino et al. [37] recently studied 763 trauma patients from the Cambridge retrospective database to establish critical thresholds for PRx, ICP and CPP that could predict death and disability. PRx thresholds for survival and favorable outcome were, respectively, 0.25 and 0.05; thresholds for ICP and CPP were, respectively, 22 and 70 mm Hg [35]. A retrospective study in TBI has proposed a new index called the PAx (defined as the correlation of arterial blood pressure and ICP pulse amplitude) that performs well at determining outcome [38]. There is a growing interest in the use of cerebral autoregulation parameters to individualize and adapt therapeutic targets [39].

Optic Nerve Sheath Diameter Measurement By Ocular Sonography

Optic nerve sheath diameter (ONSD) measurement using ocular sonography can be used to detect elevated ICP. The optic nerve is surrounded by a dural sheath that can inflate in case of raised pressure in the cerebrospinal fluid (CSF). Hansen and Helmke [40] showed that changes in ICP induced by intrathecal injection of Ringer's lactate resulted in variations in ONSD measured by ocular sonography. Several studies were then conducted in liver transplant recipients [41] and in TBI [42, 43] and aneurysmal SAH patients [44] leading to a confirmation of the link between ICP and ONSD. Two recent meta-analyses reported a large correlation between ONSD and increased ICP [45, 46]. All studies, with the exception of one [47], reported an ONSD threshold between 5.2 and 5.9 mm to be predictive of an ICP above 20 mm Hg with a sensitivity of more than 95 % and a specificity around 80 %.

Transcranial Doppler

Aaslid et al. [48] were the first to report the use of transcranial Doppler (TCD) to investigate the flow through Willis circle arteries, by using a low frequency probe (frequency ranging from 2 to 4 MHz) (Fig. 2). Pulsed Doppler sonography allows the measurement of red blood cell (RBC) flow velocity (expressed in cm/s). Mean velocity could be a surrogate for CBF as the flow can be calculated as the product of mean velocity and the section of the vessels. The pulsatility index (PI) can be calculated as follows: PI = (peak systolic velocity – end-diastolic velocity)/mean velocity. The normal PI value is 1.0 ± 0.2. PI is independent from the insonation angle. Low velocities associated with a normal PI value are related to large insonation and not to low blood flow.

Blood flow through the middle cerebral artery (MCA) accounts for 50–60 % of the total CBF of the ipsilateral brain hemisphere. The temporal window is the best acoustic window to obtain an MCA Doppler signal because of the bone's thickness allowing good transmission of ultrasound and low Doppler insonation angle (maximum 30°).

Fig. 2 Transcranial Doppler. Arterial anatomy of the Willis polygon (*upper left panel*) and color Doppler imaging of basal cerebral arteries (*upper right panel*). The velocity spectrum of the middle cerebral artery using pulsed Doppler is shown in the lower panel ▶

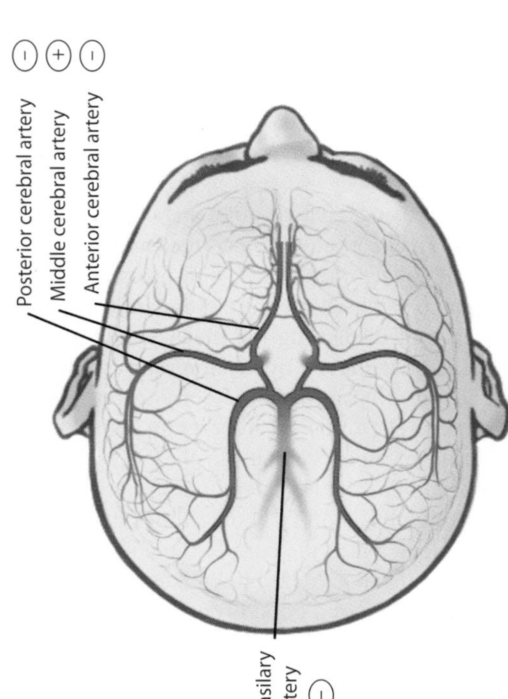

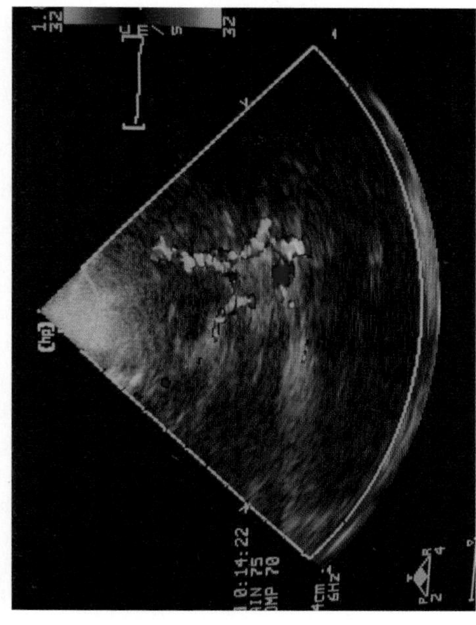

Systolic velocity: 90 cm/sec
Mean velocity: 58 cm/sec
End diastolic velocity: 42 cm/sec

Pulsatility index: 0.9

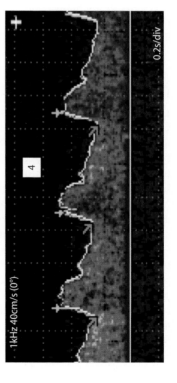

TCD to Detect Impaired CPP

If ICP increases in association with decrease in CPP, the velocity profile of large cerebral arteries can be modified to a high resistance profile (low diastolic velocity). When CPP decreases, end-diastolic velocity decreases and PI increases. Hypocapnia can also affect blood flow velocity by increasing the resistance of distal cerebral arteries [49]. In contrast, hypercapnia and anemia have the opposite effects on end-diastolic velocity and PI through vasodilation of the arterioles. Consequently, hematocrit and arterial carbon dioxide partial pressure ($PaCO_2$) have to be taken into account for valuable analysis of TCD data.

During early management of TBI before invasive cerebral monitoring is available, TCD could be of great interest to assess cerebral hemodynamic status. A prospective study of 78 moderate and mild TBI patients in the emergency room investigated the contribution of TCD for detecting patients at risk of neurological deterioration [50]. The patients who had secondary neurological deterioration had an increased PI (mean PI of 1.6) at hospital arrival. TCD goal-directed therapy was assessed in the early management of 24 severe TBI patients in order to identify high-risk patients and to prevent secondary brain injury [51]. Critical thresholds to define high-risk patients were a PI $\geq$ 1.4 and end-diastolic velocity < 20 cm/s. Early TCD, performed within 20 minutes after emergency unit admission, found that 46 % of the patients met these criteria. This group of patients was immediately (before imaging) treated with osmotherapy and mean arterial pressure increase, enabling cerebral hemodynamic impairment to be corrected.

Cerebral Autoregulation Study

Cerebral autoregulation can be investigated using TCD through static and dynamic approaches. Both have been defined by Tiecks et al. [52] as "measuring relative blood flow changes in response to a steady-state change in blood pressure" (static method) and in response to "a rapid change in blood pressure" (dynamic method). In other words, the static method consists of measuring the mean velocity in the MCA at two levels of arterial blood pressure achieved by vasopressor use, whereas the dynamic approach deals with the variation in mean velocity in response to a sudden change in arterial blood pressure. The transient hyperemic response test (THRT) consists of continuous measuring of mean velocity in the MCA ten seconds before and after a transient compression of the ipsilateral carotid artery. Correlation coefficients can be calculated on the basis of TCD recordings and arterial pressure. Mx and Mxa are respectively calculated as the correlation coefficient between mean velocity and CPP and between mean velocity and mean arterial blood pressure. A value of Mx below 0.05 is predictive of a good prognosis, whereas the prognosis is poor when Mx is above 0.3, the range between 0.05 and 0.3 being an area of uncertainty [53]. Mx seems to have a more valuable predictive value for prognosis than does Mxa [53]. The other derived indices from TCD monitoring are the dynamic autoregulatory index (ARI) and the rate of resistance (RoR) [52, 54]. Autoregulation can also be tested by studying the changes in velocities in response to changes in $PaCO_2$ (called CO_2 reactivity).

Brain Death Diagnosis

When CPP reaches zero, TCD shows an oscillating flow. TCD may be valuable when clinical brain death criteria and/or apnea testing cannot be applied [55] but careful attention must be paid to the interpretation of the TCD results. For example, persistent diastolic flow may be seen in brain-dead patients with prior craniotomy [23, 56] making the TCD less reliable. TCD is recognized by the AAN [23] as an ancillary test for the determination of brain death but cannot replace clinical examination. Circulatory arrest (i. e., flow velocities of zero) should be determined through the temporal and sub-occipital windows [23, 57, 58], a finding that confirms the diagnosis of brain death with a sensitivity of 91–100 % and a specificity of 97–100 %. In brain death patients, transient absence of flow in the MCA and preserved flow in the basilar artery account for a part of the imperfect sensitivity [58, 59]. Although TCD cannot define brain death, it may guide the timing of EEG and cerebral computed tomography (CT) angiography if required [59].

Summary

TCD may help adapt arterial blood pressure targets and management to individual physiology and help in triage at an early stage. However, TCD has the following limitations: Almost 7–10 % of patients have an inadequate temporal window that does not allow insonation. Moreover, TCD deals with large vessels and does not reflect the cerebral microcirculation, a fact that supports the need for complementary monitoring of brain oxygenation.

Brain Oxygenation Monitoring

Oxygenation monitoring is supported by the fact that brain ischemia can occur in nearly 10 % of TBI cases despite adequate ICP and CPP (i. e., values which are in accordance with recommendations) [60].

Jugular Venous Oxygen Saturation

The transverse sinuses, the petrosal inferior sinuses and the internal jugular veins provide cerebral venous drainage of near 70 % of the ipsilateral hemisphere and

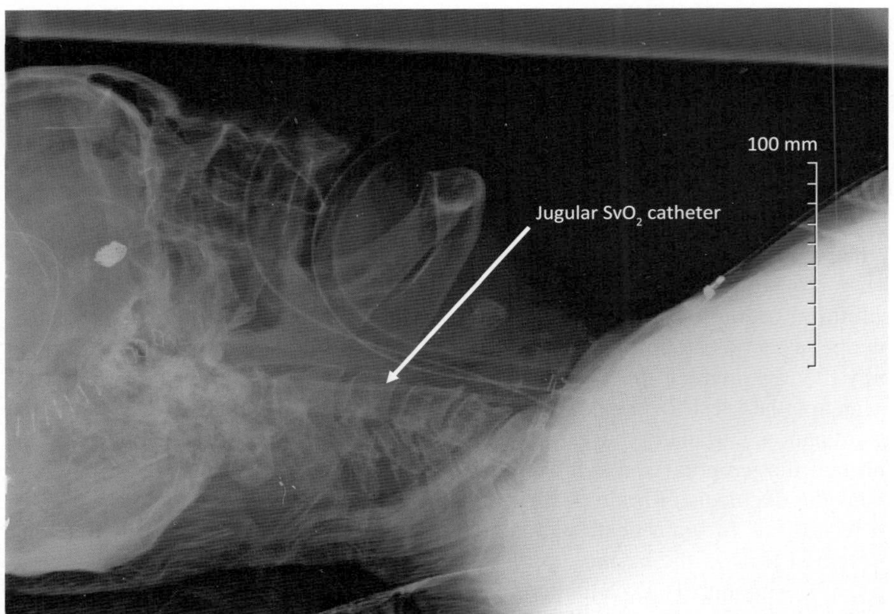

Fig. 3 Lateral X ray of the basal skull showing the correct position of the jugular venous bulb oxygen saturation catheter, with the end of the catheter superimposed on the mastoid air cells

30 % of the controlateral hemisphere. Almost 3 % of the blood flow through the jugular veins is of extra-cranial origin (coming from the superior petrosal sinus) if the catheter is correctly placed in the jugular bulb (Fig. 3). Jugular venous oxygen saturation (SjO_2) reflects the balance between brain oxygen delivery and consumption (i. e., the cerebral metabolic rate of oxygen [$CMRO_2$]). Provided that $CMRO_2$ and arterial oxygen content (CaO_2) remain unchanged, a decrease in CBF implies compensatory brain oxygen extraction, an increase in arterio-venous oxygen difference and a decrease in SjO_2. The normal SjO_2 value is 60–70 %. Values below 60 % may reflect increased oxygen extraction and possibly CBF impairment. A threshold of 50 % may be equivalent to ischemia of 13 % of the brain [61]. There are two mechanisms by which pathological conditions lead to an increase in extraction (or inadequate oxygen delivery): The first is decreased CBF as encountered with a decrease in arterial blood pressure, elevated ICP, heart failure, hypocapnia, anemia, hypoxemia, vasospasm; the second is increased $CMRO_2$ as seen with fever, convulsive status epilepticus, pain and insufficient sedation level. An increased SjO_2 is seen in hyperemia and stroke, provided that $CMRO_2$ remains unchanged. SjO_2 monitoring is able to detect ischemic episodes due to intracranial hematoma [62] or excessive hyperventilation [63]. Furthermore, in combination with TCD, it can help differentiate between hyperemia and vasospasm (a high SjO_2 may be suggestive of hyperemia). The number of episodes of SjO_2 below the ischemic threshold [64, 65] and values >75 % are both predictive of poor prognosis [66, 67].

The common complications of catheter placement are carotid artery puncture (1–3 % of cases), infection and thrombosis. Because of frequent movements of the catheter and thrombus formation, this monitoring can provide incorrect data and must be verified by venous blood gas sampling. In addition, the catheter cannot be placed for more than a few days.

Near-Infrared Spectroscopy

Near-infrared spectroscopy (NIRS) provides non-invasive real time continuous monitoring of oxygenation at the bedside. Near-infrared waves pass though skin and bone and can penetrate into the brain cortex to a depth of a few centimeters. Wave absorption by reduced hemoglobin (i. e., not bound to oxygen) is different from wave absorption by oxyhemoglobin. Quantification of wave attenuation produces an estimate of the oxygen content and the hemoglobin level in a given area of the brain. The tissue oxygen index (TOI) and the total hemoglobin index (THI) are derived from NIRS analysis using the Beer-Lambert law. It has been shown that TOI and THI reflect blood flow and blood volume, respectively [68]. TOI values $<50\%$ are considered abnormal and to correspond to ischemic tissue. NIRS has also been used to investigate cerebral autoregulation after aneurysmal SAH and severe TBI [69, 70]. NIRS technology can also estimate CBF by using the Fick principle and measurement of light absorption after indocyanine green (ICG) infusion. In theory, NIRS can assess the arterio-venous oxygen difference by using a second derivative of the signal [71, 72]. $CMRO_2$ in a given area could, therefore, be estimated as well as blood flow. The pitfalls of NIRS are the inaccuracy of measurement in presence of major cerebral edema or hematoma and contamination by extracranial measures.

Brain Tissue Oxygen Monitoring

Partial brain tissue oxygenation ($PbtO_2$) reflects oxygen delivery to the brain and its distribution in the interstitial space. The probe is typically composed of a polarographic Clark electrode. Measures must be corrected for the brain temperature. Normal values with the Licox™ system are 25–30 mm Hg in the white matter and a little higher in the cortex.

The $PbtO_2$ threshold that corresponds to the oxygen debt is still debated and appears to be near 15–20 mm Hg [73]. Occurrence of ischemic insults is also associated with the duration of episodes of tissue hypoxia. The time spent below the ischemic threshold appears to be a determining factor for irreversible damage. In TBI, van den Brink et al. [74] proposed a different ischemic threshold with respect to the time spent below the given threshold: 5 mm Hg for 30 min, 10 mm Hg for 1 h 45 min, 15 mm Hg for 4 h. Placement of the electrode – in cerebral contusion

Table 1 Neuromonitoring methods available at the bedside in the intensive care unit

Physiological determinant	Monitoring method
Brain electrogenesis	Electroencephalography Bispectral index monitoring Spectral entropy Evoked potentials
Intracranial pressure	Invasive measurement of intracranial pressure Optic nerve sheath diameter measurement with ocular sonography
Cerebral blood flow velocity	Transcranial Doppler
Brain oxygenation	Brain tissue oxygen monitoring Jugular venous oxygen saturation Near-infrared spectroscopy

versus normal tissue – is still matter of debate. $PbtO_2$ is correlated with SjO_2 when the probe is placed in a normal area [74]; it is also correlated with local CBF, CPP and partial oxygen pressure. An increase in $PbtO_2$ in response to hyperoxia is often noticed and loss of such reactivity may be a sign of cerebral autoregulation impairment [75].

$PbtO_2$ is of interest in preventing cerebral ischemia associated with normal CPP by determining the optimal target of CPP [76], a strategy called brain tissue oxygen-directed therapy (a strategy that aims at reaching the minimal CPP for which $PbtO_2$ is above the ischemic threshold). In a retrospective study, Narotam et al. [77] compared the prognosis in severe TBI (survival and neurological outcome at 6 months) before and after such a strategy using an ischemic $PbtO_2$ threshold >20 mm Hg and reported a better prognosis in the oxygen-directed therapy group than in the historical control group (management using CPP and ICP alone). In a similar study, Spiotta et al. [78] reported similar results in favor of the association of oxygenation goal with ICP and CPP management.

Conclusion

Modern neuromonitoring tools (Table 1) seem promising and will probably allow individualized management of brain-injured patients in the future. Among these strategies, autoregulation indexes and brain tissue oxygen monitoring are available at the bedside with a growing body of evidence to support their use. It seems unrealistic to claim that a specific neuromonitoring method could in itself influence neurological prognosis; rather, it is the therapeutic strategy and guided-therapy associated with the brain monitoring method that needs to be evaluated in future prospective studies.

References

1. Sharshar T, Porcher R, Siami S et al (2011) Brainstem responses can predict death and delirium in sedated patients in intensive care unit. Crit Care Med 39:1960–1967
2. Ware AJ, D'Agostino AN, Combes B (1971) Cerebral edema: a major complication of massive hepatic necrosis. Gastroenterology 61:877–884
3. Han MK, Hyzy R (2006) Advances in critical care management of hepatic failure and insufficiency. Crit Care Med 34(9 Suppl):S225–S231
4. Quagliarello V, Scheld WM (1992) Bacterial meningitis: pathogenesis, pathophysiology, and progress. N Engl J Med 327:864–872
5. Kress JP, Pohlman AS, O'Connor MF, Hall JB (2000) Daily interruption of sedative infusions in critically ill patients undergoing mechanical ventilation. N Engl J Med 342:1471–1477
6. Sutter R, Fuhr P, Grize L, Marsch S, Ruegg S (2011) Continuous video-EEG monitoring increases detection rate of nonconvulsive status epilepticus in the ICU. Epilepsia 52:453–457
7. Wijdicks EF, Hijdra A, Young GB, Bassetti CL, Wiebe S (2006) Practice parameter: prediction of outcome in comatose survivors after cardiopulmonary resuscitation (an evidence-based review): report of the Quality Standards Subcommittee of the American Academy of Neurology. Neurology 67:203–210
8. Rossetti AO, Urbano LA, Delodder F, Kaplan PW, Oddo M (2010) Prognostic value of continuous EEG monitoring during therapeutic hypothermia after cardiac arrest. Crit Care 14:R173
9. Roustan JP, Valette S, Aubas P, Rondouin G, Capdevila X (2005) Can electroencephalographic analysis be used to determine sedation levels in critically ill patients? Anesth Analg 101:1141–1151
10. Kaskinoro K, Maksimow A, Langsjo J et al (2011) Wide inter-individual variability of bispectral index and spectral entropy at loss of consciousness during increasing concentrations of dexmedetomidine, propofol, and sevoflurane. Br J Anaesth 107:573–580
11. Diringer MN, Bleck TP, Claude Hemphill 3rd J et al (2011) Critical care management of patients following aneurysmal subarachnoid hemorrhage: recommendations from the Neurocritical Care Society's Multidisciplinary Consensus Conference. Neurocrit Care 15:211–240
12. Friedman D, Claassen J, Hirsch LJ (2009) Continuous electroencephalogram monitoring in the intensive care unit. Anesth Analg 109:506–523
13. Rathakrishnan R, Gotman J, Dubeau F, Angle M (2011) Using continuous electroencephalography in the management of delayed cerebral ischemia following subarachnoid hemorrhage. Neurocrit Care 14:152–161
14. Claassen J, Hirsch LJ, Kreiter KT et al (2004) Quantitative continuous EEG for detecting delayed cerebral ischemia in patients with poor-grade subarachnoid hemorrhage. Clin Neurophysiol 115:2699–2710
15. Llinas R, Ribary U (2001) Consciousness and the brain. The thalamocortical dialogue in health and disease. Ann N Y Acad Sci 929:166–175
16. Rosanova M, Gosseries O, Casarotto S et al (2012) Recovery of cortical effective connectivity and recovery of consciousness in vegetative patients. Brain 135:1308–1320
17. Gan TJ, Glass PS, Windsor A et al (1997) Bispectral index monitoring allows faster emergence and improved recovery from propofol, alfentanil, and nitrous oxide anesthesia. BIS Utility Study Group. Anesthesiology 87:808–815
18. Avidan MS, Jacobsohn E, Glick D et al (2011) Prevention of intraoperative awareness in a high-risk surgical population. N Engl J Med 365:591–600
19. De Deyne C, Struys M, Decruyenaere J, Creupelandt J, Hoste E, Colardyn F (1998) Use of continuous bispectral EEG monitoring to assess depth of sedation in ICU patients. Intensive Care Med 24:1294–1298
20. Nasraway Jr SS, Wu EC, Kelleher RM, Yasuda CM, Donnelly AM (2002) How reliable is the Bispectral Index in critically ill patients? A prospective, comparative, single-blinded observer study. Crit Care Med 30:1483–1487

21. Riker RR, Fraser GL, Wilkins ML (2003) Comparing the bispectral index and suppression ratio with burst suppression of the electroencephalogram during pentobarbital infusions in adult intensive care patients. Pharmacotherapy 23:1087–1093
22. Cottenceau V, Petit L, Masson F et al (2008) The use of bispectral index to monitor barbiturate coma in severely brain-injured patients with refractory intracranial hypertension. Anesth Analg 107:1676–1682
23. Wijdicks EF, Varelas PN, Gronseth GS, Greer DM (2010) Evidence-based guideline update: determining brain death in adults: report of the Quality Standards Subcommittee of the American Academy of Neurology. Neurology 74:1911–1918
24. Walsh TS, Ramsay P, Lapinlampi TP, Sarkela MO, Viertio-Oja HE, Merilainen PT (2008) An assessment of the validity of spectral entropy as a measure of sedation state in mechanically ventilated critically ill patients. Intensive Care Med 34:308–315
25. Haenggi M, Ypparila-Wolters H, Bieri C et al (2008) Entropy and bispectral index for assessment of sedation, analgesia and the effects of unpleasant stimuli in critically ill patients: an observational study. Crit Care 12:R119
26. Cruccu G, Aminoff MJ, Curio G et al (2008) Recommendations for the clinical use of somatosensory-evoked potentials. Clin Neurophysiol 119:1705–1719
27. Chennu S, Bekinschtein TA (2012) Arousal modulates auditory attention and awareness: insights from sleep, sedation, and disorders of consciousness. Front Psychol 3:65
28. Faugeras F, Rohaut B, Weiss N et al (2011) Probing consciousness with event-related potentials in the vegetative state. Neurology 77:264–268
29. Boly M, Garrido MI, Gosseries O et al (2011) Preserved feedforward but impaired top-down processes in the vegetative state. Science 332:858–862
30. Miller JD, Becker DP, Ward JD, Sullivan HG, Adams WE, Rosner MJ (1977) Significance of intracranial hypertension in severe head injury. J Neurosurg 47:503–516
31. Choi SC, Muizelaar JP, Barnes TY, Marmarou A, Brooks DM, Young HF (1991) Prediction tree for severely head-injured patients. J Neurosurg 75:251–255
32. Narayan RK, Greenberg RP, Miller JD et al (1981) Improved confidence of outcome prediction in severe head injury. A comparative analysis of the clinical examination, multimodality evoked potentials, CT scanning, and intracranial pressure. J Neurosurg 54:751–762
33. Juul N, Morris GF, Marshall SB, Marshall LF (2000) Intracranial hypertension and cerebral perfusion pressure: influence on neurological deterioration and outcome in severe head injury. The Executive Committee of the International Selfotel Trial. J Neurosurg 92:1–6
34. Marmarou A, Saad A, Aygok G, Rigsbee M (2005) Contribution of raised ICP and hypotension to CPP reduction in severe brain injury: correlation to outcome. Acta Neurochir Suppl 95:277–280
35. Bratton SL, Chestnut RM, Ghajar J et al (2007) Guidelines for the management of severe traumatic brain injury. VIII. Intracranial pressure thresholds. J Neurotrauma 24(Suppl 1): S55–S58
36. Howells T, Lewen A, Skold MK, Ronne-Engstrom E, Enblad P (2012) An evaluation of three measures of intracranial compliance in traumatic brain injury patients. Intensive Care Med 38:1061–1068
37. Sorrentino E, Diedler J, Kasprowicz M et al (2012) Critical thresholds for cerebrovascular reactivity after traumatic brain injury. Neurocrit Care 16:258–266
38. Aries MJ, Czosnyka M, Budohoski KP et al (2012) Continuous monitoring of cerebrovascular reactivity using pulse waveform of intracranial pressure. Neurocrit Care 17:67–76
39. Jaeger M, Dengl M, Meixensberger J, Schuhmann MU (2010) Effects of cerebrovascular pressure reactivity-guided optimization of cerebral perfusion pressure on brain tissue oxygenation after traumatic brain injury. Crit Care Med 38:1343–1347
40. Hansen HC, Helmke K (1997) Validation of the optic nerve sheath response to changing cerebrospinal fluid pressure: ultrasound findings during intrathecal infusion tests. J Neurosurg 87:34–40
41. Helmke K, Burdelski M, Hansen HC (2000) Detection and monitoring of intracranial pressure dysregulation in liver failure by ultrasound. Transplantation 70:392–395

42. Piednoir P, Geeraerts T, Leblanc PE, Tazarourte K, Duranteau J, Vigue B (2007) Early diagnostic for vasospasm after aneurysmal subarachnoid haemorrhage. Ann Fr Anesth Reanim 26:965–972
43. Blaivas M, Theodoro D, Sierzenski PR (2003) Elevated intracranial pressure detected by bedside emergency ultrasonography of the optic nerve sheath. Acad Emerg Med 10:376–381
44. Moretti R, Pizzi B, Cassini F, Vivaldi N (2009) Reliability of optic nerve ultrasound for the evaluation of patients with spontaneous intracranial hemorrhage. Neurocrit Care 11:406–410
45. Dubourg J, Messerer M, Geeraerts T, Cour-Andlauer F, Javouhey E, Kassai B (2011) Diagnostic accuracy of ultrasonography of optic nerve sheath diameter for detecting raised intracranial pressure. Acta Anaesthesiol Scand 55:899
46. Moretti R, Pizzi B (2011) Ultrasonography of the optic nerve in neurocritically ill patients. Acta Anaesthesiol Scand 55:644–652
47. Rajajee V, Vanaman M, Fletcher JJ, Jacobs TL (2011) Optic nerve ultrasound for the detection of raised intracranial pressure. Neurocrit Care 15:506–515
48. Aaslid R, Markwalder TM, Nornes H (1982) Noninvasive transcranial Doppler ultrasound recording of flow velocity in basal cerebral arteries. J Neurosurg 57:769–774
49. Czosnyka M, Richards HK, Whitehouse HE, Pickard JD (1996) Relationship between transcranial Doppler-determined pulsatility index and cerebrovascular resistance: an experimental study. J Neurosurg 84:79–84
50. Jaffres P, Brun J, Declety P et al (2005) Transcranial Doppler to detect on admission patients at risk for neurological deterioration following mild and moderate brain trauma. Intensive Care Med 31:785–790
51. Ract C, Le Moigno S, Bruder N, Vigue B (2007) Transcranial Doppler ultrasound goal-directed therapy for the early management of severe traumatic brain injury. Intensive Care Med 33:645–651
52. Tiecks FP, Lam AM, Aaslid R, Newell DW (1995) Comparison of static and dynamic cerebral autoregulation measurements. Stroke 26:1014–1019
53. Sorrentino E, Budohoski KP, Kasprowicz M et al (2011) Critical thresholds for transcranial Doppler indices of cerebral autoregulation in traumatic brain injury. Neurocrit Care 14:188–193
54. Panerai RB (2009) Transcranial Doppler for evaluation of cerebral autoregulation. Clin Auton Res 19:197–211
55. Hadani M, Bruk B, Ram Z, Knoller N, Spiegelmann R, Segal E (1999) Application of transcranial Doppler ultrasonography for the diagnosis of brain death. Intensive Care Med 25:822–828
56. Dosemeci L, Dora B, Yilmaz M, Cengiz M, Balkan S, Ramazanoglu A (2004) Utility of transcranial Doppler ultrasonography for confirmatory diagnosis of brain death: two sides of the coin. Transplantation 77:71–75
57. White H, Venkatesh B (2006) Applications of transcranial Doppler in the ICU: a review. Intensive Care Med 32:981–994
58. Sloan MA, Alexandrov AV, Tegeler CH et al (2004) Assessment: transcranial Doppler ultrasonography: report of the Therapeutics and Technology Assessment Subcommittee of the American Academy of Neurology. Neurology 62:1468–1481
59. Sharma D, Souter MJ, Moore AE, Lam AM (2011) Clinical experience with transcranial Doppler ultrasonography as a confirmatory test for brain death: a retrospective analysis. Neurocrit Care 14:370–376
60. Eriksson EA, Barletta JF, Figueroa BE et al (2012) Cerebral perfusion pressure and intracranial pressure are not surrogates for brain tissue oxygenation in traumatic brain injury. Clin Neurophysiol 123:1255–1260
61. Coles JP, Fryer TD, Smielewski P et al (2004) Incidence and mechanisms of cerebral ischemia in early clinical head injury. J Cerebral Blood Flow Metab 24:202–211
62. Robertson CS, Gopinath SP, Goodman JC, Contant CF, Valadka AB, Narayan RK (1995) SjvO2 monitoring in head-injured patients. J Neurotrauma 12:891–896

63. Coles JP, Minhas PS, Fryer TD et al (2002) Effect of hyperventilation on cerebral blood flow in traumatic head injury: clinical relevance and monitoring correlates. Crit Care Med 30:1950–1959
64. Struchen MA, Hannay HJ, Contant CF, Robertson CS (2001) The relation between acute physiological variables and outcome on the Glasgow Outcome Scale and Disability Rating Scale following severe traumatic brain injury. J Neurotrauma 18:115–125
65. Gopinath SP, Robertson CS, Contant CF et al (1994) Jugular venous desaturation and outcome after head injury. J Neurol Neurosurg Psychiatry 57:717–723
66. Stocchetti N, Canavesi K, Magnoni S et al (2004) Arterio-jugular difference of oxygen content and outcome after head injury. Anesth Analg 99:230–234
67. Cormio M, Valadka AB, Robertson CS (1999) Elevated jugular venous oxygen saturation after severe head injury. J Neurosurg 90:9–15
68. Budohoski KP, Zweifel C, Kasprowicz M et al (2012) What comes first? The dynamics of cerebral oxygenation and blood flow in response to changes in arterial pressure and intracranial pressure after head injury. Br J Anaesth 108:89–99
69. Zweifel C, Castellani G, Czosnyka M et al (2010) Continuous assessment of cerebral autoregulation with near-infrared spectroscopy in adults after subarachnoid hemorrhage. Stroke 41:1963–1968
70. Zweifel C, Castellani G, Czosnyka M et al (2010) Noninvasive monitoring of cerebrovascular reactivity with near infrared spectroscopy in head-injured patients. J Neurotrauma 27:1951–1958
71. Tichauer KM, Elliott JT, Hadway JA, Lee DS, Lee TY, St Lawrence K (2010) Using near-infrared spectroscopy to measure cerebral metabolic rate of oxygen under multiple levels of arterial oxygenation in piglets. J Appl Physiol 109:878–885
72. Tichauer KM, Hadway JA, Lee TY, St Lawrence K (2006) Measurement of cerebral oxidative metabolism with near-infrared spectroscopy: a validation study. J Cereb Blood Flow Metab 26:722–730
73. Littlejohns L, Bader MK (2005) Prevention of secondary brain injury: targeting technology. AACN Clin Issues 16:501–514
74. van den Brink WA, van Santbrink H, Steyerberg EW et al (2000) Brain oxygen tension in severe head injury. Neurosurgery 46:868–876
75. van Santbrink H, Maas AI, Avezaat CJ (1996) Continuous monitoring of partial pressure of brain tissue oxygen in patients with severe head injury. Neurosurgery 38:21–31
76. Marin-Caballos AJ, Murillo-Cabezas F, Cayuela-Dominguez A et al (2005) Cerebral perfusion pressure and risk of brain hypoxia in severe head injury: a prospective observational study. Crit Care 9:R670–R676
77. Narotam PK, Morrison JF, Nathoo N (2009) Brain tissue oxygen monitoring in traumatic brain injury and major trauma: outcome analysis of a brain tissue oxygen-directed therapy. J Neurosurg 111:672–682
78. Spiotta AM, Stiefel MF, Gracias VH et al (2010) Brain tissue oxygen-directed management and outcome in patients with severe traumatic brain injury. J Neurosurg 113:571–580

Transcranial Magnetic Stimulation Coupled To EEG: A New Tool to Assess Brain Function in Coma

O. Gosseries, M. Boly, and S. Laureys

Introduction

Over the last decade, there has been a growing interest in the scientific and clinical literature concerning non-communicating patients who survive severe brain injury, referred to as patients with disorders of consciousness [1]. To date, the gold standard to assess the level of consciousness in these patients is behavior. Diagnosis is based on a patient's responsiveness or lack of response to command. After the comatose phase, during which patients lie with eyes closed and cannot be aroused, some patients regain full consciousness while others progress to a state of preserved wakefulness in the absence of awareness (i. e., vegetative state or unresponsive wakefulness syndrome) [2]. Others show fluctuating signs of awareness, such as visual pursuit, localization to pain or reproducible response to command but they remain unable to communicate consistently; this state is called minimally conscious state [3] and has been recently subcategorized into minimally conscious state plus (presence of response to command, verbalization or intentional communication) and minus (presence of signs of consciousness not related to language processing, such as visual pursuit) [4].

O. Gosseries
Coma Science Group, Cyclotron Research Center and Neurology Department,
University of Liège and University Hospital of Liège, Sart Tilman B30, Allée du 6 Août 8,
4031 Liège, Belgium

M. Boly
Coma Science Group, Cyclotron Research Center and Neurology Department,
University of Liège and University Hospital of Liège, Sart Tilman B30, Allée du 6 Août 8,
4031 Liège, Belgium

S. Laureys (✉)
Coma Science Group, Cyclotron Research Center and Neurology Department,
University of Liège and University Hospital of Liège, Sart Tilman B30, Allée du 6 Août 8,
4031 Liège, Belgium
E-mail: Steven.laureys@ulg.ac.be

J.-L. Vincent (Ed.), *Annual Update in Intensive Care and Emergency Medicine 2013*,
DOI 10.1007/978-3-642-35109-9_63,

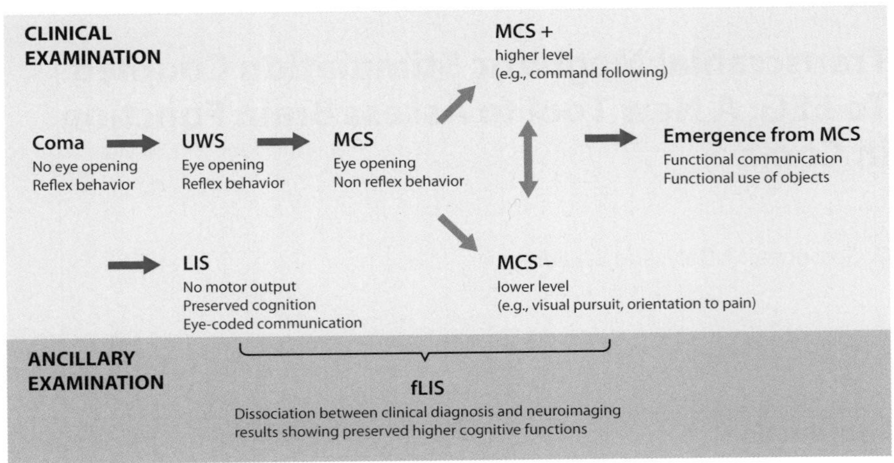

Fig. 1 Current classification of the diagnostic entities than can be encountered following coma. UWS: unresponsive wakefulness syndrome; MCS: minimally conscious state; fLIS: (functional) locked-in syndrome

Currently, the diagnostic decision-making process is extremely challenging leading to a diagnostic error of up to 40 % when not assessed with standardized scales [5]. Patients may have limited motor dysfunction (e.g., paralysis, spasticity, hypotonic status), sensory deficit (e.g., deafness, blindness), impaired cognitive processing (e.g., language deficits, apraxia), fluctuation of vigilance (from the disorder of consciousness itself or from drugs) and/or pain that can prevent voluntary responses. Lack of repeated evaluations or evaluations over too short a time-span can also lead to misdiagnosis [6]. The Coma Recovery Scale-Revised [7] seems to be the most appropriate scale to assess patients with disorders of consciousness as it searches for subtle signs of consciousness and is now widely used throughout the world [8]. However, even with the best clinical assessment, patients with disorders of consciousness can still be underestimated in terms of residual brain function and conscious awareness. Indeed, behavior can sometimes be dissociated from consciousness itself as it has been shown that a minority of totally unresponsive brain damaged patients, considered clinically to be in an unresponsive wakefulness syndrome/vegetative state can be conscious [9–11]. For example, such patients may activate specific brain areas and reliably generate appropriate electroencephalographic (EEG) responses when performing a motor imagery task (e.g., imagine moving the toes), similar to those observed in healthy controls [11]. This condition has been recently termed functional locked-in syndrome [4], whereas classical locked-in syndrome refers to patients who are fully conscious but completely paralyzed using eye-coded communication (usually caused by a stroke in the brainstem). Figure 1 summarizes the different disorders of consciousness states occurring after a coma. Paraclinical assessments are, therefore, needed to better understand these different altered states of consciousness in order to improve diagnosis, prognosis and therapeutic management.

In this chapter, we will first describe previous knowledge on patients with disorders of consciousness based on studies using positron emission tomography (PET) and magnetic resonance imaging (MRI). We will then present a novel technique, the transcranial magnetic stimulation coupled with high density EEG (TMS-EEG) and review recent studies investigating brain function in coma and in other states of altered consciousness. The last section will focus on the link between experimental results and theoretical ideas concerning the emergence of consciousness.

Ancillary Assessments to Evaluate the Brain at Rest

Advances in neuroimaging techniques have enabled brain activity at rest to be studied through functional, structural and effective connectivity. Functional connectivity refers to brain regions that act together in a coherent fashion. Structural connectivity is defined by the physical relationship between brain areas, and effective connectivity represents the direct connection between an initially perturbed area and those responding at distance, connections that must be supported both anatomically and functionally [12, 13]. Early PET studies have identified metabolic dysfunction and impaired functional connectivity in a large fronto-parietal network in unresponsive/vegetative patients [14]. The patients who recovered consciousness showed an increase in the functional connectivity within this network and a restoration of long-range thalamo-cortical connections [15, 16]. A recent PET study showed that, in minimally conscious patients, it is the intrinsic network (related to self) that seemed largely metabolically impaired, whereas the external network (related to the environment) seemed relatively preserved [17]. More group studies using functional MRI have focused on a set of brain areas that is activated at rest and called the 'default mode network' (including the posterior-cingulate/precuneus, anterior cingulate/mesiofrontal cortex and temporo-parietal junction areas), which seems to be linked to internal awareness, stimulus independent thoughts and mind wandering [18]. Unresponsive/vegetative patients showed functional impairments and severe disconnections within this default network [19]. Importantly, the functional connectivity in this network correlates with the level of consciousness in patients with disorders of consciousness [20].

Structural connectivity studies using MRI also provide valuable information on the number, nature, severity and localization of the brain lesions. Bilateral lesions in the thalamus, brainstem and basal ganglia were found to be of poor prognosis [21]. Diffusion-tensor imaging (DTI), which provides information on the structural integrity of axon tracts, correlates with the level of consciousness and distinguishes between unresponsive/vegetative and minimally conscious patients at the group level [22]. Subtle differential signs of diffuse axonal injury have also been observed in unresponsive/vegetative patients depending on the etiology (traumatic versus non-traumatic) [23]. DTI could be used as a prognostic tool, because measures in some specific brain areas (i. e., the internal capsule, the corpus callosum, the cerebral peduncle and other white matter tracts) correlate with outcome [24]. Moreover, axonal regrowth has been suggested in a traumatic patient who recovered verbal communication after 19 years in a minimally conscious state [25].

MRI and PET techniques offer a better insight into brain function in patients with disorders of consciousness but they only give information on structural and functional connectivity. They are indirect techniques in the sense that they measure the cerebral blood flow (CBF) and the diffusivity of water in the brain to determine neuronal activity and structure. They do not enable causality between brain areas *per se* to be inferred (except through new ways of complex quantitative modeling analyses, such as dynamic causal modeling [26]) and they cannot be performed at the patient's bedside. The combination of single-pulse TMS with EEG is a novel technique that overcomes these issues.

TMS-EEG: a New Tool to Assess Brain Function

TMS has been used for neurological and psychiatric research applications since the early 1980s. This technique enables the cerebral cortex to be stimulated non-invasively by generating a brief but strong magnetic pulse (<1 ms, up to 2 Tesla) through a coil applied to the surface of the scalp. The fast change in magnetic field

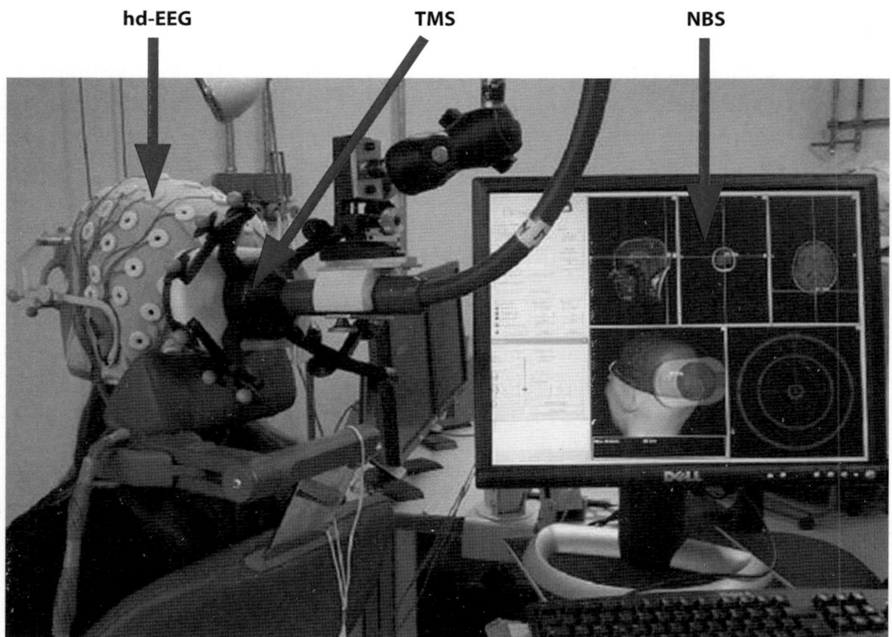

Fig. 2 Set up of the transcranial magnetic stimulation-electroencephalography (TMS-EEG) technique with a neuronavigation system (NBS). hd-EEG: high density EEG. From [13] with permission

strength induces a current flow in the tissue, which results in the activation of underlying neuronal populations [27]. These measures were first applied to the motor cortex and recorded from peripheral muscles. In the last few years, TMS has been combined with high density EEG to derive such measures directly from the cortex. In this way, TMS-EEG, combined with a neuronavigation system, enables cortical excitability and long-range cortical effective connectivity to be studied with good spatio-temporal resolution by inducing focal neuronal discharge at the cortex surface and measuring cortical electrical response both locally and at distant sites [13] (Fig. 2).

The neuronavigation system allows a selected brain area to be precisely stimulated and ensures stability of the position of the stimulation. Initial studies have demonstrated that meaningful recordings could be derived without being substantially affected by TMS-induced artifacts thanks to new hardware solutions, improved EEG amplifier technology, and advanced data processing techniques [28]. Using source modeling and statistical systems, it is currently possible to detect the effect of the focal perturbation both at distance and in time. The TMS-EEG technique offers an effective way to assess brain function at rest in patients with disorders of consciousness. It does not depend on the integrity of sensory and motor pathways, it by-passes subcortical and thalamic gates, and it does not require language comprehension or active participation of subjects [13, 29].

Application in Patients Recovering from Coma

We recently showed that when stimulating the frontal and parietal cortices of unresponsive/vegetative patients, TMS triggered either no response or a stereotyped and local slow wave response, indicating a breakdown of effective connectivity. By contrast, in minimally conscious patients, TMS invariably triggered complex activations characterized by rapidly changing and long-lasting widespread responses that sequentially involved distant cortical areas ipsi- and contralateral to the site of stimulation. This pattern was similar to those recorded in classical locked-in patients [29]. Through longitudinal measurements, when patients were in an unresponsive/vegetative state, a simple slow wave response to TMS was again recorded but when they recovered consciousness and functional communication, intracortical connectivity resurged (Fig. 3). Interestingly, one minimally conscious patient temporarily fell into an unresponsive/vegetative state the day of the experiment and showed complex and widespread brain responses to TMS even though, at the bedside, no conscious behavior could be observed; note that the patient fully recovered consciousness afterwards. This finding suggests clear-cut differences in intracortical effective connectivity, which occurred at an early stage during recovery of consciousness, before reliable communication could be established at the bedside and also before the spontaneous EEG showed significant changes [29]. TMS-EEG seems, therefore, to constitute a novel interesting tool to detect subtle differences between unresponsive and minimally conscious states as well as to track recovery of consciousness in brain-injured patients.

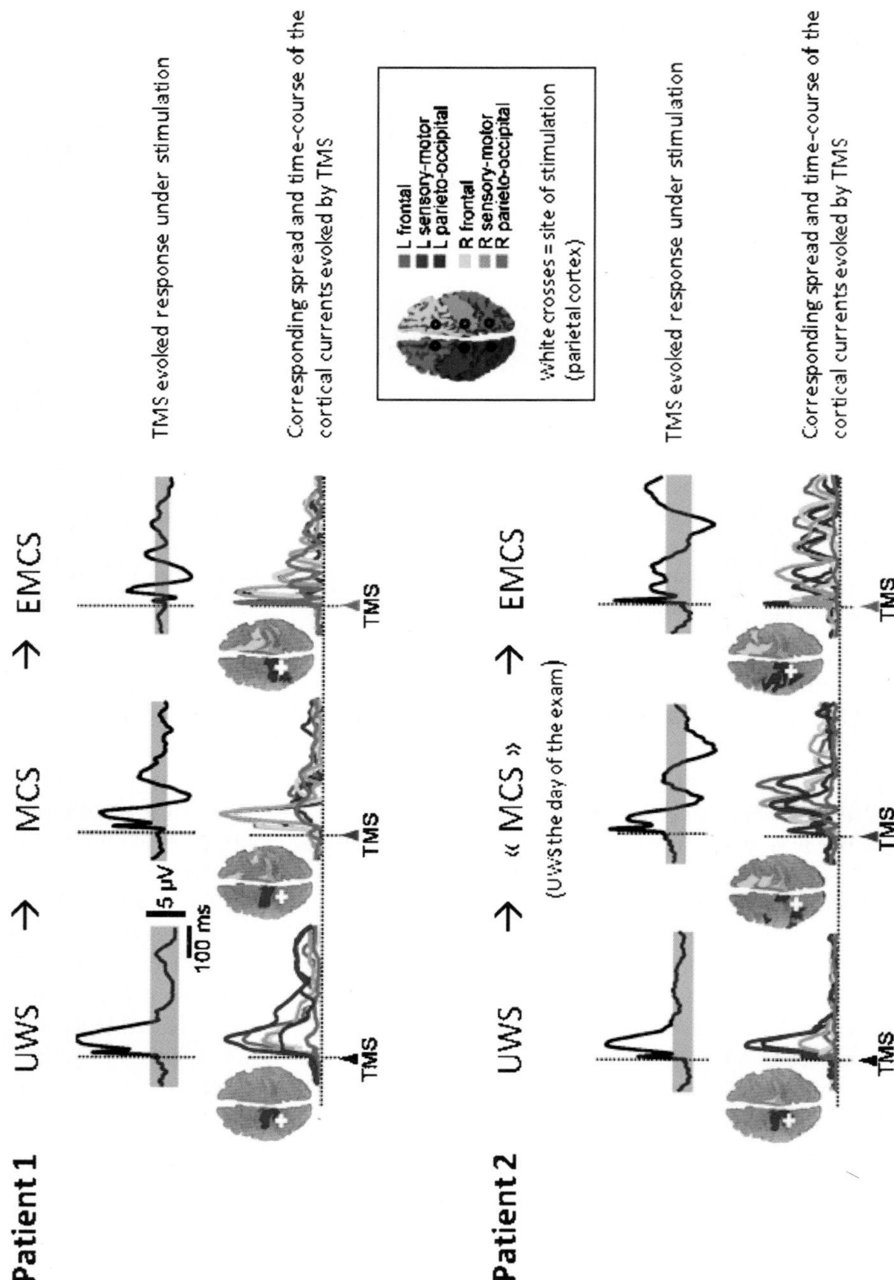

Fig. 3 Transcranial magnetic stimulation (TMS)-evoked cortical responses in patients recovering from coma. UWS: unresponsive wakefulness syndrome; MCS: minimally conscious state; EMCS: emergence from MCS. Adapted from [29]

Application in Physiological and Pharmacological States

Massimini et al. were the first to study the dynamics of TMS-evoked EEG responses in healthy subjects, during wakefulness and deep non-rapid eye movement (NREM) sleep [30]. During wakefulness, the brain is able to sustain long-range and complex patterns of activation with differentiation of brain activity depending on the site of stimulation [31]. Indeed, each cortical region tends to preserve its own natural frequency when indirectly engaged by TMS through brain connections and when stimulated at different intensities, indicating that the observed oscillations reflect local physiological mechanisms. For example, during wakefulness, TMS consistently evoked dominant alpha-band oscillations (8–12 Hz) in the occipital cortex, beta-band oscillations (13–20 Hz) in the parietal cortex, and fast beta/gamma-band oscillations (21–50 Hz) in the frontal cortex [32]. Note that these results were reproducible across individuals. In contrast, during deep sleep (when subjects if awakened report no or little conscious experience), the thalamocortical system, despite being active and reactive [33], either breaks down in causally independent modules (producing a local slow wave), or bursts into an explosive and stereotypical response due to underlying bistable dynamics of the system [13, 34] (producing a global EEG slow wave) [30, 35].

TMS-evoked responses were subsequently recorded during rapid eye movement (REM) sleep, when the brain is disconnected from the external world but consciousness comes back in the form of a dream. In this state, cortical responses to TMS propagate beyond the stimulation site and last longer than during deep NREM sleep (although still less than during wakefulness), indicating that effective cortical connectivity is largely preserved [36]. Finally, TMS-EEG was employed during general anesthesia induced by a pharmacological agent, the benzodiazepine midazolam, which provokes a state that is devoid of conscious content. Results showed that the responsiveness of a cortical area to TMS was maintained or even augmented, but the spread of activity to adjacent areas and the reverberatory reactivation of the stimulated site were quenched [37]. Similarly in many regards to what occurs in unresponsive/vegetative state and in deep NREM sleep, midazolam anesthesia also induced a local slow wave response with a breakdown of long-range brain connectivity in response to stimulation.

Together, these studies demonstrate the feasibility and potential of TMS-EEG in assessing the level of consciousness during normal, pathological and pharmacological states. These results also show that TMS-EEG permits measurement of changes in effective connectivity and corroborates the view that loss of consciousness is linked to a disconnection syndrome.

Disconnection Syndrome, Complexity and Consciousness

As suggested by theoretical and experimental studies, consciousness requires multiple, specialized cortical areas that can engage in rapid causal interactions (i. e., effective connectivity). As we have seen, experimental paradigms provide information about the probability that a patient's residual brain function can lead to consciousness. Our results and those from other recent studies have shown that coma, NREM sleep and anesthetic sedation states are commonly characterized by decreased large-scale cerebral connectivity, in proportion to the subject's impaired level of consciousness [38–42]. These observations of disconnections in long-range cortico-thalamo-cortical pathways in a widespread frontoparietal network lead to the hypothesis that these patients suffer from a "disconnection syndrome" [43–45]. However, preserved brain connectivity has also been reported during epilepsy [46], sleep [47] and anesthesia [34]. In these conditions, although connectivity was relatively preserved, a loss of cerebral activity differentiation could be observed (loss of complexity). It can, therefore, be hypothesized that consciousness emerges from both functional integration (i. e., connectivity) and preserved information capacity in the brain (i. e., differentiation responses between brain regions) [48, 49]. To achieve the most accurate estimation of the level of consciousness, theoretical approaches, such as the Information Integration Theory of Consciousness [49], aim to describe the general mechanism for conscious perception. This theory emphasizes the dynamic complexity of consciousness, which is characterized by information being simultaneously integrated and differentiated, and which is in line with what we have observed with TMS-EEG studies.

Conclusion

TMS-EEG seems to constitute a novel interesting diagnostic (and potentially prognostic) tool to detect and track recovery of consciousness in severely brain-injured patients. The use of a neuronavigation system is advised to avoid false negatives in the assessment of consciousness in patients with disorders of consciousness. It is indeed important to stimulate preserved brain regions, because stimulation of a brain lesion will induce no response. The advantage of this technique is that it can be performed at the bedside while by-passing sensory and motor pathways, and without requiring active participation of patients or language comprehension. Future studies are needed before using this tool in routine clinical practice, and these should look for compact equipment including fast, standardized data analysis software. Repetitive TMS should also be investigated for therapeutic purposes. The challenge in future years will also be to combine information coming from the different available neuroimaging techniques (e.g., functional MRI [fMRI], DTI, TMS, EEG) in order to deepen our understanding of brain (dys)function and to improve the diagnosis and prognostic assessment of this challenging population.

Acknowledgements This research was funded by the Belgian National Funds for Scientific Research (FNRS), the European Commission, the James McDonnell Foundation, the Mind Science Foundation, the French Speaking Community Concerted Research Action (ARC-06/11–340), the Fondation Médicale Reine Elisabeth and the University of Liège.

References

1. Gosseries O, Bruno MA, Chatelle C et al (2011) Disorders of consciousness: what's in a name? Neurorehabilitation 28:3–14
2. Laureys S, Celesia G, Cohadon F et al (2010) Unresponsive wakefulness syndrome: a new name for the vegetative state or apallic syndrome. BMC Med 8:68
3. Giacino JT, Ashwal S, Childs N et al (2002) The minimally conscious state: Definition and diagnostic criteria. Neurology 58:349–353
4. Bruno MA, Vanhaudenhuyse A, Thibaut A, Moonen G, Laureys S (2011) From unresponsive wakefulness to minimally conscious PLUS and functional locked-in syndromes: recent advances in our understanding of disorders of consciousness. J Neurol 258:1373–1384
5. Schnakers C, Vanhaudenhuyse A, Giacino J et al (2009) Diagnostic accuracy of the vegetative and minimally conscious state: clinical consensus versus standardized neurobehavioral assessment. BMC Neurol 9:35
6. Godbolt AK, Stenson S, Winberg M, Tengvar C (2012) Disorders of consciousness: Preliminary data supports added value of extended behavioural assessment. Brain Inj 26:188–193
7. Giacino JT, Kalmar K, Whyte J (2004) The JFK Coma Recovery Scale-Revised: measurement characteristics and diagnostic utility. Arch Phys Med Rehabil 85:2020–2029
8. Seel RT, Sherer M, Whyte J et al (2010) Assessment scales for disorders of consciousness: evidence-based recommendations for clinical practice and research. Arch Phys Med Rehabil 91:1795–1813
9. Owen AM, Coleman MR, Boly M, Davis MH, Laureys S, Pickard JD (2006) Detecting awareness in the vegetative state. Science 313:1402
10. Monti MM, Vanhaudenhuyse A, Coleman MR et al (2010) Willful modulation of brain activity in disorders of consciousness. N Engl J Med 362:579–589
11. Cruse D, Chennu S, Chatelle C et al (2011) Bedside detection of awareness in the vegetative state: a cohort study. Lancet 378:2088–2094
12. Friston K (2002) Beyond phrenology: what can neuroimaging tell us about distributed circuitry? Ann Rev Neurosci 25:221–250
13. Massimini M, Boly M, Casali A, Rosanova M, Tononi G (2009) A perturbational approach for evaluating the brain's capacity for consciousness. Prog Brain Res 177:201–214
14. Laureys S, Goldman S, Phillips C et al (1999) Impaired effective cortical connectivity in vegetative state. Neuroimage 9:377–382
15. Laureys S, Faymonville ME, Luxen A, Lamy M, Franck G, Maquet P (2000) Restoration of thalamocortical connectivity after recovery from persistent vegetative state. Lancet 355:1790–1791
16. Laureys S, Lemaire C, Maquet P, Phillips C, Franck G (1999) Cerebral metabolism during vegetative state and after recovery to consciousness. J Neurol Neurosurg Psychiatry 67:121
17. Thibaut A, Bruno MA, Chatelle C et al (2012) Metabolic activity in external and internal awareness networks in severely brain-damaged patients. J Rehabil Med 44:487–494
18. Heine L, Soddu A, Gómez F et al (2012) Resting state networks and consciousness: Alterations of multiple resting state network connectivity in physiological, pharmacological, and pathological consciousness states. Front Psychol 3:295
19. Soddu A, Vanhaudenhuyse A, Demertzi A et al (2011) Resting state activity in patients with disorders of consciousness. Funct Neurol 26:37–43
20. Vanhaudenhuyse A, Noirhomme Q, Tshibanda LJ et al (2010) Default network connectivity reflects the level of consciousness in non-communicative brain-damaged patients. Brain 133:161–171
21. Weiss N, Galanaud D, Carpentier A et al (2008) A combined clinical and MRI approach for outcome assessment of traumatic head injured comatose patients. J Neurol 255:217–223
22. Fernández-Espejo D, Bekinschtein T, Monti M et al (2011) Diffusion weighted imaging distinguishes the vegetative state from the minimally conscious state. Neuroimage 54:103–112

23. Newcombe V, Williams G, Scoffings D et al (2010) Aetiological differences in neuroanatomy of the vegetative state: insights from diffusion tensor imaging and functional implications. J Neurol Neurosurg Psychiatry 81:552–561
24. Perlbarg V, Puybasset L, Tollard E, Lehericy S, Benali H, Galanaud D (2009) Relation between brain lesion location and clinical outcome in patients with severe traumatic brain injury: a diffusion tensor imaging study using voxel-based approaches. Hum Brain Mapp 30:3924–3933
25. Voss HU, Uluc AM, Dyke JP et al (2006) Possible axonal regrowth in late recovery from the minimally conscious state. J Clin Invest 116:2005–2011
26. Friston KJ (2011) Functional and effective connectivity: a review. Brain Connect 1:13–36
27. Hallett M (2000) Transcranial magnetic stimulation and the human brain. Nature 406:147–150
28. Rogasch NC, Fitzgerald PB (2013) Assessing cortical network properties using TMS-EEG. Human brain mapping. Hum Brain Mapp (in press)
29. Rosanova M, Gosseries O, Casarotto S et al (2012) Recovery of cortical effective connectivity and recovery of consciousness in vegetative patients. Brain 135:1308–1320
30. Massimini M, Ferrarelli F, Huber R, Esser SK, Singh H, Tononi G (2005) Breakdown of cortical effective connectivity during sleep. Science 309:2228–2232
31. Rosanova M, Casarotto S, Pigorini A, Canali P, Casali AG, Massimini M (2012) Combining transcranial magnetic stimulation with electroencephalography to study human cortical excitability and effective connectivity. In: Fellin T, Michael H (eds) Neuronal Network Analysis. Springer, Berlin, p 118
32. Rosanova M, Casali A, Bellina V, Resta F, Mariotti M, Massimini M (2009) Natural frequencies of human corticothalamic circuits. J Neurosci 29:7679–7685
33. Steriade M, Timofeev I, Grenier F (2001) Natural waking and sleep states: a view from inside neocortical neurons. J Neurophysiol 85:1969–1985
34. Alkire MT, Hudetz AG, Tononi G (2008) Consciousness and anesthesia. Science 322:876–880
35. Massimini M, Ferrarelli F, Esser SK et al (2007) Triggering sleep slow waves by transcranial magnetic stimulation. Proc Natl Acad Sci USA 104:8496–8501
36. Massimini M, Ferrarelli F, Murphy M et al (2010) Cortical reactivity and effective connectivity during REM sleep in humans. Cogn Neurosci 1:176–183
37. Ferrarelli F, Massimini M, Sarasso S et al (2010) Breakdown in cortical effective connectivity during midazolam-induced loss of consciousness. Proc Natl Acad Sci USA 107:2681–2686
38. Vanhaudenhuyse A, Noirhomme Q, Tshibanda LJ et al (2010) Default network connectivity reflects the level of consciousness in non-communicative brain-damaged patients. Brain 133:161–171
39. Boveroux P, Vanhaudenhuyse A, Bruno MA et al (2010) Breakdown of within- and between-network resting state functional magnetic resonance imaging connectivity during propofol-induced loss of consciousness. Anesthesiology 113:1038–1053
40. Schrouff J, Perlbarg V, Boly M et al (2011) Brain functional integration decreases during propofol-induced loss of consciousness. Neuroimage 57:198–205
41. Martuzzi R, Ramani R, Qiu M, Rajeevan N, Constable RT (2010) Functional connectivity and alterations in baseline brain state in humans. Neuroimage 49:823–834
42. Boly M, Garrido MI, Gosseries O et al (2011) Preserved feedforward but impaired top-down processes in the vegetative state. Science 332:858–862
43. Laureys S (2005) The neural correlate of (un)awareness: lessons from the vegetative state. Trends Cogn Sci 9:556–559
44. Tononi G (2010) Information integration: its relevance to brain function and consciousness. Arch Ital Biol 148:299–322
45. Dehaene S, Changeux JP (2011) Experimental and theoretical approaches to conscious processing. Neuron 70:200–227

46. Arthuis M, Valton L, Regis J et al (2009) Impaired consciousness during temporal lobe seizures is related to increased long-distance cortical-subcortical synchronization. Brain 132:2091–2101
47. Boly M, Perlbarg V, Marrelec G et al (2012) Hierarchical clustering of brain activity during human nonrapid eye movement sleep. Proc Natl Acad Sci USA 109:5856–5861
48. Boly M, Massimini M, Tononi G (2009) Theoretical approaches to the diagnosis of altered states of consciousness. Prog Brain Res 177:383–398
49. Tononi G (2008) Consciousness as integrated information: a provisional manifesto. Biol Bull 215:216–242

Part XVIII

Physiotherapy and ICU Weakness

Diagnostic Approach to ICU-acquired Weakness: Present and Future

L. Wieske, M. J. Schultz, and J. Horn

Introduction

Since its recognition in the 1980s, many different terms and definitions have been used for weakness in critically ill patients [1]. In 2009, a consensus meeting was held to delineate terminology and provide definitions that could be used by clinicians and researchers [2]. Since then, intensive care unit (ICU)-acquired weakness has been used as an umbrella term to describe the clinical picture of weakness that develops in the setting of critical illness [2]. Using additional investigations, ICU-acquired weakness can be further differentiated into critical illness polyneuropathy (CIP), critical illness myopathy (CIM) or critical illness neuromyopathy (CINM) [2].

Many uncertainties exist regarding the diagnostic approach to ICU-acquired weakness. It is not known whether it is beneficial to diagnose this important complication early. An early diagnosis of ICU-acquired weakness may have the potential to trigger therapeutic actions. Furthermore, it is uncertain whether there is truly a need for differentiation between CIP, CIM and CINM.

L. Wieske (✉)
Department of Intensive Care, Academic Medical Center, University of Amsterdam, Room G3-228, PO box 22700, Amsterdam, The Netherlands
E-mail: L.Wieske@amc.uva.nl

M. J. Schultz
Department of Intensive Care, Academic Medical Center, University of Amsterdam, Room G3-228, PO box 22700, Amsterdam, The Netherlands

J. Horn
Department of Intensive Care, Academic Medical Center, University of Amsterdam, Room G3-228, PO box 22700, Amsterdam, The Netherlands

J.-L. Vincent (Ed.), *Annual Update in Intensive Care and Emergency Medicine 2013*,
DOI 10.1007/978-3-642-35109-9_64,

Incidence and Impact of ICU-acquired Weakness

ICU-acquired weakness is a frequent complication of critical illness, occurring in approximately 50 % of ICU patients [3]. ICU-acquired weakness develops early after onset of critical illness. Signs of nerve and muscle dysfunction have been found as early as 3 days after onset of critical illness [4]. Reliable incidences of the separate syndromes CIP, CIM and CINM are not available, because definitions have only recently been introduced and accurate delineation between these entities is dependent on the extensiveness of additional investigations; it is thought that CINM is the most prevalent [2]. The incidence of ICU-acquired weakness is likely to rise because of increased survival after critical illness [5].

ICU-acquired weakness is associated with adverse short- and long-term outcomes. Indeed, ICU-acquired weakness is an independent predictor for hospital mortality, and increased duration of mechanical ventilation and length of stay in the ICU [6–8]. After discharge, recovery of patients with ICU-acquired weakness is impeded, leading to reduced quality of life, mainly attributed to physical disability caused by muscle weakness [9, 10]. Incomplete recovery can be found up to 5 years after ICU-discharge and patients frequently fail to return to work and have high health care expenditures [11]. Weakness due to CIM is thought to have a better prognosis than CIP [12].

Risk Factors for ICU-acquired Weakness

Both sepsis and the systemic inflammatory response syndrome (SIRS) are consistent and important risk factors for ICU-acquired weakness [13]. Inflammatory mediators, metabolic stress and/or hypoxia occurring in sepsis or SIRS have been suggested to play a role in the pathogenesis of ICU-acquired weakness [14]. Other risk factors for ICU-acquired weakness include development of hyperglycemia and prolonged, but not short, use of neuromuscular blocking agents [3, 15]. Conflicting results have been reported on the role of corticosteroids [3].

Current Diagnostic Approach to ICU-acquired weakness

The diagnostic process for an ICU-patient with generalized weakness usually follows a two-step approach. First, disorders causing weakness other than ICU-acquired weakness need to be excluded. Second, if ICU-acquired weakness is diagnosed, an attempt to differentiate between CIP, CIM and CINM is made.

ICU-acquired weakness is considered the most prevalent cause of muscle weakness in ICU patients but the differential diagnosis is broad. A consensus meeting statement stresses that ICU-acquired weakness is a diagnosis of exclusion because some conditions, like Guillain-Barré syndrome or myasthenia gravis, have thera-

Table 1 Differential diagnosis of muscle weakness in the ICU [16]

	category	example
M	medications	steroids, neuromuscular blockers
U	undiagnosed neuromuscular disorder	myasthenia, mitochondrial myopathy
S	spinal cord disease	trauma, ischemia
C	critical illness	CIP, CIM, CINM
L	loss of muscle mass	cachectic myopathy, rhabdomyolysis
E	electrolyte disorders	hypokalemia, hypophosphatemia
S	systemic illness	vasculitis, paraneoplastic

CIP: critical illness polyneuropathy; CIM: critical illness myopathy; CINM: critical illness neuromyopathy

peutic consequences or prognostic implications [2]. A careful medical history (ascertaining when the weakness developed) in combination with physical examination (focusing on patterns of weakness, focal signs and brainstem functions) should confidently eliminate most differential diagnoses. Notably, ICU-acquired weakness can only be diagnosed if weakness develops *after* onset of critical illness. In cases where a medical history cannot be obtained or physical examination cannot reliably be performed, appropriate additional investigations are needed [2]. The mnemonic "MUSCLES" has been suggested to address the most prevalent causes for weakness in the ICU (Table 1) [16].

There is debate whether differentiation between CIP, CIM and CINM is necessary for daily clinical practice. Although prognostication could be a reason for differentiation, there is currently little supportive evidence for differences in outcome between CIP, CIM and CINM; data do suggest a longer length of stay in hospital and worse long-term outcome in CIP compared to CIM [12, 17].

Currently Used Diagnostic Tools for ICU-acquired Weakness

Several diagnostic modalities are used in diagnosing ICU-acquired weakness. The diagnosis of ICU-acquired weakness can be made with physical examination alone. Electrophysiological studies and/or muscle biopsies are needed to differentiate between CIP, CIM and CINM.

Physical Examination

With physical examination, weakness is objectified using the "Medical Research Council" (MRC)-scale, a subjective 5-point rating scale that scores for maximal

Table 2 The Medical Research Council scale

MRC scale score	
0	No contraction
1	Contraction palpable
2	Active movement but not against gravity
3	Movement against gravity but not against resistance
4	Movement against some but not full resistance
5	Movement against full resistance

force produced by voluntary muscle contraction [2]. The scale ranges from "no visible contraction" to "normal strength" (Table 2). For the diagnosis of ICU-acquired weakness, MRC-scores for 6 different bilaterally tested muscle-groups are summed (the so-called "MRC-sum score" or MRC-SS) [2]. An MRC-SS < 48 is used as a cut-off for diagnosing ICU-acquired weakness [2]. Generally, proximal and distal muscle-groups are tested, e.g., deltoid, biceps, wrist extensors, iliopsoas, quadriceps and ankle dorsiflexor muscles. When it is impossible to test all these 6 muscle groups, an average MRC score < 4 per muscle group is used as a cut-off. In addition to the degree of weakness, distribution of weakness is also important. In ICU-acquired weakness, weakness should be present more or less symmetrically in the upper and lower limbs [2]. Of note, facial weakness is usually not present.

The MRC scale is an easy to learn and cheap diagnostic tool, which enables repeated monitoring of neuromuscular status. In addition, the interobserver agreement for MRC testing is good [18, 19]. However, MRC testing requires an awake and attentive patient. The vast majority of ICU patients are typically sedated for shorter or longer periods. Sedated patients cannot be scored with the MRC scale. Delirium may also jeopardize the reliability of the MRC scale [18]. Thus, the MRC scale may be far from appropriate for the early diagnosis of ICU-acquired weakness. A full examination of all 6 bilateral muscle groups may be very demanding for recovering ICU patients. In these patients, a simple surrogate marker for overall strength could be obtained by assessing handgrip strength [6, 19]. Handgrip strength is measured using specific devices, like the hand-grip dynamometer.

Nerve Conduction Studies

Nerve conduction studies involve (transdermal) electrical stimulation of a motor or sensory nerve and subsequent recording of the evoked action potential over a muscle or sensory innervated area. With nerve conduction studies, several measures of muscle and nerve function can be studied.

The amplitude of the 'compound muscle action potential' or CMAP is a reflection of the number of stimulated axons and the number of muscle fibers that sub-

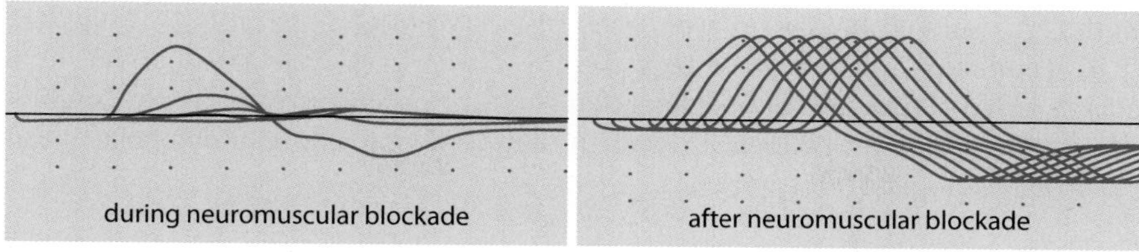

Fig. 1 Repetitive stimulation during and after neuromuscular blockade with a non-depolarizing neuromuscular blocking agent. During neuromuscular blockade, the first stimulation triggers (near-)normal compound muscle action potential (CMAP) amplitudes. Ensuing stimuli show a decrease in the amplitudes. After elimination of the neuromuscular blocking agent, repeated stimulation does not decrease CMAP amplitudes. Recorded at the Academic Medical Center, Amsterdam

sequently depolarize. A reduction in the CMAP-amplitude can be used as a marker of nerve and/or muscle dysfunction. Although reduced CMAP-amplitudes in patients with ICU-acquired weakness were often interpreted as a sign of neuropathy, this proved to be an oversimplification with the discovery that muscles are also involved in ICU-acquired weakness [2]. The amplitude of the 'sensory nerve action potential' or SNAP is the sensory homolog of the CMAP but represents solely nerve function.

CMAP and SNAP amplitudes are obtained by distal stimulation (i. e., close to a muscle or sensory area), but can also be obtained by stimulating more proximally along the course of a specific nerve. The delay in CMAP or SNAP onset between distal and proximal stimulation can be used to calculate the conduction velocity of that specific nerve. Conduction velocity is (near) normal with ICU-acquired weakness because the neuropathy is axonal, and not demyelinating [2].

Other useful nerve conduction studies include repetitive stimulation and direct muscle stimulation (DMS) [2]. Repetitive stimulation is used to examine the neuromuscular junction and is performed by repeated stimulation of a motor nerve, looking for decremental amplitudes in the CMAP; a more than 10 % decrease is considered abnormal [2]. In ICU-acquired weakness the neuromuscular junction is not affected [2]. The most frequently occurring neuromuscular junction problem is caused by neuromuscular blocking agents (Fig. 1) [2].

With DMS, CMAPs are obtained using two methods of stimulation: By conventional stimulation of the nerve or by direct stimulation of the muscle by inserting a needle into that muscle. By comparing both CMAPs, localization of the problem may be possible [2]. In case of a neuropathy, decreased CMAPs are found with nerve stimulation and normal CMAPs with muscle stimulation. Decreased CMAPs with both types of stimulation are found in cases of a myopathy. For interpretation, a nerve-to-muscle CMAP ratio is used. A ratio <0.5 suggests neuropathy, a ratio >0.5 suggests either myopathy or a combination of neuropathy and myopathy [20].

Nerve conduction studies have an advantage over physical examination in that they can be used in patients who cannot be scored with the MRC scale. Nerve conduction studies are thus proposed for the early diagnosis of ICU-acquired weakness [21, 22]. Nerve conduction studies, however, are technologically demanding in the ICU-setting. Indeed, interference caused by most, if not all ICU equipment (e.g., ventilators, renal replacement therapy devices) as well as excessive limb edema may hamper all nerve conduction studies. Moreover, some nerve conduction studies, such as DMS are relatively new and not routinely available in all electrophysiological laboratories.

Myography

With myography, a needle is placed inside a specific muscle to capture the electrical activity of that muscle. Electrical activity elicited by voluntary contraction of a muscle is most useful [2]. With voluntary contraction, myography visualizes the sequential recruitment of 'motor unit action potentials' or MUAPs (a combination of the motor neuron and the muscles innervated by that neuron). Morphology and pattern of recruitment of MUAPs can be helpful in the diagnosis of myopathy. Characteristically, in myopathy, MUAPs have a short duration and low amplitude.

For myography, an awake and attentive patient is needed to reliably evaluate MUAPs. This factor limits its applicability in sedated, unconscious or delirious critically ill patients. Clotting disorders may also be seen as a contraindication for myography. Similar to nerve conduction studies most ICU equipment may cause interference. Notably, interpretation of myography requires more experience and training compared to nerve conduction studies.

Membrane Excitability Studies

Several electrophysiological studies other than nerve conduction studies or myography have been used to investigate ICU-acquired weakness, including threshold tracking, muscle velocity recovery cycles (VRCs) and muscle fiber conduction velocity (MFCV) [23–25]. All these studies measure excitability properties of nerves or muscles. In ICU-acquired weakness, decreased excitability of muscle and nerve develops early in the pathogenesis. This is thought to occur due to a dysregulation of voltage gated sodium channels [26]. Threshold tracking measures the excitability properties exclusively of nerves, whereas VRCs and MFCV exclusively give information on muscles. A combination of these techniques may thus allow separation of neuropathy from myopathy. So far, these studies have only been used for research purposes. Clinical feasibility is uncertain.

Muscle Biopsy

Muscle tissue can be obtained via open biopsy or needle biopsy techniques. Two structural changes can be identified [27]. With ICU-acquired weakness, total muscle mass can be reduced by atrophy and/or necrosis of muscle fibers. Second, there may be loss of myosin. Loss of these so-called 'thick filaments' is a histological hallmark of CIM [2]. Myosin and actin are mandatory for contraction of muscle fibers. Selective loss of myosin in ICU-acquired weakness is thought to occur due to increased proteolysis and decreased protein synthesis [27]. Changes in histology can already be seen within five days of onset of critical illness [28]. Analysis of atrophy, necrosis and loss of myosin involves both light microscopy and electron microscopy. Quantification of the myosin-to-actin ratio using gel electrophoresis has also been used [29].

Because muscle biopsy is an invasive technique and as such carries the risk of bleeding and/or infection, its use is mostly limited to research settings. In cases of ambiguous clinical and/or electrophysiological findings or when a strong suspicion of myopathy other than CIM exists, muscle biopsy may be mandatory.

Interpretation of Electrophysiological and Histological Findings in ICU-acquired Weakness

Table 3 summarizes the diagnostic criteria for CIP and CIM [2]. For CIP, decreased CMAP and SNAP amplitudes with a normal conduction velocity (axonal neuropathy) need to be found and repetitive stimulation needs to be normal [2]. CIM is separated into probable or definitive CIM [2]. Probable CIM can be diagnosed when SNAP amplitudes are normal and either MUAPs are myopathic or the nerve-to-muscle ratio is >0.5 on DMS [2]. Probable CIM can also be diagnosed when myopathic changes are found on muscle biopsy [2]. Definite CIM is diagnosed when both sets of criteria for probable CIM are present [2]. CINM is

Table 3 Diagnostic criteria for CIP and CIM [2]

Criteria	CIP	CIM
Clinical criteria ICU-AW	+	+
CMAP	↓	
SNAP	↓	Normal
Conduction velocity	Normal	
Repetitive stimulation	Decremental response < 10 %	
Direct muscle stimulation		Nerve/muscle ratio > 0.5
Myography		Myopathic MUAPs
Muscle histology		Myopathic changes

CIP: critical illness polyneuropathy; CIM: critical illness myopathy; ICU-AW: intensive care unit-acquired weakness; CMAP: compound muscle action potential; SNAP: sensory nerve action potential; MUAP: motor unit potential diagnosed when a patient fulfills both the criteria for CIP and either probable or definite CIM [2]. Because of incomplete examinations due to technical issues, interpretation of electrophysiological results is frequently not straightforward or may even be inconclusive. Moreover, the validity of the proposed criteria has not yet been investigated.

Potential New Diagnostic Tools for ICU-acquired Weakness

Given the limitations of currently used diagnostic tools, new diagnostic tools are urgently needed. Ultrasound may be a promising diagnostic tool for ICU-acquired weakness. Ultrasound provides information on muscle structures in an easy and non-invasive way. Cross-sectional muscle area decreases rapidly with critical illness, but this has not yet been linked to development of ICU-acquired weakness [30]. Ultrasound may also be used to visualize peripheral nerves, although studies of patients with ICU-acquired weakness are currently lacking [31]. Biological markers may also be of help in diagnosing muscle and/or nerve injury. It should be noted, however, that creatine kinase levels in blood were found to be insufficient as a biological marker of ICU-acquired weakness [2]. Biological markers of nerve injury, like neurofilaments, could be useful [32].

Identification of structural nerve damage may serve as a prognosticator for long-term functional impairment. Assessing structural nerve damage using nerve biopsies seems an unattractive modality. Histological examination of nerves may also be possible through use of simple skin biopsies [33]. It is currently not known, however, whether small nerve fibers in the skin are also affected in ICU-acquired weakness.

Further understanding of the pathophysiology of ICU-acquired weakness may identify new diagnostic tools in the future. In particular, a better understanding of the transition from dysfunction to structural damage of nerves may be important. Figure 2 illustrates the progression of ICU-acquired weakness and possible time points of application of different diagnostic tools. With increasing knowledge on pathophysiological mechanisms in ICU-acquired weakness and causative disorders, the road for possible therapeutic interventions lies ahead. Properly used diagnostic tools can then also be implemented as surrogate endpoints to assess effectiveness in phase II studies.

Conclusion

Currently used diagnostic tools for ICU-acquired weakness include physical examination using the MRC scale, nerve conduction studies, myography and muscle biopsy; they all have their limitations. New diagnostic tools are urgently needed for daily clinical care and future research of therapeutic interventions aimed at

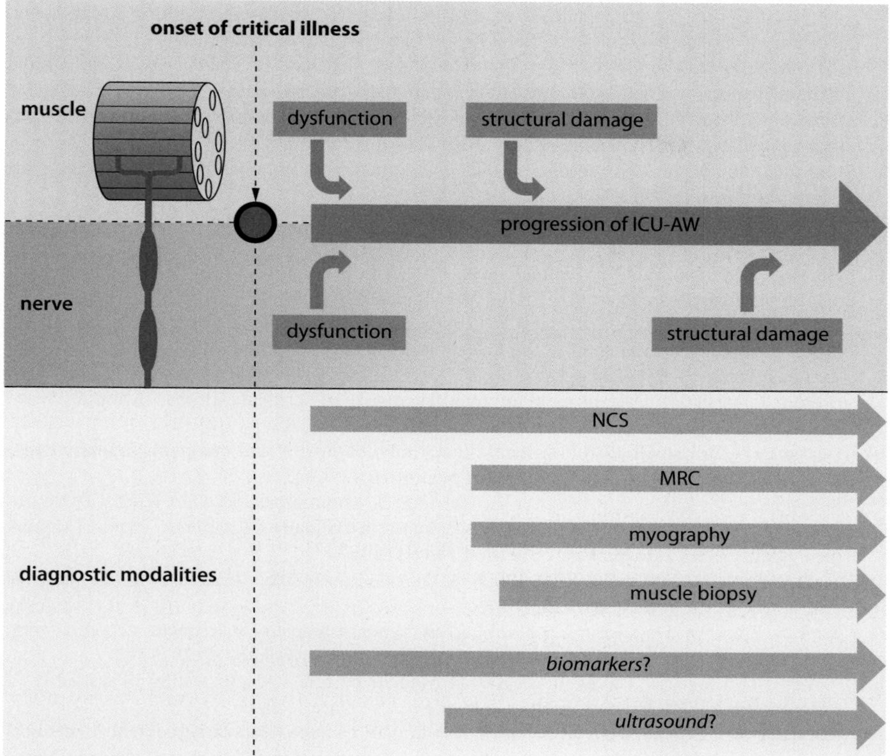

Fig. 2 Progression of ICU-acquired weakness (ICU-AW) and possible time points for use of (new) diagnostic approaches. NMD: neuromuscular disorder; NCS: nerve conduction studies; MRC: Medical Research Council

reducing ICU-acquired weakness. Ultrasound studies and biological markers may be used in the future.

References

1. Bolton CF, Gilbert JJ, Hahn AF, Sibbald WJ (1984) Polyneuropathy in critically ill patients. J Neurology Neurosurg Psychiatry 47:1223–1231
2. Stevens RD, Marshall SA, Cornblath DR et al (2009) A framework for diagnosing and classifying intensive care unit-acquired weakness. Crit Care Med 37:S299–S308
3. Stevens RD, Dowdy DW, Michaels RK, Mendez-Tellez PA, Pronovost PJ, Needham DM (2007) Neuromuscular dysfunction acquired in critical illness: a systematic review. Intensive Care Med 33:1876–1891
4. Khan J, Harrison TB, Rich MM, Moss M (2006) Early development of critical illness myopathy and neuropathy in patients with severe sepsis. Neurology 67:1421–1425
5. Needham DM, Davidson J, Cohen H et al (2012) Improving long-term outcomes after discharge from intensive care unit. Crit Care Med 40:502–509

6. Ali NA, O'Brien JM, Hoffmann SP et al (2008) Acquired weakness, handgrip strength, and mortality in critically ill patients. Am J Respir Crit Care Med 178:261–268
7. De Jonghe B, Bastuji-Garin S, Sharshar T, Outin H, Brochard L (2004) Does ICU-acquired paresis lengthen weaning from mechanical ventilation? Intensive Care Med 30:1117–1121
8. Bercker S, Weber-Carstens S, Deja M et al (2005) Critical illness polyneuropathy and myopathy in patients with acute respiratory distress syndrome. Crit Care Med 33:711–715
9. Latronico N, Shehu I, Seghelini E (2005) Neuromuscular sequelae of critical illness. Curr Opin Crit Care 11:381–390
10. Herridge MS (2009) Legacy of intensive care unit-acquired weakness. Crit Care Med 37:S457–S461
11. Herridge MS, Tansey CM, Matté A et al (2011) Functional disability 5 years after acute respiratory distress syndrome. N Engl J Med 364:1293–1304
12. Guarneri B, Bertolini G, Latronico N (2008) Long-term outcome in patients with critical illness myopathy or neuropathy: the Italian multicentre CRIMYNE study. J Neurol Neurosurg Psychiatry 79:838–841
13. Bolton CF (2005) Neuromuscular manifestations of critical illness. Muscle Nerve 32:140–163
14. Latronico N, Bolton CF (2011) Critical illness polyneuropathy and myopathy: a major cause of muscle weakness and paralysis. Lancet Neurol 10:931–941
15. Puthucheary Z, Rawal J, Ratnayake G, Harridge S, Montgomery H, Hart N (2012) Neuromuscular blockade and skeletal muscle weakness in critically ill patients: Time to rethink the evidence? Am J Respir Crit Care Med 185:911–917
16. Maramattom BV, Wijdicks EFM (2006) Acute neuromuscular weakness in the intensive care unit. Crit Care Med 34:2835–2841
17. Koch S, Spuler S, Deja M et al (2011) Critical illness myopathy is frequent: accompanying neuropathy protracts ICU discharge. J Neurol Neurosurg Psychiatry 82:287–293
18. Hough CL, Lieu BK, Caldwell ES (2011) Manual muscle strength testing of critically ill patients: feasibility and interobserver agreement. Crit Care 15:R43
19. Hermans G, Clerckx B, Vanhullebusch T et al (2011) Interobserver agreement of medical research council sum-score and handgrip strength in the intensive care unit. Muscle Nerve 45:18–25
20. Lefaucheur JP, Nordine T, Rodriguez P, Brochard L (2006) Origin of ICU acquired paresis determined by direct muscle stimulation. J Neurol Neurosurg Psychiatry 77:500–506
21. Latronico N, Bertolini G, Guarneri B et al (2007) Simplified electrophysiological evaluation of peripheral nerves in critically ill patients: the Italian multi-centre CRIMYNE study. Crit Care 11:R11
22. Weber-Carstens S, Koch S, Spuler S et al (2009) Nonexcitable muscle membrane predicts intensive care unit-acquired paresis in mechanically ventilated, sedated patients. Crit Care Med 37:2632–2637
23. Z'Graggen WJ, Brander L, Tuchscherer D, Scheidegger O, Takala J, Bostock H (2011) Muscle membrane dysfunction in critical illness myopathy assessed by velocity recovery cycles. Clin Neurophysiol 122:834–841
24. Z'Graggen WJ, Lin CS, Howard RS, Beale RJ, Bostock H (2006) Nerve excitability changes in critical illness polyneuropathy. Brain 129:2461–2470
25. Allen DC, Arunachalam R, Mills KR (2008) Critical illness myopathy: Further evidence from muscle-fiber excitability studies of an acquired channelopathy. Muscle Nerve 37:14–22
26. Teener JW, Rich MM (2006) Dysregulation of sodium channel gating in critical illness myopathy. J Muscle Res Cell Motil 27:291–296
27. Callahan LA, Supinski GS (2009) Sepsis-induced myopathy. Crit Care Med 37:S354–S367
28. Bierbrauer J, Koch S, Olbricht C et al (2012) Early type II fiber atrophy in intensive care unit patients with nonexcitable muscle membrane. Crit Care Med 40:647–650
29. Derde S, Hermans G, Derese I et al (2012) Muscle atrophy and preferential loss of myosin in prolonged critically ill patients. Crit Care Med 40:79–89

30. Puthucheary Z, Montgomery H, Moxham J, Harridge S, Hart N (2010) Structure to function: muscle failure in critically ill patients. J Physiol 588:4641–4648
31. Beekman R, Visser LH (2004) High-resolution sonography of the peripheral nervous system – a review of the literature. Eur J Neurol 11:305–314
32. Petzold A (2005) Neurofilament phosphoforms: Surrogate markers for axonal injury, degeneration and loss. J Neurol Sci 233:183–198
33. Joint Task Force of the EFNS and the PNS (2010) European Federation of Neurological Societies/Peripheral Nerve Society Guideline on the use of skin biopsy in the diagnosis of small fiber neuropathy. Report of a joint task force of the European Federation of Neurological Societies and the Peripheral Nerve Society. J Peripher Nerv Syst 15:79–92

Physiotherapy Update for the Adult ICU Patient

J.-D. Marti, G. Ntoumenopoulos, and A. Torres

Introduction

The improvement in critical care medicine and mechanical ventilation during recent decades has increased the short-term survival of critically ill patients, leading to a growing population of surviving patients needing prolonged mechanical ventilation and intensive care unit (ICU) lengths of stay [1]. However, during the ICU stay, patients often develop neuromuscular [2, 3] and pulmonary [4] complications that may deteriorate their clinical status and prolong recovery from critical illness. Additionally, patients being discharged from the ICU usually present with functional impairment and decreased quality of life that may persist for years after critical care [5].

Physiotherapy has the potential to improve pulmonary [6–8] and functional outcomes [9, 10] in the critically ill patient. However, there is a lack of robust scientific evidence resulting in variability in the delivery of physiotherapy care. The development of evidence-based recommendations and algorithms for the physiotherapy management of ICU patients aims to standardize physiotherapy delivery [11–15].

Better understanding of ICU-related complications, combined with the recent physiotherapy evidence base in the critically ill patient, should enable more appropriate implementation of physiotherapy in the ICU.

J.-D. Marti
Respiratory Critical Care Unit, Animal Experimentation Division, Thorax Institute, Hospital Clinic, Calle Villarroel 170, Esc 6/8 Planta 2, 08036 Barcelona, Spain

G. Ntoumenopoulos
Physiotherapy Department, Guys and St Thomas' NHS Foundation Trust, Kings Health Partners, London, United Kingdom

A. Torres (✉)
Respiratory Critical Care Unit, Animal Experimentation Division, Thorax Institute, Hospital Clinic, Calle Villarroel 170, Esc 6/8 Planta 2, 08036 Barcelona, Spain
E-mail: atorres@clinic.ub.es

J.-L. Vincent (Ed.), *Annual Update in Intensive Care and Emergency Medicine 2013*,
DOI 10.1007/978-3-642-35109-9_65,

Physiological Complications Associated with an ICU Stay

ICU-acquired Weakness

Critically ill patients often have neuromuscular deterioration during their ICU stay resulting in a loss of muscle mass and strength in limb and respiratory muscles [2, 3]. ICU-acquired weakness may delay return to independent functional status and increases risks of weaning failure and prolonged mechanical ventilation [3, 16]. Thus, ICU-acquired weakness results in prolonged hospitalization [16] and has been associated with increased ICU and hospital mortality [17]. Moreover, surviving critically ill patients often present with impaired functional status and decreased quality of life for many years after ICU discharge [5].

ICU-acquired weakness often results from a combination of multiple factors. Critical illness polyneuropathy (CIP), critical illness myopathy (CIM) and their usual coexistence, termed critical illness neuromyopathy (CINM), are considered the main causes for the development of ICU-acquired weakness [18]. CIP is an acute sensory-motor polyneuropathy affecting limb and respiratory muscles, whereas CIM is an acute primary myopathy not secondary to muscle denervation. CIP is associated with persistent disability, whereas a complete recovery is generally possible after CIM [18]. Although the pathophysiology of CIP and CIM is still unclear, pathophysiological metabolic mechanisms and impairment of microcirculatory and mitochondrial function have been implicated [18].

Muscle function can be assessed with tools, such as the Medical Research Council (MRC) scale [19]. Through assessment of the muscle function of three major muscle groups for each limb, ICU-acquired weakness is confirmed when the sum of the scores obtained from each muscle group is <48, from a total of 60. Respiratory muscle function is assessed by measuring maximal inspiratory and expiratory pressures [19]. However, as these volitional measures can only be performed in the neurologically responsive patient, this affects clinical accuracy and may delay time of diagnosis. The early diagnosis of ICU-acquired weakness in the neurologically unresponsive patient with differentiation between CIP and CIM can be performed through electrophysiological and morphological observations [18]. A differential diagnosis between CIP and CIM can be useful for long-term prognosis. The widely variable incidence of CIP and CIM reported in the literature, ranges from 25 % to 100 % depending on patient characteristics, risk factors, the time of assessment and the method used for diagnosis [18]. The major risk factors for CIP and CIM are systemic inflammation, sepsis and multiple organ failure. However, other risk factors, including duration of mechanical ventilation, hyperglycemia, corticosteroid administration or prolonged used of neuromuscular blocking drugs, have also been proposed in the literature [16, 18].

Prolonged bed rest is very common in the critically ill patient and may also promote muscular weakness even in the absence of systemic inflammatory changes. Indeed, prolonged immobility may alter the balance between protein synthesis and proteolysis and increases oxidative stress and apoptosis [20], starting immediately after ICU admission. Muscle impairment is significantly correlated with ICU length of stay but is generally worse during the first 2–3 weeks [21].

Finally, ICU-acquired weakness is further complicated by protein malnutrition, which is frequent in the critically ill. Indeed, protein support provided during the ICU stay is often insufficient to compensate the increased metabolic activity associated with critical illness [22], resulting in a further loss of muscle protein.

Secretion Retention and Pneumonia

Intubation and mechanical ventilation usually impairs mucociliary clearance, resulting in retention of airway secretions, lung collapse and pulmonary infections [4]. Cough, one of the main mechanisms of airway clearance, is often impaired in the mechanically ventilated patient. Airway clearance in the mechanically ventilated patient can be enhanced by respiratory flows through the two-phase gas-liquid transport mechanism [23]. Laboratory studies [24] have shown that outward mucus clearance occurs when expiratory flows are higher than inspiratory flows, although it also depends on the thickness and viscosity of the mucus. In the ICU patient, conventional ventilator settings may promote secretion retention and pulmonary infection since they predominantly deliver an inspiratory flow bias [24, 25], but this requires clinical confirmation. The use of minimal sedation during invasive mechanical ventilation can reduce the length of mechanical ventilation [26], which may lead to improved secretion clearance (e.g., improved expiratory muscle activity response to suction and spontaneous coughing), although this requires formal investigation. Moreover, the use of neuromuscular blocking agents can also predispose the patient to an increased risk of both secretion retention and pneumonia [27], which may be due to impaired secretion clearance. On the other hand, recent evidence supports the early use of neuromuscular blocking agents in acute respiratory distress syndrome (ARDS) because this approach is associated with reduced mortality, more ventilator free days, improved oxygenation and less barotrauma [28].

Ventilator-associated pneumonia (VAP) is a nosocomial pneumonia which commonly develops after 48 hours of intubation and mechanical ventilation [29]. VAP occurs in 9–27 % of all intubated patients, with the incidence initially increasing with duration of mechanical ventilation [29]. The critical event in the pathogenesis of VAP is believed to be the accumulation of contaminated sub-glottic space secretions from the oro-pharynx or gastrointestinal tract above the inflated cuff of the endotracheal tube (ETT). Semirecumbent position at > 30 degree head-up is recommended to prevent gastro-esophageal reflux and VAP in these patients, although it is uncertain whether this regime is effective or harmful with regard to the occurrence of clinically diagnosed VAP [30]. Indeed, recent animal studies have shown that gravity may have an important role in the worsening of both secretion retention and VAP during semirecumbent positioning [31, 32].

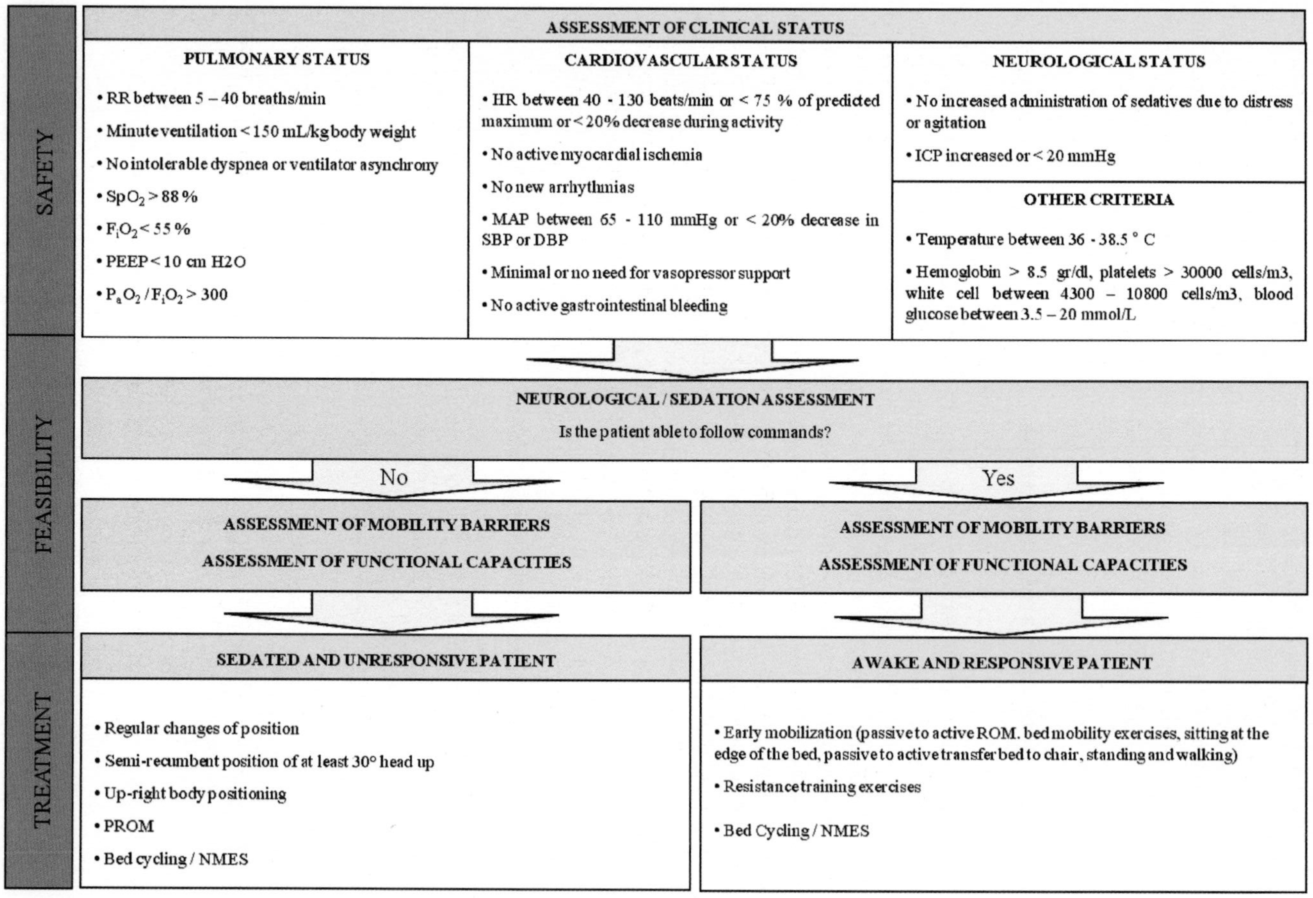

SAFETY

ASSESSMENT OF CLINICAL STATUS

PULMONARY STATUS	CARDIOVASCULAR STATUS	NEUROLOGICAL STATUS
• RR between 5 – 40 breaths/min • Minute ventilation < 150 mL/kg body weight • No intolerable dyspnea or ventilator asynchrony • SpO_2 > 88 % • F_iO_2 < 55 % • PEEP < 10 cm H2O • P_aO_2 / F_iO_2 > 300	• HR between 40 - 130 beats/min or < 75 % of predicted maximum or < 20% decrease during activity • No active myocardial ischemia • No new arrhythmias • MAP between 65 - 110 mmHg or < 20% decrease in SBP or DBP • Minimal or no need for vasopressor support • No active gastrointestinal bleeding	• No increased administration of sedatives due to distress or agitation • ICP increased or < 20 mmHg **OTHER CRITERIA** • Temperature between 36 - 38.5 ° C • Hemoglobin > 8.5 gr/dl, platelets > 30000 cells/m3, white cell between 4300 – 10800 cells/m3, blood glucose between 3.5 – 20 mmol/L

FEASIBILITY

NEUROLOGICAL / SEDATION ASSESSMENT

Is the patient able to follow commands?

No	Yes
ASSESSMENT OF MOBILITY BARRIERS **ASSESSMENT OF FUNCTIONAL CAPACITIES**	**ASSESSMENT OF MOBILITY BARRIERS** **ASSESSMENT OF FUNCTIONAL CAPACITIES**

TREATMENT

SEDATED AND UNRESPONSIVE PATIENT	AWAKE AND RESPONSIVE PATIENT
• Regular changes of position • Semi-recumbent position of at least 30° head up • Up-right body positioning • PROM • Bed cycling / NMES	• Early mobilization (passive to active ROM. bed mobility exercises, sitting at the edge of the bed, passive to active transfer bed to chair, standing and walking) • Resistance training exercises • Bed Cycling / NMES

◀ **Fig. 1** Overview algorithm for physiotherapy management of the critically ill patient. RR: respiratory rate; SpO_2: oxygen saturation; FiO_2: fraction of inspired oxygen; PEEP: positive end-expiratory pressure; PaO_2: partial pressure of arterial oxygen; HR: heart rate; MAP: mean arterial pressure; SBP: systolic blood pressure; DBP: diastolic blood pressure; ICP: intracranial pressure; PROM: passive range of motion; NMES: neuromuscular electrical stimulation; ROM, range of motion

Physiotherapy in the Critically Ill Patient

Physiotherapy may be a potential tool to counterbalance neuromuscular and pulmonary ICU-related complications. Thus, early implementation of physiotherapy in critically ill patient is gaining interest and several studies have evaluated its safety and feasibility [9, 10, 14, 33]. Generally, minimal or no serious adverse events have been reported during physiotherapy [9, 10, 14, 33]. Moreover, early implementation of physiotherapy has been associated with reduced ICU and hospital lengths of stay [14], increased ventilator-free days [10] and improved functional status [9, 10, 33]. Studies on chest physiotherapy have also reported improvement in pulmonary outcomes, such as improved clearance of airway secretions [34], decreased extubation failure [7] and incidence of VAP [6].

The criteria reported in the literature to initiate and monitor rehabilitation physiotherapy vary depending on the patient group under investigation and the specific physiotherapy treatment being evaluated. For example, specific ranges of cardiovascular, respiratory and neurological parameters have been proposed [9, 10, 14, 33] for the safe initiation and delivery of physiotherapy in critical care (Fig. 1). The daily evaluation of clinical status, functional capacities and level of sedation by the multidisciplinary team should be mandatory in order to establish safe and feasible therapy goals.

Physiotherapy services often vary across ICU settings because no definitive data concerning the adequate mode, frequency and duration of treatment have been established. The range of physiotherapy strategies also varies dependent upon a patient's clinical status, functional capacities and responsiveness (Fig. 1). For example, passive techniques are often used in deeply sedated patients, whereas more active assisted/resisted physiotherapy exercises are utilized once the patient is awake. Scientific evidence combined with expert opinion (Delphi process), has led to the important development of clinical physiotherapy algorithms for the critically ill and mechanically ventilated patient [12, 13], which may be useful to deliver more evidence based interventions.

Physiotherapy Management of the Sedated and Unresponsive Critically Ill Patient

In patients under deep sedation, physiotherapy treatment may be restricted to passive techniques because of sedation-related immobility and lack of cooperation from the patient. Chest physiotherapy to maintain airway patency or to improve pulmonary function is important and is implemented with or without active participation from the patient. However, physiotherapy for the improvement of functional status may be limited during this phase because of the acuity of illness and depth of sedation. Thus, during acute phases of the illness, physiotherapy mainly focuses on the management of respiratory system problems, although several strategies can be implemented to preserve functional capacities and to delay occurrence of neuromuscular complications.

Prevention of Functional Decline

Regular changes in a patient's body position are recommended to prevent alterations in joints' range of motion, pressure areas, prolonged compression of the nerves and soft tissue contractures, which may occur during prolonged bed rest and immobility [11, 12]. Semirecumbent positioning of at least >30º head-up is also recommended, although mainly for the prevention of VAP [12, 29, 30]. However, body positioning to approximate upright position may be used to improve gravitational stress and related fluid shifts, although the scientific evidence for this approach is limited [11]. Passive range of motion (PROM) for all limb extremity joints is recommended to preserve joint range of motion and muscle length. Although PROM has rarely been assessed separately from other physiotherapy techniques, it can be safely performed when included in a physical activity program [10, 12, 14] but may require increased dosage, for example through the use of continuous PROM devices [9].

Relatively new automated technologies, such as neuromuscular electrical stimulation (NMES), should be considered as potential tools to complement physiotherapy in the neurologically unresponsive ICU patient. However, because studies on NMES for the prevention of muscular weakness [35, 36] have recently reported contradictory results, it is unclear which patients may benefit most.

Standards to Maintain Airway Patency and Manage Secretion Retention

Detection of Airway Secretions

Research regarding the diagnosis of secretion retention in the intubated and mechanically ventilated patient is very limited [37]. A bedside method to detect secretion retention may be helpful in determining the respiratory intervention required (e.g., airway suction, chest physiotherapy, bronchoscopy or change of ETT), but is yet to be formally investigated.

Lung auscultation, although unreliable, may be useful to assist clinicians in identifying and localizing secretions and to assist with the selection of chest phys-

Signs:

- Tracheal/chest wall auscultation (transmitted coarse sounds)
- "Saw-tooth" expiratory waveform (see below)
- Chest palpation
- Visible secretions within the artificial airway
- ↑ Patient WOB
- ↑ P_aCO_2 (episodic or trends in data)
- ↓ SPO_2 (episodic or trends in data)
- Changes in ventilator parameters:
  - Pressure controlled modes = ↓ V_T, ↓ VE
  - Volume or dual controlled modes = ↑ PIP
- ↑ Rrs, ↓ Crs (episodic or trends in data)

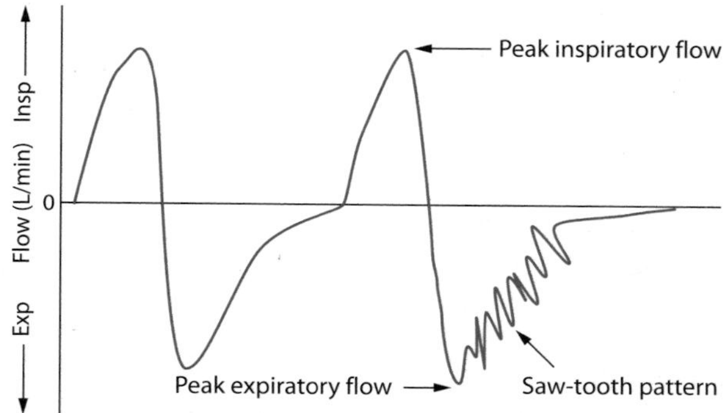

Fig. 2 Potential signs for detection of airway secretions. WOB: work of breathing; $PaCO_2$: partial pressure of carbon dioxide; SpO_2: oxygen saturation; V_T: tidal volume: VE: minute ventilation; PIP: peak inspiratory pressure; Rrs: respiratory system resistance; Crs: respiratory system compliance

iotherapy techniques. Clinical experience, patient habitus (e.g., morbid obesity), and inspiratory/expiratory flow rates are, among others, potentially important factors that may affect the accuracy of lung auscultation. Coarse respiratory sounds over the trachea on expiration and the presence of a saw-tooth pattern in the expiratory flow waveform (Fig. 2) are also good indicators of airway secretion volume greater than 0.5 ml obtained with airway suctioning [37]. Chest and ETT palpation can be also used to detect the presence of airway secretions, although the efficacy of this technique is yet to be confirmed. Moreover, the methods used to diagnose and localize secretion retention require further development.

Airway secretions can also be detected at the bedside by changes in respiratory mechanics, such as increased airway resistance and reduced dynamic lung/thorax compliance. Increased work of breathing (e.g., tachypnea, diaphoresis, accessory muscle use, paradoxical respiration), visible secretions within the artificial airway, changes in ventilator parameters and episodic or continuous hypercapnia and pulse oximetry de-saturation are also potential signs that may indicate the presence of mucus within the airways (Fig. 2). Although all these strategies are often used in clinical practice to detect airway secretions, they have not yet been validated as potential diagnostic tools. Newer technologies, such as vibration response imaging (VRI) may also be potentially useful tools to detect airway secretions [38].

Humidification

Mechanical ventilation through an ETT bypasses the normal airway humidification systems, and may cause structural and functional damage of the mucociliary escalator. Accumulation of airway secretions may also reduce ETT patency and cause obstruction. The two most common forms of humidification used in the intubated patient are the heat and moisture exchanger (HME) and the heated humidifier. A recent systematic review reported no differences in the rates of VAP, mortality and airway occlusion with either HMEs or heated humidification, although HMEs are often advocated to reduce costs and the potential risk of VAP [39]. However, HMEs are not recommended in patients with copious airways secretions because of the increased risk for airway occlusion [39]. The American Association for Respiratory Care recommended that, for intubated and mechanically ventilated patients, a humidity level between 33 and 44 mg H_2O/l should be provided by heated humidification devices and a minimum of 30 mg H_2O/l for HMEs. Moreover, respiratory gases should reach a temperature between 34–41 °C and a relative humidity of 100 % at the circuit y-piece [40].

Airway Suction

Suction of an endotracheal or tracheostomy tube is recommended for secretion clearance and to maintain airway patency. However, endotracheal suctioning can be associated with several complications (e.g., bradycardia, lung collapse, hypoxemia and increased intracranial pressure). Thus, in order to minimize the occurrence of complications, suctioning should be performed only when clinically indicated (Fig. 2) but not as routine care [41].

Endotracheal suctioning can be performed through an open suction system, which requires disconnection of the patient from the ventilator, or through a closed suction system, which uses a protected in-line suction catheter that does not require ventilator disconnection. Open suction systems have been demonstrated to be more effective than closed suction systems in terms of the volume of aspirated airway secretions. However, closed suction systems may facilitate the continued delivery of mechanical ventilation and, therefore, may be beneficial in patients requiring high levels of positive end-expiratory pressure (PEEP) and inspiratory fractions of oxygen (FiO_2) [41].

The American Association of Respiratory Care recommends hyperoxygenation (FiO_2 of 100 %) before and after any suctioning procedure to prevent hypoxemia [41]. In order to prevent lung collapse during the suctioning, it is recommended that the outer diameter of the suction catheter does not exceed one half the inner diameter of the artificial airway and the level of the vacuum should not be higher than 150 mm Hg [41]. Moreover, the procedure should last no more than 15 seconds after inserting the catheter into the artificial airway [41]. The use of saline instillation before suctioning to induce cough and dislodge secretions remains controversial, but has been reported to reduce the rate of VAP [42]. No significant differences in the amount of retrieved secretions have been shown between shallow and deep suctioning (when applied during open suctioning), although more adverse events may be associated with deep airway suctioning [41].

Additional Techniques to Optimize Secretion Clearance

Manual techniques, such as chest wall compressions or vibrations, can augment expiratory flow and may facilitate outward transport of mucus via a two-phase gas-liquid mechanism [23]. To date, only a few clinical studies [43, 44] have evaluated the effects of manual chest wall compressions/vibrations during mechanical ventilation, reporting contradictory results. These studies however used surrogate measures of secretion removal (weight of secretions aspirated, lung/thorax compliance, and arterial oxygenation), which have not yet been validated as a diagnosis of secretion retention or clearance. Manual chest wall compressions combined with vibrations improve expiratory flow rates, particularly when applied at the beginning of the expiration [45]. Interestingly, chest wall vibrations have also been associated with a significant reduction in VAP and improvements in weaning time when combined with side lying/head-down tilt [6] or with manual hyperinflation [8], respectively.

Manual hyperinflation is commonly used to recruit collapsed lung and to enhance clearance of airway secretions in intubated and mechanically ventilated patients unable to produce an effective cough [34]. Manual hyperinflation is performed by using a manual resuscitation bag to provide a larger tidal volume, followed by an inspiratory hold and a sudden release of the bag [34]. Manual hyperinflation has been shown to be a safe maneuver with short-term benefits in terms of airway secretion clearance, pulmonary compliance and oxygenation [34]. However, manual hyperinflation is not recommended in patients requiring high levels of PEEP and/or FiO_2 since the procedure requires disconnection from the mechanical ventilator. In-line pressure manometers should be used during manual hyperinflation to attain and monitor appropriate airway pressures.

Ventilator hyperinflation through adjustment of the ventilator settings (increased tidal volume or inspiratory pressure) is an alternative procedure to manual hyperinflation. To date, there are no significant differences between ventilator hyperinflation and manual hyperinflation in terms of safety, improvement in lung/thorax compliance or the wet weight of sputum cleared [46].

Mechanical insufflation-exsufflation, delivered through a variety of mechanical devices, can insufflate the lungs by applying a positive pressure to the airway, then rapidly shift to a negative pressure to create increased expiratory flows and simulate a more effective cough. Mechanical insufflation-exsufflation is often used in patients with poor peak cough expiratory flow due to severe respiratory muscle weakness (e.g., neuromuscular patients) to improve expectoration of airway secretions. There is no robust scientific evidence assessing the use of mechanical insufflation-exsufflation for intubated and mechanically ventilated patients and recent *in vitro* evidence has challenged its use through the artificial airway. Indeed, it has been demonstrated that for a same level of set pressure, peak expiratory flow decreases as the inner diameter of the artificial airway narrows [47]. Mechanical insufflation-exsufflation has recently been shown to be a potentially useful tool to prevent reintubation after extubation when applied early in patients with acute respiratory failure [7].

High-frequency airway clearance techniques such as intrapulmonary percussive ventilation or high-frequency chest wall compression can create high-frequency changes in respiratory airflows to alter the rheological properties of mucus and enhance the expiratory-inspiratory flow bias [48]. Intrapulmonary percussive ventilation rapidly delivers endobronchial bursts of gas, whereas high-frequency chest wall compression applied via a vibratory vest generates external compressions to the thorax [48]. Scientific evidence assessing the safety and efficacy of these devices to clear airway secretions is scarce but it may also be presumed that they interfere with the delivery of mechanical ventilation.

Physiotherapy Management of the Awake and Responsive Critically Ill Patient

Critically ill patients may obtain major benefits from physiotherapy once the use of sedation is reduced or stopped; indeed, this facilitates active therapy and feedback from the patient, which may improve treatment outcomes, particularly for neuromuscular complications. Increased general activity (e.g., sitting at the edge of the bed), increased use of respiratory muscles during spontaneous breathing and coughing, may assist to prevent the occurrence of pulmonary complications, but this requires confirmation. Chest physiotherapy may still be required to assist with airway secretion clearance especially when there is respiratory muscle weakness and limited cough effectiveness. Therefore, in the neurologically responsive patient, physiotherapy mainly focuses on the rehabilitation of neuromuscular status to achieve functional independence and, consequently, promote lung recruitment, optimize gas exchange and secretion clearance.

Early Mobilization

Early mobilization includes a variety of exercises that should be adapted to the patient depending on clinical status, functional capacities, responsiveness and cooperation. Indeed, mobilization includes mobility exercises in bed, limb exercises (i. e., active-assisted movements to training against resistance), sitting on the edge of the bed with or without support, passive to active transfers from bed to chair, standing and walking with or without support or devices. Moreover, the use of devices, such as NMES or a bedside cycle ergometer, can be safely used to complement early physiotherapy treatment. Indeed, bedside cycle ergometry in intensive care has been shown to significantly improve functional capacities and quadriceps muscle strength at hospital discharge [9].

The development of several structured evidenced based flow algorithms [10, 12, 14] should assist to standardize the clinical practice of physiotherapy in critical care. These evidence-based algorithms focus on clinical status, neurological status and functional capacities of the patient to set appropriate physiotherapy intervention and goal attainment.

Rehabilitation of the critically ill patient may also be facilitated by changes in ICU culture in which early physical activity is seen as a priority. For example, the optimal titration of sedation and analgesia in the acute ICU patient has been shown to shorten time to awakening, duration of mechanical ventilation and length of ICU stay [26]. By combining weaning of sedation with early mobilization this can also improve a patient's functional outcomes, shorten duration of delirium and shorten weaning from mechanical ventilation [10].

Secretion Clearance

Chest physiotherapy techniques that are often used to clear airway secretion in the sedated and unresponsive patients may also be used in the awake and cooperative intubated and ventilated patient. The ability to generate an adequate peak cough expiratory flow may guide physiotherapists in the selection of chest physiotherapy treatment. However, the cut-off point for peak cough flow to predict requirement for assistive devices or additional techniques (i. e., chest wall vibrations, manual-assisted cough) for secretion clearance is unclear.

The inability to cough to order or a peak cough expiratory flow cut-off point of $\leq$35 l/min has been associated with extubation failure with a sensitivity of 79 % and specificity of 71 % [49]. However, the cut off point for peak cough expiratory flow may vary dependent upon the measurement method used and the patient group investigated. The concept of 'whole body physiotherapy' may have a great role in improving secretion clearance and weaning outcomes by enhancing pulmonary function and optimizing cardiopulmonary fitness. Indeed, early mobilization has been associated with more ventilator-free days [10].

In patients who had passed a spontaneous breathing trial, there was a synergistic interaction between the level of alertness and neurologic function combined with a peak cough expiratory flow (> 60 l/min) and the quantity of suctioned airway secretions (> 2.5 ml/h) on extubation outcomes [50].

Conclusion

Critically ill and mechanically ventilated patients are at high risk of developing neuromuscular and pulmonary complications, which may cause deterioration of clinical status and prolong recovery from critical illness. Physiotherapy in the critically ill patient has been suggested to be a feasible and safe strategy to improve outcomes in this population of patients. Recent evidence has shown that early physiotherapy can improve functional status and reduce time on mechanical ventilation, and ICU and hospital lengths of stay. Moreover, there is a strong body of evidence to support the role of physiotherapy for the acute management of pulmonary complications associated with intubation and mechanical ventilation, such as atelectasis and secretion retention. However, the impact of physiotherapy on other major patient outcomes is unclear.

References

1. Zilberberg MD, de Wit M, Shorr AF (2012) Accuracy of previous estimates for adult prolonged acute mechanical ventilation volume in 2020: update using 2000–2008 data. Crit Care Med 40:18–20
2. De Jonghe B, Sharshar T, Lefaucheur JP et al (2002) Paresis acquired in the intensive care unit: A prospective multicenter study. JAMA 288:2859–2867
3. De Jonghe B, Bastuji-Garin S, Durand MC et al (2007) Respiratory weakness is associated with limb weakness and delayed weaning in critical illness. Crit Care Med 35:2007–2015
4. Konrad F, Schreiber T, Brecht-Kraus D, Georgieff M (1994) Mucociliary transport in ICU patients. Chest 105:237–241
5. Herridge MS, Tansey CM, Matté A et al (2011) Functional disability 5 years after acute respiratory distress syndrome. N Engl J Med 364:1293–1304
6. Ntoumenopoulos G, Presneill J, McElholum M, Cade JF (2002) Chest physiotherapy for the prevention of ventilator-associated pneumonia. Intensive Care Med 28:850–856
7. Gonçalves MR, Honrado T, Winck JC, Paiva JA (2012) Effects of mechanical insufflation-exsufflation in preventing respiratory failure after extubation: a randomized controlled trial. Crit Care 16:R48
8. Berti JS, Tonon E, Ronchi CF (2012) Manual hyperinflation combined with expiratory rib cage compression for reduction of length of ICU stay in critically ill patients on mechanical ventilation. J Bras Pneumol 38:477–486
9. Burtin C, Clerckx B, Robbeets C et al (2009) Early exercise in critically ill patients enhances short-term functional recovery. Crit Care Med 37:2499–2505
10. Schweickert WD, Pohlman MC, Pohlman AS et al (2009) Early physical and occupational therapy in mechanically ventilated, critically ill patients: a randomised controlled trial. Lancet 373:1874–1882
11. Gosselink R, Bott J, Johnson M et al (2008) Physiotherapy for adult patients with critical illness: recommendations of the European Respiratory Society and European Society of Intensive Care Medicine Task Force on Physiotherapy for Critically ill Patients. Intensive Care Med 34:1188–1199
12. Hanekom S, Gosselink R, Dean E et al (2011) The development of a clinical management algorithm for early physical activity and mobilization of critically ill patients: synthesis of evidence and expert opinion and its translation into practice. Clin Rehabil 25:771–787
13. Hanekom S, Berney S, Morrow B et al (2011) The validation of a clinical algorithm for the prevention and management of pulmonary dysfunction in intubated adults – a synthesis of evidence and expert opinion. J Eval Clin Pract 17:801–810
14. Morris PE, Goad A, Thompson C et al (2008) Early intensive care unit mobility therapy in the treatment of acute respiratory failure. Crit Care Med 36:2238–2243
15. Gosselink R, Clerckx B, Robbeets C, Vanhullebusch T, Vanpee G, Segerset J (2011) Physiotherapy in the intensive care unit. Neth. J Crit Care 15:66–75
16. Stevens RD, Dowdy DW, Michaels RK, Mendez-Tellez PA, Pronovost PJ, Needham DM (2007) Neuromuscular dysfunction acquired in critical illness: a systematic review. Intensive Care Med 33:1876–1891

17. Sharshar T, Bastuji-Garin S, Stevens RD et al (2009) Presence and severity of intensive care unit-acquired paresis at time of awakening are associated with increased intensive care unit and hospital mortality. Crit Care Med 37:3047–3053
18. Latronico N, Bolton CF (2011) Critical illness polyneuropathy and myopathy: a major cause of muscle weakness and paralysis. Lancet Neurol 10:931–941
19. Gosselink R, Needham D, Hermans G (2012) ICU-based rehabilitation and its appropriate metrics. Curr Opin Crit Care 18:533–539
20. Chambers MA, Moylan JS, Reid MB (2009) Physical inactivity and muscle weakness in the critically ill. Crit Care Med 37:S337–S346
21. Gruther W, Benesch T, Zorn C et al (2008) Muscle wasting in intensive care patients: ultrasound observation of the M. quadriceps femoris muscle layer. J Rehabil Med 40:185–189
22. Hise ME, Halterman K, Gajewski BJ, Parkhurst M, Moncure M, Brown JC (2007) Feeding practices of severely ill intensive care unit patients: an evaluation of energy sources and clinical outcomes. J Am Diet Assoc 107:458–465
23. Benjamin RG, Chapman GA, Kim CS, Sackner MA (1989) Removal of bronchial secretions by two-phase gas-liquid transport. Chest 95:658–663
24. Li Bassi G, Saucedo L, Marti JD et al (2012) Effects of duty cycle and positive end-expiratory pressure on mucus clearance during mechanical ventilation. Crit Care Med 40:895–902
25. Ntoumenopoulos G, Shannon H, Main E (2011) Do commonly used ventilator settings for mechanically ventilated adults have the potential to embed secretions or promote clearance? Respir Care 56:1887–1892
26. Kress JP, Pohlman AS, O'Connor MF, Hall JB (2000) Daily interruption of sedative infusions in critically ill patients undergoing mechanical ventilation. N Engl J Med 342:1471–1477
27. Leone M, Delliaux S, Bourgoin A et al (2005) Risk factors for late-onset ventilator-associated pneumonia in trauma patients receiving selective digestive decontamination. Intensive Care Med 31:64–70
28. Neto AS, Pereira VG, Espósito DC, Demasceno MC, Schultz MJ (2012) Neuromuscular blocking agents in patients with acute respiratory distress syndrome: a summary of the current evidence from three randomized controlled trials. Ann Intensive Care 2:33
29. O'Grady NP, Murray PR, Ames N (2012) Preventing ventilator-associated pneumonia: does the evidence support the practice? JAMA 307:2534–2539
30. Li Bassi G, Bertral R, Marti J-D, Rodriguez-Romero D, Torres A (2012) New insights in positioning tracheally intubated and mechanically ventilated patients. Clin Pulm Med 19:174–182
31. Li Bassi G, Zanella A, Cressoni M, Stylianou M, Kolobow T (2008) Following tracheal intubation, mucus flow is reversed in the semirecumbent position: possible role in the pathogenesis of ventilator-associated pneumonia. Crit Care Med 36:518–525
32. Zanella A, Cressoni M, Epp M, Hoffmann V, Stylianou M, Kolobow T (2012) Effects of tracheal orientation on development of ventilator-associated pneumonia: an experimental study. Intensive Care Med 38:677–685
33. Bailey P, Thomsen GE, Spuhler VJ et al (2007) Early activity is feasible and safe in respiratory failure patients. Crit Care Med 35:139–145
34. Paulus F, Binnekade JM, Vroom MB, Schultz MJ (2012) Benefits and risks of manual hyperinflation in intubated and mechanically ventilated intensive care unit-patients: a systematic review. Crit Care 16:R145
35. Routsi C, Gerovasili V, Vasileiadis I et al (2010) Electrical muscle stimulation prevents critical illness polyneuromyopathy: a randomized parallel intervention trial. Crit Care 14:R74
36. Poulsen JB, Møller K, Jensen CV, Weisdorf S, Kehlet H, Perner A (2011) Effect of transcutaneous electrical muscle stimulation on muscle volume in patients with septic shock. Crit Care Med 39:456–461
37. Guglielminotti J, Alzieu M, Maury E, Guidet B, Offenstadt G (2000) Bedside detection of retained tracheobronchial secretions in patients receiving mechanical ventilation: is it time for tracheal suctioning? Chest 118:1095–1099

38. Ntoumenopoulos G, Glickman Y (2012) Computerised lung sound monitoring to assess effectiveness of chest physiotherapy and secretion removal: a feasibility study. Physiotherapy 98:250–255
39. Kelly M, Gillies D, Todd DA, Lockwood C (2010) Heated humidification versus heat and moisture exchangers for ventilated adults and children. Cochrane Database Syst Rev CD004711
40. Restrepo RD, Walsh BK (2012) Humidification during invasive and noninvasive mechanical ventilation. Respir Care 57:782–788
41. American Association for Respiratory Care (2010) Clinical practice guideline. Endotracheal suctioning of mechanically ventilated patients with artificial airways. Respir Care 55:758–764
42. Caruso P, Denari S, Ruiz SA, Demarzo SE, Deheinzelin D (2009) Saline instillation before tracheal suctioning decreases the incidence of ventilator-associated pneumonia. Crit Care Med 37:32–38
43. Unoki T, Kawasaki Y, Mizutani T et al (2005) Effects of expiratory rib-cage compression on oxygenation, ventilation, and airway-secretion removal in patients receiving mechanical ventilation. Respir Care 50:1430–1437
44. Avena Kde M, Duarte AC, Cravo SL, Sologuren MJ, Gastaldi AC (2008) Effects of manually assisted coughing on respiratory mechanics in patients requiring full ventilatory support. J Bras Pneumol 34:380–386
45. Shannon H, Stiger R, Gregson RK, Stocks J, Main E (2010) Effect of chest wall vibration timing on peak expiratory flow and inspiratory pressure in a mechanically ventilated lung model. Physiotherapy 96:344–349
46. Dennis D, Jacob W, Budgeon C (2012) Ventilator versus manual hyperinflation in clearing sputum in ventilated intensive care unit patients. Anaesth Intensive Care 40:142–149
47. Guerin C, Bourdin G, Leray V et al (2011) Performance of the cough assist insufflation-exsufflation device in the presence of an endotracheal tube or tracheostomy tube: a bench study. Respir Care 56:1108–1114
48. Chatburn RL (2007) High-frequency assisted airway clearance. Respir Care 52:1224–1235
49. Beuret P, Roux C, Auclair A, Nourdine K, Kaaki M, Carton MJ (2009) Interest of an objective evaluation of cough during weaning from mechanical ventilation. Intensive Care Med 35:1090–1093
50. Salam A, Tilluckdharry L, Amoateng-Adjepong Y, Manthous CA (2004) Neurologic status, cough, secretions and extubation outcomes. Intensive Care Med 30:1334–1339

Part XIX

Organization and Outcomes

Nighttime Intensivist Physician Staffing in the ICU

D. J. Wallace, D. C. Angus, and J. M. Kahn

Introduction

The first published study to demonstrate the benefit of specialized physician staffing in the intensive care unit (ICU) took place almost thirty years ago [1]. Since that time over 25 studies have examined the association between the intensity of daytime physician staffing in the ICU and outcomes [2]. Two systematic reviews of these studies showed a consistent relationship between high-intensity daytime staffing (defined as either 'closed units' or ICUs where all patients are co-managed with an intensivist) and reduced ICU length-of-stay, reduced hospital length-of-stay, reduced ICU mortality and reduced hospital mortality compared to lower intensity daytime staffing [3, 4]. Several multicenter studies subsequent to these reviews largely, though not universally, confirmed these findings [5, 6]. These results attracted the attention of not only physicians, but also hospital administrators, policy analysts and insurance providers, leading to an expansion of the high-intensity staffing model in ICUs worldwide [7].

The strong relationship between daytime intensivist staffing and patient outcomes provides a compelling rationale for extending intensivist staffing around the clock; that is, staffing the ICU with an intensivist physician not only during the

D. J. Wallace
Department of Critical Care Medicine, University of Pittsburgh School of Medicine, 602B Scaife Hall, 3550 Terrace Street, Pittsburgh PA 15261, USA

D. C. Angus
Department of Critical Care Medicine, University of Pittsburgh School of Medicine, 602B Scaife Hall, 3550 Terrace Street, Pittsburgh PA 15261, USA

J. M. Kahn (✉)
Department of Critical Care Medicine, University of Pittsburgh School of Medicine, 602B Scaife Hall, 3550 Terrace Street, Pittsburgh PA 15261, USA
E-mail: kahnjm@upmc.edu

J.-L. Vincent (Ed.), *Annual Update in Intensive Care and Emergency Medicine 2013*, DOI 10.1007/978-3-642-35109-9_66, © Springer-Verlag Berlin Heidelberg 2013

day but at night as well. Indeed, in recent years many ICUs have introduced nighttime intensivist staffing as a strategy to improve the quality of care at night [8]. Furthermore, work-hours reductions for housestaff created additional pressure to provide attending coverage in the ICU at night [9]. However, unlike the data in support of daytime intensivist staffing, the data for nighttime staffing are much less clear [10]. In this chapter, we review the evidence for nighttime intensivist staffing, discuss the potential mechanisms for any observed benefits, and consider the potential adverse unintended consequences of nighttime staffing that might limit the benefit in the ICU.

Review of the Evidence

Existing studies of nighttime intensivist staffing are summarized in Table 1. The first study came in 2000 from an ICU in Norfolk, England that adopted 24-hour intensivist staffing [11]. Compared to risk-adjusted historical controls, patients admitted to the ICU when an intensivist was present around the clock had lower in-hospital mortality (standardized mortality ratio of 0.81 vs. 1.11, $p<0.05$). A second study of nighttime intensivists from the Mayo Clinic was published in 2008, similarly describing the experience of a single ICU in the year after adoption of 24-hour staffing [12]. Unlike the situation in Norfolk, this ICU was already staffed with in-house trainees (a junior resident, a senior resident and an ICU fellow) at all times before the addition of nighttime intensivist physicians. Although improvements were observed in non-adherence to evidence-based care processes (24 % vs. 16 %, $p=0.002$) and rate of procedural complications (11 % vs. 7 % per patient-day, $p=0.023$), these authors did not observe a reduction in in-hospital mortality after the addition of nighttime intensivists (17 % vs. 19 %; $p=0.33$). A subsequent study examining long-term outcomes in this cohort again showed no mortality benefit after nighttime intensivists were added to baseline high-intensity daytime staffing (adjusted hazard ratio of 1.05, 95%CI: 0.95–1.16; $p=0.3$) [13].

In the setting of these two single-center studies, our research group performed a multicenter evaluation of 24-hour intensivist staffing in United States hospitals participating in the Acute Physiology and Chronic Health Evaluation (APACHE) clinical information system [14]. We linked a prospective survey of ICU staffing patterns to patient-level risk-adjusted outcomes data. The final analysis included 65,752 patients admitted to 49 ICUs, and indicated that the benefit of nighttime intensivist staffing depended on how ICU staffing was organized during the day. For patients admitted to ICUs with low-intensity daytime staffing (in this cohort, these were all ICUs with optional intensivist consultation – no ICUs had no intensivists available), there was improvement in hospital mortality when intensivists were present at all times compared to only during the day (odds of death 0.62, $p=0.04$). For patients admitted to ICUs with high-intensity daytime staffing, there was no improvement in hospital mortality in 24-hour units (odds of death 1.08, $p=0.78$). These relationships were consistent in five pre-specified subgroup anal-

Table 1 Studies of nighttime intensivist staffing in the intensive care unit (ICU)

Reference	Country	ICUs	Daytime staffing model	Findings
Blunt, 2000 [11]	UK	1	Low-intensity	Lower mortality
Gaijic, 2008 [12, 13]	USA	1	High-intensity	Improvement in evidence-based practice, but no change in mortality
Wallace, 2012 [14]	USA	49	Both	Lower mortality in low-intensity daytime staffed ICUs and no change in mortality in high-intensity staffed ICUs
Wallace, 2012 [14]	USA	112	Both	Lower mortality in low-intensity daytime staffed ICUs and no change in mortality in high-intensity staffed ICUs

yses: Patients undergoing active treatment on admission, patients undergoing mechanical ventilation, patients admitted at night, patients in the highest third of acute physiology scores and patients with a diagnosis of sepsis on admission.

The primary analysis was repeated in a second, separate cohort of 107,319 patients admitted to 112 medical ICUs in the state of Pennsylvania. The results were generally similar. Among ICUs with low-intensity daytime staffing, patients admitted to units with nighttime intensivists had improved in-hospital mortality (odds of death 0.83, $p=0.049$). In ICUs with high-intensity daytime staffing there was no association between nighttime staffing and mortality (odds of death 0.97, $p=0.86$). Together, these multicenter studies reconcile the findings of the two previous single-center studies. Nighttime intensivist staffing appears to be associated with lower mortality in ICUs with low-intensity daytime staffing; but nighttime intensivist staffing does not improve outcomes in ICUs with high-intensity daytime staffing.

Possible Mechanisms of Mortality Findings

There are several reasons why nighttime intensivist staffing improves mortality in ICUs with low-intensity daytime staffing. Some patient exposure to an intensivist is almost certainly better than none, a notion that is consistent with the majority of studies on daytime staffing. When problems arise during the day in an optional consult ICU, the nurse is likely to call the primary physician, but at night the nurse may tend to call the in-house intensivist, affording that patient at least some exposure to the intensivist's expertise. Additionally, nighttime intensivists may be more adept at early resuscitation and treatment for time sensitive conditions, such as sepsis, which could impact outcomes particularly when the patient is admitted at night [15]. Indeed, the strongest signal in the APACHE study was in patients with a primary diagnosis of sepsis (odds ratio for death 0.46, $p<0.01$).

At the same time, there are plausible reasons why there might be no benefit of nighttime intensivists in ICUs with high-intensity staffing during the day. The overall benefits of intensivists derive from more than just the resuscitation of hemodynamically unstable patients or the ongoing titration of complex care. ICUs staffed with intensivists are more likely to use protocols, conduct daily multidisciplinary rounds and implement routine evidence-based care processes, such as deep-vein thrombosis (DVT) prophylaxis and head-of-bed elevation for pneumonia prevention [16]. In fact, evidence suggests that daily multidisciplinary rounding can achieve nearly the same improvement in mortality as closing the ICU [17]. It is possible that as long as intensivists are available to provide the routine best-practices associated with improved outcomes, there is little marginal benefit from more timely resuscitation and titration of complex care at night.

Several other studies support this concept. A systematic review of the effect of nighttime ICU admission on outcomes concluded that patients admitted at night were generally not at a higher risk of death compared to patients admitted during the day [18]. This finding indicates that the risks of nighttime admission are small. Additionally, a recent study of ICU telemedicine indicated an improvement in mortality that was largely mediated by increased implementation of routine evidence-based practices like DVT prophylaxis and beta-blockade after high-risk surgery – treatments that in theory are just as easily implemented during the day as at night [19].

That being said, the absence of an obvious mortality benefit in high-intensity ICUs should be interpreted with caution. Intensivists might reduce mortality for a small number of very sick patients, such as those in severe shock or cardiac arrest. Thus nighttime staffing might improve mortality at the margins, even if no impact is discernible for patients on average. Developing evidentiary support for this type of rare event mitigation is challenging because of the large samples needed to achieve statistical significance, analogous to interventions such as rapid response teams [20] or public-access automated external defibrillators [21].

Other Potential Benefits

In addition to the mortality benefit in some types of ICUs, nighttime intensivist staffing may be associated with other important benefits (Table 2). Intensivists who are physically present in the unit are more accessible for clarification on the plan of care, which in turn may translate into better nurse satisfaction [22]. For academic ICUs that train medical students and residents, nighttime intensivists might contribute to the education of medical students and residents through direct supervision at night. Supervision of procedures might also lead to fewer medical errors, albeit in a way that does not translate to reduced mortality in all ICUs.

Table 2 Mechanisms of potential benefits and harms of nighttime intensivists

Benefit	Harm
Earlier resuscitation	Invasive procedures performed on patients with lower risk of mortality
Titration of complex care	Increased handoffs
Supervision of invasive procedures	Substitution of nighttime staffing for other quality improvement efforts
Bedside clarification on plan of care	Decreased autonomy for physician trainees
Teaching opportunities for housestaff and nursing	Workforce strain
Second opinion on management	Physician burnout
Around-the-clock palliative care	
Leadership of rapid response teams	

Another potential benefit is the role that nighttime intensivists might play in the quality of death and dying [23]. ICU physicians increasingly play an active role in the palliative aspects of critical care [24]. Critical care physicians who are present at night may be more likely to initiate early discussions with patients or surrogates regarding their values and preferences [25–27]. These discussions could lead to early withdrawal of life-sustaining therapy in patients who would not want it, as well as increased family satisfaction if surrogate decision makers are reassured by the presence of an intensivist during this most difficult time. Importantly, the role of nighttime intensivists in palliative care may obscure the overall mortality signal in the ICU, if any reductions in mortality due to high quality care are offset by an increase in mortality in the setting of appropriate palliative care.

Finally, some ICUs may implement nighttime staffing in response to a societal imperative, in which the rule of rescue dictates that the sickest patients should have access to intensivists at all times. Similar decisions are present in other areas of healthcare, such as the Oregon Health Plan in the United States. Initially the plan refused to support hematopoietic stem cell transplantation, based on criteria of quality of life and cost-effectiveness. After public outcry, the position of the health plan changed to include specific diagnosis-treatment pairs [28]. Nighttime staffing may receive the same embrace – as a provision that should be granted as long as it is not associated with harm.

Potential Adverse Consequences

It is also important to consider the potential adverse consequences of nighttime intensivist staffing (Table 2). For example, nighttime intensivists may be more likely to perform invasive procedures than other physicians [1, 6]. Some procedures, such as insertion of pulmonary artery catheters, may increase costs and complications without actually improving outcomes [29]. This is especially true in lower-acuity patients, in which invasive procedures may not have a substantial role in guiding management. If still performed, these procedures would expose lower-acuity patients to potential complications without benefit.

Nighttime intensivists could also paradoxically worsen the education of future physicians. In one study of 24-hour staffing there was evidence that nighttime intensivists may lead to less perceived autonomy by critical care physicians in training [30]. Periods of autonomy followed by performance review are part of the classic model of physician education [31]. Although supervision is clearly important for inexperienced physicians, completely removing all episodes of autonomy may negatively impact the educational experience, leading to downstream harm once those physicians are forced to practice autonomously after their training ends.

Costs are also an important consideration. Critical care already comprises an outsized proportion of hospital costs. In health systems in which physicians are paid by the hospital, the costs of nighttime intensivists will increase the fixed costs of hospital care without concomitant increases in revenue, leading to decreased net revenue. In health systems in which physicians are paid via a fee-for-service mechanism, nighttime intensivist staffing will almost certainly result in increased billings at night, which will increase overall costs to payers and the health system [32]. Health care in industrialized nations is already characterized by overutilization and out-of-control expenditure – it is not clear that the marginal benefit of nighttime intensivists justifies these increased costs.

Workforce Issues

A final issue for consideration is the effect of nighttime staffing on the intensivist workforce. Considerable data suggest that, at least in the United States, there are not enough intensivists to meet either current or future demand [33]. Large-scale adoption of a nighttime intensivist model would further strain the already strained workforce. Few ICUs currently have nighttime intensivist staffing [34], and many ICUs do not even have intensivists present during the day [35], begging the question of whether we should staff some ICUs with intensivists around the clock while other ICUs go completely unstaffed.

Nighttime staffing also might have indirect consequences for the workforce. A high burden of night-call may lead to burnout syndrome or depression, potentially causing some intensivists to leave the workforce early [36]. The threat of remaining in the hospital at night may cause some trainees to opt for less rigorous fields that allow for more free time. Trainees already cite concerns about work-life balance among the reasons not to consider a career in intensive care – the addition of in-hospital night call is likely to exacerbate this problem [37]. Lastly, in academic hospitals, the burden of nightshifts may fall disproportionately on junior faculty who are early in their careers. This effect may adversely affect their ability to advance within hospital administration or compete for research grants.

Areas for Future Research

Several important questions remain to be answered with respect to nighttime intensivist staffing.

Additional Outcome Studies

The number of studies examining the impact of nighttime intensivists and outcome remains small. Additional studies are needed to confirm the mortality benefit in low-intensity daytime staffed ICUs and the lack of a mortality benefit in high-intensity daytime staffed ICUs. Moreover, research is needed into other outcomes, which, although less important than mortality, are no less patient-centered. These include family satisfaction, nurse satisfaction, physician satisfaction (including burnout), quality of death and dying, educational outcomes and costs. Ideally these evaluations should take a long-term time horizon, addressing outcomes such as long-term mortality and health-related quality of life. Additionally, these studies should attempt to delineate exactly what intensivists are doing in the ICU at night. Clearly there is nothing inherently good about the mere physical presence of an intensivist – the intensivist has to do something to affect outcome. Detailed information quantifying the supervision of procedures, number of admissions and direction of resuscitations may help clarify how intensivists improve quality and where they would be best deployed.

Role of Ancillary Staff

Increasingly ICUs are utilizing advanced care practitioners, such as nurse practitioners and physician assistants, to augment the critical care workforce [38]. Accumulating data suggest that when under the supervision of an intensivist these individuals provide care at least as good as physician trainees [39]. Often advanced care practitioners are capable of performing emergent procedures such as endotracheal intubation and central line placement [40]. In practice settings where nighttime intensivist staffing is not feasible, it is possible that advanced care practitioners may play an important role. It is telling that in our multicenter study, the strongest determinant of survival was whether or not any physician was in the hospital at night, be that individual a trainee or a trained intensivist. If resident physicians can improve the quality of nighttime ICU care, it is likely that non-physician providers can as well.

The Role of ICU Telemedicine

ICU telemedicine refers to the use of audio-visual technology to provide critical care services from a distance. Currently the most common form of ICU telemedicine involves remote monitoring at night. The data underlying ICU telemedicine are conflicting, with some studies showing a strong benefit and others showing no benefit [41]. At this time, the best evidence for ICU telemedicine is in its capacity as a quality improvement tool, used to implement best practices as an adjunct to daytime intensivists on the ground [42]. Nonetheless, there may be a role of ICU telemedicine in remote monitoring at night, especially when there is strong nurse and physician buy-in, which allows the telemedicine team to actively intervene on the ICU patients. To date, no studies have compared nighttime ICU telemedicine to nighttime intensivists on the ground. If these two strategies result in equivalent outcomes, ICU telemedicine may prove to be an efficient method of providing the experience and expertise of intensivists at night without substantially straining the intensivist workforce [43].

Conclusion

Despite strong evidentiary support for high-intensity daytime staffing in the ICU, the available data indicate that mortality benefits from nighttime staffing depend on how the ICU is managed during daylight hours. Among ICUs with low-intensity daytime staffing, nighttime intensivists are associated with lower in-hospital mortality. In ICUs with high-intensity daytime staffing, the presence of nighttime intensivists is not associated with an in-hospital mortality reduction. That being said, there may be non-mortal benefits to nighttime staffing in high-intensity daytime ICUs, such as improved family satisfaction, clinician satisfaction, quality of death and costs. Future research should address these important outcomes, as well as the role of non-physician providers and ICU telemedicine as strategies to augment the quality of critical care at night.

Given the uncertainty surrounding the effectiveness and costs of nighttime intensivists, blanket staffing recommendations at this time are premature. Nonetheless, there are several guiding principles that can help ICUs determine how best to staff their ICUs at night. First, ICUs with no physician presence at night should consider the various ways to add some physician presence through the addition of either residents, advanced care practitioners or, if resources allow, trained intensivists. Second, ICUs that are well staffed during the day should carefully consider the advantages and disadvantages of nighttime staffing. Hospitals with particularly high acuity or hospitals wishing to invest in efforts to reduce mortality at the margins among a few very sick patients may wish to adopt nighttime staffing. At the same time, all hospitals should consider alternate approaches to improving patient safety at night with the understanding that the benefits of nighttime intensivist staffing may not be worth the costs.

References

1. Li TC, Phillips MC, Shaw L, Cook EF, Natanson C, Goldman L (1984) On-site physician staffing in a community hospital intensive care unit. Impact on test and procedure use and on patient outcome. JAMA 252:2023–2027
2. Gajic O, Afessa B (2009) Physician staffing models and patient safety in the ICU. Chest 135:1038–1044
3. Young MPM, Birkmeyer JD (2000) Potential reduction in mortality rates using an intensivist model to manage intensive care units. Eff Clin Pract 3:284–289
4. Pronovost PJ, Angus DC, Dorman T, Robinson KA, Dremsizov TT, Young TL (2002) Physician staffing patterns and clinical outcomes in critically ill patients: a systematic review. JAMA 288:2151–2162
5. Treggiari MM, Martin DP, Yanez ND, Caldwell E, Hudson LD, Rubenfeld GD (2007) Effect of intensive care unit organizational model and structure on outcomes in patients with acute lung injury. Am J Respir Crit Care Med 176:685–690
6. Levy MM, Rapoport J, Lemeshow S, Chalfin DB, Phillips G, Danis M (2008) Association between critical care physician management and patient mortality in the intensive care unit. Ann Intern Med 148:801–809
7. Manthous CA (2004) Leapfrog and critical care: evidence- and reality-based intensive care for the 21st century. Am J Med 116:188–193
8. Burnham EL, Moss M, Geraci MW (2010) The Case for 24/7 In-house intensivist coverage. Am J Respir Crit Care Med 181:1159–1160
9. Pastores SM, O'Connor MF, Kleinpell RM et al (2011) The Accreditation Council for Graduate Medical Education resident duty hour new standards: history, changes, and impact on staffing of intensive care units. Crit Care Med 39:2540–2549
10. Kahn JM, Hall JB (2010) More doctors to the rescue in the intensive care unit: a cautionary note. Am J Respir Crit Care Med 181:1160–1161
11. Blunt MC, Burchett KR (2000) Out-of-hours consultant cover and case-mix-adjusted mortality in intensive care. Lancet 356:735–736
12. Gajic O, Afessa B, Hanson AC et al (2008) Effect of 24-hour mandatory versus on-demand critical care specialist presence on quality of care and family and provider satisfaction in the intensive care unit of a teaching hospital. Crit Care Med 36:36–44
13. Reriani M, Biehl M, Sloan JA, Malinchoc M, Gajic O (2012) Effect of 24-hour mandatory vs on-demand critical care specialist presence on long-term survival and quality of life of critically ill patients in the intensive care unit of a teaching hospital. J Crit Care 27:421.e1–e7
14. Wallace DJ, Angus DC, Barnato AE, Kramer AA, Kahn JM (2012) Nighttime intensivist staffing and mortality among critically ill patients. N Engl J Med 366:2093–2101
15. Rivers E, Nguyen B, Havstad S et al (2001) Early goal-directed therapy in the treatment of severe sepsis and septic shock. N Engl J Med 345:1368–1377
16. Kahn JM, Brake H, Steinberg K (2007) Intensivist physician staffing and the process of care in academic medical centres. Qual Saf Health Care 16:329
17. Kim MM, Barnato AE, Angus DC, Fleisher LA, Fleisher LF, Kahn JM (2010) The effect of multidisciplinary care teams on intensive care unit mortality. Arch Intern Med 170:369–376
18. Cavallazzi RR, Marik PEP, Hirani AA, Pachinburavan MM, Vasu TST, Leiby BEB (2010) Association between time of admission to the ICU and mortality: a systematic review and metaanalysis. Chest 138:68–75
19. Lilly CMC, Cody SS, Zhao HH et al (2011) Hospital mortality, length of stay, and preventable complications among critically ill patients before and after tele-ICU reengineering of critical care processes. JAMA 305:2175–2183
20. Hillman K, Chen J, Cretikos M et al (2005) Introduction of the medical emergency team (MET) system: a cluster-randomised controlled trial. Lancet 365:2091–2097
21. Winkle RA (2010) The effectiveness and cost effectiveness of public-access defibrillation. Clin Cardiol 33:396–399

22. Baggs JG, Schmitt MH, Mushlin AI, Eldredge DH, Oakes D, Hutson AD (1997) Nurse-physician collaboration and satisfaction with the decision-making process in three critical care units. Am J Crit Care 6:393–399
23. Lynn J (2000) Quality of life at the end of life. JAMA 284:1513–1515
24. Curtis JR, Treece PD, Nielsen EL et al (2008) Integrating palliative and critical care: evaluation of a quality-improvement intervention. Am J Respir Crit Care Med 178:269–275
25. Stelfox H, Hemmelgarn B (2012) Intensive care unit bed availability and outcomes for hospitalized patients with sudden clinical deterioration. Arch Intern Med 172:467–474
26. Prendergast TJ, Claessens MT, Luce JM (1998) A national survey of end-of-life care for critically ill patients. Am J Respir Crit Care Med 158:1163–1167
27. Curtis JR, Engelberg RA (2011) What is the "right" intensity of care at the end of life and how do we get there? Ann Intern Med 154:283–284
28. Bodenheimer T (1997) The Oregon Health Plan – lessons for the nation. First of two parts. N Engl J Med 337:651–655
29. Harvey SS, Harrison DAD, Singer MM (2005) Assessment of the clinical effectiveness of pulmonary artery catheters in management of patients in intensive care (PAC-Man): a randomised controlled trial. Lancet 366:472–477
30. Garland A, Roberts D, Graff L (2012) Twenty-four-hour intensivist presence: A pilot study of effects on intensive care unit patients, families, doctors, and nurses. Am J Respir Crit Care Med 185:738–743
31. Rotem A, Godwin P, Du J (1995) Learning in hospital settings. Teaching and Learning in Medicine 7:211–217
32. Gosden T, Pedersen L, Torgerson D (1999) How should we pay doctors? A systematic review of salary payments and their effect on doctor behaviour. QJM 92:47–55
33. Angus DC, Kelley MA, Schmitz RJ, White A, Popovich J, Committee on Manpower for Pulmonary and Critical Care Societies COMPACCS (2000) Caring for the critically ill patient. Current and projected workforce requirements for care of the critically ill and patients with pulmonary disease: can we meet the requirements of an aging population? JAMA 284:2762–2770
34. Parshuram CSC, Kirpalani HH, Mehta SS, Granton JJ, Cook DD (2006) In-house, overnight physician staffing: a cross-sectional survey of Canadian adult and pediatric intensive care units. Crit Care Med 34:1674–1678
35. Angus DC, Shorr AF, White A, Dremsizov TT, Schmitz RJ, Kelley MA, Committee on Manpower for Pulmonary and Critical Care Societies COMPACCS (2006) Critical care delivery in the United States: distribution of services and compliance with Leapfrog recommendations. Crit Care Med 34:1016–1024
36. Embriaco NN, Papazian LL, Kentish-Barnes NN, Pochard FF, Azoulay EE (2007) Burnout syndrome among critical care healthcare workers. Curr Opin Crit Care 13:482–488
37. Lorin S, Heffner J, Carson S (2005) Attitudes and perceptions of internal medicine residents regarding pulmonary and critical care subspecialty training. Chest 127:630–636
38. Gershengorn H, Johnson M, Factor P (2011) The use of non-physician providers in adult intensive care units. Am J Respir Crit Care Med 185:600–605
39. Gershengorn HB, Wunsch H, Wahab R et al (2011) Impact of nonphysician staffing on outcomes in a medical ICU. Chest 139:1347–1353
40. Kleinpell RM, Ely EW, Grabenkort R (2008) Nurse practitioners and physician assistants in the intensive care unit: An evidence-based review. Crit Care Med 36:2888–2897
41. Wilcox ME, Adhikari NK (2012) The effect of telemedicine in critically ill patients: systematic review and meta-analysis. Crit Care 16:R127
42. Kahn JM (2011) The use and misuse of ICU telemedicine. JAMA 305:2227–2228
43. Kahn JM, Hill N, Lilly C et al (2011) The research agenda in ICU telemedicine. Chest 140:230–238

Prognostication in Cirrhotic Patients Admitted to Intensive Care

S. Patel, T. Pirani, and J. Wendon

Introduction

Liver cirrhosis is an independent risk factor for death [1, 2]. Admission of patients with liver cirrhosis to intensive care units (ICU) because of complications of acute decompensation has traditionally been associated with poor outcomes [3], and various studies have demonstrated mortality rates varying between 44–71 % [4–8]. The incidence of liver disease is increasing. Liver disease is now the 5th leading cause of death in the UK [9], and is responsible for more than 25,000 deaths per year in the USA [10]. Patients are frequently admitted with sepsis, multiorgan failure (MOF), including respiratory and circulatory failure, renal failure and hepatic encephalopathy, as well as severe variceal hemorrhage, malnutrition and cachexia. Extremely high mortality rates have been observed in patients requiring mechanical ventilation or vasopressors. Cholongitas et al. observed 90 % mortality in patients with 3 or more organ failures [5], a finding replicated recently by O'Brien et al. [4]. It is, therefore, evident that these patients represent a significant burden on ICUs, both economically and in terms of bed occupancy [4], leading many physicians to question the appropriateness of admitting cirrhotic patients with established MOF to the ICU [4]. Despite such high mortality rates, the outcome of cirrhotic patients admitted to the ICU has improved significantly in the last decade [4, 5, 11], and cirrhotic patients admitted to the ICU in a timely fashion early in their disease, with single organ failure and without sepsis, have been

S. Patel
Dept of Intensive Care, King's College Hospital, Denmark Hill, London SE5 9RS, UK

T. Pirani
Dept of Intensive Care, King's College Hospital, Denmark Hill, London SE5 9RS, UK

J. Wendon (✉)
Liver Intensive Care Unit, Institute of Liver Studies, King's College Hospital, Denmark Hill, London SE5 9RS, UK
E-mail: Julia.wendon@kcl.ac.uk

J.-L. Vincent (Ed.), *Annual Update in Intensive Care and Emergency Medicine 2013*,
DOI 10.1007/978-3-642-35109-9_67, © Springer-Verlag Berlin Heidelberg 2013

shown to have acceptable survival rates [4, 8]. As a result, several scoring systems have been developed over the years to predict which patients may benefit from admission to the ICU, and in addition, to help determine resource utilization by allowing appropriate patient selection for admission to the ICU [8]. The scoring systems have been validated extensively in the general ICU population, and subsequently, more specific risk stratification scoring systems have been developed and studied in the liver disease sub-group. This chapter will look at the various prognostication tools available and their efficacy.

General ICU Scoring Systems

Several scoring systems for the prognostication of critically ill patients admitted to general ICUs exist, primarily looking at evaluating mortality in the first 24 hours of admission. These models have been found to be useful in the general population but their applicability in specific patient subgroups has been questioned. Several studies have been conducted assessing the validity of using general scoring systems in cirrhotic patients, and the majority have found them to be appropriately prognostic. Discriminatory power of the various tools is determined using the area under the receiver operating characteristic curve (AUROC).

Sequential Organ Failure Assessment (SOFA) Score

The sequential organ failure assessment (SOFA) score [12] has repeatedly been demonstrated to be a valuable tool for prognostication in cirrhotic patients. Several studies have demonstrated that as a single tool it has the best discriminative power of all the scores, including the liver specific scores. Cholongitas et al. evaluated 412 patients admitted to a single ICU and detected an AUROC of 0.85, exceeding the discriminative power of other general scoring systems, such as the acute physiology and chronic health evaluation (APACHE) II score, and the liver specific tools [13] (Table 1). These findings were replicated by Levesque et al. (AUROC = 0.92) who found a statistically significant difference when compared to the liver specific models ($p < 0.01$) [14]. With increasing numbers of failing organs, as defined by the SOFA score, there was an increased risk of mortality, ranging from 2.8 % in patients with no organ failure to 90.6 % with three or more organ failures. A score cut-off value > 10.5 determined a mortality risk of 80.6 % vs. 19.3 % if < 10.5 [14]. Das et al. used a modified SOFA score (excluding hematologic failure as it was not associated with mortality) and found it to be highly prognostic and superior to the other tools (AUROC = 0.84, $p < 0.05$). In addition, they found that the AUROC of the modified SOFA score after 3 days was significantly greater than the AUROC of scores calculated on day 1. Cut-off values of ≥ 15 on day 1 or ≥ 12 on day 3 predicted in-hospital mortality with specificities between 90–100 % [1]. Ferreira et al. similarly found that SOFA scores at 48 hours performed better than scores at admission [15]. Even with regard to liver transplantation outcomes, SOFA scores, not liver specific tools, were statistically significant predictors of 3-month and 1-year mortality [16].

Table 1 Evidence comparing the different prognostication scores

Prognostic Model and Evidence	No. of Patients	AUROC	Cut-off value	Mortality[a] (%)	p value
SOFA					
Das [1]	138	0.84 (0.84)[b]	15 (12)[b]	>90	<0.0001
Tu [25]	202	0.872	8	59.9	<0.001
Levesque [14]	377	0.92	10.5	80.6 vs 19.3	<0.0001
Cholongitas [13]	412	0.85	10	80 vs 27	–
Cholongitas [21]	128	0.81 (0.88)[c]	10	–	–
SAPS II					
Das [1]	138	0.78	–	–	<0.05
Levesque [14]	377	0.89	47.5	75.3 vs 17.5	<0.0001
Lehner [19]	117	0.72	–	–	<0.05
APACHE					
O'Brien [4]	16,096	0.77	–	1.24[d]	NS
ICNARC					
O'Brien[4]	16,096	>0.8	–	1.12[d]	NS
CHILD-PUGH					
Das [1]	138	0.76	–	–	<0.05
Levesque [14]	377	0.79	Child C[e]	51.8 vs 15.7[e]	<0.0001
Cholongitas [13]	412	0.67	10 (Child C)	75 vs 37	–
Cholongitas [21]	128	0.75 (0.78)[c]	–	–	–
Lehner [19]	117	–	Child C	44.83 vs 1.76	<0.01
Lim [32]	205	0.934	10 (Child C)	21.089[g]	<0.001
MELD					
Das [1]	138	0.77	–	–	<0.05
Jiang [28]	166	0.712, 0.708, 0.689[f]	–	–	<0.001
Cavallazzi [24]	441	0.77	26	64	–
Tu [25]	202	0.865	24	59.9	<0.001
Levesque [14]	377	0.82	28.5	71.8 vs 21.1	<0.0001

Table 1 *Continued*

Prognostic Model and Evidence	No. of Patients	AUROC	Cut-off value	Mortality[a] (%)	p value
Cholongitas [13]	412	0.80	21	77 vs 31	–
Cholongitas [21]	128	0.78 (0.86)[c]	–	–	–
Lehner [19]	117	0.77	–	–	<0.01
Lim [32]	205	0.751	17	4.596[g]	0.03
MELD-Na					
Das [1]	138	0.75	–	–	<0.05
Jiang [28]	166	0.766, 0.738, 0.714[f]	20	–	<0.001
Cavallazzi [24]	441	0.77	–	–	–
Levesque [14]	377	0.79	–	–	<0.0001
Cholongitas [13]	412	0.75	25	83 vs 52	–
iMELD					
Jiang [28]	166	0.841, 0.806, 0.783[f]	40	–	<0.001
Levesque [14]	377	0.81	–	–	<0.0001
Cholongitas [13]	412	0.76	43	83 vs 45	–
MESO					
Jiang [28]	166	0.723, 0.715, 0.694[f]	1.6	3.32[h]	<0.001
Levesque [14]	377	0.82	–	–	<0.0001
MAYO Model					
Kim [34]	160	0.832, 0.803, 0.822[f]	–	–	NS
Reweighted MELD					
Cholongitas [13]	412	0.79	4.3	81 vs 32	–
$AKIN_{48\text{-}Hr}$					
Tu [25]	202	0.814	Stage 1	–	<0.001
$RIFLE_{0\text{-}Hr}$					
Tu [25]	202	0.725	RISK	–	<0.001

[a] Mortality above versus below cut-off value; [b] Values at Day 1, and in brackets at Day 3; [c] Values at Day 1, and in brackets at 48 hours; [d] Mortality ratio; NS: not statistically significant between actual mortality and predicted, i. e., model valid; [e] Cut-off Child C grade, mortality comparison therefore Child C vs. Child A or B; [f] Values at 3-, 6 months and 1 year; [g] odds ratio; [h] relative risk of mortality

One reason why SOFA scores may be such a good tool for predicting mortality in cirrhotic patients is that outcome following admission to intensive care is predominantly determined by the severity of a patient's extra hepatic organ dysfunction as opposed to liver dysfunction being the primary driver. Thus, although in a ward and outpatient based setting a liver-based score, such as MELD and Child-Pugh, is prognostic of 3-month survival with reasonable accuracy, the onset of extra-hepatic failures determines outcome for any given degree of liver dysfunction in a critical care arena. It is of note that Das et al. excluded the platelet count to improve the modified SOFA score (as it was not an independent predictor of mortality). Interestingly, SOFA score has also recently been shown to be highly predictive of outcome in patients with acute liver failure who have taken a staggered overdose of acetaminophen, a situation when standard prognostic models perform poorly [17].

Simplified Acute Physiology Score (SAPS)

The SAPS [18] is another general ICU tool shown to have good prognostic capabilities. Levesque et al. demonstrated, as with the SOFA score, superior prognostication with the SAPS II score (AUROC = 0.89) than with the liver specific tools. Cut-off values of ≥ 47.5 were associated with a mortality of 75.3 %, vs. 17.5 % for values < 47.5 [14]. An AUROC value of 0.78 was established by Das et al., but when evaluated after 3 days, the prognostic capability diminished (AUROC = 0.63) [1]. Lehner et al. [19] did not detect as great a predictive capability, but still found that the score had some prognostic value (AUROC = 0.70). These authors examined the 15 sub-parameters comprising the SAPS II score and found that only three – bilirubin, the Glasgow Coma Scale (GCS) score and urine output – were able to predict outcome, thus possibly explaining the lower predictive capabilities [19].

Acute Physiology and Chronic Health Evaluation (APACHE) Score

The APACHE scores (versions I–IV) [20] were designed and validated for use in the first 24 hours of admission to the ICU. Cholongitas et al. evaluated their use in cirrhotic patients at 24 and at 48 hours after admission [21]. They determined that the APACHE II score had AUROC values of 0.75 and 0.78 at 24 and 48 hours respectively, demonstrating that the APACHE II score had better discriminative power at 48 hours, a previously unevaluated finding. O'Brien et al. also assessed the discriminative power of APACHE II in their UK study and found an AUROC value of 0.77, but concluded that the score under-predicted mortality and lacked calibration [4].

APACHE scores have generally been found to be inferior prognostic tools compared with the organ dysfunction tools, but remain of some prognostic value, and their use, therefore, should not be dismissed.

The Intensive Care National Audit and Research Center (ICNARC) Risk Prediction Model

The ICNARC Case Mix Program is a national comparative database of characteristics and outcomes for admissions to general ICUs across England, Wales and Northern Ireland, and a risk prediction model has been developed by the ICNARC based on physiology scores. This model was used by O'Brien et al. to evaluate prognostication for cirrhotic patients admitted to UK ICUs over a 12-year period. These authors found that the score under-predicted mortality, but had an AUROC value of >0.8 (superior to APACHE II), and concluded that the ICNARC scores should not be used to guide decision making [4]. Interestingly, they found that cirrhotic patients had worse outcomes compared to chronic renal failure patients (mortality 55 % vs. 42 %) despite similar characteristics. Little can be gleaned from this study with respect to the utility of ICNARC models for prognostication in cirrhotic patients admitted to the ICU, because patients were included if they had a diagnosis of cirrhosis as their primary cause of admission, or if it was a diagnosis in their past medical history. With limited data available on the use of ICNARC as a risk prediction tool for cirrhotic patients, further studies need to be conducted to assess its validity before its use can be promoted.

Liver-Specific Scoring Systems

Model for End-Stage Liver Disease (MELD) Score

The MELD score (Box 1) was originally designed as a prognostic tool for patients undergoing insertion of a transjugular intrahepatic portosystemic shunt (TIPSS) [22]. Its use has since been extrapolated into various settings in cirrhotic patients, in particular determination for liver transplantation [23]. The model incorporates bilirubin, creatinine and the international normalized ratio (INR) into a mathematical formula (Box 1) [23]. Cavallazi et al. performed a retrospective study of 441 patients with cirrhosis [24] and determined that each unit increase in MELD score was significantly associated with a higher risk of death ($p<0.001$) and had an AUROC value of 0.77. MELD scores <11 were associated with only 3 % mortality risk, whereas for scores ≥ 11 mortality significantly increased to 28 %. The highest mortality rates were associated with scores of 36–40. The authors surmised that a cut-off value >26 maximized the accuracy of the MELD score for prediction of in-hospital death [24]. Levesque et al., on the other hand, determined a cut-off value of 28.5 as being associated with a significantly higher risk of death, 71.8 % if ≥28.5 versus 21.1 % if <28.5 [14]. Tu et al. compared outcome scoring systems in 202 critically ill cirrhotic patients in Taiwan and found that the MELD score on the first day of admission was statistically significant for prognostication and, therefore, had a good discriminative power [25]. Cholongitas et al. also found the MELD score to have strong discriminative power in their experience of 412 patients admitted to the ICU, with an AUROC of 0.80 [13], and Das et al. reported an AUROC of 0.77 in 152 cirrhotic patients admitted to their medical ICU [1]. Interestingly, in an earlier study, Cholongitas et al. found that a MELD score at 48 hours had better discriminatory power than the score at baseline on admission to the ICU (AUROC 0.86 vs. 0.78) [21].

Box 1

Components for Model for End-Stage Liver Disease (MELD) score calculation

MELD

MELD = 10 {0.957 Ln [Serum creatinine (mg/dl)] + 0.378 Ln [Total bilirubin (mg/dl)] + 1.12 Ln(INR) + 0.643}

MELD-Na

MELD-Na = MELD + 1.59 × (135 – Na) (Max Na value 135, Min Na value 120)

iMELD

iMELD = MELD + (0.3 × age) – (0.7 + Na) + 100

MESO

MESO = MELD/Na (mmol/l) × 10

MELD-Na: MELD-sodium; iMELD: integrated MELD; MESO: MELD to sodium index

MELD-Sodium (MELD-Na) Score

Hyponatremia is frequently associated with cirrhosis. Impaired solute-free water excretion secondary to splanchnic vasodilation and a subsequent reduced circulating volume results in vasopressin release, renal hypoperfusion and reduced glomerular filtration rate (GFR) [26]. This condition is associated with an increase in morbidity and in-hospital mortality, primarily through the development of complications, such as hepatorenal syndrome, ascites, immune compromise and sepsis, and neurological disorders [26]. Serum sodium concentration has also been shown to correlate with survival in cirrhotic patients awaiting liver transplantation [27], and as such several studies have investigated the merits of combining sodium levels with the MELD score to improve prognostication accuracy.

Cavalazzi et al. determined that the MELD-Na score was associated with significantly higher odds of in-hospital death ($p = 0.007$), and AUROC value of 0.77; however it was not superior to the MELD score in predicting in-hospital mortality [24]. Similarly, Cholongitas et al. found no benefit from the combined MELD-Na score (AUROC = 0.8 vs. 0.75) [13]. Various other investigators also reflect these findings [1, 14, 17] (Table 1). The only studies demonstrating superior prognostication with the MELD-Na score were conducted by Jiang et al. who looked at mortality at 3 months, 6 months and 1 year (AUROC = 0.766, 0.738 and 0.714 vs. 0.712, 0.708 and 0.689 for the MELD, respectively) [28], and Choi et al. who found that inclusion of Na in the MELD score improved its performance [29].

Integrated MELD and MELD to Sodium Index

Further mathematical models have been developed based on MELD and MELD-Na. These include the integrated MELD (iMELD) score [30] and the MELD to sodium index (MESO) [31]. These models were compared to MELD and MELD-Na by Jiang et al. who performed a study in 166 patients, comparing the four models with regard to prognostication [28]. At 3 months, 6 months and 1 year, they found that iMELD had the highest AUROC value at 0.841, 0.806 and 0.783, respectively, whereas the MESO AUROC values were 0.723, 0.715 and 0.694, respectively. iMELD and MESO cut-off values were 40 and 1.6, respectively. A MESO index > 1.6 was shown to have a relative risk of 3.32 for mortality ($p < 0.001$). The authors concluded that iMELD was a better prognostic model than the MELD score alone [28].

Child-Pugh Score

The Child-Pugh score (Table 2) comprises five clinical and biological parameters and was originally designed to predict mortality in decompensated liver cirrhosis, where its predictive capabilities are well validated. Lehner et al. determined that the score correlated well for outcome and that with increasing scores, mortality increased [19]: Mortality was 0 % for Child A, 11.76 % for Child B and 44.83 % for Child C ($p < 0.01$). Lim et al. found the Child-Pugh score to be of high prognostic value in patients with sepsis, with an AUROC value of 0.934 with a cut-off value ≥ 10, consistent with Child C cirrhosis ($p < 0.001$) [32]. In contrast, Levesque et al. found that the Child-Pugh score had the lowest AUROC value of all the models they assessed, 0.79, and concluded that this may be due to the score not incorporating other organ dysfunctions known to contribute to mortality in cirrhotic patients [14].

Table 2 Child-Pugh Score

	1	2	3
Bilirubin μmol/l	< 34	34–51	> 51
Albumin g/l	> 35	28–35	< 28
INR	< 1.7	1.7–2.3	> 2.3
Ascites	None	Controlled	Refractory
Hepatic encephalopathy	None	Grade 1–2	Grade 3–4
Score		**Child-Pugh Grade**	
5–6		A	
7–9		B	
10–15		C	

INR: international normalized ratio

The general consensus for the liver specific models is that the Child-Pugh score is inferior to the MELD score for short- and long-term outcome predictions.

Mayo Clinic Model

The Mayo clinic model was developed in 2007 [33] as a predictive tool in postoperative patients. It incorporates the Child-Pugh score, MELD score and the American Society of Anesthesiologists (ASA) physical status classification to quantify postoperative mortality risk. Kim et al. studied the validity of the model in 160 Korean cirrhotic patients and determined that the model was valid with an AUROC value of 0.832, 0.803 and 0.822 for 30-, 90-day and 1 year mortality, respectively, but that it overestimated mortality in the 1-year group [34]. The model is attractive as it incorporates 3 scoring systems but there is a lack of evidence with regard to its prognostic capabilities as it has only been used in the original paper and in a small Korean study.

MBRS Score

The MBRS score (mean arterial pressure [MAP] + bilirubin + respiratory failure + sepsis) was developed in Taiwan by Fang et al. [35] looking at outcome predictors for critically ill cirrhotic patients with acute renal failure. This group looked at 111 cirrhotic patients with acute renal failure and assessed 32 variables as potential independent markers for outcome. Of these, four were identified by multiple logistic regression analysis as being significantly related to mortality, and were assimilated into a new model for prognostication. Interestingly, serum creatinine was not found to be associated with in-hospital mortality. The authors found that the MBRS score had an excellent AUROC value (0.898, $p<0.001$) and had a predicted mortality of >90 % if the score was ≥2. A score of 1 was given if the patient had an MAP<80 mm Hg, serum bilirubin >80 μmol/l (or 4.7 mg/dl), or had respiratory failure or sepsis. The new model was found to have greater discriminatory power than the Child-Pugh score, MELD, APACHE II and III, and SOFA scores. However, this score is limited in its applicability to only those patients who have established renal failure and further studies are required to establish its validity in more heterogeneous populations worldwide.

Alcoholic Hepatitis Scoring Systems

The Glasgow alcoholic hepatitis score (GAHS) was derived by Forrest et al. [36] from five variables found to be independently associated with mortality in alcoholic hepatitis. This scoring system has been validated and found to have far superior specificity and overall accuracy relative to the modified Maddrey discriminant function in predicting 28 and 84 day outcomes. It is equivalent to MELD in predicting 28-day mortality [36]. The variables included in GAHS are patient age, blood urea (mmol/l), peripheral blood white cell count (10^9/l), serum bilirubin (μmol/l), and prothrombin time. The GAHS is calculated as the sum of the scores derived giving a score between 5 and 12. A score of ≥9 was shown to be associated with a 28-day survival of 41 % while a score <9 gave a 28-day survival of 73 % in a subgroup analysis of patients randomized to receive corticosteroid treatment [37]. Alcoholic hepatitis is an increasingly common reason for hospital admission, and patients with severe alcoholic hepatitis are recognized to have a high short-term mortality [37].

The Lille model incorporates age, renal insufficiency, albumin, prothrombin time, bilirubin, and the evolution of bilirubin on day 7 to predict 6-month mortality in patients with severe alcoholic hepatitis who have received corticosteroid therapy [38]. Boursier et al. looked at various prognostic scores for acute alcoholic hepatitis and cirrhosis in alcoholic liver disease patients treated with corticosteroids: Lille score ≥0.45 and GAHS≥9 were the most accurate models for the prediction of mortality [39].

Despite their utility in identifying high-risk patients with alcoholic hepatitis, GAHS and Lille scores have not been assessed as potential prognostic tools for cirrhosis in intensive care settings

Sepsis

Infection is a common complication of cirrhosis as patients are relatively immunocompromized, and thus more susceptible to developing sepsis. Various studies have confirmed that sepsis is associated with an increased risk of mortality, and is an independent predictor of death in its own right. Levesque et al. observed that the presence of infection was associated with poor outcome at 2 months, with a mortality of 68 % at this time compared with 19.2 % for those patients who did not have infection at time of admission to the ICU [14], whereas O'Brien et al. noted that mortality was 65–90 % in cirrhotics with severe sepsis compared to 33–39 % in those without [4]. Lehner et al. performed microbiological analyses in all their patients and detected a mortality of 25 % in the subgroup with no pathogens identified, and 39.5 % in those in whom pathogens were cultured, but interestingly this was not statistically significant in contrast to previous studies [19]. Lim et al. recently conducted a retrospective study of 205 admissions in 153 patients who had confirmed sepsis [32]. They observed an in-hospital mortality of 24.4 %, and identified 4 factors significantly associated with mortality. These factors were the presence of infection at more than one site, pneumonia, Child's C status (AUROC = 0.934) and a MELD score ≥ 17 (AUROC = 0.751). Patients who exhibited < 3 risk factors had a significantly lower risk of mortality than those who had ≥3 risk factors (7 % vs. 91 %). Patients who developed respiratory failure with pneumonia had a higher mortality than those who did not develop respiratory failure (79 vs. 50 %). In addition, a recent meta-analysis revealed a four-fold increase in mortality for patients with cirrhosis and concurrent infection [40]. The most commonly cultured pathogens include methicillin-resistant *Staphylococcus aureus* (MRSA), coagulase negative *Staphylococcus aureus*, *Escherichia coli*, *Klebsiella pneumonia*, *Acinetobacterbaumanii*, and *Pseudomonas aeruginosa* [19, 32].

Liver Disease Severity

There is significant evidence to demonstrate that liver disease severity does not correlate with mortality. This observation is supported by the fact that the general scoring systems appear to be superior prognostic tools compared to the liver specific tools, in particular SOFA and SAPS scores. However, there does appear to be a role for the Child-Pugh and MELD scores, tools traditionally used to define liver disease severity. Their ability to predict outcome may be due to the incorporation of INR, creatinine, albumin and bilirubin into the tools, variables identified as independent predictors of mortality in their own right [1, 14, 24]. On this basis, these scores may, therefore, be acting as organ-failure specific scores [1].

Serum Markers and Other Factors

Several studies have determined the value of serum markers as independent risk factors for mortality. Bilirubin, prothrombin time, activated partial thromboplastin time (aPTT), INR, creatinine, urea, Na and lactate have all been found to have prognostic value [19, 21, 26]. An INR > 1.5 at baseline was shown to be associated with a mortality of 59 % vs. 21.7 % for INR < 1.5 ($p < 0.001$), and creatinine > 1.5 mg/dl at baseline associated with mortality rates of 66.2 % vs. 30.1 % for lower values ($p < 0.001$) in one study [24]. However, creatinine as a measure of renal function may lack clinical applicability in many situations. This is because measurement of serum creatinine is based on the Jaffe reaction by many analyzers and unless an immediate correction is performed it can be underestimated in the context of hyperbilirubinemia [41]. Serum sodium concentration < 130 mmol/l increases the risk of developing complications secondary to cirrhosis and is associated with a significantly higher incidence of ascites, renal failure, encephalopathy and mortality [26]. Serum sodium levels < 135 mmol/l were associated with significantly higher mortality than lower sodium levels (73 % vs. 56 %, $p = 0.043$). When correlated with MAP or arterial pH, mortality rates differed significantly below and above cut-offs of MAP of 80 mm Hg (84.6 % vs. 33.3 %, $p < 0.001$), and pH 7.35 (84.2 % vs. 58.6 %, $p = 0.027$) [26]. However, an AUROC value of 0.728 means that as a single parameter, serum sodium levels demonstrate inferior discriminative capabilities compared to SOFA scores.

Age has also been postulated to be an independent risk factor for mortality. A systematic review of 118 studies looking at prognostication in cirrhotic patients confirmed previous study findings that age is indeed an independent prognostic factor [42]. Das et al. confirmed that age > 50 years was an independent risk factor for in-hospital mortality [1].

Conclusion

Patients with liver cirrhosis are perceived as having an extremely poor prognosis, in particular when associated with MOF and sepsis. The need for accurate prognostic models is, therefore, desired to aid in patient selection and determination of appropriate levels of care either on the ICU or on the ward. However, prognostication in liver failure patients remains difficult. It appears that general prognostic ICU scoring systems are superior to liver-specific models when comparing AUROC values, and that, of these, the SOFA score appears to be the most discriminatory. Specific, organ dysfunction models, such as SOFA, are superior to illness severity scoring systems such as SAPS and APACHE scores. This can be explained by the fact that development of organ dysfunction, and not progression of the underlying liver disease, is the most important independent risk factor for in-hospital mortality. The high mortality associated with 3 or more organ failures, however, should not preclude admission to the ICU, but rather the severity of organ failure is best assessed after 48–72 hours on ICU [1, 14, 15, 21]. What has not been yet assessed is the relevance or otherwise of the precipitant for admission to critical care: Does a variceal bleed carry the same prognostic outlook as sepsis, for example. Use of MELD and Child-Pugh scores alone cannot be considered to be sufficiently accurate to assess prognosis and guide on the decision to admit to the ICU or not, nor on progression over time in the ICU. However, they, with or without a lactate score, may be used in conjunction with SOFA or SAPS scores, and applied in the days following admission when considering the merits of limitations to or withdrawal of treatment [4, 14]. In addition, it is essential that any prognostic scores are calibrated and shown to perform in derivation and validation sets and across various centers, both speciality and non-speciality based.

References

1. Das V, Boelle PY, Galbois A et al (2010) Cirrhotic patients in the medical intensive care unit: early prognosis and long-term survival. Crit Care Med 38:2108–2116
2. Foreman MG, Mannino DM, Moss M (2003) Cirrhosis as a risk factor for sepsis and death: analysis of the National Hospital Discharge Survey. Chest 124:1016–1020
3. Wehler M, Kokoska J, Reulbach U, Hahn EG, Strauss R (2001) Short-term prognosis in critically ill patients with cirrhosis assessed by prognostic scoring systems. Hepatology 34:255–261
4. O'Brien AJ, Welch CA, Singer M, Harrison DA (2012) Prevalence and outcome of cirrhosis patients admitted to UK intensive care: a comparison against dialysis-dependent chronic renal failure patients. Intensive Care Med 38:991–1000
5. Cholongitas E, Senzolo M, Patch D et al (2006) Risk factors, sequential organ failure assessment and model for end-stage liver disease scores for predicting short term mortality in cirrhotic patients admitted to intensive care unit. Aliment Pharmacol Ther 23:883–893
6. Ho YP, Chen YC, Yang C et al (2004) Outcome prediction for critically ill cirrhotic patients: a comparison of APACHE II and Child-Pugh scoring systems. J Intensive Care Med 19:105–110
7. Mackle IJ, Swann DG, Cook B (2006) One year outcome of intensive care patients with decompensated alcoholic liver disease. Br J Anaesth 97:496–498
8. Shawcross DL, Austin MJ, Abeles RD et al (2012) The impact of organ dysfunction in cirrhosis: survival at a cost? J Hepatol 56:1054–1062
9. Review of the Registrar General on deaths by cause, sex and age in England and Wales, 2005. Available at: http://www.ons.gov.uk/ons/rel/vsob1/mortality-statistics-cause-england-and-wales-series-dh2-discontinued-/no-32-2005/index.html Accessed Nov 2012
10. Schuppan D, Afdhal NH (2008) Liver cirrhosis. Lancet 371:838–851
11. Galbois A, Trompette ML, Das V et al (2012) Improvement in the prognosis of cirrhotic patients admitted to an intensive care unit, a retrospective study. Eur J Gastroenterol Hepatol 24:897–904
12. Vincent JL, Moreno R, Takala J et al (1996) The SOFA (Sepsis-related Organ Failure Assessment) score to describe organ dysfunction/failure. On behalf of the Working Group on Sepsis-Related Problems of the European Society of Intensive Care Medicine. Intensive Care Med 22:707–710
13. Cholongitas E, Agarwal B, Antoniadis N, Burroughs AK (2012) Patients with cirrhosis admitted to an intensive care unit. J Hepatol 57:230–231
14. Levesque E, Hoti E, Azoulay D et al (2012) Prospective evaluation of the prognostic scores for cirrhotic patients admitted to an intensive care unit. J Hepatol 56:95–102
15. Ferreira FL, Bota DP, Bross A, Melot C, Vincent JL (2001) Serial evaluation of the SOFA score to predict outcome in critically ill patients. JAMA 286:1754–1758
16. Wong CS, Lee WC, Jenq CC et al (2010) Scoring short-term mortality after liver transplantation. Liver Transpl 16:138–146
17. Craig DG, Zafar S, Reid TW et al (2012) The sequential organ failure assessment (SOFA) score is an effective triage marker following staggered paracetamol (acetaminophen) overdose. Aliment Pharmacol Ther 35:1408–1415

18. Le Gall JR, Lemeshow S, Saulnier F (1993) A new Simplified Acute Physiology Score (SAPS II) based on a European/North American multicenter study. JAMA 270:2957–2963
19. Lehner S, Stemmler HJ, Muck A, Braess J, Parhofer KG (2010) Prognostic parameters and risk stratification in intensive care patients with severe liver diseases. J Gastrointestin Liver Dis 19:399–404
20. Knaus WA, Draper EA, Wagner DP, Zimmerman JE (1985) APACHE II: a severity of disease classification system. Crit Care Med 13:818–829
21. Cholongitas E, Betrosian A, Senzolo M et al (2008) Prognostic models in cirrhotics admitted to intensive care units better predict outcome when assessed at 48 h after admission. J Gastroenterol Hepatol 23:1223–1227
22. Malinchoc M, Kamath PS, Gordon FD, Peine CJ, Rank J, ter Borg PC (2000) A model to predict poor survival in patients undergoing transjugular intrahepatic portosystemic shunts. Hepatology 31:864–871
23. Kamath PS, Wiesner RH, Malinchoc M et al (2001) A model to predict survival in patients with end-stage liver disease. Hepatology 33:464–470
24. Cavallazzi R, Awe OO, Vasu TS et al (2012) Model for End-Stage Liver Disease score for predicting outcome in critically ill medical patients with liver cirrhosis. J Crit Care 27:424
25. Tu KH, Jenq CC, Tsai MH et al (2011) Outcome scoring systems for short-term prognosis in critically ill cirrhotic patients. Shock 36:445–450
26. Jenq CC, Tsai MH, Tian YC et al (2010) Serum sodium predicts prognosis in critically ill cirrhotic patients. J Clin Gastroenterol 44:220–226
27. Kim WR, Biggins SW, Kremers WK et al (2008) Hyponatremia and mortality among patients on the liver-transplant waiting list. N Engl J Med 359:1018–1026
28. Jiang M, Liu F, Xiong WJ, Zhong L, Chen XM (2008) Comparison of four models for end-stage liver disease in evaluating the prognosis of cirrhosis. World J Gastroenterol 14:6546–6550
29. Choi PC, Kim HJ, Choi WH et al (2009) Model for end-stage liver disease, model for end-stage liver disease-sodium and Child-Turcotte-Pugh scores over time for the prediction of complications of liver cirrhosis. Liver Int 29:221–226
30. Luca A, Angermayr B, Bertolini G et al (2007) An integrated MELD model including serum sodium and age improves the prediction of early mortality in patients with cirrhosis. Liver Transpl 13:1174–1180
31. Huo TI, Wang YW, Yang YY et al (2007) Model for end-stage liver disease score to serum sodium ratio index as a prognostic predictor and its correlation with portal pressure in patients with liver cirrhosis. Liver Int 27:498–506
32. Lim LG, Tan XX, Woo SJ et al (2011) Risk factors for mortality in cirrhotic patients with sepsis. Hepatol Int 5:800–807
33. Teh SH, Nagorney DM, Stevens SR et al (2007) Risk factors for mortality after surgery in patients with cirrhosis. Gastroenterology 132:1261–1269
34. Kim SY, Yim HJ, Park SM et al (2011) Validation of a Mayo post-operative mortality risk prediction model in Korean cirrhotic patients. Liver Int 31:222–228
35. Fang JT, Tsai MH, Tian YC et al (2008) Outcome predictors and new score of critically ill cirrhotic patients with acute renal failure. Nephrol Dial Transplant 23:1961–1969
36. Forrest EH, Evans CD, Stewart S et al (2005) Analysis of factors predictive of mortality in alcoholic hepatitis and derivation and validation of the Glasgow alcoholic hepatitis score. Gut 54:1174–1179
37. Forrest EH, Morris AJ, Stewart S et al (2007) The Glasgow alcoholic hepatitis score identifies patients who may benefit from corticosteroids. Gut 56:1743–1746
38. Louvet A, Naveau S, Abdelnour M et al (2007) The Lille model: a new tool for therapeutic strategy in patients with severe alcoholic hepatitis treated with steroids. Hepatology 45:1348–1354
39. Boursier J, Demy M, Moal V (2008) Prediction of outcomes in patients with severe acute alcoholic hepatitis treated by corticosteroids. Hepatology 48:S636A (abst)

40. Arvaniti V, D'Amico G, Fede G et al (2010) Infections in patients with cirrhosis increase mortality four-fold and should be used in determining prognosis. Gastroenterology 139:1246–1256
41. Lolekha PH, Sritong N (1994) Comparison of techniques for minimizing interference of bilirubin on serum creatinine determined by the kinetic Jaffe reaction. J Clin Lab Annal 8:391–399
42. D'Amico G, Garcia-Tsao G, Pagliaro L (2006) Natural history and prognostic indicators of survival in cirrhosis: a systematic review of 118 studies. J Hepatol 44:217–231

Delayed Neuroprognostication After Cardiac Arrest and Temperature Management

T. Cronberg, J. Horn, and N. Nielsen

Introduction

The majority of patients who reach the intensive care unit (ICU) following a cardiac arrest are unconscious. For the comatose cardiac arrest survivor, the chances for a good neurological recovery diminish with time after return of spontaneous circulation (ROSC). Neurological assessment is usually performed within days after cardiac arrest as a foundation for decisions concerning limitation of care and interventions. The clinical neurological examination is central in prognostication and is usually combined with neurophysiological, neuroradiological and occasionally biochemical investigations to estimate the extent of permanent brain injury. The predictive values of the different methods have been investigated in numerous trials and incorporated into clinical guidelines [1–3].

Treatment with mild hypothermia has been widely implemented as a neuroprotective strategy for cardiac arrest survivors, but may alter the recovery pattern and the predictive value of prognostic markers. Current guidelines do not provide specific instructions on how to evaluate hypothermia-treated patients but recommend delayed prognostication [3] based on multiple instruments [1]. As a poor prognosis statement usually results in withdrawal of supportive treatment and, subsequently, death of the patient, the method for prognostication clearly has the power to affect the outcome of clinical trials in comatose cardiac arrest survivors.

T. Cronberg
Department of Neurology, Skåne University Hospital, Lund, Sweden

J. Horn
Department of Intensive Care, Academic Medical Center, Amsterdam, The Netherlands

N. Nielsen (✉)
Department of Anesthesia and Intensive Care, Helsingborg University Hospital, Helsingborgs lasarett, 25187, Helsingborg, Sweden
E-mail: niklas.nielsen@telia.com

J.-L. Vincent (Ed.), *Annual Update in Intensive Care and Emergency Medicine 2013*,
DOI 10.1007/978-3-642-35109-9_68, © Springer-Verlag Berlin Heidelberg 2013

This is particularly relevant when blinding is difficult, as with different temperature regimes.

In this review, we discuss how mild hypothermia may affect neuroprognostication, how this issue was dealt with in previous trials of cardiac arrest, and finally we present a novel model for delayed neurological prognostication applied in a large ongoing trial on target temperature management after cardiac arrest, the Target Temperature Management after Out-of-Hospital Cardiac Arrest Trial (TTM)-trial (NCT01020916).

Cardiac Arrest

Out-of-hospital cardiac arrest is a common cause of mortality and morbidity in the western world and in Europe it has an annual incidence of 38 cases per 100,000 inhabitants [4]. Although increased survival from all-rhythm out-of-hospital cardiac arrest has been reported in several studies [5, 6], mortality is still approximately 90 % for the whole group and at least 50 % following hospital admission [7, 8]. Because of a high metabolic ratio and very limited energy reserves, the brain is particularly vulnerable to circulatory arrest and ischemic damage occurs after only a few minutes. Consequently, brain injury accounts for two-thirds of all deaths after admission to the ICU following out-of-hospital cardiac arrest [9] and the majority of survivors suffer some degree of cognitive impairment [10].

Mild Hypothermia

Mild hypothermia to 33 °C has a robust neuroprotective effect in animal models of global ischemia [11]. Following one randomized [12] and one quasi-randomized clinical trial [13] hypothermic treatment has been included in international guidelines as a recommended therapy for patients in coma after cardiac arrest [1]. However, a systematic review of previous trials concluded that the evidence in favor of hypothermia is weak and that earlier trials were associated with substantial risk of potential systematic as well as random error [14].

Neuroprognostication After Cardiac Arrest

A global ischemic brain injury following cardiac arrest manifests itself as persisting coma, myoclonic seizures and loss of brain stem reflexes. Patients who improve their level of consciousness after withdrawal of sedative and analgesic substances usually have a good outcome [15]. For those who remain in coma, the prognosis becomes gradually worse with increasing time from cardiac arrest. Recovery of brain-stem functions, such as the pupillary light reflex, corneal reflex and spontaneous breathing usually occurs during the first days after cardiac arrest. This effect is also found in the majority of severely injured patients. Therefore, bilateral lack of pupillary light reflexes or corneal reflexes has a high specificity but low sensitivity for the prediction of a poor prognosis at 72 hours after cardiac arrest [16, 17]. A complete loss of brain stem functions on the other hand might signal complete brain infarction and brain death [18].

Neurological prognostication is usually based on repeated clinical neurological examinations and electrophysiological investigations (electroencephalography [EEG] and somatosensory-evoked potentials [SSEP]). It may be further supported by neuroradiological examinations (computed tomography [CT] and magnetic resonance imaging [MRI]) and biomarkers (neuron specific enolase [NSE] in particular) but the evidence for these methods is less solid [1, 2]. Because the specificity of clinical and neurophysiological findings increases with time, a well-founded judgment of prognosis can usually be made at 72 hours after cardiac arrest in a patient who has not been treated with hypothermia [2, 16]. Hypothermic therapy has been found to make a clinical neurological examination less reliable [19–21], possibly related to increased use [18] and decreased clearance [22] of sedative medication. Delayed neuroprognostication has, therefore, been recommended in patients treated with hypothermia [3].

SSEPs are less sensitive to sedative medication than are EEGs and a bilateral loss of the cortical N20-potential at 24 hours or more after cardiac arrest, predicts a poor outcome with a very high accuracy [17, 23]. The high specificity of SSEP appears to be retained for hypothermia-treated patients if the examination is performed after rewarming, but sporadic false predictions have been reported with SSEP performed during hypothermia [20], and even after rewarming [24]. Furthermore, interobserver variability in the interpretation of SSEPs has been reported [25].

Severely pathological EEG-patterns, including burst-suppression, generalized status epilepticus and α-coma, are associated with a poor prognosis after cardiac arrest. The EEG-pattern is very sensitive to sedative medication and false predictions may therefore occur [2]. The prognostic implications of the supposedly pathological EEG-patterns are not fully known. Specifically, the occurrence of postanoxic status epilepticus has been reported in some patients with good outcome following hypothermia-treated cardiac arrest [26].

Status myoclonus, i. e., generalized myoclonic seizures for more than 30 minutes and usually occurring in facial and axial limb musculature, has been considered a reliable predictor of a poor prognosis if it occurs within 24 hours after cardiac arrest of a primary cardiac origin [27]. After the introduction of hypothermia, survival with good outcome despite early status myoclonus has been reported [28]. A small fraction of cardiac arrest patients develop a total brain infarction with massive edema leading to herniation and may be diagnosed as brain dead [18]. The accuracy of clinical tests to diagnose brain death in cardiac arrest survivors treated with hypothermia has recently been questioned [29].

Neuroprognostication and Outcome of Clinical Trials

The neurological assessment of prognosis following cardiac arrest is critical for outcome because a 'poor-prognosis-statement' often leads to withdrawal of life-sustaining treatment and death of the patient. Early prognostication after hypothermia-treated cardiac arrest is associated with a high rate of false predictions of poor outcome [30]. It has recently been suggested that prognostication that is performed too early may have introduced bias into clinical trials of neuroprotective strategies after cardiac arrest and, thus, may have led to negative results, because a delayed recovery process may have been missed [31].

Neuroprognostication in Previous Cardiac Arrest Trials

The Brain Resuscitation after Cardiac Arrest Trial (BRCT) 1 [32] and BRCT II [33] studies were conducted prior to the introduction of hypothermia and included comatose adult cardiac arrest patients. BRCT I studied the effects of thiopentone and BRCT II the experimental calcium entry-blocker, lidoflazine. The reports of both studies do not describe any rules for treatment decisions in patients who remained in coma due to severe brain injury. In 1994, Edgren et al. [16] used the 262 patients from the BRCT I study to investigate whether it was possible to reliably predict a permanent vegetative state a few days after cardiac arrest. Variation in treatment of patients who remained in coma existed in this group, as the authors report in the results: "For ethical and economic reasons it was not possible to require indefinite intensive care in the protocol, and local variations in decision making were permitted. Although most patients were given unlimited therapy, some in the Scandinavian centers were changed to intermediate care as early as 2–5 days after cardiac arrest." No further details on treatment limitation or withdrawal were reported.

In 2002, the Hypothermia after Cardiac Arrest (HACA) [12] group and Bernard et al. [13] reported on the positive effects of treatment with hypothermia after cardiac arrest. After enrolment of 275 patients, the HACA study stopped inclusion because of a lower than expected inclusion rate. Of the included patients, 132 died during follow-up. In the manuscript on this study, nothing is described on how decisions on treatment limitations or withdrawal were made. In the Bernard study, active life support was withdrawn from most patients who remained deeply comatose at 72 hours. Patients with an uncertain prognosis underwent tracheostomy and were discharged from the ICU. Of the 84 included patients, 45 died during follow-up. The cause of death was cardiac failure in nine, brain-death was diagnosed in both groups in one patient. The remaining deaths (34) resulted from severe neurologic injury and withdrawal of all active therapy. In the discussion, the authors state "this was always a consensus decision of the treating medical and nursing staff, made in consultation with the family of the patient". Which diagnostic methods were used and how the results of these tests were weighed in treatment decisions is not described.

More recently, a pilot study on the effect of high dose erythropoietin was reported [34]. Nothing is reported about treatment decisions and prognostication in this study. The protocol of the currently ongoing phase III study (clinicaltrials.gov identifier NCT00999583) is not clear about the diagnostics used for prognostication and rules for limitation or withdrawal of treatment.

Is There an Optimal Time-Point for Neuroprognostication After Cardiac Arrest?

Before the introduction of hypothermia as a treatment strategy, relatively strong evidence supported the 72 hour time-point after cardiac arrest as a reasonable moment for prognostication [2, 16]. By this time, the majority of patients with a favorable prognosis will have woken and the risk of a false prediction from clinical findings (absent or extensor motor response to pain, bilaterally absent pupillary or corneal reflexes) or test results (absence of N20-potential on SSEP) will be minimal. Hypothermia appears to have effects on the reliability of the clinical neurological examination and possibly other methods of neuroprognostication as well. Whether this is a result of an altered recovery process or a protracted effect of sedative drugs is not clear. Evidence from further studies will, therefore, need to accumulate until a new algorithm for prognostication after hypothermia-treated cardiac arrest can be formulated.

When therapeutic hypothermia for cardiac arrest was introduced at the Skane University Hospital in Lund (2003), decisions were made to postpone neurological prognostication for patients who remain in coma until 72 h after rewarming to account for a possibly delayed recovery process. In a report of this strategy, 52 % of hypothermia-treated patients awoke before prognostication, 17 % died early and 31 % were still in coma 72 h after rewarming (4.5 days after cardiac arrest) [35]. Only 6/34 patients who were in coma at prognostication awoke at some time-point and 28/34 remained in coma until death. In the majority of the deceased patients, clinical, neurophysiological, biochemical (NSE) and neuroradiological findings supported a massive brain injury and this was confirmed by post-mortem examinations. However, a sub-group of 8/34 patients with low-range NSE ($\leq$20 μg/l) was identified. All examined patients had normal MRI (5/8) and normal SSEPs (6/8). All had a generalized status epilepticus pattern on EEG and a lack of motor or extensor response to pain. Only one patient recovered and with a neurological handicap (Cerebral Performance Category [CPC] 3). Whether more active treatment would benefit the sub-group of cardiac arrest patients with status epilepticus has never been tested in clinical trials, but several authors have reported a prolonged recovery-phase with subsequent good outcome [36, 37], which is in accordance with our own recent experience of four patients (T. Cronberg, unpublished observations).

From a clinical trial perspective, the ideal would be to refrain from prognostication and await the natural course of the postanoxic encephalopathy. However, this approach has practical and ethical limitations. When prognostication is done at 72 hours after rewarming, i. e., 4 to 5 days after cardiac arrest, almost all patients breathe spontaneously after withdrawal of supportive care and extubation. These patients usually die during the following 1–2 weeks, mainly due to respiratory complications (I Dragancea, personal communication). If a high level of care is maintained and no treatment limitations are implemented, the majority of patients who remain in coma up to several days can be expected to end up in a persistent vegetative state.

Given the uncertainty about the optimal moment after cardiac arrest for prognostication and the serious consequences if the window of opportunity for withdrawal of care is missed, the time-point of prognostication in a modern cardiac arrest-trial needs to be conservative enough to allow recovery of patients and strict enough to avoid unnecessary resource utilization and possible suffering.

The Target Temperature Management Trial

In an attempt to better investigate the optimal target temperature management strategy for comatose survivors after cardiac arrest, the TTM-trial was launched in November 2010. In the trial, outcomes of survival, neurological function and safety are compared for two strict target temperatures of 33 °C and 36 °C for 24 hours after return of spontaneous circulation, with a minimum follow up of 180 days. The sample size will be 850 to 950 patients with cardiac arrest of presumed cardiac origin and according to current inclusion rates, the trial will be finished mid-2013. The aims when designing the TTM-trial were to investigate temperature management in a sufficiently large and general population with two temperature regimes both avoiding fever and where possible sources of bias would be minimized. A standardized and transparent protocol for prognostication and withdrawal of life sustaining treatment was regarded as one of the key components of a low-risk-of-bias trial.

Neuroprognostication in the TTM-Trial

The principles of neurological prognostication for patients enrolled in the TTM-trial have been protocolized [38]. A manual is available and investigators have been instructed concerning principles of prognostication at investigator meetings. The following overruling principles have been adopted:

1. The person who performs the prognostication has to be blinded to the intervention.
2. All patients have to be regarded as if they were treated with hypothermia to 33 °C.
3. Rules for prognostication are to be conservative.

As a general principle, all patients in the trial will be actively treated until 72 hours after the end of the intervention period/rewarming. Neurological prognostication is performed at this time-point or later for all patients who remain unconscious. Earlier prognostication is indicated if: (1) the patient becomes brain dead; (2) the patient has an early myoclonus status; or (3) if there are strong ethical reasons to withdraw intensive care.

In the study protocol, it is defined that: "the neurological evaluation will be based on a clinical neurological examination (including Glasgow Coma Scale [GCS] motor score, pupillary and corneal reflexes), median nerve SSEP and EEG". A conventional EEG is performed in all unconscious patients 12–36 h after rewarming and SSEP at 48–72 h after rewarming at centers where this technique is available. In addition, information from neuroimaging (MRI and CT) may be used but cannot constitute the sole reason for withdrawal of intensive care. Biochemical markers for brain damage should not be used for prognostication for patients included in the TTM-trial. Instead a biobank is collected for later analyses.

One of the following recommendations should be made by the physician performing prognostication:

- Continue active intensive care
- Do not escalate intensive care
- Withdraw intensive care

Findings allowing for discontinuation of life support have been specified in the protocol (Box 1). In the case-record-form, findings from all examinations, recommendations and decisions are recorded.

Box 1

Findings allowing for discontinuation of life support in the Target Temperature Management after Out-of-Hospital Cardiac Arrest Trial (TTM)-trial

1. Brain death.
2. Early myoclonus status# (<24 h from sustained return of spontaneous circulation) and bilateral absence of N20 peak on somatosensory-evoked potential (SSEP) after rewarming.
3. Seventy-two hours after rewarming: Glasgow Coma Scale-motor (GCS-M) score 1–2 and bilateral absence of N20 peak on SSEP performed 48–72 hours after rewarming, or later.
4. Seventy-two hours after end of intervention period: Treatment refractory status epilepticus* and GCS-M 1–2.

Generalized myoclonic seizures in face and extremities and continuous for a minimum of 30 min.

* Status epilepticus defined by electroencephalogram (EEG) as sequences (> 10 s) of repetitive epileptiform discharges with an amplitude > 50 μV and a medium frequency ≥ 1 Hz,

constituting >50 % of a 30 minute period in a patient with or without clinical manifestations. Treatment refractory, defined as unresponsive to treatment with propofol, midazolam or thiopental for at least 24 h in combination with at least one intravenous antiepileptic substance (including valproate and/or fos-phenytoin) in adequate dose for at least 24 h. Free use of further antiepileptic substances and combinations at the discretion of the attending physician.

Rationale for Prognostication in the TTM-Trial

Despite international and national guidelines, the practice of neurological prognostication and withdrawal of life support varies considerably and may often adhere poorly to recommendations [30, 39]. By strictly regulating the time for prognostication and criteria allowing for withdrawal of life support we aimed to avoid false and premature predictions. The majority of patients with a favorable prognosis will wake up during the first three days after cardiac arrest [16] and we decided to postpone prognostication an extra 1.5 days to account for the effects of sedation during cooling and a possible delay in the recovery process by hypothermia. Recently published studies have showed that although awakening itself may not actually be delayed by hypothermia [40], effects of sedation probably explain why clinical examination at 72 h after the arrest is less reliable after hypothermia-treated cardiac arrest [18]. Clinical examinations may still be unreliable at 4.5 days after cardiac arrest and data supporting this time-point are admittedly scarce. Therefore, an extensor or absent motor response to pain at 4.5 days must be combined with absent SSEPs or treatment refractory status epilepticus to allow for withdrawal of life sustaining treatment in the TTM-trial and, if any of these two conditions, is not fulfilled, at least an extra day of observation is demanded.

We have defined minimal therapeutic efforts to define status epilepticus treatment as refractory, but we recognize that there may be potential for recovery in some patients if more aggressive treatment and/or a longer observation time are allowed. Clearly, this is an area where more knowledge is urgently needed. Moreover, the TTM-protocol defines when withdrawal of life sustaining treatment is allowed but the decisions are made by the treating physician and continued intensive care is always an option.

Most intensivists would consider it unethical to continue intensive care in a patient with generalized myoclonus after cardiac arrest, but false predictions may occur from status myoclonus both with and without hypothermia [28]. To solve this dilemma, we combined early myoclonus status with another strong predictor, SSEP, and allowed for SSEP to be performed earlier in patients with status myoclonus, immediately after rewarming. Early prognostication is also allowed for the small fraction of patients who become brain-dead and they should be diagnosed according to national legislation. However, we recommend that the clinical diagnosis of brain death should be avoided during the first 24 hours after resuscitation and that radiological evidence of herniation and loss of intracerebral blood flow is sought when there is any doubt about the diagnosis to avoid misdiagnosis [29]. Finally, strong ethical reasons for early withdrawal of care may include generalized malignant disease or a clearly stated wish not to be resuscitated. Such reasons may become evident only after the patient has arrived in the ICU.

Several recently published reviews deal with the issue of neuroprognostication after cardiac arrest in the era of hypothermia treatment [41–43] and detail the reliability of individual prognostic instruments. From the large amounts of comparative data in the TTM-trial, we will be able to learn how different prognostic instruments are affected by cooling. Until we learn more, it is the authors' opinion that a reasonable clinical praxis is to delay prognostication and to avoid decisions to withdraw care based solely on clinical findings and use the model outlined in Box 1. In our experience, such an approach has not resulted in patients with chronic vegetative state [35].

Conclusion

Timing of neuroprognostication and decisions on further life-sustaining therapies are crucial for outcome after cardiac arrest. Hypothermia and concomitant sedation make a clinical neurological examination less reliable even at 72 h after cardiac arrest. We therefore recommend postponing neuroprognostication further until at least 72 h after rewarming and in the proposed model a liberal use of adjunctive methods to support a decision on withdrawal of intensive care is advocated. In the model, the EEG has a central role to diagnose and adequately treat status epilepticus, while SSEP may be used to allow for earlier withdrawal in patients with status myoclonus or confirm poor prognosis at 72 h after rewarming. Neuroimaging is not a part of the model other than to give further support for a clinical diagnosis of brain-death. The role of biomarkers for neuroprognostication after cardiac arrest is currently unclear but a large biobank is being created within the TTM trial. In future cardiac arrest trials, it is imperative to protocolize timing and methods for prognostication to avoid possible bias and imbalances among study groups.

References

1. Deakin CD, Nolan JP, Soar J et al (2010) European Resuscitation Council Guidelines for Resuscitation 2010 Section 4. Adult advanced life support. Resuscitation 81:1305–1352
2. Wijdicks EF, Hijdra A, Young GB, Bassetti CL, Wiebe S (2006) Practice parameter: prediction of outcome in comatose survivors after cardiopulmonary resuscitation (an evidence-based review): report of the Quality Standards Subcommittee of the American Academy of Neurology. Neurology 67:203–210
3. Peberdy MA, Callaway CW, Neumar RW et al (2010) Part 9: post-cardiac arrest care: 2010 American Heart Association Guidelines for Cardiopulmonary Resuscitation and Emergency Cardiovascular Care. Circulation 122:S768–S786

4. Atwood C, Eisenberg MS, Herlitz J, Rea TD (2005) Incidence of EMS-treated out-of-hospital cardiac arrest in Europe. Resuscitation 67:75–80
5. Adielsson A, Hollenberg J, Karlsson T et al (2011) Increase in survival and bystander CPR in out-of-hospital shockable arrhythmia: bystander CPR and female gender are predictors of improved outcome. Experiences from Sweden in an 18-year perspective. Heart 97:1391–1396
6. Lund-Kordahl I, Olasveengen TM, Lorem T, Samdal M, Wik L, Sunde K (2010) Improving outcome after out-of-hospital cardiac arrest by strengthening weak links of the local Chain of Survival; quality of advanced life support and post-resuscitation care. Resuscitation 81:422–426
7. Herlitz J, Engdahl J, Svensson L, Angquist KA, Silfverstolpe J, Holmberg S (2006) Major differences in 1-month survival between hospitals in Sweden among initial survivors of out-of-hospital cardiac arrest. Resuscitation 70:404–409
8. Langhelle A, Tyvold SS, Lexow K, Hapnes SA, Sunde K, Steen PA (2003) In-hospital factors associated with improved outcome after out-of-hospital cardiac arrest. A comparison between four regions in Norway. Resuscitation 56:247–263
9. Laver S, Farrow C, Turner D, Nolan J (2004) Mode of death after admission to an intensive care unit following cardiac arrest. Intensive Care Med 30:2126–2128
10. Cronberg T, Lilja G, Rundgren M, Friberg H, Widner H (2009) Long-term neurological outcome after cardiac arrest and therapeutic hypothermia. Resuscitation 80:1119–1123
11. Che D, Li L, Kopil CM, Liu Z, Guo W, Neumar RW (2011) Impact of therapeutic hypothermia onset and duration on survival, neurologic function, and neurodegeneration after cardiac arrest. Crit Care Med 39:1423–1430
12. The Hypothermia after Cardiac Arrest Study Group (2002) Mild therapeutic hypothermia to improve the neurologic outcome after cardiac arrest. N Engl J Med 346:549–556
13. Bernard SA, Gray TW, Buist MD et al (2002) Treatment of comatose survivors of out-of-hospital cardiac arrest with induced hypothermia. N Engl J Med 346:557–563
14. Nielsen N, Friberg H, Gluud C, Herlitz J, Wetterslev J (2011) Hypothermia after cardiac arrest should be further evaluated – A systematic review of randomised trials with meta-analysis and trial sequential analysis. Int J Cardiol 151:333–341
15. Schefold JC, Storm C, Kruger A, Ploner CJ, Hasper D (2009) The Glasgow Coma Score is a predictor of good outcome in cardiac arrest patients treated with therapeutic hypothermia. Resuscitation 80:658–661
16. Edgren E, Hedstrand U, Kelsey S, Sutton-Tyrrell K, Safar P (1994) Assessment of neurological prognosis in comatose survivors of cardiac arrest. BRCT I Study Group. Lancet 343:1055–1059
17. Zandbergen EG, Hijdra A, Koelman JH et al (2006) Prediction of poor outcome within the first 3 days of postanoxic coma. Neurology 66:62–68
18. Samaniego EA, Mlynash M, Caulfield AF, Eyngorn I, Wijman CA (2011) Sedation confounds outcome prediction in cardiac arrest survivors treated with hypothermia. Neurocrit Care 15:113–119
19. Al Thenayan E, Savard M, Sharpe M, Norton L, Young B (2008) Predictors of poor neurologic outcome after induced mild hypothermia following cardiac arrest. Neurology 71:1535–1537
20. Bouwes A, Binnekade JM, Kuiper MA et al (2012) Prognosis of coma after therapeutic hypothermia: A prospective cohort study. Ann Neurol 71:206–212
21. Rossetti AO, Oddo M, Logroscino G, Kaplan PW (2010) Prognostication after cardiac arrest and hypothermia: a prospective study. Ann Neurol 67:301–307
22. Tortorici MA, Kochanek PM, Poloyac SM (2007) Effects of hypothermia on drug disposition, metabolism, and response: A focus of hypothermia-mediated alterations on the cytochrome P450 enzyme system. Crit Care Med 35:2196–2204
23. Zandbergen EG, de Haan RJ, Stoutenbeek CP, Koelman JH, Hijdra A (1998) Systematic review of early prediction of poor outcome in anoxic-ischaemic coma. Lancet 352:1808–1812

24. Leithner C, Ploner CJ, Hasper D, Storm C (2010) Does hypothermia influence the predictive value of bilateral absent N20 after cardiac arrest? Neurology 74:965–969
25. Zandbergen EG, Hijdra A, de Haan RJ et al (2006) Interobserver variation in the interpretation of SSEPs in anoxic-ischaemic coma. Clin Neurophysiol 117:1529–1535
26. Rossetti AO, Oddo M, Liaudet L, Kaplan PW (2009) Predictors of awakening from postanoxic status epilepticus after therapeutic hypothermia. Neurology 72:744–749
27. Wijdicks EF, Parisi JE, Sharbrough FW (1994) Prognostic value of myoclonus status in comatose survivors of cardiac arrest. Ann Neurol 35:239–243
28. Lucas JM, Cocchi MN, Salciccioli J et al (2012) Neurologic recovery after therapeutic hypothermia in patients with post-cardiac arrest myoclonus. Resuscitation 83:265–269
29. Webb AC, Samuels OB (2011) Reversible brain death after cardiopulmonary arrest and induced hypothermia. Crit Care Med 39:1538–1542
30. Perman SM, Kirkpatrick JN, Reitsma AM et al (2012) Timing of neuroprognostication in postcardiac arrest therapeutic hypothermia. Crit Care Med 40:719–724
31. Geocadin RG, Peberdy MA, Lazar RM (2012) Poor survival after cardiac arrest resuscitation: a self-fulfilling prophecy or biologic destiny? Crit Care Med 40:979–980
32. Brain Resuscitation Clinical Trial I Study Group (1986) Randomized clinical study of thiopental loading in comatose survivors of cardiac arrest. N Engl J Med 314:397–403
33. Brain Resuscitation Clinical Trial II Study Group (1991) A randomized clinical study of a calcium-entry blocker (lidoflazine) in the treatment of comatose survivors of cardiac arrest. N Engl J Med 324:1225–1231
34. Cariou A, Claessens YE, Pene F et al (2008) Early high-dose erythropoietin therapy and hypothermia after out-of-hospital cardiac arrest: a matched control study. Resuscitation 76:397–404
35. Cronberg T, Rundgren M, Westhall E et al (2011) Neuron-specific enolase correlates with other prognostic markers after cardiac arrest. Neurology 77:623–630
36. Hovland A, Nielsen EW, Kluver J, Salvesen R (2006) EEG should be performed during induced hypothermia. Resuscitation 68:143–146
37. Sunde K, Dunlop O, Rostrup M, Sandberg M, Sjoholm H, Jacobsen D (2006) Determination of prognosis after cardiac arrest may be more difficult after introduction of therapeutic hypothermia. Resuscitation 69:29–32
38. Nielsen N, Wetterslev J, Al-Subaie N et al (2012) Target temperature management after out-of-hospital cardiac arrest – a randomized, parallel-group, assessor-blinded clinical trial-rationale and design. Am Heart J 163:541–548
39. Busch M, Soreide E (2008) Prognostication after out-of-hospital cardiac arrest, a clinical survey. Scand J Trauma Resusc Emerg Med 16:9
40. Fugate JE, Wijdicks EF, White RD, Rabinstein AA (2011) Does therapeutic hypothermia affect time to awakening in cardiac arrest survivors? Neurology 77:1346–1350
41. Blondin NA, Greer DM (2011) Neurologic prognosis in cardiac arrest patients treated with therapeutic hypothermia. Neurologist 17:241–248
42. Friberg H, Rundgren M, Westhall E, Nielsen N, Cronberg T (2013) Continuous evaluation of neurological prognosis after cardiac arrest. Acta Anaesthesiol Scand 57:6–15
43. Oddo M, Rossetti AO (2011) Predicting neurological outcome after cardiac arrest. Curr Opin Crit Care 17:254–259

Burn Trauma in the Elderly: Treating those with a Chance

O. Jeanjaquet, Y. A. Que, and M. M. Berger

Introduction

The characteristics of critically ill burned patients follow the same trends as the general intensive care unit (ICU) patient population. The age of patients requiring ICU admission has increased in parallel with increased life expectancy in Western countries, and the mean age of patients in the ICU is now often close to 65 years. Age impacts on mortality rates after burn trauma: Already after 60 years, the risk of death increases, even with small burns [1]. Several factors explain this increased risk of death: Lower wound healing capacity [2], increased susceptibility to infections and metabolic complications, and the increased likelihood of suffering from multiple comorbidities, such as alterations in vital organ function. Moreover, in this 'frail' population, the likelihood of trauma increases, as shown by the WHO statistics [3]. Not only are the elderly more likely to die in residential fires because of their frequently limited mobility, they are also more likely to succumb to thermal injury complications. In US burn centers during the decade 1999–2008, in-hospital mortality was 9 % for the seventh decade of life, 16 % for the eighth, and 25 % for those over 80 years old compared to the 3 % mortality rates for adults from 20 to 50 years of age [4]. In addition, the elderly are at higher risk of death after burns because they suffer larger burns. For example, although two-thirds of

O. Jeanjaquet
Medical School, UNIL, Lausanne, Switzerland

Y. A. Que
Service of Adult Intensive Care Medicine & Burns, University Hospital (CHUV) & UNIL, Lausanne, Switzerland

M. M. Berger (✉)
Service of Adult Intensive Care Medicine & Burns, University Hospital (CHUV) & UNIL, Lausanne, Switzerland
E-mail: Mette.Berger@chuv.ch

J.-L. Vincent (Ed.), *Annual Update in Intensive Care and Emergency Medicine 2013*,
DOI 10.1007/978-3-642-35109-9_69,

children under age two are hospitalized for treatment of burns affecting less than 10 % of their body surface area (BSA), nearly 60 % of the elderly over 60 years of age are hospitalized for burns greater than 10 % BSA [4].

Elderly burn trauma patient also experience increased morbidity, which is not restricted to physical damage. Survivors often suffer psychological and physical sequelae that are severe enough to cause permanent disability [5]. At the time of the burn injury, all patients experience shock, pain and anxiety that translate into an increased incidence of confusion and delirium states. The overwhelming emotional trauma may cause withdrawal, loss of interest in food and activity, and further limits movement. This lack of activity in turn exacerbates the speed at which the healing burn wound causes wound contractures to occur, and heightens the survivor's disability. After burn scalds, only 10 % of elderly patients are able to return home alone [6].

In some cases, it is obvious from the severity of the initial injury and condition that the patient will not be able to survive the burn marathon: In these cases, additional criteria are not needed to institute palliative care. As in other age categories, progress in critical care has increased survival rates in the early phase of burn trauma. At the same time, studies show that the likelihood that these patients will return to autonomy is very low.

Ethical concerns arise from these observations [7]. Whom should we treat? Is it humane and appropriate to treat elderly burn patients for prolonged periods in the ICU, if the result is a very poor quality of life or even death? If autonomy cannot be achieved is it worth the suffering?

What Do We Know?

Several studies have addressed the issue of age-specific risk factors for outcome after burn injury [5, 6, 8–10] (Table 1). Among identified factors, the most prominent are age, presence of inhalation injury, comorbidities (cardiac, respiratory, renal, neurological), pre-injury nutritional status, length of ICU stay, the severity of the injury and more specifically the magnitude of burn injury and the surgical requirements. Among these factors, age is the strongest predictive factor with burns exceeding 40 % BSA, which is reflected in the two most frequently used burn severity scores (Baux and Ryan scores [1]). But age is neither a sensitive nor a specific outcome predictor in the elderly. It is clear that additional predictive factors are needed to identify elderly burn patients with a poor outcome, either because of a high risk of death, or because of poor likelihood of achieving autonomy.

In an attempt to find additional objective criteria, we scrutinized our database, including only elderly patients admitted within a few hours after injury to our Burn Center and requiring ICU treatment. We further concentrated on those surviving the initial resuscitation phase (>48 hours).

Table 1 Factors potentially associated with poor outcome in critically ill elderly burn patients

Known burn injury characteristics and comorbidities	Known burn ICU variables	Potential additional factors
Burned body surface (BSA), depth of burn injury [12]	Abdominal hypertension and abdominal syndrome [13]	Fluid delivery of the first 24 hours and per day
Extension of surgical grafting [14]	Hemoglobin <70 g/l [15] Blood transfusion requirements	Increasing fluid balance
Gender, age [16]	Infections and antibiotic treatment [17]	Hypo- and hyperglycemia [18]
Ryan score [1]	Early, low albuminemia [19, 20]	Sedation (over-) and delirium
Baux scores (age + BSA and revised for inhalation) [21]	Acute renal failure any time [22]	Weight increase
Abbreviated burn severity index (ABSI)	Intolerance to enteral feeding [23] (high gastric residual volumes)	Protein intake (low or high)
Multiple injury [24]	Leukocyte count <3 or >20 g/l [25]	Non-albumin colloids
Burn mechanism [5]	Length of mechanical ventilation	Hyperlactatemia >2 mmol/l [26]
Comorbidities [27, 28]	Length of ICU stay [14]	SAPS II [29]
Ischemic heart disease [30]		
Renal failure [22]		

Survey Characteristics

A 10-year retrospective study including any admission for burn trauma between 2001 and 2010 was carried out using our computerized ICU database. In a preliminary search, we observed increasing cardiovascular complications in patients of the 6th decade. We, therefore, included patients aged ≥ 50 years. One hundred and one patients were analyzed out of 363 consecutive admissions: 17 were excluded due to short stay <48 hours (dead or alive), and one due to admission several days after injury. Sixteen of the 101 patients died (16 %).

Preadmission status (age, weight, body mass index), details of injury severity, and comorbidities, such as heart diseases (ischemia, hypertension), chronic obstructive pulmonary disease (COPD), diabetes, renal and liver disease, neurological and psychiatric diseases, and autonomy limitation were recorded. We also looked at ICU variables, such as SAPS II score, fluid resuscitation details, mechanical ventilation, and occurrence of complications, such as intra-abdominal hypertension or renal failure (Table 1). Screening was limited to the first 10 days.

Clinical Management

A standardized resuscitation protocol has been used for several years: The Parkland equation is considered indicative of the first 24-hour fluid requirements, and resuscitation is guided by hemodynamic variables aimed at achieving a mean arterial pressure (MAP) >65 mm Hg, urine output ≥ 0.5 ml/kg/h, cardiac index ≥ 3.0 l/m^2, and a stable lactate. Albumin is only infused after 12 h post-injury if albuminemia is <18 g/l. Enteral feeding is initiated within 3–12 h after injury and the energy target is monitored by indirect calorimetry. Glycemic control aims at blood glucose values between 5 and 8 mmol/l: The protocol is nurse driven. Antibiotics are delivered only in case of microbiologically proven infection.

Anything New? Preliminary Observations

Previously identified risk factors of poor outcome were confirmed (Table 2), except for the presence of malnutrition, multiple injury or COPD, which were too rare in our cohort to be significant. The non-survivors were older and more severely burned, requiring more surgery. The SAPS II score, which has never been validated for burn injuries, performed well, but without being discriminant. The problem with the previously identified variables was that there was a considerable overlap between the values in survivors and non-survivors, with no clear cut-off value, making them of little use in the individual patient.

There were no significant differences in fluid intake during the first 10 days (Fig. 1), with only a trend to more fluid in the more severely burned patients. On the other hand, fluid handling, i. e., fluid elimination, seemed to be an unsolvable issue in non-survivors. This handicap leads to the persistence of abnormally high weight because of persistent generalized edema. Without weight determinations, the calculated cumulated fluid balances may be a potential surrogate variable reflecting problems.

In addition, non-surviving patients more frequently had comorbid ischemic heart disease and/or renal failure before admission, which reduced their functional reserves. Occurrence of intra-abdominal hypertension seemed prohibitive: 5 of the 6 patients with pathological elevated pressures (i. e., intra-abdominal pressure [IAP] >20 mm Hg) died. Among laboratory variables, there was a significantly steeper decrease in the albumin values within the first 48 hours and creatinine values were higher, with little overlap, with those patients with creatininemia >170 mmol/l doing poorly.

Associations strongly predictive of poor outcome were renal failure, ischemic heart disease, massive early decrease in albuminemia (delta >15 g/l) (requiring more substitution), and very positive creeping fluid balances (Fig. 1), with or without intra-abdominal hypertension. Those patients developing acute renal failure (or suffering from chronic renal failure), handled the fluid resuscitation poorly, resulting in particularly positive cumulative fluid balances (Fig. 1), and abdominal hypertension in 5 of those who died (31 %), which further worsened their renal condition.

Table 2 Patient characteristics and outcome variables

Variable	All N = 101	Survivors N = 85	Non-survivors N = 16	p
Sex (F/M)	44/57	36/49	8/8	ns
Age (years)	66.6 ± 12.0	65.7 ± 11.6	71.7 ± 13.1	0.06
BMI (kg/m^2)	25.7 ± 5.3	26.0 ± 5.4	23.8 ± 4.3	ns
TBSA %	21.5 ± 14.9	19.1 ± 12.0	34.6 ± 21.6	<0.0001
% full thickness burn	15.3 ± 14.5	12.5 ± 10.9	30.1 ± 21.5	<0.0001
Inhalation injury	51 (51 %)	43	8	ns
Carbon monoxide poisoning	9 (9 %)	9	0	0.07
SAPS II	39.0 ± 12.8	36.2 ± 11.2	53.7 ± 11.3	<0.0001
Baux score	88.3 ± 18.1	84.9 ± 16.1	106.3 ± 17.7	<0.0001
Baux score revised	97.2 ± 19.5	93.7 ± 17.0	115.9 ± 21.8	<0.0001
ABSI	8.0 ± 1.9	7.7 ± 1.7	9.7 ± 2.1	<0.0001
Diabetes (type I or II)	17 (17.8 %)	13	4	ns
COPD	16 (15.8 %)	12	4	ns
Renal failure # A/C/C+A/N	13/10/4/74	9/6/2/68	4/4/2/6	0.01
Hypertension	44 (43.6 %)	37	7	ns
Ischemic heart disease	17 (17.8 %)	11	6 (37.5 %)	0.03
Valvular heart disease	10 (9.9 %)	7	3	ns
Autonomy before injury	92 (91.1 %)	78	14	ns
Psychiatric disease	25 (24.8 %)	24	1	0.08
Neurological condition (epilepsy, dementia)	19 (18.8 %)	14	5	ns
Intra-abdominal hypertension (>20 mm Hg)	6 (5.9 %)	1	5 (31.2 %)	<0.0001
Mean intra-abdominal pressure (mm Hg)	22 ± 3	17 ± 2	25 ± 4	0.009
Length of mechanical ventilation (d)	8.4 ± 13.4	7.9 ± 12.9	11.3 ± 16.2	ns
Length of ICU stay (d)	23.2 ± 23.4	23.8 ± 23.7	20.1 ± 22.2	ns

#: A = acute, C = chronic, C + A = chronic + acute, N = none; BMI: body mass index; COPD: chronic obstructive pulmonary disease; TBSA: total body surface area; ABSI: abbreviated burns severity index; ns: not signifikant

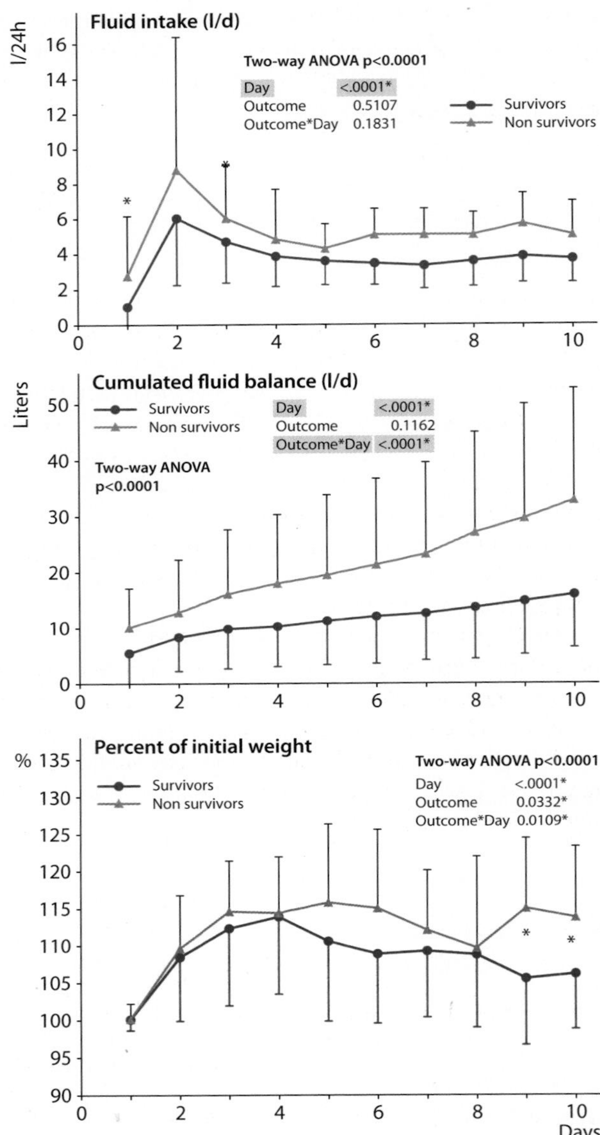

Fig. 1 Evolution of fluid intake and balance, and of weight changes over the first 10 days

We also observed for differences in glycemia: There was no case of hypoglycemia <4 mmol/l in our cohort despite a typical burn on/off enteral nutrition feeding pattern, and only a limited number of cases of toxic glycemia >10 mmol/l. No association of glycemia with outcome could be found. There was also no association of lactate levels >2 mmol/l with outcome.

Because of the relatively low number of deaths (n = 16) we could not carry out multiple logistic regression analysis as the latter requires 20 events per variable to be appropriate [11]. Perhaps with the inclusion of even older patients in a future, larger study, this type of analysis may become possible.

Conclusion

In an ageing population, the proportion of elderly burn patients requiring ICU treatment is increasing. As mortality from burn trauma increases already over 60 years of age and as the return to autonomy after this type of injury is often compromised, we need individual predictive factors: None of the currently identified factors is entirely specific. Observation of a cohort of 101 senior burn patients showed that some additional factors present during the first 10 days of treatment may help guide our decisions towards full or palliative treatment after an initial therapeutic trial. Pre-existing ischemic heart disease and renal failure prevent these patients from responding adequately to the early fluid resuscitation resulting in an irreversible accumulation of fluid that causes organ failure, including abdominal compartment syndrome.

Our observations will change our appreciation of the response to treatment of the elderly burn patient. Fluid delivery, balances and weight gain will be even more strongly monitored. Our clinical discussions will focus more on the support of renal and cardiac function. When facing severe complications, e.g., septic shock, and having to decide about the continuation of treatment, these facts will be integrated. Further investigations should focus on factors that impact on renal function and fluid handling.

References

1. Ryan CM, Schoenfeld DA, Thorpe WP, Sheridan RL, Cassem EH, Tompkins RG (1998) Objective estimates of the probability of death from burn injuries. N Engl J Med 338:362–366
2. Gosain A, DiPietro LA (2004) Aging and wound healing. World J Surg 28:321–326
3. World Heath Organisation (2004) The global burden of disease: 2004 update. Available at: http://www.who.int/healthinfo/global_burden_disease/GBD_report_2004update_full.pdf Accessed Oct 2012
4. National burn repository (2009) National burn repository 2009 report. Available at: http://www.ameriburn.org/2009NBRAnnualReport.pdf Accessed Oct 2012
5. Pham TN, Kramer CB, Wang J et al (2009) Epidemiology and outcomes of older adults with burn injury: an analysis of the National Burn Repository. J Burn Care Res 30:30–36
6. Alden NE, Bessey PQ, Rabbitts A, Hyden PJ, Yurt RW (2007) Tap water scalds among seniors and the elderly: socio-economics and implications for prevention. Burns 33:666–669
7. Eccles J (2003) Ethical considerations in the care of older people. Clin Med 3:416–418
8. Bessey PQ, Arons RR, Dimagio CJ, Yurt RW (2006) The vulnerabilities of age: burns in children and older adults. Surgery 140:705–715

9. Demling RH (2005) The incidence and impact of pre-existing protein energy malnutrition on outcome in the elderly burn patient population. J Burn Care Rehabil 26:94–100
10. Wibbenmeyer LA, Amelon MJ, Morgan LJ et al (2001) Predicting survival in an elderly burn patient population. Burns 27:583–590
11. Peduzzi P, Concato J, Kemper E, Holford TR, Feinstein AR (1996) A simulation study of the number of events per variable in logistic regression analysis. J Clin Epidemiol 49:1373–1379
12. Lionelli GT, Pickus EJ, Beckum OK, Decoursey RL, Korentager RA (2005) A three decade analysis of factors affecting burn mortality in the elderly. Burns 31:958–963
13. Ivy ME, Atweh NA, Palmer J, Possenti PP, Pineau M, D'Aiuto M (2000) Intra-abdominal hypertension and abdominal compartment syndrome in burn patients. J Trauma 49:387–391
14. Mahar P, Wasiak J, Bailey M, Cleland H (2008) Clinical factors affecting mortality in elderly burn patients admitted to a burns service. Burns 34:629–636
15. Hébert PC, Blajchman MA, Marshall J et al (1999) A multicenter, randomized, controlled clinical trial of transfusion requirements in critical care. N Engl J Med 340:409–417
16. Lundgren RS, Kramer CB, Rivara FP et al (2009) Influence of comorbidities and age on outcome following burn injury in older adults. J Burn Care Res 30:307–314
17. D'Avignon LC, Hogan BK, Murray CK et al (2010) Contribution of bacterial and viral infections to attributable mortality in patients with severe burns: an autopsy series. Burns 36:773–779
18. Preiser JC, Devos P, Ruiz-Santana S et al (2009) A prospective randomised multi-centre controlled trial on tight glucose control by intensive insulin therapy in adult intensive care units: the Glucontrol study. Intensive Care Med 35:1738–1748
19. Kumar P (2010) Grading of severity of the condition in burn patients by serum protein and albumin/globulin studies. Ann Plast Surg 65:74–79
20. Macedo JL, Santos JB (2007) Predictive factors of mortality in burn patients. Rev Inst Med Trop Sao Paulo 49:365–370
21. Osler T, Glance LG, Hosmer DW (2010) Simplified estimates of the probability of death after burn injuries: extending and updating the baux score. J Trauma 68:690–697
22. Sabry A, El-Din AB, El-Hadidy AM, Hassan M (2009) Markers of tubular and glomerular injury in predicting acute renal injury outcome in thermal burn patients: a prospective study. Ren Fail 31:457–463
23. Rimdeika R, Gudaviciene D, Adamonis K, Barauskas G, Pavalkis D, Endzinas Z (2006) The effectiveness of caloric value of enteral nutrition in patients with major burns. Burns 32:83–86
24. Santaniello JM, Luchette FA, Esposito TJ et al (2004) Ten year experience of burn, trauma, and combined burn/trauma injuries comparing outcomes. J Trauma 57:696–700
25. Rao K, Ali SN, Moiemen NS (2006) Aetiology and outcome of burns in the elderly. Burns 32:802–805
26. Okorie ON, Dellinger P (2011) Lactate: biomarker and potential therapeutic target. Crit Care Clin 27:299–326
27. Keck M, Lumenta DB, Andel H, Kamolz LP, Frey M (2009) Burn treatment in the elderly. Burns 35:1071–1079
28. Lumenta DB, Kamolz LP, Frey M (2009) Adult burn patients with more than 60 % TBSA involved-Meek and other techniques to overcome restricted skin harvest availability – the Viennese Concept. J Burn Care Res 30:231–242
29. LeGall JR, Lemeshow S, Saulnier F (1993) A new simplified acute physiology score (SAPS II) based on a European/North American multicenter study. JAMA 270:2957–2963
30. Khadim MF, Rashid A, Fogarty B, Khan K (2009) Mortality estimates in the elderly burn patients: the Northern Ireland experience. Burns 35:107–113

Index

J.-L. Vincent (Ed.), *Annual Update in Intensive Care and Emergency Medicine 2013*,
DOI 10.1007/978-3-642-35109-9, © Springer-Verlag Berlin Heidelberg 2013

D

E

Printing: Ten Brink, Meppel, The Netherlands
Binding: Stürtz, Würzburg, Germany